The Poor Man's James Bond
Volume 2

Desert Publications
P.O. Box 1751
El Dorado, AR 71731-1751
501-862-2077

ISBN 0-87947-226-X
12 11 10 9 8 7 6 5
Printed in U. S. A.

Desert Publication is a division of
The DELTA GROUP, Ltd.
Direct all inquiries & orders to the above address.

This compilation contains the original
"Poor Man's James Bond Volume 2"

SECRET— NOFORN

EXCEPT U. K., CANADA, & AUSTRALIA

Detailed Intelligence Report

Name: After Action Report

B.E. No.: 16-790-9

Date of Report: August 28, 1979

Series: Technical Evaluation

EXCLUDED FORM AUTOMATIC
REGRADING; DOD DIR 5200.10
DOES NOT APPLY.

SECRET— NOFORN

EXCEPT U. K., CANADA, & AUSTRALIA

CONFIDENTIAL

SPECIAL REPORT

DRSX - AS

29 August-1979

TO: Director - Special Operations Division, Special Assistant For Counter-Insurgency and Special Activities

FROM: Senior Field Agent David Fischer, acting for Field Agent George Neary (deceased)

SUBJECT: After Action Report - Weapons Evaluation

REFERENCE: Operation "Bridge City" (16-790-9)

DISTRIBUTION: Level 1 Section Heads Only

In accordance with Counter-Insurgency Directive 24A-156-75 the following report is forwarded. Please be advised that this initial evaluation covers only an overview of weapons and weapon systems used by and against operational personnel in the Northern districts of Mexico during August, 1979. (Bridge City 16-790-9)

For additional information on specific weapons refer to FSTC-CW-07-1-69.

David Fischer

David Fischer
Senior Field Agent

COPY NO. 2
PAGE 1 of 11

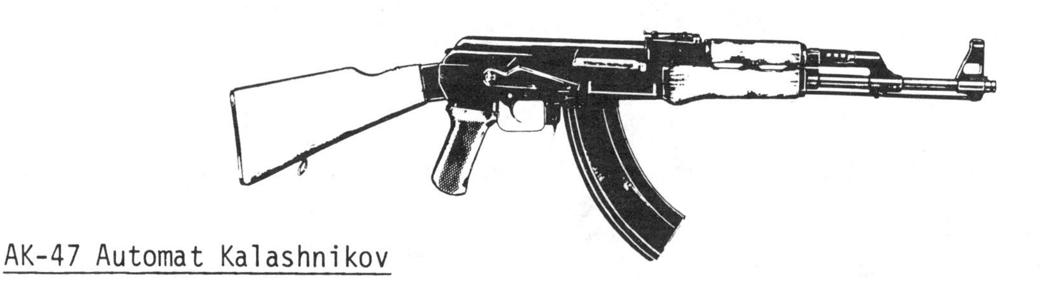

AK-47 Automat Kalashnikov

The years following W.W.II saw the Russians with the need to replace their aging submachine guns (PPSH41Y PPS43) and the variety of rifles still in service. The AK-47 filled their needs so well that more than 30 million have been produced since (the production figure includes variations)

The AK-47 is far more accurate at a longer range than the Israeli Uzi, British Sten, or U.S. M3-A1 "Grease Gun". It will hold a six inch group at 100 yards, about one-half the group size of conventional sub-machine guns. The AK-47 is usually found in two versions, one with a wooden stock and one with a folding metal stock.

The AK-47 frequently turns up in small guerilla wars around the world. One of the greatest attributes of the AK-47 is its ability to function under adverse conditions. Even when rarely cleaned and firing "corroded" ammunition it continues to be an effective weapon.

AK-Assault Rifle

Caliber: 7.62 mm
System: gas, selective fire
Feed device: 30-rd. detachable box magazine
Weight 10 1/2 lbs.
Muzzle velocity: 2330 F.P.S.
Rate of Fire 600 r.p.m.

Browning High Power 35 pistol

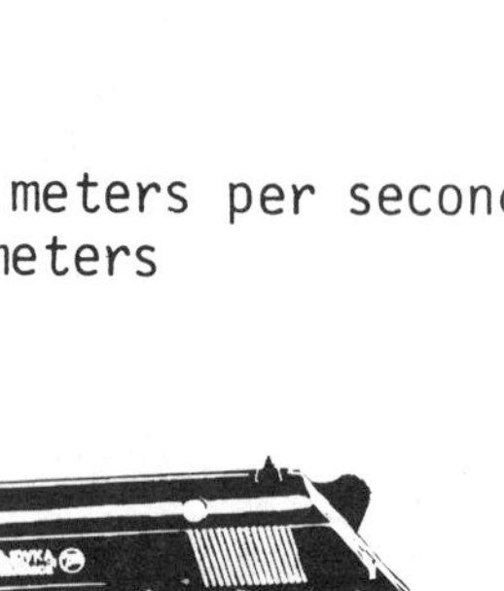

This was the last pistol designed by John Browning. Though in design and function it is very similar to the Colt .45 1911A1 (Browning designed) there are major differences. The High Power was used extensively during W.W.II by the British and Canadian governments, and is still the main service sidearm in those countries. Models are frequently found with tangential sights and detachable shoulder stocks. The effectiveness and availability of the 9 mm cartridge has made this a highly desirable sidearm in most countries outside the U.S.

Caliber - 9 mm parabellum
System - recoil
Feed device - 13 round detachable box magazine
Weight - 0.8 kg.
Muzzle velocity - 450 meters per second
Effective range - 70 meters

CZ-50 Pistol

The model 1950 pistol is no longer in service with the Czechoslovakian army. Large numbers of these weapons have been given to the "emerging" and third world nations. The CZ-50 is frequently encountered in both Africa and South America.

Caliber - 7.65 mm (pistol)
System - blowback, semi-automatic
Feed device - 8 round removeable box magazine
Weight - 1.5 lb.
Muzzle velocity - 919 feet per second
Effective range - 50 meters

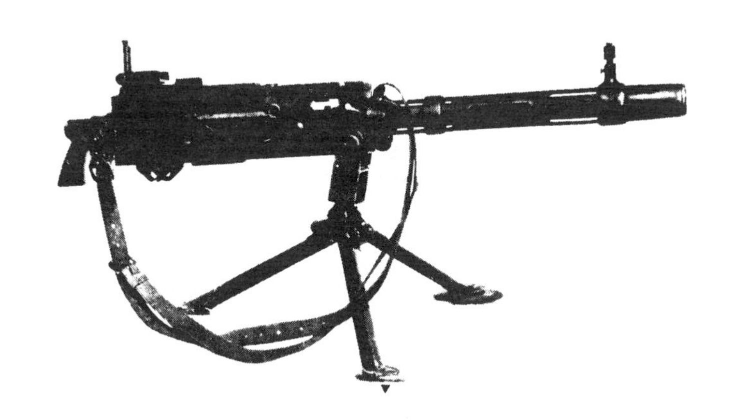

Browning .30 Cal Machine Gun

The original design dates from 1910, but the design was finally adopted by the Army in 1917. Early versions were water cooled, but these have been obsolete for years - though occasionally found in use in third world nation.

The excellent air cooled version was replaced by the M-60 machinegun in the 1960's. It is, however, still used as secondary armament in armoured vehicles or for infantry use with a wide variety of tripod mounts.

Caliber - 30 in.
System - recoil operated
Feed device - 250 round fabric belt, or disintegrating link belt
Weight - 14 kg.
Muzzle velocity - 850 meters per second
Effective range - 900 meters

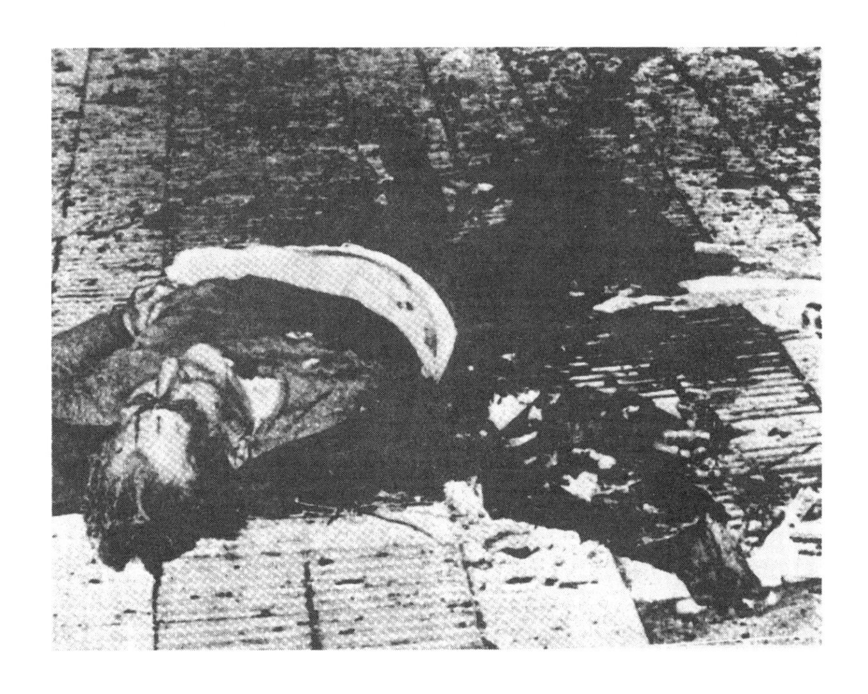

Leftist Guerilla Found Armed With AK-47

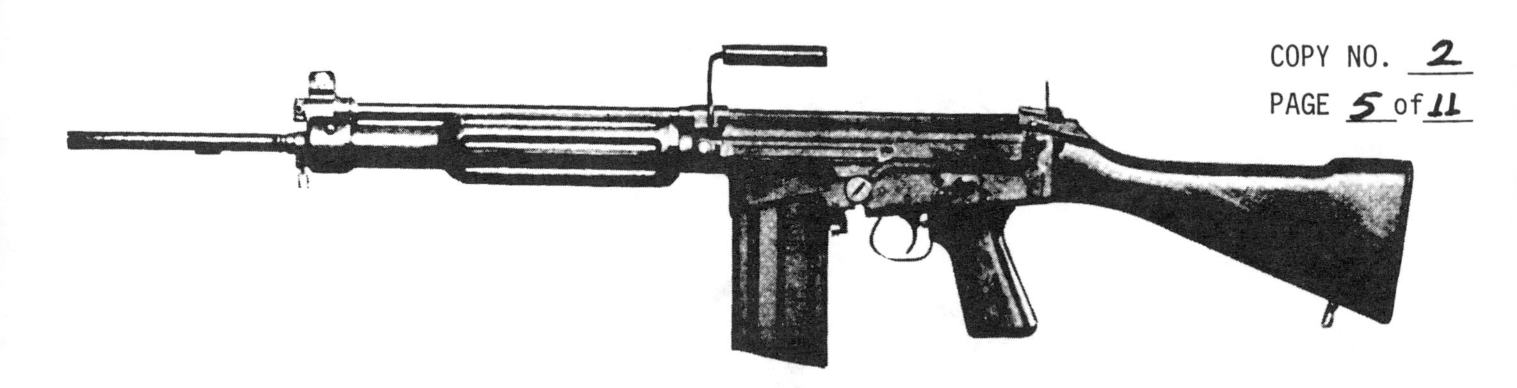

FN-FAL rifle (Fabrique Nationale Herstal Belgium)

The FAL is the most successful of all assault rifles developed since World War II. With minor modifications it is in use by more than 65 countries around the world. The FAL is a selective fire weapon that fires from a closed bolt. Two variations of the rifle are in general use - one with a fixed stock and one with a folding stock.

Caliber - 7.62mm
System - Gas
Feeding device - 20 round detachable box magazine
Weight - 4.5 kg.
Muzzle velocity - 730 meter per second
Effective range - 500 meters

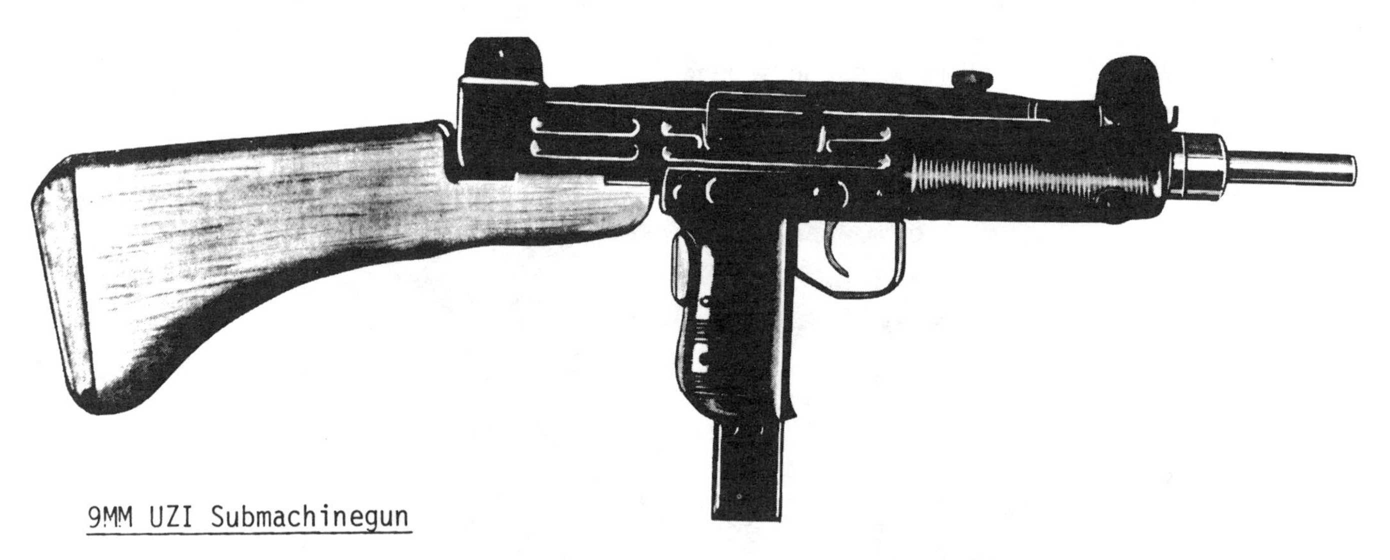

9MM UZI Submachinegun

The 9 MM UZI submachinegun was developed by an Israeli army officer during the early 1950's. The design seems to have been influenced by the Czech M-23 submachinegun; however, the UZI has several novel features for a submachinegun: A bayonet and a spigot type grenade launcher. The UZI is considered to be an extremely reliable weapon.

The UZI is manufactured in Israel and Belgium. It is a standard weapon in Israel, W. Germany and the Netherlands. It is also carried by members of the U.S. Secret Service.

Caliber - 9 mm
System - blowback
Feed device - 25 rd., 32 rd., or 40 rd. detachable box magazine
Weight - 8.8 lbs.
Muzzle velocity - 435 meters per second
Effective range - 200 meters

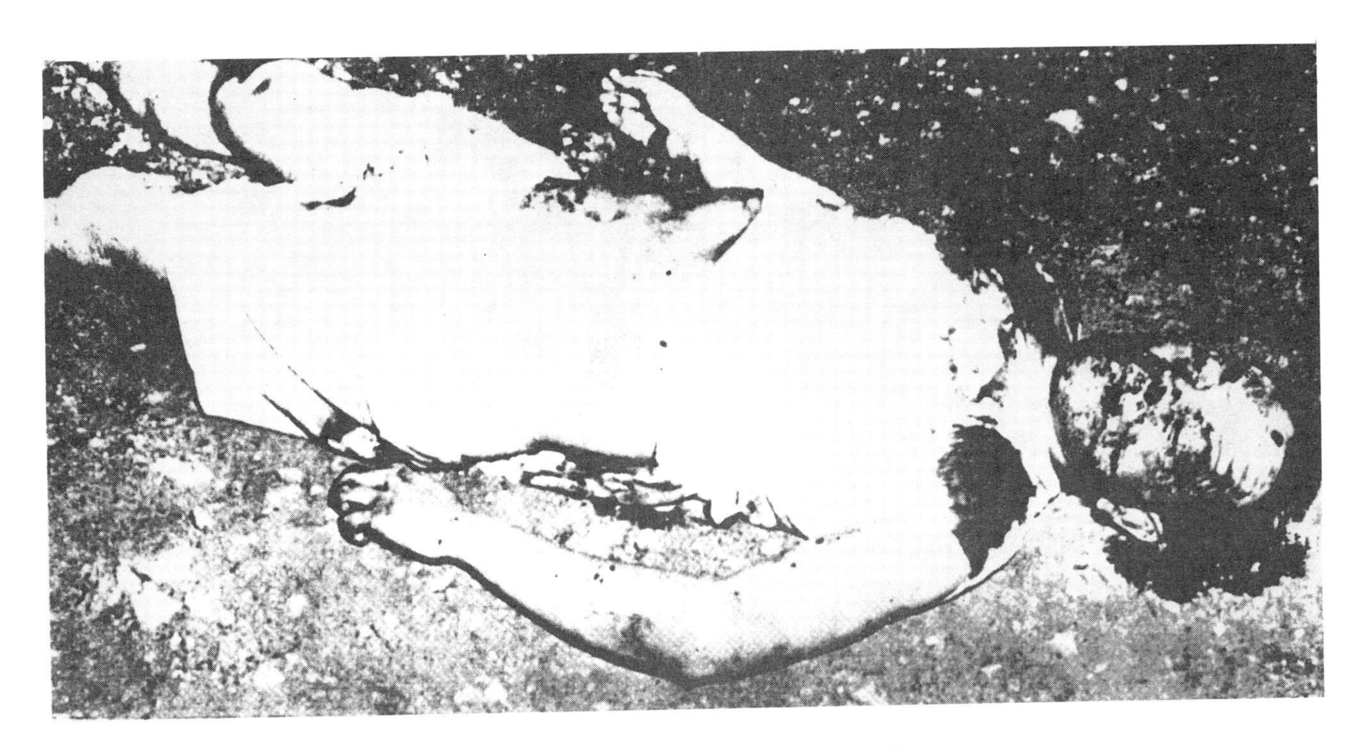

Guerilla Found Armed With UZ1

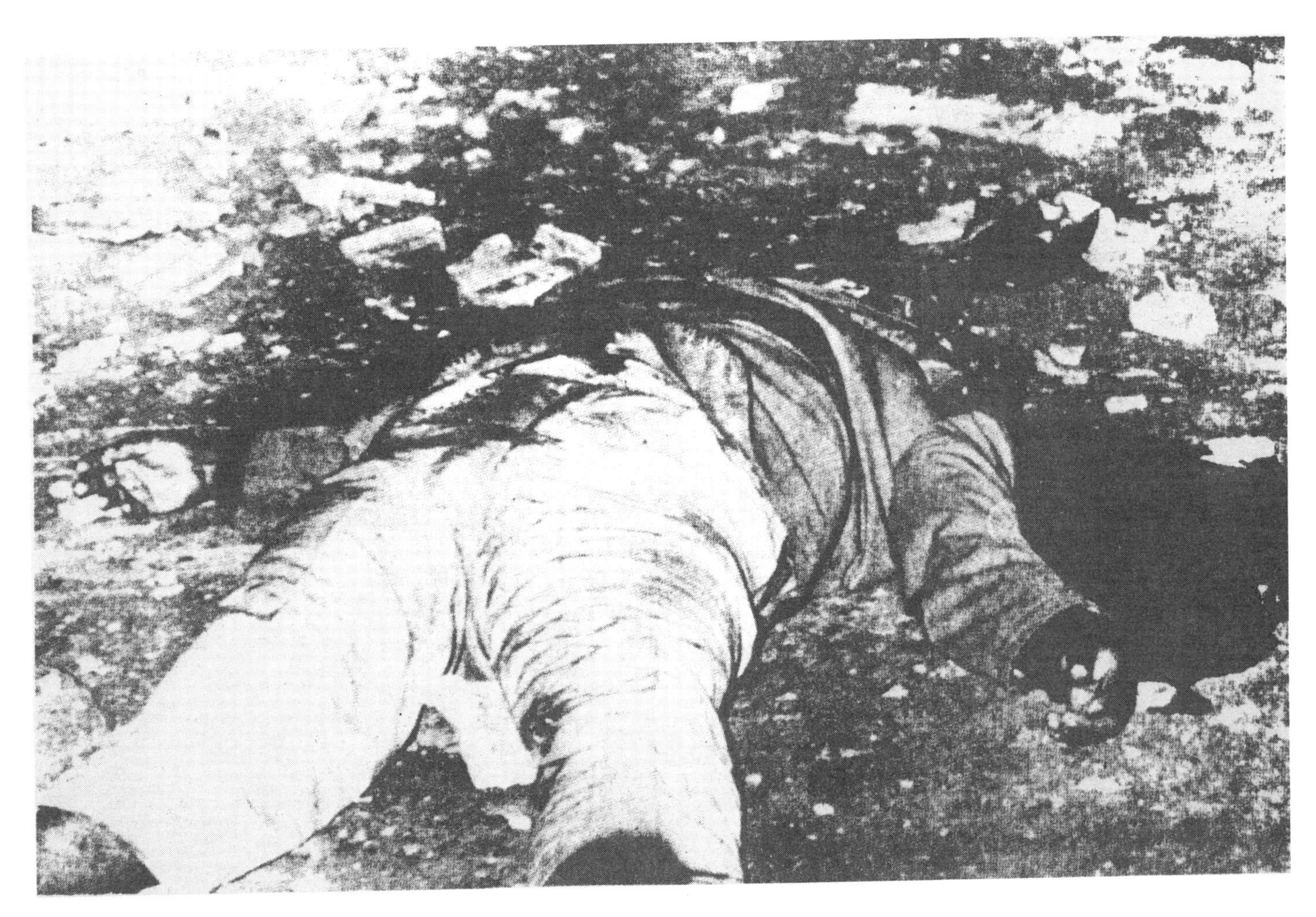

Remains Of Guerilla Found Armed With FAL

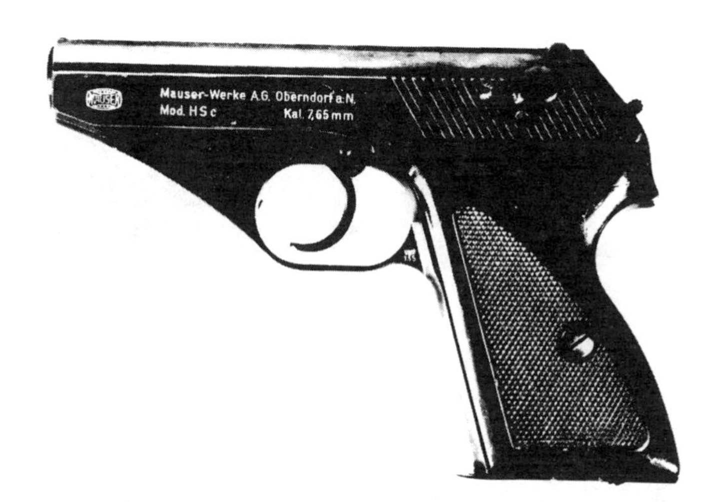

MAUSER HSC

The Mauser HSC was designed during the 1930's for use as a military-Police weapon. In general it is a well designed and effective pistol. Its primary drawback is that it is chambered for the relatively weak 7.65mm cartridge. A threaded barrel was available to attach a silencer.

Caliber - 7.65 mm
System - Blowback, automatic
Feed device - 8 round detachable box magazine
Weight - 1.3 lb.
Muzzle velocity - 950 feet per second
Effective range - 50 meters

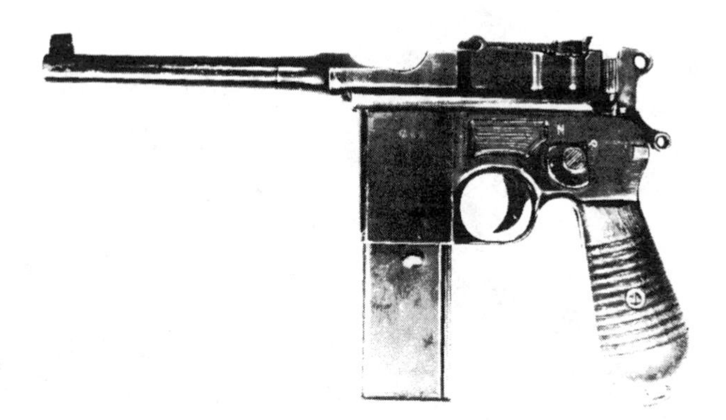

MP-6 Spanish Super AZUL, 7.63 mm

The Spanish Super Azul is an exact copy of the early mauser MP 1932 selective fire pistol without locking selector switches. The Azul was widely distributed commercially before W.W.II and many have made their way into the United States and Latin America.

Caliber - 7.63 mm
System - recoil, selective fire
Feed device - 10 rd. or 20 rd. detachable box magazines
Weight - 2.93 lb.
Muzzle velocity - 1575 feet per second
Effective range - 100 meters

VZ 61 Skorpion Machine Pistol (Czechoslovakia)

The Skorpion is a true machine pistol. The highly concealable Skorpion was designed for use by armoured vehicle crews. Though it fires a relatively weak cartridge, the weapon is highly functional and is in general service with Czechoslovakian troops. The weapon has recently began turning up in Africa and South America.

Caliber - 7.65 mm
System - blowback, selective fire
Feed device - 10 or 20 round detachable box type
Weight - 1.31 kg.
Muzzle velocity - 305 meter per second
Effective range - 50 to 75 meters

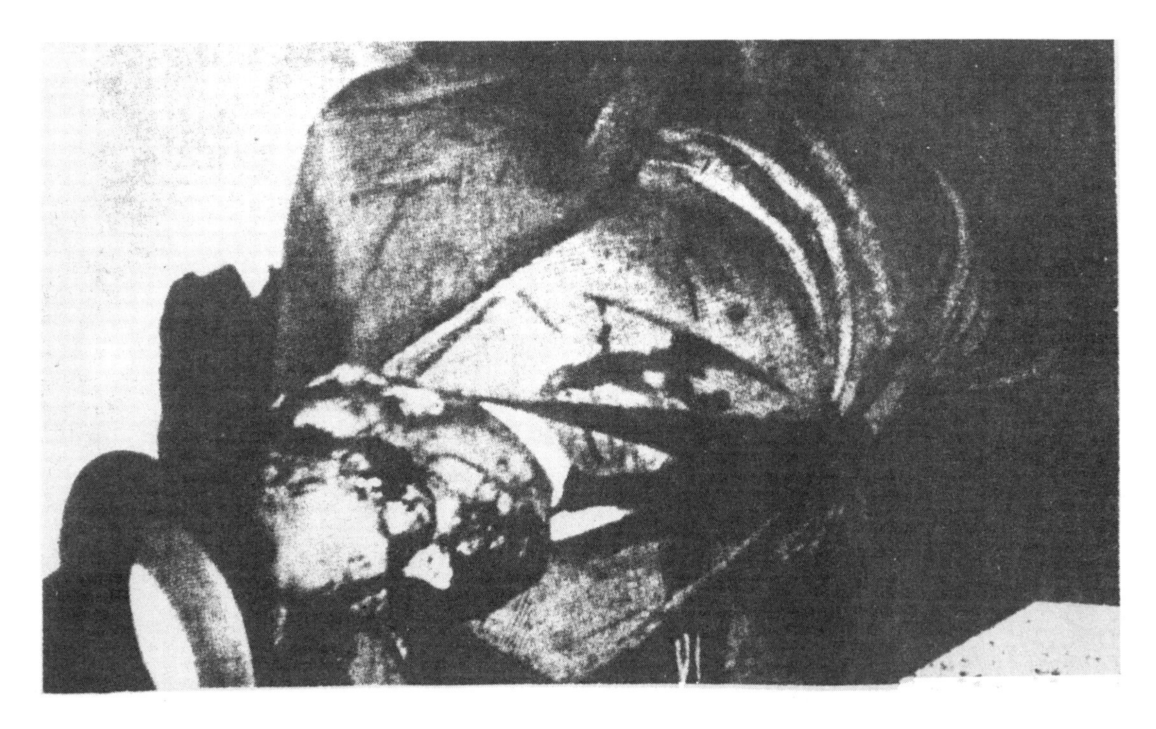

Guerilla Found Armed With CZ-50

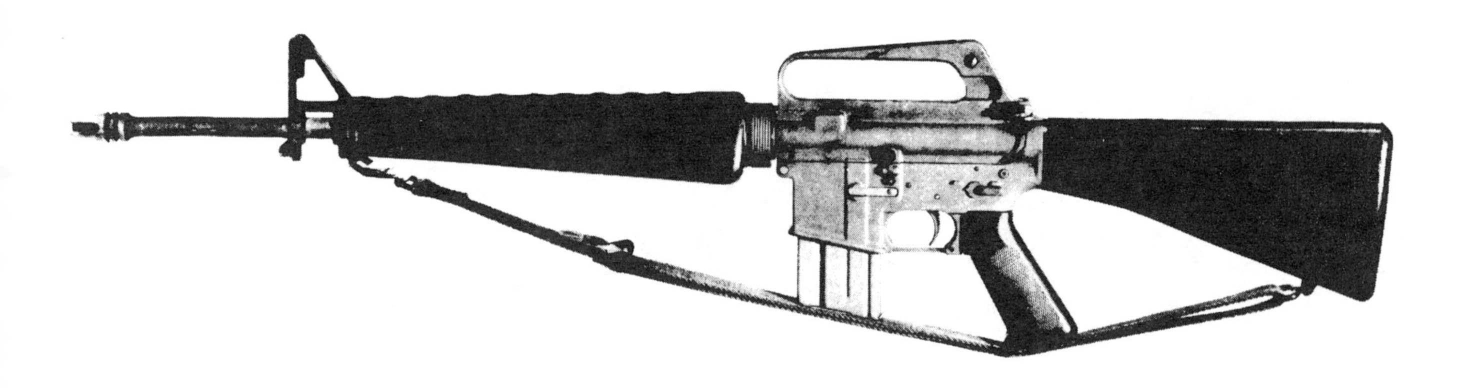

U.S. M-16 (Colt Industries)

The M-16 was developed in the late 1950's. To date more than 2 1/2 million have been produced. The U.S. Army proved its value for jungle warfare conclusively during the Viet Nam era. The rifle is now standard issue with nearly all U.S. Forces. Because of their wide spread distribution the weapons are frequently on the black market and are commonly encountered among guerilla units South of the border.

Caliber - 5.56 mm
System - Gas
Feed device - 20 rd. and 30 rd. box type
Weight - 2.9 kg
Muzzle velocity - 990 meters per second
Effective range - 400 meters

Colt .45 pistol

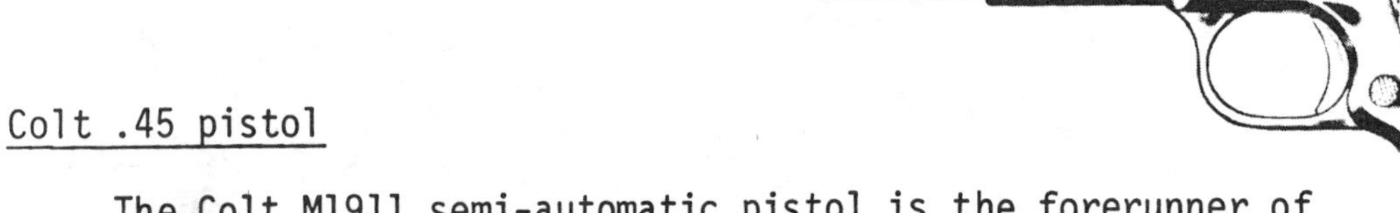

The Colt M1911 semi-automatic pistol is the forerunner of most modern military weapons - The original Browning has been copied more than any other single pistol. The weapon has seen service in every war in which the U.S. has participated since W.W.I. Modifications and improvements were made to the gun in the 1920's and the designation was changed to M-1911A1. The .45 ACP pistol is the premier military pistol in the world. It is highly accurate and hits with a punch reminicent of a slow moving freight train.

Caliber - .45 acp
System - recoil
Feed device - 7 round detachable box magazine
Weight - 1.1 kg.
Muzzle velocity - 250 meters per second
Effective range - 50 yards

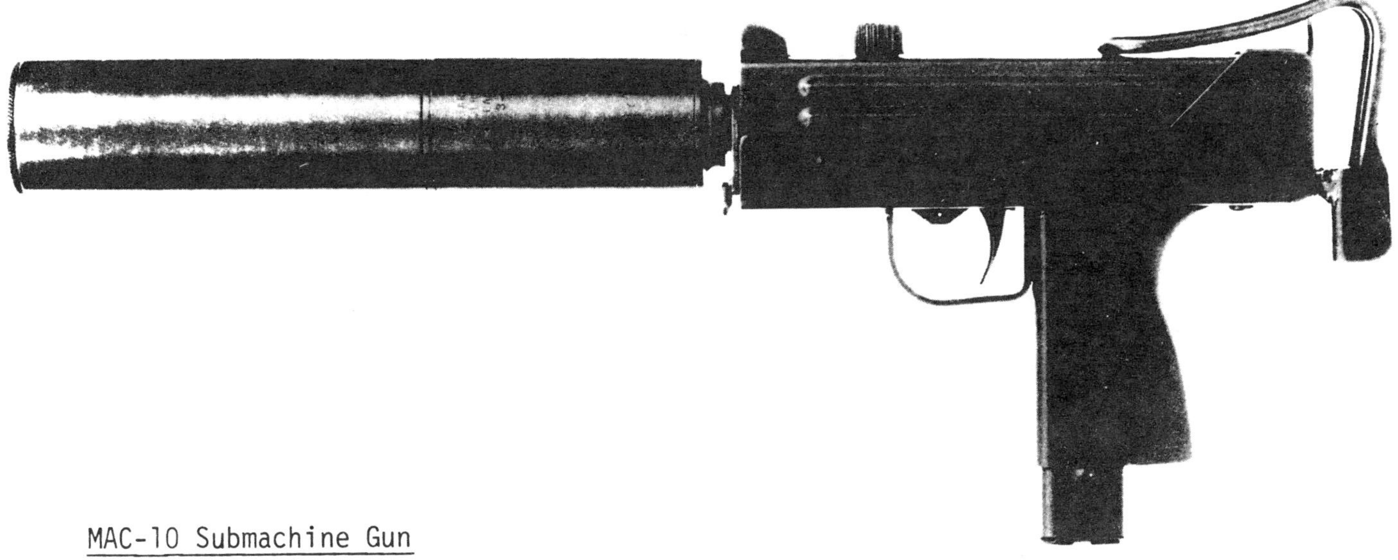

MAC-10 Submachine Gun

The MAC-10 is a light, compact, durable and accurate submachine gun. It may very possibly be the most effective submachine gun in the world. With a fitted sound and flash supressor it is an ideal personal weapon for clandestine operations. It is currently in use with agencies of the U.S. Government as well as numerous countries around the world.

Caliber - .45
System - blowback
Feed device - 30 round detachable box type
Weight - 2.8 kg
Muzzle velocity - 850 Feet per second
Effective range - 75 meters

Laco Laser Sight

The Laco sight is one of the first successful applications of laser technology to small arms sights. The self contained laser unit projects a laser beam over a long distance with a relatively minor increase in the dispersion pattern. Within the effective range of the weapon it is mounted upon the laser beam remains a small pencil head size dot.

The combination of a Laco Laser sight, teloscopic sight, and properly sighted in high powered rifle is devastating. In a properly alligned weapon system the laser beam accurately predicts the impact point of the bullet at a given range.

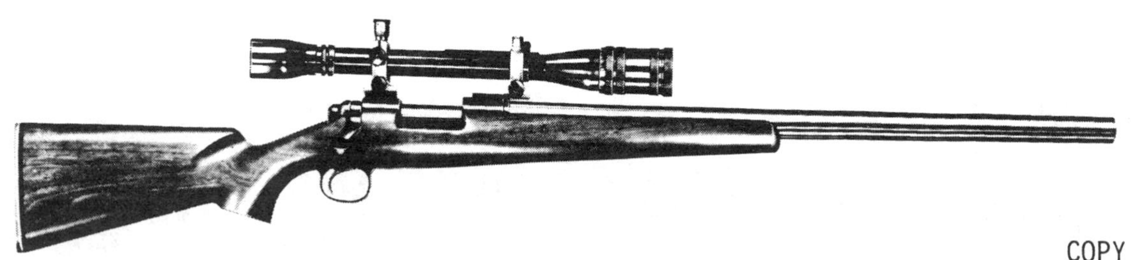

Remington 40-XB

The Remington Model 40-XB silenced rifle is completely hand fitted and tested before it is shipped. Its accuracy is guaranteed by the factory. This is perhaps the finest counter sniper weapon available for intermediate and longer ranges. The SIONICS silencer effectively muffles the report and camouflages the position of the rifleman. The Automatic Ranging Telescope provides almost certain first round hits anywhere within the effective range of the weapon.

Caliber - .308
System - bolt action
Effective Range - 600 meters

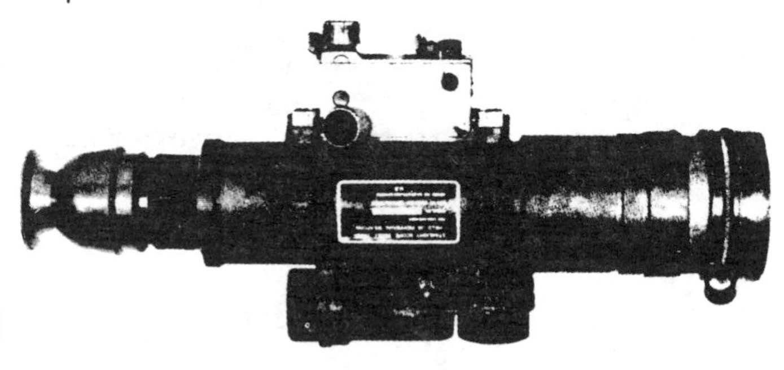

"Starlight Scope" (U.S. Army scope AN/PVS-2)

The "Starlight" scope is a portable, hand held, electro-optical instrument, designed for passive use in visual observation, and as a night sight. Even a minimal amount of starlight or moonlight is sufficient to give a surprisingly good picture. The "Starlight" scope was developed for the Viet Nam conflict. It was extensively used there in counterinsurgency operations with a great deal of success. The scope may also be fitted to most current military weapons for use as a night sight.

Weight - 2.7 kg.
Magnification - 4 power
Range - 400 meter moonlight
300 meter starlight

Smith and Wesson Model 58

The .41 magnum model 58 is a vicious and effective weapon. While made ostensibly for the military police in the U.S., its main purpose is as a combat weapon. The .41 magnum is an ideal compromise between the .357 magnum and .44 magnum. It retains the strong points of each cartridge and few of the drawbacks. As a "man killer" it is frequently the choice of mercenarys and other professional gunmen.

Caliber - 41 magnum
System - double action revolver, 4" barrel
Feed device - 6 shot cylinder
Weight - 2 1/2 lbs.
Muzzle velocity - 1200 feet per second
Effective range - 50 yds.

DON'T BE AN IDIOT! READ THIS FIRST

This book is power. Whether you apply it against your enemies or yourself is up to you. The best way to insure your safety and your ability to use this power is to study each book in this volume before trying any process.

Otherwise, you might spend a long time in the hospital pondering your stupidity, as I did. On September 29, 1969, I wanted to re-prime some shotgun shells. I wanted a powder which exploded by concussion. The ingredients for paper caps seemed the ideal medium.

I looked up the formula for paper caps in Weingart's Pyrotechnics, under "Japanese or Cap Torpedoes". The formula called for potassium chlorate, sulphur, chalk and amorphous (red) phosphorous. The formula plainly said to moisten the ingredients before mixing. In my ignorance, I believed this was necessary only so as to drop the mixture on paper so it would dry in little mounds.

Since I wanted it as a dry powder to pour into holes made in the primers, I used no water. While holding a plastic medicine bottle in my left hand I mixed less than a half ounce of potassium chlorate with sulphur, chalk and a small amount of red phosphorous. Suddenly my left hand was fingerless hamburger and I was also legally blind for several awful months.

Had I read the whole book before trying to make the priming powder, I would have learned that potassium chlorate can often explode spontaneously by dry mixture with sulphur; and with dry red phosphorous, every time. I learned the hard way and I don't want you to share any such experience. I didn't have the overview then that I have now.

I'm often bothered by readers of my works who have not completely read the book they are working from. They say they tried a process and it didn't work. They're like the man who doesn't know his way around the kitchen but tries to bake a three layer cake, with icing yet. He follows the recipe from the cookbook but still winds with a terrible mess and an enraged wife. No overview.

Another example of a fool who acts without an overview is the religious fanatic. This is the person who has never really read the Torah, Bible, Koran, etc., and pondered all its concepts before inflicting himself on others. No. Although he reads avidly, he is merely scanning the material looking for passages to reinforce his own prejudices.

The best example of this lack of an overview is the Moslem terrorist. Islam is actually a peaceful religion. But this dope has never really read the Koran and pondered its concepts. He gets his religion from power-mad, hypocritical mullahs and so tries to bomb the world back to the seventh century. If every sand monkey would read the Koran from cover to cover, learning what it says, rather than what others say it says, there would be no Islamic terrorism.

Possibly more important than anything you might learn from this book is how to study it. First, read every word in the index. Unconciously, this will feed data into your brain and give you a subconcious overview of the subject. It will also help you later to find subjects which are not cross-indexed to your satisfaction.

Next, read the entire book from the first page through to the last. Do this even if you don't think you can understand it. It's like studying a foreign language you can't understand and don't think you ever will. At a certain point, and all of a sudden, ideas and concepts start falling into place and you know. You'd be surprised how much your brain can absorb, and will by the time you've finished the book. And don't just breeze through it. When you come to a word you don't understand, look it up.

When you come to a paragraph you don't understand, read it over. Maybe it will become clearer if you reread the previous paragraph. If that doesn't help, read the next paragraph. At any rate, try and then go on. Your brain will work on the unregistering concept as you forge ahead.

By the time you've struggled through the whole book you will know much more about the subject than you did when you started. Also, your higher conciousness will then send an alarm if you are drastically mistaken during working a process, unless you are pre-programmed to self-destruction in the first place.

Although a college course in chemistry is helpful, it is not essential. Also, college courses tend to be based on high school chemistry courses which you might not have had, and with a teacher who has no patience with beginners.

Most of my books contain material written years ago for people with no higher education. Better to teach yourself from them than to quit in confusion and frustration because of classes for those used to formal study.

Of course, if you are young, get all the formal education on those studies you have time for. But whether formally or self-educated, read every word in the book. Otherwise you'll be like the karate student who gets thrashed by a street punk, or other educated fools who learn only enough to impress the ignorant, including themselves.

KNOWLEDGE IS POWER

Knowledge sets man apart from the beasts and above them all. It is knowledge alone, not money nor force, which secures money and force for the knowledgeable man, while the dull-witted lose whatever they've come by through luck or conniving.

As world civilizations decline and the presently powerful and affluent are reduced to beggery and helplessness, the owners of these volumes holding a veritable storehouse of both industrial and military power will survive to form dynasties.

Pages 3 and 4 are, intentionaly omitted

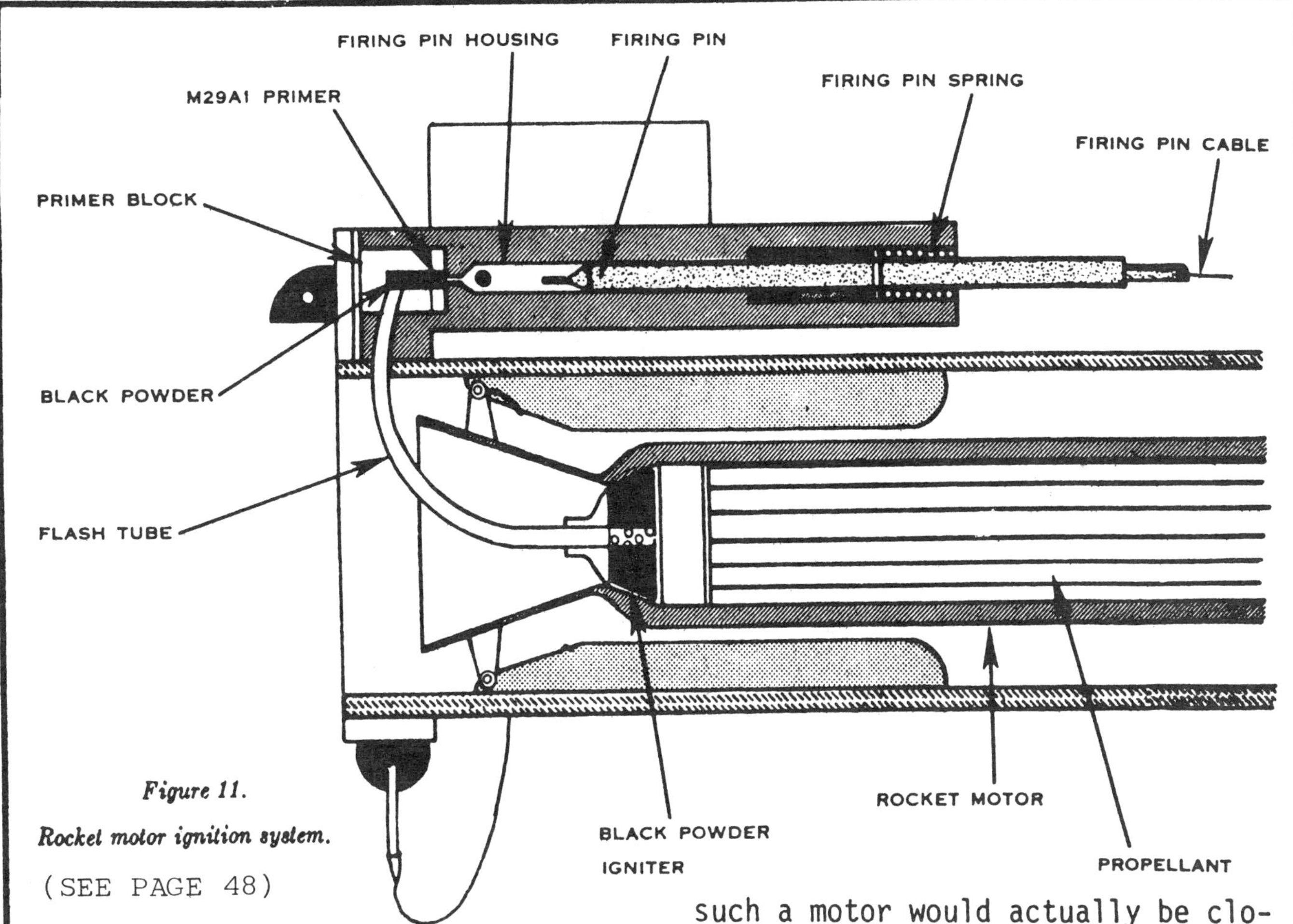

Figure 11.

Rocket motor ignition system.

(SEE PAGE 48)

Optimum accuracy for bazooka rockets is achieved when the motor's entire thrust occurs while the rocket is still within the launch tube. When it leaves the launcher, the rocket is then coasting toward the target, without power, much like a bullet fired from a conventional firearm. This eliminates the wobble that results from a sudden increase in the motor's thrust while the rocket is in free flight.

This "ideal" system is not practical for use with one man recoilless shoulder launchers for one or more of the following reasons; it requires an extremely long and cumbersome launch tube, an ultra light rocket that may be easily deflected by crosswinds, or a motor that delivers its entire thrust almost instantaneously. Ignition of such a motor would actually be closer to a small explosion. This is dangerous, unnerving, and hard to regulate.

The next best solution in terms of both safety and accuracy is the blowout igniter system used on the LAAW Rocket M 72A1 and M72A2 (see PMA Vol.1 #4/pp 64).

In this type of system, the nozzle of the rocket motor is sealed with an ignitor plug that pops out when the motor generates a predetermined amount of pressure. Although the motor is still burning when the rocket exits the tube,it has reached both peak thrust and a steady burning rate. This steady thrust will tend to push the rocket in a relatively straight line without the sudden bursts of power that destabilize conventional bazooka rounds.

The Only Magazine Of Improvised Weaponry . . .

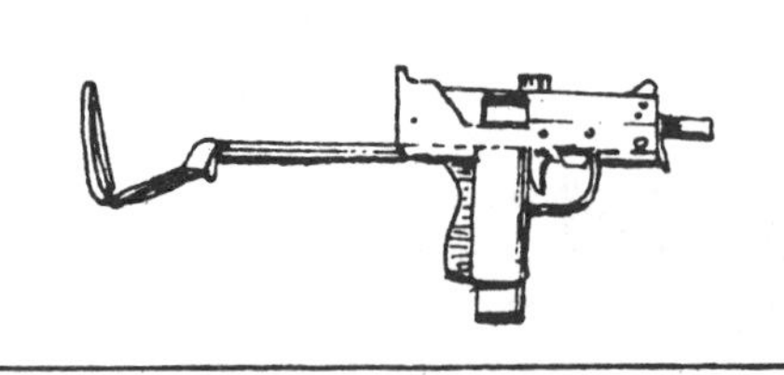

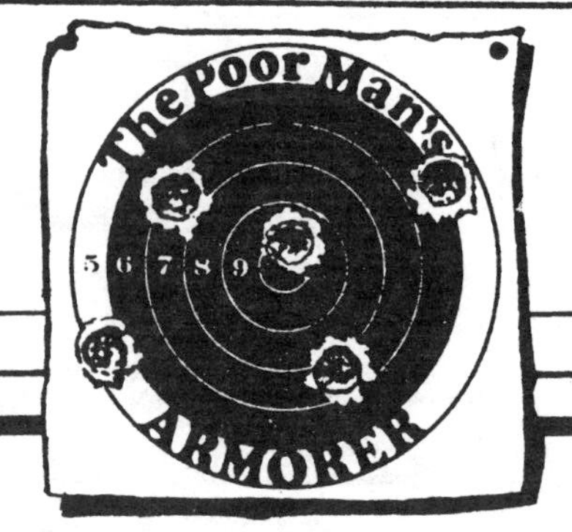

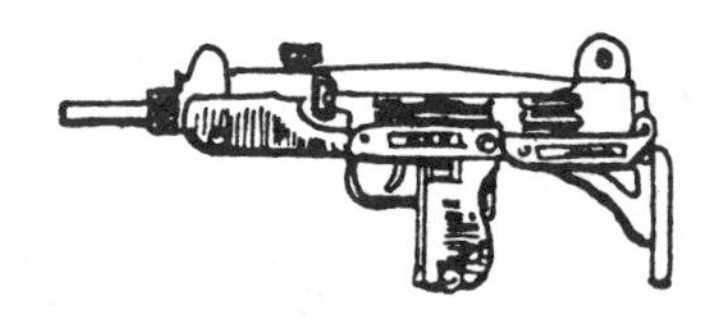

Editor - Clyde Barrow

Publisher - Kurt Saxon

Volume I, No. 1

COMBAT PISTOL TARGET

By Clyde Barrow

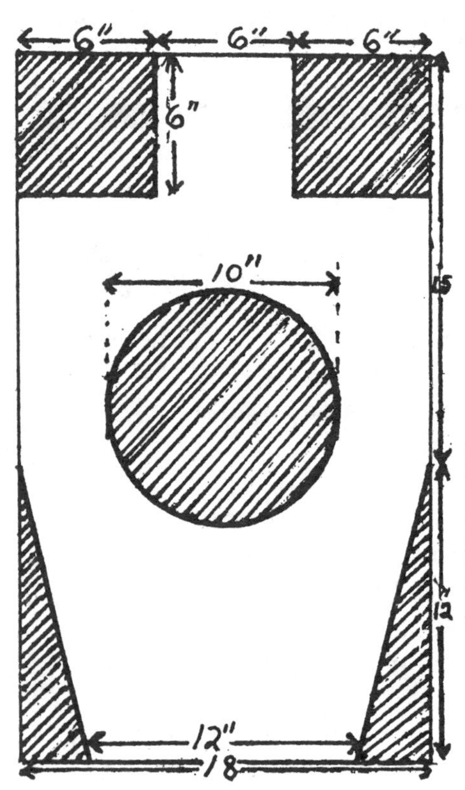

Pictured is a diagram of an excellent target to use when practicing defensive shooting with a pistol. A wide black felt tip pen is used to lay out several targets on 18 inch X 30 inch pieces of corrugated cardboard, following the measurements given in the drawing.

These targets are hung from a piece of clothesline about 25 yards from the shooter. The silhouettes may be used singularly, in groups of two or three, or even more if you anticipate a gun fight with a band of desparados.

Any hit in the 10 inch circle is a score, as this is the area containing the majority of the vital organs of the human body. .

After each round of shooting, bullet holes can be repaired with pieces of masking tape and the lines touched up with a felt pen.

The diagonal lines increase the visibility of the target in poor light, and unlike the solid black of conventional targets, each hit can be easily seen, even several feet from the target.

POPULAR MECHANICS 1913

To Explode Powder with Electricity

A 1-in. hole was bored in the center of a 2-in. square block. Two finishing-nails were driven in, as shown in the sketch. These were connected to terminals of an induction coil. After everything was ready the powder was poured in the hole and a board weighted with rocks placed over the block. When the button is pressed or the circuit closed in some other way the discharge occurs. The distance between the nail points—which must be bright and clean—should be just enough to give a good, fat spark.—

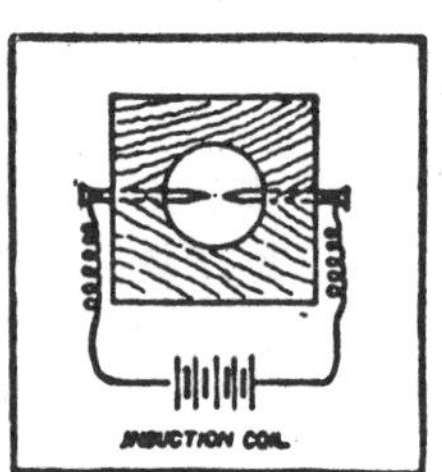

A Small Bench Lathe Made of Pipe Fittings

POPULAR MECHANICS 1913

The most important machine in use in the modern machine or wood-working shop is the lathe. The uses to which this wonderful machine can be put would be too numerous to describe, but there is hardly a mechanical operation in which the turning lathe does not figure. For this reason every amateur mechanic and wood-worker who has a workshop, no matter how small, is anxious to possess a lathe of some sort. A good and substantial homemade lathe, which is suitable for wood-turning and light metal work, may be constructed from pipe and pipe fittings as shown in the accompanying sketch.

The bed of this lathe is made of a piece of 1-in. pipe, about 30 in. long. It can be made longer or shorter, but if it is made much longer, a larger size of pipe should be used. The headstock is made of two tees, joined by a standard long nipple as shown in Fig. 1. All the joints should be screwed up tight and then fastened with $\frac{3}{16}$-in. pins to keep them from turning. The ends of the bed are fixed to the baseboard by means of elbows, nipples and flanges arranged as shown. The two bearings in the headstock are of brass. The spindle hole should be drilled and reamed after they are screwed in place in the tee. The spindle should be of steel and long enough to reach through the bearing and pulley and have enough end left for the center point. The point should extend about $1\frac{1}{2}$ in. out from the collar. The collar can be turned or shrunk on the spindle as desired. The end of the spindle should be threaded to receive a chuck.

The tailstock is also made of two tees joined by a nipple. The lower tee should be bored out for a sliding fit on the bed pipe. The upper one should be tapped with a machine tap for the spindle which is threaded to fit it. The spindle has a handle fitted at one end and has the other end bored out for the tailstock center.

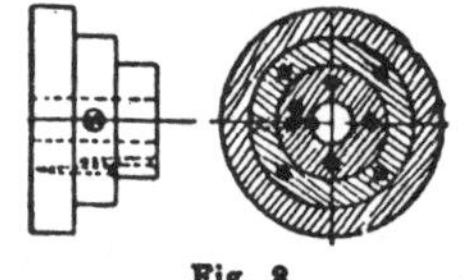
Fig. 2

Both the tailstock and the headstock centerpoints should be hardened. A clamp for holding the tailstock spindle

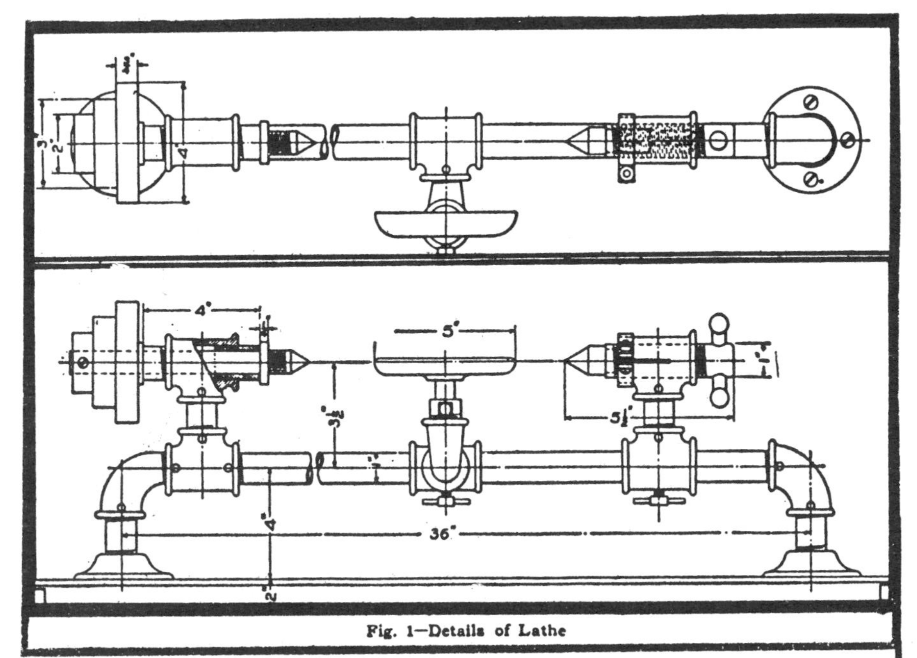

Fig. 1—Details of Lathe

is made of a piece of strap iron, bent and drilled as shown. It is held together by means of a small machine screw and a knurled nut. The tee should have a slot cut in it about one-half its length and it should also have one bead filed away so that the clamp will fit tightly over it.

The hand rest is made from a tapering elbow, a tee and a forging. The forging can be made by a blacksmith at a small expense. Both the lower tees of the handrest and the tailstock should be provided with screw clamps to hold them in place.

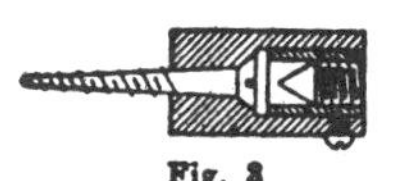
Fig. 3

The pulley is made of hardwood pieces, ¾ or 1 in. thick as desired. It is fastened to the spindle by means of a screw, as shown in Fig. 2, or a key can be used as well.

Care must be taken to get the tailstock center vertically over the bed, else taper turning will result. To do this, a straight line should be scratched

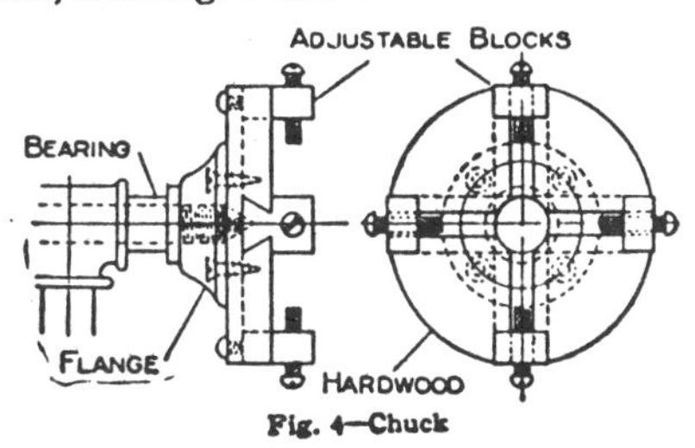

Fig. 4—Chuck

on the top of the bed pipe, and when the tailstock is set exactly vertical, a corresponding line made on this. This will save a great deal of time and trouble and possibly some errors.

The two designs of chucks shown in Figs. 3 and 4 are very easy to make, and will answer for a great variety of work.

BARGAIN BUGGING

By Clyde Barrow

When it is necessary to record your conversation with another person or his conversation with a third party after your departure, a "bug" can be hidden in your pocket and may be left at the scene. The bug transmits to a receiver/tape recorder setup in your nerarby parked car or carried by your associate who places himself as close to the scene of conversation as possible; outside an office, in an adjoining room, etc.

The simplest method uses two walkie talkies. Adequate ones are available for about $25 from any radio and electronics store. These units are small enough to carry in a coat pocket or may be taped to your leg. The transmit button is taped down, and your conversation is broadcasted to the companion unit which receives the signal and transfers it to the tape machine either by microphone or wire connection. If the walkie talkie is too bulky to hide on your person or leave at the scene, a "wireless mini mike" can be used. These units are available for $25 from security suppliers or for $14 direct from the manufacturer. These units are miniature radio transmitters that broadcast on the FM band. The "mike" should be tuned to broadcast on an unused portion of the band, thus lessening the chance that the conversation might be monitored. The chances of being overheard are slight anyway, as the range is only about 300 feet outside and less than 100 feet if the signal must pass through the walls of a building.

After an open spot on the FM band is found and the transmitter tuned (complete instructions are included with the mike) a portable FM radio is tuned to the same frequency. The radio is turned on and is connected to a tape recorder with a phone jack. One end is plugged into the speaker outlet on the radio. The other end is plugged into the input jack on the tape machine. Insert a blank 120 minute tape (60 min./side) and press the "record" button. Professional surveillance people use modified cassette machines that turn very slowly, allowing about 9 hours of recording. An existing machine can be so modified by installing a rheostat switch to control the speed of the motor in the tape recorder.

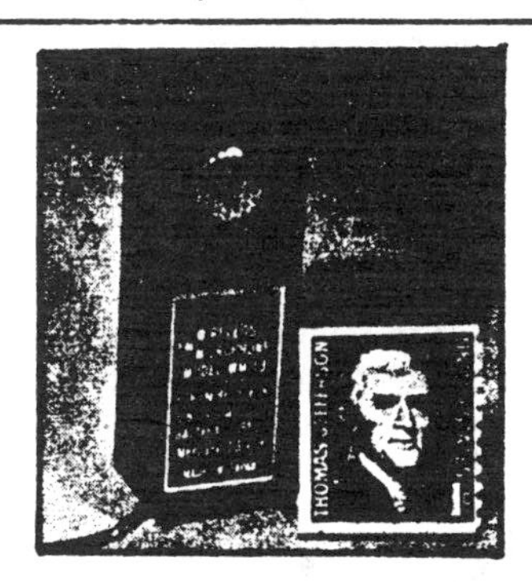
NEW SUBMINIATURE FM WIRELESS MICROPHONE

If left on the scene the wireless mike will continue to transmit for about 80 hours. It can be attached to the bottom of a desk or chair with a piece of tape or ribbon epoxy or hidden in a paper bag and placed in a convenient waste basket.

The one drawback to this transmitter is the short battery life. This is a result of the unit being constantly "on" as long as the battery is in place. Anyone with a fair amount of electronic skill can tap into the battery circuit of the mike and install a voice activated switch on the bug. This adds little bulk and allows the bug to function for weeks. The bug transmits only when conversation in the room triggers the voice activated switch. When the conversation ceases, the unit remains on for five seconds and then switches off. This is the type of system Dick Nixon used to cut his own throat during the days of Watergate. A similar voice activated switch can be installed between the radio and tape machine. This will allow the tape machine to remain off until a signal is received from the radio.

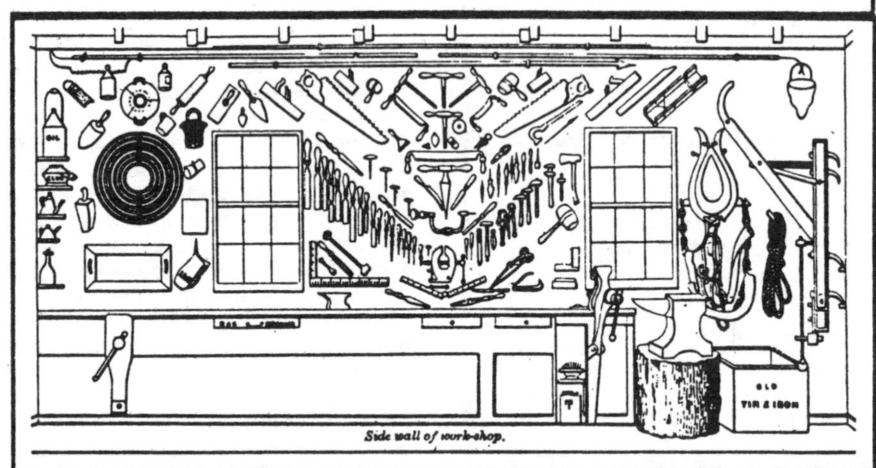

Side wall of work-shop.

HOW TO BLACKEN METAL

By Clyde Barrow

Many of your knife and gun parts, belt buckles, and various other pieces of hardware are probably made of polished metal. You may look like a walking signal mirror as you stalk through the woods or sleaze around in dark alleys.

Any metal surface can be blackened temporarily with G96 Gun Sight Black. This is a spray on dull black paint that washes off with gun solvent. Sight Black leaves no residue and won't harm the surface. It rubs off easily and must be constantly touched up.

Chrome and stainless steel can only be blackened with epoxy paint. Get the best you can afford. Epoxy does chip off and must be retouched periodically.

Aluminum can be blackened permanently only by anodizing. It is expensive and few metal shops do this type of work. (How to anodize at home will appear in a later issue.) Several gun accessory firms sell Aluminum Black. This product contains tellurium dioxide, fluoboric acid, nickel sulfate and copper sulfate. The solution produces a chalky black surface that looks great, but scratches and wears off easily. Parts that receive a lot of handling or abrasion will have to be touched up every few days.

Carbon Steel and brass parts can effectively blackened with one of the commercial touch up blues currently on the market. These are a cold type bluing, wipe on and rinse off, and should not be confused with commercial hot bluing which requires large tanks of chemicals and assorted paraphenalia. Cold blue is designed to be used to touch up scratches and worn spots on an existing blue job. If cold blue is used to color a large area, such as a knife blade, it will often appear blotchy and uneven. This is not good at gun shows, but matters little for our purposes here. Cold blue will wear off in time, but a coat of Pledge or similar furniture polish will seal the surface and help to protect the finish. A light coat of oil will also protect a new cold blue from the elements.

The traditonal military finish for steel is a black or gray matte finish known as Parkerizing. A complete article on this process will appear in a future issue.

CO2 BOMB

By Clyde Barrow

Empty CO2 cartridges can be used as mini bombs or grenades, either singly or in groups attached to a central pipe bomb or grenade device.

A 3/16 inch diameter hole is drilled into the neck of the cartridge. A small funnel is used to fill the bomb with black or smokeless powder. A section of 3/16 inch diameter cannon and hobby fuse is now glued into the hole Be sure to cut the ends on a diagonal. This will assure positive ignition of the powder. If a fragmentation effect is desired, a layer of finish nails or tacks is taped to the outside of the cartridge. The nails may first be dipped in poison if desired. A fragmentation device capable of large distribution can be made by taping several of these small bombs to a central pipe bomb or grenade. The fuses of the individual bombs are trimmed to the same length and the ends to be lit are held together loosely with a rubber band. These fuses should be set to burn several seconds longer than the main bomb or grenade fuse. After all fuses are lit, the unit is thrown or shot from a launcher. When the main bomb explodes, the mini bombs will be scattered through the air over a wide area, and then a few seconds later, each bomb will explode individually. Each of these mini bombs will in turn spray their respective areas with shrapnel.

The fuse should always be tested beforehand to determine the specific burning rate. Each new roll of fuse should be tested, as the burning rate may vary from one roll to another.

Nunchaku

By Darvis McCoy

When Japan invaded and occupied Okinawa some 350 years ago, possession of any weapon by an Okinawan was forbidden. So the Okinawans had to turn to improvising weapons from common tools, as Americans will someday have to do. One such weapon was the nunchaku, a tool used by the farmers to pound their grain. It consisted of two sticks tied together by a rope or cord, making it the most versatile and wicked hand-to-hand weapon ever devised. The nunchaku can be used as a club, a flail, or a garrote, and can be mastered at home with only a few hours practice. It can be made with materials easily had from any lumber yard or hardware store. When used as a flail or whiplash club, the striking end reaches speeds of over 100 m.p.h. When used as a garrote, each stick uses the other for leverage, creating a viselike garrote.

To make one, take a piece of 1 1/2 inch diameter dowel 31 inches long and cut in half, each piece then being 15 1/2 inches long. Now drill a hole into the end of each piece to a depth of about three inches. The hole should be just wide enough to accommodate a nylon rope, which is the best for this purpose. Now drill into the side of the dowel to intersect the end of the other hole, but big enough to hold the rope doubled. You should now have one "L" shaped hole. Now insert the end of the rope through the end of the dowel and pull through the larger hole. Double the rope end and fuse the doubled strands together with a match. Now repeat the process with the other stick, using the other end of the rope, leaving about five inches between the two sticks. The fused strands should fit into the hole, leaving nothing sticking out. A simple knot could be tied in the ends of the ropes instead of burning them with the matches.

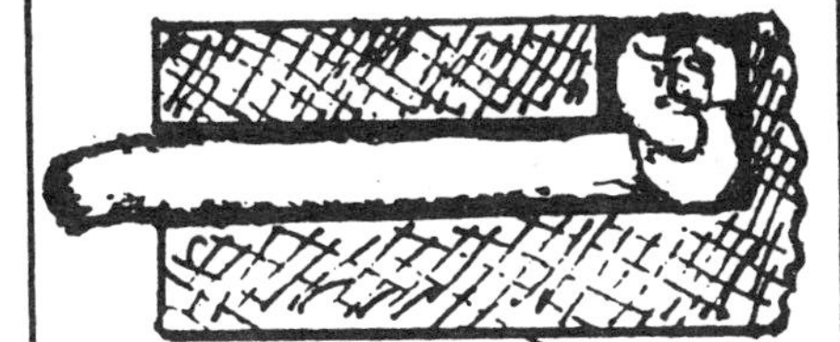

The nunchaku is used as a flail by holding one of the sticks about midway, thumb pointing toward the rope. It can be swung from a hanging position, with the other end either hanging backward over the same shoulder, or from the under arm position, like in the movies. For the under arm position, the striking end is held firmly in the armpit, and released with a sudden snap at the victim's temple or ribs. Your own imaginations is the limit to the number of ways and methods of striking that can be used.

Most store-bought nunchakus come with chains instead of rope, but chains are noisy and are not worth the effort.

When you have practiced enough to keep from bashing yourself in the forehead, take a block plane and plane off the roundness of the dowel, making it into a hexagon. When these edges hit a victim, the pounds per square inch are much deadlier than those delivered by a round object.

The nunchaku is very superior to the yawara stick for several reasons. It has a much greater reach, it hits harder due to the whiplash effect, and it does more damage because of the edges left after planing off the curves. It can be used as a regular club by holding the two sticks together; and when you realize that the club you are holding is also effective as a garrote, with no modification, you begin to realize that you hold the world's most effective hand-to-hand weapon.

SWITCHES
By Clyde Barrow

A simple pull switch for use in burglar alarms, booby traps and for arming bombs can be made from a spring clothespin, a wood or plastic wedge, and a pull wire or string. (See drawing #1)

First strip the insullation from the ends of the two circuit wires and wrap them tightly around the two jaws of the clothespin. The bare wires should touch and close the circuit when the clothespin is in a relaxed position. To hold the circuit in an open position, a wedge of some non-conductive material such as wood or plastic is inserted between the jaws. A pull wire is attached to the wedge. When the wire is pulled, the wedge is pulled free and the clothespin snaps shut, completing the circuit. The switch is mounted to a solid surface by driving a nail through the hole in the clothespin spring.

The one drawback to the above system is the easewith which it can be disarmed. If the subject should spot the wire, he can simply cut it and proceed about his business. A failsafe switch to foil these sneaky types is shown is drawing #2.

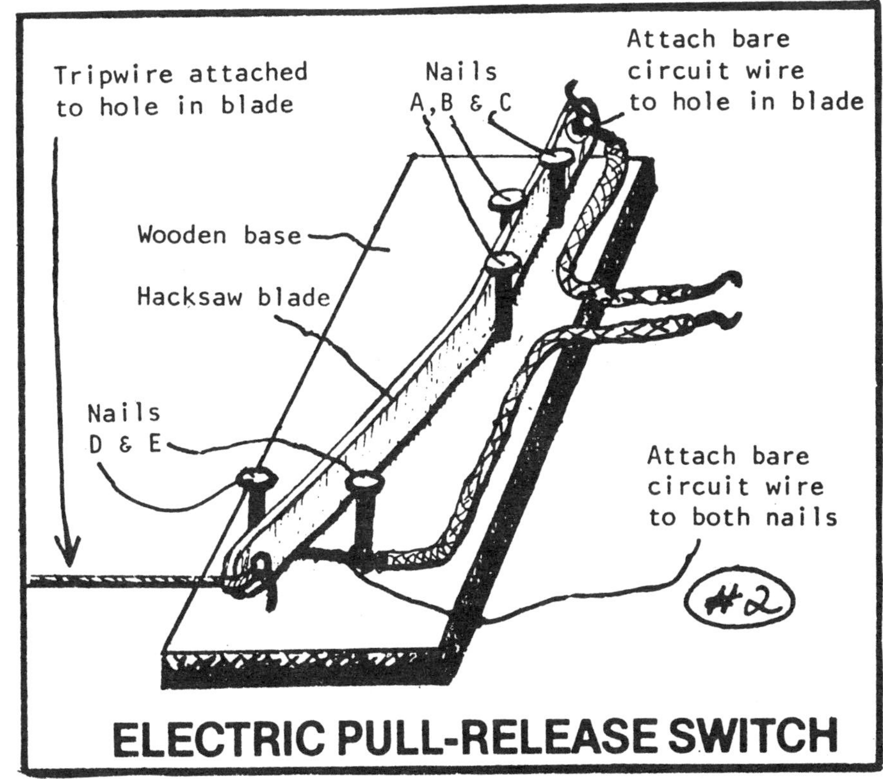

ELECTRIC PULL-RELEASE SWITCH

A hacksaw blade or similar flexible strip of conductive metal is secured to a board with three nails (a, b, and c) as shown. One of the two circuit wires is now attached to this end of the metal strip.

Nails D & E are driven into the board about 1 inch apart. The second circuit wire is now attached to these two nails as shown. In this manner the circuit will be closed if the metal strip touches either nail D or E.

The trip wire is attached to the D/E end of the metal strip. Adjust the tension to suspend the strip between the two nails.

If the wire is pulled in a trip wire fashion, the metal strip will touch nail D but if the wire is discovered and cut it will spring open and contact nail E. Either way, the circuit will be completed. This is a popular anti distrubance device for bombs because it is almost impossible to cut the wire and maintain the correct tension to prevent touching the contacts.

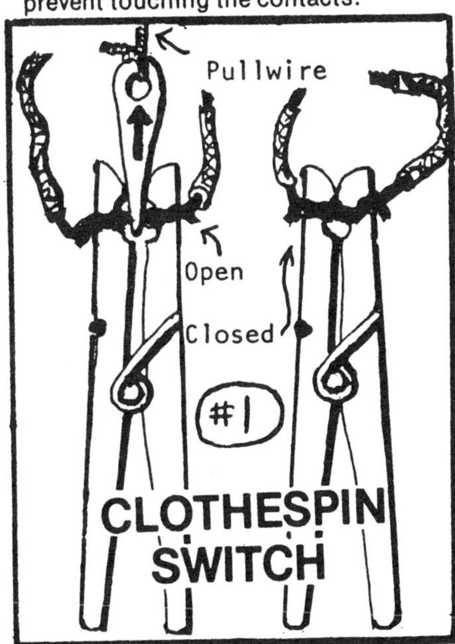

CLOTHESPIN SWITCH

Hit-Men's Silenced .22 Weapon

New York

The type of gun used recently to silence so many informers and mob dissidents would have never been used by professional gangland assassins until two years ago.

"The mob has always preferred the 9mm; the .38 revolver, a Baretta automatic, or a shotgun in the past," a federal source said. "What it looks like is that some mob assassin squads have stolen a page from our spy agencies."

The .22-caliber automatic was a favorite of agents of the Office of Strategic Services during World War II. It has been a long-time favorite of the CIA. Light, compact, highly accurate from close range, its one-ounce slug, when muffled by a silencer, gives a "pop-pop" noise that can barely be heard. Made even more efficient in recent years, it has attracted the mob.

Both police and federal ballistics experts note that high-velocity ammunition can now be fired by the .22 and that hollowed-out heads that splatter and rip apart after hitting a victim leave no traceable ballistics.

In at least several instances in the mob purge that is believed to have been going on for the past two years hollowed-out copper heads were used, but most of the hit victims have left a ballistics trail. In New Jersey and New York, for example, the murders of two men have been traced to the same, but unrecovered weapon

The interest of the mob and others in the .22 as a murder weapon was recently exemplified by the conviction of George Nathaniel Garrett in Miami. Garrett, an associate of a Carmine Galente crime family soldier, had been peddling do-it-yourself assassination kits for $600 apiece.

The kits included a Luger-type automatic .22, a silencer, and an attache case through which the gun could be fired: a pull-ring near the handle that, when tugged, automatically fired a clip of eight to ten rounds with deadly accuracy.

Garrett was arrested in October by undercover agents of the federal Alcohol, Tobacco and Fire arms bureau but not before an undetermined number of the assassin kits were believed sold to the mob.

Garrett, however, was only a minor source of the weapons. Variations of the gun can be bought through gun stores around the nation, in Mexico or from foreign sources, and many gun buffs have similar weapons for target practice. "Its value is in its compactness, lightness, high velocity, accuracy and availability," a police source said.

A silencer cannot be bought in a gun store, but there are mob gunsmiths available, willing and able to provide them at from $75 to $200 depending on quality.

San Francisco Chronicle Newsday

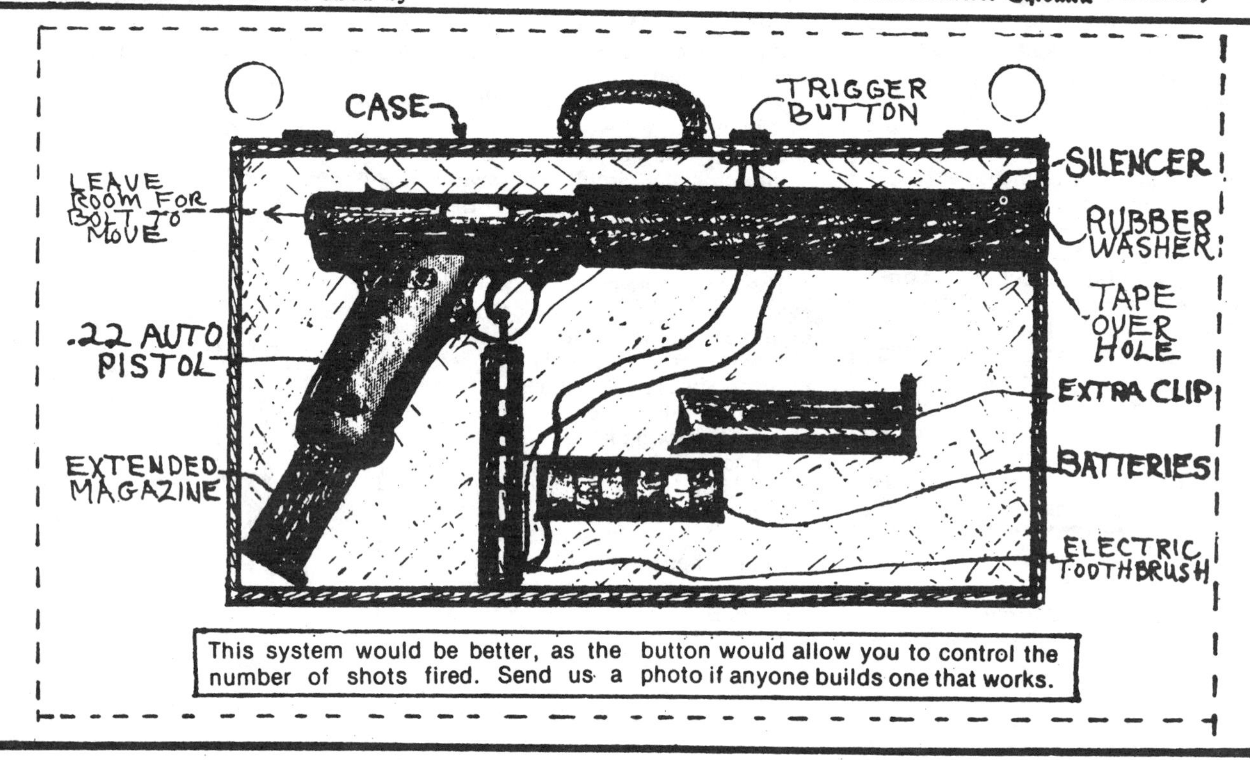

This system would be better, as the button would allow you to control the number of shots fired. Send us a photo if anyone builds one that works.

THE SILENCERS

By Clyde Barrow

Of all 20th century small arms developments, the firearm silencer is probably the most mysterious and the least understood. Invented in 1908 by Hiram Maxim, the firearm silencer was one of Maxim's early contributions to the field of noise pollution control. By the 1930s, poachers, gangsters, strike breakers and stickup men had made "silencer" a dirty word. The silencer had become so steeped in intrigue the it was included in the restrictive "destructive devices" category of the National Firearm Act of 1934. Since 1934, possession, use, or manufacture of a silencer has been a serious felony. Silencer possession for private citizens is currently restricted to those who can meet the following requirements.

1. Pay a $200 Federal Transfer Tax.
2. Receive transfer approval from the Federal Bureau of Alcohol, Tobacco, and Firearms. (ATF)
3. Comply with all state and local restrictions on silencer possession.

Silencer production is restricted to holders of a $500 Federal Firearms Stamp that designates them as "manufacturers of destructive devices."

In general, the modern commercial silencer is a metal tube, 1 inch to 3 inches in diameter and about a foot long. The tube is mounted on the muzzle end of the barrel and is aligned with the axis of the bore, i.e. the bullet travels down the exact center of the tube. The front of the tube is covered with an endplate, the center of which has a hole that is slightly larger than the diameter of the bullet to be fired. The interior of the silencer tube contains a series of baffles and chambers which catch and delay the rapidly escaping gases produced by the propellant powder as it burns.

The major source of gun blast and noise from conventional weapons is this escaping gas slamming into the atmosphere upon exiting the barrel. The remaining sources of gun noise are as follows:

A. A supersonic crack is produced if the bullet reaches a speed greater than 1120 feet per second, the speed of sound.

B. Mechanical noise is produced by the functioning of the weapon upon firing. This attendant clatter is most pronounced in semi and full automatic weapons.

Some noise also escapes through the unlocked breech area of these autos. A bolt action rifle will produce little if any mechanical noise when fired and no sound escapes from the breech area.

Contrary to what you see on TV, the revolver is not suitable for silencer use. Considerable noise is generated by the gas escaping from the gap between the barrel and cylinder. To make matters worse, those mini silencers, a couple of inches long, are a twisted joke on the part of Hollywood prop men.

In addition to noise suppression, the forward pressure of the gas in the silencer equalizes and virtually eliminates the recoil experienced with unsilenced weapons. A silencer also doubles as an effective flash hider for night shooting.

When a silencer is used on a high powered firearm, the supersonic crack experienced with these weapons can be eliminated in one of the three ways:

A. Standard ammunition will not produce a crack if fired in weapons with shortened barrels. The burning powder is unable to generate the necessary pressure to drive the bullet faster than 1120 f.p.s.

B. Similar results are obtained with standard ammo when it is fired through a conventional length barrel that has had a series of tiny holes drilled along its length. These holes bleed off a portion of the propellant gases, again reducing bullet speed.

C. A special milder load may be used in unaltered weapons. These are referred to as sub sonic loads. These rounds contain less powder and do not propel bullets to super sonic speeds. Some semi and full auto weapons need to be altered to function reliably with subsonic rounds.

In addition to commercially produced and federally regulated silencers, several other types are available:

1. Commercial units smuggled in from other countries.
2. Underground production in domestic factories.
3. Individually produced, home made silencers.
4. Improvised or one shot silencers.

Examples of this last type of silencer

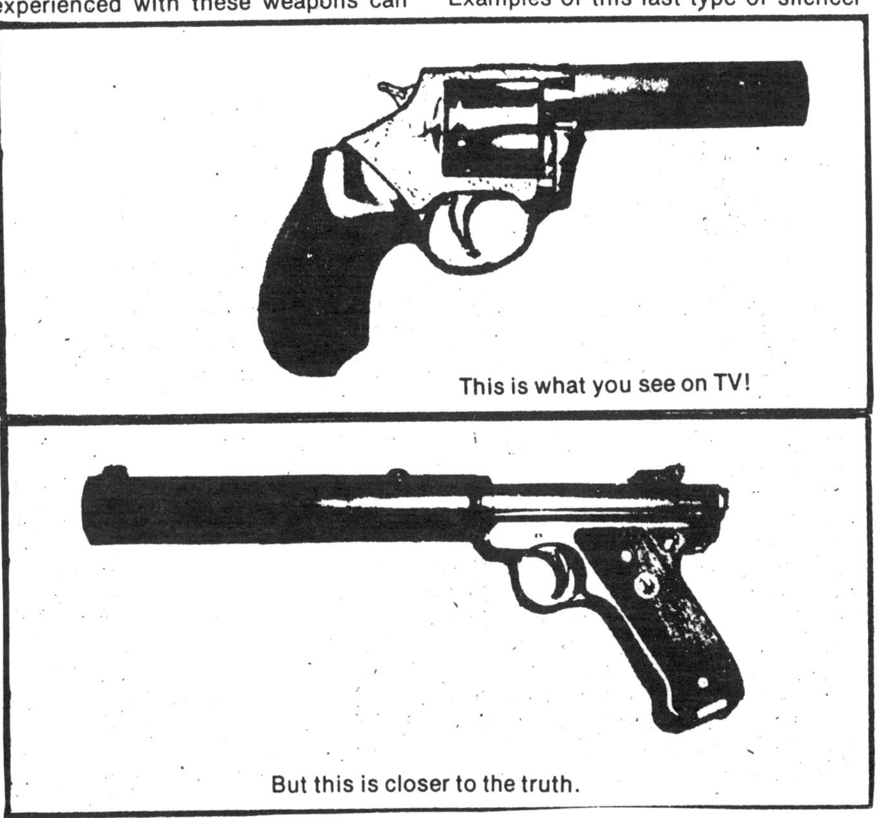

This is what you see on TV!

But this is closer to the truth.

are: balloons, rubbers, baby bottle nipples, etc. These are stretched over the end of the barrel and taped in place. A small hole or "X" is cut in the end. They expand to contain a portion of the propellant gases. These units may or may not hold up to repeated firing. The overall effect is sort of half-assed but then half quiet is better than no quiet at all. Pillows, heavy coats, foam rubber, etc. can be wrapped around a firearm to reduce firing noise. Even with a excellent silencer, most autos need to be wrapped in something that will muffle the mechanical noise of operation.

THE POOR MAN'S JAMES BOND by Kurt Saxon contains plans for a silenced box with a handgun inside. Just reach inside and blast away.

Most individually produced or "hand made" silencers soon meet a common fate. At some point the silencer loses proper alignment with the barrel. The next round catches on a baffle and the entire interior of the unit is destroyed. As a bonus, the tube is often launched 50 feet down range. You can imagine how embarrassing this is to a young guy just starting out. The key then is aligning the tube with the bore, then everything else falls into place.

Alignment and mounting of the tube can be handled in several different ways, but one basic rule holds true for all of them. To assure constant alignment with the bore, the silencer tube must be supported by at least two points on the barrel.

The simplest method is to tape the barrel at two points to support the tube (see improvised silencer mount article). This method works well for a while and is extremely accurate. If care is taken when wrapping the tape, the resulting unit will be no more than two tape thicknesses out of alignment. The one drawback to this system is a tendency for the tube to slowly crawl off the barrel, a little more with each successive shot. It is a good idea to hang on tight to this type of unit, always maintaining a constant rearward tension on the tube while firing.

Tubing

The two types of metal tubing generally used in homemade silencer construction are thick walled aluminum tubing and thin walled brass drain pipe. Both are light, inexpensive, and available at most hardware and plumbing stores. The aluminum comes in 6 foot lengths and sells for about $3.00 each. Brass drain pipe is sold in straight sections 12 inches long, both plain brass and chrome plated. These sections cost about $2.00 each.

Thin walled brass tubes are easily joined together with silver solder. Aluminum tubing can't be soldered but is easily held together with screws because the wall thickness is sufficient to hold threads. The holes can be drilled and tapped in the conventional manner or simply drilled with a hand drill and threaded with self tapping machine screws.

The following are construction plans for two 22 caliber silencers. The first one uses brass tubing and is silver soldered together. The second is made from aluminum and is held together with machine screws. Both units are simple, trouble free and quite effective. These construction proceedures can be easily modified for building silencers in larger calibers.

A. Brass Tubing Silencer

Materials needed.

- 1 piece Brass drain pipe (plain or chromed) 12 inches long, 1 1/4 inch diameter.
- 12 fender washers—1 3/16 inch diameter.
- 1 piece 9/32 inch brass tubing—sold in 12 inch sections (8 inches are needed).
- 9/32 inch drill bit and drill.
- 1/16 inch drill bit.
- silver solder and propane torch
- hacksaw
- file or grinder
- C clamp

Step 1

Grind down all twelve washers until they will slide into the tube. A file or bench grinder may be used. Take care that the washers remain round and that the hole is in the exact center.

Step 2

Enlarge the hole in the washers to 9/32 inches.

Step 3

Cut the 9/32 inch brass tubing to eight inches long. Remove the burrs from the ends with a file, knife, or piece of sandpaper.

Step 4

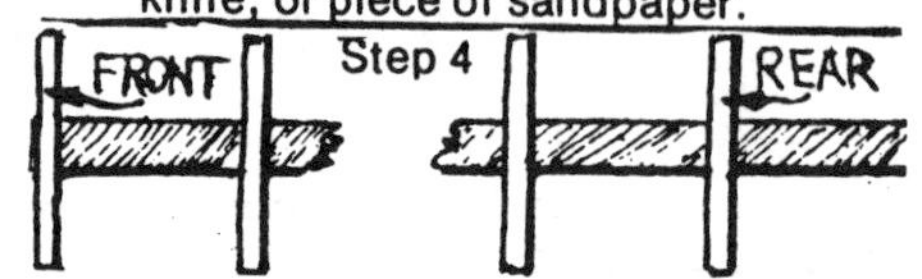

Ten of the twelve washers are now slipped over the 9/32 inch tube. The front washer (end cap) should be flush with the front end of the tubing. The rear washer is placed one inch from the rear of the tube. The remaining eight washers are spaced equally between the front and rear. Solder all ten washers in place.

Step 5

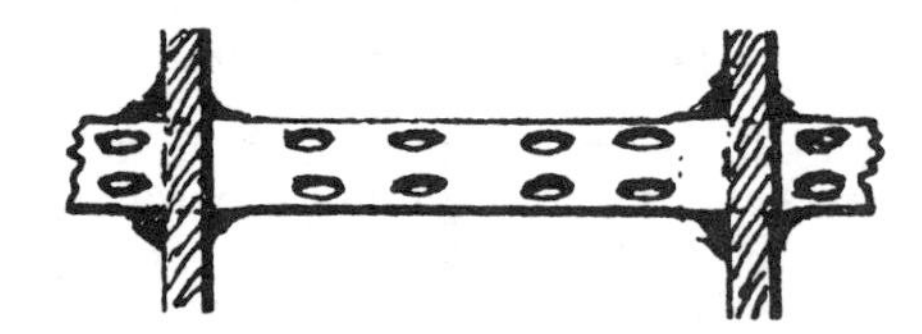

Drill two rows of four 1/16 inch holes between each set of washers. Drill completely through the tube. This will result in four rows of four, a total of sixteen holes between each baffle. Remove any burrs or metal chips from the interior of the tube with a thin file or a rolled up piece of sandpaper.

Step 6

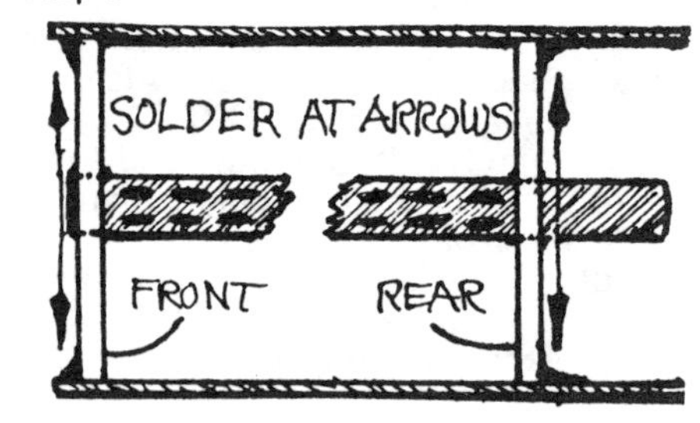

Install the baffle assembly into the outer tube. The front baffle (end cap) should be recessed about 1/16 inch. The spaces between the washers may be filled with steel wool or rolls of brass screen before installing in the outer tube. This is optional as there is some disagreement about the value of these materials as baffling devices. Solder the baffle assembly in place.

Step 7

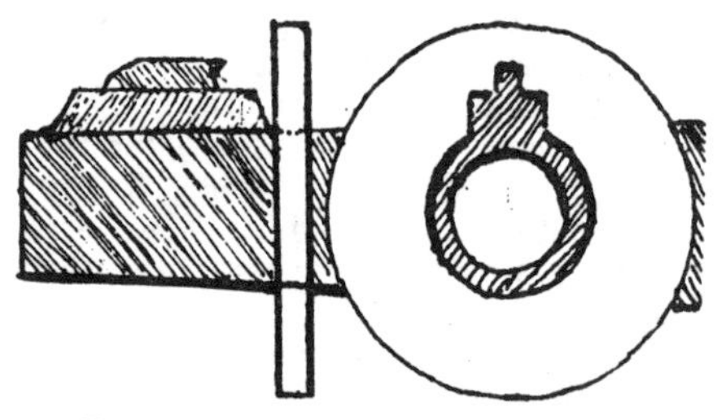

The two remaining washers are used as the mounting assembly. The front washer is modified to slip over the barrel and rest at a point directly behind the front sight base. This requires reaming, drilling or filing out the hole to match the diameter of the barrel at this point. A cut out is made in the washer to allow it to slip past the sight base. The washer is now slipped over the barrel and turned 180 deg. If the above was done properly, the washer will be held from forward movement by the sight base. The taper of the barrel will prevent it from moving to the rear.

Step 8

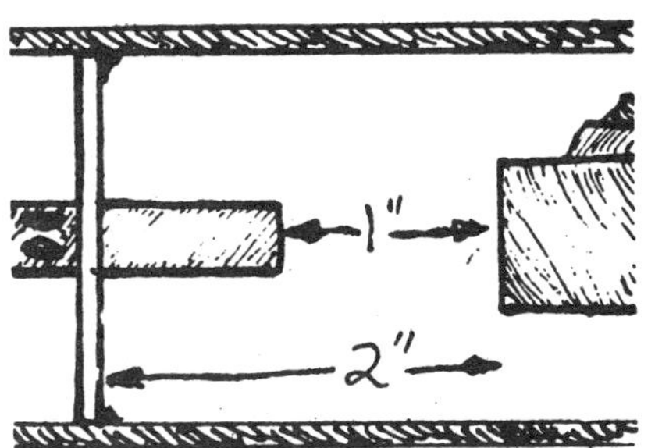

With the front mount washer in place on the barrel, slip the silencer onto the gun as far as possible. The gun's muzzle will be resting against the rear end of the silencer's inner brass tube. The silencer is now moved forward one inch. This creates a two inch chamber between the muzzle and the rear baffle. This space is necessary for the initial expansion of gas as it leaves the muzzle. Place a mark on the barrel that corresponds to the rear edge of the silencer tube.

Align the silencer with the bore of the gun. This may be done visually or with a tight fitting stick. When the unit is aligned, place a C clamp around the silencer directly over the front mount washer and tighten the C clamp in place. Remove the silencer from the barrel. Take care not to disturb the position of the washer in the tube. This washer is now soldered in place to the silencer interior. Remove the C clamp.

Step 9

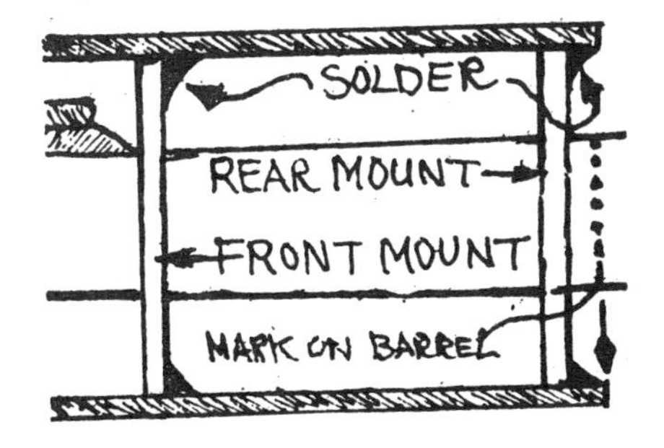

The rear washer is now notched and drilled until it will slide onto the gun and come to rest at a point 1/16 inches in front of the mark on the barrel. This washer doesn't lock onto anything, it: functions as a rear support only. Slide the silencer over the barrel and onto the rear washer. It should extend 1/16 inch beyond the washer. Solder the washer to the silencer. The completed silencer/mount assembly can now be installed and removed in seconds.

Step 10

If for some reason the silencer is not in correct alignment when installed, it may be adjusted. Clamp the gun into a padded vise. Sight down the silencer and bend it into proper alignment while heating the soldered joints of the two mount washers.

Improvised Silencer Mount

This device can be used to mount a commercial or improvised silencer, attaching it firmly to the barrel of the weapon and maintaining perfect alignment with the bore.

The Mount can be used with several sizes of silencers and is designed for quick installation and removal. It is made from a metal or hard plastic tube 1-1 1/2 inches inside diameter and about 9 inches long.

Four 1 inch deep hacksaw cuts are made in each end of the tube. This will produce 8 evenly spaced slots, 1 inch deep. Bevel the inside edges of both ends of the tube with a round file or sandpaper. Place a hose clamp on each end of the tube and screw down finger tight.

The barrel is now wrapped with black plastic electrical tape at 2 points, the first directly behind the front sight and the second about 5 inches behind the muzzle. On barrels shorter than 5 inches, the tape is wrapped at the rear of the barrel. Continue to wrap the tape until both rolls are a snug fit when the tube is pushed onto the barrel.

Slide the mount tube onto the barrel until the rear clamp is directly over the rear roll of the tape. Tighten the rear clamp with a penny or screwdriver. The tube is now in almost perfect alignment with the barrel.

The silencer is now taped in two places until it is also a snug fit in the tube. The front clamp should correspond to the front roll of tape on the silencer.

This mount will not interfere with the slight pattern on a scoped rifle, but sights must be installed for use on a handgun.

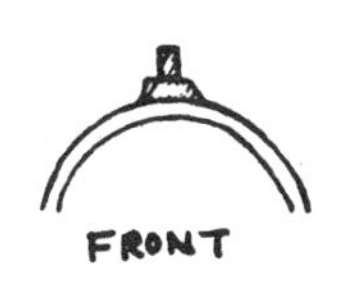

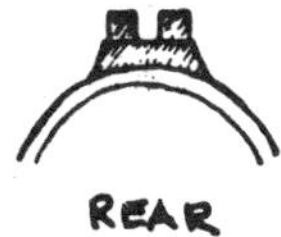

Sights may be fabricated from metal or plastic and soldered or epoxyed in place. Ready made commercial sights may also be used.

When the mount is completed it may be blued, painted, or covered with black plastic tape.

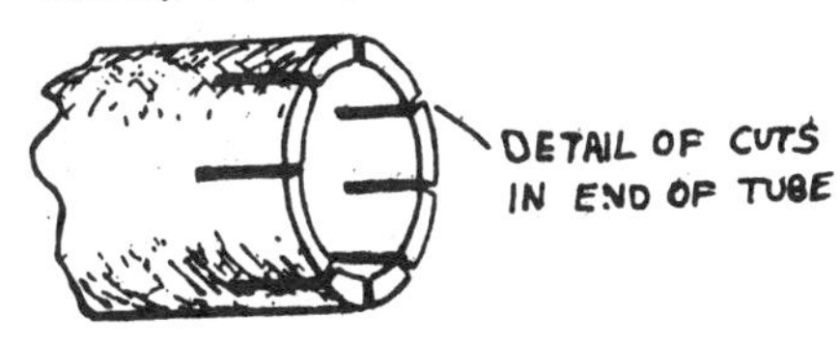

See finished silencer next page.

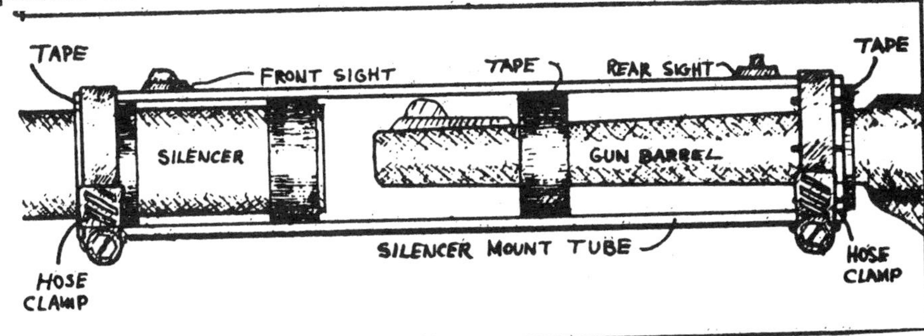

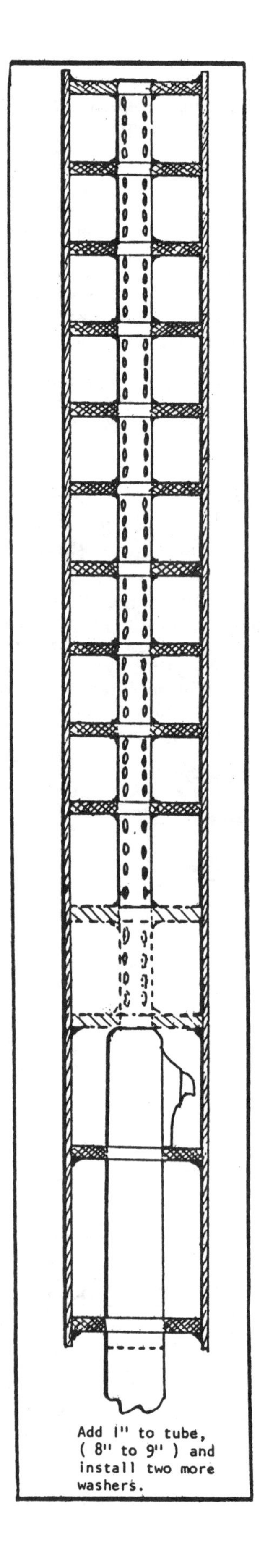
Add 1" to tube, (8" to 9") and install two more washers.

SHARP KNUCKLES

BY M. OHNO

An inexpensive, convenient, and legal pocket weapon has long been known in the guise of the ordinary household scissors. However, the new folding type in stainless steel won't rust if gotten wet, are compact, handy, fit any budget at under $3, and they are available from most any camping, hardware, or discount store. Most importantly, the folding feature insures against inadvertant misadventures such as castration or disembowelment when sitting down quickly (it pays not to be your own most dangerous enemy,believe me). What is more, they should pass muster at airport or police shakedowns. While they may not believe that your fingernails grow so fast you have to clip them all day, you're quite safe from concealed weapons hassles.

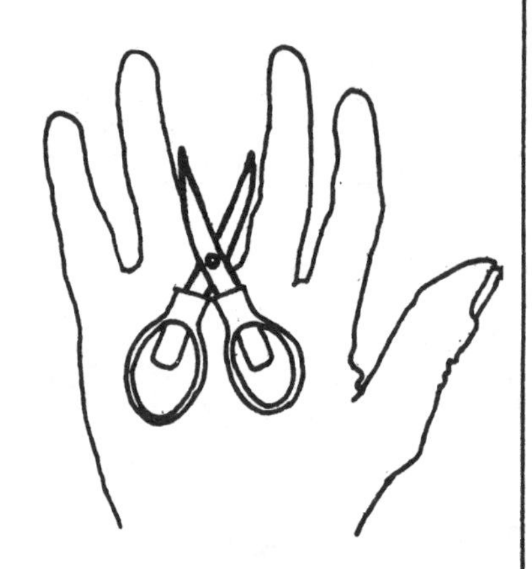

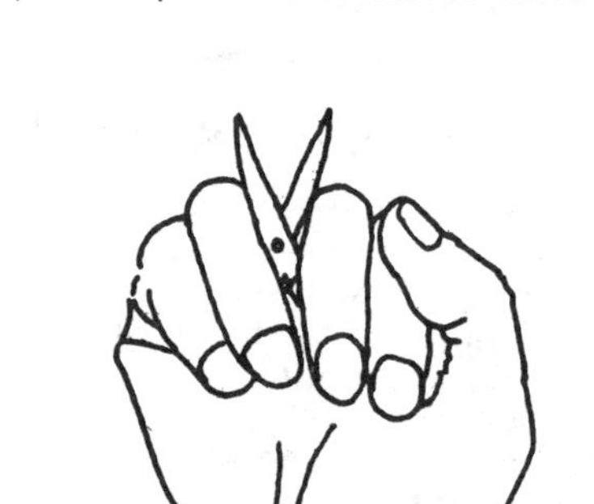

Finally, their use is as natural as throwing a punch— more important than one might think. A weapon is only as good as one's ability to use it under stress. Many a top notch pistol shot has been known to miss targets across the room due to the involuntary"heeling" and muscular tension experienced while under stress. Just place the scissors in the fist as shown and you are all set to throw a punch with some real authority in it.

THE HANDY NO IMPACT REQUIRED FIREBOMB

By The Firebug

I came up with this devilish little device one day while pondering the best way to torch piles of hay. It uses a minimum amount of fuel, is silent (no bottles breaking), and cheap to build. Take an empty soft drink can and remove the top. Stuff with some sort of absorbant material. Pour in a few ounces of gas and pour out excess. To use, all you have to do is light the top and throw on a flammable substance. A little sand in the bottom of the can helps it throw farther.

HARPER'S YOUNG PEOPLE JUNE 19, 1894.

THE SAME THING OVER AGAIN.

BY JAMES BARNES.

LONG years ago a knight who rode forth to battle was supposed to be the bravest of the brave. Perhaps he was. We read of valorous deeds in every old bit of verse, and the history of the age of chivalry is full of him. He slew foemen by the score, he was always in the thickest of the fray, and there was only one thing he could not do—get up if he fell down. Some of the deadly blows that struck him rang off his heavy armor in much the same way that the blows of a hammer would ring off an iron boiler. Now perhaps all this had something to do with his valorous deeds, and may account for the many foemen slain, and it certainly does account for his remaining alive so very often. They say that a knight in armor was as good as twelve men without it, and that as long as he could stay on his horse or keep his feet he was safe from the ordinary weapons of those days. It is proof enough to say that in a battle in France fifty armed knights on a side fought throughout an afternoon, and not a single one was killed. Therefore we must infer that they stopped from lack of breath, or perhaps the game may have been called "on account of darkness"; who knows?

With the advent of gunpowder things changed. Armor gradually went out of fashion. It was no use. Bullets went through it, and came out the other side; so helmet and cuirass, shield, targe, buckler, greaves, and chain-shirt were used only for show, or to decorate armorial halls. Nothing could stand before the swift-speeding unseen bullet—and perhaps the knights became braver than ever—many more were killed in battle.

In naval circles, after the little iron-clad *Monitor* fought the iron-clad *Merrimac* wooden ships of war practically ceased to be built. Every nation turned its attention to building impenetrable bulwarks, and then guns were built to pierce them, and then thicker armor was made, and then heavier guns, and so on, hammer and tongs, they are fighting it out to this day. Now they are building ships fast enough to run away from each other, which seems the only way to stop this game of Everlasting.

But the powers of invention are most wonderful. What do you think of a steel-pointed bullet that penetrates two feet six inches of solid oak being stopped by a stiff pad of felt and some other composition; not only stopped, but all crumbled out of shape? This has been done, and a little tailor of Manheim, Germany, is the inventor.

His name is Dowe. Like almost all inventors no one believed him at first, and every one was too busy to listen to his talk. When he wished to put on his bullet proof vest, and stand up to be shot at, they all laughed, and thought that the tailor was crazy. At last he persuaded some one to take a shot at him, and lo, and behold, there was Herr Dowe bowing through the smoke of the rifle all unharmed, and as smiling as an Aunt Sally at a fair. Of course people believed him after that, and everybody said, "We thought there was something in it; but we did not know." Lots of other people wrote letters saying that they had invented the same thing years before, and scores of imitators started up on every side. Before very long the army people—who hate to have other persons invent things—took up the subject, and Herr Dowe was given an official trial before prominent German officers. They were most sceptical, and would not let the anxious little tailor don his heavy waistcoat, and make a target of himself. They carefully put it on a plaster statue, and blazed away. "Ach!" said the German officers, when the smoke cleared—"ach! the tailor does not lie." Then they put the shield on a horse, and fired directly at his side. The animal went on eating, all unconscious that a great many spectators expected him to pitch forward and die on the spot; he was as unmoved as a deaf man at a pathetic sermon. It was Mr. Dowe's turn after that, and they shot at him, and he smiled, and they shot again, and he smiled again.

The breast-plate that Herr Dowe invented is made of felt and metal, it is supposed, but of course he doesn't tell any one just how it is made; it weighs about ten pounds, and is inflexible. The bullet does not glance, but tears itself to pieces in the cloth, and the blow is softened by the gradual impeding of the speed, so that there is little shock to the wearer; in fact, Herr Dowe says he *knows* when he

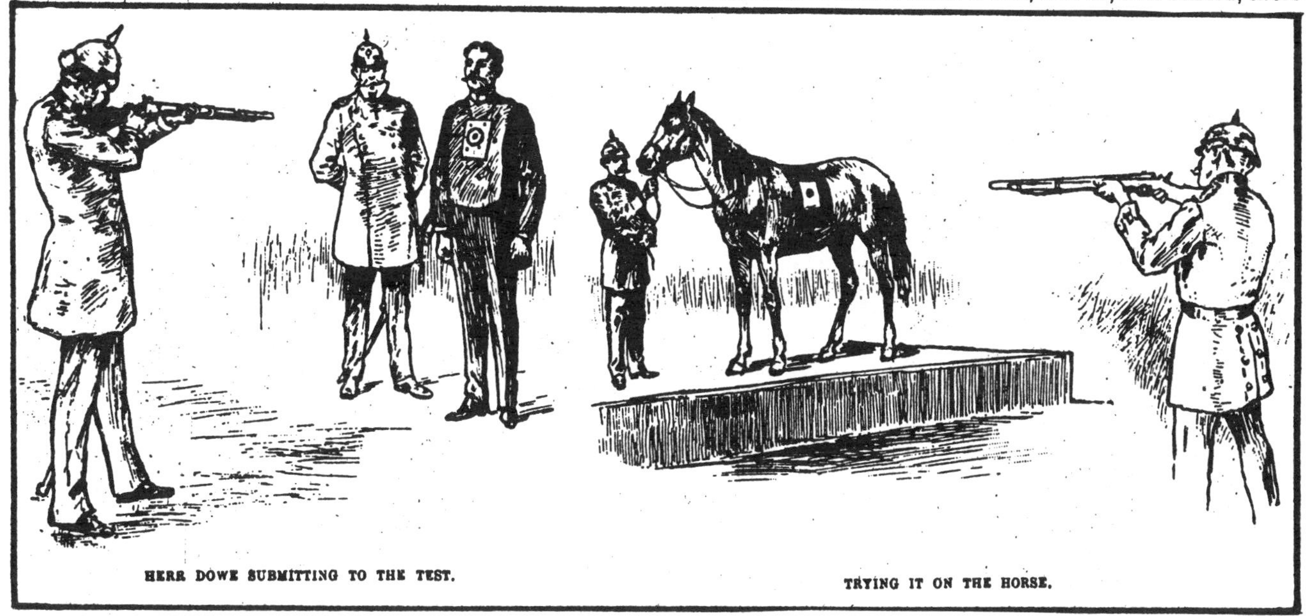

HERR DOWE SUBMITTING TO THE TEST. TRYING IT ON THE HORSE.

is hit, and that is all. What the German army will do with the shield remains to be seen. Its inventor is now in England, and the other day gave an exhibition in London. Several Englishmen wished to try their own pet rifles, and many supposed that a bullet that would go through the tough hide of an elephant would certainly pierce three inches of anything but solid steel. Elephant rifle, express rifle, Martini-Henry, and Lee-Metford (the two latter being the army rifles of Great Britian), each one proved ineffectual, and the experiment (so far as Herr Dowe goes) was a great success. The Duke of Cambridge, who was present, refused to allow any one to be shot at, although Admiral Saumerez, one of the committee, volunteered to stand up like a man and run the risk. The little tailor almost shed tears of disappointment because they would not let him take his favorite role. The horse, however, was again brought on, and I suspect wondered what it was all about, for he never seemed to know whether to go to sleep or to prance about; and the bullets did not alarm him.

What they will do with this new invention is a problem; if they can make it light enough to wear, it may change the style of fighting, and they will have to build rifles to pierce it. Then comes the thicker armor again, you see. In Berlin in the great army museum there is a cuirass (a breast-plate and back-plate) that is perforated through and through by thirteen bullets. They took it off a poor French cavalryman, who was dead on the field where his squadron had charged on a line of intrenched infantry. If he had had on a Dowe shield he might have thought it a joke. Perhaps they may get tired spending money on war, and armor, and great guns, and stop fighting. I say again—who knows?

POPULAR SCIENCE MONTHLY 1937

Flight Bow

PULLS INSTEAD OF PUSHES THE ARROW

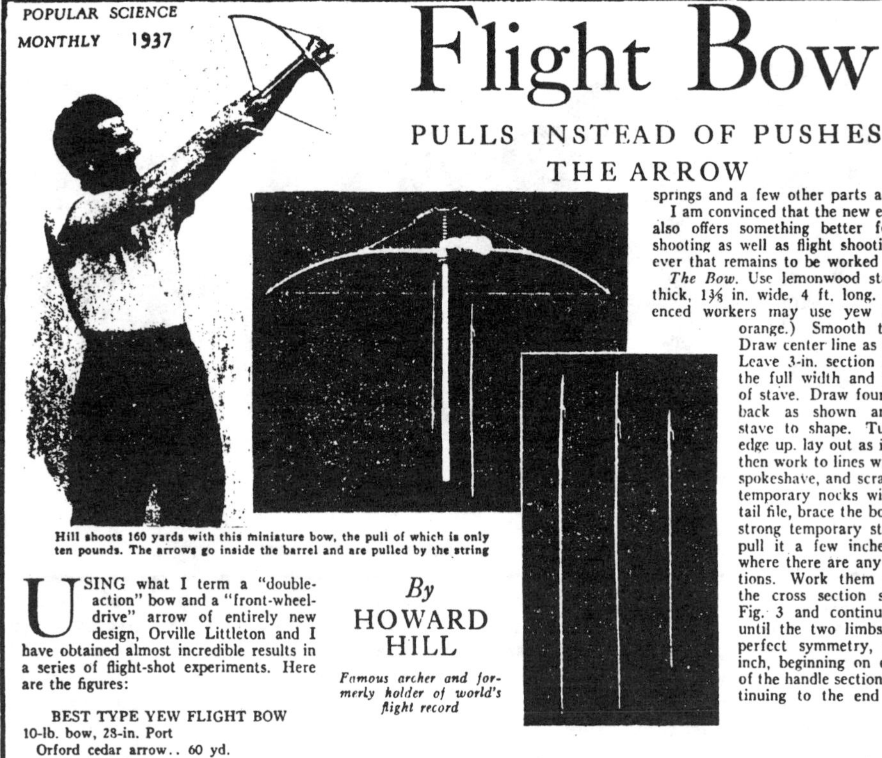

Hill shoots 160 yards with this miniature bow, the pull of which is only ten pounds. The arrows go inside the barrel and are pulled by the string

By HOWARD HILL

Famous archer and formerly holder of world's flight record

USING what I term a "double-action" bow and a "front-wheel-drive" arrow of entirely new design, Orville Littleton and I have obtained almost incredible results in a series of flight-shot experiments. Here are the figures:

BEST TYPE YEW FLIGHT BOW
10-lb. bow, 28-in. Port Orford cedar arrow.. 60 yd.
30-lb. bow, 28-in. Port Orford cedar arrow..209 yd.
65-lb. bow, 28-in. Port Orford cedar arrow..304 yd.

BOW AND ARROW OF NEW DESIGN
10-lb. bow, spring type, front-drive arrow ...160 yd.
30-lb. bow, spring type, front-drive arrow ...328 yd.

The term "30-lb. bow" means that a pull of 30 lb. is required to draw back fully whatever length of arrow is intended to be used with it. Note therefore that the new 30-lb. bow and arrow gave a greater flight than a 65-lb. bow of the finest type heretofore developed for flight shooting.

Conventional arrows are difficult to make successfully, but those used with the new bow, which are pulled instead of pushed, are simplicity itself—a piece of squared umbrella rib, a nail, and a sliver of bamboo. The new double-action bow is made like other bows, but three springs and a few other parts are added.

I am convinced that the new equipment also offers something better for target shooting as well as flight shooting; however that remains to be worked out.

The Bow. Use lemonwood stave 1 in. thick, 1⅜ in. wide, 4 ft. long. (Experienced workers may use yew or osage orange.) Smooth the back. Draw center line as in Fig. 1. Leave 3-in. section in center the full width and thickness of stave. Draw four lines on back as shown and plane stave to shape. Turn stave edge up. lay out as in Fig. 2; then work to lines with plane, spokeshave, and scraper. Cut temporary nocks with a rat-tail file, brace the bow with a strong temporary string, and pull it a few inches to see where there are any stiff sections. Work them down to the cross section shown in Fig. 3 and continue testing until the two limbs bend in perfect symmetry, inch for inch, beginning on each side of the handle section and continuing to the end of each limb. Round the belly, but keep the back perfectly flat. Sandpaper well.

Barrel. Bore a ¾-in. hole as in Fig. 1. Use a 30-in. length of ⅝-in. conduit pipe for barrel. Make bracket of 1/16-in. thick flat steel as in Fig. 4. Solder it to barrel 4 in. from one end. Make handle as in Fig. 5, slip the eye over short end of barrel, add the spring, and solder a washer (Fig. 6) to end of barrel. Drill a series of ⅛-in. holes through both sides of the pipe as indicated and cut a short slot with a thin-bladed chisel; then insert a hack saw blade and saw the entire slot as in Fig. 6. Round off sides of slot so string will not be cut. Slip pipe through hole in bow, glue pipe inside the hole, and fasten bracket.

The bow when fully drawn

Springs. Make two clips from brass or heavy tin (Fig. 8) to fit limbs of bow about 8 in. from tips as in Fig. 7. Put loop of booster wire through hole in clip and insert pin or nail. Be sure both clips are the same distance from ends of limbs. Fasten a 1-in. section of ¾-in. diameter coil spring in each hole in washer. Run ends of booster wires through the hooks of springs. Pull wire taut and make fast so that when the bow is drawn, the springs will be stretched as in Fig. 9.

The size of springs given are for a bow of from 30 to 40-lb. pull, but the springs should be selected to suit the pull.

Strings. Form clips (Fig. 8) for bow tips from tin or brass, solder the joints, and place on bow so the overlapped portion is toward the back. Glue on. The wire loops may then be put on and the bow braced. (The bow may be given a coat of white shellac, rubbed down with steel wool, and finished with spar varnish before the clips and booster wire are made fast.) The size of the music wire to be used as a string will vary according to the pull.

Arrow. Take a 4-in. piece of hollow umbrella rib and drill a small hole in the closed side ¼ in. from one end as in Fig. 10. Bend and sharpen an eightpenny finishing nail, insert through hole, and solder. Make shaft of bamboo or very tough wood and insert in umbrella rib up to hole. Glue it in and slightly crimp the sides of the rib. Taper the shaft gradually to the end.

Shooting. Drop arrow through the pipe so that the nock or hook will straddle the string. The nock should fit snugly on the string.

The arrow and parts from which it is made

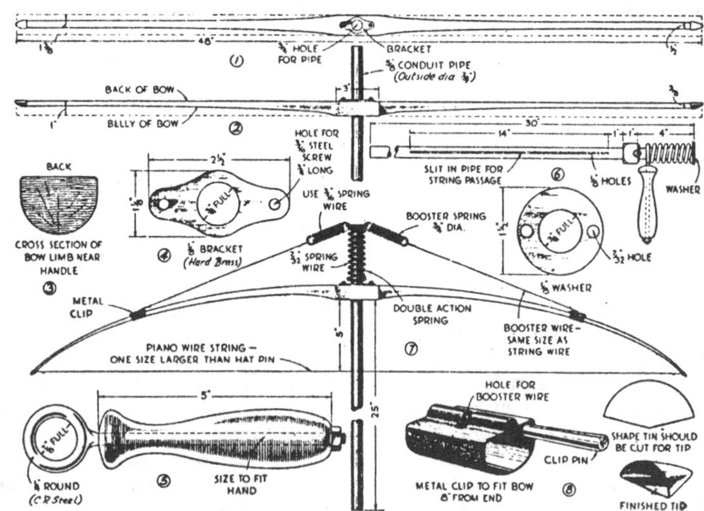

A bow with a pull of thirty to forty pounds. The handle slides on the barrel back of the large spring

Five Dollar Boot Knife and Push Dagger

By Clyde Barrow

Boot Knife

Most boot knives cost between $35 and $100. An excellent 8 inch boot knife (4 inch blade) can be made for about five dollars. The basis for the knife is the Sykes-Fairbain Commando Knife. A genuine S/F knife from England may be used, but they cost about $15. A well made copy of the knife, manufactured in Germany is available from American Colonial Armament: P.O. Box F, Chicago Ridge, Illinois 60415. The price is $4.95 plus shipping.

Drawing A shows the orginal configuration and B the finished boot knife. A simple way to shorten the blade is to grind and reshape the blade. Although this method works, the resulting knife is rather shoddy looking and hard to resharpen.

A more desirable method is to remove the handle and shorten the blade from the rear, leaving the sharpened edges and point intact. The handle was originally secured to the blade by peening (mushrooming) the end of the tang. To remove the handle it is necessary to grind off the top 1/8 inch of the handle to remove this peened over material.

The blade is now secured in a vise after wrapping it in several layers of masking tape to protect the edge and your fingers. Tap gently against the finger guard with a hammer and the handle should slide off the tang.

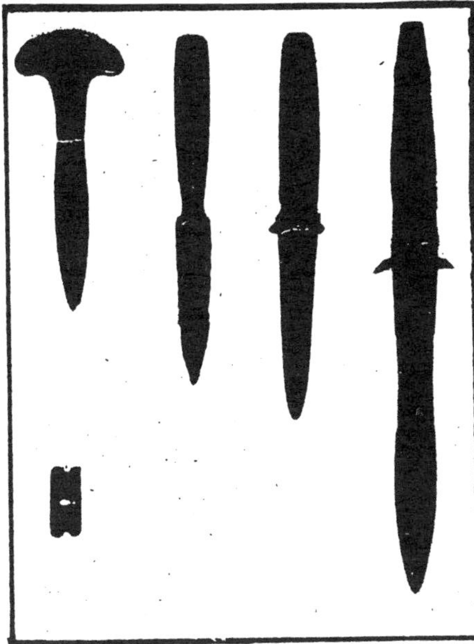

FIGHTING KNIVES L to R [Push Dagger, Throwing Knife, Boot Knife, Gerber MK II Survival Knife.]

Using a bench or hand grinder, remove the material indicated with diagonal lines in drawing D. Continue to grind until the handle can be hammered back onto the tang. The excess tang protruding from the handle is now hacksawed or ground off. The handle is secured in its new position by repeening the end of the tang with a center punch. It may also be epoxyed in place. Grind end of handle smooth and reblacken with firearm touch up bluing or black paint.

The handle is solid steel and rather heavy. It is also slippery when wet or bloody. The handle may be lightened by grinding the front and back flat before reinstalling on the blade. A more secure grip is obtained by wrapping the handle in wet linen twine. When the twine dries it will shrink tight to the handle. This wrapping should be sealed with linseed oil to prevent it from becoming frayed and unraveled. About 12 feet of twine are used. The linen is very strong and can be removed from the knife and used as fishing or snare line in an emergency. It would also make an excellent garrot if the need should arise.

The knife may be carried in a sheath sewn to the inside of your boot or the scabbard supplied with the knife can be shortened to fit the new blade length.

Push Dagger

The push dagger, like the derringer, was a popular backup or hideout weapon for the American traveler in the 1800s. Riverboat gamblers would often produce a push dagger to settle a gambling argument, and many gentlemen carried a dagger as a discrete means of protection for encounters with the local riff-raff.

Many of these early push daggers were works of art. One of the more popular designs was produced by Will and Finck of San Francisco. Their push daggers featured engraved blades and handles of german silver and walrus tusk. The knife was supplied in a german silver sheath

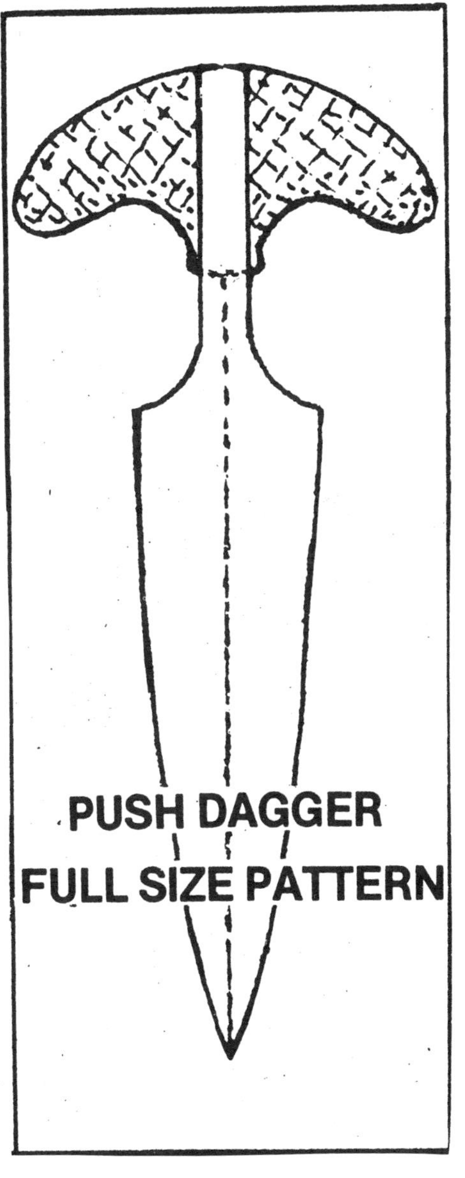

with a fancy clip for attaching to the belt. In recent years, the push dagger has become a popular concealed weapon. Two basic designs are currently available, the traditional push dagger with palm shaped curved handle, and a relatively new design, the belt knife. All traditional type push daggers now being produced come from custom knife makers. These beautiful knives can cost anywhere from 50 to several hundred dollars.

The belt knife design is available from several manufacturers. The price range in $10 to 30 dollars. Quality is governed by price. The cheaper plated steel knives are supplied with vinyl belts, while the high priced units are stainless steel with belts of high quality saddle leather.

An excellent push dagger of the traditional design can be made from the five dollar Commando knife used in the boot knife project. The original handle is removed in the same manner as before. It will not be used on the completed push dagger, but should be saved, as it makes an excellent file handle. Excess material is removed from the blade with a grinder. Use the full size pattern, Drawing E, as a guide and be sure to keep the blade cool by periodically dipping it in a can of water. This will preserve the temper of the blade.

The handle can be made from any traditional knife handle material or it can be machined from aluminum or brass bar stock. When completed, a hole is drilled in the center of the handle and the blade is epoxyed in place. Use a quality brand of epoxy and allow 24 hours curing time before using the knife. A good way to determine the optimum handle shape is to first carve it from soft pine or balsa wood. When the right shape is found, it is copied in the final material.

EDITOR'S NOTE:
If the combined weight of the dowel and projectile are much greater than the weight of the original shot charge, excessive chamber pressure is created, which may damage the shotgun. The clandestine military services use a similar improvised system, but they recommend removing ½ of the powder charge. I suggest starting with the reduced load, and carefully work up to the full power charge that Bob describes. Clyde

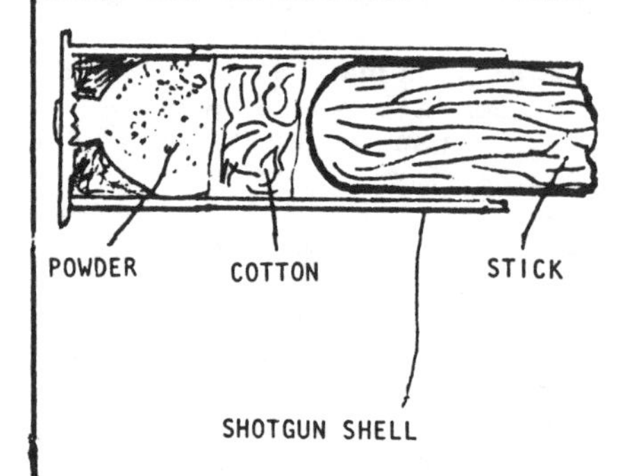

A HOME-MADE MORTAR

By Robert Maybeth

A simple mortar can be made from a shotgun of any gauge. It can deliver almost any type of bomb, including incendiaries, pipe bombs, molotov cocktails even the CO_2 bomb detailed in issue #1.

First, a regular shotgun shell is converted for use in the mortar. The shell is opened and the pellets are removed; the wadding is pulled out and replaced by a wad of cotton.

Next, obtain a piece of round wood stick or dowel. When the stick is loaded in the gun, it should be long enough to protrude from the gun's muzzle about six inches.

Attaching the ordnance to be launched is done in various ways. The bomb can be taped to the stick with good, strong tape. Or the mount can be partly built into the bomb itself. If it's something like the potato masher grenade shown on page 37 of the POOR MAN'S JAMES BOND, it can be screwed right onto the stick. Or, design your own.

The weapon can be fired from the shoulder, like a conventional grenade launcher; but bracing the unit against the ground like a conventional mortar is better as the recoil is severe. A pair of legs are attached to the shotgun as shown, and the gun is set at a 45 degree angle. It is aimed by adjusting the angle of the shotgun. Before firing, a sandbag is placed under the shotgun's butt to prevent stock damage from repeated firings.

To use, the shell is chambered and the stick, with armament attached, is pushed into the barrel to contact the shell. Then the bomb's fuse is lit and the thing is fired. A great home defense weapon if there ever was one.

* * * * *

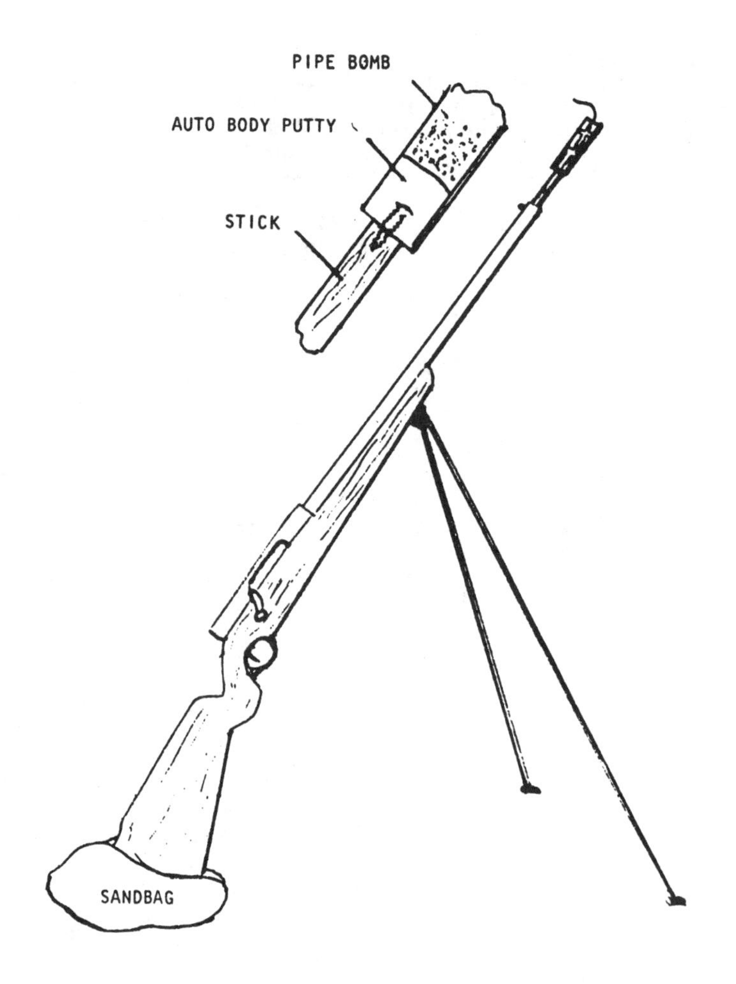

Eye Popper

By Fritz the Cat

Set guns are a dandy way to protect yourself and your property. Correctly rigged, they can kill or maim an intruder, and, if you are around, announce the intruder's tresspasses. If push ever comes to shove in our uncertain future, set guns will provide cheap, (they can be improvised) reliable, and effective insurance for a broad variety of security problems. For the present, they must be used with the greatest discretion. The authorities and their minions frown upon the use of firearms in general and set guns in *particular*. Juries have been known to award huge sums to burglars who were maimed in the process of breaking into or looting the home of a set gun user. The gun is being increasingly portrayed as a villan in our society by those who wish to ban them, and the use of set guns has decreasing sympathy with juries.

There is an alternative solution available to us: a non-lethal, yet devastating weapon-the EYE POPPER. It is simple to make and use; it consists of a flashbulb(s), battery, and a victim activated circuit. It makes use of the following fact: even a single, small flash bulb, can cause permanent and serious damage, when fired from close range at a dark adapted eye (iris dilated).

Several flashbulbs fired simultaneously at close range would instantly and permanently blind an intruder, putting an end to his activities of the moment and rendering him incapable of organized activities-hostile action or easy escape.

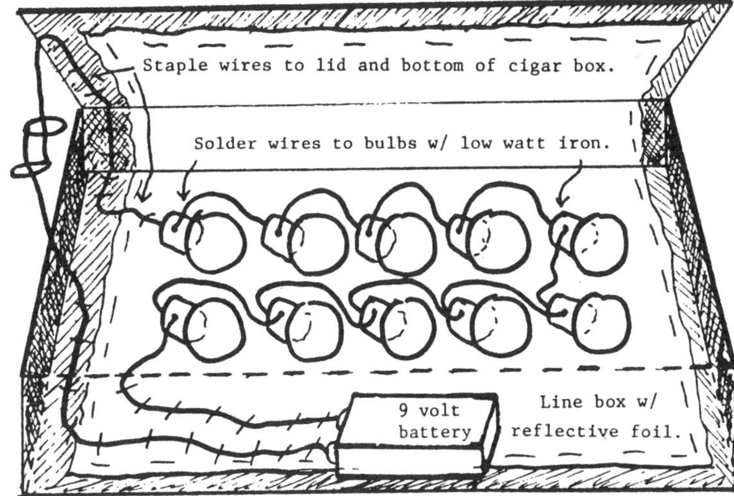
Staple wires to lid and bottom of cigar box.
Solder wires to bulbs w/ low watt iron.
9 volt battery
Line box w/ reflective foil.

The main fly in the ointment with the set gun is the gunshot wound which is proof in itself that a firearm was used; with the EYE POPPER, the jury has only the burglar's word that something you rigged up blinded him and the chances are he never got a look at the device before it was activated (and promptly lost his chance forever). Why, the poor slob simply fired the electronic flash on your camera as he was stealing it-what could you do? The diagram illustrates one simple method of using an EYE POPPER. It is by no means the only way; you are limited only by your imagination. A cigar box (or jewelry box: it makes an irresistable bait that takes burglars out early in the game) is rigged with a double wire pull, a 9 volt battery, and four flash bulbs, all in series. Opening the box does the trick! Use as many flash bulbs as you wish, or have room for, or your battery will fire—the more the better. Always use aluminum foil to reflect and concentrate the maximum amount of light out of the box and into the burglar's face. But make sure your wires are insulated so they do not short out on the foil. I used the double pull switch because it is simple, others are possible. Try to keep wires short enough that the circuit can fire before it is recognized as a "trap" or camouflage it. The CLOTHESPIN SWITCH, page 14 of PMA Vol. 1 #1 is a good one to use in boxes for any purpose.

Flash bulbs offer many possibilities. They are still easy to come by and will probably be amoung the last items to be serialized, registered, and eventually banned.

BOLAS

By Darvis McCoy

For centuries, the Indians of South America have used a weapon called the bola, or bolsadero, for hunting and warfare. It was used widely in tribal disputes, and was very effective against the Spanish cavalry. Today the gauchos who inhabit the pampas use them to snare the feet of livestock on the run, but their value as a weapon has not diminished. The bola of old was made by wrapping a stone in a leather pouch, tying a leather thong about three feet long to the pouch, then tying three of these together. The stones were of unequal weights so when they were thrown, they circled at different speeds, spreading out to form a six foot line that wrapped around anything in its path. The centrifugal force caused the stones to whiplash into whatever the line had caught with unbelieveable force.

A modern version of the bola can be made with three fishing sinkers (a 12 oz., an 8 oz., and a 10 oz.), and some leather thongs. First, drill a hole in each sinker just wide enough to allow passage of the cord. Then round off the edges of the hole with a sharp knife so there won't be any sharpness to cut the cord. Now feed the cord through the hole and tie a knot on each side of the sin-

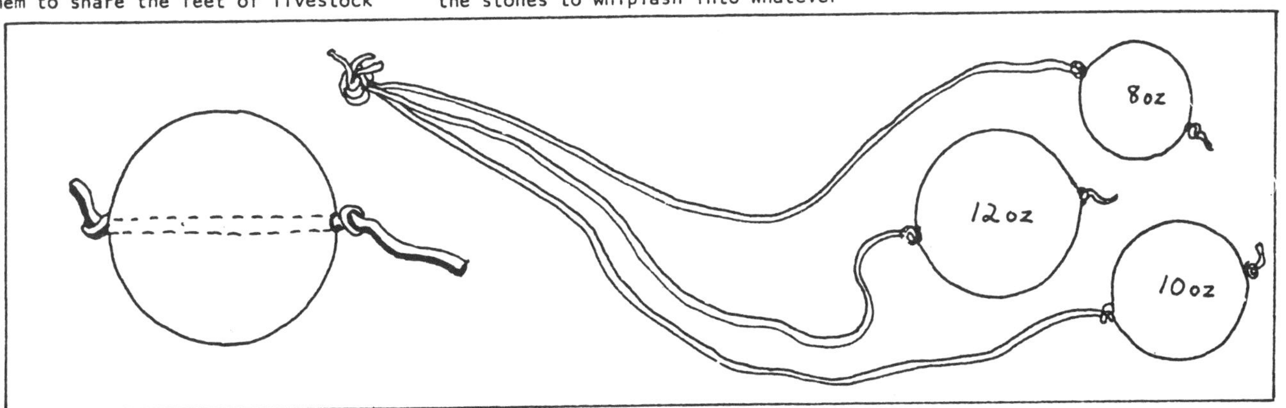
8oz
12oz
10oz

ker so it can't slide either way. Make sure the knots are tight. You don't want the sinker coming off and flying around as you swing the bola. (It might be even more hazardous to your health than smoking!) Tie the other end of the cord to the ends of the other two cords, about 3 feet from the sinker. Follow the same procedure with the other two sinkers.

To throw the bola, start out holding the smallest weight in the last three fingers, with the index finger hooked through the fork of the other two cords. Swing these clockwise around your head, then let go of the fork, while keeping the smallest weight tightly in your hand. The bola will now be circling at its full six foot length, and can be thrown. Find a secluded spot and practice on a tree trunk until you are confident in your new skill.

The bola is not a close quarters weapon, but is effective on any victim within throwing distance. It really comes into its own when coupled with the element of surprise, or when used against horsemen or bikers. It is not easily mastered, but it's deadly in experienced hands.

War-making is not the only capacity in which the bola is useful. As the Indians have shown for many years, medium-sized game can be brought down consistently by an experienced thrower. The common method of hunting is to cast the bola at the legs of the prey, snaring them together, making it possible for the hunter to cut the throat of the animal while it lies helpless on the ground.

Long after ammunition has disappeared from the face of the earth, primitive hunters of the future will be putting meat on the table with their leather-thonged death. * * *

Legal But Lethal

By Boyd Hill

In their rush to regulate firearms use, our legislators have apparently forgotten to control the ownership or carrying of one particular silent, deadly and easily concealed weapon. This is the common rubber, spring, or CO_2 powered spearfishing gun beloved by snorkle and scuba divers

Although designed for underwater work, a speargun will throw its heavy, pivot barbed, metal "arrow" through the air for at least 30 yards with considerable accuracy and enough force to penetrate 6 inches or more into a coco palm tree. At 15 yards it will probably put the spear completely through a man.

Normally these are powered by a length of surgical tubing. If this tubing is doubled, the power should be increased by about 1/2. Most of these guns run between 2 feet and 30 inches long. Generally they are light, in the neighborhood of 1 1/2 pounds. The two pistol grips are compact. Such a gun can be hidden up a raincoat sleeve, or inside an ordinary jacket. Almost all of them have a safety catch, which means they can be carried cocked and ready without too much danger of accidental discharge.

Such a gun, with several shortened spear "arrows," can be carried around wrapped in a brown paper cover, tied with a string. And, unless its employment has been demonstrated previously in action, it should pass as a simple tool for recreational sport. * * * * *

UNCONCEALED CONCEALED WEAPON

By Clyde Barrow

In NYC, California, and several other areas of the US it is illegal to carry any weapon, concealed or not. I assume this is to protect the poor misguided criminal from savage citizens who have the gall to defend themselves when mugged on their doorstep.

One legal weapon available to those who choose to obey these laws is an improvised fighting stick made from a rolled up magazine. This weapon is devastating when the end is jabbed full force into the "victim's" throat, stomach, kidneys or groin. When held two handed, it will also serve to block or deflect a punch, kick, or knife thrust.

The stick is 1 inch diameter, 11 inches long and costs about one dollar, depending upon the quality of your reading material. Roll the magazine up as tight as you can, paper edges first so the stapled edge is exposed. Secure the ends with rubber bands. The stick is carried in the hand or back pocket. If your local laws are so twisted that the mere presence of the rubber bands could place the stick in the dangerous weapons category, just roll up the magazine and hang on to it.

It would be hilarious to watch the action at the local precinct after some overzealous police officer had arrested a citizen for carrying a deadly magazine.

Note: If you don't read, a discarded newspaper can be rolled and secured in a similar manner.

NINJA TOOLS

BY DARVIS MC COY

In feudal Japan there existed an organization of assassins known as Ninja. They were adept in the use of all weapons of their day. The one we are interested in here is the weighted chain, or manrikigusari. Different versions of this weapon existed, such as the long rope, with a ring on one end and a knife on the other, or the chain with a weight on each end. The most appropriate for modern street defense is the latter.

The weighted chain is a versatile fighting tool. It can be snapped at the face or groin (like a wet towel) swung like a flail, used as a garrote, or thrown like a bola. When swung like a flail, it is very difficult to block because it continues to whiplash around the block, striking the target behind anyhow.

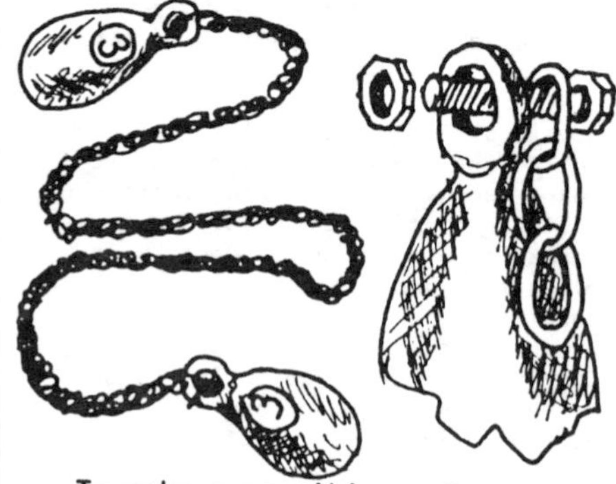

To make a manrikigusari, you need a chain (the dog leash type works well), two bolts with nuts, and two fishing sinkers (I used 3oz. sinkers). The chain should be from 2 to 3 feet long. The bolts have to be small enough to fit through the holes in the sinkers and the links in the chain, but the head and nut should be too big to slip through. Drill a hole through the center of each sinker, just wide enough for the bolt. Put the bolt through the end link of the chain, then through the sinker, then screw the nut up tight to the sinker. Cut off any excess length of bolt and mess up the threads to prevent the nut from working off.

As with any weapon, it is necessary to practice in order to become proficient. This is especially true with the manrikigusari, because of the tendency for the chain to keep swinging after you are ready for it to stop. Once you do master it, you have a highly concealable, extremely potent weapon in your arsenal.

Exploding Mortar Bombs

By James L. Robertson

Mortars are not really very impressive or effective unless they fire an explosive projectile. Here is one that is easy to make and really works.

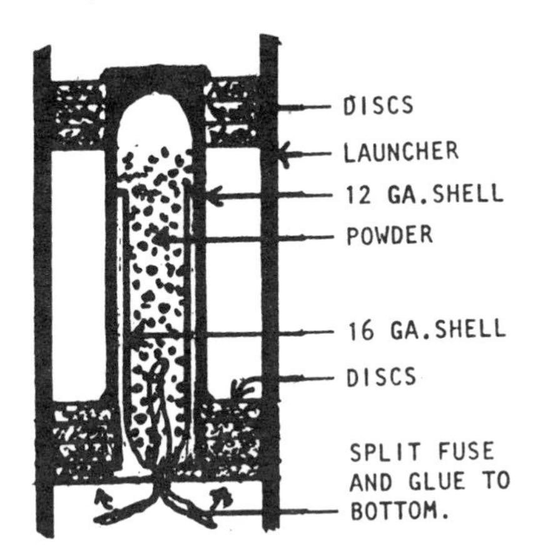

First cut a number of discs from cardboard that are the same size as the inside diameter of your mortar. Next obtain some empty (fired) 16 ga. and empty 12 ga. shotgun shells Punch the primer out of the 16 ga. shell, insert a length of firecracker fuse and fill the remainder of the primer hole with tissue paper. Seal the fuse in with glue. Be sure the fuse comes back into the empty shotgun shell 1/2" or so. Fill the 16 ga. shell with black powder, or better yet, flash powder. Slide the empty 12 ga. shell over the 16 ga. shell containing the powder. The two shells will fit tightly together. Be careful not to damage the fuse while you are putting the shells together. You should now have two shotgun shells fitted together, filled with powder and with a fuse about 1" long projecting from the 16 ga. end.

Next, punch a small hole in the middle of several of the cardboard discs. Slip them over the fuse carefully and glue to the 16 ga. shell. Glue a couple of discs to the other end, so that the projectile looks like a dumbell. Then split the fuse almost to where it enters the disc. Spread the split ends apart carefully so as not to dump out any more powder than necessary. Glue the fuse to the cardboard and drop a pinch of black powder on the glue before it dries.

The fire from the propelling explosion will ignite the fuse. You can adjust the length of time before the projectile explodes by adjusting the length of the fuse and the number of cardboard discs. Remember there can be no wadding between the powder in the mortar and the fuse. The cardboard discs serve as wadding, so they should be a reasonably good fit. I have made quite a few of these and I have never had one that failed to ignite.

EXPLOSIVE CHARGE

BY

FRED BILELLO

1. Using scotch tape, make a tube out of a paper grocery bag about 2" long by 1" wide. Cut a 1" circle of paper and tape it to one end.
2. Pick and scrape the explosive off of about a thousand stick matches. Add a little water to them and crush them up in a glass ashtray.
3. Pack the tube full for about 3/4".
4. Take a 1/4" wood dowel and insert it into the center of the tube. Then pack the rest of the explosive around it. When it starts to harden carefully remove the dowel so that you have a hole 1/4" wide by 1-1/4" long in the center of the charge. The purpose of the hole is to allow the interior to dry, and it is also there to insert your detonator.
5. After a few days, peel off the scotch tape and gently remove as much of the paper bag as you can. Some of it will probably stick to the charge. Set it in a warm, dry area and let it dry completely.

This explosive charge will cost about a dollar and its size and shape can be modified to suit your particular job. It should be great for making bombs and as a propellant for light artillary and rockets. When utilizing it for a bomb, a booster charge such as gunpowder should be placed in the hole. The device is another step in standardizing your ordinance for mass production. ⚜

EXPLOSIVE CHARGE

HOW TO USE WIRE-DRAWING PLATES

FEW mechanics, amateur or otherwise, know much about wire-drawing plates, yet these tools are most useful, and once tried, are hard to get along without. They are particularly useful to model makers and in the long run save considerable time and money.

The plates are made in several styles. With them wires of copper and similar soft metals, and even mild steel, can be made round, square, knife-edged, or half-round. With two plates in the round variety, it is easy to reduce ⅛-in. wire to 1/64 in. with almost no loss of material and an increase of length of almost 6,400 percent. The plates are obtainable at jewelers' supply houses and cost only about $1.50 each.

The operation is this: Clamp a plate upright in a vise, name-face to the front. Sharpen one end of the wire to be drawn, making a long point. Insert the point in a hole small enough to bind, grasp it with pliers, and pull it through, using a smooth, steady force. Repeat with the next smaller hole, and so on. After being reduced in several holes, the wire will need to be annealed by heating it to redness.

The drawing, it will be noticed, not only reduces the diameter, but straightens the wire so that there are no local kinks whatever. This in itself is an advantage in most kinds of work. Besides, the exact degree of hardness and stiffness can be obtained to suit the requirements of the work in hand. The principal advantage, however, is that the owner of such plates needs to stock but one or two sizes of the metals he commonly uses as he can quickly make any smaller size necessary.

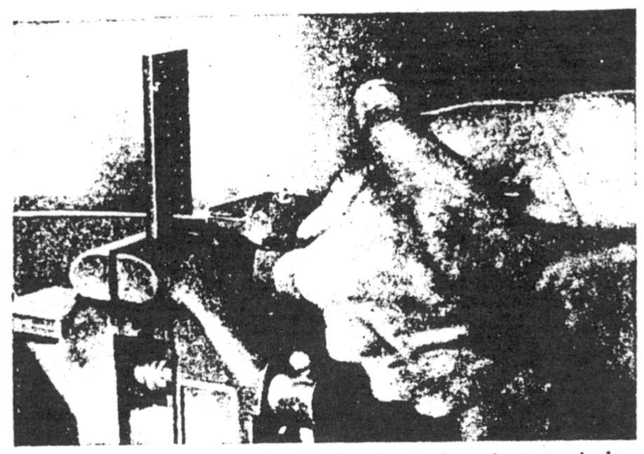

The wire is reduced in size by drawing it through successively smaller holes in the plate, which is clamped upright in a vise

The usefulness of the plates does not end with shaping, sizing, hardening, and straightening wire. They can be used for making tubing. Simply cut a strip of sheet metal of a width approximately 3 1/7 times the outside diameter of the tube required, snip a taper at one end, bend lengthwise into a shallow trough, and draw like wire to close the joint.

$10 SILENCER

By Clyde Barrow

$10 mailorder silencers are now available, for your motorcycle, of course. These units may also be used to quiet portable power plants, lawn mowers, pumps, chainsaws and any other noisy item with a barrel of 3/4" OD or more.

The silencer is formed from welded steel tubing with a flat black painted finish. The body is 7¼" long and 2" OD. Total silencer length when assembled is 8".

The interior contains a 1" ID perforated steel core and a roll of fiberglass packing. A spring loaded baffle maintains core alignment and a sturdy snap ring holds the steel endcap in place.

The rear mounting area is slotted for easy installation with the hose clamp provided. For a more permanent installation, the unit may be welded in place.

The J&R silencer may be disassembled for cleaning or packing replacement. Disassembly requires a pair of snap ring pliers, available from any hardware or auto parts store.

The $2 replacement kit contains a new baffle spring, perforated core and a piece of yellow fiberglass packing material.

Be sure to specify barrel OD when ordering.

BOY MECHANIC VOL.3

A Crossbow Magazine Gun

A new type of bow gun that a boy can make, and which will give him plenty of good sport, is one of the repeating or magazine variety. To make the gun, cut a soft pine board, 40 in. long and 5 in. wide. With a saw and knife, cut the gun form as shown. Cut a groove along the top of the barrel, where the arrow will lie ready to be shot out when the hickory bow is released. The magazine holding the five arrows is made of thin boards, 24 in. long, and is held in place by four small strips. The magazine is 3 in. deep, thus permitting the five arrows to lie evenly in it without crowding. The bow is of seasoned hickory and is set into the end of the barrel. The notch in which the bowstring catches, should be cut just under the rear end of the magazine. The trigger is an L-shaped, pivoted piece, and pushes the cord off the notch when ready to fire. As soon as the first arrow leaves the gun the one just above it drops down into the groove when the bowstring is again pulled back into place behind the notch. Pressure on the trigger shoots this arrow, another takes its place, and the cord is pulled back once more. The arrows should be of light pine, 22 in. long and ½ in. square, the rear end notched and the front pointed. To make the arrow shoot in a straight course, and to give it proper weight, the head end should be bored with a 5/16-in. bit, 3 in. deep, and melted lead run into the hole.—

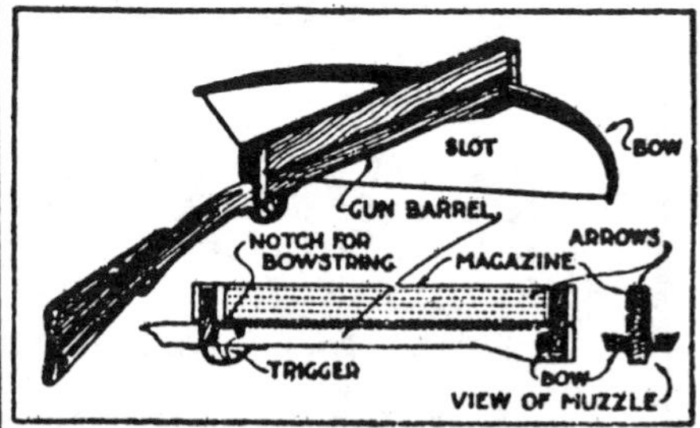

The Arrows are Stacked in the Magazine and Fired in Succession by the Bowstring Released at the Trigger

J & R has developed a silencing device to be used on expansion chambers. A considerable reduction in the noise level is now possible with no loss in power. The principle of operation is much the same as a gun silencer. After much use, the silencer can be easily taken apart for cleaning. After extended usage a replacement kit is available which includes new deadening material and a new perforated core which will bring your silencer back to new operation.

J & R
7738 Scout Ave.
Bell Gardens,
CAL - 90201

SILENCER REPLACEMENT KIT

XC1 to fit XC Silencers from .709 through .937	$2.00
XC2 to fit XC Silencers from 1.000 through 2.000	2.00
XC3 to fit all XXC Silencers	2.00

MODEL XC (Black) .... **each $9:95**

ORDER BY DECIMAL SIZE

SIZES OF SILENCERS AND SPARK ARRESTERS

FRACTION	DECIMAL	MM	DESCRIPTION
	.709	18	Early Harley Davidson/Baja
3/4"	.750	19	Kawasaki 100, G31M Green Streak, Honda 250
	.789	20	Sachs and Penton
13/16"	.812		———
	.827	21	———
7/8"	.875	22	Suzuki 90, Honda CT70, Suzuki 90/125 GitKit, 90 Yamaha MX
	.906	23	Yamaha (early DT1), Early Suzuki 250
15/16"	.937	24	Yamaha 125MX, Yamaha 100MX, Suzuki TM250
1"	1.000	25	Hodaka 100, Honda C100, 105, 110, S90, CL90, SL90, C200, CT90, Suzuki
1-1/16"	1.062	27	———
	1.102	28	———
1-1/8"	1.125		Hodaka 100 Super Rat, Yamaha 250, 360, RT1-MX, DT1-MX, 71 Greeves 250
1-3/16"	1.187	30	———
1-1/4"	1.250		Kawasaki 250, Honda CB, CL, SL100, CB, CL, 125, 160, SL175, Suzuki TM400
	1.259	32	Maico 250, 360, 400, 501
1-5/16"	1.312		———
1-3/8"	1.375	35	Bultaco 250, 360, Montessa 250, Honda CB, CL175 to K4, Ossa 250
	1.417	36	CZ250, 360, 400
1-7/16"	1.437		———
1-1/2"	1.500	38	Triumph BSA, Honda CB, CL 72. 77, CB, CL, SL 350, A11 ,CB, CL 450
	1.574	40	Husky 250, 360, 400, 450, Montessa 360
1-5/8"	1.625		———
	1.654	42	72 Harley Baja
1-3/4"	1.750		Greeves 250, 360, 1970
2"	2.000	50	Kawasaki 100 Trail Boss, Yamaha 1971, RT1-B DT1-E
	Open End		To be welded on pipe

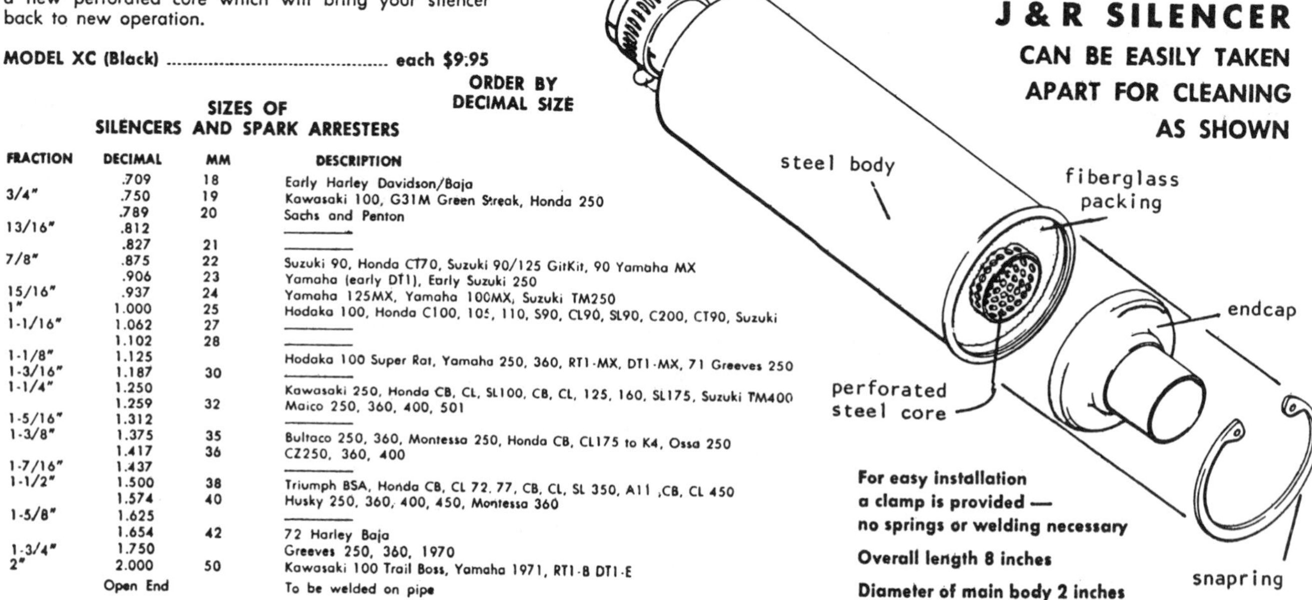

BOOBY TRAP

BY THE KENTUCKY RIFLEMAN

A very effective and versatile exploding booby trap can be made from parts available at any hardware store.

This device can be used as a fragmentation mine, flare launcher, tear gas projector, or as a directional mine or set gun.

Cut the breechblock down until it will just fit into the coupling and make it just long enough to make the barrel (long pipe nipple) fit snugly when loaded with the shotgun shell. Take the breechblock out and drill a 1/8" hole through the exact center. Cut the nail to

All that's left is to load the shotgun shell into the barrel and screw the barrel into the other end of the coupling.

CAUTION !!

This device fires as soon as the pin is pulled! For safety, don't load the shotgun shell until you have the trap set up.

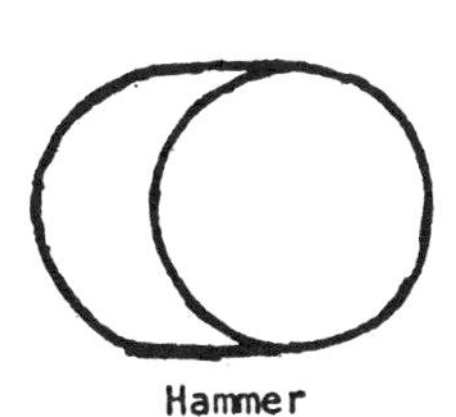

Hammer

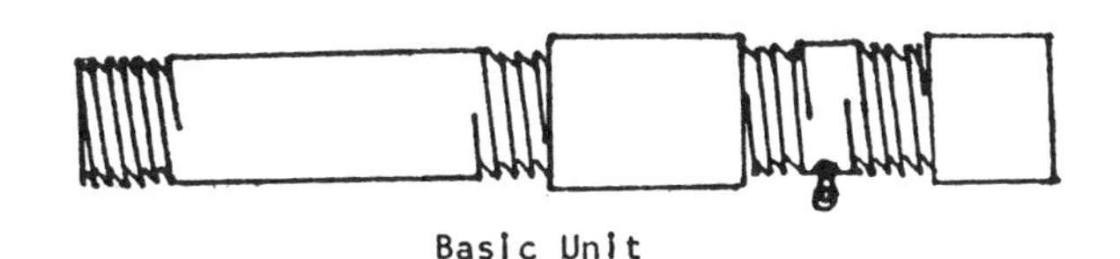

Basic Unit

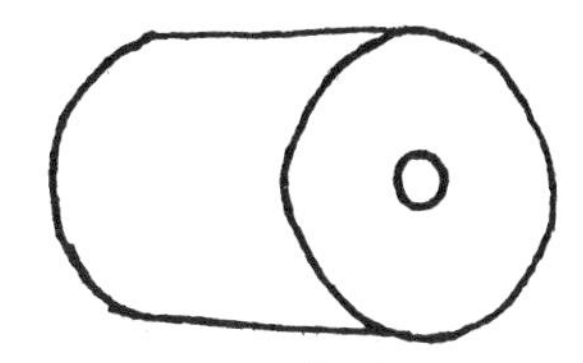

Breechblock

You will need these items:

1 - 3/4" pipe nipple 2" long.
1 - 3/4" pipe cap.
1 - nail approx. 1/8" thick.
1 - 3/4" pipe coupling.
1 - 3/4" pipe nipple 4" long (or longer).
1 - cotter pin.
1 - spring, any size as long as it's strong enough.
1 - round steel piece approx. 1" x 1".
1 - round steel piece approx. 3/4" x 1/2".
1 - 12 ga. shotgun, flare, or tear gas shell.

The cut-a-way drawing shows how the device is put together. Start by screwing the coupling to the end of the 2" pipe nipple as tightly as possible.

1/8" longer than the breechblock and file the end round and smooth so that it will hit the exact center of the shotgun shell primer, otherwise the shell won't go off.

Drill a 1/8" hole in the side of the 2" nipple about 1/2" behind where the nipple and coupling join.

Make the spring long enough to push the hammer against the breechblock.

To assemble:

Start with the coupling-short nipple assembly, and install the breechblock. Next, push the cotter pin into the hole in the short nipple, then slide the hammer down the nipple to rest against the cotter pin. Now set the spring against the hammer, and compress it with the cap and screw the cap down tight.

You can set this one off yourself by a pull wire, or rig trip wires or use your own ideas.

A good way to mount this device is to weld or braze a large wood screw to the cap and screw it to a tree, fence post, or corner of a building (see drawing). A muffler clamp can be used to mount to metal posts and fences.

To make a fragmentation bomb, saw, file, or grind grooves in the barrel and put a second pipe cap on the end (see drawing).

The range and spread of the shot can be varied by making the barrel longer.

If you handload shotgun shells, you can make the whole thing much more powerful by overloading the shell with powder.

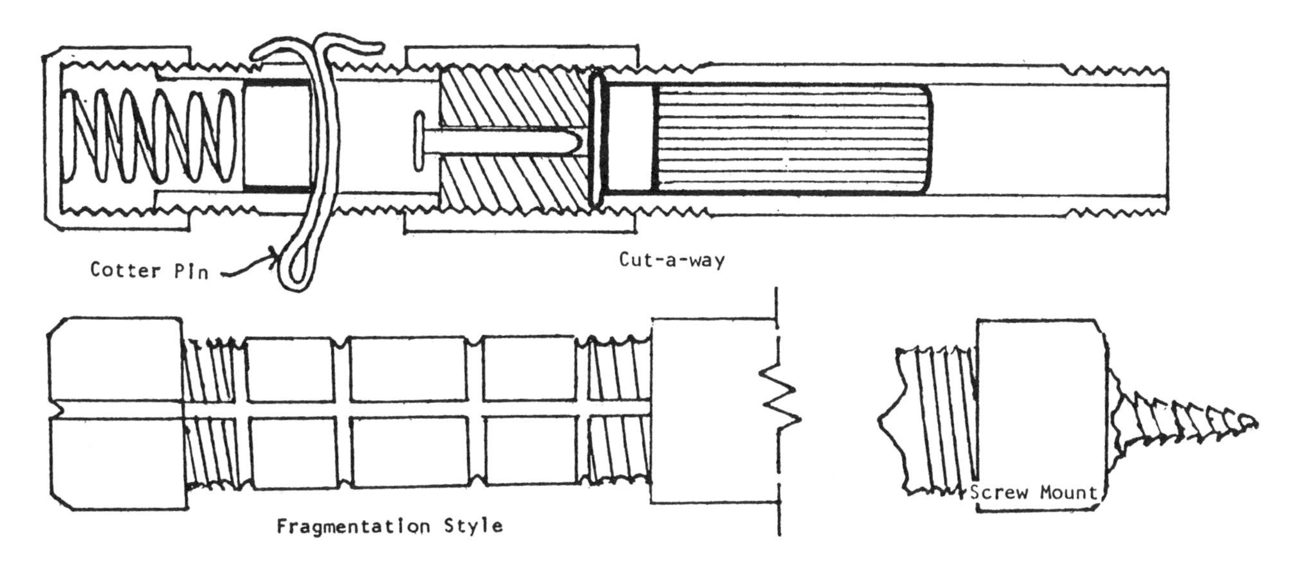

CHLORINE

Chlorine gas is generated when chlorine bleach is mixed with sodium bisulfate (Sani-Flush). Pour a can of Sani-Flush in a baking pan, and level off the top of the pile. Punch a hole near the bottom of the plastic bleach jug and place the jug in the center of the pan. A steady cloud of gas will be generated, the actual duration depending upon the rate of bleach flow. If it is necessary to direct the gas to a specific area, the generator can be covered with an airtight top fitted with a hose.

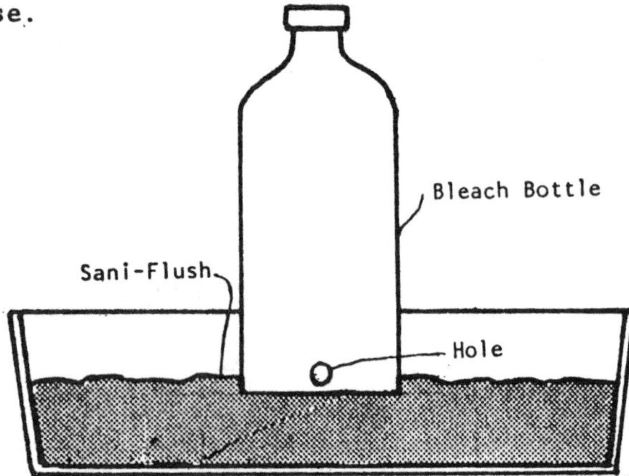

PLASTIC BOMBS

Hand grenades and antipersonel mines can be easily and cheaply constructed from polyester casting resin, auto body putty, ABS and PVC pipe, plexiglass, vacumn formed styrene sheet etc. These plastic devices won't produce shrapnel fragments or concussions equal to the power of conventional bombs, but they do have two unique and noteworthy features; they are both non metallic and x-ray transparent.

The first feature allows these devices to be carried through airports, government buildings and other controled areas where a magnometer check might be encountered.

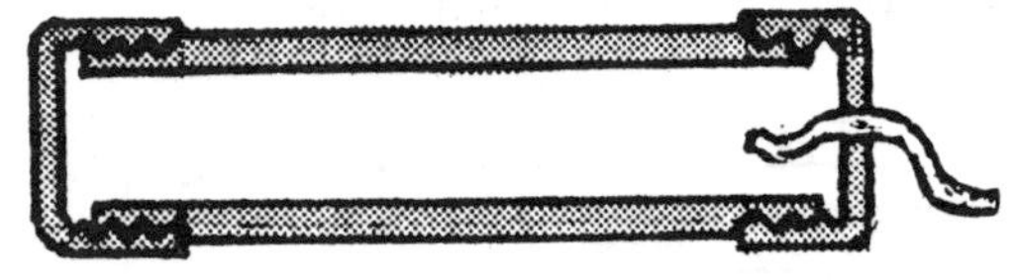

Pipe Bomb-made from prethreaded plastic tube

The inability to detect plastic fragments with x-rays will require that each fragment be probed for and will complicate surgical treatment.

Mortar Bomb-cast halves in mold and join together

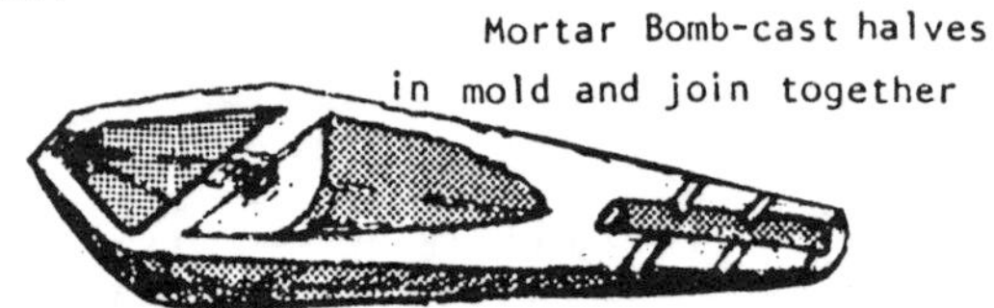

Plastic shrapnel filler can be coated with poison before it is added to the bomb to increase the kill rate of the explosion.

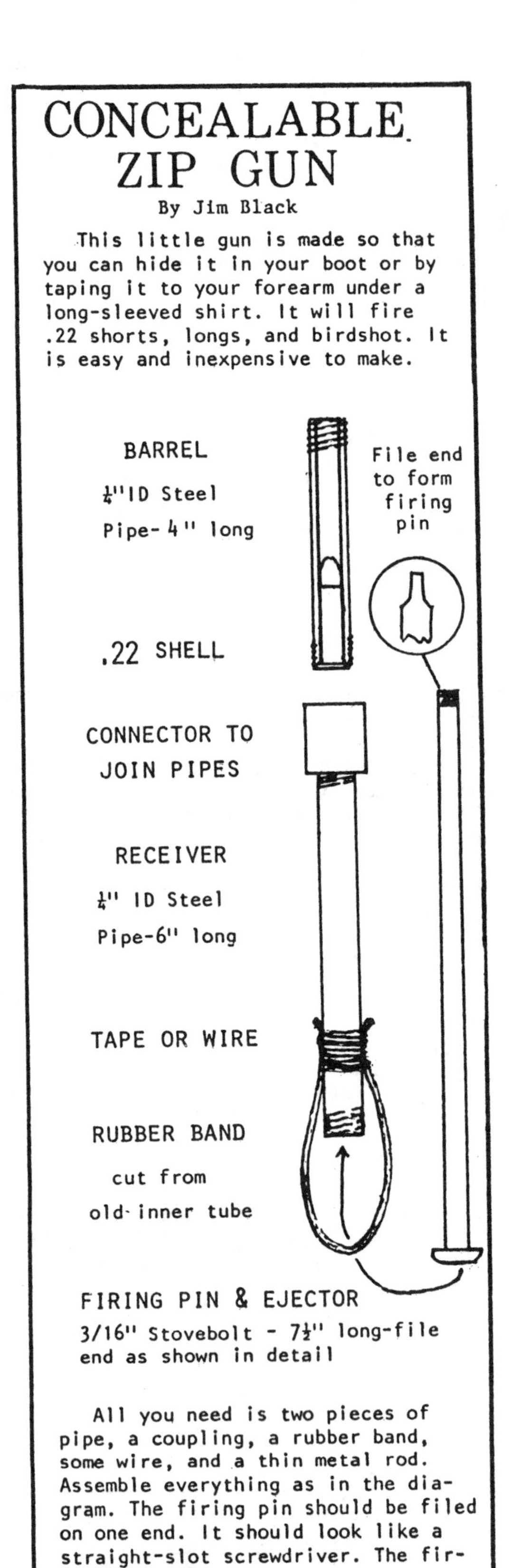

CONCEALABLE ZIP GUN

By Jim Black

This little gun is made so that you can hide it in your boot or by taping it to your forearm under a long-sleeved shirt. It will fire .22 shorts, longs, and birdshot. It is easy and inexpensive to make.

All you need is two pieces of pipe, a coupling, a rubber band, some wire, and a thin metal rod. Assemble everything as in the diagram. The firing pin should be filed on one end. It should look like a straight-slot screwdriver. The firing pin is used to both fire the .22 and to poke out the fired shell.

TAKEDOWN ROCKET LAUNCHER

by Clyde Barrow

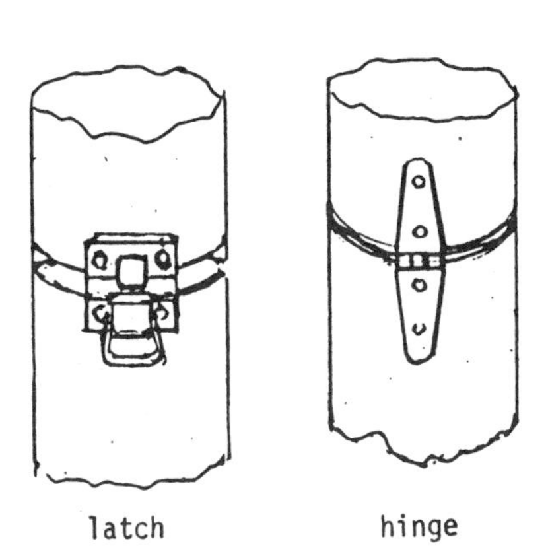

Materials:

three - 3" aluminum irrigation tubes, 18" long.
two - small gate hinges.
two - luggage latches.
pop rivets and gun.
suitcase approx. 18"x10"x6", inside dimensions.

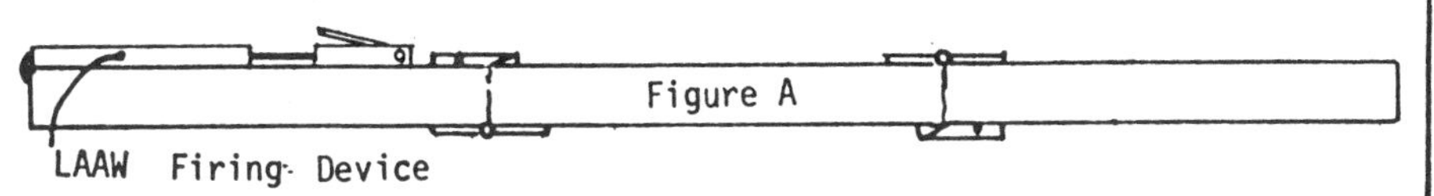

Figure A shows a 48" long x 3" dia. launcher.

When extended, the tube is sufficiently rigid for firing. When folded, it measures a compact 18" x 10" x 3". The folded launcher will easily fit in a small suitcase

The rear section, X, carries a LAAW rocket type percussion firing device (see PMA Vol.1 #8).

If an 18" x 10" x 6" case is used, three complete rockets can also be carried with the launcher.

Note: To flatten the pop rivets that extend into the tube, clamp a heavy pipe in a vise and peen flat as shown.

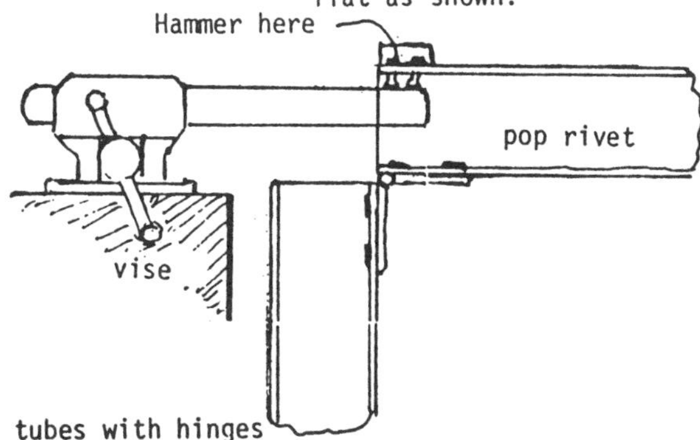

Join the three tubes with hinges and pop rivets at points 1 and 2 as shown. Attach latches at points 3 and 4.

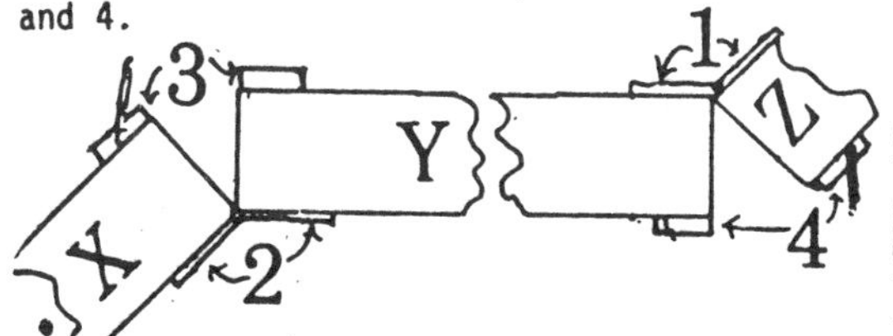

All dimensions are arbitrary as is the choice of aluminum as the tube material. Modify this example to suit the materials most available to you.

MAKING PROPORTIONAL DIVIDERS

Popular Mechanics 1937

IF ONE'S drafting kit does not include proportional dividers, an efficient substitute for this rather expensive instrument may be easily made by the method illustrated. The dividers will be found very useful for enlarging or reducing a drawing or sketch.

The blades may be made of cardboard, brass, aluminum, or even thin wood. If

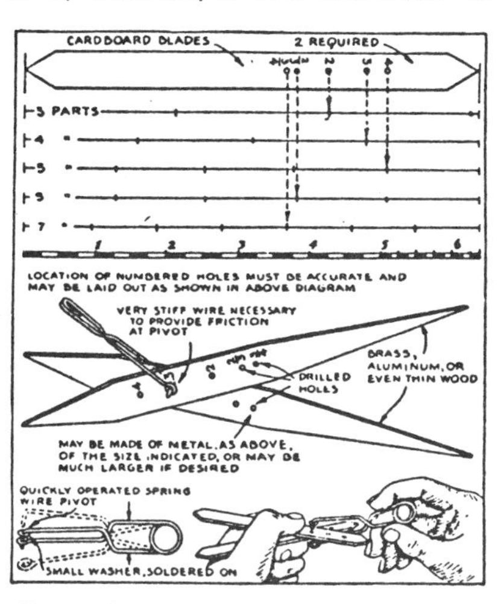

How to lay out blades for proportional dividers, and a quick acting spring wire pivot

of cardboard, cut the two blades to the shape shown in the upper diagram; if of stronger material, taper them as suggested in the larger perspective drawing. Then mark the blades as accurately as possible for the holes. The principle of laying these out is made clear by the divisions on the five lines drawn immediately below the pattern for the cardboard blades.

If, for example, it is desired to enlarge a drawing to exactly twice its size, the blades should be divided lengthwise into three parts and the hole made at one of the divisions so that, when the instrument is assembled, the distance from the pivoted joint to the one end will be exactly twice the distance from the joint to the other end. Similarly, to enlarge three times, the blades must be divided into four parts and the pivot hole placed at a point one quarter the length of the blades from one end. Other divisions can be worked out in the same way. For small work, a good length to make the blades is 6⅜ in., as indicated by the inch scale placed beneath the lines upon which the divisions have been marked.

The pivot should be quickly removable for setting the blades. The wire design shown has given satisfaction and is not difficult to make.

FIRE-BALL CANNON

by Joe Brown

Materials Needed:

3 Beer Cans	Can Opener
Black Electric Tape	Lighter Fuel
Slow Burning Fuse	Tennis Ball
Gasoline	

Cut out the tops and bottoms from 2 beer cans leaving clean edges. Then cut out the top of a third beer can and make a fuse hole in the center of the can bottom. Fig.1

Tape the three cans with electric tape to form them into a tube, making sure that the walls are smooth.

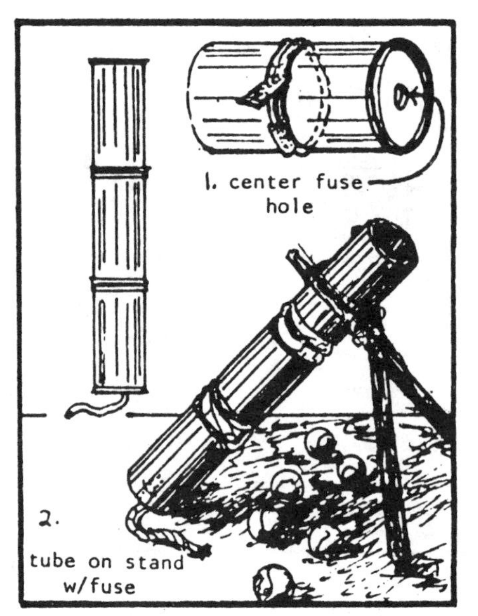

Fig.2

Line the walls of the tube with a thin coating of lighter fuel, insert fuse and tennis ball. While I know of a few who have launched dry tennis balls holding the tube in their hands, I feel that a stand should be made.

Fire-Ball - Soak a tennis ball in a container of gasoline for several hours or until it fills with gas. The ball will fit snugly into the tube, but may have to be gently pushed down with a stick. This ball of gasoline may reach as far as a city block, flatten out upon impact, and spread flaming gasoline.

Measuring Split Hundredths

WITH AN ORDINARY SCALE

Reprinted From Popular Mechanics 1937

DO YOU realize what can be done in the way of accurate measuring with an ordinary, high-grade steel scale? The hundredth of an inch divisions were not put on the scale as an ornament or to impress you with the quality of the tool. They are for use, and with a little patience and practice you can split the hundredths and make linear measurements correctly within a few thousandths of an inch.

Hair-splitting precision like this is easy. All you need is the scale, a small magnifying glass, a reasonable supply of patience, and above all, confidence in the fact that it can be done and that you can do it.

As an example, look at the two tiny slotted-head brass studs in the palm of the hand shown in the photograph above. The original pieces, of which these are copies, were located in such a position on the apparatus of which they are a part, that it was not possible to get at them even to measure the head diameter with an ordinary micrometer. All measurements were taken from the originals with the aid of nothing but a steel scale and a small magnifying glass.

Under a magnifying glass it is relatively easy to make measurements within .01 inch

Then a small brass rod was chucked in the lathe and two slots sawed in it sufficiently far apart to make the two pieces. A diamond pointed tool was then adjusted in the lathe tool holder at an angle so that the sides of the point cleared both the lengthwise and crosswise faces. Cuts were taken with great care, using the saw cuts as reference points, and the same scale and magnifying glass were used for the measurements.

On this job the critical dimension happened to be the distance from the upper edge of the saw cut to the shoulder on the stud. The second photograph shows one of the studs placed against the edge of the scale. This illustrates how coarse and easily read the hundredths of an inch divisions appear under a magnifying glass. It is clear, even from the photograph, that the dimension in question is a trifle over six and one half divisions and is, therefore, approximately .066 in., the required size. A check-up after the studs were finished showed one of them calibrated .0668 in., the other .0672 in.

The matter of getting proper light is extremely important. Have the light evenly diffused from both sides, and check each measurement from two positions if possible.

Special Purpose Shotgun Ammo

By Clyde Barrow

Birdshot, buckshot and the rifled slug are three standard rounds available for the 12 gauge shotgun. While these loads are adequate for most applications, certain situations call for special ammo. Each of the five following loads is designed to overcome a shortcoming found in the standard 12 gauge rounds. 16 or 20 gauge shells may also be used. The procedures are oriented to non reloaders who will be buying and modifying preloaded ammo. The processes should be easy to modify for those of you who have reloading setups.

A

The factory loaded rifled slug is adequate to stop most medium size game and penetrate most thin metal barriers. Large bones and steel over 1/8" thick will cause the soft lead slug to rapidly mushroom and stop before it has penetrated the target. A round headed steel wood screw in the tip of the slug will increase the degree of penetration by delaying this mushrooming action. Drill a hole in the exact center of the slug and turn the wood screw in flush with the slug's tip. It is important to keep the screw from projecting past the end of the shotshell case. If a shell with an exposed point were loaded in a tubular magazine, the gun's recoil could cause the point to detonate the primer of the shell in front of it. This is the reason all lever action rifle ammo is of the round nose type.

B

This load is used to penetrate a steel armor plate, Kevlar body armor and bullet proof glass. It would also be useful against tempered aluminum alloy armor found on current riot control vehicles. A standard shotshell is cut in half lengthwise with a razor blade. The cut should extend from the front end to the edge of the brass base. Carefully peel the two case halves back and remove the shot or slug and the large cardboard wad. The lower wad and powder charge are left intact. Carefully drill a hole in the center of the large wad and insert a carbide or hardened steel burr or grinder bit into the hole in the wad. This projectile should not weigh more than the original slug or charge of pellets. Additional weight can cause excessive chamber pressure and may damage you or the gun. If you are a reloader, it's a simple chore to weigh the new projectile on a bullet scale and then charge the case with the appropriate amount of powder. After the wad and tool bit are inserted, the case is sealed with a soldering gun. Just touch the cut to reseal it. Seal the sides only as the end should be free to unfold when the shell is fired. It is sometimes possible to seal the case with scotch tape but this causes feeding problems in some shotguns.

C

Standard rifled shotgun slugs have a usable range of only 100 yds. If a lighter rifle bullet is substituted for the slug, the range is increased several times. This is accomplished by encasing the bullet in a 3 piece collar called a sabot(sa-bō) defined as a thrust-transmitting carrier that positions a projectile in a tube). The sabot travels down the barrel with the bullet and falls aside a few feet after leaving the muzzle. This principle was first used with artillery rounds and is the basis of the new Accelerator rifle round. The Accelerator carries a 22 cal. bullet with a surrounding plastic sabot. The bullet/sabot combo is fired from a standard 30.06 case. The .22 bullet reaches a velocity of about 4,000 feet per second. This is currently the highest velocity round available in small arms ammo. Several years ago a 12 gauge shotshell/sabot load was available commercially. The sabot carried a 50 cal. machine gun bullet. This round is now out of production and is no longer availble. An in depth look at the Accelerator and 50 cal. sabot loads will appear in a future issue.

To make a 12 gauge sabot load, first cut a shell as in B. Remove the large wad and drill about 2/3 way through the wad's center. The wad is now cut into 3 equal pieces with a razor blade. Assemble the 3 sections around the bullet and install the unit in the case. Reseal the case as in B. The bullet will have a range of several hundred yards. As with all 5 of these loads, adjustable rifle sights should be installed to utilize the full potential of the round.

D

Commercial rifled slug loads are often hard to obtain. An improvised slug load can be made from any regular shotshell. The end is first heat-sealed with a soldering gun. This will prevent the end from unfolding when the shell is fired. The case is now cut almost through with a razor blade. Cut along a line just above the brass base. Leave only enough uncut material to hold the case together. These loads should be handled carefully as they may break open while being fed through a pump or gas auto action. When the shell is fired, the case breaks along the cut and the entire front of the shell travels as a unit. These improvised slugs usually stay together on impact but could be modified to break open after striking the target.

E

Riot shotguns with 18" or 20" barrels are ideal for slug shooting but tend to allow buckshot to scatter in too wide a pattern for long shots. Buckshot patterns can be controlled by tying the individual balls together with piano or picture framer's wire. This type of load is known as grapeshot and originated during the Civil War. To make a grapeshot load, pry open the end of a buckshot shell and empty out the individual balls. A small hole is drilled in each ball. They are now strung like beads on the wire which should be about 12" long. Tie the ends of the wire to form a circle about 4" in diameter. A simpler method is to substitute an equal amount by weight of fisherman's split shot. Tie the wire loop as above and then crimp on each split shot with a pair of pliers. The completed grapeshot is now installed in the case. It may be necessary to remove a portion of the wad in the case to make room for the increased volume. When the shot is in place, refold the end of the shell and spot seal or glue the end closed. Do not seal the end completely as was done in D, as this case is supposed to open normally when fired. The shot remains attached to the wire loop and travels to the target as a unit.

NOTE: Please remember not to greatly increase projectile weight without

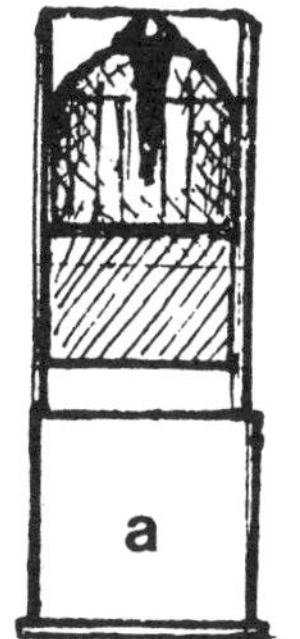

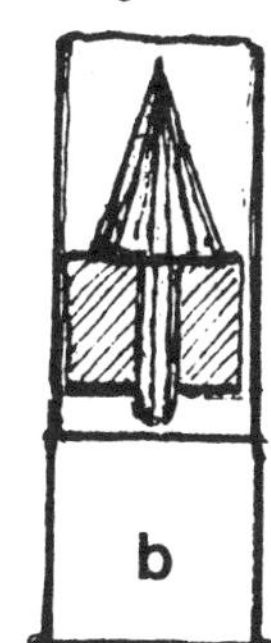

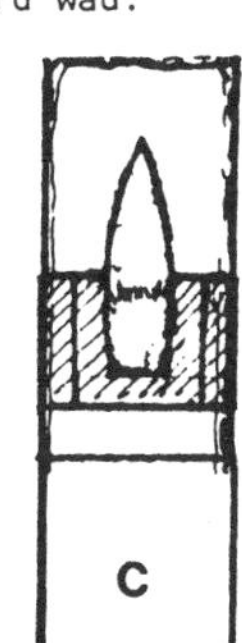

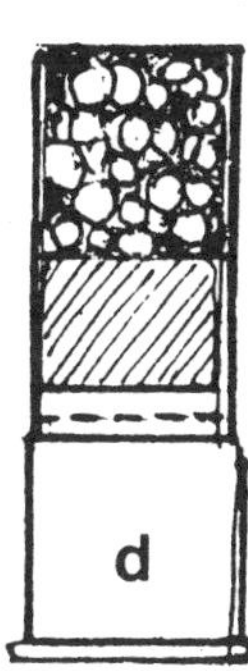

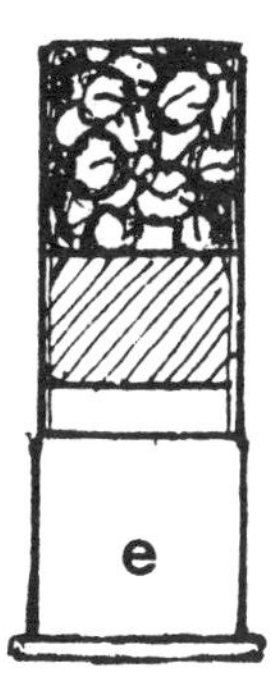

A. Round headed wood screw in end of rifled slug.
B. Hardened steel or tungsten carbide tool bit in wad.
C. Rifle bullet encased in three piece sabot.
D. Improvised slug made from regular shotshell.
E. Grapeshot load - lead balls and wire.

CHEAP TARGET

Reprinted From Popular Mechanics 1937

ARCHER ROLLS TARGETS FROM PASTEBOARD

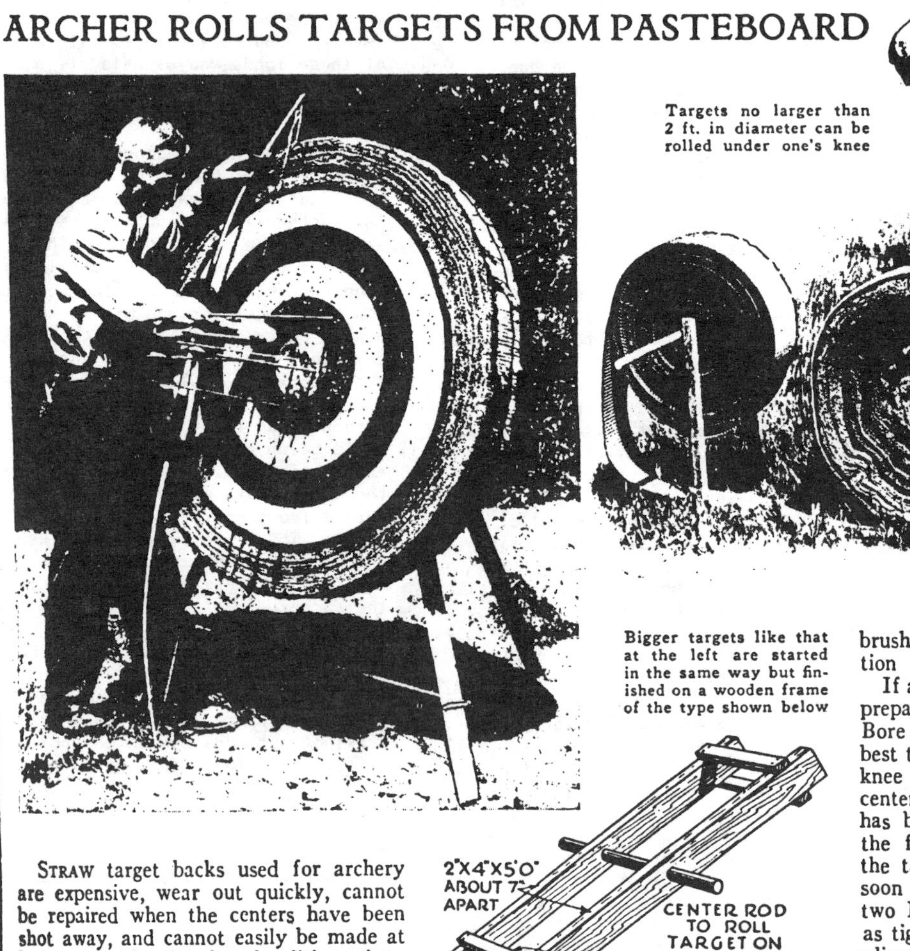

Targets no larger than 2 ft. in diameter can be rolled under one's knee

Bigger targets like that at the left are started in the same way but finished on a wooden frame of the type shown below

STRAW target backs used for archery are expensive, wear out quickly, cannot be repaired when the centers have been shot away, and cannot easily be made at home even in the few localities where suitable rye straw is to be obtained. An excellent substitute, however, can be made from ordinary single-faced corrugated pasteboard, which is sold in large rolls for packing purposes. A target back of any size can be rolled from this material. The cost is low, it lasts well, and it can be repaired easily.

Saw the roll of corrugated board into 5- or 6-in. lengths and crush the strips as flat as possible by running them between the rollers of a wringer, by flattening them with a lawn roller, or in any other convenient way. If the target is to be no larger than 2 ft. in diameter, it is now necessary only to roll the strips as tightly as possible under your knee and bind with wire as described a little later on. It will improve the target to brush the pasteboard heavily with a solution of sodium silicate (water glass).

If a standard 4-ft. target is to be made, prepare a frame as shown in the drawing. Bore the center for a wood roller. It is best to start rolling the target under your knee (with the wooden roller in the center) until a diameter of about 18 in. has been reached and then mount it in the frame and continue rolling. Make the target from 4- to 6-in. oversize. As soon as the rolling is completed, place two No. 6 or 8 wires around the target as tight as possible and crimp them with pliers. Insert a small, hard roll of pasteboard in the center.

When the center has been hit so many times that it "leaks," loosen the wires, push out the damaged part, and roll and insert a new center. It may then be desirable to cut out a wedge-shaped segment from the old part of the target, starting at the new insert and widening out to about 4 in. at the outer edge. Apply new wires and tighten until this space closes.

reducing the powder charge. Always wear tempered shooting glasses and hearing protectors when firing experimental loads. I recommend their use for all shooting, but they are a necessity when firing improvised weapons or ammunition. * * * * * * * * * * *

Grenades

ARMING GI PRACTICE GRENADES

by Clyde Barrow

Surplus practice grenades can be easily converted to live status in the home workshop. These converted units have several advantages over improvised grenades. The completed unit is waterproof, the cast iron body shatters well into deadly fragments, the shape and weight are handy for both hand throwing and rifle launching. The fuse is lit with no smoke, flash and relatively little noise. Probably most important is the lever/pin system. The unit is absolutely safe until the pin is removed. After pin removal, the armed grenade can be loaded in a launcher or carried in the hand, in both cases it's ready for immediate use. This eliminates fumbling around with lighters, strikers and friction igniters. This is also the type of grenade that TV terrorists carry in their hand, without pin. "Shoot me and we all die" etc.

These practice grenades are identical to the fragmentation units diagramed on P. 12 PMA Vol. #1, except for the following:

A. The filler hole at the bottom of the body has not been threaded, and is left open. No plug is supplied.

B. The fuse assembly is supplied with a fired primer and burnt out fuse, usually corroded in place.

C. Some examples have had the striker and striker spring removed, others are supplied with the above parts intact.

D. No ignitor or explosive charge is supplied.

Several military surplus suppliers are currently selling these "inert" grenades. Ads may be found in Shotgun News and in several gun magazines. Many examples of these grenades are rusty, dinged up and are missing the striker and spring. Some are of recent manufacture, while others date back to the early 1950's.

The finest example we've seen is currently available from Sherwood Distributors. Price for a single unit is $4.95. A lower price is available for case lot orders. These grenades are clean, with no rust and are of recent manufacture. The striker assembly is intact.

When ordering grenades from Sherwood, or any other surplus outfit, be sure to specify ' moveable parts' as most dealers also sell training grenades. These are cast in one piece, contain no firing apparatus & are useful as paper weights only.

CONVERSION PROCEDURE

A. Body

The unthreaded hole in the bottom of the cast iron body varies from 3/8" to 5/8" diameter. (The example from Sherwood was 3/8" dia.) The prefered procedure is to thread this hole and install a removable filler plug. This allows the fuse assembly to be installed and waterproofed on the empty grenade body. The unarmed grenades can be safely stored in this manner and filled with powder prior to use. If threading the hole is not possible, it may be sealed permanently by soldering a plug in place. A glob of auto body plastic filler may also be used. The only other work required on the body is to true up the top surface where the fuse assembly screws in. A file should be used to make this surface as flat as possible. This will allow a tight, moisture proof fit between body and fuse assembly. The rubber washer supplied is often cracked and should be replaced with a new one of similar size.

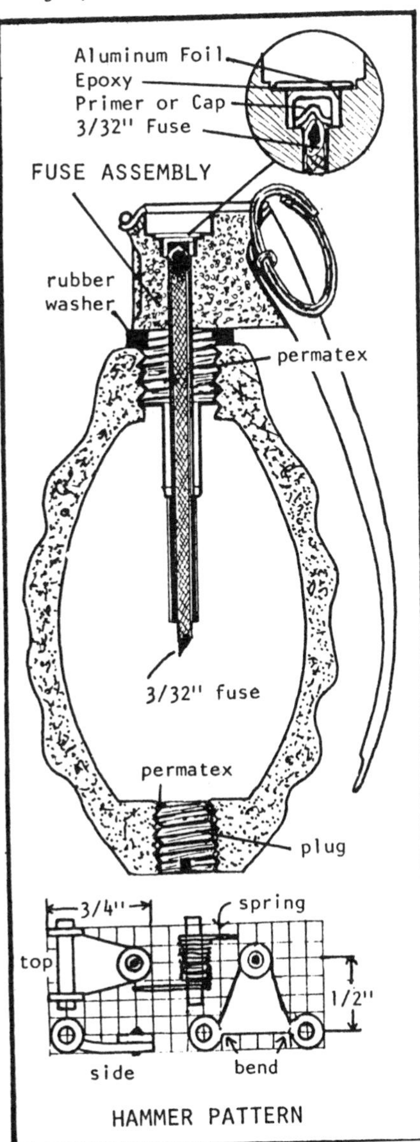

NOTE: *Cock the striker, install the safety lever and pin before proceeding on the fuse assembly.*

B. Fuse Assembly

Insert a long punch or nail, about 1/16" diameter, in the bottom of the fuse assembly. Drive out the spent primer and powder residue from the tube. Use a 1/8" drill to clean out and enlarge this tube. Enlarge the primer pocket to accept a small or large pistol or rifle primer, which ever is available to you. A black powder cap may also be used. The primer or cap should be flush with the top of the fuse body when installed. The hole should be large enough to allow the primer or cap to be pressed into the hole with finger pressure only.

Cut a circle of aluminum foil about 7/16" in diameter and epoxy in place over the primer or cap. This acts as a moisture barrier and allows the grenade to be carried in foul weather without worrying about misfires due to damp primers.

Test various lengths of 3/32" cannon fuse, available from Zeller Enterprises @ 15 ft. for $1.00. The test should determine reliability and the specific burning rate for that particular roll. This is important because although fuse is consistant within each roll, the burning rate may vary greatly from one roll to the next.

Cut a length of fuse which will give the proper delay. Five seconds is generally accepted as a good duration, but the actual time may be varied to suit your individual needs. The Nazis often left grenades lying around with no delay fuse at all. When a GI pulled the string on what he thought was a 5 second delay fuse, he was greeted with an instantaneous explosion. If for some reason you make up a batch of fuse assemblies with various time delays, it's imperative that you color code or otherwise mark them for your future identification.

When the proper length fuse is determined, cut both ends on a diagonal for maximum exposure of the black powder center. This insures both good ignition from the primer and a nice fat spark to detonate the explosive filler. Coat the fuse except the ends, with epoxy, and press into place inside of the fuse assembly. If the grenade body will be filled with black or smokeless powder or match heads, (potassium chlorate) the spark from the fuse itself will be sufficient to detonate the filler. If the entire body will not be filled, a wad of paper should be used to ensure that a quantity of filler is held in place around the fuse. The spark cannot be counted on to make a jump. If a more sophisticated explosive filler is to be used, be sure to use the correct companion booster or ignitor charge. Most high explosives cannot be detonated by fuse only.

When the epoxy is dry, coat the threads of the grenade body with Permatex or a similar non drying gasket sealer. This will form a waterproof seal between the body and fuse assembly, yet allow for later disassembly if necessary. After addition of the explosive filler, the filler plug should also be coated with Permatex before installing. If the filler hole has been permanently sealed instead of threaded for a plug, the explosive must be added before the fuse assembly is installed. Wipe all powder grains from the threads before installing the fuse assembly. The grenade is now ready to use (see Grenades Part I for procedure).

NOTE: *If your particular fuse body has been made "safe" by removal of the striker and spring, the full size pattern enclosed may be used to fabricate a replacement.*

HOW TO SAFELY STORE DYNAMITE

BY TODD W.

Anyone who has read The Poor Man's James Bond knows something about dynamite. The section on p.6 of the PMJB has some good information on dynamite, however, the part about storage of this high explosive is rather vague, and also somewhat incorrect.

Contrary to what is written in the PMJB, gelatin dynamite CAN leak nitroglycerine just like the sawdust-clay type dynamite. Last year, a friend of mine, who is a road construction contractor and uses dynamite in his work, began a series of experiments on storing dynamite. He experimented with gelatin dynamite by storing it in different places to find out if it would leak nitroglycerine. Two sticks of 40% gelatin dynamite were stored in his workshop at room temperature. After eight months, some nitroglycerine had leaked out of both sticks and the milk carton that they were stored in had quite a bit of the unstable liquid in the bottom of it.

Another two sticks of gelatin 40% were stored in a cool place under his workshop. After eight months, the nitroglycerine had just started to seep through the seams in the paper wrapping on the outside of the sticks.

The third group was stored under the workshop in a cool spot, laid out on a piece of plywood. Once a month, he simply rolled each stick over 180 degrees. After twelve months the dynamite was just like new; no leakage at all.

After his experiment was complete, I asked my friend how to safely store dynamite and what happens to dynamite when it becomes unstable. I found out that the more dynamite is handled, the more unstable it becomes. One important thing about dynamite that has leaked and become unstable is that the explosive power is greatly reduced.

If you are going to store dynamite, a good idea is to store it in a cool place and turn it over once a month. It will take more than a month to start leaking, but it is better to be safe than sorry. Also it is a good idea to store it in a leak proof carton, such as a milk carton, so that in case it does leak, the nitro will be contained and it won't run out all over the place.

Disposing of unstable dynamite is a problem that has to be faced if you are careless about storing it. There is no safe way to dispose of it, but a good idea is to carry it very carefully away from all buildings and then get clear of the area and set it off under a pile of newspapers. If you do this, it is very likely that the newspapers will catch on fire, so you should be prepared to douse the fire. If you do not want to blow it up, you can burn it. Burning dynamite is very dangerous because if you bump it or give it any kind of a jolt while it is burning, it will most likely blow up.

Unstable dynamite is very tricky and dangerous, so if you store it right in the first place, you won't have to worry about it. And, when someone tells you that gelatin dynamites don't leak nitroglycerine, you will know the facts.

Flameless Molotov

BY F.B.

Step 1

Take a wine bottle with a concave bottom and fill it with 30% Sulphuric Acid, 20% Motor Oil, and 50% Gasoline. Seal the top and thoroughly wipe the bottle clean and dry, especially the concave bottom.

Step 2

Pack the bottom full of Potassium Chlorate. Cut a circular piece of cardboard so it snugly fits over the bottom and tape it in place to keep the Potassium Chlorate in. Slip a plastic baggie over the bottom and wrap a rubber band around it. This is to keep moisture out.

When the bottle is broken, the Sulphuric Acid will set off the Potassium Chlorate which in turn, will explode the gasoline.

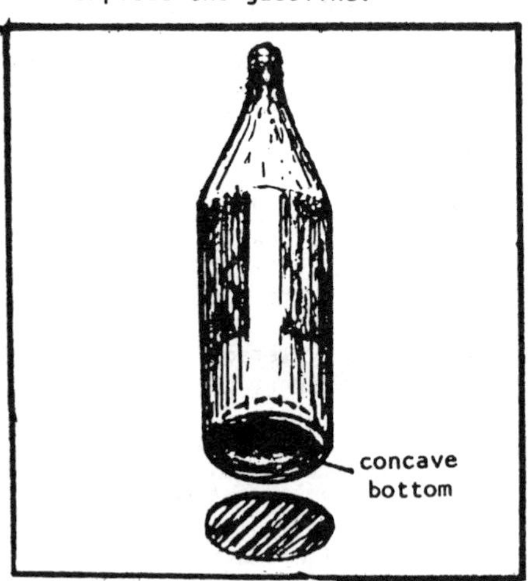

HYDROCHLORIC ACID GENERATOR

by William Segal

When foil is dropped into hydrochloric acid, the result is a gaseous substance which can effectively clear a room. Occasionally, however, the gas may need to be emitted a short distance, in which case an acid-filled coffee can with foil placed inside, would be of no help.

A simple generator to aid in emitting this gas can be easily and inexpensively constructed. This generator can be used in instances where the smoke may need to be issued through a ventilation system, through a screen, or generally in situations where the gas is to be directed to one certain area.

The materials needed are; a jar, a metal funnel, a small electric motor, one D size battery, a propeller smaller than the diameter of the jar, a tube of desired length (preferably metal, though heavy plastic will do for a limited duration before it melts), some hydrochloric acid, and aluminum foil.

First, the jar lid is cut to shape using tin snips (as shown in drawing). The center strip is cut in the middle and its ends folded downwards--the gap between the folds should match the diameter of the motor. The propellor is connected to the shaft and the motor is then inserted between the two metal folds, held in place by wire and electrical tape.

Onto this improvised jar lid is fastened a metal funnel, carefully sealed to avoid gas leakage. A small opening is made between the funnel and lid to allow space for the wires connected to the motor.

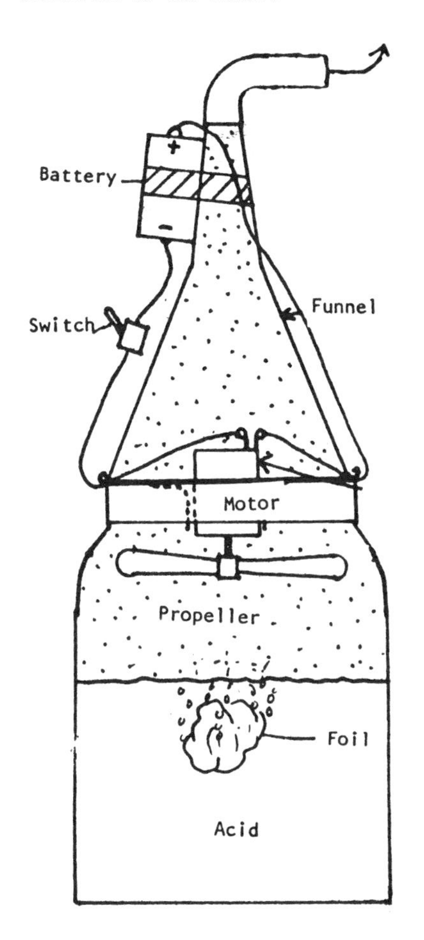

The D size battery is taped to the side of the funnel and the motor wires attached to it. A switch is connected to the wiring and the polarity should be such that the propeller

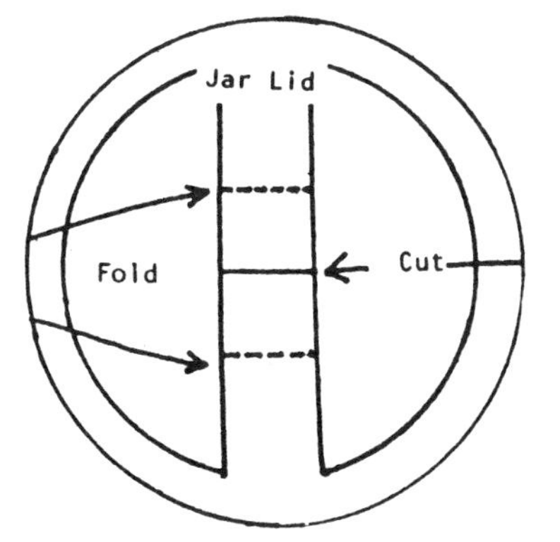

turns in the direction to suck up the gas and push it out of the tube. If the propeller spins the wrong way, the device's purpose will be defeated.

The tube is then connected to the small, open end of the funnel and should also be sealed with black tape or epoxy to prevent leaks.

When ready to use, the jar is filled with hydrochloric acid and a wad of aluminum foil is dropped inside. It takes a few moments for the foil to begin creating the smoke, providing ample time for the lid to be tightly screwed on and the propeller activated.

Depending on the size of the device and the motor's torque, the gas can reach from three to six feet. This generator would be excellent for bug extermination and, if carried inconspicuously in a case, for keeping agressive dogs at bay--to say nothing of assailants.

5 Homemade Spearguns

BY

WILLIAM SEGAL

While it is true that the speargun is an effective and legal weapon, it is also true that the speargun can be expensive; the cheapest of which being in the price range of 20 to 30 dollars. However, once the basic principle is understood, they can be constructed easily and inexpensively (certainly much less than you would spend on a factory made one).

The most simple kind of speargun can be made using a six inch long piece of bamboo, a steel shaft, and a replacement rubber for a wrist rocket. The ends of the surgical tubing are attached to one end of the bamboo, using strong twine or string. This attachment should be made especially strong, as much tension will be applied to this area. The steel shaft is slid into the bamboo and the non-pointed end placed inside the rubber pouch. The pouch is grasped between the thumb and fingers as if you were firing an average wrist rocket, then pulled back as far as possible. When it is released, the spear is forced through the bamboo and into the water (or air, depending on how you are using it).

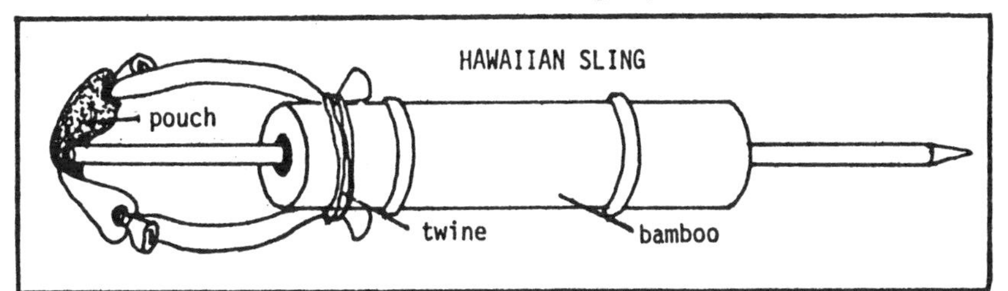

The above version is fine but if you wish to have the luxury of a handle and a trigger mechanism, then a more complicated design must be employed. First, a piece of wood (preferably oak or birch--one which will not warp) is cut to shape as shown in the drawing. The holes drilled through the two tower-like protrusions at the top should be made especially level, for much of the gun's accuracy will depend on this.

A trigger is then cut from a thin piece of wood or a thick piece of plastic. Strong wire is used for the second part of the trigger mechanism which is placed through a hole in the rear tower to match the height of the trigger top. The steel shaft should be about 1/4 " in diameter with a notch filed in it, allowing for the wire mechanism to fit snugly inside. A wrist rocket replacement rubber is again used to provide the power for the speargun. The pouch is fastened onto the top of the first tower using a thick, bent nail as shown in the drawing; this arrangment will reduce the tension from the tower. On the ends of the surgical tubing is tightly wrapped a thick piece of wire in the form of a V shape. A notch is made on the end of the spear shaft and the middle of the V is fit tightly into it. The first notch is secured onto the trigger assembly and the tubing is pulled back and placed on the end notch. When the trigger is pulled the wire drops from the first notch, thereby releasing the shaft to be pushed with the surgical tubing.

Another kind of aquatic weapon, (though not exactly a speargun), can be made at home. Devices similar to these in commercial use are called shark darts and are different from spearguns in that they force a dart into the opponent rather than a spear. For this weapon to work the dart must be pushed directly against the marauding animal.

An empty CO2 capsule is obtained and the open end drilled through to allow for a valve. The valve stem from a bicycle inner tube can be cut off and cleaned thoroughly of the remaining rubber. Using a hacksaw, half of the thread portion of the valve is carefully cut off. In the center of the end of the valve is a valve release in the form of a small pinhead like protrusion. With half of the surrounding thread wall gone, the valve release is readily accessible. The valve stem is then pushed through the hole in the capsule and soldered or epoxyed around the rim to ensure an air-tight seal. Once dry, an air pump (preferably one with a quick release) is attached and the cartridge filled with air until the pumping strokes become difficult. After the pump is released, a hollow metal tube about 3" long is prepared with inside threads to match those of the valve stem. This tube is then screwed onto the end of the valve and a dart (without the fins) is slid inside. The dart should protrude at least half an inch from the tube so that when the dart point is pushed against an attacking shark (or whatever) it will release the compressed air, forcing the dart out of the tube and into the victim.

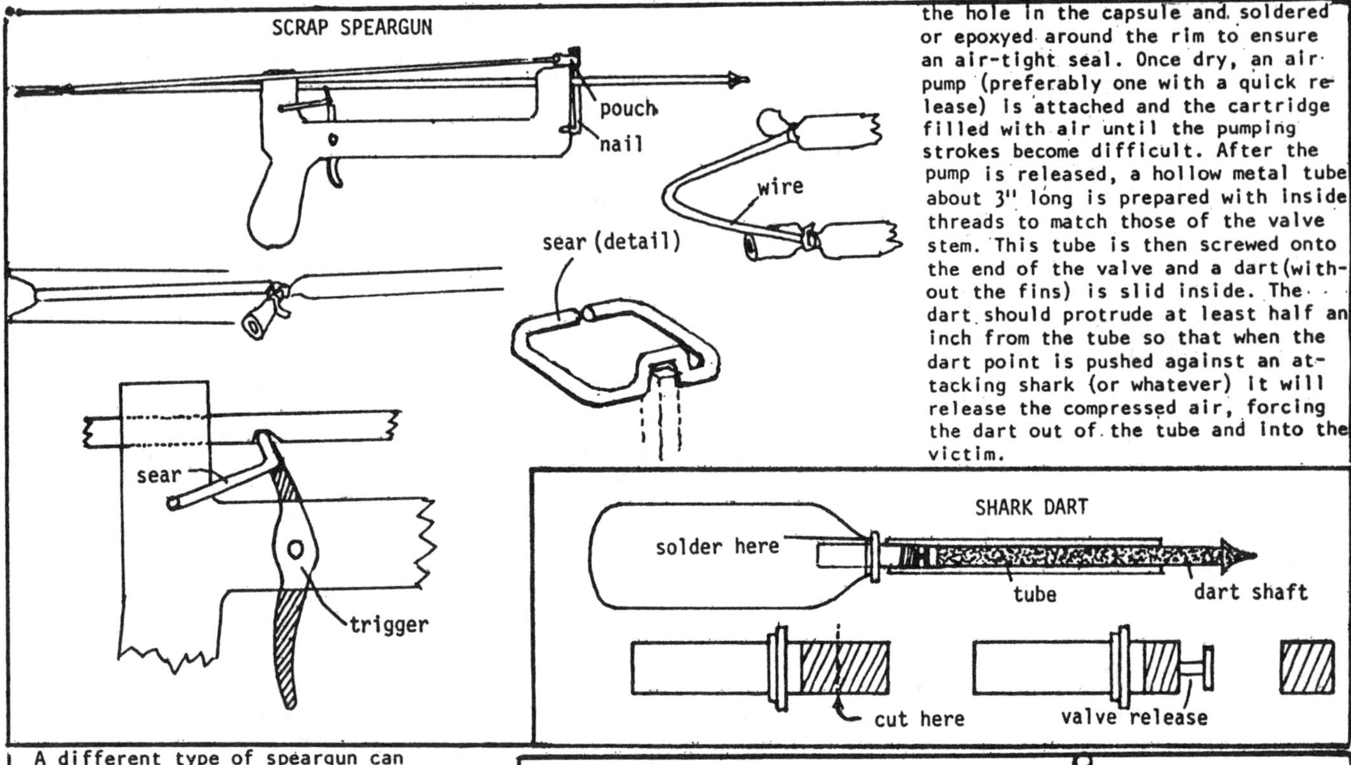

A different type of speargun can be made cheaply using an old tree lamp; the kind of lamp fixture which encases a spring and extends from floor to ceiling. Three feet from the end is marked off and then cut using a hacksaw, though careful not to damage the spring inside. The long spring is removed and some form of pouch is made on the end of it. A knob from an old radio or television works fine as a pouch when it is attached upside down on the end of the spring. A wooden plug to match the diameter of the lamp pole is cut to shape about an inch apart in the top of the wooden plug and through them is pushed a wire which will serve as a trigger.

After the spring is placed back inside the pole the wooden plug is fit tightly onto the end. A notch near the end of the spear will serve to hold it in place with the wire trigger. When the wire is pushed down it leaves the notch and releases the shaft.

wooden plug

trigger

knob

pushed up into notch

SPRING-LOADED SPEARGUN

The last kind of speargun requires little alteration and works on the same principle as gas powered spearguns. On the small home fire extinguishers there is usually a nozzle through which the fire extinguishing substance is emitted. On some units there is a cone shaped pipe connected to this, which can easily be taken off, leaving nothing but the short nozzle. If this nozzle is plastic, a strong plastic sealant can be used to attach a hollow tube about 2 feet (or longer or shorter depending on the extinguisher's length) and bent at a right angle near the end. If the nozzle is metal, an aluminum tube, also at a right angle, can be fitted with threads and fitted onto the nozzle. Care should be taken when bending the metal tube so that there are no cracks or folds to allow for gas to escape. A steel shaft, slightly smaller and thinner than the tubing's inside diameter, is slid into the tube as far as it will go. Depending on how your extinguisher is designed, a handle or trigger will release the gas and force the spear out of the tube.

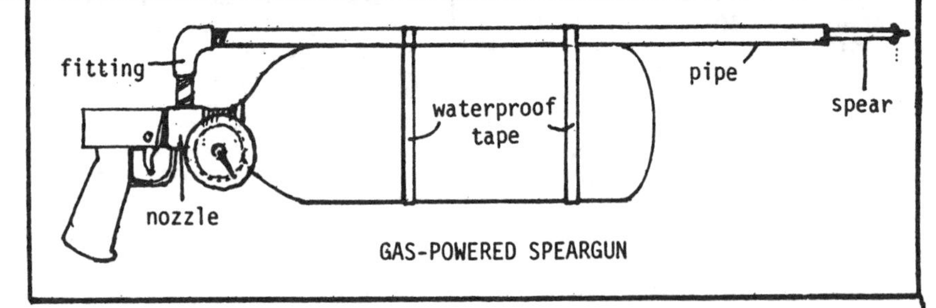

GAS-POWERED SPEARGUN

All spearguns are legal to own, however, it is illegal to load or fire one while on a public beach. The gas powered spearguns should not be left out in the sun, as it is possible the tank might explode.

Silenced Ruger Pistol

By Clyde Barrow

This silenced pistol design is a simplified version of the AWC Silenced Ruger manufactured by S & S Arms Co. The AWC unit is available to Class 3 dealers for $225 and retails for $275, plus a $200 Federal Transfer Tax when sold to private individuals. Included is a reprint of the instructions that accompany the pistol. Qualified buyers should contact the manufacturer for further information.*

The basis of this unit is a Ruger RST 22 autopistol, with a 4-3/4" barrel. The Ruger was chosen for both its reliability and relatively low mechanical noise. An earlier version of this design was used by the OSS in W W II and is still available to CIA and National Security Agency (NSA) personel. This early version was built on a High Standard pistol and contained a compressed stack of brass screen washers instead of shreaded copper and fiberglass.

All measurements and procedures are based on the S & S drawing and they may differ slightly from the actual unit. Note that the instructions call for two sizes of spanner wrenches. This has been simplified to the use of a large screwdriver and hand tightening. If taps and dies aren't available, a system of shims, collars and set screws may be substituted. This type of attachment is covered in the short barreled silencer article in PMA, page 58. If you don't have access to a lathe, a large drill may be clamped into a vise. Support the other end of the work with a wood block or similar steadyrest.

The simplest method is to drill the 4 rows of holes in the barrel and install a removable silencer mount on the muzzle. These mounts are ½"x20 male thread at the front. They are available for $25 from D.A.Q.* Mounts for several other guns are also available. The bushings and aluminum tube work can be farmed out to a machine shop.

Materials Used

1 - Ruger RST 22 cal. pistol w/4-3/4" barrel
1 - 7/8" ID-1" OD brass tube; sold in most hardware and plumbing shops as a toilet tank overflow tube, about 12" long.
1 - 2-3/4" long aluminum tube ¼" ID, ½" OD
2 - 1 " OD washers
2 - Drills - 1/8" and 1/4" diameter
3 - Taps; 15/16-5/8 and 3/8
3 - Dies; 15/16-5/8 and 3/8
2 - Threaded bushings
1 - Set screw w/allen wrench.

The above taps, dies, bushings and set screw may be of any thread pattern you choose and the sizes can be altered to fit the materials available.

Packing Material

See enclosed S & S instructions for description of packing material and procedure.

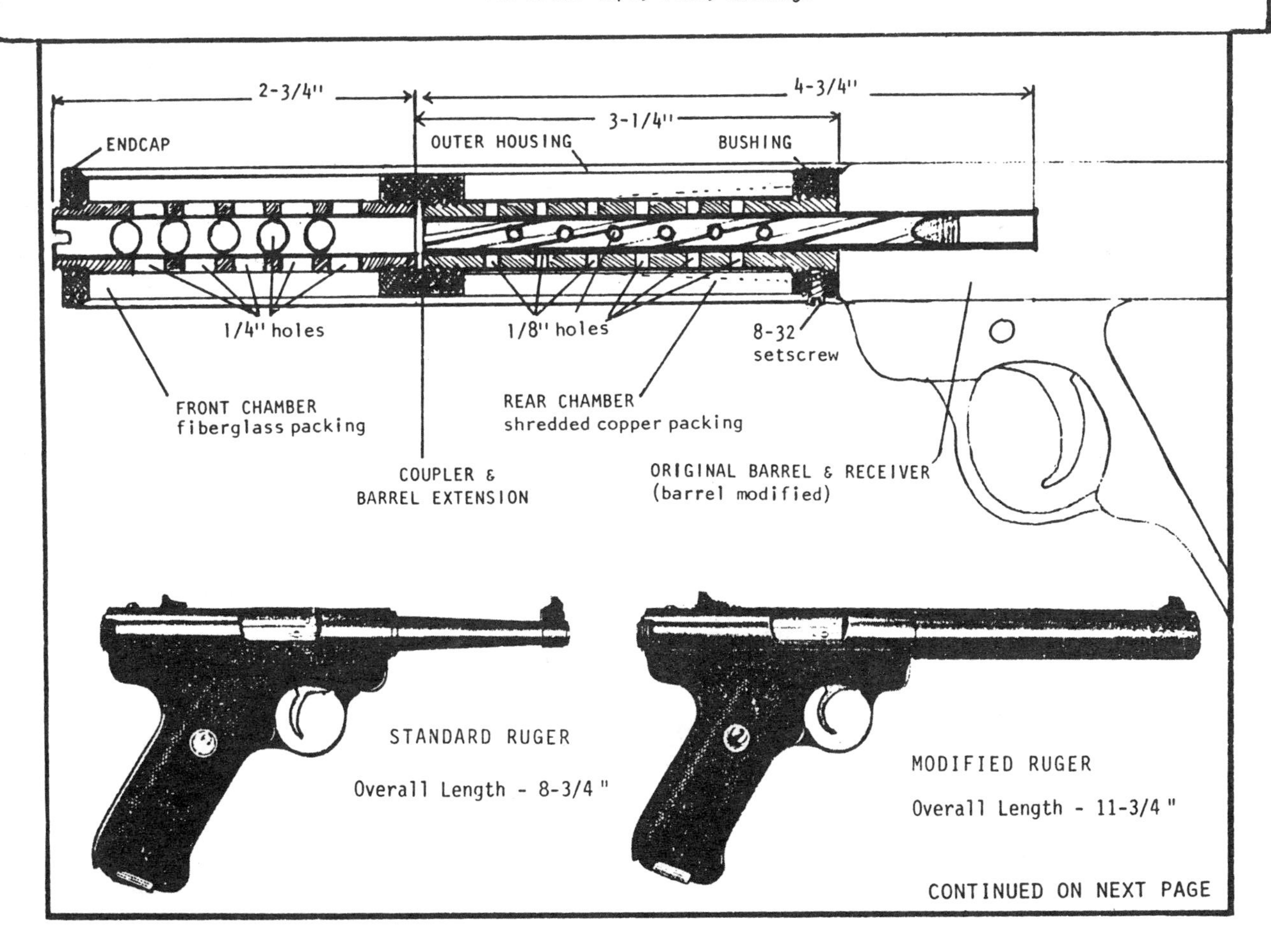

CONTINUED ON NEXT PAGE

Construction Procedure

A. Disassemble the pistol and clamp the receiver-barrel assembly in a lathe.
B. Measured from the front of the receiver, the first 3/8" of barrel is turned down to 5/8" OD. The remainder is turned down to ½" OD.

C. A piece of ¼" ID aluminum tubing is cut to 2-3/4" long and is turned to a ½" OD.
D. Thread both ends of the aluminum tube and the front of the barrel with a ½" die. The thread pattern is up to you. Use ½-20 threads with the D.A.Q. mount.
E. Thread the 5/8" OD area of the barrel and install a 3/8" long bushing - 5/8" ID,15/16" OD.
F. Drill and tap the bushing for a 8-32 set screw. Drill a shallow corresponding hole in the bottom of the barrel.
G. Cut a screwdriver slot in the front end of the barrel extension and join the barrel and extension with a 5/8" long bushing-½"ID, 7/8" OD. This bushing is threaded on the inside only. The outside should slip snugly into the 7/8" ID brass tube.
H. Drill four rows of holes in both the barrel and barrel extension.Six 1/8" holes per row in the barrel and five ¼" holes per row in the extension. Refer to drawing for placement of holes.
I. To build the endcap, reduce a 1" washer to 15/16" OD on one side and taper to 7/8" on the other. Solder this washer to a second 1" washer. Drill the center hole to ½" ID and thread. Use a file to serrate checker or knurl the edge of the 1" washer. This allows a good grip and eliminates the need for a spanner wrench.
J. Screw the endcap onto the barrel extension. Measure the distance from the front of the receiver to the front of the tapered area on the endcap. This distance is about 6", but will vary with each individual installation.
K. Cut the 1" OD brass tube to the length arrived at in step J. The inside rear of the tube is threaded to fit the bushing. Bevel the inside front of the tube until the tapered edge of the endcap will slip snugly inside. This taper is important because it aids in realignment of the tube mounted front sight when the unit is reassembled after each repacking.
L. Follow the instructions below for packing and assembly.
M. If additional sound or flash suppression is needed, an endcap w/baffles may be installed. Construct and mount the unit as detailed in the AR 7 silencer plans on page 58. The endcap may also be based on the MAC design-see ("The Removable Endcap") elsewhere in this issue.

Suppressor Disassembly:

1. After field stripping the pistol, remove the trigger-frame assembly (it slides slightly to the rear) and the bolt. Using the allen wrench in the end of the packing guide (see drawing), remove the 8-32 Allen set screw from the bottom of the suppressor housing.
2. Use the spanner wrench to unscrew the Front Assembly Nut.
3. Clamp the suppressor outer housing in a vise. It is recomended that either a block of wood drilled with a 1" hole, two blocks of wood with a "V" slot, or several layers of rubber inner tube be used to prevent marring of the blueing.
4. Using the Packing Guide barrel extension spanner, unscrew the barrel extension. It will unscrew about 1/2 inch.
5. Remove the barrel extension. If stuck, you may screw the spanner wrench onto the front of the barrel extension to give you a handle to pull with. DO NOT use pliers, as the barrel extension is aluminum. You will note that the coupler remains attached to the rear of the barrel extension. Do not separate the two.
6. Unscrew the receiver from the suppressor tube. This may require a bit of force, and it has been found that a rod (or large Phillips screwdriver) makes a good wrench when inserted in the holes in the rear of the receiver.
7. Discard all packing.Clean all parts thoroughly and lubricate thoroughly with a light rust inhibiting grease. If the barrel holes are plugged with lead, clean with a sharp instrument, such as an icepick.

Packing and Reassembly:

1. Punch or cut out the rivet in the copper scouring pads. Unfold the pads. Each pad is made of a sleeve of copper mesh about five inches diameter and slightly over a foot long. Cut crossways into five pieces and then twist each piece into a "rope" about 1/4" diameter and 7-8 inches long. With 2-1/2 pads, you will have twelve of these copper "ropes."
2. Screw the suppressor tube onto the barrel-receiver after lubricating the barrel and tube with a rust inhibiting grease. Align the index marks on the bottom of the housing and receiver near the setscrew hole. Replace the setscrew.
3. Stand the unit upright on the workbench with the open end of the suppressor tube pointing up. Insert the narrow end of the packing guide into the end of the barrel (the Allen wrench will be pointing up). This is used to guide the copper packing into the rear suppression chamber.
4. Wrap one of the copper "ropes" made in step 1 aound the packing guide and push in with the white plastic tube supplied (1/2" PVC water pipe). Hammer the end of the plastic tube to drive the copper rope in as far as possible. After partially hammered in, it may be necessary to temporarily remove the packing guide. Packing the copper in tightly is critical to the effectiveness of the suppressor, and remember that you are going to pack 12 ropes (2-1/2 copper scouring pads) in the rear chamber alone! In a similar manner, pack in the other 11 ropes of copper. After the 2-1/2 scouring pads have been hammered in, you should still be able to see portions of the threads on the end of the barrel. Note: 2-1/2 to 2-3/4 pads appears to be optimal. Never use over 3 pads.
5. Looking down the bore of the pistol, you may have seen several small wisps of copper packing protruding throught the holes in the barrel. Several passes of an oiled brass bore brush should clean out most of these strands of copper. The rest will disappear after the first shooting.
6. Install the coupler/barrel extension assembly. Use the spanner on the packing guide to tighten the assembly.
7. In a manner similar to step 4 above, pack the fiberglass around the barrel extension in the front suppression chamber. The fiberglass does not have to be packed quite as tightly as the copper, but light blows with a hammer are recommended. Fill the front chamber with fiberglass to the front end of the suppressor outer housing.
8. Screw on the front assembly nut using the spanner wrench provided. Screw hand tight only.
9. Shoot the weapon to check the point of impact, and adjust the sights if necessary. Point of impact may change slightly with repacking.

NOTES:

1. NEVER use a thread sealant (such as Loctite).
2. Factory repacking service is availble, but shipping the weapon requires transfers.Repacking can be done while you wait, if you bring the weapon.
3. Repacking kits (copper pads and fiberglass) are available for $2 ppd. Obtaining the materials locally is cheaper.

AWC SERIES SOUND SUPPRESSED RUGER PISTOLS -

Description: The unit consists of a standard Ruger model RST-4 pistol in cal .22LR with an integral sound suppressor. The barrel of the pistol has been modified for use with the sound suppressor by having been drilled to port hot gasses into the rear suppression chamber (see drawing). By bleeding the gasses within two inches of the chamber, velocity is slightly reduced, keeping the bullet subsonic. The rear chamber is packed with dense shredded copper, which cools the hot gasses quickly reducing both their temperature and volume. Copper has been found to be exceptionally effective as a heat conductor. The front suppression chamber is packed with fiberglass and acts similar to a "Glasspack" automobile muffler, helping to further muffle the report, expand the gasses, and spread out the sound pressure peak. The suppressing principles are not new, but the combination is effective. The barrel extension coupler and front assembly nut both help keep the outer tube (which carries the front sight) concentric with the bore of the barrel.

Ammunition: Because of early porting of the gasses in the barrel reducing recoil, the recoil spring of the pistol has been modified by having three turns removed from the spring. This functions well with all types and brands of ammunition with the exception of CCI Standard Velocity, which occasionally fails to eject. All other CCI ammuniiton works well. Velocity measurements range from 825 f.p.s. to 875 f.p.s. (Standard & HV) in the suppressed weapon as compared to 1,050 to 1125 f.p.s. in an unmodified pistol. The velocity of the CCI Stinger ammunition is reduced froml,440 to 930 f.p.s. There is a slight loss in effectiveness of the suppressor using HV ammunition, and we recomend standard velocity .22LR ammunition for backyard and basement shooting.

Sights: The standard model suppressed Ruger uses the original fixed sights which came with the pistol. The front sight is attached to the suppressor housing, and is normally supplied somewhat high, making the weapon shoot low. This is done in case the purchaser wishes to install adjustable rear sights. If the standard sights are to be used, the front sight may be lowered by filing during the sighting in process. Windage can be adjusted by drifting the rear sight. We can provide adjustable sights at a slight additional charge if ordered at the time of ordering the weapon. There are many excellent sights which can be field installed, including Micro and Miniature Machine Company (MMC) adjustable rear sights. Interestingly, the MMC sight requires a front sight lower than the original non-adjustable sight. Sighting radius on the suppressed pistol is approximately 10", and the suppressor adds only about three inches to the overall length of the pistol.

Cleaning: It is recomended that only minimal cleaning of the weapon be performed between repacking intervals. Routine cleaning should consist of using a brass brush dipped in solvent to scrub the bore, followed by a dry patch and a lightly oiled patch. The receiver and bolt can be cleaned with powder solvent and lightly oiled. We use WD-40, and have been satisfied, although any light oil will work. Whenever repacking of the sound suppressor is performed, then a thorough disassembly and cleaning of the weapon is recommended.

Loss of Efficientcy: With time, minute lead shavings and powder residues will obstruct the ports in the barrel leading to the rear suppression chamber, and the weapon will become noisy, requiring repacking. It is estimated that repacking will have to be performed every 400-800 rounds. Materials are available locally, and after the first time about an hour will be required. For owners in the Albuquerque area, we can provide this service at the factory for a nominal fee.

Packing Materials: Total cost will be slightly less than a dollar. The shredded copper for the rear suppressors chamber is available at most supermarkets as "Chore Girl Pure Copper Scouring Pads." Buy three, as you will use 2-1/2 pads. Cost as of April 1977 was 20¢ per pad. DO NOT USE STEEL WOOL; IT BURNS. For the front suppression chamber you will use a piece of one inch thick fiberglass about 6" by 15". This is available in hardware stores in 6" wide rolls for insulating pipes.

THE REPLACEABLE ENDCAP

by Clyde Barrow

This design for replaceable silencer endcaps was developed by Mitchell Werbell, head of Military Armament Corp (MAC). The design resulted from silencer research conducted during the Vietnam era.

The endcap contains two hard rubber baffles, a spacer and a retaining washer which is staked in place. The undersized holes in the baffles become enlarged and ineffective after several hundred rounds. The unit is then removed by hand and a fresh replacement is installed. The worn caps can be discarded or may be returned to an arsenal for rebuilding.

Replacement baffles can be made from amber squeegee rubber, available from art supply shops and janitorial suppliers.

INTERIOR VIEW

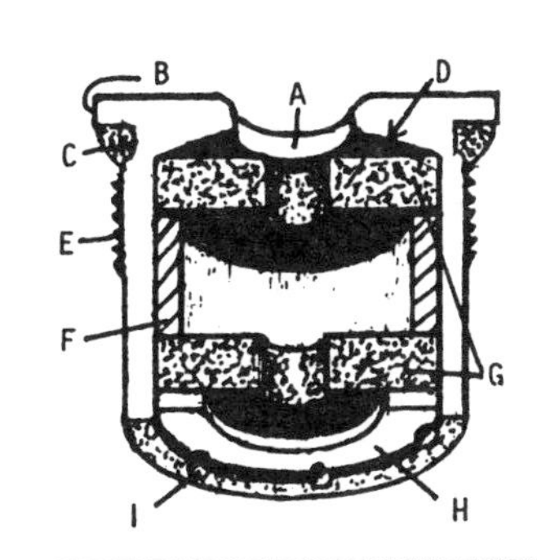

ENDCAP COMPONENTS

A. Hole 5/8" ID
B. Knurled Rim 1-3/4" OD x 3/32"
C. Undercut 1-7/16" OD x 1/8"
D. Undercut For Baffle Expansion
E. Male Threads 1-9/16" x 20 NC x 3/8" long
F. Spacer - Aluminum Tubing 1-1/4" OD x 1" ID x 1/2" long
G. Plastic Baffle 9/32" ID x 1/4" thick x 1-1/4"OD
H. Aluminum Retaining Washer 1-1/4" OD x 3/4" ID x 1/16"thick
I. Indentation From Staking Punch (1 of 6)

These caps will fit tubing with the following specs: 1-3/4" OD - 1-1/2" ID (1/8" wall) Threads-20 per inch NC - (thread depth 1/32")

Available in .45, 9mm, or .380 sizes, the caps are sold to anyone for $17.50 each or $150 per dozen plus UPS shipping. (you can mix sizes for a dozen.) Order from;

Tim D. Bixler Firearms Co.
Box 1455, Gretna LA 70053

Specify: MAC Suppressor Wipe Assemblies and include caliber desired when ordering.

Ringed Shotgun Slug

By Martin Kruse

Photos by M.Kruse

Back on page 27 of the Armorer an article appeared under the title "Special Purpose Shotgun Ammo." This article dealt with improvised techniques for modifying regular shells to perform specialized functions.

In discussing this with Clyde, he informed me that several readers had written him questioning the use, functionability, and safety of these loads. He wondered if I could shed any light on the use of any of them.

Well, I havn't tried all of them, but I have had a great deal of experience with the one designated in the article by the letter "D". This is an improvised slug made from a regular shot shell. This really is an old hillbilly trick. We call it "ringing a load" or "cutting a ringed load." Its use goes back to the time when the first brass based paper shells came out, and in some parts of the country it's been a pretty common practice ever since.

To make a ringed load, all you need is a shotshell and a good sharp knife. Just cut through the shell at the wad column leaving only a narrow strip, maybe about 1/16 of an inch, of shell casing holding the two sections together. I've never bothered to heat seal the end of the shell casing so I guess it really isn't necessary, but you can if you want to. However, most of the time this is used in a pinch, or as a survival measure and a soldering iron just isn't handy.

When a shell treated in this manner is fired, the entire shot load remains intact within the shell casing and wadcolumn, impacting the target as a single projectile. Fragmentation takes place during penetration.

For this reason, the ringed load does far more damage in many cases than a conventional rifled slug.

I've taken wild pig and several coyotes with them and I know guys in Alaska who've used them on moose and bear. They're a little too destructive for regular meat or hide hunting but they sure do the job in a pinch.

The explosive nature of their construction as well as the accuracy and performance of the ringed load makes this a good choice for defensive use. They should be one hell of a manstopper, and certainly better than a birdshot load used in the conventional manner. What's more, their accuracy and shooting characteristics are such that you may choose the ringed load over the conventional rifled slug for many anti-personnel applications.

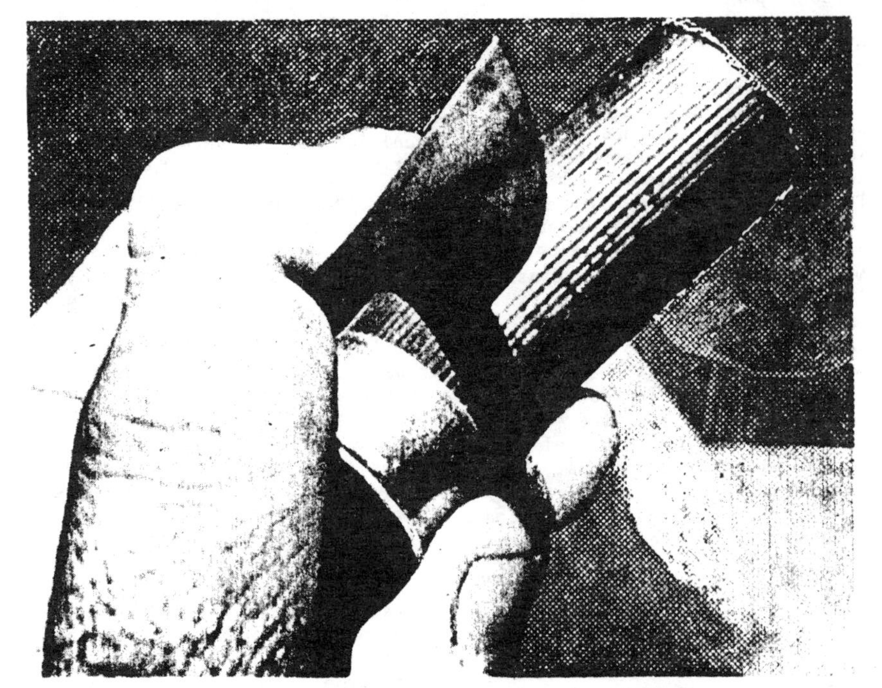

"Ringing or cutting the shell for ringed load.

Some time ago, in preparing an article for one of the more conventional gun magazines, I ran extensive tests comparing the accuracy and performance of the ringed loads and regular factory rifled slug loads.

Comparisons were made in 12,16, and 20 gauges through a wide range of barrel lengths and chokes. Tests were made for both ballistic performance (effect on the target) and accuracy of the the projectiles. In side by side comparisons, the ringed loads' performance was truly surprising. This 'field conversion' actually outshot the factory load.

The biggest plus I found for the ringed load was that they shoot much flatter than the rifled slug. The greatest difference occured when both types of projectiles were fired through full choked barrels of standard 28" length.

One reason for the great difference in the trajectories of the 2 loads is that the constriction at the end of the barrel has more slowing effect on the rifled lead slugs than on the slick hull casings. This is born out by the fact that both loads shoot flatter in more open-choked barrels, but the amount of difference was greater with the slugs.

The Remington factory chart for their 12 ga. rifled slugs gives a drop figure of 10.4" at 100 yds. This figure is established using a test barrel designed and choked specifically for rifled slugs. Firing these rifled slugs through several full-choked barrels, I got between 33 and 37" drop at 100 yds. Ringed loads fired from the same barrels dropped from 15 to 18" below the point of aim.

Both loads gave their best performance through special slug barrels, or riot guns. Barrels of this type were tried in lengths of 18, 20,22, and 24", with chokes of imp. cyl. bore.

The 12 ga. slugs dropped an average of 12 " at 100 yds. (an acceptable amount of deviation between factory claims and actual performance.) The ringed loads came in with an average of 9" through the same guns at that distance.

No special slug guns were available for testing in 16 and 20ga., so all testing was done with regular field guns. They seemed to shoot a little flatter than the 12 ga, but the same descrepancy occurred between loads. The flatter trajectory means a decrease in necessary holdover. This reduces the possible error at unknown distances and greatly improves chances for a clean kill under field conditions.

In addition, the ringed loads showed considerably less lateral dispersion. Test groups were fired from a bench rest at 25, 50, and

100 yards. The ringed load groups were about 30% tighter in all gauges and through every barrel. This is due, in great degree, to the fact that the ringed loads fit the bore (about .69 in 12 ga., which is .72 caliber). The slugs pitch and yaw, wobbling down the barrel and in flight. Also, their short, almost round shape, is not conducive to great inflight stability.

These characteristics are evidenced by the fact that rifled slugs occasionally keyhole on target at 100 yds. and frequently at 150 yds. (The latter distance is too great a range for their effective use but proved very revealing for test purposes.)

The ringed loads with their tighter fit and greater weight and length seem to leave the bore on a true line and stabilize well. No keyholing occurred with ringed loads even out to the somewhat impractical range of 200 yds. They cut a neat, full-caliber, wad-cutter like hole.

The other factor which may lead to your choice of the ringed load for some application is that, due to their greater weight, (573 gr. for a ringed load cut from a Western 1-1/4 oz. 12 ga. load of fours with fiber and card wads opposed to 382.8 gr. for a Winchester factory rifled slug), they hit a hell of a lot harder. And as I mentioned earlier, their construction makes these projectiles highly destructive. They'll make a hell of a mess out of anything which is more easily penetrable than steel plate.

If you have to use a shotgun for that purpose (car bodies, for example) make a batch of the loads designed by the letter 'A' in the afore-mentioned article in Vol.1#2 PMA. But for face to face anti-personnel applications, the ringed load should do one hell of a job. And they are, contrary to some of the warnings I've heard from several armchair experts, safe to fire.

Chamber pressure does not become excessive. The projectile wt. is the same as if the uncut shot load had been fired. I've never experienced any barrel problems as a result of using ringed loads, but I'm told, and suppose it is conveivable, that it may blow the chokes out of some European shotguns which have extremely thin tubes.

You may come into one problem though. Back when this trick came into use, the shotguns around were mostly break actions, either singles or doubles, that you could feed anything into without a hitch. Some repeaters are a bit more finicky. In all the pumps I've tried, the ringed loads feed into the chamber smoothly. But on some of them, the ejector missed the shortened piece of casing and it smokestacked in the action. This necessitated tipping the gun while the action was open to dump the fired base before closing the breach on a new round. As with the pumps, some autos functioned smoothly. Others gave varying degrees of headaches, with cures ranging from simply clearing the action to complete disassembly. If you shoot an auto, try it out first before you put it on the line.

At any rate, check out how the ringed loads shoot through your own gun. There's no substitue for knowing first hand. **Editor's Note:**

If you are concerned about possible gun or shooter damage, make your first batch of ringed loads from low power dove and quail loads.

Comparison photo shows difference in size between ringed load projectile on left and twelve gauge rifled slug.

THREE SHOT PLASTIC PISTOL

The Troika pistol, designed by the Soviets as an assassination weapon, is comprised of as little metal as possible. This allows the user to conceal the weapon on his body and hopefully pass through a magnetometer check at airports, guarded government installations, etc. The pistol shown is not an exact copy of the Troika, but it is based on the same general principle.

The body is made of plexiglass, with a thin brass liner in each barrel. A plastic or fiberglass bullet, about 30 caliber, is muzzle loaded over a charge of black powder.

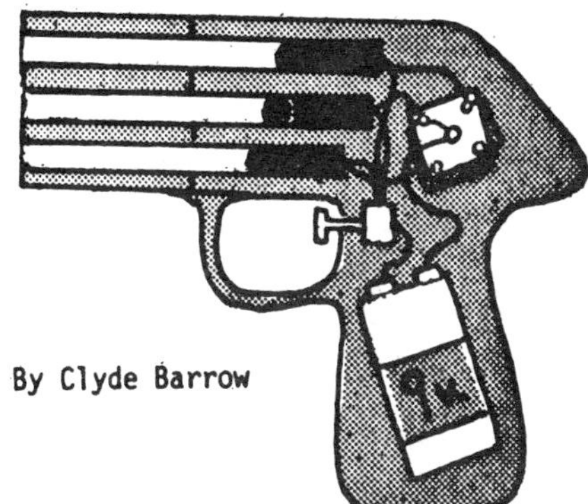

By Clyde Barrow

The black powder is ignited by a light bulb filament located at the rear of each barrel. A rocket ignitor would also work. The three filaments are wired to an on/off trigger and a four position selector switch. Settings A, B, & C will allow the corresponding barrel to fire. Setting D is wired to A, B&C so all three barrels may be fired at once if desired. Power is supplied by a 9 volt radio battery

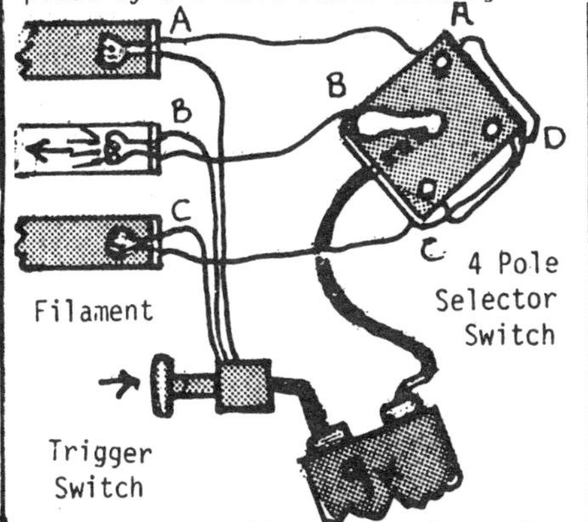

The projectiles have a low relative stopping power and should be poisoned to insure a kill. This pistol is intended for point blank use only. It would have little accuracy at any great distance.

FLASHBULBS AS DETONATORS

By Fred Bilello

Inserted in explosives, a flashbulb will prove to be an effective detonator for mines and bombs. To test your equipment, scotch tape a match to your flashbulb and perform the experiment as illustrated in Fig.1. The bulb should go off, igniting the match. A good bulb to use is Sylvania model AG1. They come in a small flat box.

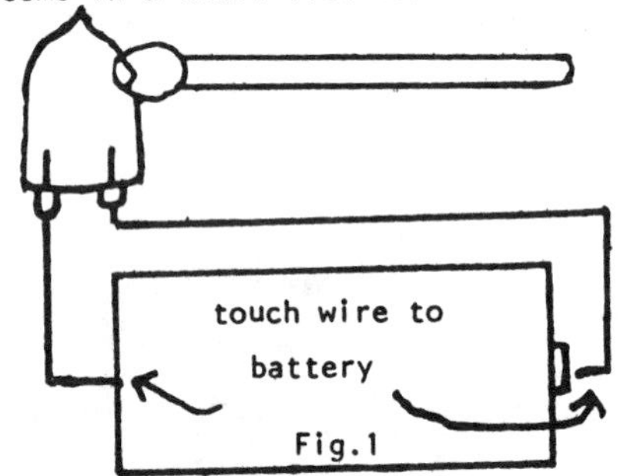

Fig.1

Once your experiment is successful, you can build your control box.

SUPPLIES:

4 - dry cell batteries.
1 - Light copper strip, 1/2" wide x 4" long .
3 - Lightweight springs, inside diameter about 3/8", length 1/4" .
3 - Flashbulbs.
3 - Wood dowels, 1/4" diameter, 1" long .
3 - Lightweight electrical terminal lugs .
3 - Small wood screws .
3 - Pieces of heavy bare copper wire, each piece 1/2" long .
6 - Headless nails, 3/4" long.
2 - Pieces of wood, about 1-1/2" wide by 4" long.
2 - Pieces of wood, about 2-1/2"x 4".
2 - Pieces of wood, about 2-1/2" x 1-1/2" .
2 - Small hinges & wood screws.
1 - Strip rubber or plastic, 1-1/2" x 4" .
4 - Lengths of different colored bell wire. Colors A,B,C & D will be used in the diagrams.
Glue
Electricians tape
Small screws or nails (optional)

STEP 1 - POWER PACK

1. Tape the 4 batteries together in a row.
2. Strip the insulation off of about 6" of bell wire, color D. Then make 4 double loops in the wire as illustrated, spacing the loops so that the center bottom of each battery will touch one.
3. Lay the copper strip on the contact points of the battery. Then, with the looped wire on the bottom, tape the strip and wire securely to the battery pack. Be sure there is at least a 1/4" space of bare copper strip between each taping. See Fig. 2.

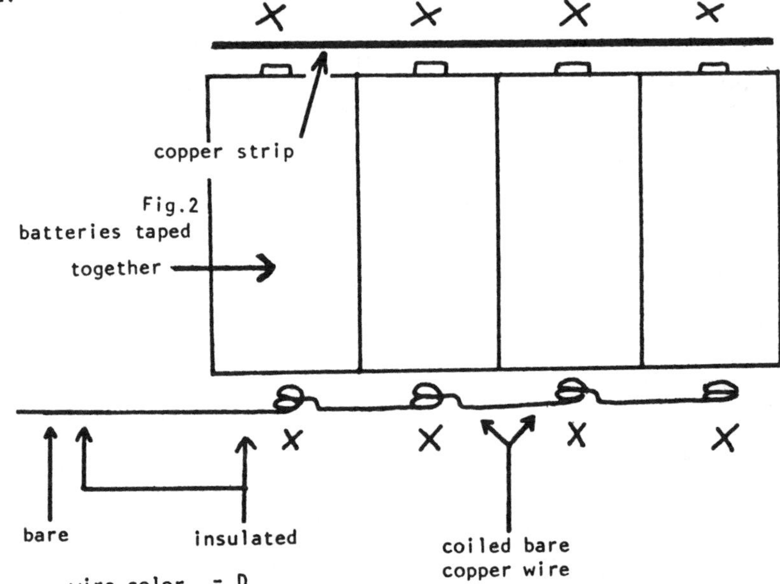

STEP 2 - PUSH BUTTON CONTROL PANEL

1. Cut 3 5/16" holes in one of the 1-1/2" x 4" pieces of wood. The holes should be lined up to allow contact with the bare space between the tape on the copper strip on the power pack.
2. Screw the electrical terminals in the bottom side as illustrated in Fig. 3.

3. Connect three different colored lengths of bell wire, each length about 12" long.

STEP 3 - PUSH BUTTON

1. Drill a 1/4" hole in the bottom of each dowel.
2. Take the 6 nails and bend them at right angles so the lengths will be 1/2" x 1/4". Glue 2 of the bent nails to each side of a dowel with the 1/4" end protruding.

3. Put a drop of glue on an end of the heavy copper wire and insert into each dowel hole. Be sure that no glue gets on the opposite end. See Fig. 4.

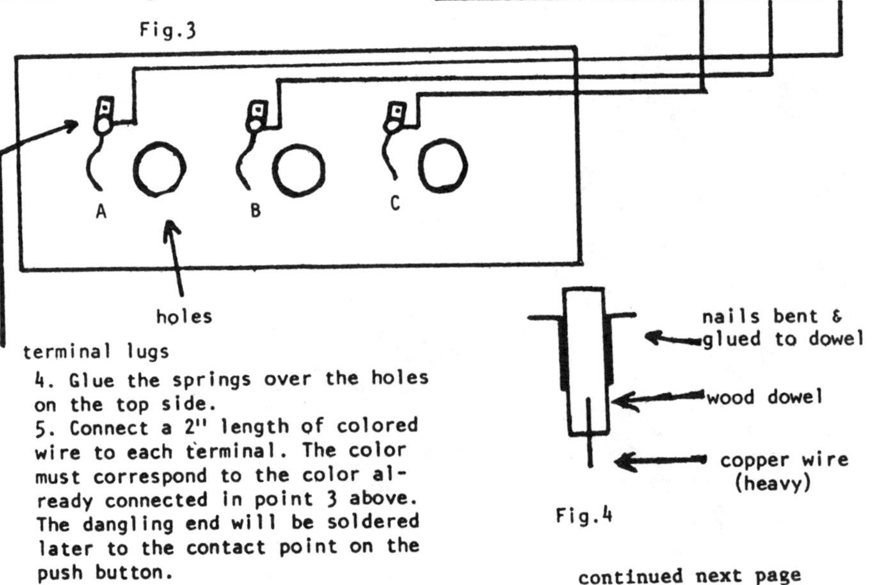

4. Glue the springs over the holes on the top side.
5. Connect a 2" length of colored wire to each terminal. The color must correspond to the color already connected in point 3 above. The dangling end will be soldered later to the contact point on the push button.

continued next page

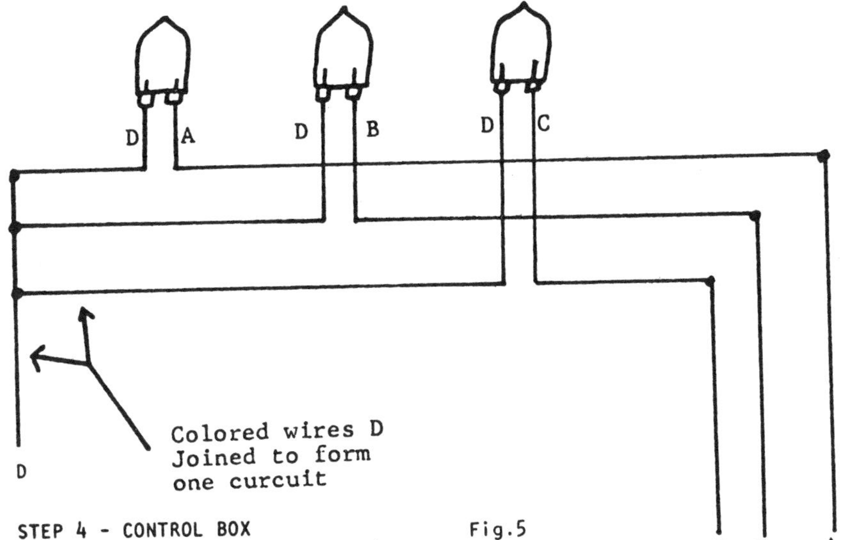

Fig.5

STEP 4 - CONTROL BOX

1. Glue the rubber or plastic strip to the other 1-1/2" x 4" strip of wood. This will be the bottom of the box. When assembling, the plastic or rubber will be facing up.
2. Screw the hinges to one of the 2-1/2" x 4" pieces of wood and attach the other side of the hinge to the side of one of the 2-1/2" x 1-1/2" pieces of wood.
3. Drill a 1/16" hole in the bottom of the other 2-1/2" x 1-1/2" piece of wood, which will be the left side of the box, and a 1/8" hole in the top right hand corner of the other 2-1/2" x 4" piece of wood, which will be the back wall of the box.
4. Using nails, screws or glue, assemble the box. There will be no top to it.

STEP 5 - ASSEMBLY

1. Take 3 flashbulbs and attach a length of wire, color D, to one terminal on each bulb. Then take one length each of wire colors A, B & C and attach one of the colored wires to the remaining terminal. Follow the hookup diagram in Fig.5. Insert the bulbs into the explosive of your mine or bomb.
2. Slide the push buttons over the springs and glue the springs to the bent nails.
3. Solder the dangling ends of wire from the control panel to the contact points.
4. Rest the power pack on the rubber strip, and feed the wire (D) through the hole.
5. Secure the control panel to the top of the box and feed wires A, B & C through the hole at the top right back of the box. There should be a space of about 1/8" separating the contact points on the push button from the copper strip on the power pack.
6. From Fig. 5, connect wire D to wire D on the control box and then connect wires A, B, & C to wires A, B, & C from the control box. See Fig. 6 for completed assembly.

The instructions and diagrams listed here will give you a control box capable of detonating 3 mines or bombs. Using your imagination, you can modify the design and make a switchboard holding a hundred or more buttons.

If you decide to build a bigger switchboard, it would be a good idea to keep the control buttons in groups of 3 for easy hookup, repair, and replacement of batteries. Be sure to label each button so you can identify it with your target. If you plan to hook up your defenses against a future attack, you should protect the wires running from the control box to the mines. Either coat them with a spray or paint to avoid deterioration of the insulation, or encase the wires in tubes like BX cable.

Besides the switchboard hookup for manual detonation, flashbulbs are great for all sorts of contact mines, trip wires, and bombs to combat tree climbing snipers.

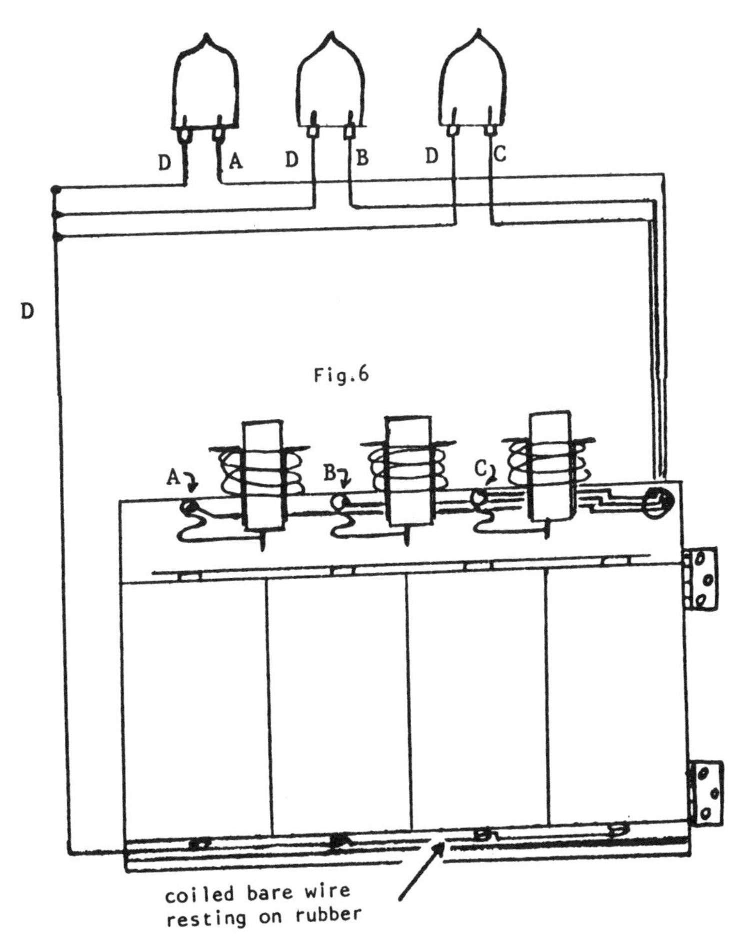

Fig.6

Improvised Claymore Mine

By Raymond J. Larner

Black Powder Squib:

Obtain a 12 volt lamp bulb (with a flange on it [head or tail light bulb]). Carefully break the glass off of the bulb. Solder wire leads to the rear and the side of the bulb. You can check the filament by very quickly attaching the wire leads to a 12 volt battery. Glue the bulb into the rear of the claymore casing with the flange inside the case and the wire leads out the back. Make a paper cylinder that is large enough and long enough to protect the filament of the bulb. Glue this cylinder to the inside of the casing so that it protects the filament.

Casing:

This can be made of almost anything, but 1/8 inch thick plexiglass is one of the easiest materials to work with. Make a small box that is 3 inches wide by 6 inches long by 1 inch deep. You need 4 sides and a bottom but no top. Use solvent type glue to put the box together.
Note: the box can be made any size. The larger it is the more damage you can do with it but also the more explosive it will take to fill it.

Drill a hole in the middle of the bottom of the casing large enough to put the base of the light bulb thru. Install the black powder squib in the casing as shown in the drawings.

Casting:

Make a mold with an outside length and width slightly less than the inside dimensions of the casing. This should be approx. 1 inch deep. This mold can be made with body putty or with plaster of paris. Let it cure and then use spray paint to coat the inside of it until the mold is smooth to the touch.

To Cast:

Spray the inside of the mold with a casting release agent. Mix and pour liquid casting plastic into the mold until it is approx. 1/4 inch deep. Now pour in 3/16" or 1/4" steel ball bearings until you have a layer of them covering the bottom of the mold. Add casting plastic if needed so that the layer of balls is barely covered. Set the mold aside and let the plastic cure. NOTE: Plaster of Paris or body putty can also be used to cast the balls in. The ball bearings are the easiest to work with but any metal can be used (nuts, bolts, screws, nails, etc.).

When the casting has cured, remove it from the mold. Use alcohol to remove the wax residue from the casting.

Now carefully pour black powder into the paper cylinder that protects the filament of the bulb in the casing. Lightly shake the casing to settle and pack the black powder around the filament. Now fill the rest of the casing with black powder until you have a level layer of black powder slightly above the top of the paper cylinder.

Place the casting inside the casing on top of the layer of black powder. Now use a silicone or plastic sealing compound to seal around the 4 edges of the casting. Once it dries your claymore mine is ready to be used. NOTE: for concealment use colored plexiglass or paint the claymore after you've put it together.

Emplacement:

To place the claymore, tape it to a tree, pole or what ever is handy. Make sure the ball bearings point toward the enemy. Remember that this type of weapon produces a mean back blast so make sure you are under cover when you set it off.

You can make up a control board to control a number of claymores that you have in place. Or you can simply string wires from each of your mines to a central location and touch the ends of the wires to the poles of a 12 volt battery.
NOTE: This weapon can be made more effective (cover a larger area) by making the casing and the casting slightly curved.

THIS WEAPON CAN ALSO BE MADE USING THE EXPLOSIVE AND FUSE BELOW.

Explosive:
Mix three (3) parts Potassium chlorate and one (1) part granulated sugar. Confine in a container (in this case the claymore mine) and use time fuse to set it off.
Time Fuse:
Boil equal parts of potassium chlorate and granulated sugar in water. Dip cotton string in the solution and let dry. Buring rate is approx. sixty (60) seconds per foot. Test some to make sure!

This weapon can also be used on the side of a truck or tractor. This was done in Vietnam and was found to be highly effective in ambush situations where the enemy was at close quarters to the vehicle being attacked.

Make a steel box approx. 6" deep and 12 by 12" on the sides. Just sides & bottom, no top. Solidly attach the box to the side of a vehicle with bolts or weld it in place. Make sure it is attached to something solid - remember that back blast! Make up 2 sand bags, one 6 x 12 and the other about 10 x 12. Set the small bag in the bottom of the box and the larger bag into the back of the box. (The open end of the box should point outwards from the vehicle). Now set the claymore into the box so that it is sitting on top of the small bag and against the large bag. Securely fasten the mine into the box with wire or what ever is handy so it won't fall out as you drive down the road.

A switch set into the dash is the easiest way to set this placement off. Wire a lead from the battery thru a breaker or a fuse to the switches and them to the claymores.

CLAYMORE

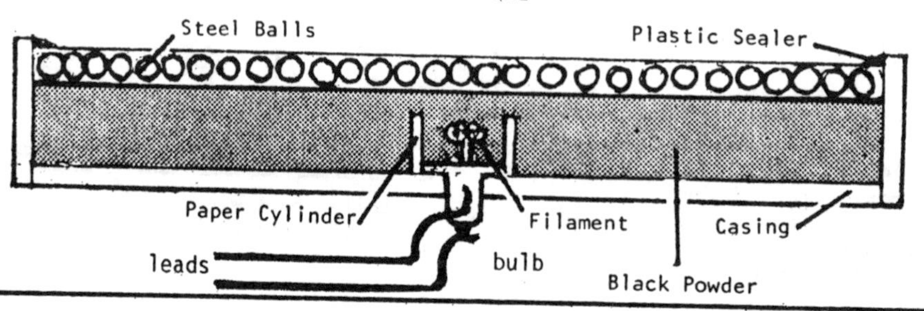

SILENCER

This silencer design is an improvement of the OSS silencer from WW II and is the forerunner of the silenced Ruger design from issue #4 PMA.

Aug. 31, 1948. **W. P. MASON** **2,448,382**

SILENCER

Filed Oct. 26, 1944

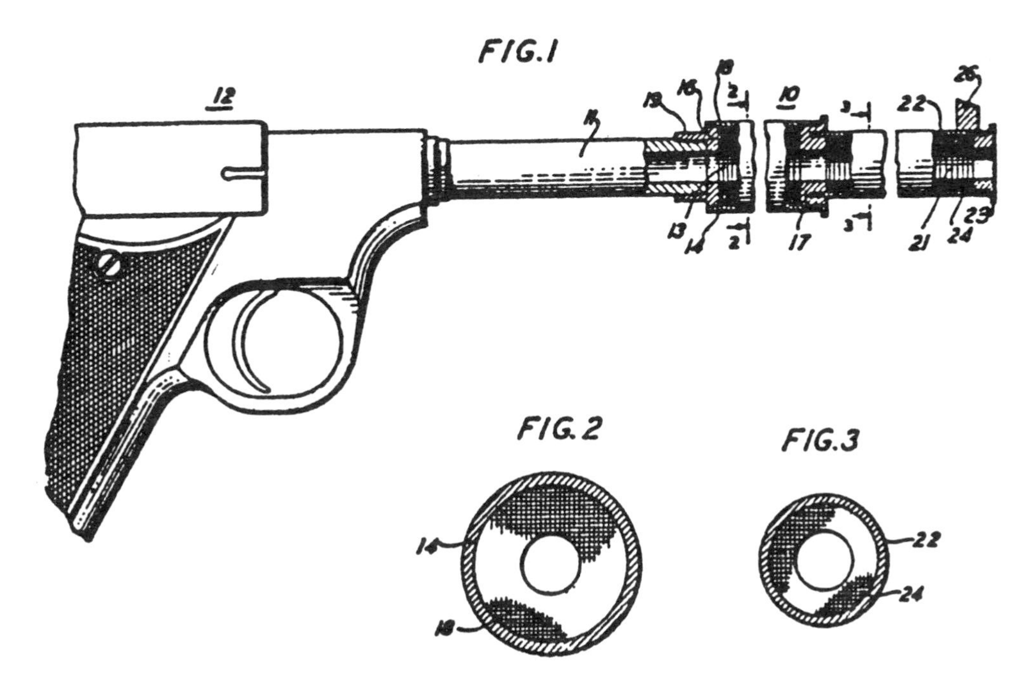

This invention relates to firearms and more particularly to a silencer for reducing the muzzle blast.

The principal object of the invention is to reduce the noise associated with the muzzle blast of a firearm. Other objects are to reduce the weight, size and cost of a silencer and improve the stability of performance.

Important factors in silencing the muzzle blast of a firearm are the rapid cooling of the power gases and the reduction of pressure before they emerge. An effective silencer utilizing these principles comprises a chamber containing heat absorbing material through which the bullet passes. The effectiveness of such a device depends, amoung other things, upon its cross-sectional area. Applicant has discovered, however, that the importance of having a large cross-sectional area diminishes considerably toward the front end of the silencer.

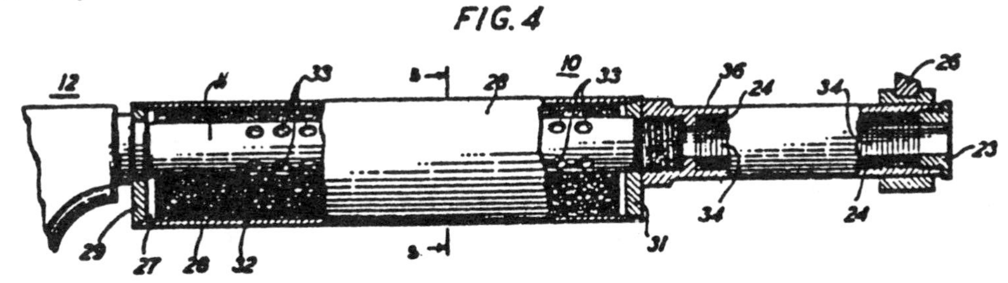

FIG.5

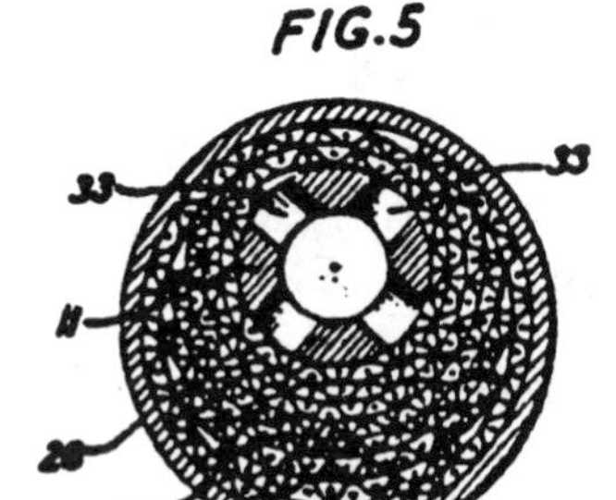

INVENTOR
W.P. MASON
BY
Ralph T. Holcomb
ATTORNEY

In accordance with the invention, therefore, the chamber has at its front end a section of reduced cross-sectional area. Weight, size and cost are reduced without seriously affecting the efficiency of noise reduction. The silencer may be built as an attachment or, preferably, the rear portion of the chamber may be built around the barrel of the firearm, with communicating holes through the barrel. The heat absorbing material may be metal screen , which may take the form of apertured discs, stacked one upon another and preferably held in compression. Plating the screen with some metal such as tin before punching the discs will increase the stability of performance.

Flash Powders and their Production

By Dan Moore

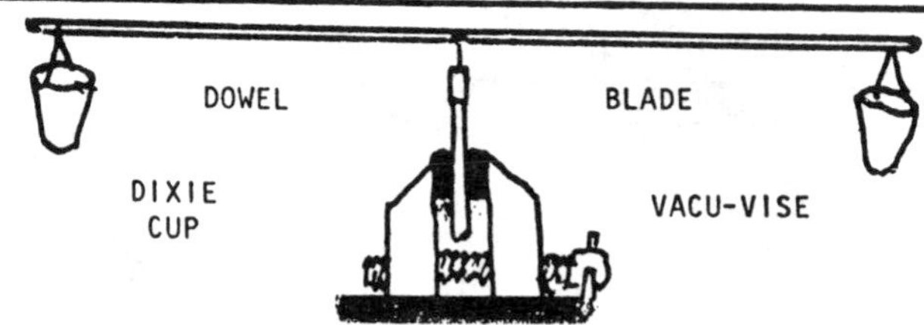

Flashpowders are some of the most explosive kinds of powders known. In fact, Lenz* even regards flashpowder as high explosive due to its tremendous power. In addition to this, flashpowders are both easy and safe to manufacture. It is because of this that I have decided to explain in detail the manufacture of these powders.

*Lenz, Robert R., Explosives and Bomb Disposal Guide.

The most common of these powders is "Photoflash" powder or just simply "Flash" powder. This powder is the easiest to manufacture and the least expensive. The equipment needed to make photoflash powder is a mortar and pestle, a scale or balance, and several plastic containers. The chemicals required are; powdered aluminum (Al), sulphur (S), and potassium permanganate ($KMnO_4$). These chemicals should all be finely powdered for best results. (It is best to buy finely powdered aluminum as it cannot be ground. Sulphur and potassium permanganate should be ground separately in the mortar and pestle to a consistancy of flour.) The ratio of weight of these chemicals is: one (1) part sulphur, one (1) part powdered aluminum, and eight (8) parts potassium permanganate. After powdering, these chemicals should then be placed in a plastic container and shaken thoroughly for ten (10) minutes to insure even mixing. The flashpowder should then be kept in a plastic container and stored in a cool dry place.

Another explosive powder which even surpasses photoflash powder is chlorate flashpowder. Chlorate flashpowder is much more powerful than photoflash powder and also much more sensative. The reason for its increased strength is the use of potassium chlorate (a very powerful unstable oxidizing agent). The equipment needed for making chlorate flashpowder is the same as for photoflash powder with one minor exception. A flat metal pan and a hammer are used to powder the potassium chlorate as the friction from a mortar and pestle could cause an explosion. The chemicals required to manufacture chlorate powder are; potassium chlorate ($KClO_3$), sulphur (S), and powdered aluminum (Al). The ratio by weight of these chemicals is: one (1) part sulphur, one (1) part powdered aluminum, and two (2) parts potassium chlorate. Once again all chemicals should be finely powdered and thoroughly mixed for best results. Chlorate powder should be kept in a plastic container and stored in a cool dry place.

One other flashpowder is a derivative of chlorate powder. This flashpowder is manufactured in the same way as chlorate powder, however instead of using potassium chlorate, sodium chlorate is used. This may offer an alternative to survivalists as sodium chlorate can be obtained from Solidox(See The Survivor Vol.2, issue #9).

Although I have just listed the basic flashpowders and their manufacture, there are several things that one should know before manufacturing them. To start with, the equipment meeded for producing these powders is very basic in nature. Really, the piece of equipment that needs to be purchased is the mortar and pestle, as it would be hard to improvise. The plastic containers can come from just about anywhere. For example, the plastic containers I found to work best were nothing more than plastic butter dishes. The balance that is required can be makeshift just as long as it is reasonably accurate. The balance I used was constructed as such:

A notched wooden dowel is used for the main beam of the balance while a Vacu-vise and an Exacto knife are used as a base. Dixie cups can be used for containing the chemicals during weighing and fishing sinkers are used for weights. I have found this kind of balance to be very successful for the measuring purposes in this article.

One final note about manufacturing these powders is the emphasis on safety, as it should be with any article on explosives production. Although these powders are not as sensitive as conventional explosives, there is always the chance of an accidental detonation. To lessen or eliminate this possibility, certain precautionary steps should be taken. A list of these steps is as follows;

1. Mix flashpowder in no more than 3 ounce batches to lessen the explosive potential.
2. For chlorate powders, add a small amount of bicarbonate of soda to desensitize the chlorate powders.
3. Never mix or store powders near an open flame.
4. Keep the work area clean and well-organized.
5. Mix only enough powder for immediate use.

Provided these steps are taken, the manufacture and use of flashpowders will be both safe and simple.

IMPROVISED SMOKE/ GAS GRENADES

BY "Q"

To those readers who've built Dan Moore's "Super Bazooka" on page 53 and have spent the past few months' free time by blasting away at trees and fenceposts in sessions of secret target practice, the question has probably arisen as to what to do with all those empty rocket engines. Fervent Survivalists needn't discard them as useless; because I have just the information you need to turn those little tubes into some of the best smoke 'n stink bombs available.

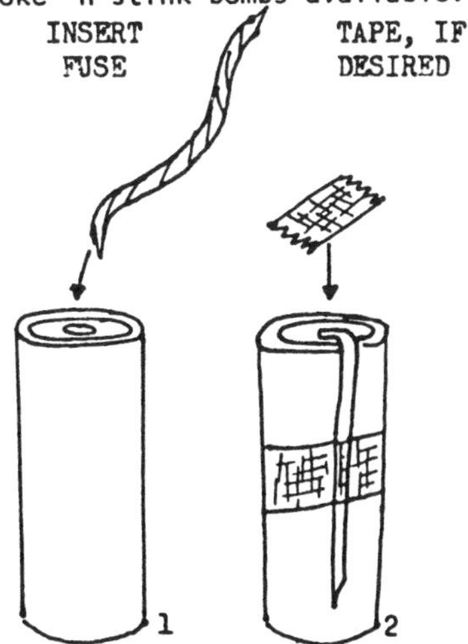

Start by examining your supply of spent engines: select those which havn't had their walls burnt thin and with their nozzles still intact. Open up the venturi in any of the clay nozzles which have been fused shut.

Place a piece of reliable fuse in the nozzle, use any length of delay you wish but have at least 1-1/2" inside the casing. Zeller's 3/32" cannon fuse works fine. Bend and tape the fuse over to the side of the engine, to keep it out of the way, and apply a square of tape over the fuse/nozzle junction. This will help keep the filler from leaking from the fuse end during manufacture-you can remove the tape when they're finished, though that's not essential.

I might point out here that it's a good idea to simplify your work by setting up an "assembly line" and by performing each step on a number of casings at the same time.

Next, place either 3-4 scoops (use a .22 LR case as a measure) of Fuzee powder, the black ignitor portion from the body of a railroad flare; or 3 to 4 paper match heads inside the inverted casing. If you use Fuzee, carefully tamp it down with an unsharpened pencil.

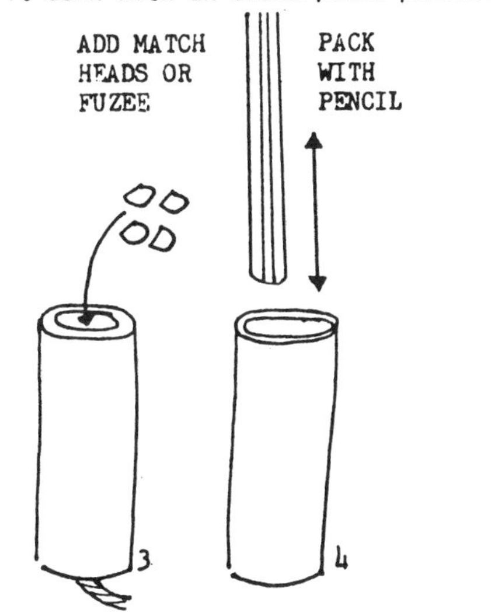

Next, fill with the smoke powder mixture to the end of the casing and tamp down with a dowel the same size as the inside of the engine. (You can first start packing using the pencil, in order to avoid scrunching the fuse.) Fill to the top again and tamp in. We have used either a vise or a hammer in order to insure that the mix is tightly packed, without a single mishap. Repeat this until there is about 1/4" distance left to the end of the case. Note: depending upon a number of variables, which include the exact composition of your mix, your ability to construct them and local weather/atmospheric conditions, your grenades may work better left relatively loose, or rammed down tight; so a bit of experimentation is in order here.

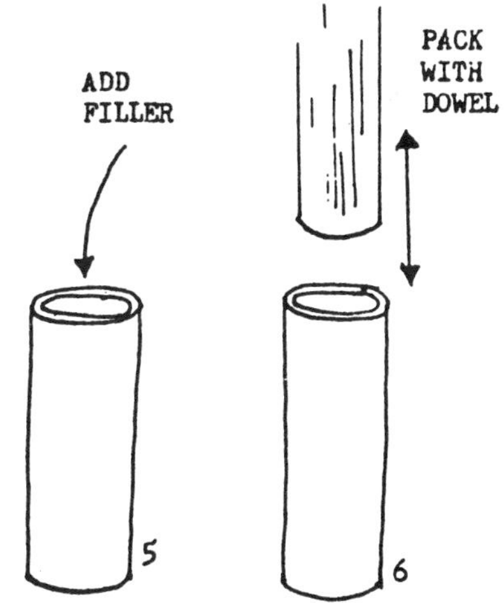

Finally, wad up some 4X4" scraps of paper (newspaper or magazine stock is what we prefer) and tamp them down in on top of the powder charge. Use several pieces to bring up the level to about 1/8" from the end of the casing. This paper serves both as a primary end seal and as a heat-sink to prevent possible damage to the mix by the final wax seal. With that done, seal the end by pouring melted wax over the paper; allowing it to pool in the recess. We just let the wax drip from a candle. This is better than using epoxy to seal the cases, as it enables one to use the grenades immediately after production, as well as permitting you to dig out the seal on a used/dud unit in order to use the casing for several more reload-

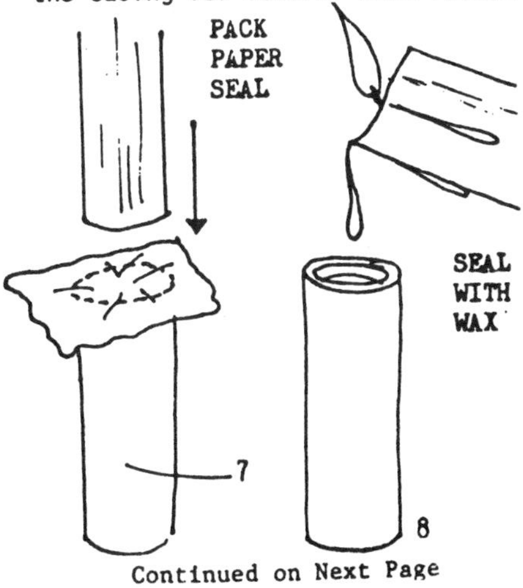

Continued on Next Page

ings and practice "firings". Once the wax has cooled your little wonder is ready for use.

Our most successful demonstration indicated that one of these goodies would produce enough Ammonia-Sulferish smoke, in the 5 to 7 minutes they last, to contaminate the interior of a suburban-type ranch house. Outside, especially on damp nights, they will produce a foul-smelling white cloud which just Blankets a 50X50' area. These were made from a "C" size engine. Naturally a "D" engine would be proportionally more effective-or, make regulation "Police" size grenades from cardboard tubes, forming your own nozzles.

Various chemical fillings will work, but the mixes we found most effective run as follows:

75% NH_4NO_3 Ammonium Nitrate

15% C Carbon (finely grqund charcoal briquettes will work

10% S Sulfur

This will produce a "seeper" that will slowly function over a 10 minute period; good for the situations where you wish to leave before much of a stink is started. For a more devastating filler that will actually BILLOW, use about 5% less NH_4NO_3 and add 5% KNO_3 (Potassium Nitrate) or homemade black powder.

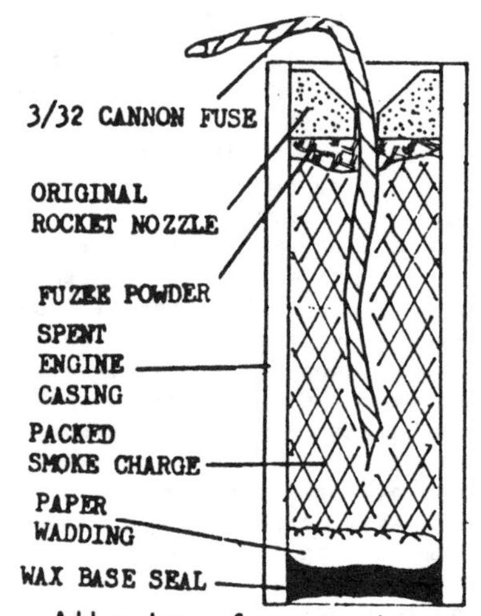

Add a drop of wax to the nozzle/fuse junction or store your completed grenades in a ziplock bag, as the mix is somewhat hygroscopic and may take on some moisture from the air or moist surroundings. For your first test firing it is best not to hand-hold the grenade, although this is possible once you can predict its functioning. Not only may it get quite hot, but it may malfunction dangerously if you prepared the filler incorrectly. Wedge it into the ground and stand upwind to watch the action. When you're satisfied that your construction is safe you can proceed to throwing or otherwise delivering the rest of that batch to your target. ⚜

Interchangeable Powder Cartridge

By Martin Kruse

The .32 Winchester special,which was introduced in 1895 and chambered until recently in the Model '94 Winchester level gun, was originally designed as a smokeless powder cartridge suitable for reloading with black powder.

It was found that the .320 caliber and a rifling twist of one turn in 16 inches would accomplish this idea better than the .30 caliber bore with one turn in 12 inches twist found in the .30/30. The faster rifling twists found in rifles chambered for smokeless cartridges foul so badly when used with black powder (especially in bores of .30 caliber and smaller) that they are rendered totally inaccurate after just a few rounds.

If you think smokeless powder just might not be here to stay, an old .32 Winchester special may be your kind of gun.

CALTROPS

and IMPROVISED BARRIERS

By Clyde Barrow

The traditional Caltrop is a four pointed device that was originally scattered on roads in ancient times to injure the hooves of horses being ridden by the opposing army. These devices are equally effective against today's automobile tires.The four points are arranged in a manner that guarantees that one point will stick straight up no matter how the caltrop is placed on the ground. This allows the devices to be scattered from a fleeing auto, thrown by hand or dropped from the air.The road can be opened only after the caltrops are picked up one at a time by hand. The cleanup personnel are susceptible to sniper fire during this cleanup period. A pileup of several disabled vehicles will of course add to the problem of reopening the roadway, especially if all available tow trucks have received multiple flat tires,as there is usually only one spare tire per truck. Imagine several hundred of these devices on a major freeway during rush hour traffic.

A.A simple caltrop can be made as follows. They are easier to make than describe. If the following does not make sense, try it first with a couple of pieces of coat hanger or welding rod, and play with the design until you come up with the right shape. A dimestore protractor is useful in determining the correct number of degrees for each bend.

The completed units should be painted flat black or dark gray.They will blend in with the color of the roadway and will be almost impossible for drivers to spot and avoid, even if they are on the lookout for them.

1. Cut two pieces of iron or steel rod, ¼" to ½" diameter, to a length of 3½".

2. Sharpen all four ends to a sharp point with a file or grinder.

3. Weld or braze the pieces into and 'X' shape.

4. With the 'X' lying flat on the bench, bend one leg until it is straight up in the air, i.e. at a right angle to the bench.

5. The remaining three legs are now bent until they are at 120 deg. angles to one another. If placed on a circle, the legs would divide that circle into three equal parts. All 3 legs should still be flat on the bench.

6. Each of the three legs is now bent until they rest at a 30 deg. angle from the surface of the bench. The fourth leg should still be vertical.

Each of the four legs should now be 120 deg. from its two adjacent legs. The caltrop should now rest solidly on any combination of three legs, with the fourth pointing straight up.

Several variations of the caltrop design exist. The following are the most useful and easily improvised.

B. The spike board (see PMA Vol.1#3).

C. The spiked hazard used at drive-in movies. These allow normal traffic to exit, but cars trying to make an unauthorized entry are impailed on the spikes, which protrude at about

45 deg. from the ground. Those spikes are mounted on a weighted axle which pivots flush with the roadway on exit but locks solidly in place during an attempted entry.

D. The borders between European countries are equipped with movable road blocks that resemble the folding gates often used to prevent toddlers from falling down stairs or from entering 'off-limits' rooms. The device has a sharpened spike at each pivot point and is anchored at one side of the road. A guard extends the obstacle into one or both lanes to block the road, and folds it out of the way to allow authorized vehicles to pass.

E. A Caltrop like device that requires no welding or bending can be constructed from short sections of pipe and six bolts and nuts. If welding equipment is available, the same device can be constructed using six large nails. The advantage of this type of caltrop is that several of the units can be strung onto a chain or cable. This assembly can be stretched across a roadway and anchored to solid material, i.e. boulders, trees, wrecked vehicles, etc., at each end. The road can be reopened only by cutting the chain or cable with a torch or bolt cutters. The personnel attempting to remove the obstacle are again open to sniper fire.

The pipe caltrop is constructed follows. The measurements can be altered to suit the materials on hand. Each individual caltrop is made from a six inch long section of 1-1½" diameter pipe, and six 3" bolts w/nuts.

a. Drill 6 sets of holes through the pipe, in 3 rows of 2 holes each. Pipe will contain total of 12 holes. IE., six sets of holes, one set for each bolt (See drawing).

b. Use a grinder or file to sharpen the ends of the bolts.

c. Pass the bolts through the holes and install and tighten the nuts.

d. If welding equipment is available, large nails may be installed in the holes and welded in place.

Dear Clyde,

Just got PMA #5 and saw your little article on Caltrops. There's an even easier way to make them out of about 1/32" sheet steel that needs only a pair of tinsnips (although compound leverage aviator's snips would be easier to use). Just cut a piece of sheet steel to the shape shown in Figure 1, then twist 90° across the narrow waist, see Figure 2. The Caltrop will sit on one edge and one point with the remaining point sticking up. See Figure 3. The 1/32" thickness is okay for passenger cars, but heavier metal should be used for trucks and other large vehicles. With nothing but scrap steel, a pair of tinsnips, and a couple of hours, you can have hundreds of these little devils!

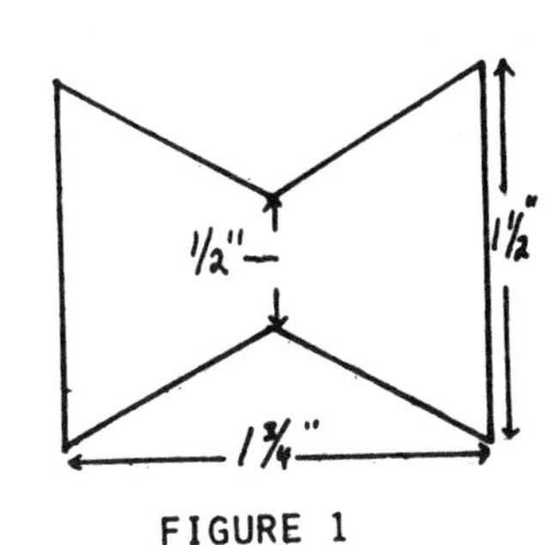

FIGURE 1

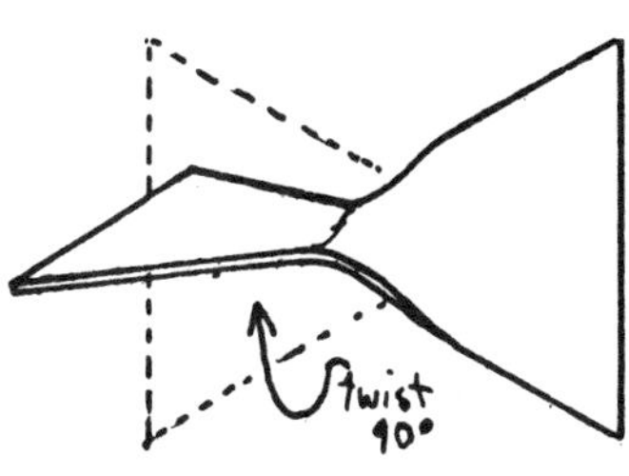

FIGURE 2

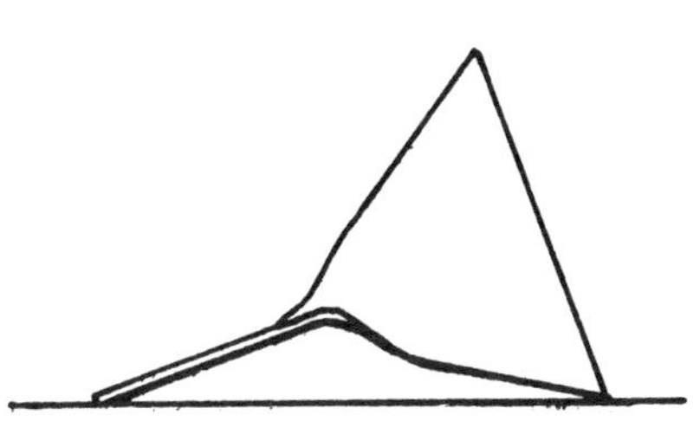

FIGURE 3

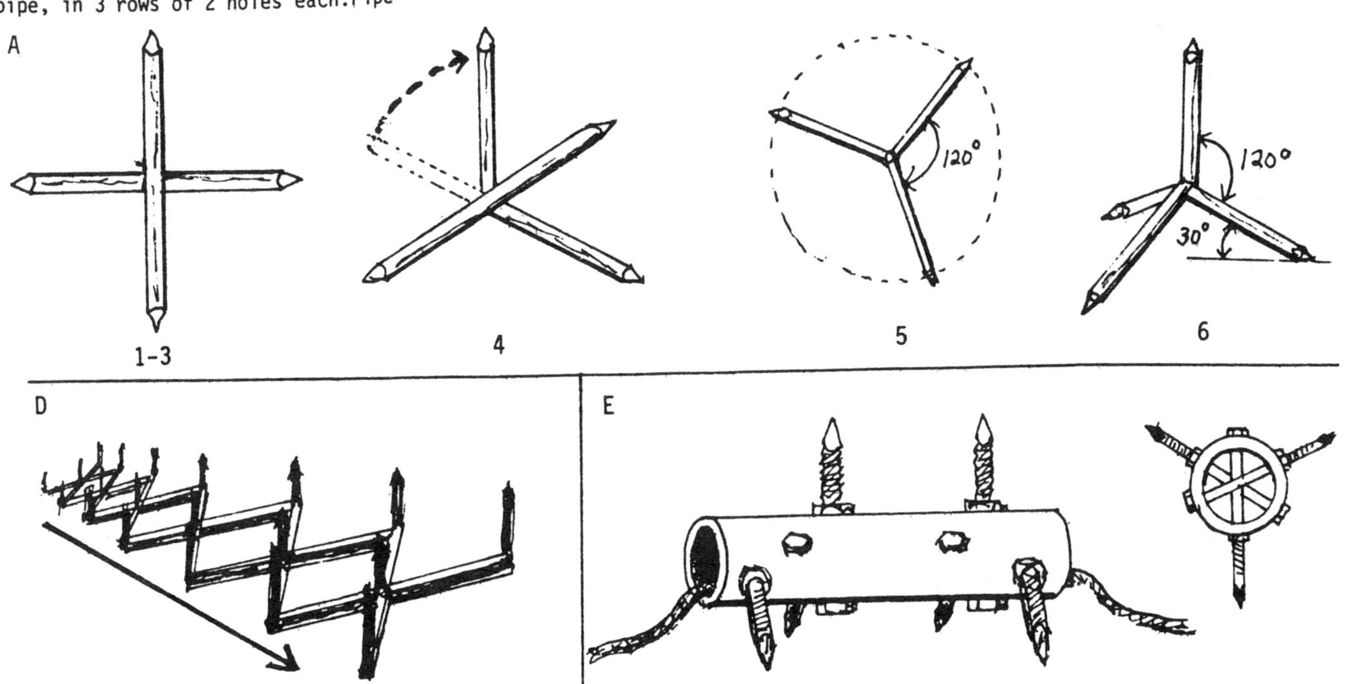

The Truth About Knife-Throwing

By Martin Kruse

Throwing knives is an enjoyable way to pass idle time. It's an interesting and challenging sport,and it's a skill which may save your life in a pinch.But don't count on it. Knife throwing is not nearly as efficient a means of dispensing death as paperback novels, television, and movies would lead us to believe.

The fact is, even if you devote the time and effort required to develop the skill, it's of very limited value.

First off, it's strictly a close range proposition. Most men I know get a range of 12-15 feet maximum with any degree of reliability.I know a few men who stick a blade consistently and accurately out to 30 ft. When I hear a man claim he can do any good with a blade beyond that distance,well,I may not call him a liar, but I sure want to see it before I believe him.

Another thing, your range isn't just limited by a maximum distance. Unless you take the time to develop a high degree of skill and practice regularly,your effectiveness may be limited to one or two specific distances. This is because the knife turns in the air and there are only a few points along it's line of travel at which it will be point first at the target.

The more common throwing techniques cause the knife to turn once every six feet.(It varies with the individual.I'm planning a slow motion film study on the subject.If I ever get around to it I'll report the findings in the Armorer.) This means that while you may be sudden death at 6 or 12 feet, you're probably S.O.L. from 8 to 10 feet. That's not a favorable prospect for use in combat.

You can improve your odds with practice,however.If you're good at accurately judging distances you may be able to change your throwing style to turn the blade faster or more slowly and thereby increase the span of your effective ranges.

But, throwing a knife is still an iffy proposition at best. The only 'throwing knife' which has a high degree of reliability is the Oriental Shirken or Throwing Star. These wicked little gems are nothing but points and stick no matter how they are turned.All the thrower need worry about is accuracy. (I also hope to report on the shirken and how they're made and used in a later issue.) This isn't the case with a conventional blade,however.

I would like to state here and now that in further discussions of edged weapons, any mention of a blade's throwing characteristics is merely an evaluation of the weapon,not an endorsement for using the technique in combat.

Just about any knife can be thrown. The balance point of a knife means very little in most cases.Once you have learned to get the feel of a knife just shift the position of your grip accordingly and you'll be able to stick almost any knife in a target.

Being able to throw a knife is impressive, especially to someone who's tried it a couple of times without success.It's a great way to win a few beers and it may save your ass someday.I've never regretted having taken the trouble to acquire the skill. But at no time should you allow yourself to forget the limitations of this in practical applications. While it is definitely worthwhile to be able to throw any blade which presents itself as a weapon of opportunity, if there is a serious intent to your practice,knife selection becomes critical.

Stay away from the so-called throwing knives that are supposedly made for the purpose.As weapons,they're not worth a tinker's damn and most of them actually don't throw well anyhow. Stilettos and daggers also make poor choices.While they throw nicely,they are generally too light to do much good as an attack stopping projectile.

For defensive or combat use,it is best to stick with a heavier blade whenever possible. For my money the large Bowies are the best bet. The Marine Corps combat knife is an excellent choice.I believe this represents about the minimum size and heft for a real fighting blade. I consider anything smaller and lighter,including the ever popular British Fairbairn to be inadequate.They may be fine for a surprise attack where one or two quick thrusts will do the job.But when it comes down to a real brawl,I want something with some heft to it to slash and even cleave bone if necessary.

The Marine Corps knife is also about the largest blade that most people can wear concealed.A butt down underarm carry works well as does positioning it in the center of the back butt down.Depending on where you live you may be able to just strap it on in plain sight as I often do.The respectful looks you'll see on the faces of the street corner punks will enrich your soul and restore your faith in humanity.

These knives possess excellent throwing characteristics and have enough weight to give at least some penetration,thereby giving you at least some chance to put your man down. It probably won't do the job, but it is a chance,and if it's the only one you've got, take it!

Where knife throwing is concerned, if you have time to think about it, think of something else.You're probably better off hitting someone with a brick or a good heavy rock. But when all the bets are on the table, you play the cards you've got and hope they're good enough.Sometimes all rules of thumb are meaningless. Just act quickly and relentlessly. And stay alive!

If the bastard's about to pull the trigger on you and the knife is in your hand, then have with it,pitch away.Take your best shot and follow through with it.It probably won't take him down,but it may divert his attention long enough to close the distance and kick his head in.

Follow through is important in any knife attack. A simple stab or slash is seldom enough to put an attacker down. Especially a thrown blade which may not have penetrated deeply.

Follow your blade in. (Unless you're one hell of a knife thrower,you'll only be two jumps away.) Jump on the sonofabitch and push the blade in the rest of the way. Then twist it. Or, follow it up with a swift hand-to-hand attack using every dirty trick you know or every weapon at your disposal. Do so regardless of whether your throw went true or not.

Any opening you can create in your opponent's defense (or balk in his attack-which is actually the same thing) should be exploited with all the fury and force you can muster.

* * * *

YAWARA STICK WITH .410 PUNCH

BY DARVIS MC COY

The walking-stick shotgun described in issue #1 PMA can easily be turned into a yawara stick that is deadlier than any martial arts weapon ever taught in self-defense schools.

The materials needed are the same as described in issue #1, except that the point of a nail makes a more efficient firing pin than a bolt. The .410 shotgun shell fits the half in. size of the pipe very nicely, while 3/4 inch lead pipe works well as the outside sleeve. Wrap the 1/2 inch section in duct tape until there is enough friction to keep the inner section from sliding around freely inside the outer sleeve. The 3/4 in. piece should measure about 4 in., while the 1/2 in. section should measure an inch longer.

Drill a shallow hole from the inside of the pipe cap, exactly in the center of the cap. The diameter should be the same as an eight penny nail or a little larger. Don't drill all the way through the cap, just deep enough to form a recess that will hold the shaft of the nail. Now cut off the point of the eight penny nail, giving you a quarter inch section of shaft with a sharp point. Put epoxy on the blunt end and insert into the hole. The assembly of the yawara stick is described in issue #1.

Either end of this stick can be used for its respective purpose: the cap end for striking, as with a regular yawara stick, or the protruding end of the half inch section for deadlier intentions. Care should be taken to wrap enough duct tape around the inner section so there will be no danger of the .410 shell going off when the cap end is struck forcefully. It should only detonate when the small end is smashed against its target. The end can also be securely taped together to prevent the sections from separating while it's being carried.

To test your stick, empty a .410 shell of shot and powder, and load it into the stick. Smash the business end into the dirt, slanting it away from you to protect your eyes from flying particles. If the primer detonates, success! If not, make sure the firing pin (nail point) is in the center of the cap. * * *

WATER PIPE SHOTGUN SAFETY

BY MARTIN KRUSE

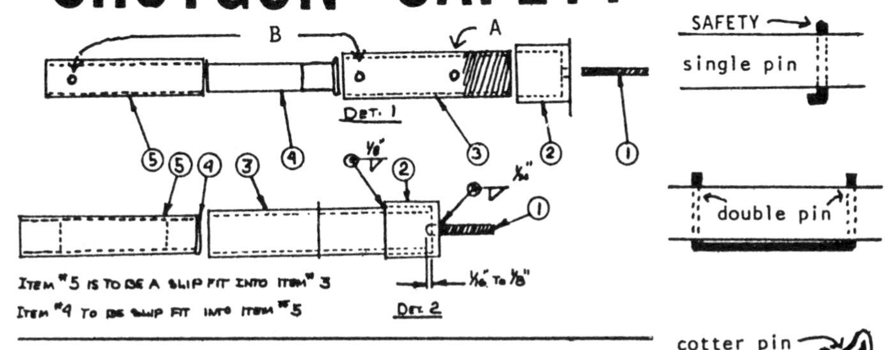

1. MACH. BOLT W/HEAD CUT OFF. 1/8" DIA. x 2" LONG. (ROUND ONE END)
2. PIPE CAP 3/4 - 1/8" HOLE DRILLED IN END (TAP HOLE FOR ITEM #1)
3. PIPE x 4" LONG (THREAD FOR ITEM #2)
4. SHOTGUN SHELL (410 3 MAG. WORKS NICE)
5. PIPE x 6" LONG

The walking stick shotgun made from water pipe which was featured in PMA #1 could be a very handy weapon, except that it's unsafe to carry. Besides the danger, it could be very embarrassing as well as a detriment to your continued freedom to have your 'walking stick' either fall apart or go off at the wrong time.

You can eliminate this potential hazard by putting in a pin type safty lock. This is simply a piece of 1/8" or 3/16" drill rod slightly longer than the diameter of piece number three and bent at a right angle at one end for a stop. By drilling a hole through piece three at Point A and inserting the safety pin there you will block the shell from the firing pin. It won't, however, prevent the weapon from sliding apart.

If you don't trust tape not to let go at the wrong time, you may run the pin through both pieces #3 and #5 by placing it at position B. This placement requires section #3 to be longer than your shell. Keep in mind that section #5 must be longer than section #3 for the mechanism to fire.

The pin through both pieces at point B will prevent the mechanism from sliding apart or closing to the firing position. But the shell can still come into contact with the firing pin and possibly discharge. The best method, I think, would be to use a double safety shaped like a large staple which would engage at both points. This would not be any slower to remove for firing than the single pin, and is truly double safe.

If you worry about the pin falling out and the weapon 'arming', you can drill the open ends of the staple-shaped pin and fit them with small removable cotter pins. This step will, however, greatly increase the time needed to take the weapon 'off safe' and make it ready to use.

Editor's Note: A rubber band around piece #3 would also hold the 'U' shaped safety in place.

UNCONCEALED CONCEALED WEAPON

BY MARTIN KRUSE

The good old-fashioned blackjack is still one of the best hand-to-hand weapons around for real close quarter work. Unfortunately, however, our lawmakers have seen fit to make this fine defensive weapon illegal. In most states, now, the laws are so warped that the blackjack is not only illegal to carry, but it's even prohibited to own one (unless you're a police officer). This has made this fine weapon relatively hard to come by.

As usual, though, the law is really pointless, since there are several improvised types you can make yourself which work just fine. The handiest, least conspicuous, and most "bust proof" is an English style cap

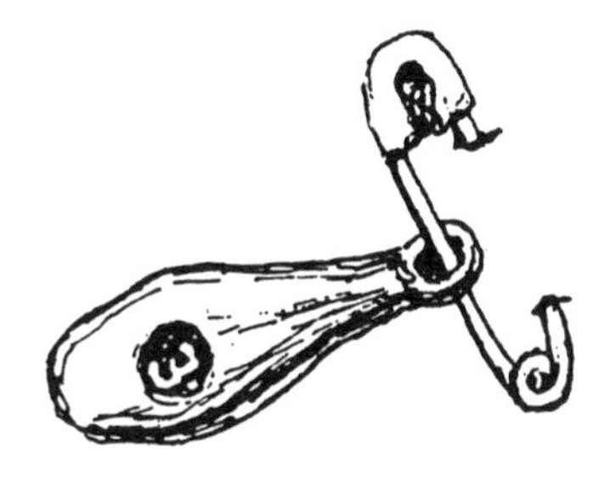

with a one to three ounce fishing sinker in it. Just attach the sinker inside the back of the cap with a large safety pin.

This is perhaps the best kind of concealed weapon in that it is disguised rather than hidden. You can "legitimize" the weapon by pinning in a small packet of fishhooks and maybe even some line with the sinker. As far as I know, there is no law against carrying any fishing gear in your hat. And, it will do double duty if you do happen to be a fisherman (fishperson?).

When needed, the weapon can be brought into play in a hurry. No digging into pockets, boot-tops or sleeves. Just grab the brim and swing. It's extremely quick and effective. Catch an attacker across the side of the head with a good swing and he'll go out like a light.

The English cap is a comfortable and practical piece of headgear which has come back into style in recent years. It's just the thing for a late stroll in any neighborhood!

HOMEMADE MISSILE

By Clyde Barrow

INTRODUCTION (SEE PAGE 5)

The missile plan detailed in this article is a sythesis of several antitank missile designs used by NATO forces during the last 15 years. The construction data has been broken down into three sections: airframe/motor assembly; guidance unit; and payload/detonator section.

This design is intended as a general guideline only and there are many areas where alternative materials may be substituted. All materials described are available from either model rocket suppliers or firms that sell radio control airplane accessories. A sample list of these firms and their addresses has been included at the end of the article.

Actual construction information has been kept to the basics. Those familiar with building model planes and rockets will be able to improve upon the design and come up with a more sophisticated product. For those unfamiliar with radio control or model rocketry I suggest buying a copy of 'Basics of Radio Control Modeling' by Marks and Winter and 'The Handbook of Model Rocketry' by Stine. These and similar publications are available at the local library, hobby shop, or bookstore. There are also several radio control plane magazines available at the local news stand.

As cost is a factor, it should be noted that these missiles can be built for about $50 each. This compares favorably with the Soviet SAM missile, currently used by third world terrorists.SAM missiles are known to cost about $1000 each to produce.

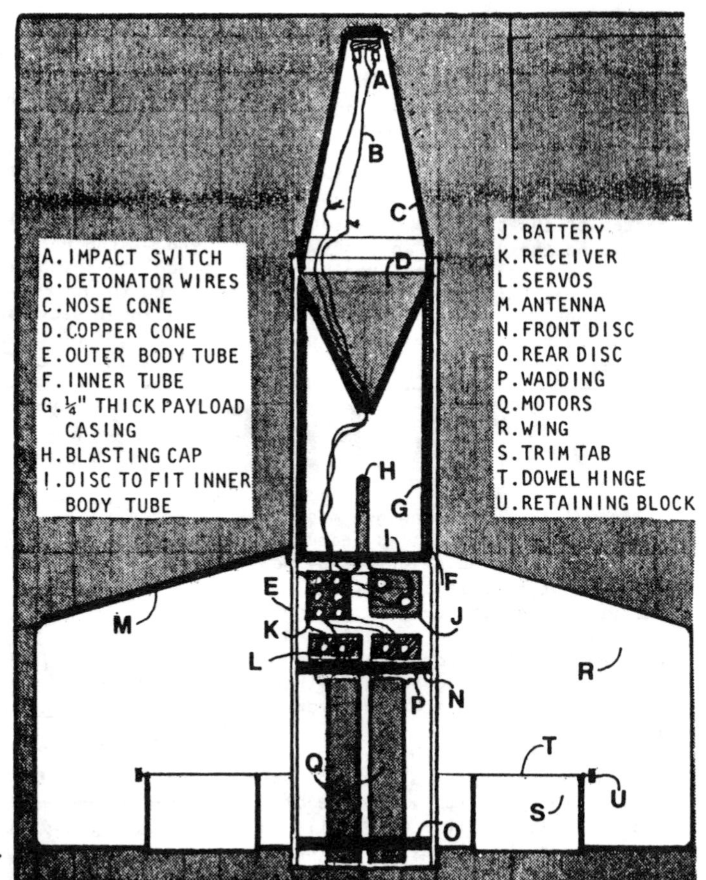

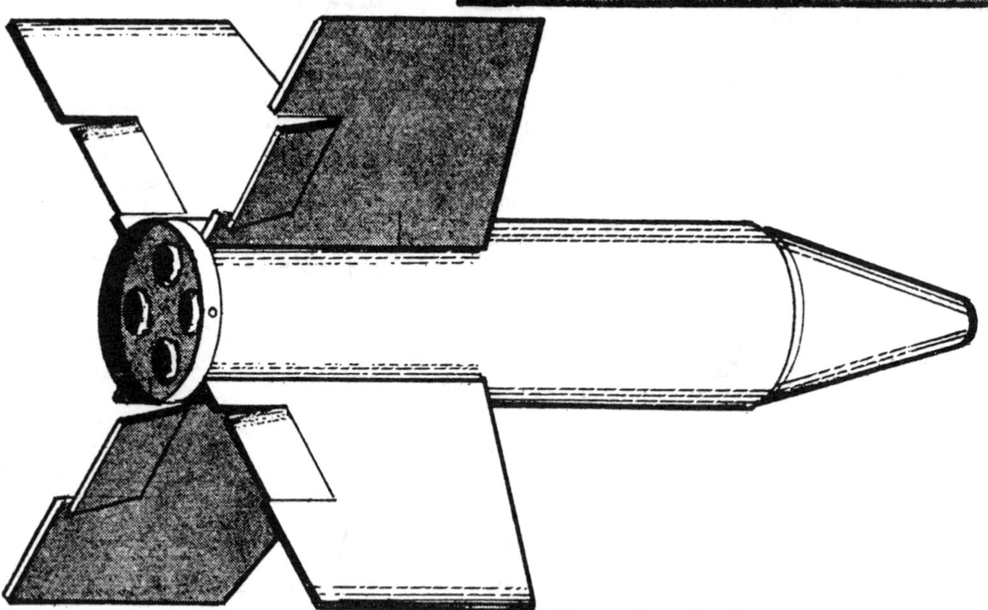

GENERAL DATA

Type: surface to surface antitank missile.

Configuration: length, 24"; diameter, 4"; wingspan, 18"; solid balsa cruciform wings, spiral wound paper tube body and nosecone.

Propulsion type: 4 solid propellant single stage motors - burning time - three seconds, maximum combined thrust - 36 lbs - average combined thrust - 8 lbs.

Payload: high explosive shaped charge approx. two lbs. of explosive.

Guidance type: two channel radio control, visually guided to target. 4 movable trim tabs on wings for steering.

Detonation: impact switch in nose activates electric detonator.

Launching: launch frame has rail to accept tee shaped launch lug on missile body. frame is adjustable for height and has top mounted handle for carrying.

MATERIALS

Section One - Airframe/Motor Section

balsa - three pieces 4" x 36" x ¼".
hardwood dowel - 1/8" x 36".
spiral wound paper tube - two pieces 3 7/8" diameter x 16½" long available from Estes.
motors - 8 " D " motors by Estes.
ignitors - 4 Estes "solar ignitors".
fireproof wadding - 1 piece Estes.

Section Two - Guidance Unit

R/C receiver, two servo units and an on board battery for missile. Compatable transmitter for ground direction. These units are available from numerous suppliers of R/C gear. Only two channels are needed. The two channel setups are available complete for as little as $75. Several frequencies are available. Any frequency will work but those within the CB radio range (27 MHz) should be avoided to eliminate the possibility of outside interference.

NOTE: #1
As a backup to the impact detonation system, a third channel may be added to allow manual firing of the missile. This type of system is known as COMMAND DETONATION.

NOTE: #2
If an airburst fragmentation charge is used, it will be necessary to use a command detonator type of system.

NOTE: #3
A variation of this missile can be built without the control mechanism or movable trim tabs. Launch angle and point of impact can be figured with the tables and related information contained in The Handbook of Model Rocketry by Stine or with the artillery range calculation tables available in many military publications. Trial and error will also be a factor in achieving accuracy.

Section Three - Payload / Detonator

doorbell button.
4 feet of bell wire.
electric blasting cap or improvised electric initiator.
commercial high explosive or improvised plastic explosive filler - about 2 lbs.
1/16" copper sheet to make cone-approx. 3 7/8" diameter x 4" long.

Accessories

motorcycle battery
two channel radio control unit. (transmitter)
launch frame.

CONSTRUCTION INFORMATION

Section One - Airframe/Motor

Wings:

A. Glue two pieces of balsa, 36"x4"x¼" together to form a piece 36"x8"x¼".

B. Cut this piece in half to obtain two pieces 18"x8"x¼".

C. Cut these two pieces as shown in Fig.1. Note that one wing should have a 2¼" slot from point A to point B, while the other wing's slot is cut from point C to B. The two wings will then fit together as shown in Fig.2. Test fit and disassemble for step D.

D. Cut a slot in each wing for the 1/8"x13" dowel hinge. Note that the slot in one wing is offset 1/8" to allow the dowels to cross each other when the wings are assembled. See Fig.3.

E. Glue the four trim tabs to the two dowels and install these assemblies into the wings. Glue a small retaining block over the ends of the dowels to hold them in place. Test the movement of the trim tabs in the wings. They should turn freely.

F. Apply glue to the 2¼" slot in each wing and assemble the wings as shown in Fig.2. Allow this assembly to dry before continuing.

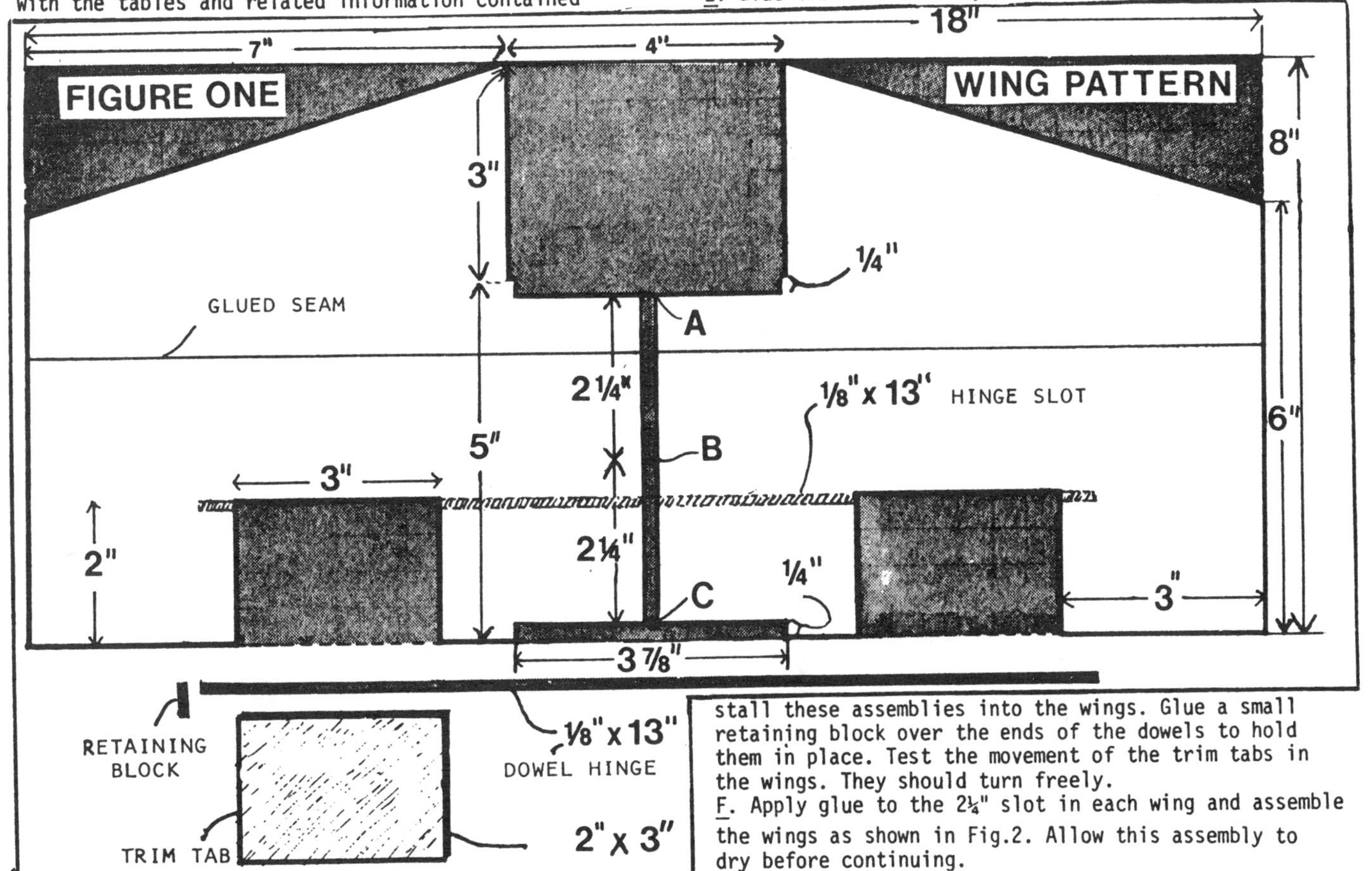

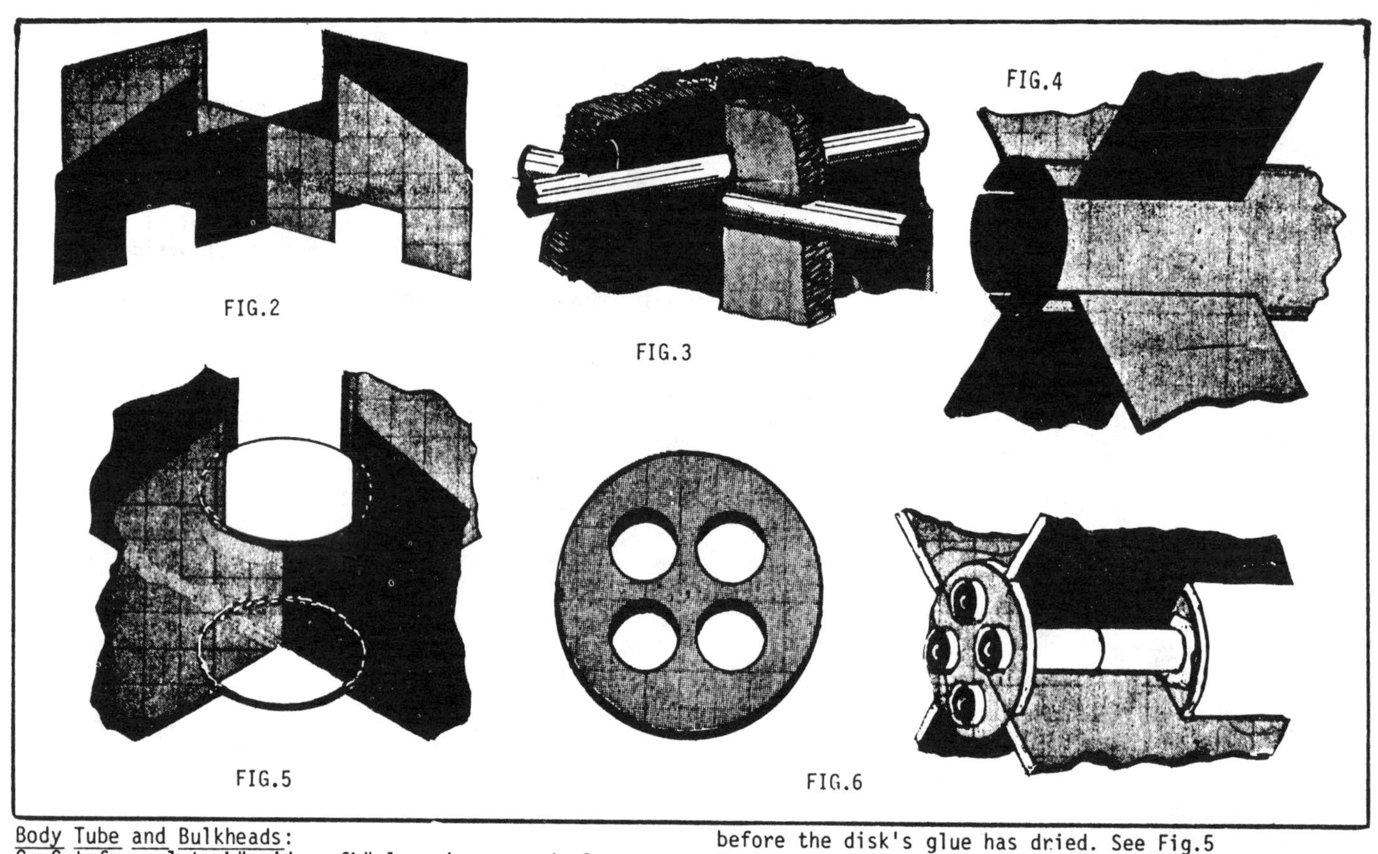

FIG.2

FIG.3

FIG.4

FIG.5

FIG.6

Body Tube and Bulkheads:

G. Cut four slots ¼" wide x 6½" long in one end of the body tube. The tube should now slip over the wing assembly. The rear of the tube should extend ½" beyond the rear of the wings. (see Fig.4)

H. Cut two 3 7/8" diameter disks (measure the ID of the body tube for exact size) out of the remaining ¼" thick balsa sheet. Glue one disk into the front and one into the rear of the wing assembly. Check to be sure the body tube will still slip over the wings before the disk's glue has dried. See Fig.5

I. Cut two ½" wide rings from the other 3 7/8" tube. Split the rings and use tape to join them into one 7 3/4" long strip. Wrap this strip around the body tube and apply glue to the portion of the strip that

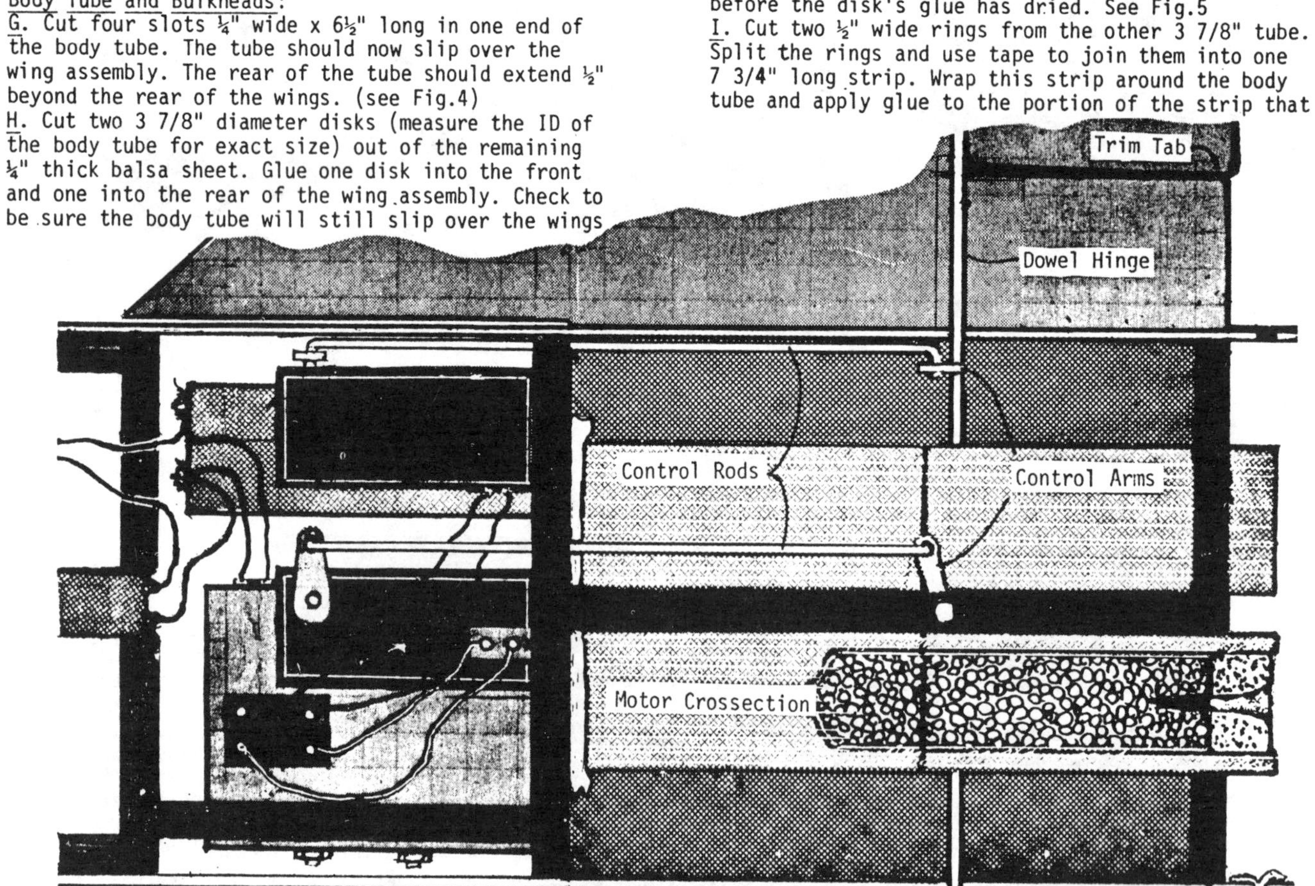

overlaps itself, but not to any portion that touches the body tube. Remove the completed collar from the tube. It will be used to hold the wings in place.
J. Cut four one inch diameter circles in the rear disc as shown in Fig. 6.
K. Cut ¼" off of the eight "D" motors (remove material from the end w/o the nozzle). The black powder grains should now be exposed. Glue these ends together to form four 5" long motors. Apply glue to the paper tube only, not to the black powder area. Wrap tape around the motors until they are almost 1" in diameter. They should be a snug fit in the holes of the rear of the wing assembly.
L. Place three or four layers of fireproof wadding (Estes) between the front bulkhead and each motor and glue motors in place.

Section Two - Guidance

The guidance system is comprised of a receiver, two servo units and a battery. (The battery will also be wired into the detonator system).Specific details will depend upon the size and type of servos you buy. A general outline of the system is shown in Fig. 7. The two control rods are attached to the servos, extend through the bulkhead and are hooked to two arms that extend from the dowel hinges on the trim tabs. Most servos have about 45 degrees of travel, and will turn the trim tabs about 23 degrees in either direction. This is more than enough to steer the missile in flight.

The control rods and arms can be purchased from radio control model companies or can be fabricated from brass sheet, nylon, etc. Mount the above components so that the body tube will slip over them. Mounting tips are included with the servo/receiver set. The antenna for the receiver should be mounted on the front edge of one of the wings.

Section Three - Payload and Detonator

A. Form a 4" tall cone out of the 1/16" copper sheet and solder it together. The cone should slip into the body tube without resistance. Leave a 1/8" diameter hole at the point of the cone.
B. Cut 7½" from the spare 3 7/8" diameter tube.Split this tube lengthwise and overlap the edges so that it will slip into the 16½" long body tube. Apply glue to the overlap area, hold together with rubber bands, and set aside to dry. After the glue has set, glue the copper cone from Step A to this inner tube as shown in Fig. 8.
C. Cut a ¼" thick balsa disc to slip into the rear of the inner tube from Step B. Glue a blasting cap or improvised electric initiator to this disc.
D. Cut three or four ¼" x ¼" x 3" balsa strips to be used to join the front bulkhead of the wing section and the disc from Step C. The strips should be glued into notches cut in the two discs. Placement will again depend upon the arangement of the radio components. Cut the four feet of bell wire in half and attach to battery and blasting cap as shown.

NOTE: For building and testing purposes, a small light bulb should be used in place of the blasting cap. Unhook one set of wires after testing. These wires are reconnected when it is time to arm the missile prior to use.

E. Use several shopping bags or a long piece of wrapping paper to make a tube about 7" long with walls about ¼" thick. This tube should fit into the inner tube and cone. Glue this tube in place.

NOTE: The purpose of this thick walled tube is to resist the force of the explosive and direct it toward the copper cone at the front. The cone melts and a narrow jet of flame is then directed to the target. This focused jet will burn through several inches of steel armor. This type of charge is known as a shaped charge and the principle behind it is called "The Monroe Effect."

F. Feed the two free ends of bell wire through the hole in the copper cone. Pack the 7½" tube/copper cone assembly with about two pounds of high explosive or potassium chlorate/vaseline filler. (See Improvised Munitions Handbook section for instructions on making this improvised plastic explosive.) Glue the tube assembly to the disc on the front of the wing assembly. The copper cone should now be recessed about ½" from the front end of the 16½" body tube when the body tube is in place. The missile is now complete except for the nose cone assembly. The nose serves to streamline the missile in flight and also creates the correct "standoff" distance from the target.

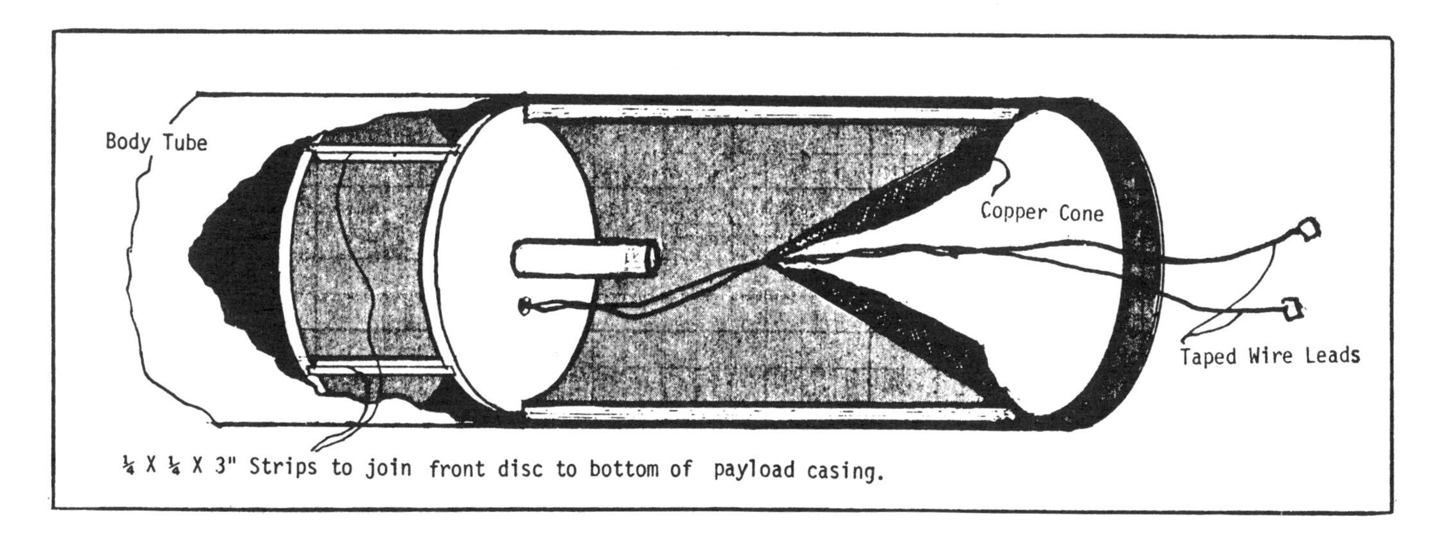

G. Nosecone

Cut a 1" wide ring from the spare 3 7/8" diameter tube. Slit it and overlap the edges to make a ring that will fit into the body tube. Use the remainder of the 3 7/8" tube to make a cone that will fit into the ring. The cone should be about six inches tall with a one inch diameter hole at the point. Use tape and glue to assemble the cone and ring into one piece. See Fig. 9..

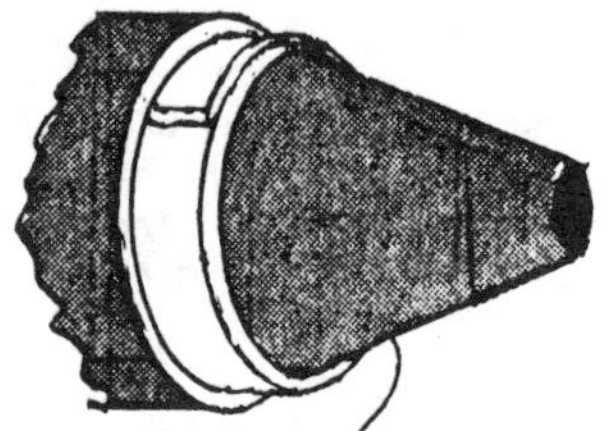

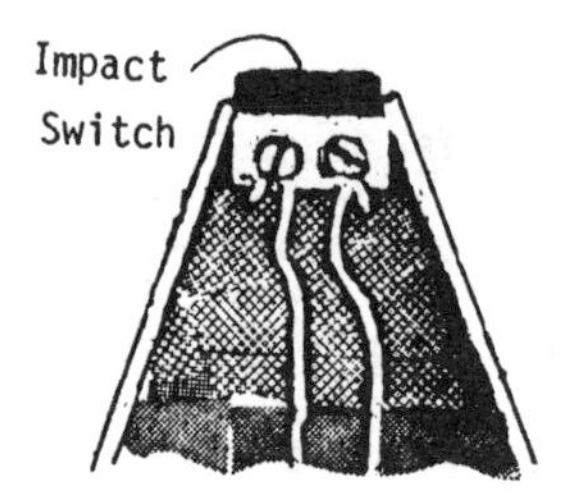

H. Cut an 8" long piece from each of the wires extending through the copper cone. Attach one wire to each terminal of the doorbell switch. Glue the switch into the front of the cone so the button is exposed. If the switch is too large to allow the button to be exposed, it is necessary to glue a block of balsa to the button.

I. Make a small cone that can be slipped over the nose to protect the switch. Use tape to hold the cone in place.

LAUNCHER

Two basic types of launchers are shown. The first unit is a disposable, one shot affair which also serves as a shipping and carrying container. Inside measurements are 13 inches x 13 inches x 24 inches long. The two back flaps are spread at a 90° angle to stabilize the launch box. The front flap is folded

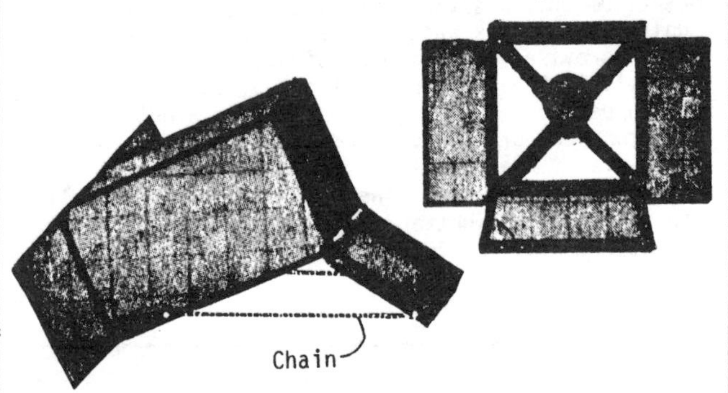

down in front of the box to elavate the launcher for firing. The four corners of the box guide the missile as it leaves the launcher. Cardboard, wood, or light metal sheets can be used.

The second launcher is a bit more complex and is intended for multiple launchings. It features a carrying handle for repositioning and transport and a screw type elevation adjustment.

The launch switch, motorcycle battery and a spare parts box can all be attached to the back of the launcher. With this unit a two man team can carry the launcher and a minimum of three missiles. One man handles the launcher with one missile strapped in place and the second man carries one or more missiles in each hand. A wraparound carrying strap would be helpful in this instance.

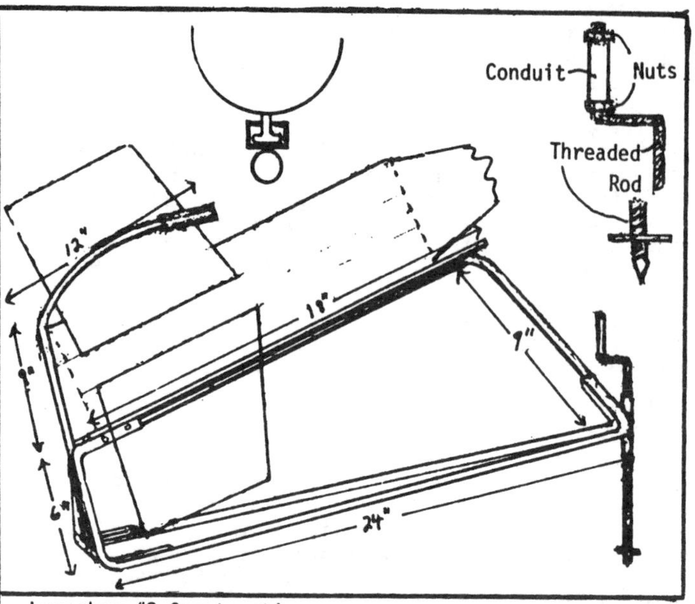

Launcher #2 Construction:

A. Cut pieces of electrical conduit to the dimensions shown, and weld or braze together. Bolts and nuts may also be used.

B. Braze or weld a nut, preferably a 2" long "tall" nut, to the inside of the front joint. Bend a piece of threaded rod or a long carriage bolt as shown. Slip a piece of conduit between the nuts for a handle. The bottom of the threaded rod should be ground to a point to bite into hard surfaces. Braze or weld a large washer about 1" from the point to prevent the rod from sinking in soft or muddy ground. Two nuts may also be used to "jam" the washer in place. The optional blast shield can be made from any type of thin sheet metal. It is screwed or spot welded to the rear of the launcher. Screw the Estes "C" launch rail to the underside of the top arm of the launcher. A "bunji" strap or length of rubber tubing can be used to hold the missile in place for carrying.

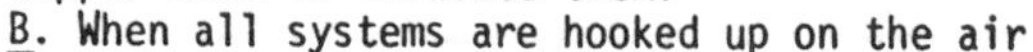

FINAL ASSEMBLY AND FIRING

A. The body tube remains removable to allow the battery to be installed, R/C units to be serviced etc. Before installing or hooking up the battery, tape the ends of the wires extending from the copper cone to insulate them.

B. When all systems are hooked up on the air

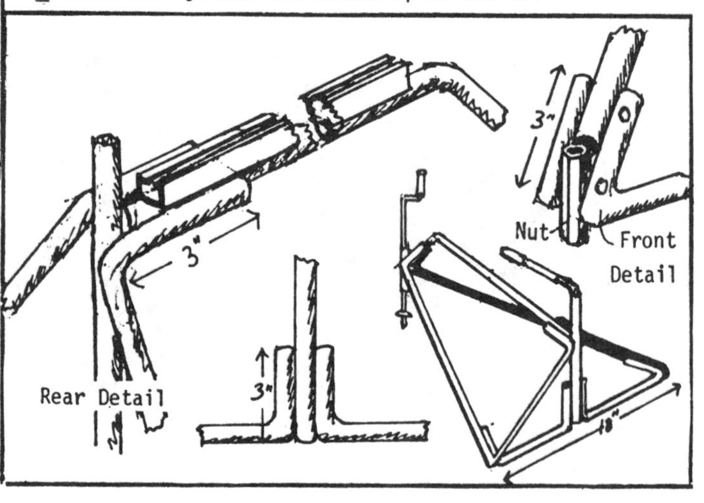

frame, slip the body tube in place. Slip the one half inch wide collar over the rear of the body tube. Use a paperpunch to make four holes, one in each of the four body tube sections. Punch four corresponding holes in the retaining collar. Use four wire shank paper fasteners to hold the collar in place.

C. Carefully attach the nose cone wires to the two wires that were taped off in Step A. Tape the connections well to insulate them from the copper cone. Install the nose cone and use glue or tape to hold it in place.

D. Slide the missile onto the launcher. Adjust the launcher for elevation.

E. Install the ignitor bundle into the four motors. Follow the instructions provided with the motors. Connect the ignitor bundle to the battery and firing circuits *AFTER PLACING THE FIRING SWITCH IN THE OFF POSITION.*

F. Turn on the R/C transmitter and test the function of the trimtabs.

G. Stand behind the optional blast shield or to one side of the launcher, and fire the rocket motors by turning the switch to the *LAUNCH POSITION.*

H. Visually steer the missile to the target. Gain some initial altitude and then allow the missile to approach the target on a shallow glide path.

MODEL ROCKET MATERIAL SUPPLIERS

1. Centuri Engineering Co.
   Box 1988, Phoenix, AZ 85001.
2. Competition Model Rockets
   Box 7022, Alexandria,VA 22307.
3. Flight Systems Inc.
   9300 East 68th St,Raytown, MO 64133.
4. Estes Industries Inc.
   Box 227, Penrose CO 81240.
   Estes also publishes technical reports on various aspects of rocketry. Titles and prices are listed in their catalog.

RADIO CONTROL AND MODEL PLANE COMPONENTS

1. Hobby Shack, 18480 Bandilier Circle, Fountain Valley, CA 92708.
2. Orbit Electronics, 8140 Center St. La Mesa, CA 92041.
3. America's Hobby Center, 146 West 22nd St., NY, NY 10011.
4. Royal Electronics Corp., 3535 So. Irving St., Englewood, CO 80110.

BOOKS AND MAGAZINES

1. "Basics of Radio Control Modeling" by Marks/Winter. $4.50-Kalmbach Publishing Co.,1027 North Seventh St., Milwaukee WI, 53233.
2. "Handbook of Model Rocketry" by Stine. $6.95-from Follet Publishing Co., Chicago, Illinois.
3. "Armies and Weapons" Magazine
   World wide distribution. Excellent product reviews and features on new military weapons including laser guidance hardware. Many illustrated ads from all of the world's larger weapons manufacturers. Subscription information is available from :
   Sky Books International Inc., 48 East 50th Street, New York, NY 10022.
4. "The Art of Scale Scratchbuilding-A Guide to Professional Model Making" by Dario/Chivers. $6.95-Grenadier Books, 7950 Deering Ave., Canoga Park, CA 91304.

CONSTRUCTION OF A

HOMEMADE BAZOOKA

By Dan Moore

The subject of improvised weaponry has been a topic to which much thought has been devoted. However, until recent times, in the light of massive anti-gun legislation,it has been somewhat crude and ineffective.

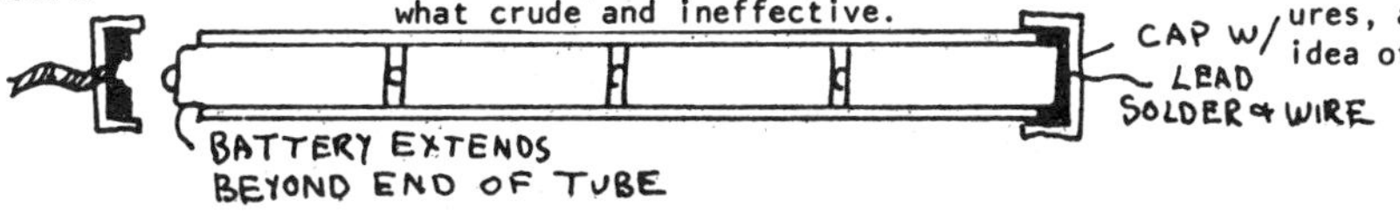

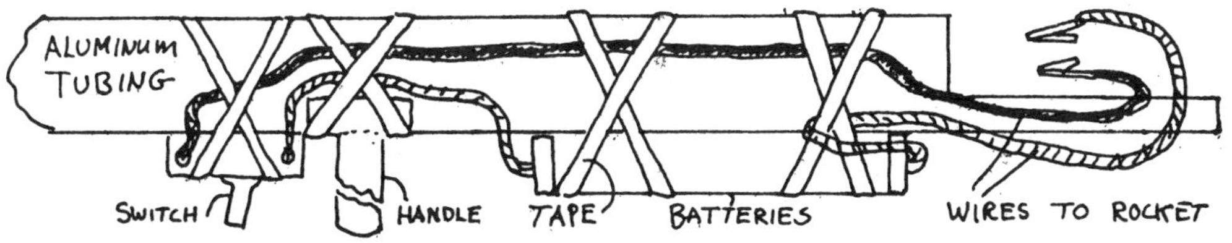

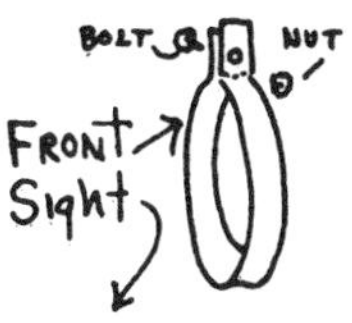

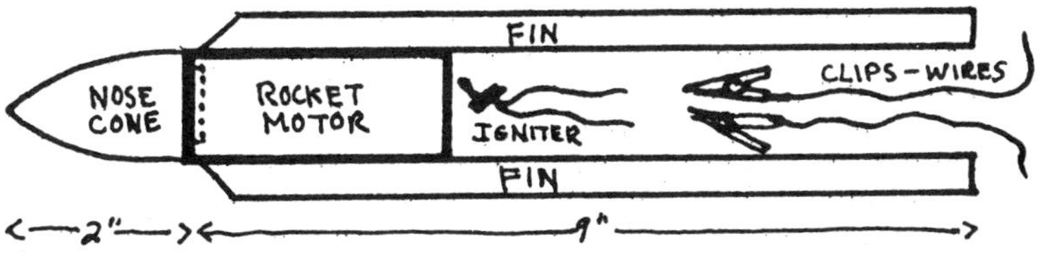

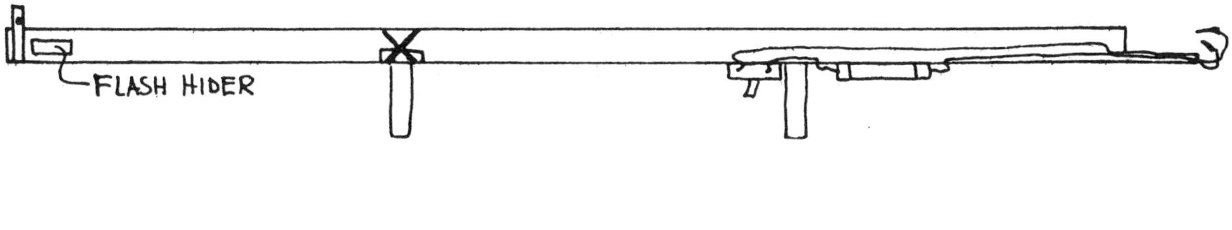

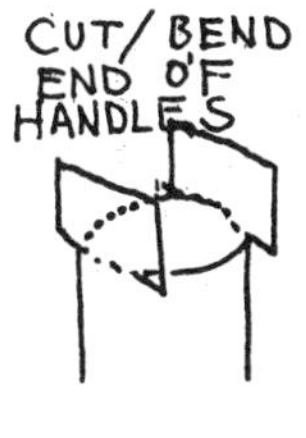

Taking these facts into mind I decided to design, build and test a weapon that would be easy to make and highly effective. Ater toying with the idea and encountering a few failures, a friend of mine developed the idea of the bazooka. He later built a working model and it was an instant sucess. Really though, it couldn't have been anything but a success, as it was so very simple in construction.

This first bazooka consisted of nothing more than an aluminum tube six feet long and 3/4 to 1 inch in diameter, a motorcycle battery (power pack), a light switch (trigger), and the necessary wiring and electrical connections. These parts were all taped together for easy assembly and disassembly. The assembly goes as follows: The wiring goes from the rocket shell to the switch. From here the wiring then goes to the power pack (set on ground when firing) and then back to the rocket shell. To fire this bazooka the firer simply has to sight his target and pull the trigger. The shell will then speed out of the tube at amazing velocities and then onward to the target.

The next refinement on the bazooka was developed by another friend. This improvement was one that would prove to be very important at a later time. This consisted of placing the battery pack in a canvas satchel. The motorcycle battery was replaced with a 6 volt lantern battery which was much less expensive, about $2.50. Now a firer simply slings the satchel over his shoulder and he has a completely portable weapon.

The final improvements on the bazooka came when I took the other designs and added some ideas of my own.

First, I redesigned the battery pack which was rather bulky and expensive. To improve it, I took four alkaline penlight cells and wired them in series, thus producing the needed six volt current. To make this battery pack I found a length of tubing slightly larger in diameter than the batteries. Next I cut the tubing slightly shorter than the lengthwise measurement of the batteries. (see diagram) Finally I took two plastic caps, placed the lead wires in them and filled the caps with a layer of solder. These caps were then placed firmly on the battery tube completing the unit. The next improvement was the placement of handles on the bazooka tube. These handles proved invaluable as they aided not only in holding the bazooka, but they also helped to improve the firer's accuracy. When placing the handles on the bazooka tube, I divided the tube into two foot measurements and taped the handles in place. (see diagram). When taping any of the parts, black electrical tape or friction tape should be used.

My final improvements on the bazooka were the adaption of a flash guard, a loading breech and an open sight. The flash guard was nothing more than a set of slots cut into the forward end of the aluminum tube. These are used to prevent the rocket flash from being seen, thus improving concealment. The loading breech was nothing more than the opposite end of the bazooka tube with the top end removed for a distance of six inches. This is used to hold the trailing fins of the rocket shell steady during firing. This causes the shell to travel much straighter out of the tube. Finally, the open sight was constructed in this way: a thin piece of sheet metal 1/4" wide is bent around the end of the bazooka tube. Then the additional metal pointing outward from the tube is bolted solid and this is used as a sight. (For the listed improvements see diagram).

Now that the improvements were made, I had to put the bazooka together. The final assembly goes as follows: First the bazooka tube is outfitted with a flash guard, loading breech and open sight. Secondly the trigger switch is wired and taped in place along with the battery pack. Next the handles are firmly taped in place and then covered with friction tape to insure a good grip. Lastly the wire leads at the end of the bazooka tube are fitted with alligator clips. The bazooka is then ready for firing. (see diagram)

Once you have completed these assemblies,your bazooka or "Super Bazooka" as I call it, will be finished. This weapon is very powerful as it is very similar to a gun in range and velocity

It will take several dozen firings before you become familiar with the bazooka and are able to fire it quickly and accurately. It took me several weeks of firings before I could use it with any proficiency. Among some of the targets I have hit accurately are tree trunks (within a six inch radius), two foot diameter targets (within a one foot radius), and most recently fence posts (within a six inch diameter). As far as ranges are concerned, my bazooka has a range of somewhere between 100 yards (used in target shooting) and 1,000 feet (maximum arc of fire).

Of course if you plan to fire your bazooka you will need to know how to make up rocket shells for it. These shells are easy to make and generally imexpensive, although my designs are not the only ones you can use. To make these shells you will need a few essential items. They are; an Estes "T" rocket motor, 3 - 1/4"X1/16"X9" balsa fins, a nose cone and an Estes solar igniter. In order to construct the rocket you do as follows.

First, you glue the fins onto the rocket motor so that they are evenly spaced. Next, glue the nose cone onto the front end of the motor. Lastly, put the igniter into the nozzle of the rocket motor as stated in the igniter instructions. Now the fins and nose cone are sanded smooth and the bazooka shell is ready. (see diagram) These shells can then be stored for later use or fired immediately.

You can also use other types and sizes of rocket motors like the larger Estes rocket motors, Astron or 'D', by increasing the diameter of your bazooka tube. You can even use a homemade or modified rocket. These are not reccommended though, as they can be very dangerous. An example of a motor modification is taking the Estes rocket engine and boring carefully through the propellant. Upon firing, all of the propellant burns at one time producing an unbelieveable amount of thrust.

Other methods of altering your rocket shells are equiping them with warheads or similar explosive devices. The simplest way to accomplish this is to fill the front end of the rocket motor with black powder, matchheads, broken glass or anything your heart desires. You then glue or epoxy (reccommended) the nose cone out of some material other than balsa. I have found that plastic, metal, and auto body filler work best. These types of nose cones work best against walls, targets and even people, as the penetration with them is very good. I have used this same kind of nose cone to pierce 1/2 " plaster board and it is extremely hard. The last modification to the design of the completed rocket, is employment of an impact ignition system to detonate the rocket's warhead. These shells will penetrate window glass, windsheilds, walls and even people at considerable distance.

You can start fires (matchhead warheads) and detonate explosives with it. The main advantage to causing this kind of mayhem with the bazooka are that the firer can remain concealed (many firing places are within 1000 ft. radius) and the firer can easily carry and use the bazooka.

In closing, I would like to add these last few points. You should treat your bazooka with respect as it is capable of devastating damage. Most likely it is illegal everywhere in the U.S.

BOY MECHANIC VOL. 1

A Gas Cannon

If you have a small cannon with a bore of 1 or 1½ in., bore out the fuse hole large enough to tap and fit in a small sized spark plug such as used on a gasoline engine. Fill the cannon with gas from a gas jet and then push a

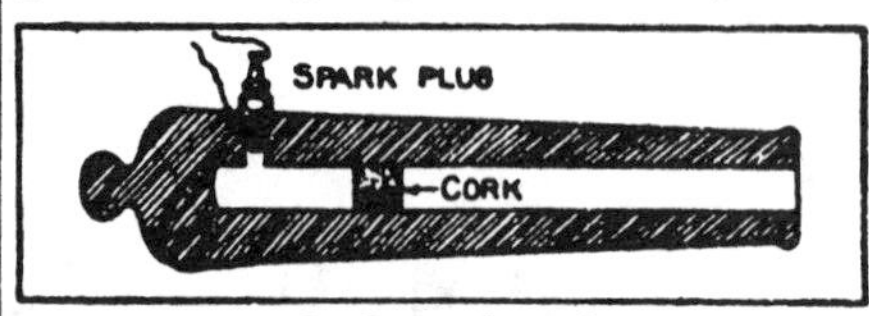

Gas Cannon Loaded

cork in the bore close up to the spark plug. Connect one of the wires from a battery to a spark coil and then to the spark plug. Attach the other wire to the cannon near the spark plug. Turn the switch to make a spark and a loud report will follow.

Briefcase Weapons System

By Clyde Barrow

Basic Pistol Grip Folding Stock

The AR-7 Rifle is handy to carry around when the parts are stored inside of the 16 1/2" plastic stock, but it's rather inconvenient to reassemble the rifle every time you want to shoot When assembled, the rifle is 34 1/2" long. This length, combined with the fat bulky stock, make the AR-7 unmanuverable in tight spaces such as cars, boats, narrow hallways etc. The weapon is also uncomfortable to shoot one handed.

Any rifle may be shortened to the minimum legal length of 26". It's best to be on the safe side and maintain a total length of 26 1/2". 16" of this length must be barrel. The AR-7 barrel has already been made to the minimum length, so you cannot legally shorten it.

A custom folding stock will reduce the length of the standard weapon by 8". When extended, the stock is the original length.

Several types of folding stocks will be featured in future issues but this stock is probably the simplest and easiest to construct.

Materials List

- 1 pc. 5/8" plywood 4"x6"
- 1 pc. 5/8" balsa-same dimensions (opt.)
- 2 pcs. 1"x12"x1/6" brass strip
- 1 pc. 12"x13/32" inside diameter (ID)-7/16" OD brass tubing
- 2 pcs. 12"x3/8" ID - 13/32" OD brass tubing
- 8 pcs. 7/8"x1/8" machine screws w/nuts
- 1 pc. 3/8" OD brass rod length 18"
- 1 pc. 1 1/4"x7/16" coarse thread screw (same thread as takedown screw in standard stock)
- 2 pcs. 1 1/2"x4x1/4" wood or plastic material for grips

Tools Needed

Hacksaw - fine tooth blade
File
Drill w 1/8" and 7/16" drill bits
Propane torch
Silver solder and flux

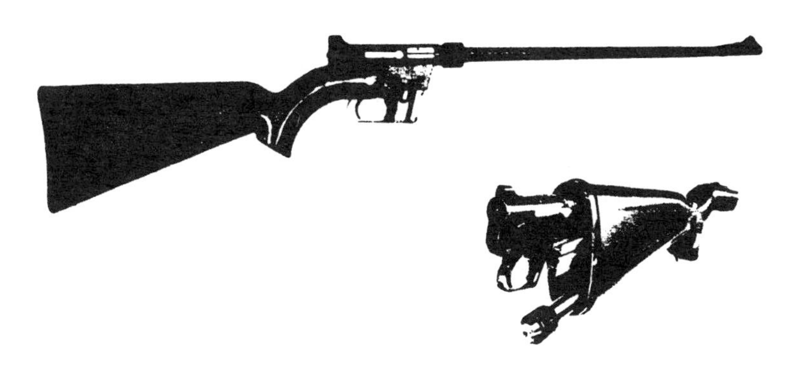

CHARTER ARMS, AR-7, Rifle
Automatic: .22 LR; eight round detachable box magazine; adjustable ramp front, adjustable peep rear sights; barrel and action dismantle without tools and stow in stock; overall length, 34½ inches. Weight, 2½ lbs.
$75.00

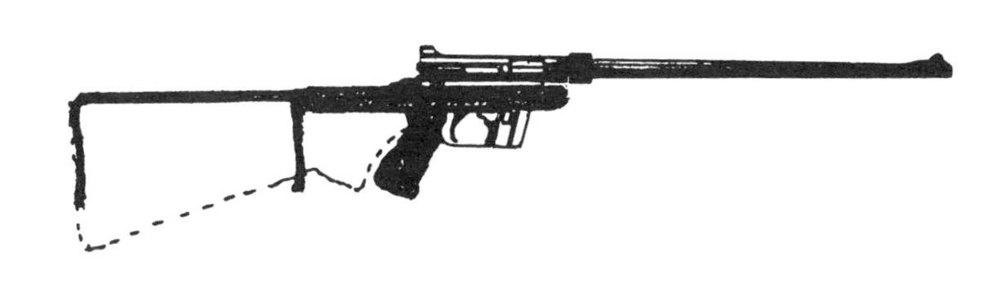

STEP 1
Cut grip frame out of 5/8" plywood, using pattern #1. It is a good idea to first make this piece out of balsawood. This allows you to make changes in grip shape or angle. When the entire stock is completed and you are comfortable with the final shape, it is duplicated in plywood. Drill four 1/8" holes and 7/16" takedown screw hole as shown. Taper the rear of the hole to accomodate the head of the screw. Drill hole for stock latch.

STEP 2
Drill seven holes in brass side plates as shown in pattern #2. Clamp the two pieces together in a vise when drilling holes. This will insure that the holes will be properly aligned.

STEP 3
Cut two 4" pieces of 13/32" ID tubing and silver solder in place as shown in pattern #2. Be sure to ream out the ends of the tubing to ensure smooth operation of the sliding stock.

STEP 4
Use the hacksaw and file to round off corners of the side plates and cut off excess material.

STEP 5
Cut front and rear spacer blocks out of 5/8" plywood, using patterns #3 and #4. Drill 1/8" holes where indicated.

STEP 6
Assemble grip frame, side plates and two spacer blocks with six 1/8" machine screws. If you are right handed, the nuts should be on the right side to reduce snagging on clothing. Reverse for left handers.

STEP 7
Insert takedown screw into grip frame and install stock assembly onto receiver

STEP 8
Cut two pieces 3/4" long of the 3/8" OD brass rod and solder into one end of each 3/8" ID brass tube. File notch as shown in pattern #5.

STEP 9
Bend 3/8" brass tod as shown in pattern #5. Solder two 3/8" ID tubes in place.

STEP 10
Build stock latch as shown in pattern #6.

STEP 11
After final sanding, the stock is wiped down with alcohol and painted with black enamel primer. All small holes should first be filled in with plastic wood putty or body putty. Do not paint the stock tubes or the stock will not be able to slide freely. It can be blackened with touch-up blue or with one of the formulas on page 11, issue #1. The stock tubes should have a light coat of oil to insure smooth operation.

STEP 12
Cut out two grips, using pattern #7. Shape to suit and install on grip frame. The area under the grips can be cut out and used to store spare parts. Use dotted lines on pattern #7 as a guide.

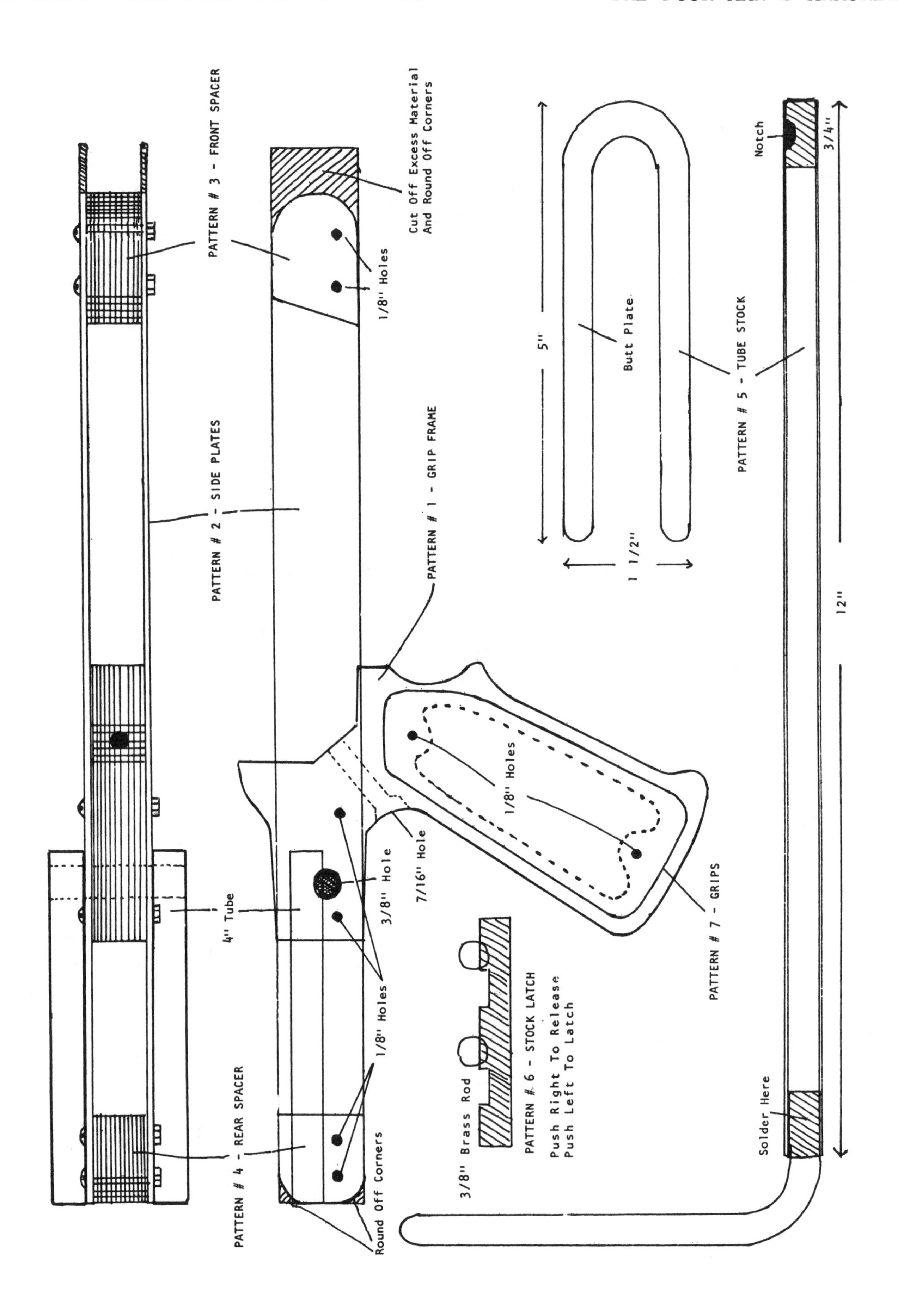
PATTERN # 3 - FRONT SPACER
Cut Off Excess Material
And Round Off Corners
1/8" Holes
5"
Butt Plate
1 1/2"
Notch
3/4"
PATTERN # 5 - TUBE STOCK
12"
PATTERN # 2 - SIDE PLATES
PATTERN # 1 - GRIP FRAME
1/8" Holes
7/16" Hole
3/8" Hole
4" Tube
PATTERN # 7 - GRIPS
1/8" Holes
PATTERN # 6 - STOCK LATCH
Push Right To Release
Push Left To Latch
3/8" Brass Rod
PATTERN # 4 - REAR SPACER
Round Off Corners
Solder Here

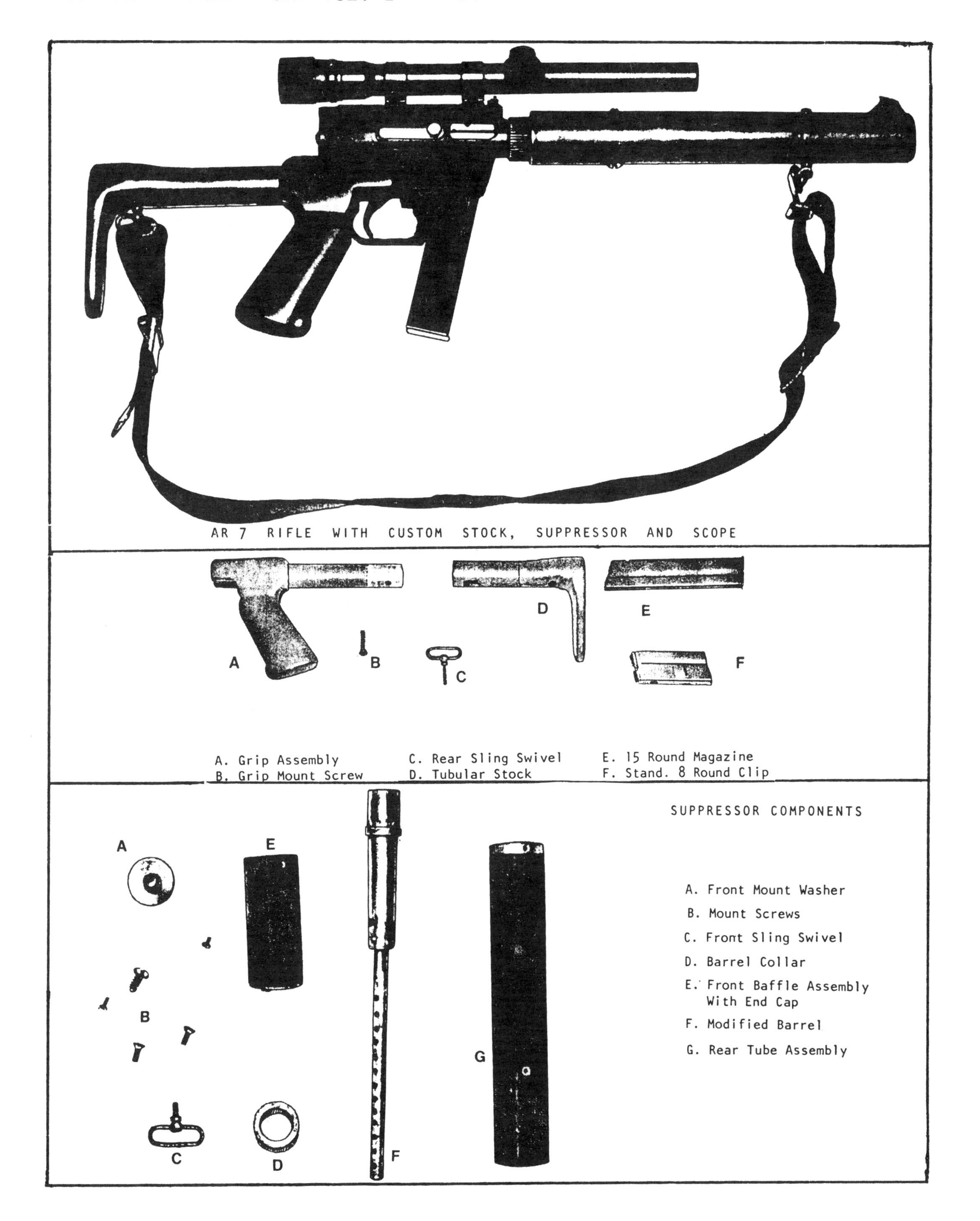

AR 7 RIFLE WITH CUSTOM STOCK, SUPPRESSOR AND SCOPE

SUPPRESSOR COMPONENTS

AR 7 SILENCED BARREL

Note: The components pictured in PMA page 14 are for a general purpose design. That design is altered here to allow the option of maximum concealment at short ranges (short barrel), or maximum accuracy for long range use (long barrel). The long barrel version will be covered on page 33.

SHORT BARRELED VERSION

Materials Needed:

1 - extra AR 7 Barrel w/Barrel Nut. See your rifle's parts list for ordering instructions from the factory-about $12.00

1 - 3/4" Shaft Collar - 3/4"ID-1¼"OD This is a ½" thick collar with a ¼" NC or NF thread set screw. The collar is used to retain pulleys and gears on a 3/4" diameter arbor shaft. Available from hardware stores and tool suppliers. About 50¢.

1 - pc. Metal Screen - 4½"x24". Found at hardware and plumbing stores. Material from an old screen door may also be used. Plastic screen is unacceptable.

2 - pcs. Brass Drain Pipe - either plain brass or chromed. Actual size is 1-3/8" OD - 1-5/16" ID. Drain pipe is usually sold in 8" and 12" sections. Found at hardware, plumbing and building stores. 2 - 8" sections are enough. Cost is about $2.00 each. Cut tubing to the following lengths:

- 1 pc. 8 in.
- 1 pc. 4 in.
- 1 pc. 1 in.
- 1 pc. 3/4 in.
- 3 pcs. 1/2 in.

17- 1¼" OD Washers. If possible, buy thin washers with a 3/16" diameter hole. These are known as fender washers and are available from hardware and auto supply stores. Drill all the washers out to an ID of 3/8" and sand all galvanizing off of them (be sure to degrease with alcohol before soldering).

1 - Knurled Knob, Thumbscrew, or Bolt with at least 1/2" of threads. This should thread into the shaft collar, which is either ¼" NC or ¼" NF thread.

6 - Screws/ 4 Nuts and assorted baffle material-described in article.

Tools Needed:

- Hacksaw w/fine tooth blade.
- Drill motor or hand drill with the following drill bits; 1/16", 1/8", 3/8", 15/64" or 1/4" (15/64" is preferred)
- Center punch
- Tubing cutter - not necessary but handier than the hacksaw for cutting drain pipe. The hacksaw is still needed for other cutting.
- Propane torch and silver solder or acid core general purpose solder.
- Large pair of vise grips or pliers.
- Various flat and round files, depending upon what is available to you. A machinist's scraper or a sharp knife is also helpful for removing burrs from inside the tubing.
- Bench vise - a clamp on vise for the kitchen table is fine.

Procedure:

STEP A

Measure 2½" from rear of barrel and mark with a file.

STEP B

The barrel is composed of a steel liner 3/8" OD and an aluminum outer sleeve that is 3/4" OD at the mark. You want to cut through the outer barrel only, so draw a line on the hacksaw blade 3/16" above the teeth. Cut the barrel at the file mark, rotating it as you go, until the entire cut is 3/16" deep. If you saw slowly, you can feel when you reach the steel liner.

STEP C

The liner is epoxied into the outer barrel, so you remove it by heating the outer barrel with the torch, expanding it and breaking the epoxy bond. (Epoxy breaks down at about 300°) Clamp the rear of the barrel in the vise, and use the vise grips or large pliers to slowly twist and pull the outer barrel section off the liner. If it won't turn when heated, go back to the cut, remark the hacksaw blade and find the spot that is not completely cut through. Go easy when removing the outer barrel, it's easy to bend the inner liner.

Note: If you want to be able to disguise the barrel with the silencer removed, save the outer barrel. A small set screw can be installed in the bottom of the rear, with a corresponding hole in the barrel liner. The outer barrel can then be slipped over the barrel and screwed in place.

STEP D

With the outer barrel removed, mark a point 5" from the rear of the barrel and cut off the excess 11" of liner. Cut a piece 3½" long from the discarded 11" piece. This is the support for the baffles.

STEP E

Draw 2 lines along the exposed liner of the barrel-one along the side, and one along the top of the barrel. (Measure from the rear of the barrel.) Mark and center punch the following points along each line; 4",4¼",4½", and 4-3/4". With a 1/8" drill bit, drill at the punch marks, going all the way through the barrel. You should now have four rows of 1/8" holes, ¼" apart.

STEP F

Wrap a piece of tape around the 15/64" drill bit, 1-1/8" from the front. Carefully drill out the barrel to the depth of the tape mark. Use plenty of oil and don't let the hole become out of round. This drilling won't enlarge the barrel, it just removes the lands which cause the bullet to spin. It also removes the burrs caused by drilling the 1/8" holes. The undrilled portion of the barrel will still impart the needed spin, when the bullet reaches the drilled portion, it is better to have the surface smooth to minimize bullet distortion as it passes the drilled holes. If a 15/64" drill is not available, a ¼" may be used.

STEP G

Remove the piece of tape from the 15/64" or ¼" drill bit, and completely drill out the 3½" long piece of barrel liner from step D.

STEP H

The shaft collar is now installed on the barrel. The outer barrel is tapered; it measures about 3/4" OD at the hacksaw cut and is about 1/16" larger, ½" back (2" from the rear of barrel). Carefully file this ½" wide area until the shaft collar will snugly slip over the outer barrel and rest flush with it. The collar itself may be filed to fit if the original outer barrel is going to be used to cover the liner when the silencer is not in place.

STEP I

With the collar in place, turn it until the screw hole points down when the barrel is on the gun. Remove the screw and use a center punch to mark the location of the hole on the barrel.

STEP J

Remove the collar and drill a ¼" diameter hole at the mark. The hole should be about 1/8" deep. Take the knob, thumbscrew or bolt you bought, and install it in the shaft collar. Slide the collar onto the barrel and tighten the knob until it seats into the hole in the barrel. The hole may need to be slightly enlarged or the end of the screw may have to be ta-

CONTINUED ON NEXT PAGE

pered with a file to obtain the correct fit. The collar should now be a tight fit on the end of the outer barrel; straight, with no wobble.

STEP K

Cut a piece of the drain pipe 8" long. Use a scraper or sharp knife to remove any inside burrs and a file or sandpaper to smooth up the outer edge. Drill a ¼" hole 1" from one end. Cut a second piece of pipe ½" wide, and drill a ¼" hole in the center of the side. Split one edge and file or cut out enough material to allow the ½" piece to fit snugly into the 8" piece. Remove all burrs and sharp edges and install the ½" shim and 8" rear tube over the collar. Line up the ¼" holes and install the screw. The rear of the tube is now centered on the barrel.

STEP L

The front barrel mount is made by drilling a 1¼" washer to an ID of 3/8", then drill 8 - 1/8" holes around its edge. A 4" section of pipe is split and trimmed as in step K, and is soldered together, one half at a time, with the remaining half slipped into the 8" tube. This completed tube, when filed smooth, should slide snugly into the 8"tube, without wobbling. Don't make it so tight that you can't slide it in and out. A 1¼" washer is now installed flush with the end of the 4" tube and is soldered in place. Remove the 4" tube and washer assembly from the 8" tube.

STEP M

The 4½"x24" piece of screen is now folded in half to form a 2¼"x24" strip. Roll the screen tightly around a pencil and carefully slip it into the front of the 8" tube and over the barrel. It should rest against the shaft collar and about ¼" of barrel should protrude from the forward end. The 4" tube, with the drilled washer to the rear, is now slipped into the 8" section and is compressed against the screen until the front is recessed ½" into the 8" tube. The 8" tube should now be perfectly centered on the barrel with no wobble.

STEP N

A 1" piece and a ½" piece of brass pipe are used to make the endcap assembly. Split the 1" piece and trim as before until it will slip into the ½" piece, flush with one end. Solder in place. A 1¼" washer is slipped into this end and is soldered in place. The endcap should now slide into the front end of the 8" tube and come to rest against both it, and the front of the 4" tube. Tape the endcap in place for step O.

STEP O

Mark a center line on the top rear of the 8" tube. Measure 5/8" down each side from the center line and mark the tube. Measure 1" from the rear of the tube and mark again, intersecting the first 2 lines. These two points are the location for the tube support screws. They can be drilled and tapped for machine screws or simply drilled for self tapping screws or pop rivets. Be sure that whatever fasteners used do not extend through the collar into the barrel itself. This allows the collar/tube assembly to be removed from the barrel by loosening the bottom screw only.

STEP P

The spiral baffle and front barrel assembly is made as follows. It will be contained inside the 4" tube.

Stack 12 washers, with the edges aligned, and clamp together in the vise with the top of the center hole exposed. Cut with hacksaw through the stack of washers from the outside edge to the center hole. The cut should be at a right angle to the washers. Remove the stack of washers from the vise, and replace them, this time with one side of the cut in the vise and one side exposed. Use a hammer or the vise grips to bend the stack until the outside cut of the first washer lines up with the inside cut of the third washer. Remove the stack from the vise and slide it onto the 3½" front barrel liner section. Solder a solid washer flush with one end (front),and a washer with 8 -- 1/8" holes, ½" from the other end, (rear). Build up the rear of the barrel/washer area with solder as shown in the diagram. This increases gas flow to the 8 - 1/8" holes.

STEP Q

The 12 split washers are now spaced evenly between the front and rear unsplit washers and soldered in place. The edges should line up to form a spiral.

STEP R

Drill a row of 1/16" holes in the front barrel liner tube, between each of the spirals.

STEP S

Pass the 15/64" (or ¼") drill through the front barrel/spiral section to remove the burrs from drilling the 1/16" holes. Taper the hole in the rear with the 3/8" drill.

STEP T

The 3/4" long piece of drain pipe is used to make a spacer for the area between the rear of the 4" tube and the spiral assembly. Split the edge of the 3/4" tube and overlap the edges, reducing the size until it will fit into the 4" tube. Slide it into the tube until it rests against the barrel support. The spiral assembly is now installed into the 4" tube.It should fit flush with the front of the tube.

STEP U

The remaining piece of brass tubing, ½" wide, and the remaining 1¼" washer, are used to hold the nuts for the mount screws that secure the endcap to the 8" tube. Split the ½" brass tube and trim until it will fit into the endcap. Solder the seam and solder the tube to the washer.Prior to inserting the mount assembly into the endcap, insert a ½" spacer of rolled cardboard or paper. The ½" spacer will hold the mount assembly in position while drilling the mounting holes. The mount assembly is now inserted into the endcap, washer to the front. The rear should be flush with the rear of the endcap.

STEP V

Insert the endcap into the 8" silencer tube. Mark the 8" tube at 4 points; top, bottom, and the center of both sides. Each point should be ¼" to the rear of the front edge of the tube. Drill one of the holes and insert a screw. This will prevent the mount assembly from moving when the other 3 holes are drilled. Drill the 3 remaining holes as marked. Remove the screw, take the endcap off, and remove the mount assembly. The ½" roll of cardboard in the endcap can now be discarded. Four nuts are now soldered or epoxied in place under each of the holes in the mount assembly. The bottom nut may be used to mount a sling swivel if desired. Reinstall the mount assembly and endcap in the front of the silencer and check that the 4 screws will all fit.

Endcap Packing Procedure:

Various materials can be used as flexible baffles to fill the endcap. These baffles are intended to allow the bullet to pass, but to partially seal off the end of the silencer and help to slow the release of gas. Flexible plastic, nylon, and red or black rubber may all be used.

The front half of the endcap will take a baffle with a 1¼" OD, while the rear ½" of baffles must be notched to clear the nuts from the mount assembly. If soft rubber is used, a small 'X' cut in the center is sufficient to allow the bullet to pass. If harder plastic or nylon is used, a tapered hole ¼" at the rear and about 1/8" at the front must be made. Don't try to make a hole in a baffle by firing a bullet through it, you will probably destroy the endcap. A 1/8" stack of wire screen discs can also be used as part of the endcap packing material. The stack of screen discs should have ¼" holes in the centers. Regardless of the baffle material used, they will wear out after several hundred rounds and will have to be replaced. After the end-cap is packed with baffles, it is reinstalled on the 8" tube. The unit is now completed. If a front sight is needed, a sight blade can be soldered in the notch of the top mount screw, or a conventional sight ramp can be mounted on the 8" tube.

The completed unit can be painted with conventional spray paint or MG Coat (see article elsewhere in this issue). If the unit will be used extensively, it will get quite hot. A handguard to protect your hands can be made by wrapping the silencer in several layers of asbestos gasket material. The asbestos is covered with a layer of black plastic electricians tape.

After extensive use, the silencer should be disassembled and cleaned. The screen should be scrubbed clean or replaced, as well as the baffles in the endcap. Be sure to inspect the spiral baffle assembly for any breaks in the soldered washer spiral, and resolder them.

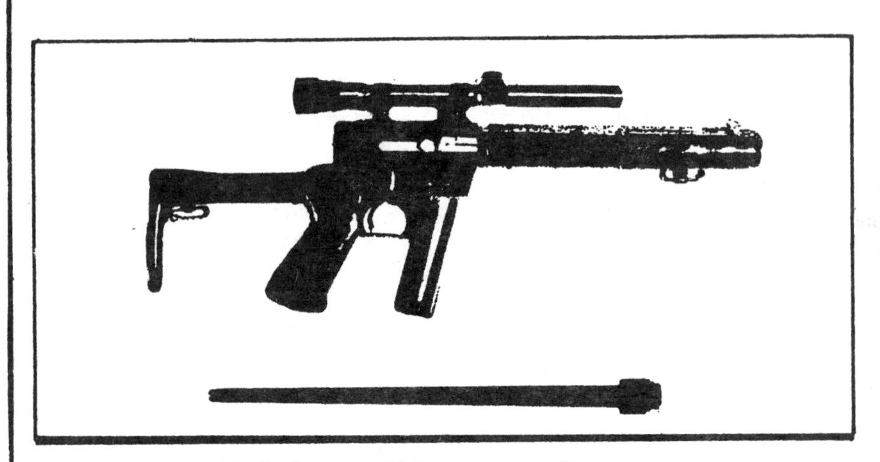

Briefcase Weapons System

The AR-7 survival rifle is a light, compact, 7 shot, 22 caliber semi automatic rifle that is popular with hikers, campers, and pilots. First produced in the early 1960s by the Armalite Corp., the AR-7 was originally designed as a survival weapon for downed Air Force crews. A silenced version was also built by the government during the Viet Nam War.

The rifle is currently manufactured by Charter Arms Corp. and retails for $75. FFL holders can buy the rifle wholesale for about $54.

There are four major parts to the rifle: the barrel, stock, receiver, and the magazine. When disassembled, all parts are contained in the floating, waterproof stock.

The AR-7 rifle can be used as the basis of a complete mini weapons system designed to be carried in a small attache' case.

The original stock and 7 shot magazine are not used with this system, but should be retained for possible future use.

In addition to the basic receiver and barrel assembly, the following parts are needed to build the new system.

1. Several 15 round magazines
2. One extra barrel assembly
3. 22 Caliber rifle scope with scope rings and base
4. Custom scope mount
5. Pistol grip with collapsible, tubular stock
6. Silencer mount tube
7. Silencer
8. Cleaning and tool kit with spare parts
9. Small attache' case or instrument case

The system allows a variety of weapons to be assembled.

1. Full length rifle with scope
2. Rifle with short barrel and silencer
3. Pistol
4. Pistol with silencer
5. Submachine gun with silencer

The whole works can be built for about $100.

AR 7 SCOPE MOUNT

TYPE A - FIXED MOUNT

BY CLYDE BARROW

NOTE: THIS MOUNT WILL NOT FIT INTO THE CONVENTIONAL AR 7 PLASTIC STOCK. IF YOU INTEND TO USE THIS STOCK, A REMOVABLE MOUNT IS NEEDED.

Tools and Materials Needed:

1 - Weaver Scope Mount Base #T9 intended for use on Ruger 10/22 rifle. Price about $2.50

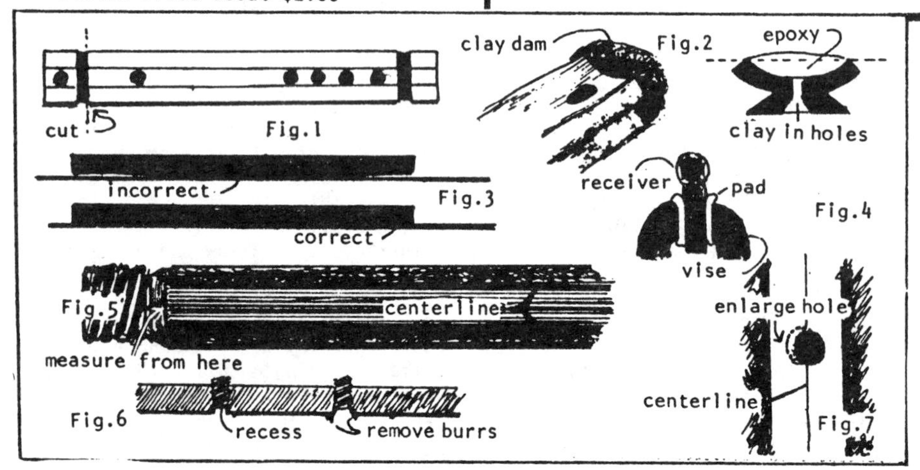

1 - 7/64" drill - 80¢
1 - 6x32 National Coarse (NC) tap. 90¢ (and a tap handle if you don't have one.)
- Oil for drilling and tapping.
- Drill motor or hand drill.
5 - 6x32 NC machine screws ½" long. about 10¢ each (flat head)
- Rubbing alcohol to degrease before gluing.
- Epoxy glue.
1 - Pc. Coarse sandpaper 36-80 grit.
1 - Pc. Wet or Dry sandpaper 220-320 grit.
1 - Small piece of modeling clay.
- Hacksaw, Padded Vise, Center Punch.

Procedure:

A. Using the hacksaw and padded vise, cut the scope mount as shown in Fig. #1. Sand all rough edges smooth.

NOTE: scratch a small ' F ' for front in the slot at the front of the mount.

B. Use coarse sandpaper to roughen the bottom (curved) surface of the mount. Wash the mount in alcohol and dry with a clean towel.

C. Place the mount on a flat, smooth surface. Fill all screw holes with clay. Clay is also used to make a small "dam" at each end of the mount.

D. Mix enough epoxy to fill up the area created by the curve and dams at each end. The epoxy should be slightly "piled up" on the mount. See Fig. #2. ALLOW TO DRY OVERNIGHT Even if it says 5 or 10 min. epoxy.

E. Glue a piece of 220- 320 grit wet or dry sandpaper to a large piece of glass. Sand off the excess epoxy from the scope mount base by sliding it across the sandpaper. Check the progress often to be sure you aren't applying all the pressure to the ends. This will create a rocking chair effect, instead of the absolute flat bottom desired. Stop sanding when a bare aluminum line appears on both sides. Check the mount for flatness on an open area of the glass. See Fig. #3. Spot sand any high areas that are found.

F. Place the mount, epoxy down, on a hard flat wood surface and drill through the mount holes and epoxy underneath. Enlarge the holes in the epoxy with a sharp pointed knife. The screws should slip through the holes in the mount without resistance.

G. Disassemble the receiver as per the gun's enclosed instruction sheet. Remove all internal parts except for the safety lever assembly which is left in place. Clamp the receiver in the padded vise. See Fig. #4. There are 10 true ribs on the top of the receiver (12 if you count the shorty on each side). Find the center groove of this area and use a scriber or knife point to scratch a line the length of the groove. It should be bright silver and constrast well with the black background. Use a center punch to mark this groove at the following points, as measured from the front edge of the groove. See Fig.5 3/4",1-1/4",1-5/8",2-1/8",3-13/16"

H. Drill at each punch mark with the 7/64" drill. Go slow and keep the drill as vertical as possible.

I. Thread each hole with the 6x32 tap. Go slow, use oil as a lubricant and again try to keep the tap in a verticle position. When finished, use a knife point to scrape away all burrs and rough edges from both the inside and outside of the tapped holes. Take care not to damage the threads. Wash the receiver in hot soap and water to remove all traces of drilling debris, oil, etc.

J. Squirt a drop of oil in each threaded hole. Place the mount on the receiver and start the five screws by hand. If one or more won't start, elongate the hole in the mount until the screw will thread into the receiver below.

K. Run all five screws down snug and check that the mount is in complete contact with the receiver without any gaps. An easy way to do this test is to hold the unit up to a window and look at the side of the mount-receiver joint. If no light is seen, fine. If large gaps appear, one or more of the screws is probably rubbing against the side of the hole in the mount, which distorts it and prevents a flush fit. Elongate any problem holes as in J. When a flat fit is obtained, all 5 screws should be tightened - BEWARE - you are plenty tough to strip all 5 holes of their threads, so use moderation when tightening.

L. About 1/16" of each screw will be protruding into the top area of the receiver's interior. Remove each screw individually and file or grind off material until the screw is slightly recessed into the top of the receiver when tightened in place. After grinding, be sure to cleanup any ragged threads on the screw ends. These will easily strip out the soft aluminum threads. With all 5 screws tightened in place, run your finger along the top inside of the receiver. You should feel nothing but 5 shallow holes. See Fig. 6.

M. Mount scope, and set both adjustment knobs to a central setting. Sight the rifle in at 25 feet, using a large white sheet of paper. When the scope is sighted in, you should still have plenty of adjustment left in all 4 directions. i.e. up, down, left, right - to later compensate for any slight alignment differences. If one or both controls is turned to it's extreme before the scope is centered, the mount will have to be adjusted. If the gun shoots too far to the left the scope base must be moved left. Ditto for right. To move the base, the holes in the mount must be altered as follows:

Enlarge the holes with a knife or round file. The tapered screw head will fill the larger hole. If the mount is to be moved to the right, make the oversized holes slightly to the left of center, do the opposite for right to left. Continue this process until the scope is sighted to center, with both scope controls in a near neutral position. Up and down is easier; a shim or series of shims is slipped under the front of the mount to correct high shooting, and under the rear for low shooting. See Fig. 7. Shims of hard plastic or metal may be used. If the shimming is very extreme, the screws will be too short, and it will be necessary to replace them with a longer unit.

N. Alignment is rarely this far off, but if you wish, an alternate method may be used. Drill and tap the front and rear holes only. Clean and reassemble the gun. Clamp the rifle in place with a portable vice or heavy sand bags. Adjust both up/down and left/right scope controls to a central position and install scope and mount on rifle. If the scope is aimed at a point fairly close to the point of bullet impact, minor adjustment is all that is necessary. Drill and tap the remaining 3 holes. If the bullet and scope are grossly misaligned right to left, the front, rear, or both holes will have to be enlarged slightly off center as in step M above. Vertical misalignment is again handled with shims. When the unit is finally aligned, drill and tap for the remaining 3 screws. Remember, when enlarging the holes for adjustment, to remove the excess screw length that may now protrude into the inside of the receiver.

NOTE: If you can't fire the rifle, do step N by removing the bolt and rear sight screw. The scope is aligned with the point that is seen when looking through the rear of the receiver and sighting down the barrel. This is a crude form of BORE SIGHTING.

O. When you are satisfied with the mount's alignment, roughen the receiver and mount contact areas with coarse sandpaper. Clean all parts, especially the screws and the threaded holes with alcohol. Epoxy the mount to the gun, as well as each screw into it's appropriate hole. Replace any shims that had been in place before cleaning. Let it dry AT LEAST 24 HOURS before firing. If in the future you need to remove the mount, the epoxy bond is broken with heat: Take off the scope and disassemble the receiver. Heat the mount and receiver to about 300° or until the epoxy melts.

TYPE B - REMOVABLE MOUNT

BY CLYDE BARROW

Three years ago, I began to design modifications for the AR - 7 rifle. I asked several gunsmiths about a provision for mounting a scope, either by screwing on a base or cutting a dovetail directly into the receiver. "Can't be done, too soft, insufficient wall thickness, threads will strip out, etc.etc." After some experimenting it was discovered that by using coarse threaded screws, they resisted stripping of the threads. This led to the design presented in issue #3. As stated, this unit is unacceptable if the storage feature of the original stock is to be retained. A number of so-so clamp-on removable mounts were then produced, and were to be the basis of this article. For the hell of it, I also revived the integral dovetail idea, and cut one in an old AR 7. If nothing else, I wanted to see where it would crack. It didn't crack. It works perfectly. The horizontal top surface of the receiver is even close enough to bore alignment to allow the slight error to be corrected with the internal scope adjustments.

It's so simple a 'how-to' article isn't even necessary.

Just clamp the receiver in a padded vise and file a 'V' along both sides of the ribbed top of the receiver. A small amount of the vertical rib behind the chamber on the right side must also be filed away, but no loss of strength was noted. Continue to file until standard claw mount .22 scope rings can be installed. Before reassembling the gun, bore sight it as described in issue #3, and adjust as needed.

The scope is easily removed for storing the rifle in the stock and the original sights remain intact. This is especially nice in a survival rifle. When the scope breaks or malfunctions, a back-up sighting system is invaluable.

A Home-Made Hand Vise

A very useful little hand vise can easily be made from a hinge and a bolt carrying a wing nut. Get a fast

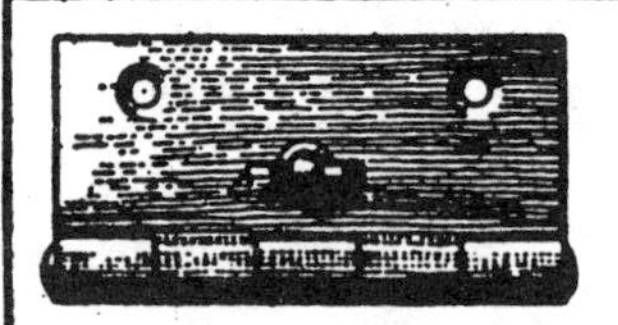

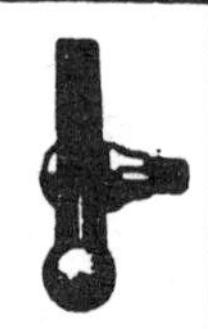

Hand Vise Made from a Hinge

joint hinge about 2 in. or more long and a bolt about ½ in. long that will fit the holes in the hinge. Put the bolt through the middle hole of the hinge and replace the nut as shown in the drawing. With this device any small object may be firmly held by simply placing it between the sides of the hinge and tightening the nut.

velEX the EXPLODING BULLET

VELEX EXPLODING AMMO
A PRELIMINARY REPORT

by Clyde Barrow

A new line of pistol ammunition with exploding bullets is now manufactured and marketed by Velex Inc., N. 6809 Lincoln, Spokane, Washington 99208. (509) 326-5283 phone.

The line is called Velex and is currently available in the following calibers:

380 Auto/	87 grain	bullet
9mm /	92 "	"
38 spec /	101 "	"
357 mag /	101 "	"
45 ACP /	200 "	"

44 magnum, 38 super auto and 44 special loads are currently being tested and will be available from Velex in the near future.

Dealer prices are as follows. A $50.00 minimum order is required for the wholesale price break. Include FFL with your order or have a licensed dealer order for you.

Caliber	pack of:	Retail	Whlse
380 auto	10	8.00	5.75
9mm	10	8.00	5.75
38 spec	8	7.00	5.05
357 mag	8	9.50	6.85
45 ACP	10	9.50	6.85

Standard semi and full jacketed hollow point ammo is the basis for the Velex load. The hollow point bullets are redrilled until the cavity is 3/16" in diameter. The hole extends to the base of the copper jacket. This enlarged cavity is filled with what appears to be Pyrodex, a modern black powder substitute. It may be conventional black powder, however.

The detonator (discriminating impact fuse) is a brass cup 3/16"x3/16". The wall thickness is about half that of a conventional primer. The interior of the cap is coated with a shock sensitive explosive, probably the same composition found in toy pistol caps (Pottasium Chlorate, Red Phosphorus and Black Antimony Sulfide). The volume used is also about that of a toy cap. The cup is seated open end to the rear and is recessed about 1/32" from the front edge of the bullet. This recess prevents the round from detonating on auto pistol feed ramps.

A thick layer of red sealant, possibly laquer, is used to seal the cup from moisture, and is also intended to act as an impact buffer.

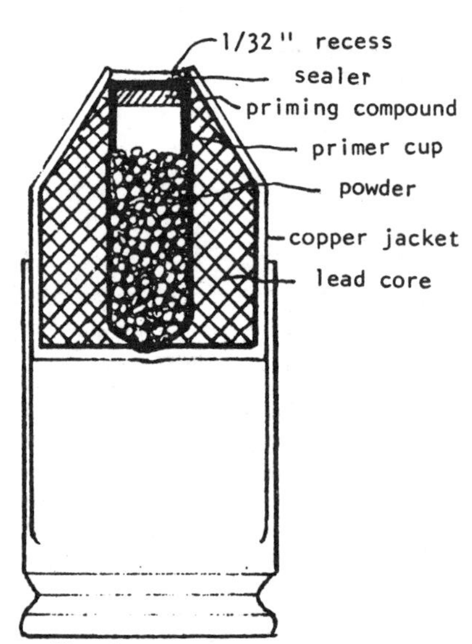

The few test rounds I was able to obtain, 45 ACP and 380 auto, were fired into large pink grapefruits. In each case the Velex detonated and the bullet mushroomed to approx. twice it's original diameter. We'll present an indepth look at Velex in a future issue after more extensive testing is completed.

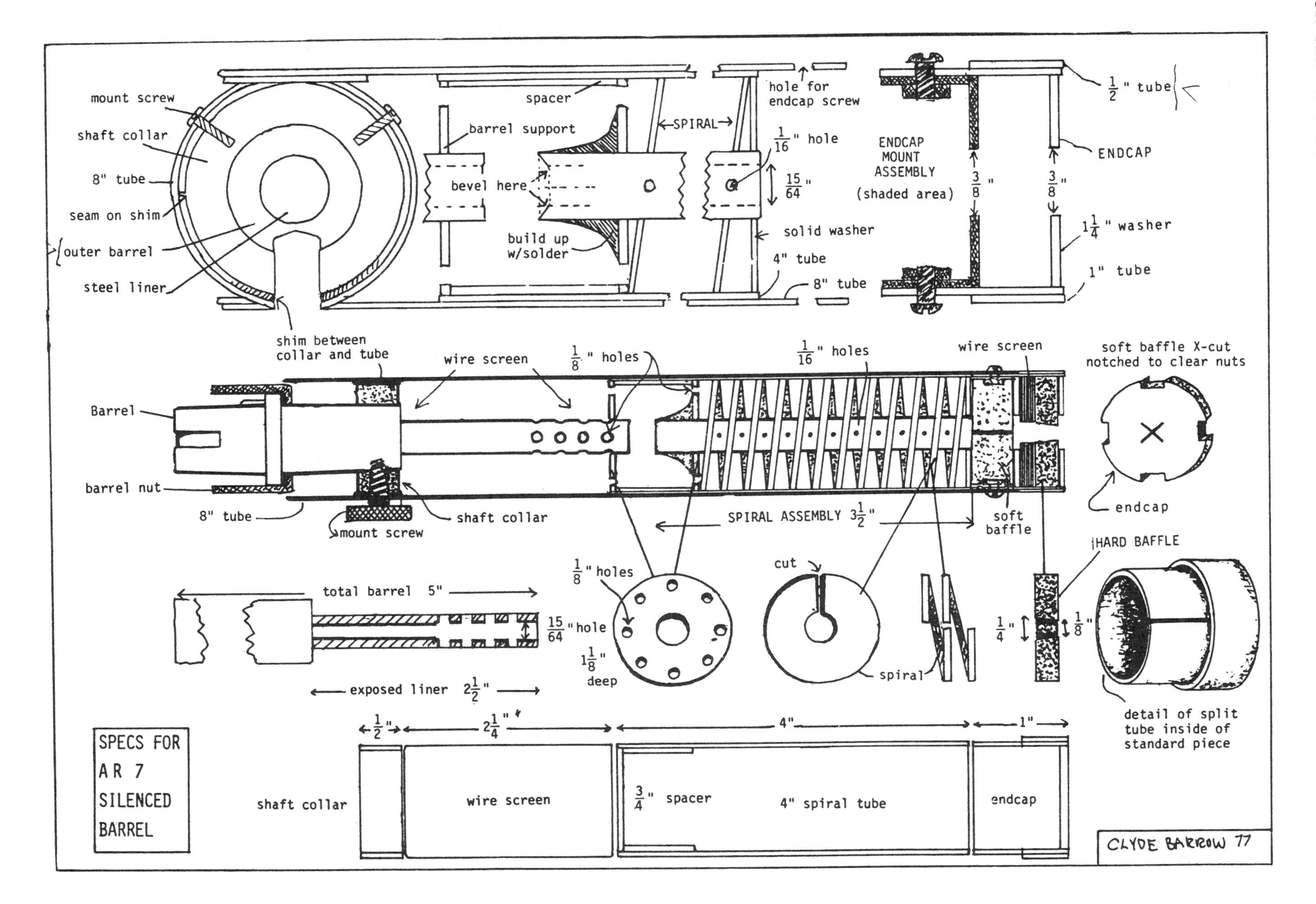
mount screw
shaft collar
8" tube
seam on shim
outer barrel
steel liner
spacer
barrel support
bevel here
build up w/solder
SPIRAL
hole for endcap screw
1/16" hole
15/64"
solid washer
4" tube
8" tube
ENDCAP MOUNT ASSEMBLY (shaded area)
3/8"
3/8"
1/2" tube
ENDCAP
1 1/4" washer
1" tube
shim between collar and tube
wire screen
1/8" holes
1/16" holes
wire screen
soft baffle X-cut notched to clear nuts
Barrel
barrel nut
8" tube
mount screw
shaft collar
SPIRAL ASSEMBLY 3 1/2"
soft baffle
endcap
HARD BAFFLE
total barrel 5"
1/8" holes
15/64" hole
1 1/8" deep
cut
spiral
1/4"
1/8"
exposed liner 2 1/2"
detail of split tube inside of standard piece
1/2"
2 1/4"
4"
1"
SPECS FOR AR 7 SILENCED BARREL
shaft collar
wire screen
3/4" spacer
4" spiral tube
endcap
CLYDE BARROW 77

SMGs

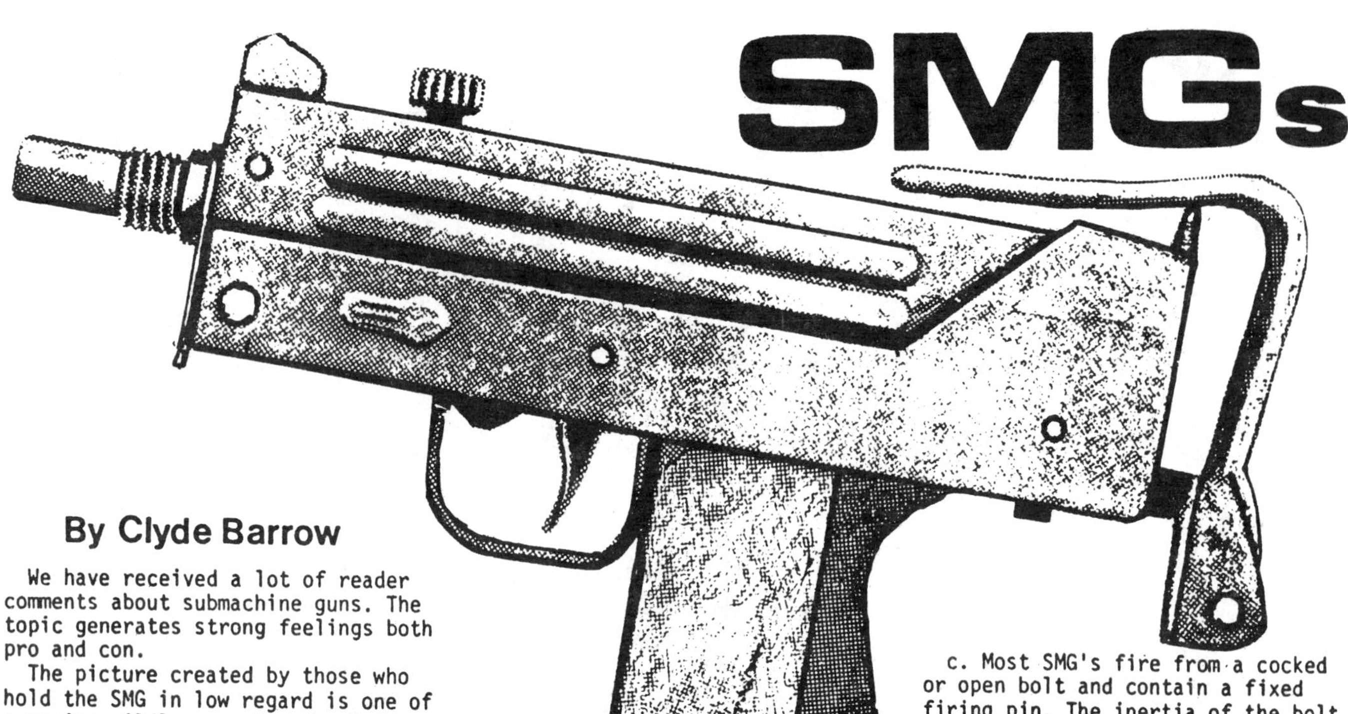

By Clyde Barrow

We have received a lot of reader comments about submachine guns. The topic generates strong feelings both pro and con.

The picture created by those who hold the SMG in low regard is one of a maniac wildly spraying the landscape, firing entire 30 round magazines with each burst. "My god, he's wasting ammo!"

Proponents will describe special combat firing techniques, relate tales of hits at incredible distances and swear that the SMG has rendered the autopistol and light assault rifle obsolete.

As usual, the truth falls somewhere between these two extremes. To most people, SMG means full auto. This is only one of the characteristics of these weapons, and need not be considered a detriment. Most modern SMG designs also allow for semi auto fire, full auto being used only selectively, as the need arises.

The primary attractions of SMGs are one handed use, large magazine capacity and simplicity of design which allows for low cost production in small home workshops, without the need to resort to investment castings, milling machines, and other exotic manufacturing techniques and equipment.

The basic SMG type of weapon is ideal for small group or individual manufacture for the following reasons.

a. The receiver is usually based on either easily obtained and worked round steel tubing, or is designed around a square or rectangular box shape. Examples of the round type of receiver include the Sten, Sterling, S & W M76, M3 Grease Gun, and the German MP40. The square or box receiver is used in both the Israeli UZI, and the Ingram M10 & M11 submachine pistols.

b. SMG's are designed to be cheap and easy to produce and are geared to a military market. Therefore, the design can be based on practical considerations alone, without the need to make concessions to appearance. Appearance is a major factor when designing a commercial gun for commercial sales, and can greatly increase the cost and complicate the manufacturing process.

c. Most SMG's fire from a cocked or open bolt and contain a fixed firing pin. The inertia of the bolt moving forward eliminated the necessity for complex breech locking mechanisms or stiff recoil springs found in commercialy available semi auto guns. This open bolt firing allows the weapon to be both lighter in weight and simplier in design. The open bolt or slam-bang type of action does jar the weapon upon firing, and therefore some concession is made to target type accuracy.

The next few PMA issues will feature material on some of the more popular modern SMGs.While we haven' yet been able to purchase a set of plans for PMA publication, we have found sources of several excellent designs geared toward home manufacture. (See Roy Mc Laughlin's ad this issue and The Void's ad for Holmes' Home Workshop Book in previous issues, both are good sets of plans.)

If you have a design for sale, want to buy or sell specific SMG components, or would like to see material on some specific SMG, drop me a card care of PMA and we'll see what we can do.

The issue features a reprint of the patent for Gordon Ingram's M10 and M11 (MAC) Machine Pistols. All parts for these guns are available except the lower receiver, and we hope to have a set of construction plans for the lower unit in a future issue. If you are interested in the MAC 10 or 11 unit drop George Liu a line (see classified ads this issue). He sells complete registered SMGs to qualified buyers as well as all replacement parts and several reprints of articles that have been written about the M10 and M11.

3,651,736

BOLT HANDLE AND PISTOL GRIP MAGAZINE FOR AN AUTOMATIC FIREARM

Automatic weapons of the submachine gun type are sometimes referred to as machine pistols and such weapons must be light in weight and efficient in operation.

According to this invention weight of the weapon is kept to a minimum by constructing certain elements so that they perform two or more functions. For example, the trigger guard of this invention is arranged in such manner as to afford protection for the outwardly protruding trigger and also so as to function as guide means whereby rounds of ammunition are directed into the breech end of the gun barrel. According to another feature of the invention, the bolt handle is arranged so as to provide manual means for operating the bolt from its closed to its open position and vice versa and in addition the bolt handle is movably mounted on the bolt so as to form a locking relationship with an enlarged end of the slot formed in the receiver and in which the bolt handle is slidable. In addition, the bolt handle is provided with a sight path which accommodates the passage of liquid in alignment with the front and rear sights when the bolt is unlocked but which precludes sighting when the bolt is locked. In this manner a visual indication of the locked and unlocked condition of the bolt is afforded.

For a better understanding of the invention reference may be had to the following detailed description taken in conjunction with the accompanying drawing in which

FIG. 1 is a side view of a sub-machine gun constructed according to the invention;

FIG. 2 is a top view of the gun shown in FIG. 1;

FIGS. 2A and 2B are views taken along the line designated 2—2 in FIG. 2 and which respectively depict the bolt handle in locked and unlocked condition;

FIG. 3 is a side view partially sectioned and similar to FIG. 1;

FIGS. 3A and 3B are views taken along the line designated 3—3 in FIG. 3 and depict respectively the bolt handle in locked and unlocked positions;

FIG. 4 is an enlarged side view partially in section and which shows the bolt in its extreme open position ready for the initiation of a firing operation by the trigger;

FIG. 5 is a view similar to FIG. 4 but showing the bolt in an intermediate position;

FIG. 6 is a view similar to FIGS. 4 and 5 but showing the bolt in its closed firing position;

FIGS. 7 and 8 are enlarged views partially in section of the mechanism which depict the extractor and the ejector at the beginning of an ejecting operation and at the completion thereof respectively and in which

FIG. 9 is a sectional view taken along the line 9—9 in FIG. 1.

In the drawings the numeral 1 designates the frame structure of the weapon to the bottom portion of which a magazine housing designated by the numeral 2 is affixed. A hand gripping portion 3 forms a part of magazine housing 2 and the numeral 4 designates a conventional removable magazine structure.

The trigger is of conventional construction and is designated by the numeral 5. Trigger 5 is pivotally mounted on pin 6 secured to frame 1 in a manner well known in the art. The numeral 7 generally designates a trigger guard which is affixed at one end to the frame 1 as by welding designated by the numeral 8. Trigger guard 7 is provided at the other end with an inwardly extending portion 9 which serves not only as a portion of the trigger guard but which also serves as guide means whereby rounds of ammunition from the magazine 4 are directed into the breech end of the barrel. The numeral 10 designates an intermediate portion of the trigger guard 7 which protrudes outwardly and functions in the conventional manner as a guard for trigger 5.

In order to facilitate secure holding of the gun by the user, a strap 11 is mounted on bracket 12 to the frame of the weapon.

The barrel of the weapon is fixedly mounted to the frame and is designated by the numeral 13. Barrel 13 is arranged to extend inwardly into the receiver 14. As is apparent from FIG. 9 the receiver 14 is supported at 14*a* and at 14*b* by lateral portions of the trigger guard 7.

Front sight 15 is affixed in conventional manner to the forward end of receiver 14 and rear sight 16 is affixed by pins 17 and 18 to the frame 1.

A retractable stock 19 is mounted on a pair of rods 20 which are slidable into and out of the frame structure 1.

Bolt 21 is slidably mounted within receiver 14 and is provided with a cavity at its lower right hand portion as viewed in FIG. 3 which is reciprocal relative to the breech portion 22 of barrel 13. Bolt 21 is biased toward the right as viewed in FIG. 3 by recoil spring 23 which is disposed about rod 24. Rod 24 is affixed at its left hand end as viewed in FIG. 3 to the frame structure 1 and is received within a passage formed in bolt 21 so that the rod 23 is slidably related to bolt 21.

For the purpose of manually operating bolt 21 from its open to its closed position and vice versa, a manually operable handle 25 is provided in accordance with one feature of this invention. Handle 25 is rotatable about its vertical axis and is held in a particular position by means of locking pin 26 which is biased toward the left by a spring 27 and which seats within recesses formed on the sides of handle 25 such as are indicated by the numerals 28 and 29. It will be understood that recesses such as 28 and 29 are disposed about the periphery of handle 25 and preferably are four in number. Handle 25 extends through slot 30 formed in the upper portion of receiver 14. Slot 30 is constructed with enlarged end portions 31 and 32.

As is apparent from FIGS. 2A, 2B, 3A and 3B, the part of handle 25 which is slidable within slot 30 is formed with a major axis and a minor axis so that when the major axis is disposed in perpendicular relationship to slot 30 and with the handle 25 disposed within the enlarged portion 31 or 32 of slot 30, the bolt 21 is locked in position. Of course the bolt is locked in its closed position when handle 25 is locked within the enlarged portion 32 of slot 30. On the other hand, when the handle 25 is disposed in its locked position in enlarged portion 31 of slot 30, the bolt is locked in its open position. With the bolt handle rotated to the unlocked position as shown in FIGS. 2B and 3B, the bolt 21 is freely slidable from left to right and vice versa.

Bolt handle 25 is provided with a sight passage 33 which allows sighting along the front and rear sights 15 and 16 when the bolt handle 25 is disposed in an unlocked position.

On the other hand, when the bolt handle is arranged in locked position, the sight passage in handle 25 is disposed in transverse relationship to the line of sight defined by front sight 15 and rear sight 16 thereby affording a ready visual indication of the locked condition of the bolt.

For the purpose of securing the removable magazine 4 in position within magazine housing 2, a rotatable latch 34 is pivotally mounted on pin 35 within the hand grip portion 3 of magazine housing 2. Furthermore latch 34 is biased in a clockwise direction toward latching position by a compression spring 36 to cause the latching surface 37 of latch 34 to ride underneath the latching surface 38 formed in magazine 4. Thus as shown in FIG. 3, the magazine 4 is held in its service position.

In order to remove magazine 4, manual pressure is applied to projecting portion 39 of latch 34 to cause the latch to rotate in a counterclockwise direction about pin 35. This action releases latching surface 37 from latching surface 38 and allows the magazine 4 to be removed downwardly in conventional fashion.

For the purpose of biasing ammunition rounds upwardly in a conventional manner, a spring 40 is provided which is of the compressional type and which functions in known manner as is obvious from FIG. 3.

For controlling the operation of bolt 21 by means of trigger 5, a sear 41 is provided with a latching surface 42 which engages the lower right hand corner 43 of bolt 21 to hold the bolt in its extreme left hand position. Sear 41 is pivotally mounted on pin 44 supported on frame 1. Sear 41 is biased in a clockwise direction about pin 44 by means of compression spring 45. A pin 46 is mounted on sear 41 and affords a surface for engagement by trigger 5. Thus in order to fire the weapon and with the parts disposed in the positions depicted in FIG. 4, it is simply necessary manually to rotate trigger 5 in a clockwise direction about its pin 6. This action causes the trigger 5 to rotate sear 41 in a counterclockwise direction about pin 44 due to the engagement of trigger 5 with pin 46. Rotation of sear 41 causes its latching surface 42 to disengage the lower right hand latching surface 43 of bolt 21. When the bolt is thus released, recoil spring 23 drives the bolt 21 toward the right causing the round of ammunition designated R1 to slide upwardly and toward the right along guide portion 9 of trigger guard 7 as shown for example in FIG. 5. With round R1 seated within the breech portion 22 of barrel 13, firing pin 47 engages the cap portion of round R1 and fires the round. The projectile P1 proceeds outwardly toward the right in conventional fashion. The pressure developed urges the cartridge case C1 toward the left which action drives the bolt 21 toward the left against the action of recoil spring 23. Of course the weapon continues to fire automatically in known manner as long as trigger 5 is depressed.

Cartridge case such as C1 is extracted from the breech 22 of barrel 13 by an extractor designated for example in FIG. 7 by the numeral 48. As the cartridge case such as C1 moves toward the left in unison with the bolt 21, ejector pin 49 strikes the cartridge case C1 and drives the case downwardly and outwardly through the ejector opening 50 formed in frame 1. This action is depicted in FIG. 8. Of course the ejector pin 49 is disposed within a passageway 51 formed in bolt 21 so that there is a slidable relationship between the bolt 21 and ejector pin 49 which pin is fixed in position relative to frame 1. The extreme right hand end 52 of ejector pin 49 simply engages the lower side portion of cartridge case C1 and forces the case to swing out of contact with the jaws of the extractor 48.

The stock 19 as explained above is retractably mounted on the frame 1 by virtue of the slidable relationship of rods 20 with the frame 1. Rods 20 are provided with a pair of notches which cooperate with manually controlled transversely disposed locking rods. For example, outwardly protruding manually engageable pin 53 is engageable with transversely disposed locking rods 54 and 55 which cooperate with a transverse notch formed in rods 20. Rods 54 and 55 together with the manually operable element 53 are biased downwardly by compression spring 56 which is mounted within manually operable element 53. Spring 56 at its upper end is seated against plate 57 secured at its forward and rear portions to transversely disposed rods 58 and 59 which are mounted at their ends in fixed relationship on frame structure 1. Thus with the stock 19 disposed in its retracted position as shown in FIG. 3, upward pressure on manually operable release element 53 elevates the transversely disposed locking rods 54 and 55 and causes those rods to disengage the notches formed in rods 20 and allows the rods 20 to be withdrawn toward the left. When the right hand notch of rods 20 (not shown) engages the downwardly biased locking rods 54 and 55, the stock 19 is locked in its outwardly extended position. In this position the weapon may be fired by resting the stock 19 against the shoulder hip, chest or the like of the user. In order to retract the stock 19, the element 53 is pushed upwardly and the stock pushed inwardly into the locking position shown in FIG. 3.

Safety element 60 is movable by pin 61 manually in a transverse direction about pin 62 as a center so as to engage the sear 41 at the rear thereof thereby to prevent bolt releasing movement of the sear.

The embodiments of the invention in which an exclusive property or privilege is claimed are defined as follows:

I claim:

1. A firearm comprising a frame, a receiver mounted on said frame, a barrel mounted on said receiver, a bolt mounted in said receiver and telescopically movable relative to the breech end of said barrel, a firing pin fixedly positioned on a portion of the bolt so located relative to the breech end of the barrel as to come into contact with the free end of a cartridge of a round of ammunition in the breech end of the barrel upon release of the bolt from its open position, recoil spring means arranged to bias said bolt toward firing position, means including a trigger and sear movably mounted on said frame and operable to release said bolt from its open position to initiate a firing operation, a magazine mounted on said frame with its discharge portion adjacent the breech end of said barrel, a trigger guard fixedly mounted on said frame and having an intermediate portion extending from said frame outwardly and in enveloping relation to said trigger, said trigger guard being arranged with one end thereof disposed adjacent the discharge portion of said magazine and extending toward the breech end of said barrel for guiding rounds of ammunition into the breech end of said barrel prior to firing, and a bolt handle

movably mounted on said bolt and protruding outwardly through a longitudinal slot formed in said receiver, said slot and said bolt handle being configured so as to prevent movement of said bolt relative to said receiver for one position of said bolt handle relative to said bolt and so as to accommodate movement of said bolt relative to said receiver for another position of said bolt handle relative to said bolt.

2. A firearm comprising a frame, a receiver mounted on said frame, a barrel mounted on said receiver, a bolt mounted in said receiver and telescopically movable relative to the breech end of said barrel, recoil spring means arranged to bias said bolt toward firing position, means including a trigger and sear movably mounted on said frame and operable to release said bolt from its open position to initiate a firing operation, a magazine mounted on said frame with its discharge portion adjacent the breech end of said barrel, and a trigger guard fixedly mounted on said frame and having an intermediate portion extending from said frame outwardly and in enveloping relation to said trigger, said trigger guard being arranged with one end thereof extending inwardly into the interior portion of said frame through an opening formed therein and disposed somewhat to the rear of the breech end of said barrel and said one end of said trigger guard being configured to define an upwardly inclined path for guiding rounds of ammunition into the breech end of said barrel prior to firing.

3. A firearm according to claim 2 wherein the other end of said trigger guard is fixedly mounted on said frame immediately forward of said trigger.

4. A firearm comprising a frame, a receiver mounted on said frame, a barrel mounted on said receiver, a bolt mounted in said receiver and telescopically movable relative to the breech end of said barrel, recoil spring means arranged to bias said bolt toward firing position, means including a trigger and sear movably mounted on said frame and operable to release said bolt from its open position to initiate a firing operation, a magazine mounted on said frame with its discharge portion adjacent the breech end of said barrel, and a trigger guard fixedly mounted on said frame and having an intermediate portion extending from said frame outwardly and in enveloping relation to said trigger, said trigger guard being arranged with one end thereof disposed adjacent the discharge portion of said magazine and extending toward the breech end of said barrel for guiding rounds of ammunition into the breech end of said barrel prior to firing and said one end of said trigger guard being provided with lateral portions for engaging lower parts of said receiver and for affording support therefor.

5. A firearm comprising a frame, a receiver mounted on said frame, a barrel mounted on said receiver, a bolt mounted in said receiver and telescopically movable relative to the breech end of said barrel, recoil spring means arranged to bias said bolt toward firing position, a bolt handle movably mounted on said bolt and protruding outwardly through a longitudinal slot formed in said receiver, said slot and said bolt handle being configured so as to prevent movement of said bolt relative to said receiver for one position of said bolt handle relative to said bolt and so as to accommodate movement of said bolt relative to said receiver for another position of said bolt handle relative to said bolt, and a sight passage being formed in said bolt handle and arranged to accommodate sighting when said bolt handle is disposed in unlocked condition but not when said bolt handle is in a bolt locking position.

6. A firearm according to claim 5, further comprising at least one sight aligned with the bolt handle.

7. A firearm according to claim 5, further comprising front and rear sights aligned with the bolt handle.

• • • • •

Continued On Next Page

25mm Flare Gun Conversion

BY THE AMATEUR

Here are the plans for modifying a flare gun to fire .22 long rifle ammo.

Articles Needed:

1. a .25 mm to 12 gauge adapter or reducer, this converter is available from Olin Corp., Box 107, Peru Indiana 46970. Price $3
2. a 12 gauge to 22 LR shell shrinker, price $12.95, available from Shell Shrinker Industries, Box 462, Fillmore, California 93015. (They also make a neat gun storage safe)
3. a .25 mm flare gun. Olin Corp. sells one for about $40. A.C.A. Inc. Box F, Chicago Ridge, Ill. 60415 sells one for $19.95. Either one works equally well, but the cheaper one needs an assist from a rubber band after the first few shots.

By simply taking a hacksaw and sawing the .25 mm adapter just above the ridge on the inside, you are halfway home. Olin made the adapter with the ridge so that it would accomodate a 12 gauge flare but not a 12 gauge shot-shell. If you saw it below the ridge, you will find the adapter will accommodate a shotgun shell. This is not advised because then you have an N.F.A. weapon which is unsafe to use. If you saw if off just above the ridge, it will still not accept a 12 gauge shotgun shell, but you can hammer the stainless steel shell shrinker into the aluminum adapter. It will not easily come apart this way, but to play it safe you may want to weld or solder it in place. You then place the adapter, the shell shrinker, and a 22 rim fire bullet in the flare gun as you would if you were going to fire a flare. You now have a sanitized, single-shot .22 LR pistol, with a possible bell-type sound depressor. (contact silencer) It is easy to make, requires only a hacksaw as a tool, and uses easily available materials. The disadvantages are that it is single-shot, possibly illegal

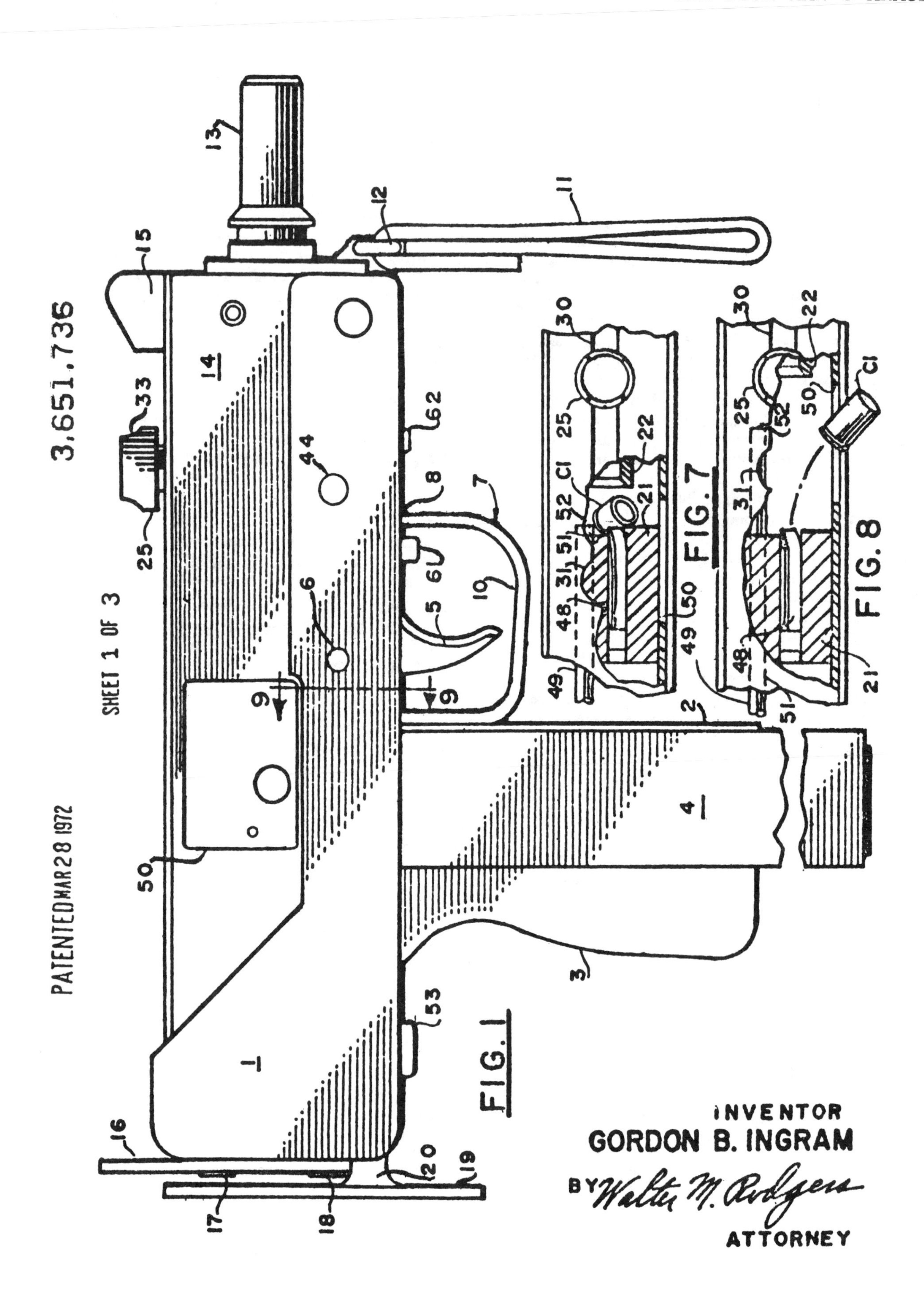
PATENTED MAR 28 1972
SHEET 1 OF 3
3,651,736
FIG. 1
FIG. 7
FIG. 8
INVENTOR
GORDON B. INGRAM
BY Walter M. Rodgers
ATTORNEY

PATENTED MAR 28 1972 3,651,736

SHEET 2 OF 3

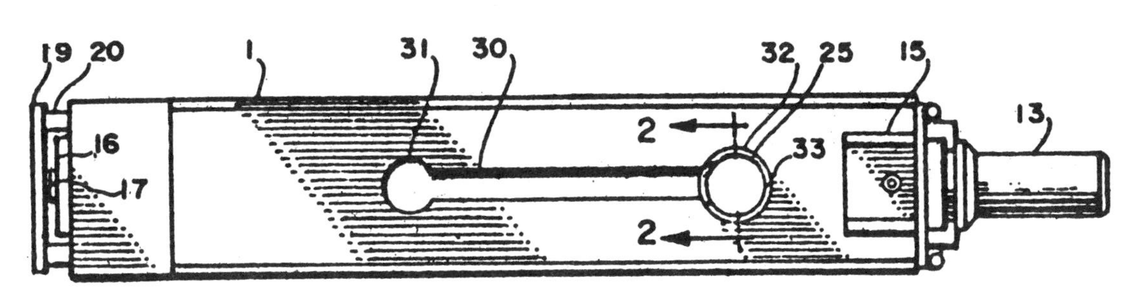

FIG. 2

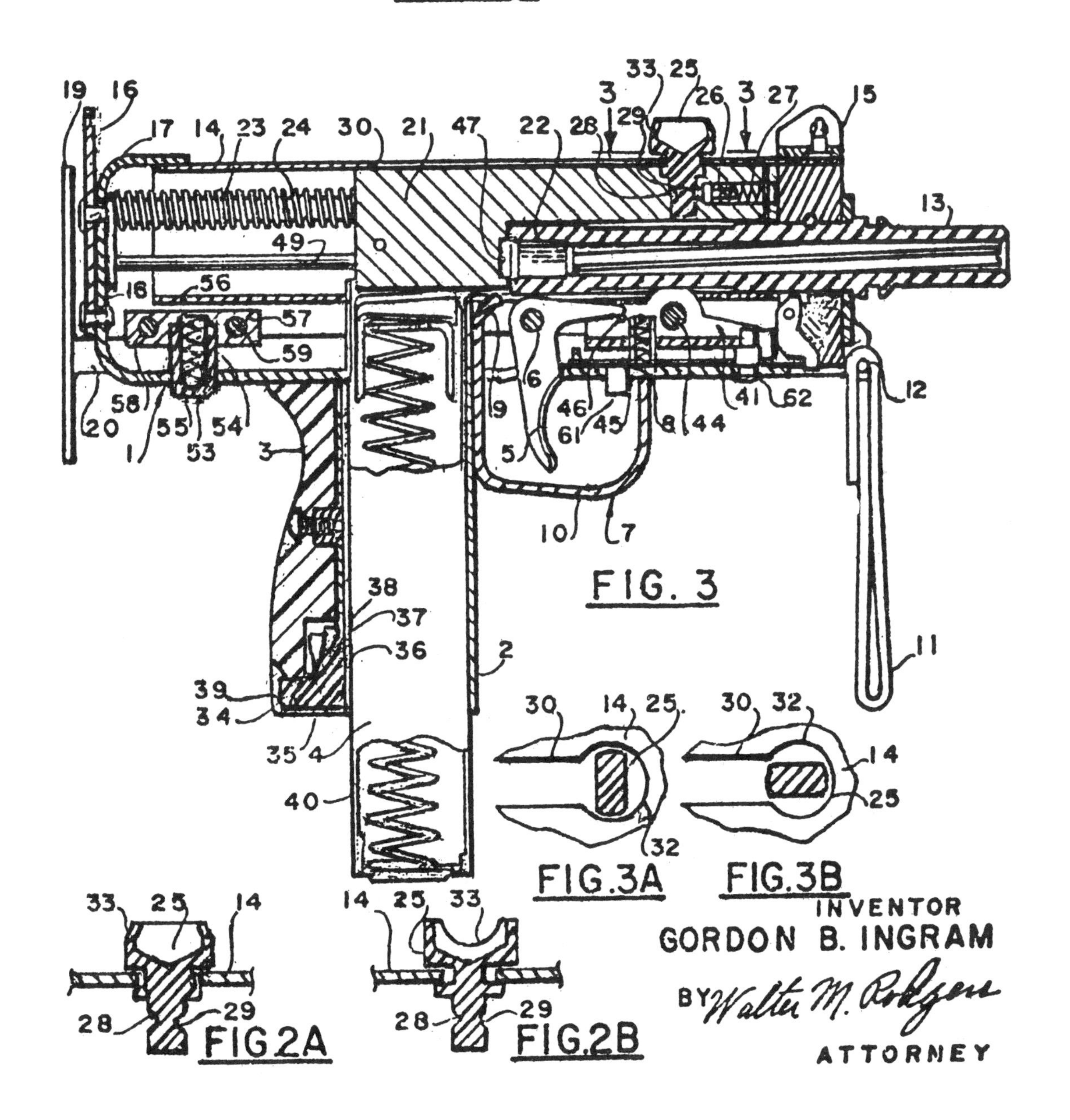

FIG. 3

INVENTOR
GORDON B. INGRAM

BY *Walter M. Rodgers*

ATTORNEY

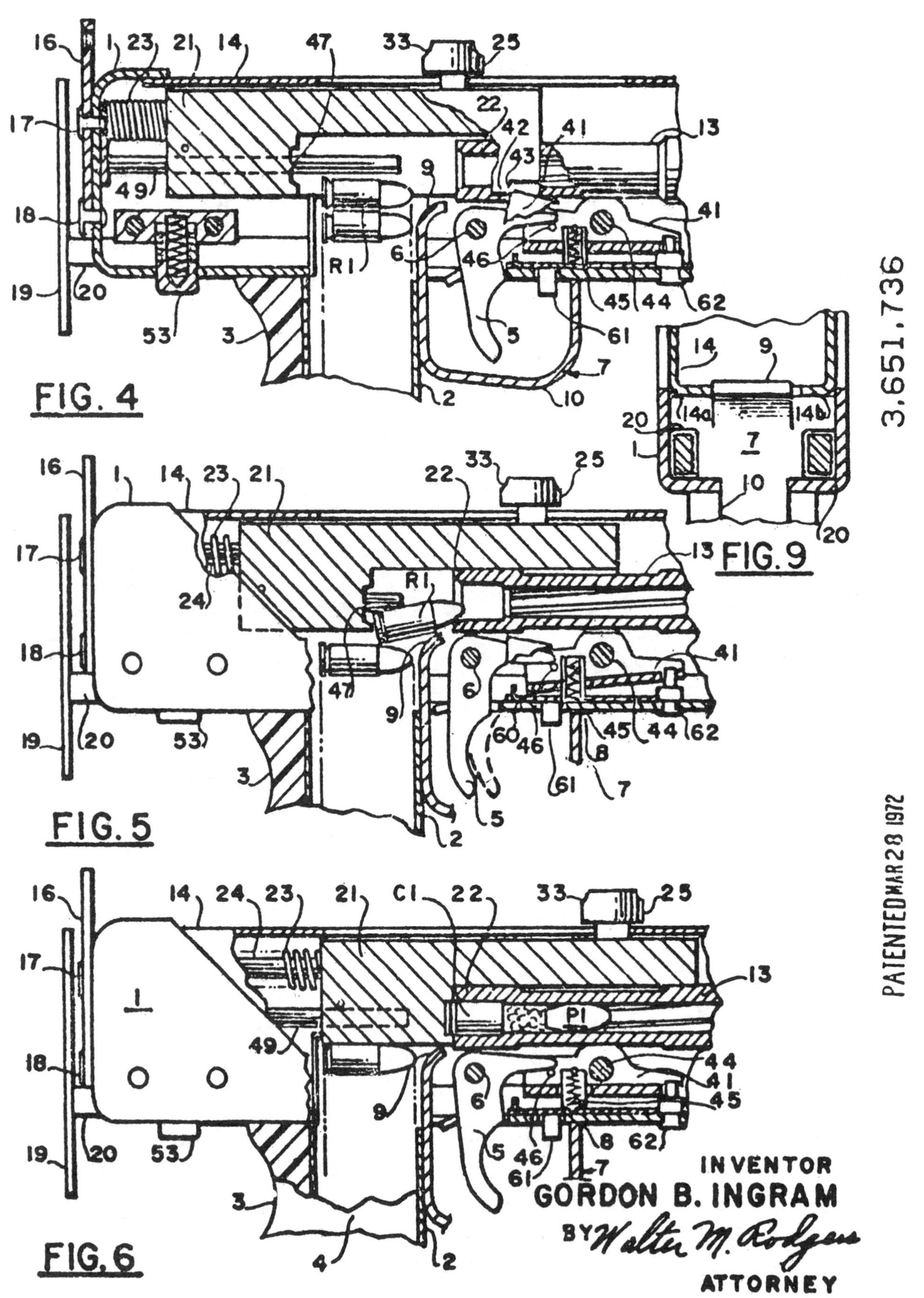
FIG. 4
FIG. 5
FIG. 6
FIG. 9
3,651,736
SHEET 3 OF 3
PATENTED MAR 28 1972
INVENTOR
GORDON B. INGRAM
BY Walter M. Rodgers
ATTORNEY

United States Patent

Ingram

[15] **3,651,736**

[45] **Mar. 28, 1972**

[54] **BOLT HANDLE AND PISTOL GRIP MAGAZINE FOR AN AUTOMATIC FIREARM**

[72] Inventor: **Gordon B. Ingram,** Studio City, Calif.

[73] Assignees: **Michael H. Adair; Rosser S. Reeves, III,** c/o Tiderock Corporation, New York, N.Y., attorneys-in-fact

[22] Filed: **June 11, 1969**

[21] Appl. No.: **832,083**

[52] **U.S. Cl.** ....89/132, 42/16, 89/1 K, 89/195

[51] **Int. Cl.** F41d 11/02

[58] **Field of Search** 42/7, 16.3, 72; 89/27.3, 136, 89/132, 180, 194, 195, 197

[56] **References Cited**

UNITED STATES PATENTS

710,660	10/1902	Bennett et al.	42/16.3 UX
786,099	3/1905	Clement	89/195 X
1,502,676	7/1924	Kewish	42/16.3 UX
1,869,911	8/1932	Reising	42/16.3 UX
2,297,693	10/1942	Dicke	89/180
2,424,194	7/1947	Sampson et al.	42/72
3,039,366	6/1962	Linthurn et al.	42/7 X
3,276,323	10/1966	Dieckmann	89/195
3,318,192	5/1967	Miller et al.	89/185 X

Primary Examiner—Benjamin A. Borchelt
Assistant Examiner—Stephen C. Bentley
Attorney—Nolte & Nolte

[57] **ABSTRACT**

An automatic firearm comprises a frame, a receiver mounted on the frame, a barrel mounted on the receiver, a bolt disposed in the receiver and telescopically movable relative to the breech end of the barrel against the action of a recoil spring, the bolt being controlled by a sear which is movable in response to movement of the weapon trigger. A trigger guard is mounted on the frame and disposed in enveloping relationship to the trigger and arranged with one end protruding inwardly of the frame and adjacent the breech end of the barrel so as to aid in guiding rounds of ammunition into the breech end of the barrel. A bolt handle is movably mounted on the bolt and arranged to extend through a longitudinal slot formed in the receiver. The bolt handle is constructed so as to form a locking relationship with enlarged ends of the longitudinal slot when moved relative to the bolt and a sight passage is formed in the outwardly protruding portion of the bolt handle which allows sighting therethrough in line with the front and rear sights when the bolt handle is in an unlocked condition but precluding sighting when the bolt handle is in locked position.

7 Claims, 13 Drawing Figures

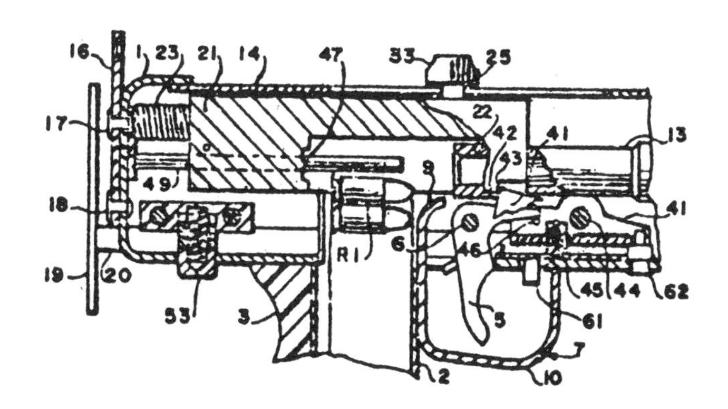

U.S. Patent No. 3,651,736 was issued on March 28, 1972, to GORDON B. INGRAM. It covers the basic design of the Ingram M10 and M11 Submachine Guns formerly manufactured by the Military Armament Corporation of Marietta, Georgia.

MOSSBERG FULL AUTO PLANS

BY ROY Mc LAUGHLIN

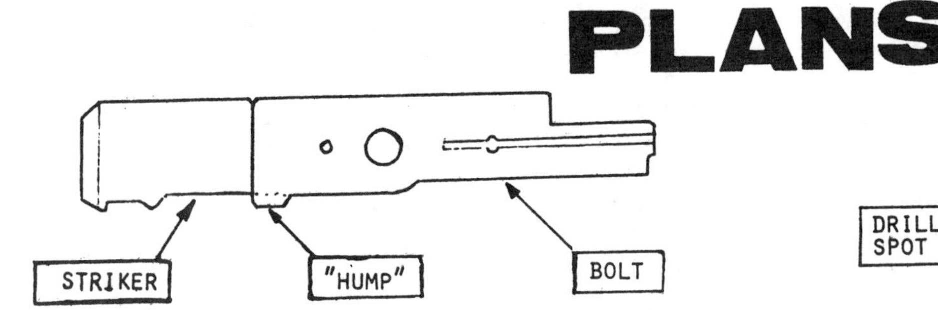

BOLT ASSEMBLY

DRILL OUT SPOT WELDS

MAGAZINE GUIDE PLATE

S/A MOSSBERG 7-SHOT .22LR MAGAZINE

Converting the Mossberg .22 semi-auto rifle to full-automatic is very easily accomplished.

The rear bottom of the bolt must be filed flat (see diagram). This "hump" activates the sear; causing engagement of the striker on recoil. Removal of the "hump" allows continuous firing for the time the trigger is held to the rear; full-automatic fire of the weapon until trigger is released.

The Atchisson M-16/AR-15 .22 lr CONV. MARK II 30-shot magazine is used for the Mossberg in this conversion. The magazine is available from BINGHAM LTD, 1775-C Wilwat Dr. Norcross, GA. Price $17.95 + postage.

See diagrams for all instructions below.

Dis-Assemble magazine:

First remove upper rear of magazine for 1 13/16" from the top. File flat with body of magazine. Braze or solder the magazine guide (with extensions removed) from a 7-shot Mossberg magazine in this location so that bottom of magazine guide is 1 5/8" from top of magazine.

Next, file the magazine feed lips to the configuration shown: leaving enough metal to keep feed plate from exiting magazine at top.

After filing, clean magazine completely and oil inside lightly. WD 40 is fine for this purpose. Re-assemble magazine; load 1 round and check feeding manually.

Magazine guide arm extending down from bottom of receiver may have to be bent "slightly" forward or rearward. This is actually un-likely, but possible.

Once (1) round feeds successfully, load (10) rounds and repeat manual operation. Successful operation of (10) rounds suggest a completed job.

Congratulations!

MAGAZINE GUIDE

1-5/8"

SERVES AS MAGAZINE STOP

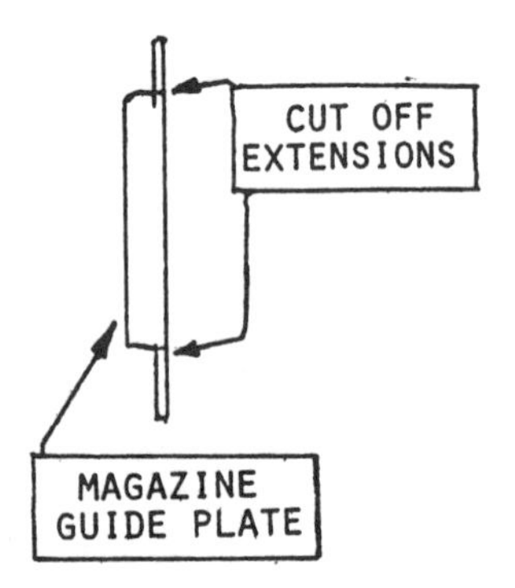

Continued Next Page

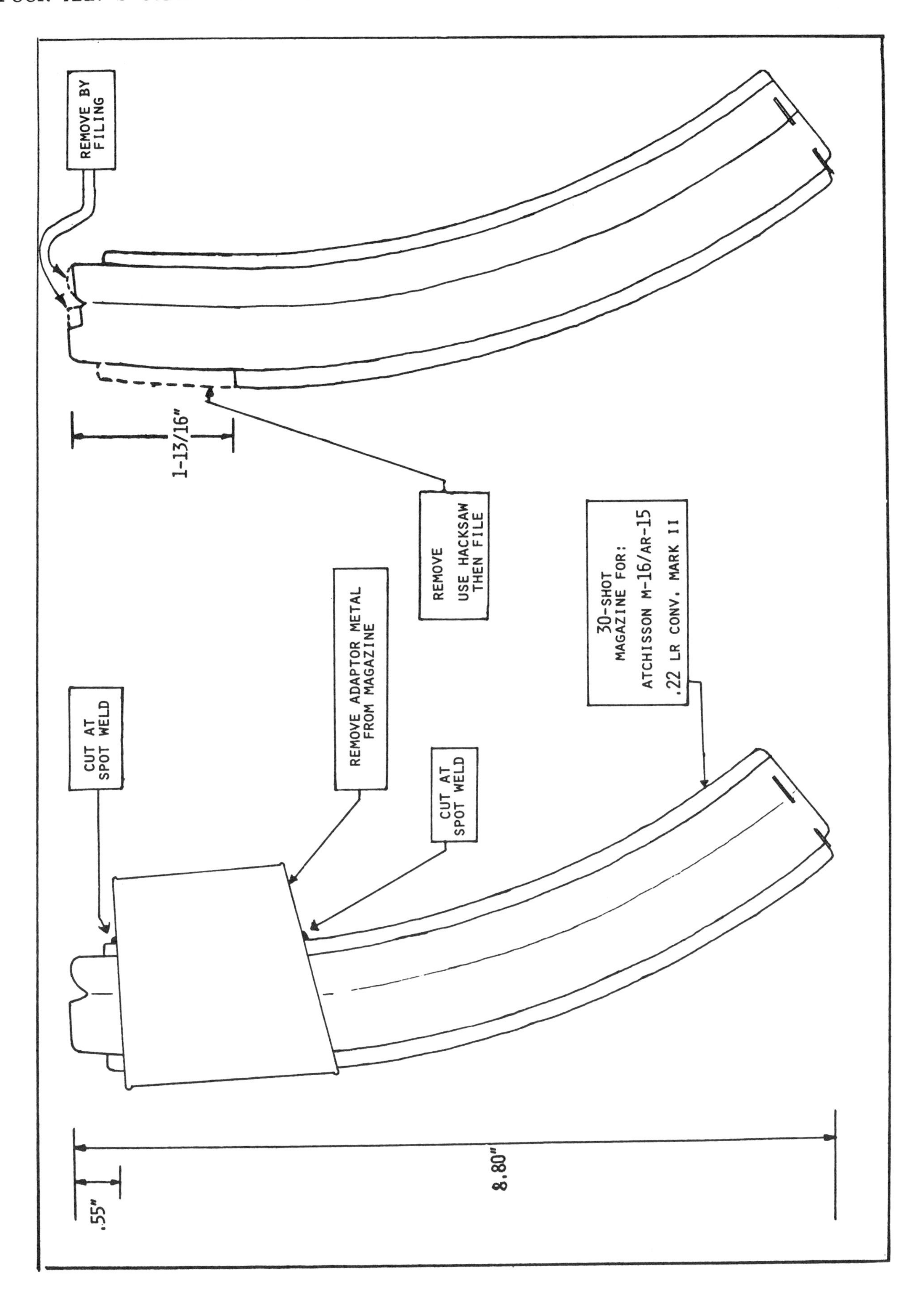
REMOVE BY FILING
1-13/16"
REMOVE
USE HACKSAW THEN FILE
30-SHOT MAGAZINE FOR:
ATCHISSON M-16/AR-15
.22 LR CONV. MARK II
REMOVE ADAPTOR METAL FROM MAGAZINE
CUT AT SPOT WELD
CUT AT SPOT WELD
.55"
8.80"

DO-IT-YOURSELF MACHINE PISTOLS

BY THE KENTUCKY RIFLEMAN

Building an SMG from scratch is not an easy job for most people, even though excellent plans are available from various sources. Not everyone has the shop, tools or skill required. Converting a semi-auto pistol would seem to be a more practical approach.

These conversions still appear to be difficult to most folks, who believe that complex machine work and hard to get parts are needed.

All of these objections are true sometimes, for instance, to change an M-1 carbine to M-2 (a favorite) requires a set of parts that are costly, rare, and watched by the Federal boys.

The AR 15 rifle needs the lower receiver re-machined plus new parts before it will fire fully auto.

The new Thompson M1927A1 looks like a natural, but it would be a difficult job indeed to convert it because it was designed just to stop such a project.

But take heart! There is a way out for the resourceful individual. There are weapons that can be altered to be useful, useable, and in some ways, about ideal.

Many modern automatic pistols are easily and cheaply convertable to full auto, and in a lot of cases no one can tell the difference unless they shoot it.

After examining many pistols I can offer the following list of suitable guns, along with a few comments.

Walther P-38

An easily converted pistol with good handling and reliability. It's biggest disadvantage is it's high cost, both new and used.

Browning Hi-Power

Very good design with large magazine and larger ones available. Very strong.

Mauser HSc

Compact size, easily converted, large capacity magazines available. Disadvantage is 32 ACP cal.

Llama 45:

See Colt 45

Colt 45 M 1911

Easily converted to full auto with parts and magazines available. My choice for a big bore sub-machine gun.

Sauer M-38

A high quality pistol easily converted to full auto, a compact size. Easy to work on.

To put together your custom gun, you will need a long barrel, an oversize magazine (I suggest at least 25 rounds), a custom-made shoulder stock, and the time and desire to put them together.

The long barrels are available from various parts dealers for some pistols. Other guns may need custom made ones. Check around and read the Shotgun News. Lots of places carry the magazines, again, check around. The stock is easily made from a piece of steel or aluminum strap (see drawings).

The Colt M1911 in any cal is a natural because of simplicity and ruggedness.

After you have your pistol and the new parts, you must do the alterations.

The first order of business is to strip the pistol. If you are working on a Colt 45, a military manual can be a big help. For any make or model of gun, a copy of Small Arms of the World by W.H.B.Smith is invaluable in helping you to understand the works.

After you have the slide, barrel and spring off your 45, notice the disconnector sticking up from the frame just behind the magazine well. This is the part that must be shortened to convert the 45 to full auto. Remove the disconnector and shorten it by either filing or grinding it just enough to be flush with the frame. Then re-assemble the pistol using the longer barrel (if you wish) and if you wish, a buffer unit and a stronger recoil spring to insure reliability.

All that is left is to install the new shoulder stock, give the whole thing a good safety test and you're in business!

The Sauer M-38 is even easier to alter than the Colt. Start by stripping the gun. The Sauer is stripped by pulling down the latch in the trigger guard, then pulling the slide all the way back and up, then letting it go forward off the frame. Then remove the grips.

To start the conversion, remove the trigger bar (see drawing) by gently prying out of the frame.

Then locate the hump on the outside of the bar that acts as a disconnector by fitting into a cutout in the slide. This hump must be filed down until it no longer makes the contact with the slide.

There is a pin at the front of the barrel mount that locks the barrel in place. Remove this pin by carefully driving out with a hammer and punch. Then gently heat the barrel with a propane torch or soldering gun or iron until it can be pulled free. Your new long barrel is installed by first tinning the barrel (heating until a thin layer of solder adheres) then inserting into the barrel mount. Then replace the pin and heat to melt solder.

The beauty of this type of barrel mount is that since the barrel is solidly fixed, you can mount just about anything on the end (such as a silencer), just be sure it is removable so you can strip to clean.

To reinstall the trigger bar, simply insert the round lug at the front into the trigger, making sure that the trigger spring end that is facing to the rear gets placed over the pin in the trigger bar.

When you have re-assembled your pistol, attached your shoulder stock, inserted the long magazine, and test fired, you have the poor man's MAC 11.

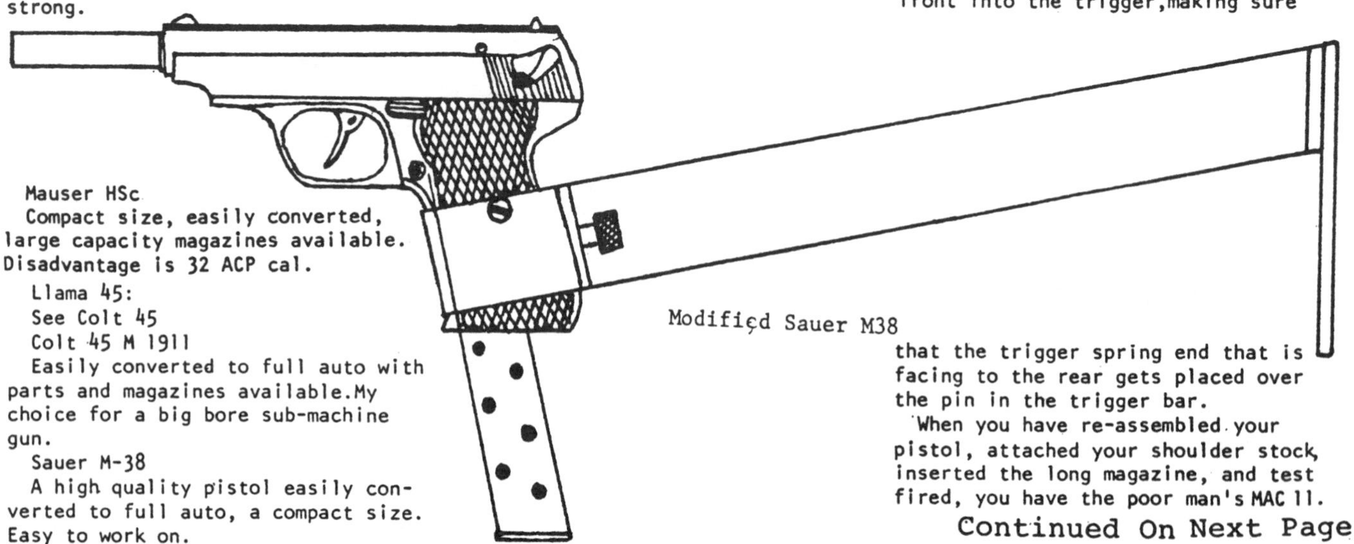

Modified Sauer M38

Continued On Next Page

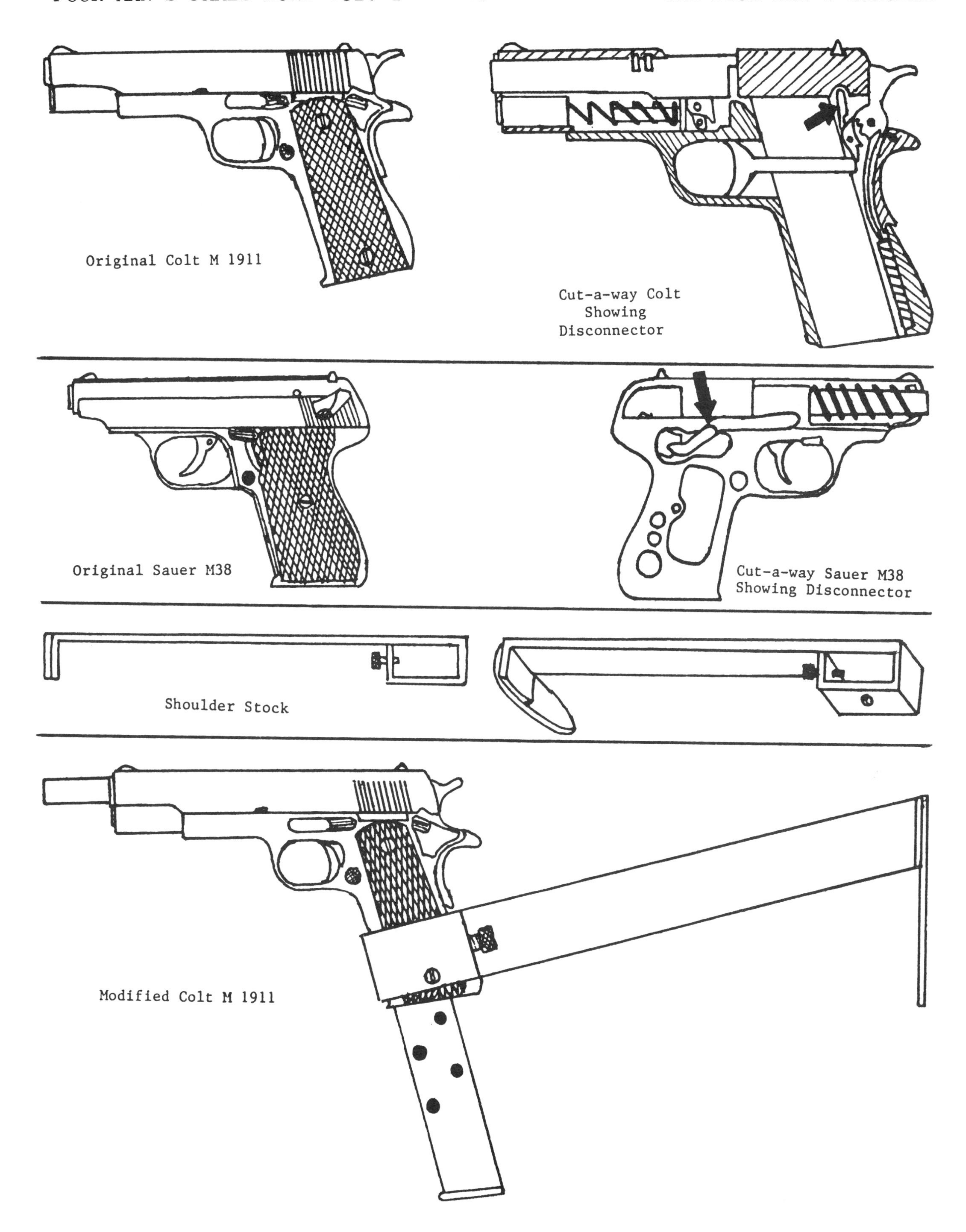
Original Colt M 1911
Cut-a-way Colt
Showing
Disconnector
Original Sauer M38
Cut-a-way Sauer M38
Showing Disconnector
Shoulder Stock
Modified Colt M 1911

IMPROVING THE BASIC CROSSBOW

BY ROBERT MAYBETH

The crossbow is one weapon no arms buff should overlook. It is silent, powerful, and more accurate than the long bow, given equal time to practice with both weapons. And best of all, many city penal codes completely ignore any mention of the crossbow.

A simple crossbow is detailed on p. 31 of the Survivor. It's a good design, but like most other crossbows it can only be used to shoot arrows or bolts. A crossbow with an enclosed 'barrel' is better because one, steel balls and other round ammo can be used and two, rifle sights can be mounted on top of the stock. A crossbow of this kind can be made by anyone at all skilled in woodwork for about $15.

If you're the type who wants the best, get walnut for the stock; for most of us, though, maple or ash is more realistic. You should get an unwarped, knot-free piece of wood 34" long, 7" wide and 1-1/2" thick. If the thickest wood you can find is only 3/4" thick, then buy 2 pieces and glue them together.

To make the crossbow, first the outline of the stock is drawn on the wood and cut out with a jig saw or a coping saw. After the stock shaping is done with a rasp or files, the top section of the barrel is cut off and set aside. Next the 2 slots, for the trigger assembly and the bow, are cut. The smaller slot in front of the bow opening is for the wedges that will hold the bow in place.

The next step is to make the barrel. The top section (that was previously set aside) and the bottom section of the barrel are both planed flat, and a 5/8" barrel channel is roughly gouged out to less than final diameter with a chisel. The barrel is finished by wrapping a foot long steel bar with sandpaper, and sanding both barrel sections to final diameter.

You will then need to cut away 1/8" from the inside surface of the upper barrel section for the bowstring slot. The cut starts at a point 3" behind the muzzle and ends at the same point that the barrel does, at the end of the trigger slot.

Metal Strip
Barrel
3/4"
5/8
1"
1 1/2"
bow slot
FRONT

Bowstring Slot
Upper Block
TRIGGER ASSEMBLY
Trigger
Trigger Stop
Trigger Spring
Lower Block

COMPLETED CROSSBOW

The barrel sections are not joined together until the bow and trigger assemblies are put in.
The trigger return spring is mounted, on the one end, in a shallow hole drilled in the rear of the trigger, and on the other end, between the two small blocks.

The third step is making the bow. It is a compound bow, made of 3 strips of yew or ash 1" wide by 1/4" thick. During this particular step, some guys go overboard and use steel for the bow, along with a wire bowstring. This arrangement is fine for punching holes in panzer tanks but the bowstring wears the crossbow rapidly. So, if you must make such a monster, use a high-test dacron bowstring.

Getting back to the bow: the last and longest strip is 33" long, with the ends tapered and nocked for the bowstring. The second strip is 27", the first 25". The strips are held together with 1" wide metal bands. The bands are bent around the strips as shown in the diagram, and held to the longest strip, only, with short screws. The other two strips of wood must be able to move freely within the metal bands.

The bow is put together as follows: one band is attached to the left side of the bow; then the bow is slid into its slot in the stock and the other band is put on the right side. Lastly, the wedges are spread with glue and driven into the appropriate slot to hold the bow in place.

The diagram for the trigger assembly should be self explanatory. The trigger is cut from 1/8" thick steel or brass, and holes are drilled in the trigger and stock for the trigger pivot screw. All parts of the trigger that will touch the bowstring are well rounded with a file or grinder.

The assembly procedure for the trigger is as follows: the upper block, with the bottom rounded to accept the spring, is smeared with glue and

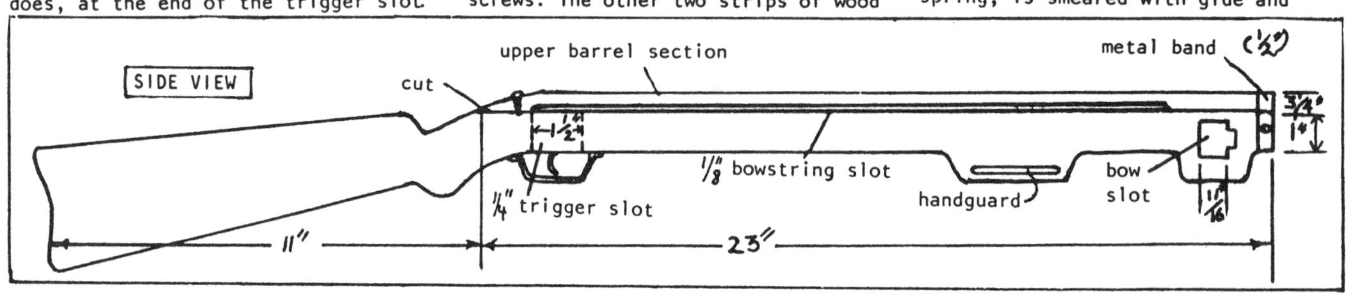

pushed into the trigger slot. Then the trigger, with trigger spring attached, is pushed into the slot and the trigger pivot screw is added. The lower block is spread with glue and pushed in place under the spring. Lastly, the trigger stop block is added.

This completes the trigger assembly. Now, the upper section of the barrel is attached; a screw holds the rear, and a thin metal strip 1/2" wide holds the front section together. The completed crossbow is then stained and varnished, if desired. Any design of homemade sights can be attached, leaf, peep sight, or any commercial rifle sights.

After the bowstring is strung, you can test the thing with a variety of ammo. Regular arrows can be used, but the feathers may need to be trimmed to fit the barrel. The best ammo to feed it is 1/2" steel ball bearings, but you can even use nuts, bolts, marbles, etc. When shooting any kind of round ammo, cotton wadding is tucked in to hold the pellet in place.

HOW TO CONVERT A FILE INTO A HUNTING KNIFE

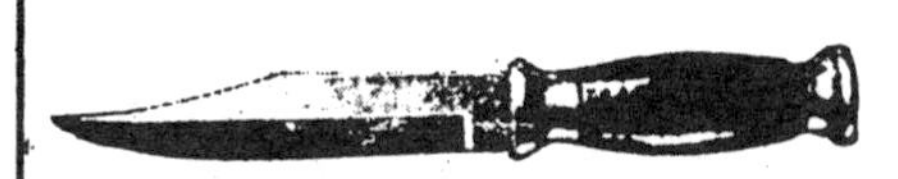

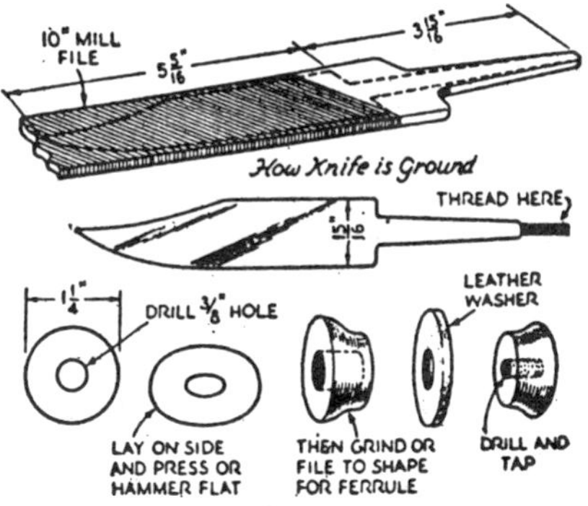

ALL that was required to make the high-grade hunting knife shown above was a worn-out 10-in. mill file, 10 cents worth of scrap sole leather from a shoe repair shop, and a piece of scrap brass 1¼ in. in diameter.

Place the file in a forge or bury it in a roaring bed of live coals in a furnace or stove and bring to a white heat. Remove and let cool gradually. This will leave just the right temper.

Now place the file in the vise with 5 in. above the jaws, and break it off with a hammer. Grind the file down to shape on a coarse wheel as shown in the drawings, and finish on a fine wheel, but do not put a knife edge on the blade until the whole is completed. Thread the end of the tang as indicated.

Shape the ferrules on a lathe or by grinding. Anneal the front ferrule by heating to a cherry red and plunging it into cold water. Then drill a ⅜-in. hole through the center. Place the piece on the anvil and drive down flat so that it will slip into place on the tang.

Cut the sole leather into approximate sizes. Drill or punch holes through the centers and slip them onto the tang. Drill and tap the end ferrule, and screw it tightly on the end of the shaft, which has previously been threaded.

Let the knife stand for a few days until the leather has thoroughly shrunk; then turn up the end ferrule as tightly as possible.

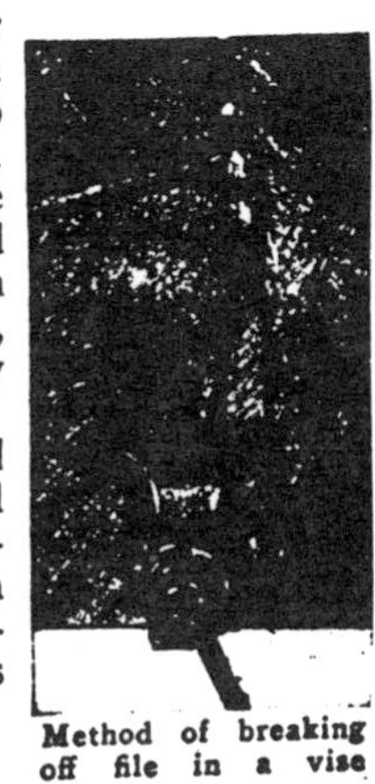

Method of breaking off file in a vise

RIGGING YOUR COMMAND POST

BY F.B.

4 5 6

tree stump 4 5 6 wood pile

Command Post

Place your manually detonated mines in spots that can be readily identified by you. If you put one in a tree stump, run the string into your command post, put a little tag on the pulling end that says 'tree stump'. If you have a big project like a long wall that you want to dot with mines, put numbers on the wall facing you and tag your strings accordingly. By doing this, you just sit back and wait for someone to take his position, and then finish him off. If you are being stormed, pull all the strings at once. * * *

CONTACT MINE

BY F.B.

Materials:

1. One Bullet
2. Nails
3. One 1" metal tube that will snugly hold the bullet.
4. One lightweight spring about 1" diameter.
5. One 6" length of broomstick.
6. One circular piece of wood 2" diameter.
7. One metal tube, about 6" long, diameter being wide enough to allow the broomstick to pass through.
8. Glue, solder, and aerosol spray sealant.
9. Large plastic bag.

1. Nail the circular piece of wood to one end of the broomstick. Drill a hole in the other end. Insert a nail into the hole, point showing, and glue it firmly in place. Slip the spring over it. This is the plunger.
2. Drill several holes in the side of the small metal tube, 1/4" from the end. This is the detonator housing.
3. Solder the detonator housing to the bottom mid-section of your mine, drilled holes down.

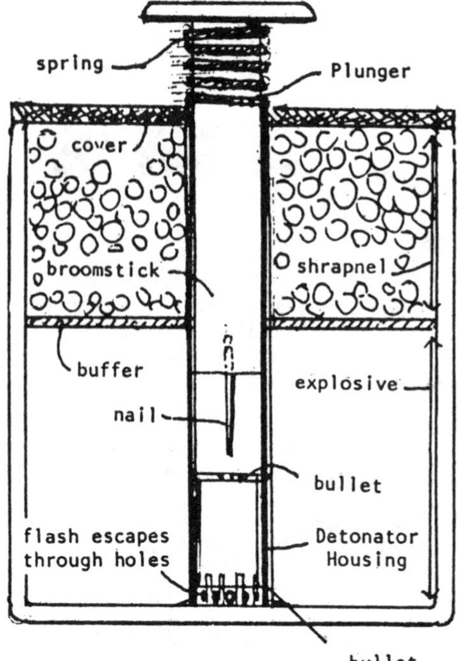

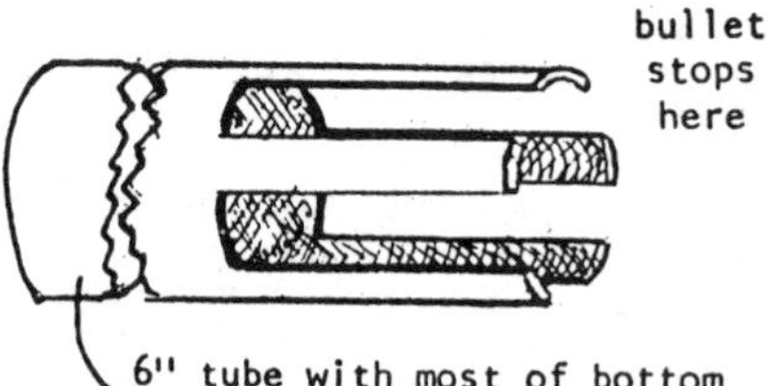

6" tube with most of bottom removed-insert over housing

4. Remove the slug from the bullet. Insert a light wad of paper into the cartridge so the gunpowder does not run out. Invert the cartridge and insert it in the tube.
5. Cut a hole in the buffer that will be used to separate the explosive from the shrapnel.
6. Take the 6" tube and cut 1/2" of one end away so that only 4 thin pieces of metal remain. Insert it over the detonator housing and secure it in place with glue or some other adhesive.
7. Fill the mine with explosive, slide the buffer over the tube, secure it, and fill with shrapnel.
8. Cut a hole in the mine cover, placing it over the tube so that about 1/2" of the tube extends above the mine.
9. Seal any spaces between the mine cover and tube with an aerosol sealant to keep moisture out. Do the same to all corners and cracks.
10. To arm the mine, carefully slide the plunger into the tube so that the nail is about 1/8" from the cartridge primer.
11. Carefully place a plastic bag over the plunger and secure it to the tube with a rubber band to keep water and dirt out. Then take the rest of the bag and slip it over the mine and tie it around. This will provide further resistance to the elements.

BOOBY TRAPS

BY BILLY L. NIELSEN

In the event of an extreme emergency or catastrophe, the urge to survive will be the one most uppermost instinct in all men. As we prepare for an eventual crisis, we begin stocking up on food, water, defense firearms and ammunition.Having made the above provisions, we next must consider keeping and protecting these precious supplies, as well as keeping alive. Booby traps will not only help protect one against unwelcome intruders, but can also serve as an alarm system. It should be stressed that all of the following are extremely dangerous and can and will cause extreme harm and death. They are definitely not toys to play with, nor to be used as a prank. As anyone who has been to Viet Nam will tell you, these devices have been used against our Forces with deadly effectiveness.

The first group of Booby Traps are classified as 'Stationary' traps, which means that no movement on the part of the trap itself is required to cause a resulting action. The first and simplest to make is the ordinary 'Spike Board' trap. This device consists of a wooden board of any convenient size, and has a number of long nails or spikes driven through it. A most typical size is a board of about 3/4" thickness and about 1 ft. square. The nails should be spaced about 2 to 3 inches apart, and have the points sharpened after being driven through the board.Fig.1

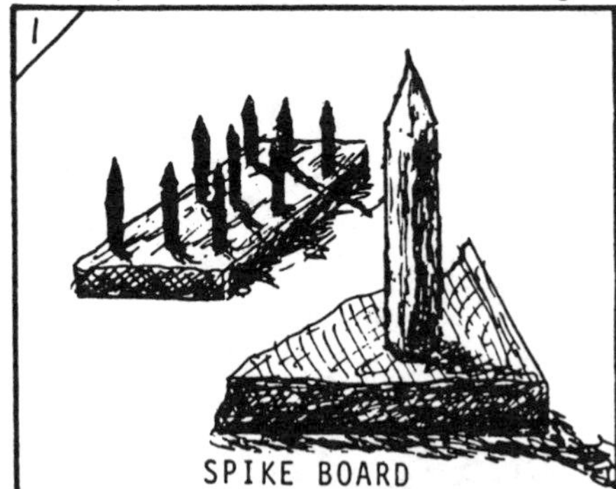

SPIKE BOARD

A variation of the 'Spike Board' is one called the 'Barbed Spike Bd. The construction of this one is similar to the plain 'Spike Board' except that the points of the nails are flattened and filed to a barb after being driven through the board. Fig. 2 The purpose of the 'Barbed Spike Board' is to prevent immediate withdrawl of the spikes, thereby requiring the victim to be carried back to a modern facility and to give the defender more time to escape.

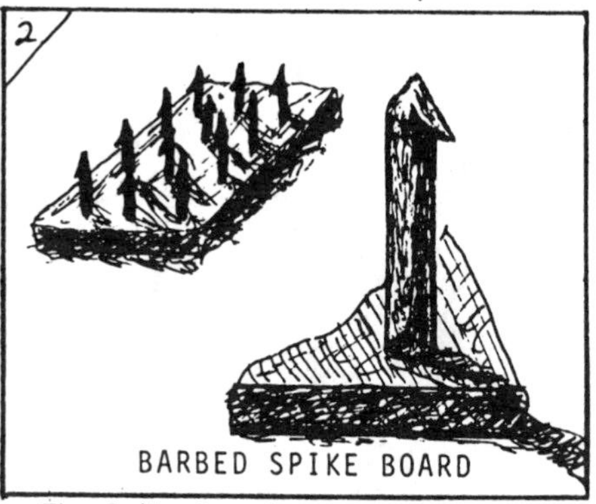

BARBED SPIKE BOARD

The Spike Boards are mostly used as a harassment or delaying device and are usually placed in a small pit about 10 to 12 " deep.They are placed on well traveled trails or paths.

A good place to place these traps is on the main path to the survival shelter or hideout. I should like to mention at this time that some method of marking your booby traps should be used so that you won't become a victim of your own trap. Some suggestions are, a twig broken or bent, a piece of string or yarn placed on a tree near the trap to mark its location. Do not make your marking too obvious, or it will re-

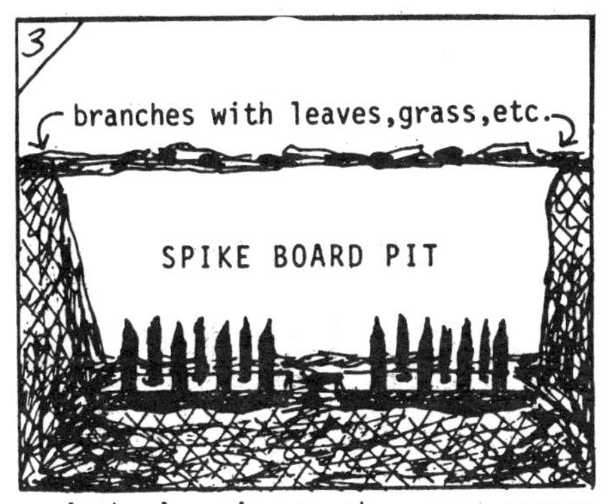

veal the location to the wrong person.

The next type of trap is the 'Punji Pit', borrowed from the North Vietnamese. The Punji Pit is a pit or hole dug into the ground approximately 4 ft. square and 5 to 6 ft. deep. Several small saplings or long stakes are driven into the bottom of the pit and the tips of the stakes are sharpened. The entire pit is covered with interwoven small twigs or branches and covered with grass or leaves, depending on placement of the pit. This one can really be deadly! Fig. 4 A simpler use of the Punji is sometimes very effective when used in fields where tall grass or weeds grow. In this trap the sticks are driven into the ground at an angle of about 30 to 40°. Anyone walking or running through the field will run into these stakes.

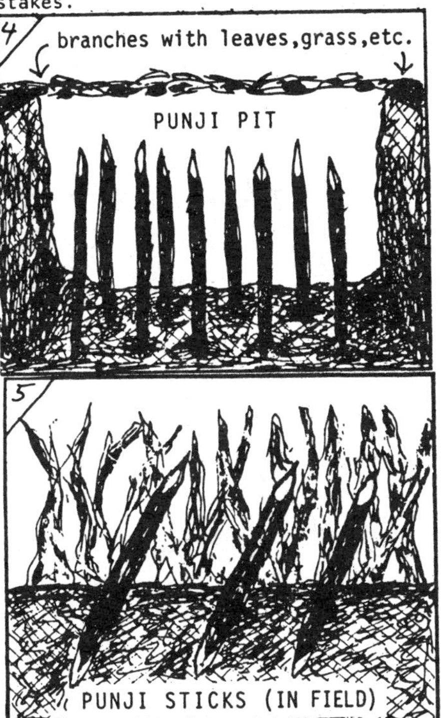

Fig.6 illustrates using the Punji stick in a small creek or stream. Again, these should be placed at a site that would normally be used for a crossing place in line with a path

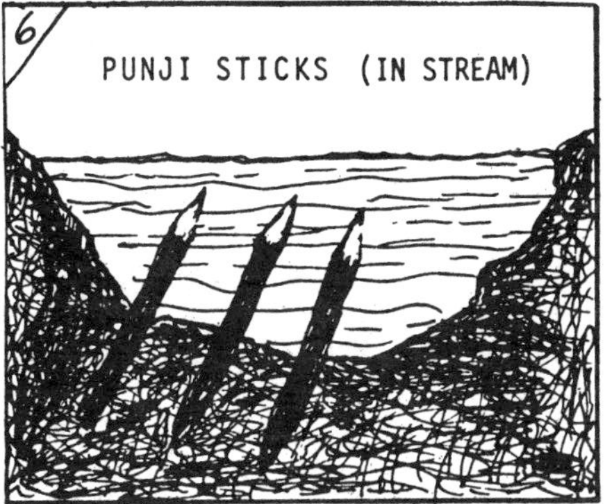

or trail. As with all booby traps, any variations on these ideas should be tried and in almost all cases will be effective. The main point is to conceal or camouflage the trap in such a manner as to make it blend in with the natural surroundings.

Remember that a trap which is easily spotted can be avoided. All steps should be taken to make the trap look as natural as possible. Don't forget to periodically check the traps to ensure that the cover is still effective and also to determine whether or not someone or something has not sprung the trap. The weather or wild animals can sometimes bare the trap, and as we said earlier, a trap not well camouflaged is not a trap.

BOOBY TRAPS PART 2

by Billy Nielsen

In Part I of this article we discussed the construction and installation of stationary booby traps, traps that require no motion to cause damage. In Part II we are going into some ideas on 'Moving Booby Traps', or traps that cause damage due to their movement. Note that placement of these traps as in Part I requires a location that is a well traveled foot path or an avenue of approach to your hideout or survival shelter. In both instances, camouflage is the key factor to installing an effective trap. I would like to point out that the traps illustrated in this article were all used very effectively against out Armed Forces in Viet Nam, and can be very deadly. They are definitely not toys to play with.

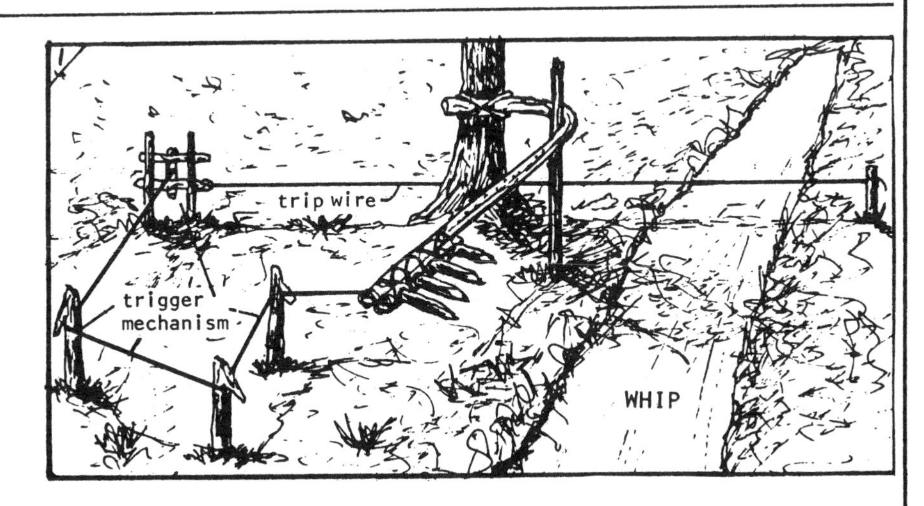

The first type of trap is called the 'Whip.' In this device, a young sapling, about 1-1/2 to 2 inches in diameter, is tied crossways to a sturdy tree along the side of a well traveled path or approach and is positioned so that it's end will be about chest high in the sprung position.. Fig.1 A Spike Board similar to the one that was used in the Spike Pit Trap (PMA vol.1 #3) is tied to the sapling in such a manner that it will strike whomever trips the wire in either the chest or back; depending on their direction of travel. The sapling is then bent back away from the trail and secured with the trip-wire mechanism. When the trip wire is pulled, it removes one of the retaining sticks and allows the Whip to spring towards the trail striking anyone in it's path. Notice in Fig.2, how simple the trigger mechanism is to construct. The various traps described here all use a similar trip mechanism which is readily constructed from materials at hand. The principle of keeping the trip mechanism as simple as possible and the use of one type of mechanism for several trap designs reduces the amount of equipment that a person may have to carry in the construction and placement of these traps.

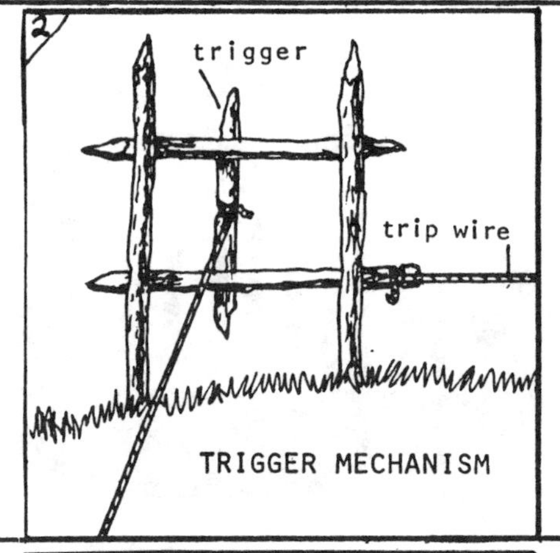

The next device is called the 'Angled Arrow' trap. It is constructed and placed in a pit in the ground which has a sloping bottom. Fig.3 The arrow platform is constructed from a piece of board about 1 in. thick, 3 ft. long, and about 12 in. wide. A guide channel, such as a piece of tubing, is fastened to the board to direct the arrow in the desired direction. Two spikes are driven into the board on a line across one end of the tube and are used to secure the rubber bands. The rubber bands can be made by cutting up an old inner tube or you can use surgical tubing. The trigger mechanism is constructed out of steel rod or a large nail, and uses the same principle as that of the crossbow. Remember that the rubber bands exert a constant strain on the trigger mechanism and therefore must be the strongest part of the trap. Fig.4 Note that the trigger wire is set into a small hole in the board as well as being held in place by the pivot rod. Any tension on the trip wire rotates the trigger wire on the pivot axis, releases the rubber bands and causes the arrow to fly out of the tube.

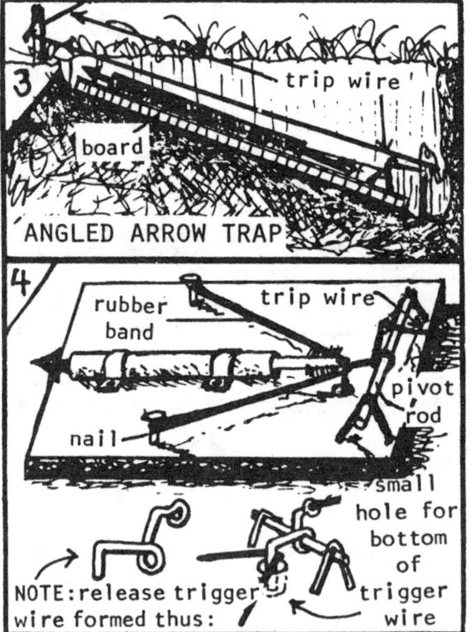

The third trap is called the 'Pivot Spike Board'. This one is used in conjunction with a foot pit. When a person steps on the treadle, the board with spikes, Fig.5, pivots about an axle and strikes the victim in the leg. A variation of this trap is called the 'Sideways' trap and is shown in Fig.6. This one is usually placed at the top of a pit about 4 feet deep and is camouflaged. As a person steps on the trap, he dislodges the prop stick, which releases the rubber bands, causing the sides of the trap to close. As the victim is falling, the spikes rake his body, arms, and legs, causing much damage.

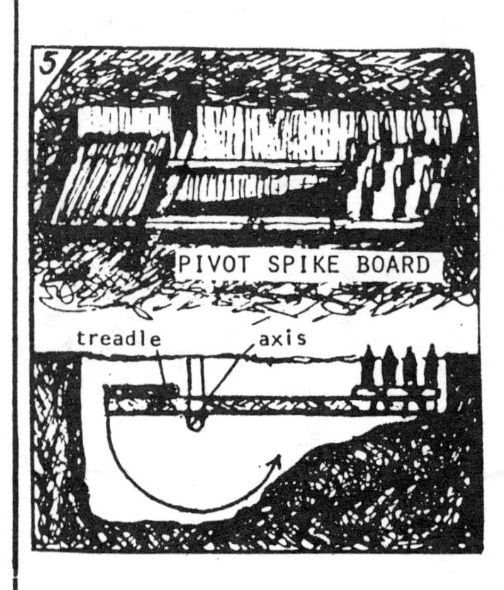

The final group of moving traps are suspended above the trail or path. The first is a 'Log Mace', a small diameter log 8 to 10 feet long with spikes driven into it. It is suspended from an overhead tree so that the spikes are about chest high, and then pulled back up into a second tree and fastened to the trip mechanism. When the trip wire is sprung, it swings down along the path hitting anyone in the way. Fig.7 Two variations of the Log Mace are the 'Spike Ball', which is a large cement ball with spikes in it, and the 'Suspended Spike Board'. Figs. 8 & 9 With the Suspended Spike Board, the device falls straight down on the person springing the trip wire. It has also been known as the 'Tiger Trap'. This one can really be deadly. Again, I remind you that these devices can cause severe injuries and care should be taken when building and setting them up.

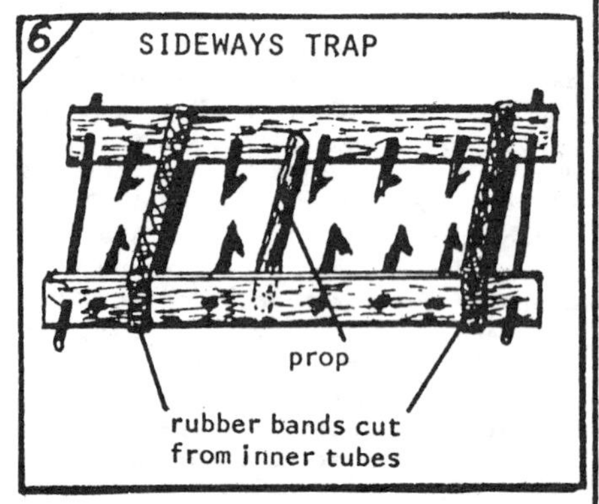

Continued next page

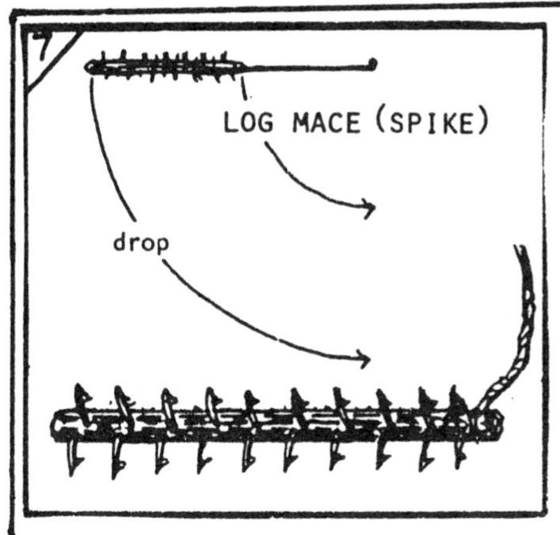

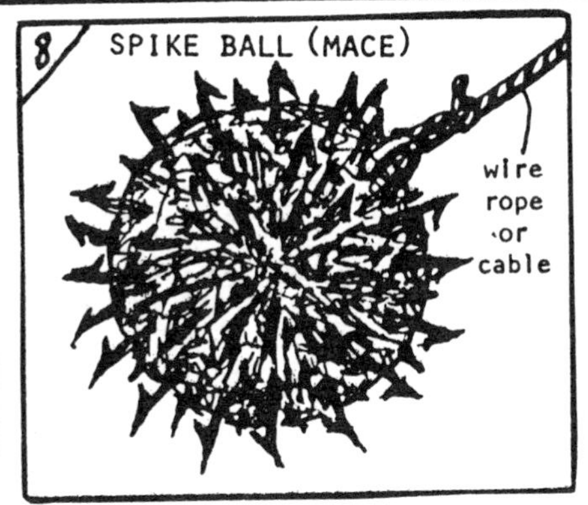

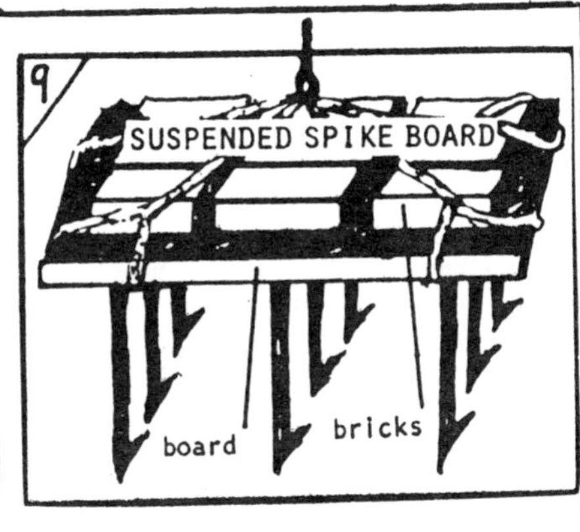

SWINGING GRENADE LAUNCHER

by

A.D.CRANFORD

Here's a neat little device that can launch a 2 lb. pipe bomb 100 yards or more, depending upon the thrower. Use a pipe bomb with a 10-15 second fuse and tie a string 2-3 feet long around one end, as shown in Fig.1.

Using this method of launching, you shouldn't find it too difficult to throw accurately at surprisingly long distances. The grenade that wouldn't reach a nearby hill can now be thrown over the next one as well. There are several times when you'll need a grenade to reach something hidden behind cover where your rifle or shotgun cannot reach.

This launcher has the advantage of silence, is cheap, and is simple to build and operate. This device requires a bit of practice in order to be used accurately and a little room is required to swing it. The correct throwing method is shown in Fig.2. If you are tall, perhaps the method I use, shown in Fig.3, will produce better results. The object is to swing it over your head like a cowboy swings a lasso, and by releasing the string at the right moment, get the pipe close enough to the target to destroy it. I prefer to swing it along my side. For me, it gives better accuracy and more range, but it is a matter of personal preference.

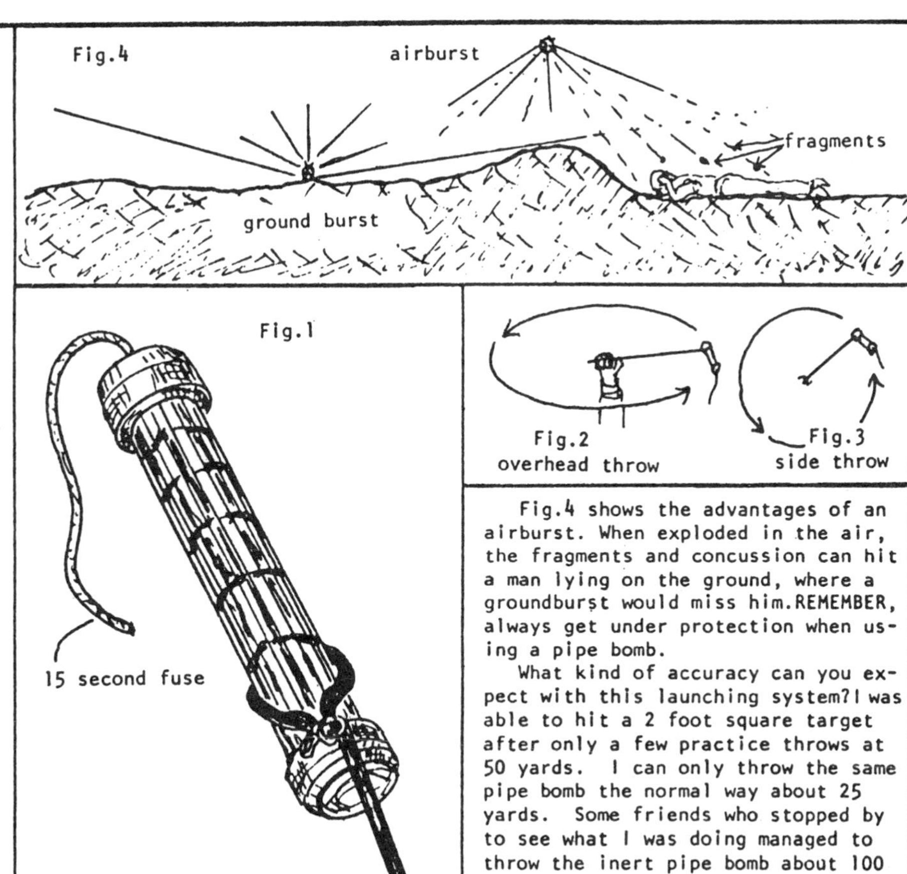

Fig.4 shows the advantages of an airburst. When exploded in the air, the fragments and concussion can hit a man lying on the ground, where a groundburst would miss him. REMEMBER, always get under protection when using a pipe bomb.

What kind of accuracy can you expect with this launching system? I was able to hit a 2 foot square target after only a few practice throws at 50 yards. I can only throw the same pipe bomb the normal way about 25 yards. Some friends who stopped by to see what I was doing managed to throw the inert pipe bomb about 100 yards. Your performance will vary under different conditions and will improve with practice. Use sand instead of explosives for the filler when practicing.

SIMPLE RELOADING & Special Purpose Ammo

By
J. Richard Young

Part I
Introduction:

Many readers will probably wonder if material dealing with reloading belongs in this magazine of improvised weaponry. The answer is yes. All firearms, either bought or made by you, need ammunition in one form or another. Many of you who have read Mel Tappan's book, Survival Guns, probably realize that a time may come when we will need large quantities of ammunition. Many of us, including me, cannot afford to purchase large quantities of ammunition for practice and to stockpile for when that time may come. If you run out, where will you buy ammo when a crisis is on?

A five dollar Lyman manual, ten dollar Lee Loader, and powder, primers, and bullets for a hundred rounds of ammo will all cost about the same as buying a hundred rounds of factory ammo.

Begining Reloading:

Please, if you are going to improvise ammunition for conventional firearms, buy or borrow a copy of Lyman Reloading Handbook for Rifle, Pistol, Shotshell and Muzzle Loading. The cost is around $5. It is not the cheapest, but it is the best. You can get it from most gunshops and sporting goods stores.

Reloading is no deep, dark secret. If you obey the rules it is much safer than running a lawn mower. I have reloaded tens of thousands of rounds of conventional ammunition. It is much cheaper and better than factory ammo. I have also designed and loaded thousands of rounds of special purpose ammunition. I have yet to have an accident.

Never touch the powder or the face of the primer with your fingers. No matter how clean or dry they are, they still have enough body oil on them to ruin the primer and affect the powder.

To store handmade ammunition more than one year, buy a small can of red Lacquer paint. With a small artist brush paint a coat of lacquer around the primer and the bullet where it goes into the case. Your ammunition is now waterproofed just like military ammunition and will keep for years.

I have taught dozens of people how to reload in a few minutes. If you are interested then seek out a small gun shop in your area. Almost without exception the people are very helpful at these small shops. They sincerely try to help you solve any problems. Start out with a Lee Loader. They are complete except for a plastic mallet, cost around $10 and turn out very good ammo, although they are slow.

Bench press equipment can make jacketed bullets and change cartridge cases from one caliber to another. A 30-06 case can be made into 21 other different military and commercial cartridges. Bench equipment is 5-10 times faster at reloading than Lee Loaders.

Now that you have read the book from Lyman and understand the basics of reloading and reading signs of pressure, you can start designing your own special purpose ammunition. Remember that small and large pistol primers are the same size as small and large rifle primers. Pistol primers will show signs of pressure faster than rifle primers because the metal cap is thinner and softer. Remember this when improvising goodies using primers. Pistol primers take much less impact to set them off than rifle primers. Buy a box of shotgun primers at your gun shop. They cost about $1.50. They improvise into fantastic goodies that work by impact.

Unless you intend to commit suicide, your inventions are less than useless if they get you killed inventing them. Read Lymans book before tampering with or making any ammunition. Learn how to be safe. Test everything by remote control. Tie fishing line or stout string to the trigger. Tie or sandbag the firearm down. Stand behind a tree or something while jerking the line. Stay alive. Examine the fired rounds for sign of too much pressure as described by Lyman.

Part II
Bullets:

Now that you have learned the basics it is time to get into experimenting with homemade bullets.

To learn the basics of bullet making it is best at this point to buy a Lee Mold complete for about $10 or a set of Lyman blocks and handles, which in my opinion is far better, for about $18. Some people prefer the Lee mold. R.C.B.S. and Ohas also make molds. The instructions with the molds are excellent. I molded excellent bullets for two years without the accessories. Use a large spoon to stir and pour the lead. Tape the handle or put wood on it because it gets very hot very fast. Use any old pan found in the kitchen to melt the lead in on the stove or use a wood fire. KEEP ALL WATER OR MOISTURE AWAY FROM THE MOLD AND HOT LEAD. Water will cause the melted lead to explode. Scrounge lead from wheelweights at the gas station, sewer pipe joints in houses being torn down, the lead sheath around telephone cable, and scraps of solder. Sometimes you can buy scrap lead from junk dealers. The hardware store sells lead in 5 lb. blocks. I scrounged 225 lbs. of lead from the last house that was torn down here.

Stand the bullets you have cast in a shallow pan and pour melted bullet lube on them. When the lube cools and hardens cut the bullets out of the lube by pressing a fired cartridge case down over the bullet. Punch the fired primer out first and use a stiff piece of wire to shove the bullet out of the case. The bullet shoots fair as is but for better accuracy, get a Lee Lube and Size kit. The lubed and sized bullets shoots very accurately with a little playing around with the powder charge. Excellent bullet lube is made by melting together a pound of parafin from the supermarket with a can of S.T.P. Better lube is made from one pound of parafin melted with one grease gun cartridge of Lithium Grease from the auto parts store. The best lube is Alox 2138 I bought at the gun shop. A stick will lube hundreds of bullets.

Now that you have loaded and shot a few hundred rounds of cheap ammo you can use blocks of plaster of paris or something to make your own molds. Use a drill or knife or something to drill holes in the plaster blocks. Pour the hot lead into the holes.

Buckshot from the gunshop costs about75¢ a lb. in 5-lb. bags and makes excellent rifle and pistol bullets for small game and practice. A 30-06 case loaded with 2-1/2 grains of Red Dot, Trap 100, or 452 AA powder and a number 1 buck sounds, shoots, and kills exactly like a 22 long rifle. #1 buck weighs 40 grains. A 22 short case holds about 2-1/2 grains of powder. You will get nearly 3000 rounds out of a pound of powder.

There are:	Works in:
340 #4 buck / lb.,	.22,.243,6mm.
300 #3 buck / lb.,	.257 or .25 cal.
175 #1 buck / lb.,	7mm to .30 cal.
145 #0 buck / lb.,	8mm & .32cal.
130 #00 buck/ lb.,	.33 cal.
100 #000 buck/lb.,	9mm,.357,&.38 cal.
50 #45 cal buck/lb.,	.44 & .45 cal.

A 22 short or 22 long rifle case full of powder is about right for nearly all cartridges. Use a fast shotgun powder. Use the buckshot as is and press it in flush with the mouth of the case.

Wood dowel rods make good bullets for close range. Saw the dowel into bullet sized pieces. They tend to explode inside the victim. Keep the the velocity down or they will explode in mid air. They seem to work best ar pistol velocities of 800-1000 feet per second.

Plastics make rotten bullets. Forget them. Bolts with the heads cut off make good bullets in a pinch but will ruin the accuracy of a rifled barrel so use them only when nothing else can be found or in zip guns.

You have probably heard of Dum-Dums. They are simply bullets with a deep "X" cut into the nose. They blow frightful holes in people and animals. They only work if the bullet is going faster than 1000 feet per second. Most pistol cartridges won't work. The lyman manual tells the velocity of factory cartridges. Hollow points seldom work below 1000 feet per second also.

Bullets with a copper or brass jacket are easy to make. Copper tubing and fired 22 rimfire cases make good jackets. You can also buy jackets. Even if you buy the jackets the bullets still cost less than one third of what bought bullets cost and are as good or better. Dave Corbin is the best expert to consult here. Send $5 to Corbin Manufacturing and Supply, Box 758, Phoenix, Oregon 97535 for their Bullet Swedge Manual and Catalog. Their manual tells it in plain language how to begin.

Now that you have done some reloading for your rifle, pistol, or shotgun, you can start dreaming up your own special purpose loads with a reasonable amount of safety.

An excellent Velex type special purpose round can be made by drilling a 7/32 inch or number 2 drill bit hole in the nose of a .30 cal. or larger bullet. Pull the bullet from a 22 rimfire cartridge. Press the 22 case, powder and all, into the nose of the bullet until the rim of the case touches the bullet. A 22 short works best and is a must for short pistol bullets but a 22 long rifle will work in long bullets. For a bigger bang put some more explosive in the 22 case. Be careful of the explosive that you use. Sensitive explosives may go off in the barrel of the gun. The four that I like are nitrocellulose, picric acid, blank powder from noise making cartridges, and pistol smokeless or black gun powder. Never use blank powder for any reloading. It is the fastest burning gunpowder by far and even the lightest bullet may raise pressure high enough to blow up the gun. The Velex type bullet will explode on impact yet is safe enough to carry.

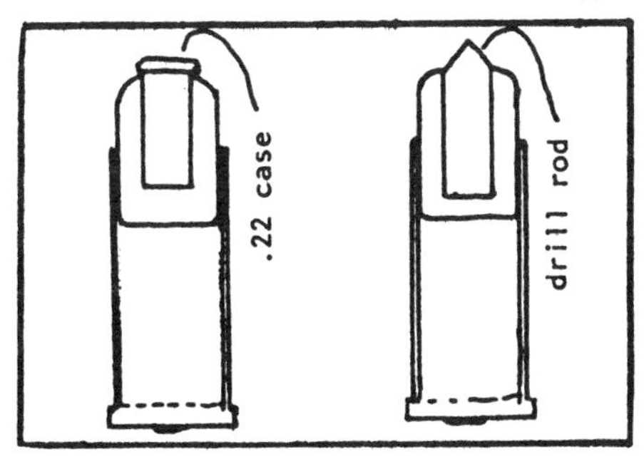

An excellent armor piercing round is made as follows: .22 cal. = 3/16" drill rod. .30 cal.=1/4" drill rod. 8mm = 1/4". 9mm and 38 cal.= 5/16" drill rod. .44 &.45 cal.= 3/8" drill rod. Buy hardened drill rod from a welder or machine shop in the correct diameter. It is very hard. Nick the rod with a triangle file and hold the end in a pair of pliers or vise and snap the rod off like breaking a piece of glass. This stuff is too hard to file and will rapidly dull a file while trying to nick it. Cutting it with a cold chisel is also difficult. If you have a bench grinder carefully grind a point on the rod before snapping off the piece. Don't get the rod hot or you will soften it. Dip it in water often and work slow. Grind the point quite sharp with about a 45° angle to it. This works much much better than leaving the front flat, but you cannot file it, so if you don't have a grinder, tough luck.

Part III

Powder Charges:

Currently there are over 50 different smokeless powders on the market. Included here is a list of 42 powders that I have experimented with and arranged in their approximate burning order from fast at the top to slow at the bottom. This list is only correct by my experiences so a few powders may be slightly out of place.

Find the section in the Lyman manual running from .30 carbine to .300 magnum. Notice that the larger the cartridge case, the slower the powder that works best. Notice also that the heavier the bullet in a particular case, the slower the powder that works best. .243 Win., .308 Win., and .358 Win. all use the same cartridge case. Notice that the larger the caliber the heavier the bullet or faster the powder that works best. That is why 12 gauge shotgun which is .70 caliber, takes a very fast powder. 2-3/4" is very short for a .70 cal bore. So, the larger the case for a given caliber, the slower the powder. The heavier the bullet, the slower the powder.

The powder chart can be used for powder substitution. Say you have load data for IMR-4895 but you want to use the much cheaper H-335. H-335 is faster than IMR-4895 so you must reduce the powder charge. Most manuals will list the very popular IMR-3031. It is faster than H-335, so use the same weight of H-335 and work the load up slowly to safe limits as described in the Lyman manual. When substituting a faster powder, decrease the weight of the powder. When substituting a slower powder, Increase the powder weight.

So much for experimenting with factory smokeless powder. How about making your own. You have to be a genius to make smokeless powder. If you want to try it, read Chemistry of Powder and Explosives and Gunpowder in Britannica Encyclopedia. Black Gunpowder is safe to use in all modern cartridges and most improvised cartridges. Black powder is easy to make. Many formulas are given in PMJB and the Britannica Encyclopedia. Black powder is very dangerous to make. The slightest static or metallic spark and BOOM .

Match heads and match head compositions make good gunpowder. Crush the heads if you want them to burn faster. Most firecracker compositions work fine. Some cannon cracker compositions are very fast so be careful. Flash cracker compositions are also fast. Nearly any mixture that burns violently without detonating will work. Anything that detonates like fulminates and high explosives will certainly blow up the gun.

FAST BURNING

Blank Powder
Hercules Bullseye
Hodgdon HP-38
Dupont Unique
Dupont P B
Hercules Red Dot
Hodgdon Trap-100
Winchester 452AA
Winchester 473AA
Dupont SR7625
Dupont SR4756
Alcan AL5
Hodgdon HS-6
Winchester 540
Winchester 571

Hodgdon HS-7
Hercules #2400
Winchester 296
Hodgdon H-110
Hodgdon H-4227
Dupont IMR-4227
Norma N-200
Hodgdon H-4198
Dupont IMR-4198
Dupont IMR-3031
Norma N-201
Norma N-203
Dupont IMR-4064
Hodgdon BL-C(2)

Hodgdon H-335
Hodgdon H-4895
Dupont IMR-4895
Hodgdon H-380
Hodgdon H-414
Dupont IMR-4350
Norma N-204
Hodgdon H-450
Hodgdon H-4831
Dupont IMR-4831
Norma N-205
Hodgdon H-570
Hodgdon H-870

SLOW BURNING

Editor's Note:

Velet Ammo Co. is now selling Mercury filled exploding bullets. See Issue #3, pg. 36 for address.

MINE DETONATOR

BY FRED B.

Supplies
1-piece of hardwood, about 1½"x½"x3/4"
1-piece of hardwood, about 2"x 1"x1"
1-strip of tension steel, about 3"x1"
The Bates MFG. Co. of Orange, NJ makes a steel ruler that will do. The stock # is BNR-12. It can be bought in most stores.
1-roofing nail
1-nail about 1" long
String
4-¼ " wood screws
1-bullet

1. Drill 4 small holes at the bottom of the tension steel. Drill 2 of them 3/8" from the bottom and the other 2 3/4" from the bottom. If you are using the ruler there will be no problem.
2. Snip all but ¼" off the roofing nail, and file it to a point. Solder or glue it ¼" from the top of the tension steel. This is the firing pin. See fig. 1.
3. Cut and drill the 1½" piece of wood as illustrated in fig. 2. Secure the string to it. This is the trigger.
4. Drill a 3/4" hole through the center of the other piece of wood. File ½" grooves in the front and rear of the hole. Then using the 1" nail as an axle/pivot, hammer it into the side until the point just pokes through the hole. Place the trigger into the hole and hammer the nail through the hole in the trigger. It should easily rock back and forth at least 30° each way.
5. Screw the firing pin to the front of the block.

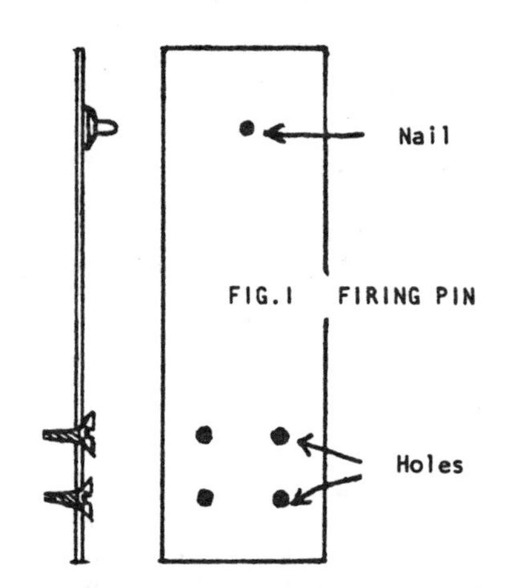

FIG.1 FIRING PIN

To utilize this device, remove the business end from the bullet and put a small wad of paper in the cartridge to keep the powder in. Then insert the cartridge into the explosive, align the firing pin so it will strike the primer, and set the mechanism. To detonate, pull the string.

FIG.2 - TRIGGER

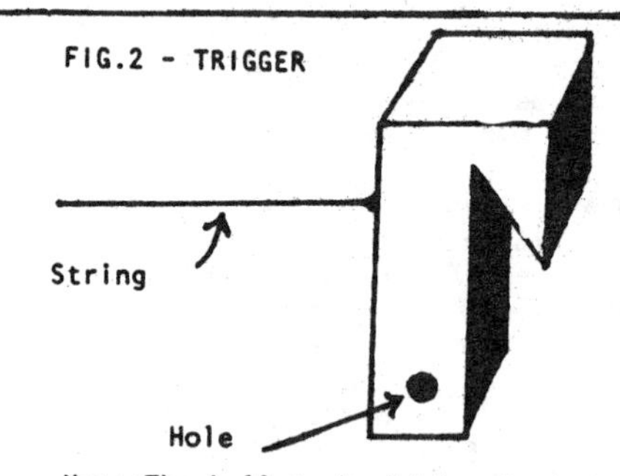

Note: The bullet should be slanted downward with a 1" metal tube extending from it, blocked at the end with paper, so that the flash sets the charge off at the bottom middle. Better yet, put the detonator below the charge so the bullet rests at the bottom.

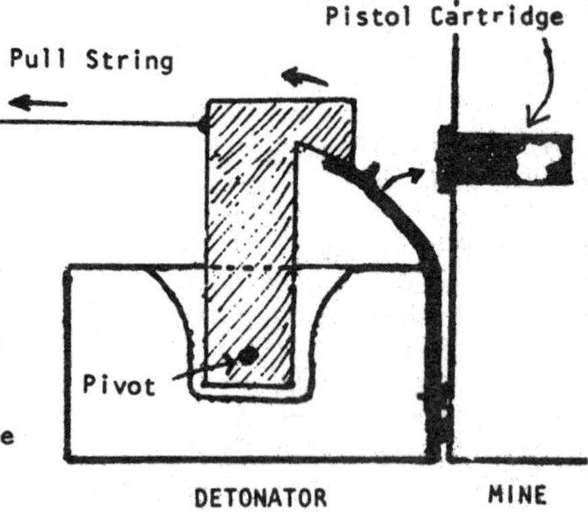

CAP-CHUR ACCESSORIES

CAP CHUR GUNS

BY CLYDE BARROW

The following material is reprinted from the 1976-1977 Nasco Farm and Ranch Catalog.

The system, including guns, blanks, charges, darts and sedatives, is intended for use in subduing or medicating both wild and domestic animals. Other possible uses are left to your imagination.

All three guns appear to be overpriced and future issues will deal with converting an air pistol to fire Cap Chur darts. The darts and Cap Chur charges are both good buys for the price, are well made and can be used as the basis of several types of improvised systems. More specific info on this in a later issue.

Note: Gun #3 appears to be a 28 gauge H & R shotgun. The adapter, part # C4425N, is basically a shell shrinker, (28 gauge to 22LR). The front carries a screw on extension that holds the darts away from the flash of the blank, thus preventing burnt tail feathers. Every item listed is available by mail from either of the two Nasco stores.

Note: The Cap Chur charges contain black powder and cannot be mailed parcel post.Catalog 50¢.

Nasco; 901 Janesville Ave, Fort Atkinson, WIS. 53538 or P.O.Box 3837 Princeton Ave., Modesto, CALIF. 95352.

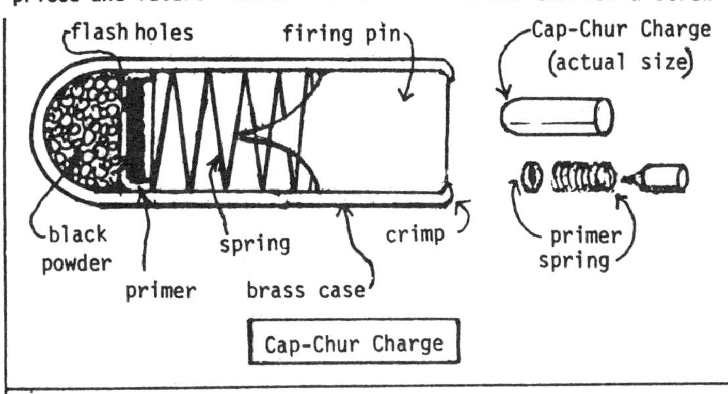

CAP-CHUR ACCESSORIES AND REPLACEMENT PARTS

PLUNGER LUBRICANT
For lubrication of rubber plunger inside of syringe.
C1601N Per tube $2.00

EXTRA PUSH ROD AND POSITIONER
For preparing syringes. Sh. wt. 1 oz.
C1223N $2.00

HEAVY DUTY VINYL GUN CASE
Fits either powder fired or pneumatic rifle. Sh. wt. 2 lbs.
C1225N $20.00

VINYL CASE
For pistol. Sh. wt. ¾ lb.
C5669N $8.80

EXTRA ADAPTER FOR POWDER FIRED GUN
C4425N $12.00

SYRINGE PARTS

NEEDLES
¾'' needle normally used on dogs, 1'' to 1½'' normally used on cattle, deer, etc.

BARBED NEEDLES
C4232N ¾'' needle — C4233N 1-1/8'' needle — C4234N 1½'' needle
Each $3.00

PLAIN NEEDLES
C4574N ¾'' needle — C4222N 1-1/8'' needle — C4223N 1¼'' needle
C4575N 1'' needle — C4224N 1½'' needle
Each $3.00

COLLARED NEEDLES
C4227N 1-1/8'' needle — C4229N 1½'' needle — C4230N 1¾'' needle
C4228N 1¼'' needle
Each $3.00

NEEDLES FOR LARGE THICK SKINNED ANIMALS
C5844N 1¼'' needle — C5845N 1½'' needle — C5846N 1¾'' needle
Each $3.80

EXTRA RUBBER PLUNGER
Fits any of the syringe sizes.
C4239N $1.50

BARRELS

C4235N 1cc	$1.45	C4236AN 5cc	$2.00
C6808N 2cc	1.55	C6810N 7cc	2.30
C4236N 3cc	1.65	C4237N 10cc	2.65
C6809N 4cc	1.80	C4237AN 15cc	6.05

TAIL PIECE
Fits any size Cap-Chur syringe.
C4238N $2.30

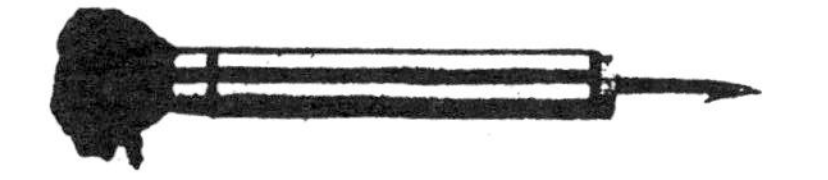

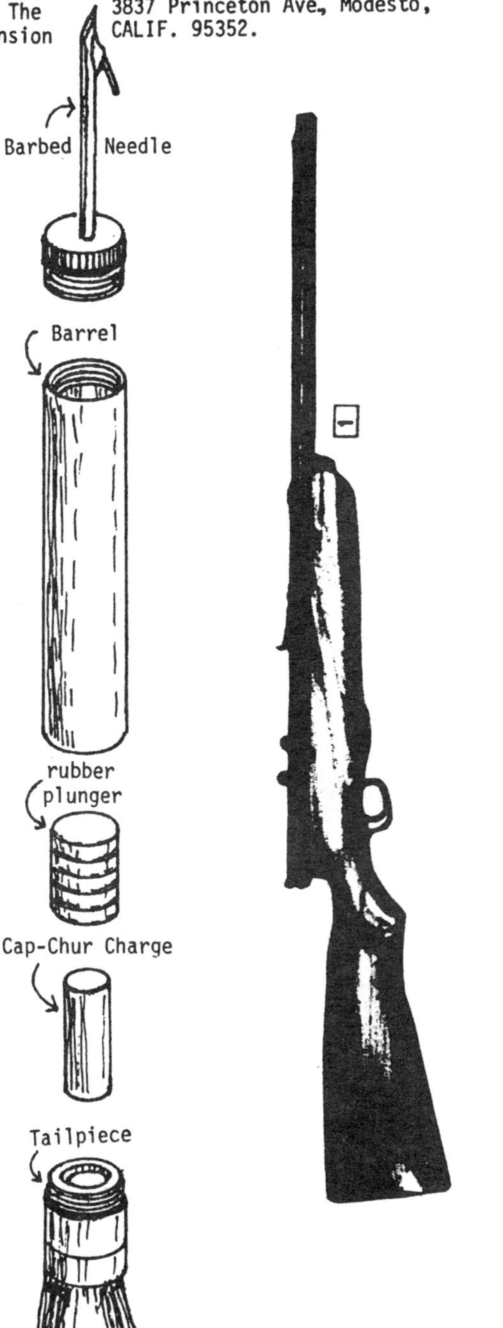

CAP-CHUR EQUIPMENT

The world famous system for immobilizing or medicating wild or domestic animals. A patented method for injecting any fluid drug into an animal from distances up to 80 yards – safely, accurately and instantaneously. The drug we offer is for the purpose of immobilizing an animal for easy capture or handling, but any liquid medicine or drug recommended by your veterinarian may be used with this equipment.

The weapons propel a unique patented syringe which carries the drug. On impact with the animal, a small explosive charge within the syringe instantaneously discharges the fluid through the needle and into the muscle tissue. Syringes are available in sizes ranging from 1cc to 15cc, and are reusable.

This equipment is being used with great success, throughout the world, on both wild and domestic animals. Dramatic and highly publicized uses tend to overshadow the fact that it is an indispensable everyday working tool for domestic livestock producers, police departments, veterinarians, wildlife managers, biologists and zoo personnel.

Three types of projectors are available: a long range projector fired by a powder charge quite similar to a conventional firearm, but with special adaption to handle the syringe; a long range pneumatic powered (CO_2) projector; and a short range pneumatic powered pistol type projector.

PROJECTORS

LONG RANGE PROJECTOR – RIFLE TYPE (CO_2 powered)

1. Specially designed pneumatic rifle that fires patented Cap-Chur syringe. The 2 small CO_2 cylinders inserted into the rifle will discharge the rifle approximately 10 times.

Can be successfully used at distances up to about 35 yards, but most effective at 25 to 30 yard range.

The lower velocity of this unit minimizes danger of injury to animals resulting from the physical impact of the syringe. Bolt Action. Specially designed barrel. Sh. wt. 8½ lbs.

C1219N $180.00

SHORT RANGE PROJECTOR – PISTOL TYPE (CO_2 powered)

2 A specially designed pistol powered by CO_2 gas. Effective range up to about 40 feet. Approximately 25 shots per CO_2 cylinder. Well balanced. Easy to load. Convenient to use. Sh. wt. 2¾ lbs.

C1220N $125.00

EXTRA LONG RANGE PROJECTOR – RIFLE TYPE (Powder fired)

3. Has the look and feel of a conventional sporting weapon. Fires any one of 3 special .22 caliber blank powder loads depending upon the range desired. The syringe is loaded at the breech and the metal adapter which holds the blank cartridge is inserted behind it. May be used at ranges from 10 to 80 yds. See description of .22 blank powder loads for ranges each will provide.

Care must be exercised to be sure the proper load is used for the range desired. The use of the heavy loads at very short ranges may cause impact damage to thin skinned or light muscled animals. Sh. wt. 9 lbs.

C4240N $175.00

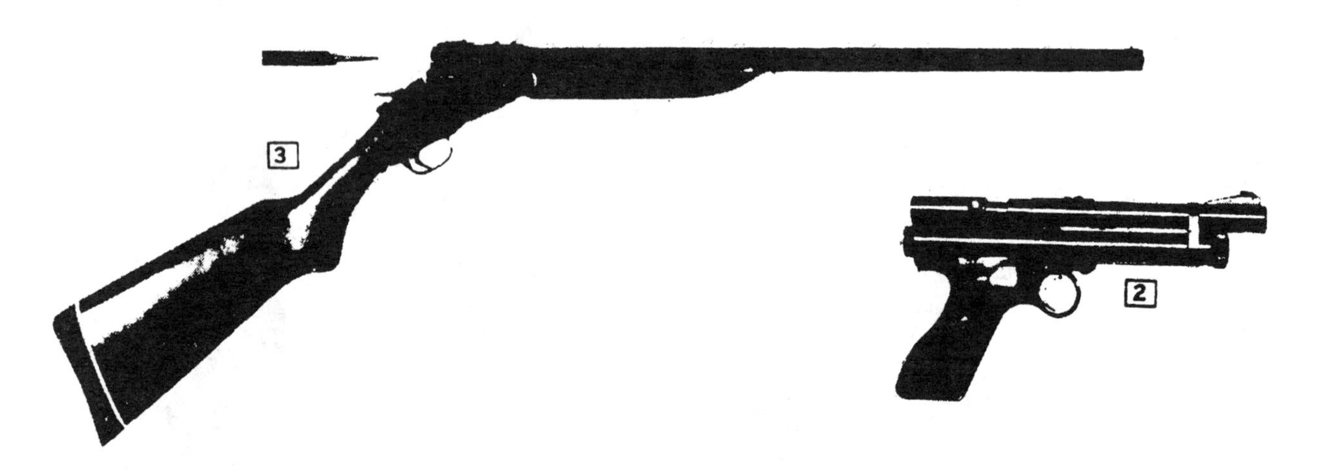

CAP-CHUR SOL – IMMOBILIZING DRUG

Cap-Chur Sol is the most rapid acting immobilizer available. Total immobilization usually occurs in from 2 to 10 minutes. Dizziness and lack of visual coordination may occur in as short a time as 30 seconds so that the animal will normally not move far after injection. Best results are usually obtained by making the injection in the muscular area of the hindquarters on larger animals. The dosages prescribed are for intramuscular or intraperitoneal injection.

Cap-Chur Sol contains nicotine alkaloids and is a poison. It is designed for intramuscular injection and should not be administered orally.

WARNING – EXTREME CAUTION SHOULD BE EXERCISED TO AVOID INJECTION OR SWALLOWING BY HUMAN BEINGS. Read instructions carefully.

The approximate correct dosage should be administered to an animal at one time. One injection of Cap-Chur Sol tends to induce a resistance to a second given very shortly after, or in some cases the second may induce a fatal reaction. 48 hours should lapse before a second injection.

Animals, just as humans, vary in their reaction to any drug. Consequently, caution must always be exercised.

This drug is offered in a wide range of concentrations in terms of milligrams per cc of the fluid, and this is then related to the weight of animals to be injected. A 1cc dose is used on small animals such as dogs, and 3cc on cattle and other large animals.

Cap-Chur Sol is effective on most animals, both wild and domestic. However, it **SHOULD NOT BE USED ON HOGS OR CATS.**

The following Cap-Chur Sol dosages are offered as a general guide for use

CAP-CHUR SOL – FOR CATTLE AND LARGE ANIMALS
30cc bottles – Sh. wt. 4 oz. – INJECTION 3cc DOSE

C1244AN 165mg per cc – for 330 lb. (150 kilos) animals $5.20
C1244BN 220mg per cc – for 440 lb. (200 kilos) animals 5.60
C1244CN 275mg per cc – for 550 lb. (249 kilos) animals 6.00
C1244DN 330mg per cc – for 660 lb. (299 kilos) animals 6.40
C1244EN 385mg per cc – for 770 lb. (349 kilos) animals 6.80
C1244FN 440mg per cc – for 880 lb. (399 kilos) animals 7.20
C1244GN 495mg per cc – for 990 lb. (449 kilos) animals 7.60
C1244HN 550mg per cc – for 1100 lb. (488 kilos) animals 8.00
C1244JN 605mg per cc – for 1210 lb. (549 kilos) animals 8.40
C1244KN 660mg per cc – for 1320 lb. (599 kilos) animals 8.80
C1244MN 770mg per cc – for 1540 lb. (699 kilos) animals 9.60

CAP-CHUR SOL – FOR DOGS AND SMALL ANIMALS
30cc bottles – Sh. wt. 4 oz. – INJECT 1cc DOSE

C1245AN 30mg per cc – for 10 lb. (5.5 kilos) animals $2.50
C1245BN 45mg per cc – for 15 lb. (6.8 kilos) animals 2.70
C1245CN 60mg per cc – for 20 lb. (9.0 kilos) animals 2.90
C1245DN 75mg per cc – for 25 lb. (11.3 kilos) animals 3.10
C1245FN 90mg per cc – for 30 lb. (13.6 kilos) animals 3.30
C1245HN 120mg per cc – for 40 lb. (18.1 kilos) animals 3.50
C1245JN 150mg per cc – for 50 lb. (22.6 kilos) animals 3.70
C1245KN 195mg per cc – for 60 lb. (27.2 kilos) animals 3.90
C1245MN 240mg per cc – for 80 lb. (36.3 kilos) animals 4.10
C1245NN 285mg per cc – for 95 lb. (43.1 kilos) animals 4.30

on animals for which we do not list specific concentrations for varying body weights.

Dosage in milligrams per pound of body weight:

Dogs	2 to 4	Sheep	2 to 4
Cattle	1 to 2	Goats	2 to 4
Deer	3 to 4		

There is no antidote for Cap-Chur Sol; however, Hydrocortisone Acetate may be used to relieve some of the shock and stress resulting from an injection. The recommended application is 50 milligrams per 100 lbs. of body weight.

Under certain circumstances an animal may be adversely affected by the Cap-Chur Sol drug. It must be remembered that the administration of any drug can be dangerous. For example, animals or humans occasionally react unfavorably to most any drug. But in general there is far less danger and stress on the animal, less cost and less danger to the operator with the use of Cap-Chur equipment than any form of mechanical restraint such as roping.

CAP-CHUR SOL – STOCK SOLUTIONS
30cc bottle – Sh. wt. 4 oz.

C6811N 100mg per cc	$3.00		C6815N 500mg per cc	$ 7.00
C6812N 200mg per cc	4.00		C6816N 600mg per cc	8.00
C6813N 300mg per cc	5.00		C6817N 800mg per cc	9.00
C6814N 400mg per cc	6.00		C6818N 1000mg per cc	10.00

MONOJECT DISPOSABLE SYRINGE WITH NEEDLE
Made of polypropylene, a nontoxic plastic, compatible with all known medications. Sterile Monoject needles and syringes are ready for use anywhere, and can be autoclaved in their sealed polypropylene containers. Capacity 3cc. Gauge & length 20 x 1". Graduation 1/10cc. Minims.
C4124N Per 100 .... $10.45

TUBERCULIN SYRINGE
Disposable 1cc syringe with 5/8" needle is excellent for measuring exact proportions to put in Cap-Chur syringes. Features 1/100th cc graduations.
C6802N-501-TB Per 10 .... $1.65

All Cap-Chur equipment and supplies are available for immediate shipment from Nasco. Your orders will be processed without delay.

Our staff is experienced in the use of this equipment and is able to answer your questions. Simply call the nearest Nasco office if you need assistance.
NASCO Fort Atkinson, Wisconsin 414 563-2446 NASCO-WEST Modesto, California 209 529-6957

Prices quoted here are from 1977 and are undoubtedly much higher now.

Unless you are affiliated with your police department or a close friend of your local veterinarian, you might have trouble getting these materials. I suggest you call one of the above numbers and claim to be your area's poundmaster. When you call, you might say something like this: "Hello. I'm (your name) the poundmaster for (your town) and we're having trouble with dog packs. Some are homeless and pretty wild and some are pets. We can't get close enough to use the noose and we don't want to shoot them. Our local vet referred you to me and I'd like a brochure on your line of capture darts and equipment". The firm will send you a brochure and you can order with no trouble. Of course, don't say exactly what I've written but put it in your own words.

FRICTION DETONATOR

BY FRED BILELLO

Supplies:
- one box of stick matches
- string
- scotch tape
- glue
- one heavy paper grocery bag

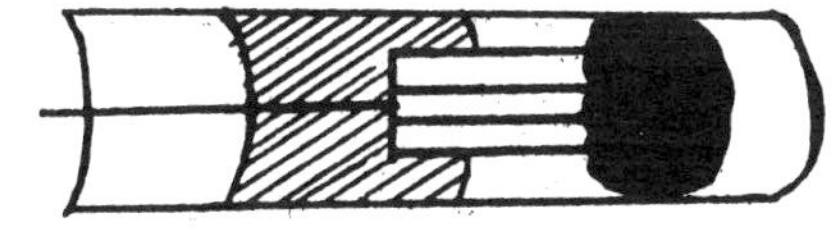

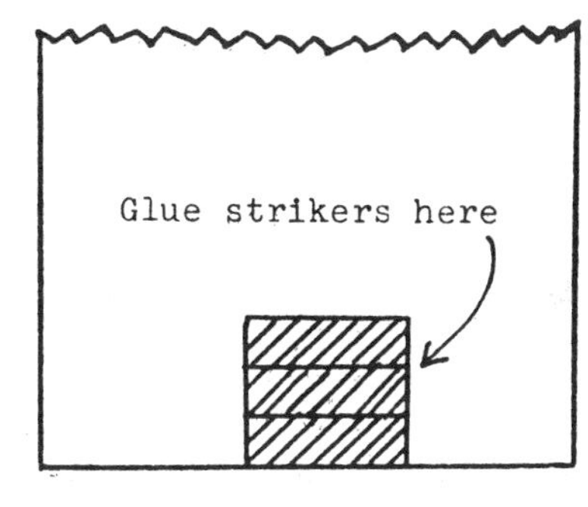

Step 1
Make a giant match by taking 3 stick matches and cut all but 1/2" of the wood off. Tie them together with a long string, wrap scotch tape around it, and set it aside. Then pick the white heads off of about 25 stick matches and put them in a glass ashtray. Add a couple of drops of water and lightly mash them with a spoon. Pack this paste around the 3 matches and set the arrangement on the ashtray like a cigarette, turning it occasionally. It will dry hard.

GIANT MATCH

string

Step 2
Cut 3 pieces of the striker into 3/4" strips and peel as much of the paper off the back as you can. Then cut a length of paper from the bag about 2 1/2" long and 6" wide. Glue the strikers, side by side, in the middle of the 2 1/2" side of the paper, starting at one side.

Step 3
Lay the match on the paper, with the match head being about 1/4" above the striker. Then roll the whole thing into a tube and glue it closed. The tube should be tight enough to hold the match in place, but not tight enough to grip the match. When you pull the string, the match will slide over the striker, ignite, and send a violent jet of flame out of the tube. Your cost is about 3¢.

This detonator should be inserted in a metal tube and is used in manually detonated mines. If you reverse the match position and lengthen the sticks, it can be used to explode flying bombs.

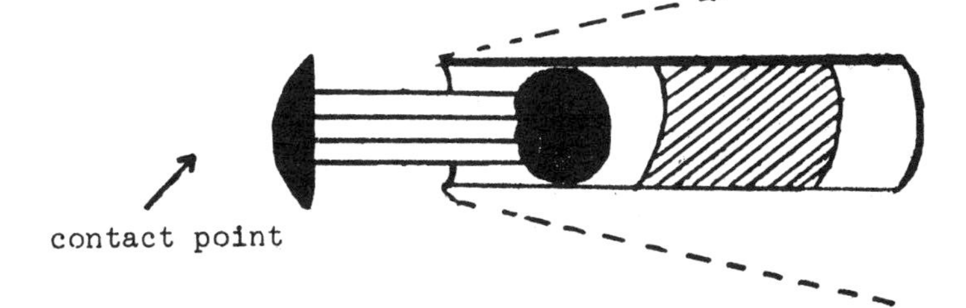

Cutaway view of friction detonator (used to detonate flying bombs)

DART CATAPULT

BY CLYDE BARROW

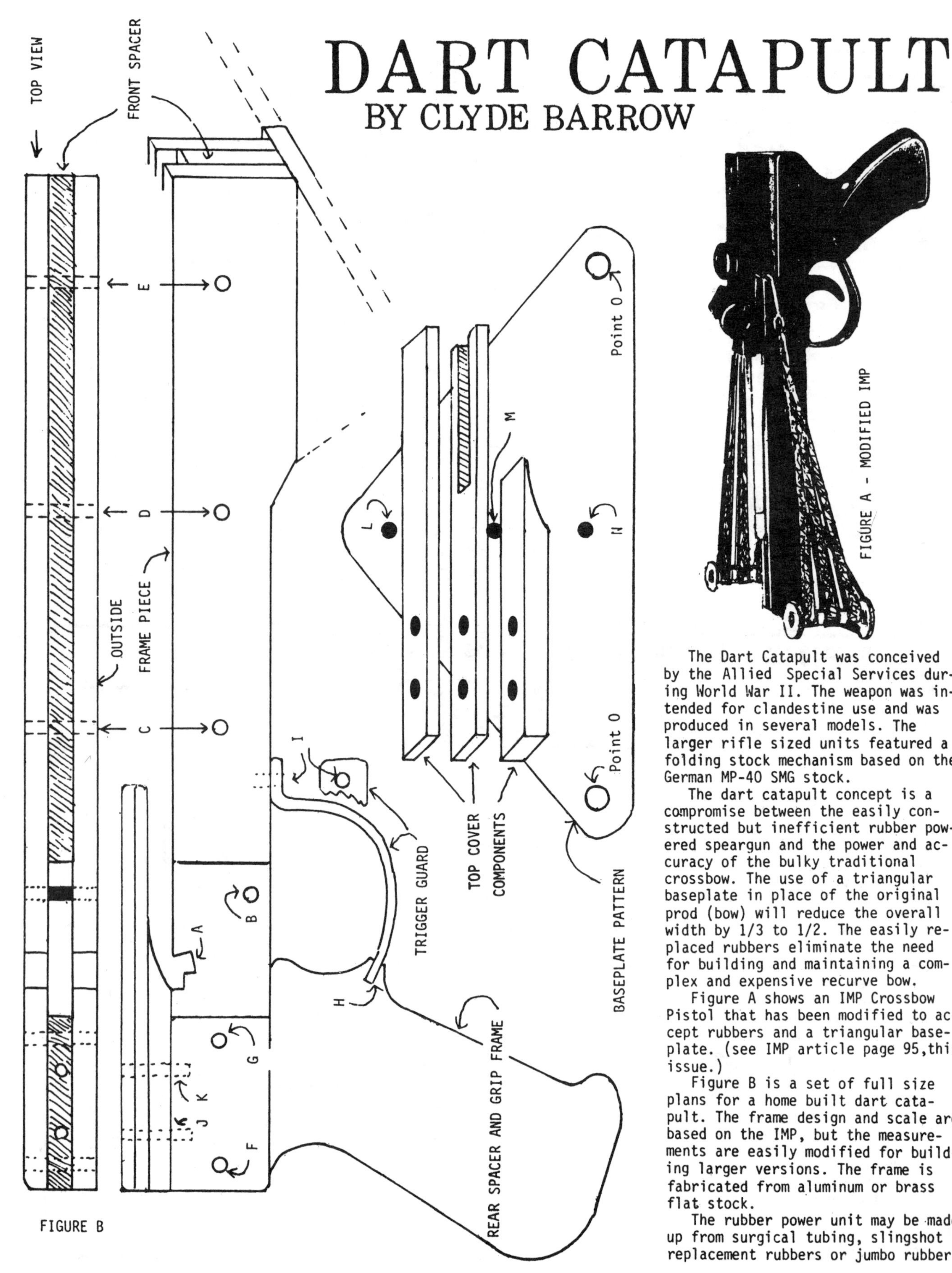

FIGURE B

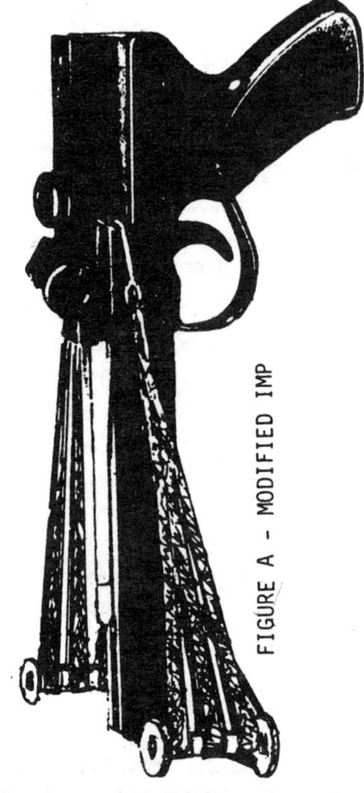

FIGURE A - MODIFIED IMP

The Dart Catapult was conceived by the Allied Special Services during World War II. The weapon was intended for clandestine use and was produced in several models. The larger rifle sized units featured a folding stock mechanism based on the German MP-40 SMG stock.

The dart catapult concept is a compromise between the easily constructed but inefficient rubber powered speargun and the power and accuracy of the bulky traditional crossbow. The use of a triangular baseplate in place of the original prod (bow) will reduce the overall width by 1/3 to 1/2. The easily replaced rubbers eliminate the need for building and maintaining a complex and expensive recurve bow.

Figure A shows an IMP Crossbow Pistol that has been modified to accept rubbers and a triangular baseplate. (see IMP article page 95,this issue.)

Figure B is a set of full size plans for a home built dart catapult. The frame design and scale are based on the IMP, but the measurements are easily modified for building larger versions. The frame is fabricated from aluminum or brass flat stock.

The rubber power unit may be made up from surgical tubing, slingshot replacement rubbers or jumbo rubber bands.

STEP 1

Cut the two outside frame pieces from ¼" flat stock. Carefully align edges and clamp together for steps 2 and 3.

STEP 2

Cut the cocking notch in the frame pieces at A. Increase the angle of the undercut for rugged field use. Decrease angle to near verticle for a target type "hair trigger."

STEP 3

The front spacer is cut from ¼" stock and is positioned between frame halves until all three bottom and front edges are aligned. (There should now be a ¼" x ¼" channel along the top edge of the frame.) Clamp pieces together and drill 1/8" diameter holes through all three pieces at points B-E. Hole B is for a press fit trigger pin so a slightly undersized drill may be used if available. Holes C-E may be threaded for machine screws or 1/8" bolts and nuts may be used to fasten the three pieces together.

STEP 4

Cut the trigger pin from 1/8" diameter drill rod. The trigger is made from ¼" flat stock. Cut two shims from an old credit card or similar plastic sheet. Use a sanding block to reduce trigger width until the trigger and two shims are a wobble free fit in the frame. Align with hole B and tap pin in place. If the pin is not a secure fit, a drop of Loctite at each end will hold it in place.

STEP 5

Build the rear spacer/grip frame from ¼" metal sheet. If the gun will receive light duty only, ¼" plywood or other non metal materials may be used. Custom grips can be used or this frame's shape may be altered to accept spare pistol grips on hand. Use a saw or file to cut slot H in grip frame before installing grips.

STEP 6

The trigger guard is cut from 1/8" stock and is ¼" wide. Bend to the shape indicated and trim off the excess length. Insert the rear of guard into slot H. Drill 1/8" hole at point I and screw guard to frame.

STEP 7

Construct top cover from individual pieces and assemble as shown. Note arrow stop slot on underside. Drill 1/8" holes at J & K and install top cover on the frame.

STEP 8

The 3"x6" triangular base plate should be cut from 3/16" (minimum) brass. Thickness should be at least ¼" if aluminum is used. Drill 1/8" holes L, M, and N in the plate. Use the base plate as a template to mark the bottom of the center piece (front spacer) on the frame. Edge of base plate should be flush with front of frame. Thread holes and coat screws with Loctite before installing plate to frame. If you are using bolts and nuts for assembly, the bolts must be inserted from the top down into the arrow track. The front spacer (bottom of the track) should be counter drilled to allow the bolt heads to fit flush and not obstruct the track.

STEP 9

Drill a ¼" hole at each end of the base plate (points O). Install the two ¼"x2" bolts with 1" OD washers and jam nuts as shown. These are the mount points for the rubber power units.

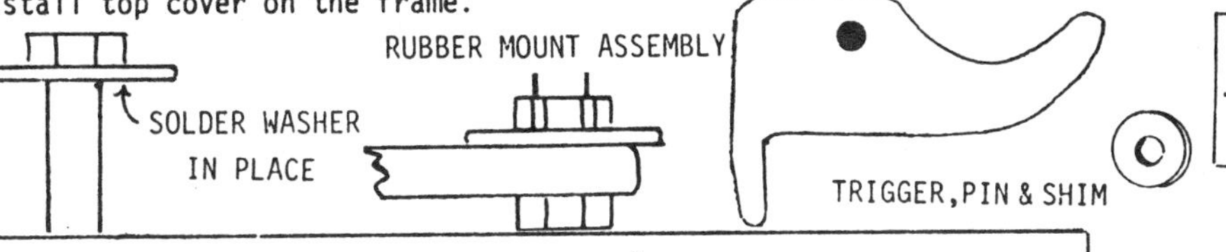

PRODUCT REVIEW

'IMP' PISTOL CROSSBOW

This compact little crossbow was originally designed for indoor use. With our new 30 lb draw weight glass-fibre prod, target and flight shooting out of doors becomes an exciting venture. The extremely fast recoil of the prod casts the bolt a minimum of 50 yards.

The IMP Pistol Crossbow features a two piece cast aluminum frame, plastic grips, fiberglass prod (bow) and fully adjustable rear sights. The aluminum trigger should be shimmed on both sides with nylon washers to eliminate wobble.

The crossbow is 10½" long and 5½" tall. The prod measures 12" across when strung and in the uncocked position. The child size grips should be lengthened about 1" by taping or gluing a wood or plastic block to the bottom. There is no provision for a safety so bolts (arrows) should not be inserted until you are ready to fire. The two bolts provided are brittle plastic and should be replaced with ones made of fiberglass or aluminum.

The design of this crossbow is the basis for the dart catapult project on page 92 and may be used instead of beginning from scratch.

The IMP Crossbow sells for about $30 and is available from one of the sources listed below. Order both catalogs as they contain info on several crossbows, books, crossbow components, replacement bolts,etc.

Crossbowman (USA), Box 2159, Petaluma, CAL 94952. Catalog 25¢.

B.&P. Barnett (Canada), 93 Ashbury Ave., London, Ont. N6E 1T3, Tel.(519) 681-6482. Catalog 50¢.

INDEX

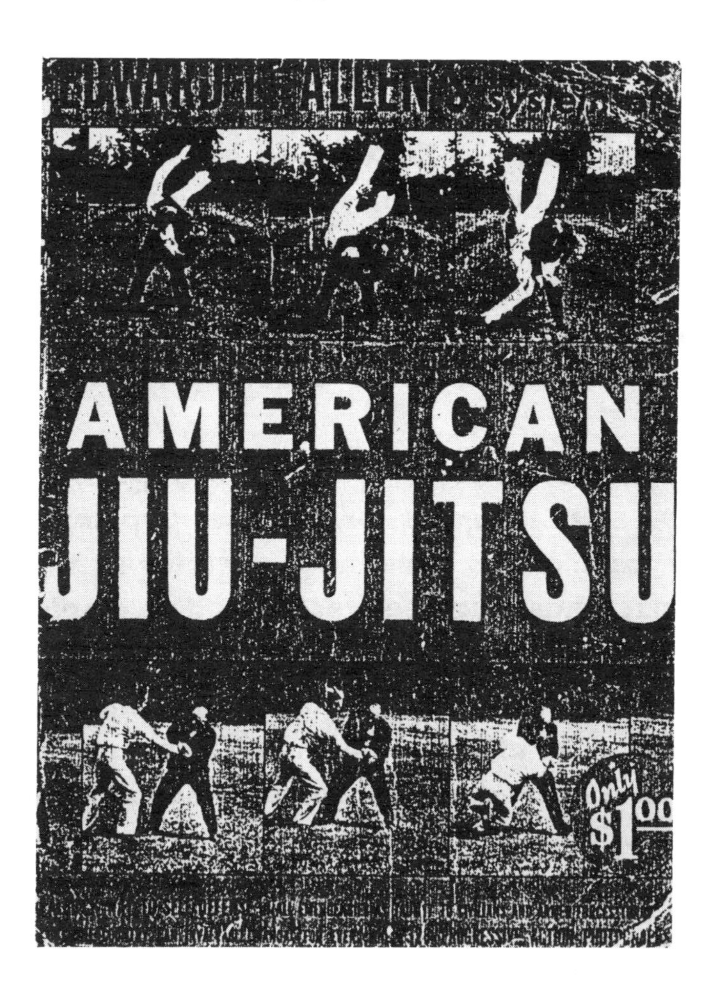

Edward L. Allen's system of Jiu-Jitsu (Now known as Judo) is one of the oldest and most basic of the martial arts. This course is the simplest, designed for the rank amateur with no previous experience in any sort of combat. It was taught in this manner to America's service men. The idea, from the Army's point of view, was to train them fast and get them to the front. It obviously worked, as many reports came back from the Pacific that in hand-to-hand encounters with the Japanese, the good big man was better than the good little man.

As was necessary in those days, this course is without frills or ceremony. Just get in there and take the man out as quickly as possible. And this is what you want, at least to start with.

When the moves in this basic course are mastered, you can handle just about any situation which might put you at risk. Later, if you want to go professional, you will find it much easier to adapt to any of the more complex martial arts.

I would suggest, at first, you make an agreement with a friend to spend at least two hours a day in practice for one month. This is all the time it should take you both to master this course. Then, you and your partner will be proficient enough to start a school. There is a pressing need for this course among all classes of our population. Most people who feel a need to protect themselves from muggers and such simply don't have the time or the inclination to go higher. This is your market.

AMERICAN JIU-JITSU

For 20 years I have studied and taught Jiu-Jitsu. My students have been city and state policemen, business men, soldiers, housewives, college students, penitentiary guards, private and industrial policemen, Y.M.C.A. classes and householders. Sixteen year old boys and girls and sixty-five year old men and women; two hundred and fifty pounders and ninety pound lightweights have gained poise and confidence by acquiring the knowledge and skill of Jiu-Jitsu.

Whether the art originated, as some historians repeat, with ancient Chinese Monks forbidden to carry weapons, or, as more popularly believed, with the physically inferior Japanese as a means of overcoming their natural handicap in bodily encounters, it has long been recognized as a potent method of attack and defense.

In this book I teach you how to master the fundamental principles of Jiu-Jitsu and to acquire a variety of attacks and counter-attacks. I have chosen lessons easily understood and learned but which cover situations some of which are all too apt to occur within the experience of any or all of us. You can master these numbers!

A person with a knowledge of Jiu-Jitsu has the one ignorant of its mysteries almost completely at his mercy. There is a method of Jiu-Jitsu defense for every attack and a Jiu-Jitsu attack for every occasion. The size of the person attacking has little bearing on the outcome; the Jiu-Jitsu operator knows that the bigger they come the harder they fall.

Regardless of your weight and size you will be able to handle anyone not familiar with Jiu-Jitsu practices. Sometimes spoken of as the "gentle art", it is as gentle or as punishing as you care to make it or as the occasion demands. I hope that you will never have occasion to use one of the defenses seriously. You may, however, someday even save your life by applying one of the lessons of this book. The confidence that knowledge of this skill gives you will in itself carry you through situations which otherwise might be dangerous or embarassing.

As you study the lessons in this book please do not use your new power carelessly. Please remember that Jiu-Jitsu is not a game or sport. It is a serious weapon which gives to you, as its possessor, an immense advantage in physical encounters. Be considerate of your partner with whom you practice. When he indicates that you are hurting him relax or release your grip for, although you may be using but the fingers of one hand, a little pressure

skillfully applied can cause intense pain.

Published by
SUN DIAL PRESS
Copyright 1942
ALLAN J. HALL
BLOOMFIELD HILLS, MICH.

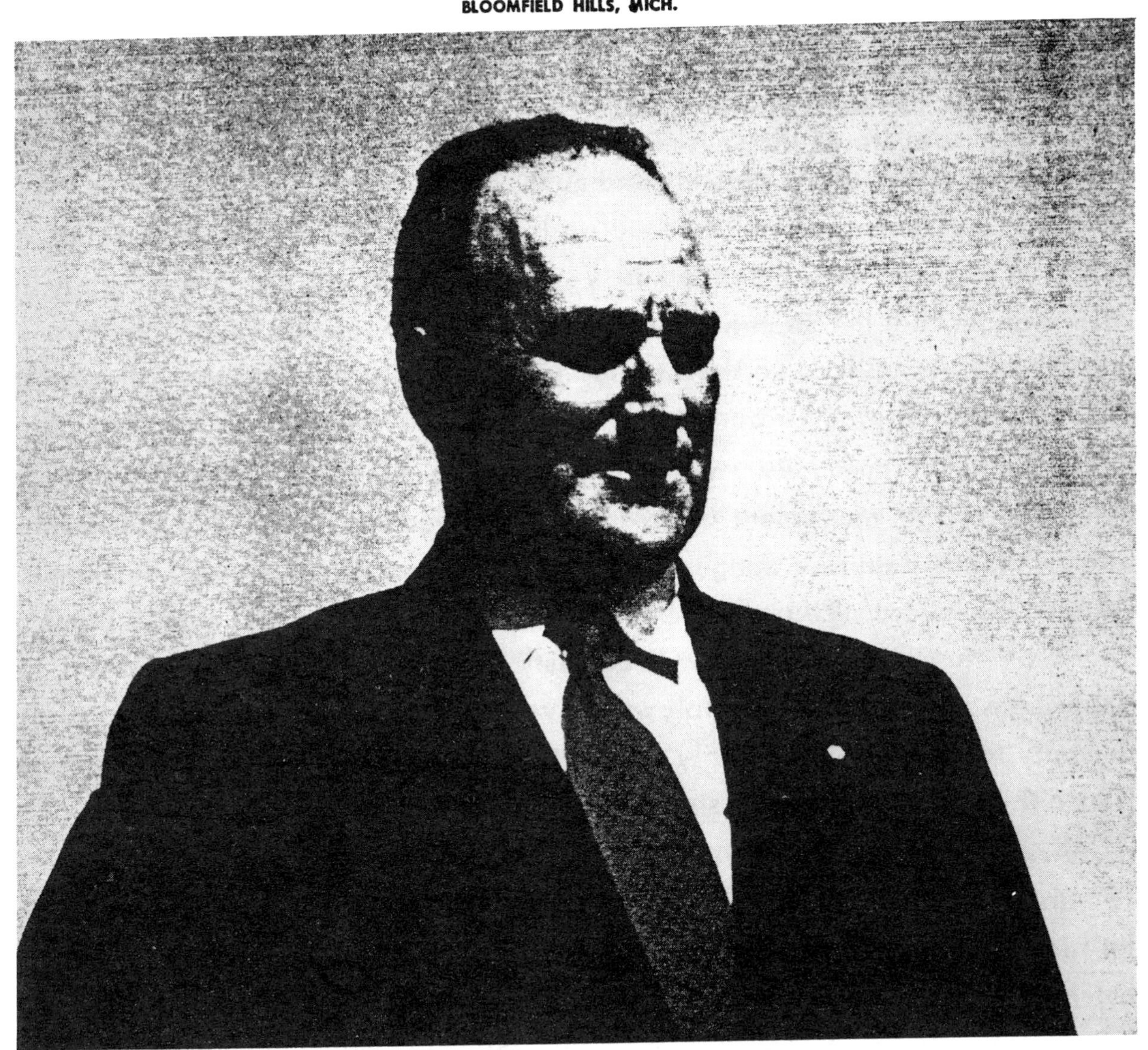

EDWARD L. ALLEN

Since Mr. Edward Allen began teaching Jiu-Jitsu twenty years ago he has taught thousands of law enforcement officers and law abiding citizens. He gives private lessons to single pupils and class lessons to hundreds. He teaches business men interested in Jiu-Jitsu as a means of keeping order in their establishments and officers eager to have this additional weapon at their command. Housewives making certain that they can repel possible intruders in their homes and soldiers preparing for foreign duty have learned Jiu-Jitsu from him.

He has instructed Y.M.C.A. classes in numerous cities, police and highway patrol officers in Pittsburgh, Detroit, and smaller cities, prison guards at the Ohio State Penitentiary, industrial guards of various large corporations, classes at the University of Michigan, many groups of business men and countless individuals.

Edward Allen, whose home is Akron, Ohio, gives many thrilling exhibitions every year to organizations interested in this ancient science. He has at his command more than two hundred different Jiu-Jitsu attacks and counterattacks which he demonstrates against any who will oppose him.

The success of his teaching efforts is attested by the many reports in metropolitan newspapers of incidents in which his students successfully used their Jiu-Jitsu to subdue unruly persons and even, on several occasions, to save lives.

Jiu-Jitsu is a system of self-defense and attack which consists of a series of holds, locks, and blows applied to various parts of an opponents' body in such manner that the strength and weight of the opponent, as well as that of the operator, is utilized so that additional movement or pressure will tend to dislocate a joint, break a bone, or otherwise cause the victim increasing pain.

The joints of the body have a distinctly limited movement. Any forced extension of this movement or pressure in a direction contrary to the normal motion means pain and danger to the joint or bone. Bend one of your fingers sharply backward. You won't bend it far before the pain becomes intense. That's all there is to Jiu-Jitsu. It consists of a well thought out system for applying such pressures and blows to your opponent. Pressure he attempts to apply to release himself only serves to make the painful grip more severe. Hence there is seldom much struggling against a lock properly applied.

Jiu-Jitsu experts depend upon three factors in subduing their assailants. The first one is "misdirection". Mislead your man as to your intentions. Do not let him anticipate your attack. The second is "off balance". Act quickly to catch and keep your opponent off balance. He'll help to throw himself if you do. It is just as important also that you keep your own balance at all times. The third factor is "leverage". Leverage makes it easily possible for a Jiu-Jitsu operator to subdue and hold an adversary twice his own size and strength.

In the lessons following I will point out the specific applications of each of these principles.

● ● ●

The two charts on the next page indicate the position of a number of the nerve centers of the body. Sharp pressure on any of these spots, if located accurately, will cause very acute pain. The pain is usually so sharp as to temporarily numb or paralize, and thus make entirely useless, the area involved. Using the knuckle of your second finger, as shown in the lower picture on page 4, give a very firm, very quick twist onto the exact nerve spot. The effect on your opponent is almost ludicrous in his violent and instantaneous reaction.

As these nerve centers are so important in this work you should spend the necessary time in becoming familiar with their exact location. With your knuckle search out each pressure point on yourself. One or two experiments will convince you that applying pressure to these nerve centers brings a very quick response. Practice locating them quickly.

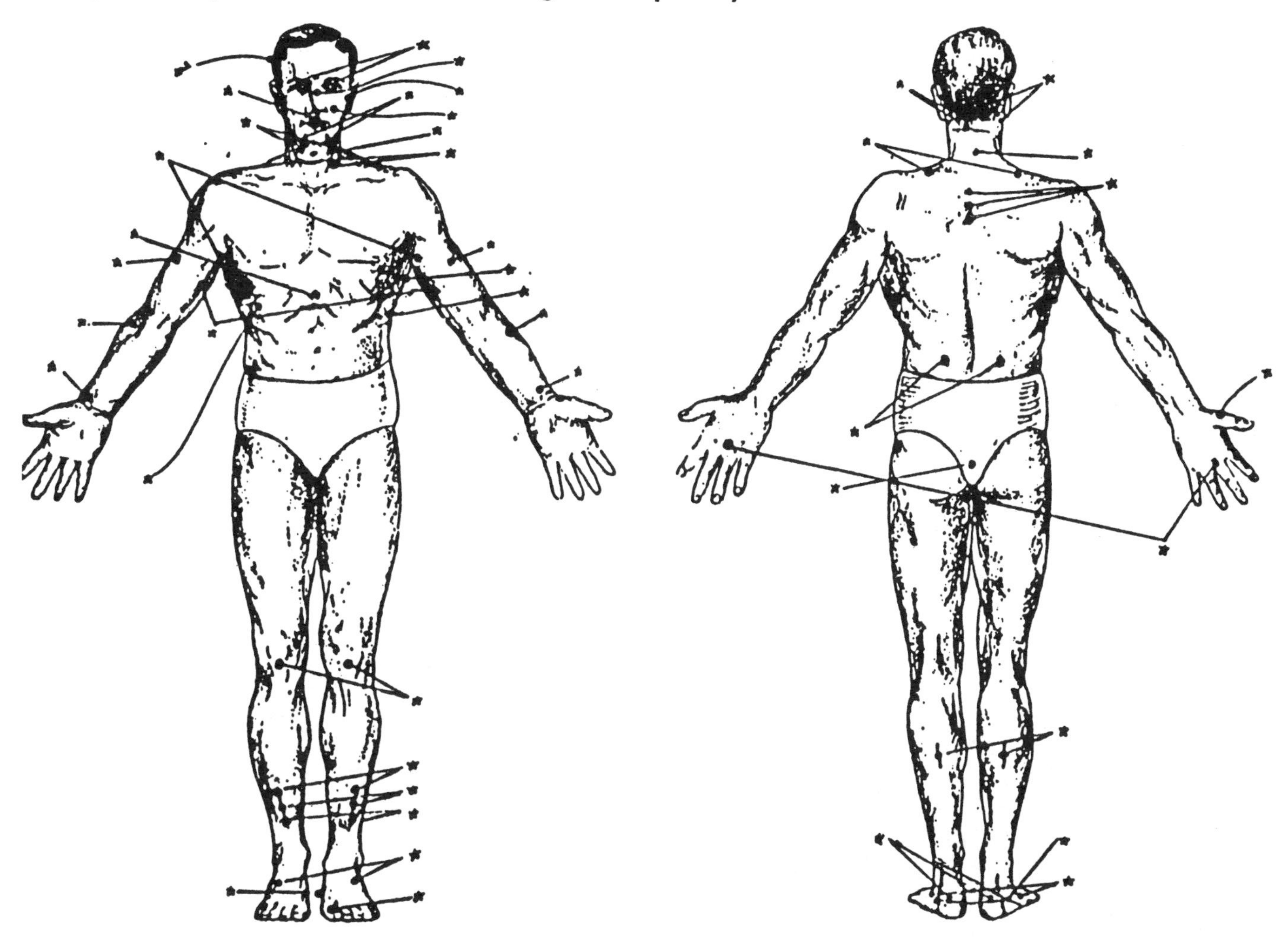

It is impossible to list, catagorically, the many situations in which a knowledge of these pressure points would come in handy. Almost any encounter would furnish opportunity for a little work on one of these spots. For instance sharp pressure on the spot shown between the second and third finger close to the second finger will open the grip of the strongest man—at once. Actually he will probably be so startled and hurt that you will have an easy opening to finish him off with any Jiu-Jitsu number you may choose. Another instance might be when the opportunity arose to deliver a short, sharp blow with the knife part of the hand to the spot where the upper lip joins the cartilage of the nose. Such a blow, properly delivered, is often enough to end all hostilities right at that point.

Be sure of the location of these nerve centers and you have, in that information alone, a very potent protection.

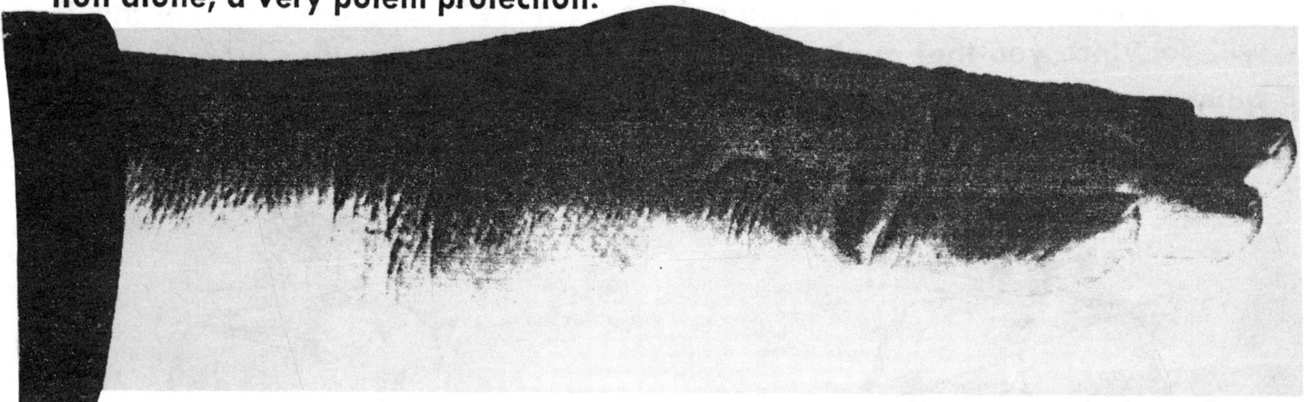

In Jiu-Jitsu we never use the fist. The knife part of the hand, as shown here, is used for all blows. As a Jiu-Jitsu operator you will have a definite location at which any blow is aimed and, using this "knife blow" you can attain that location accurately.

In exerting pressure on the nerve centers make a wedge of your hand as shown below. The second finger is thus in a position to bore into the nerve with considerable sharpness and accuracy. There is no bending tendency as there could be if you were to use your thumb or a straight finger.

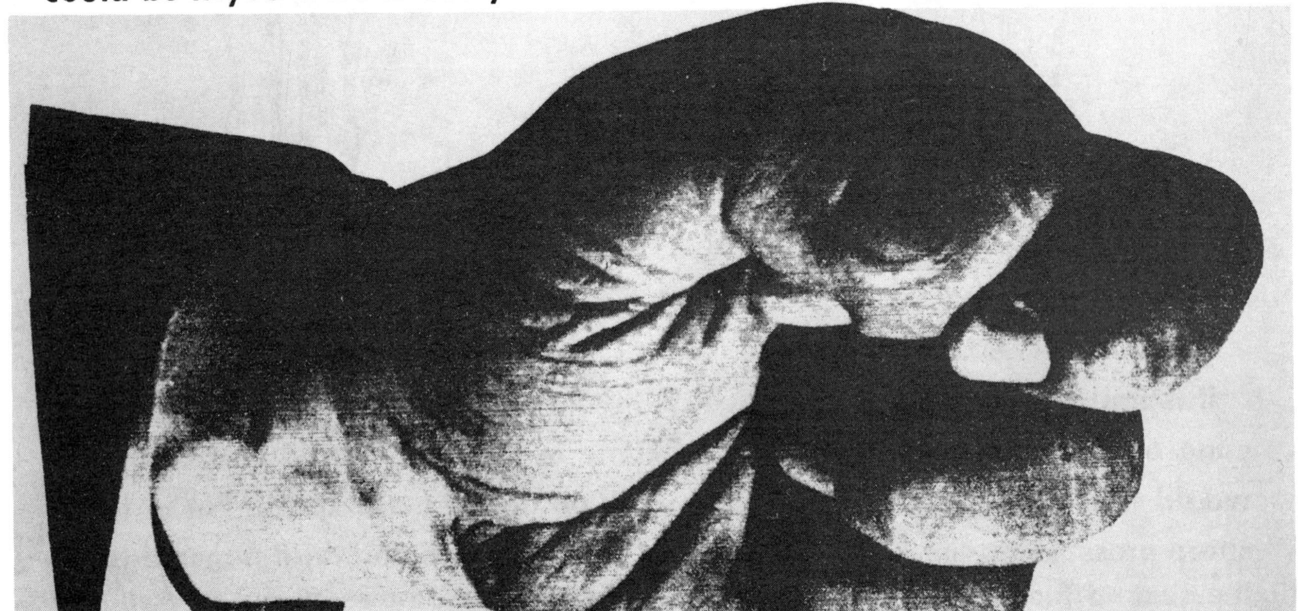

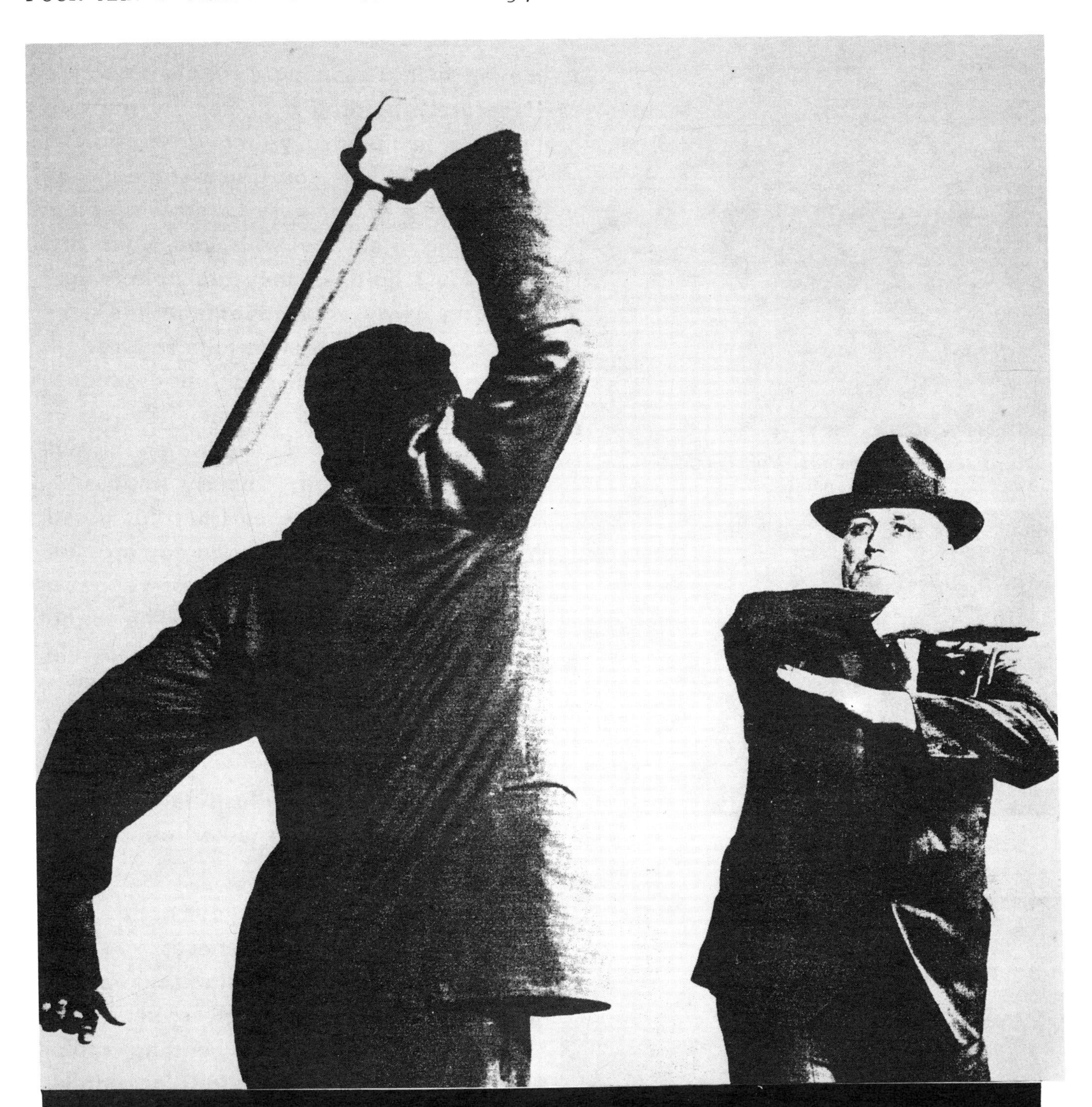

This is the perfect defense position in Jiu-Jitsu. Stand with your feet apart, one four or five inches ahead of the other. Thus you may rock forward, backward or to either side without seriously disturbing your balance. A slight crouch will allow you to rise somewhat or sink further. Your arms in this position are ready to strike to either side. Of course you may in actual use not have time to completely assume this position but if you practice it you will in an emergency tend to automatically hold yourself this way in the face of an approaching troublemaker.

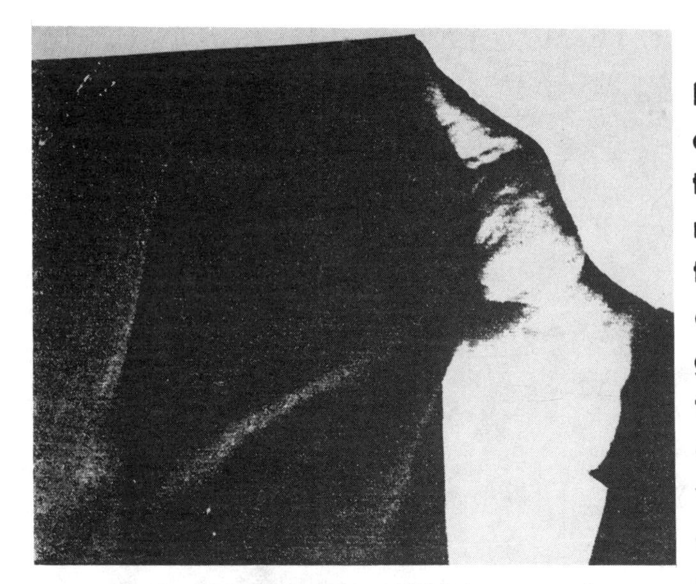

This is the correct grip. Hold the garment only, not the arm

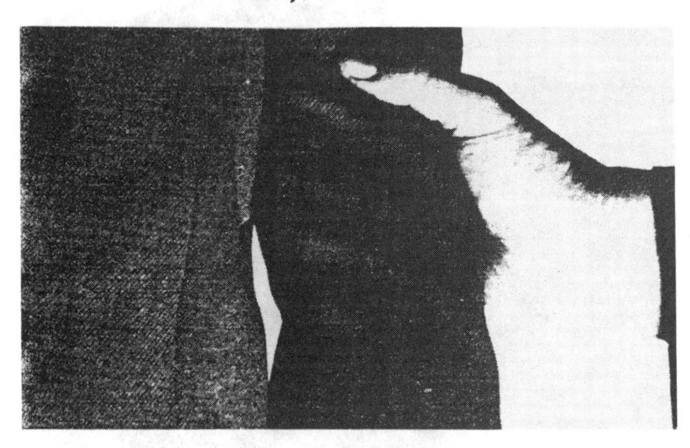

Holding the arm itself this way is very ineffective

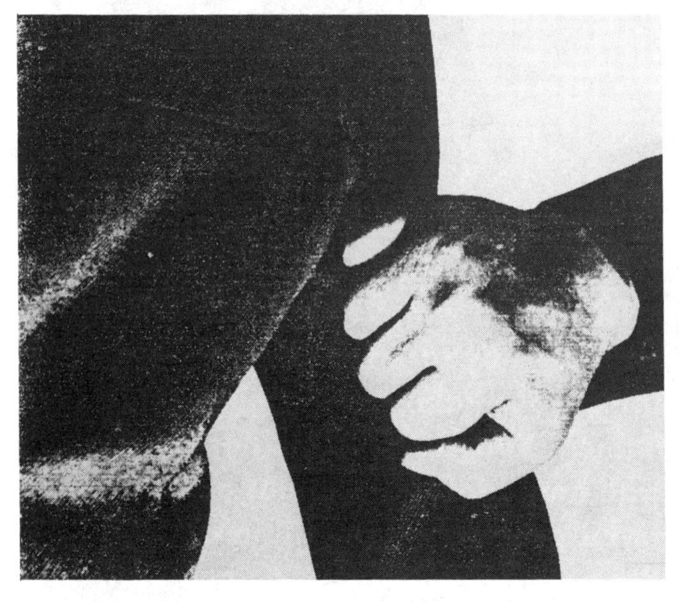

It is easy to break away when held like this

In even such a seemingly simple operation as securely holding a person by the arm there are, in Jiu-Jitsu, wrong ways and one right way. When you grasp someone by the arm as a preliminary to throwing them or making them go with you your first grasp must hold—if they are able to jerk their arm away your advantage has gone or at least has been materially reduced. It will be much harder, if not impossible, to grasp the arm a second time. It's just as easy to use and a little experimenting will convince you that it is nearly impossible for the arm to be released from this grasp. With the palm of your hand toward you grip a substantial fold or two of your subjects' coat or garment. Thus held he cannot break away. Of course this is, as a rule, only preliminary to an arm lock or other hold but as long as you hold this grip he cannot release his arm.

The two lower pictures illustrate poor grips. The arm can easily be jerked out of such holds as these.

To strengthen the grip of your hands there are several beneficial exercises you may use. While they are old standbys for this purpose they are, nevertheless, very effective. One consists of kneading rubber balls, the size of tennis balls or smaller, in your hands. Another is to stand with arms outstretched and crumple a sheet of newspaper up in each hand, starting by holding them only by the edge or corners and continuing until they are balled up in your hands. This exercise does not sound impressive but a few trials will convince you of its effectiveness.

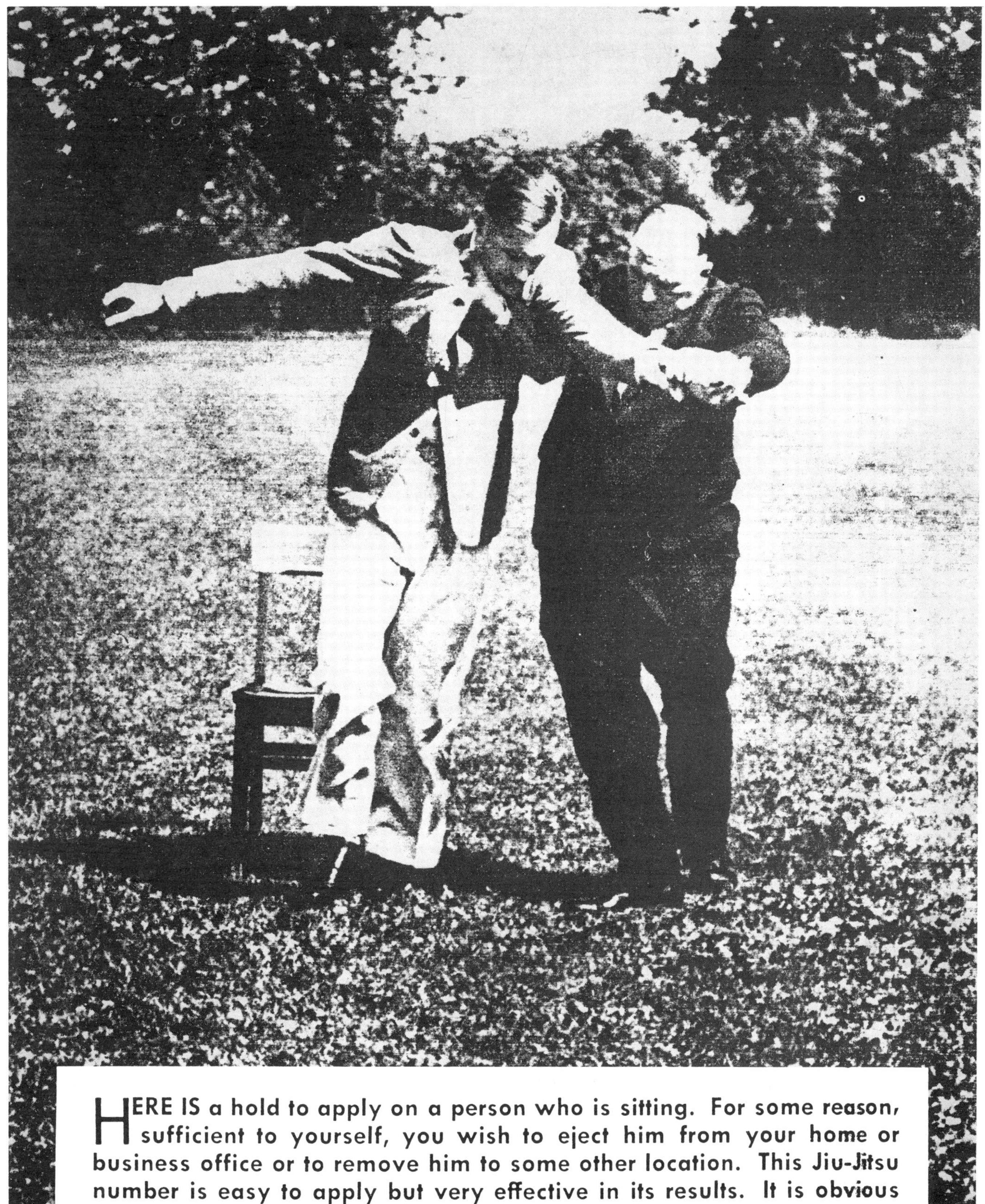

HERE IS a hold to apply on a person who is sitting. For some reason, sufficient to yourself, you wish to eject him from your home or business office or to remove him to some other location. This Jiu-Jitsu number is easy to apply but very effective in its results. It is obvious that this is only used when the subject is wearing a coat, jacket, or some such substantial garment.

In these "come along" holds you make your job easier by approaching your man without evident sign of belligerence, if possible. Remember, in Jiu-Jitsu, you are not looking for a fight, or trouble; you are bent on mastery of the situation in a neat, efficient manner.

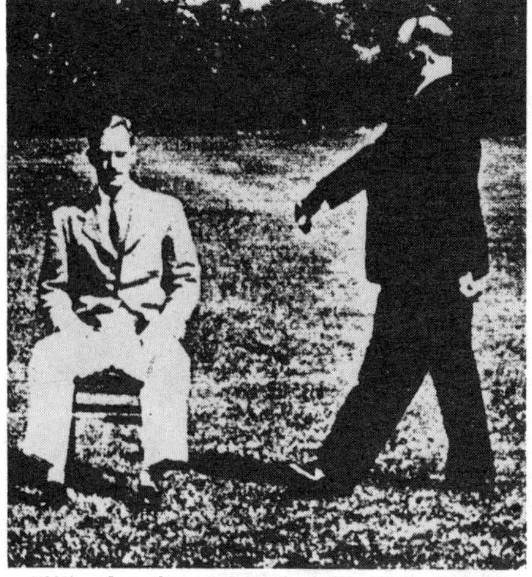

"What's the matter, old fellow, a little trouble here?" you may ask as

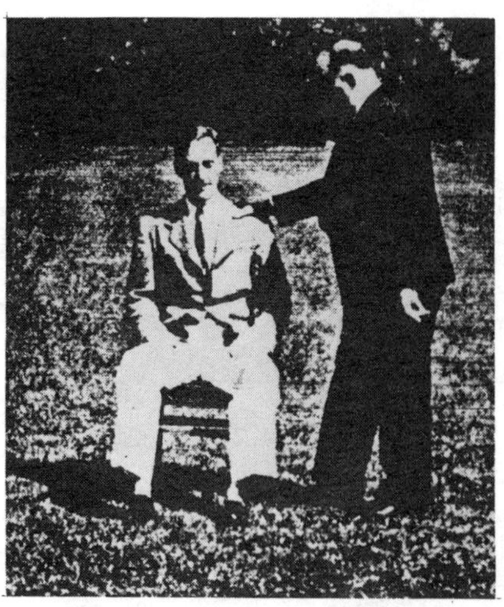

your hand is laid solicitously on his shoulder. This, of course, is an example of misdirection.

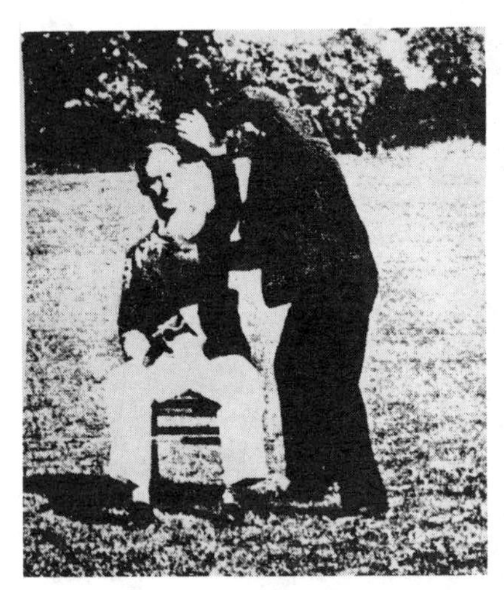

Your right hand is after a strong grip on his right coat lapel.

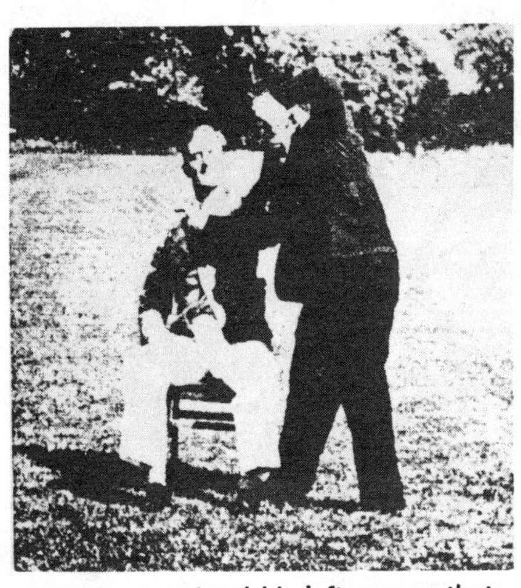

You have twisted his left arm so that the palm of his hand is straight up.

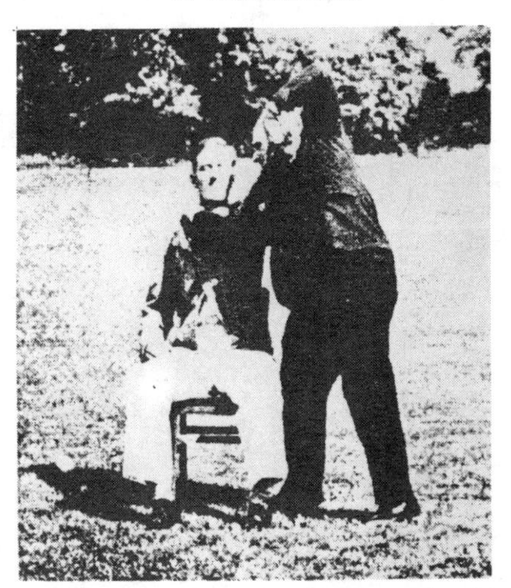

Your right arm should be under his arm exactly at or a little above his elbow.

He'll fairly jump out of his chair. Keep his left arm tightly twisted.

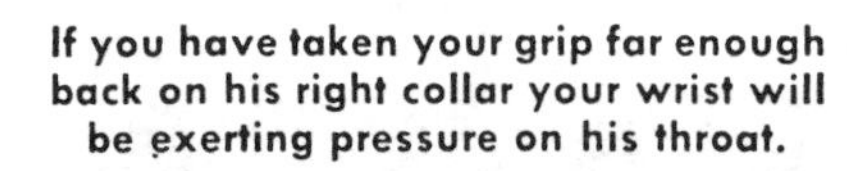

If you have taken your grip far enough back on his right collar your wrist will be exerting pressure on his throat.

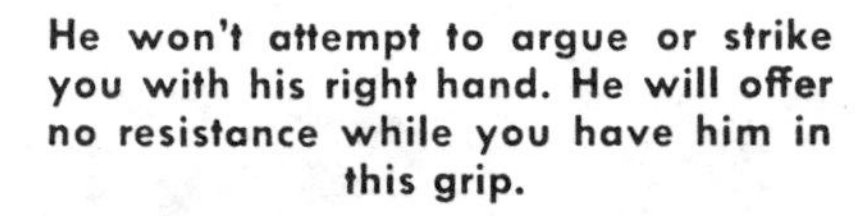

He won't attempt to argue or strike you with his right hand. He will offer no resistance while you have him in this grip.

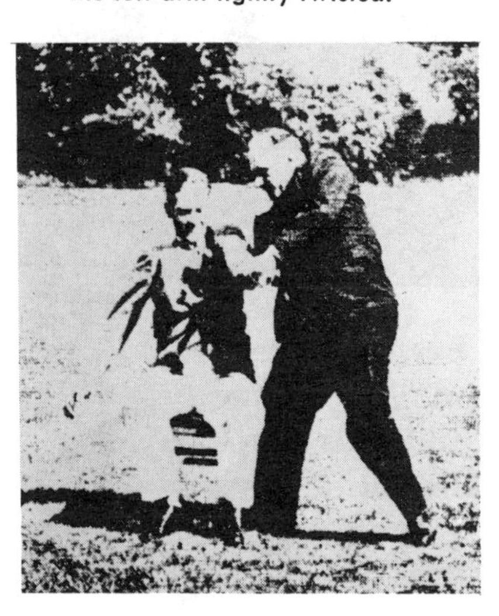

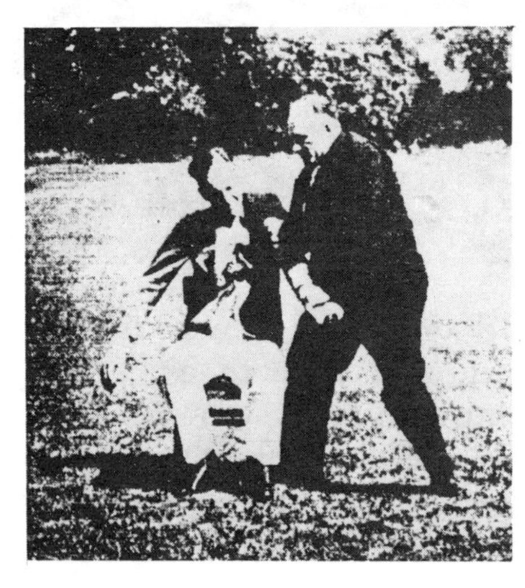

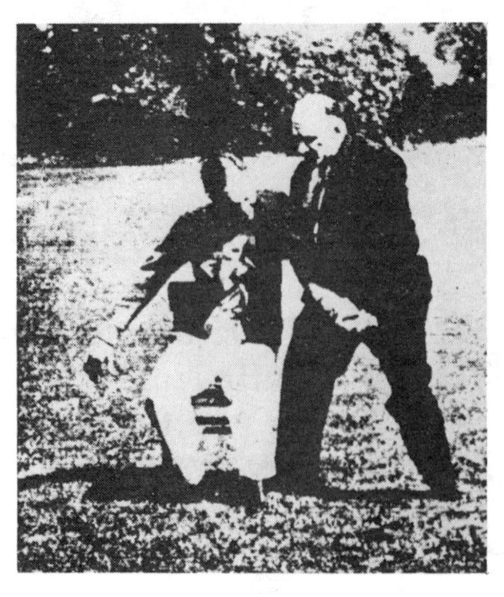

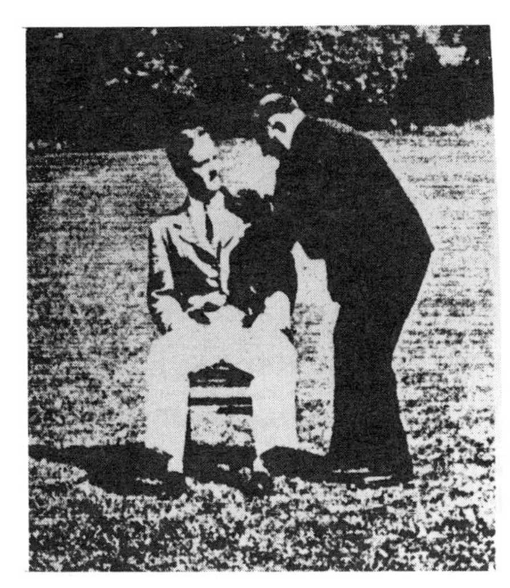

Grasp for his left wrist. Great speed is now essential.

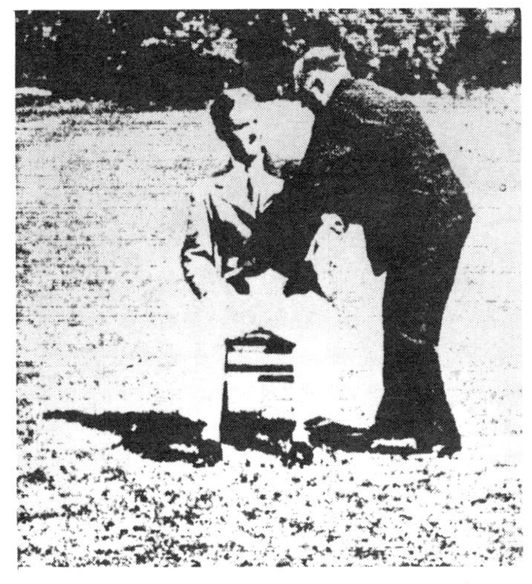

You grip far around his wrist in order that you may easily twist his arm toward you

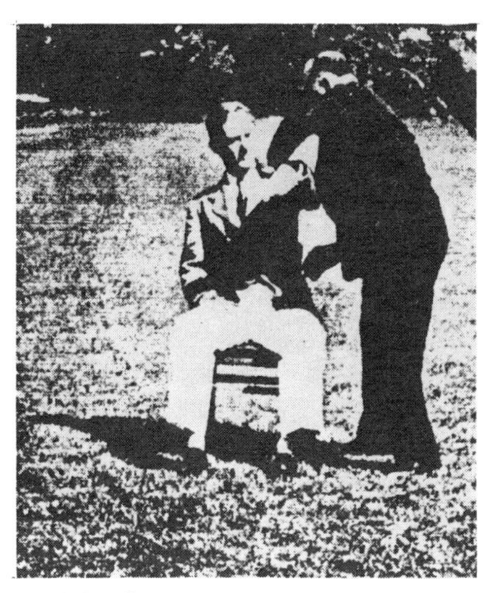

raising his arm as you twist it. Your right arm goes underneath his left arm.

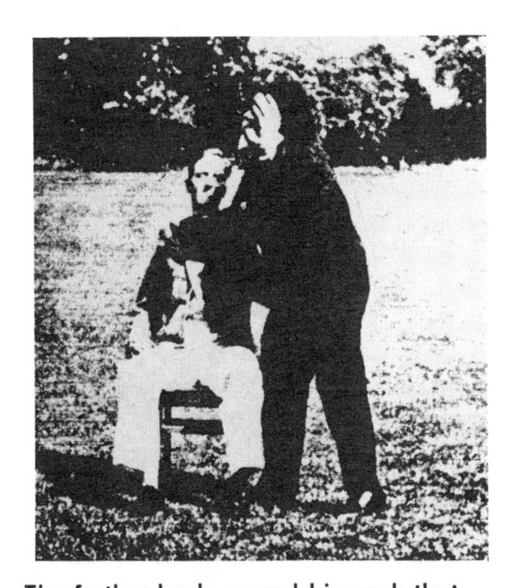

The farther back around his neck that you grip his coat collar the more effective your control.

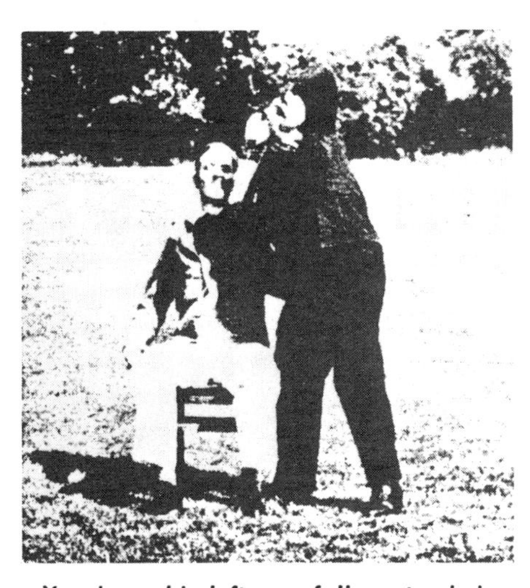

You have his left arm fully extended now, palm of hand up, and a firm grip on his right collar.

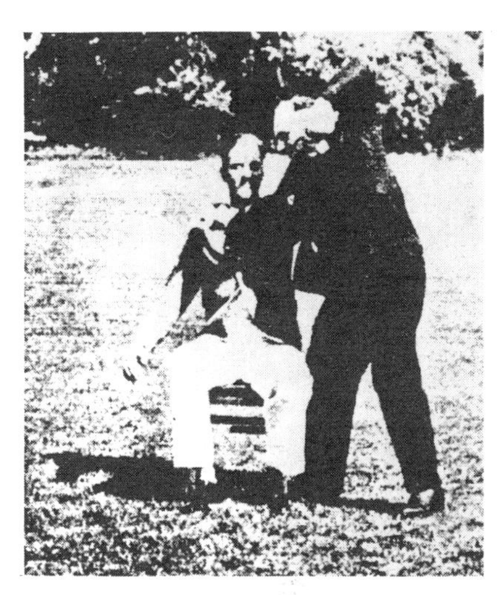

Now using your right arm as the fulcrum, you exert leverage by forcing his left wrist sharply downward.

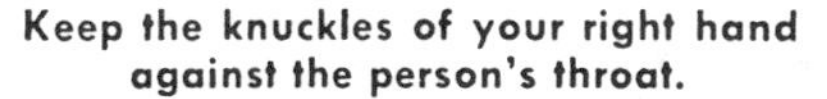

Keep the knuckles of your right hand against the person's throat.

The leverage you are exerting on his arm causes him great pain.

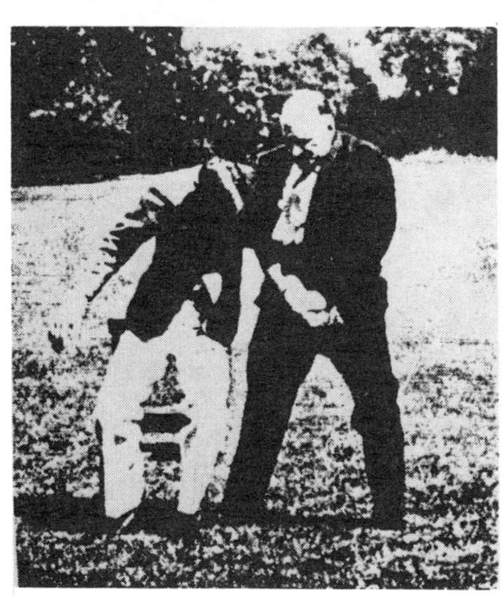

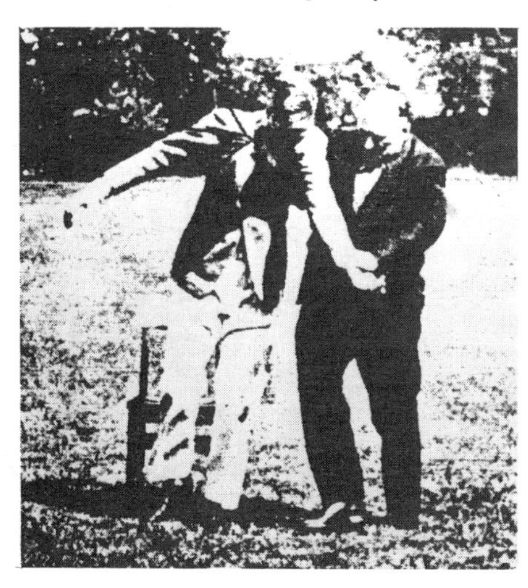

All the action shown here took place within three seconds. It looks slow in pictures but speed is actually the very essence of successful Jiu-Jitsu. The pictures on the next page review the most important movements of this number.

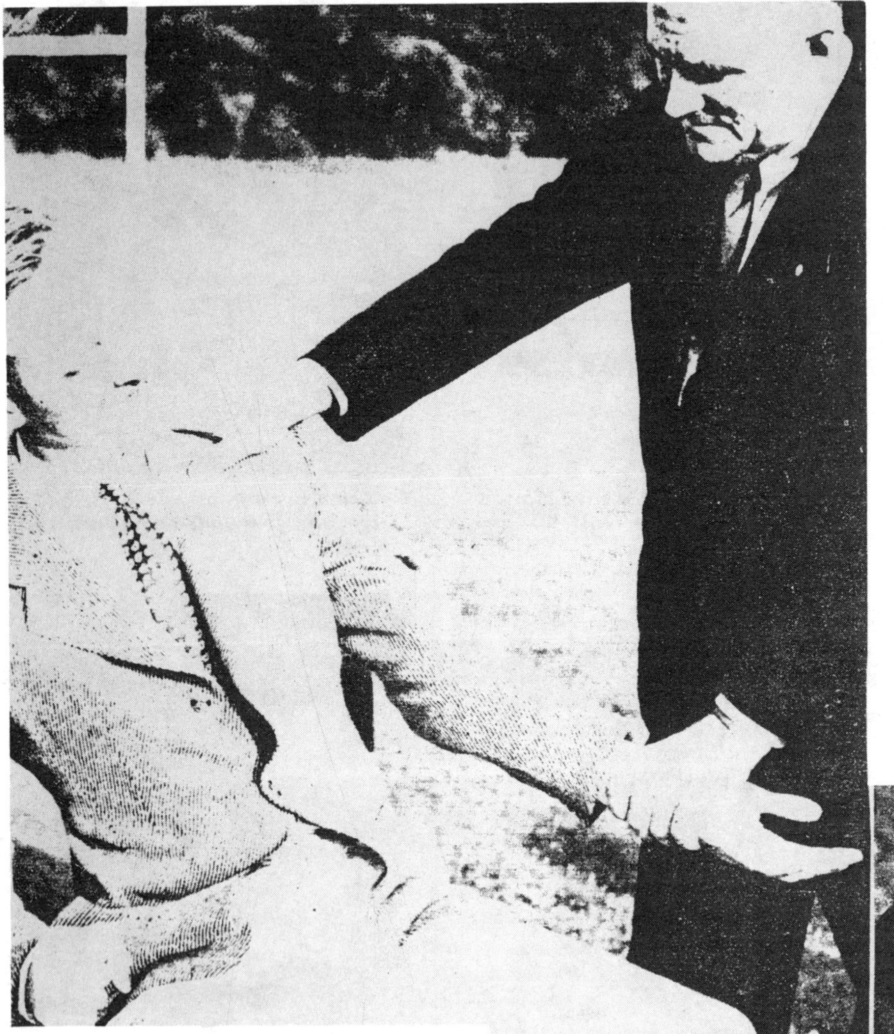

In reviewing the foregoing number you can see that the importance of the twist given the man's arm cannot be over emphasized. Unless it is turned at least enough to bring his hand palm-up the entire action will be unsuccessful. And when correctly twisted a slight additional turn is an effective way to coax a little snappier action from your captive.

The other very essential portion of this "come along" hold consists of the part played by the hand and arm holding the victim's coat collar. The grip on the collar must be very solid and it should be far around the person's neck. This will make the knuckles of your hand press against his neck or collarbone.

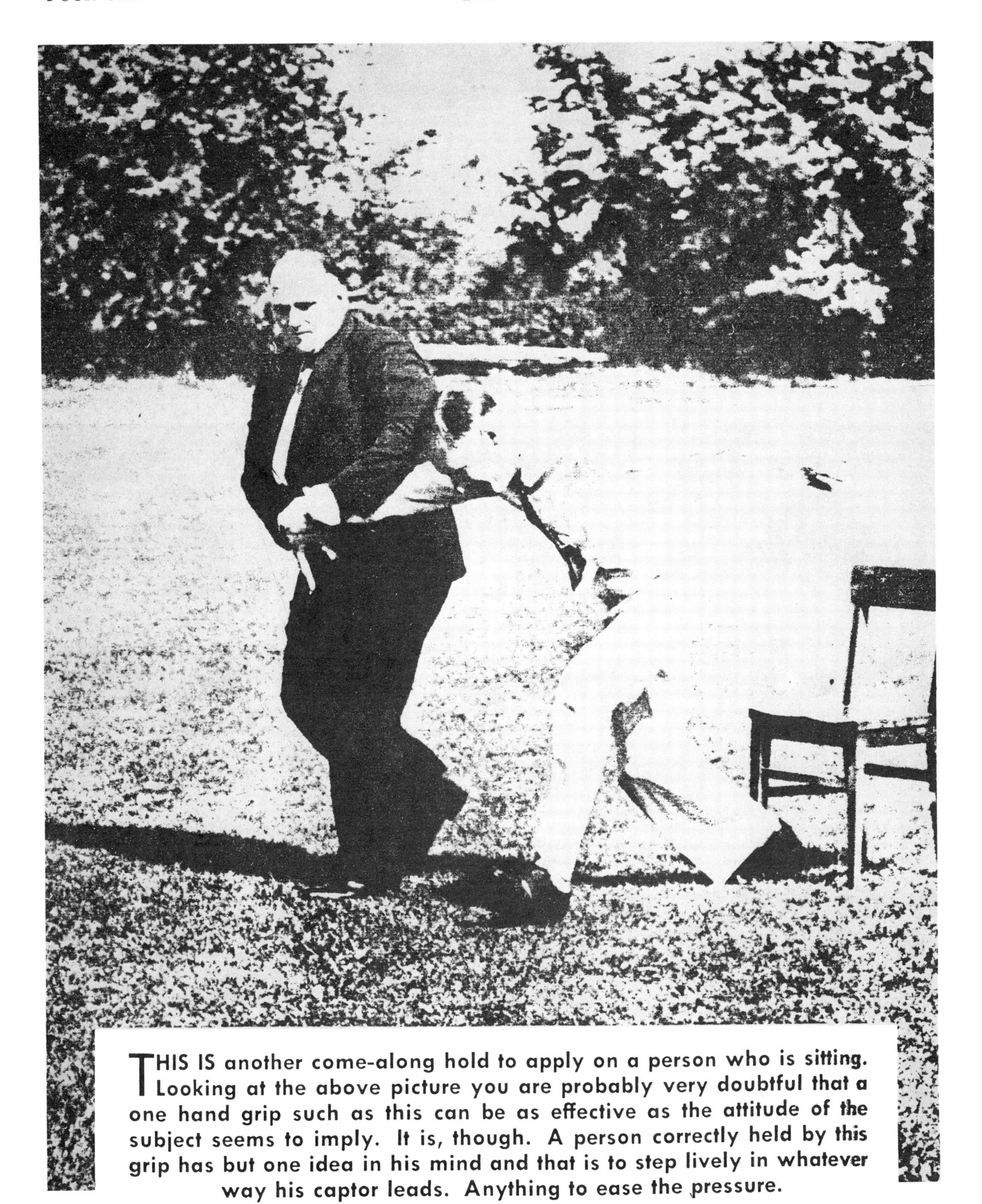

THIS IS another come-along hold to apply on a person who is sitting. Looking at the above picture you are probably very doubtful that a one hand grip such as this can be as effective as the attitude of the subject seems to imply. It is, though. A person correctly held by this grip has but one idea in his mind and that is to step lively in whatever way his captor leads. Anything to ease the pressure.

This number is easy to use if you have the chance to grasp the subject's wrist firmly for one half a second.

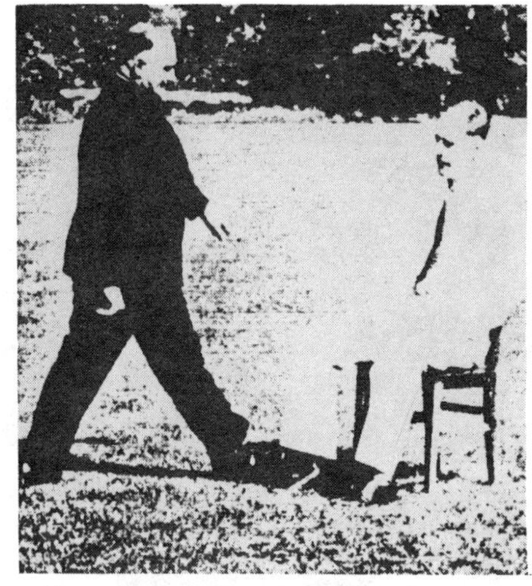

Therefore try to approach in a manner which will not put him on his guard at once.

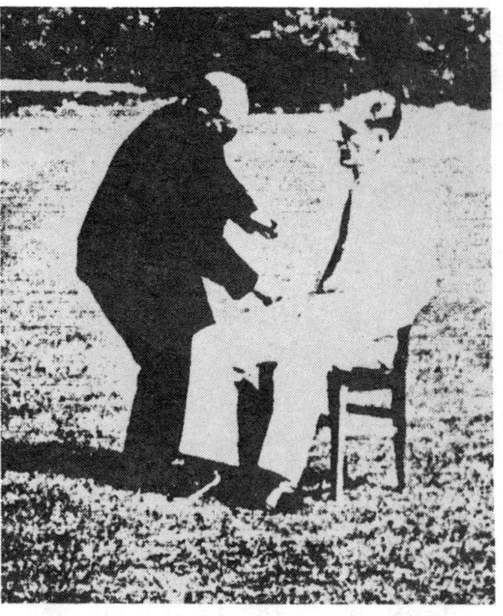

Even while taking hold of his wrist you may ask him if "these people are bothering him."

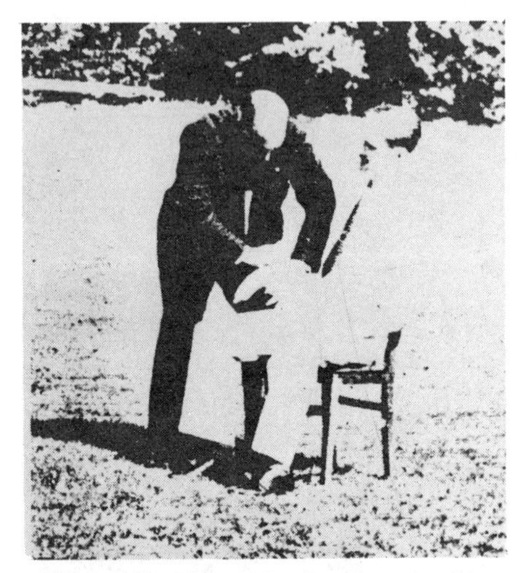

Still holding his wrist firmly, raise his arm as you pull his thumb back.

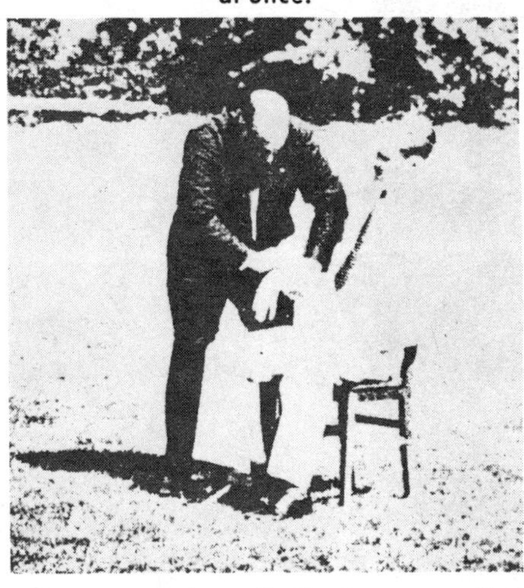

You are doing all this in one swift motion depending on misdirection, speed, and surprise.

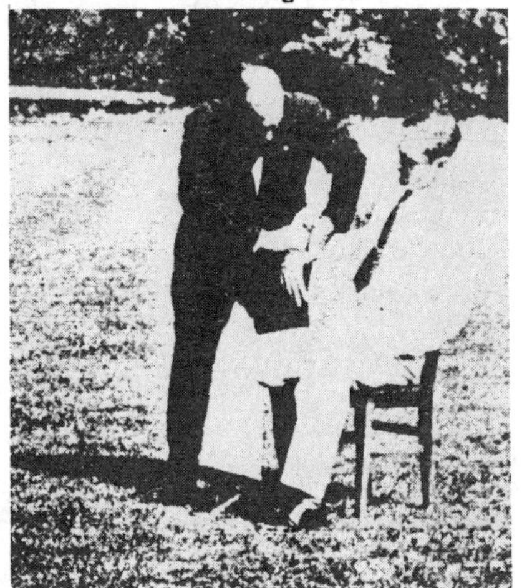

But if he should attempt to strike you with his free hand you can hit him with the knife part of your left hand on the nerve spot just below his nose.

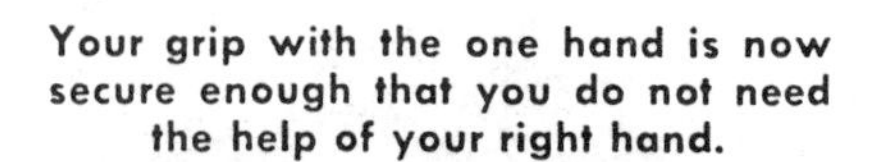

Your grip with the one hand is now secure enough that you do not need the help of your right hand.

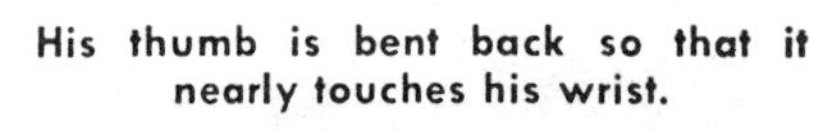

His thumb is bent back so that it nearly touches his wrist.

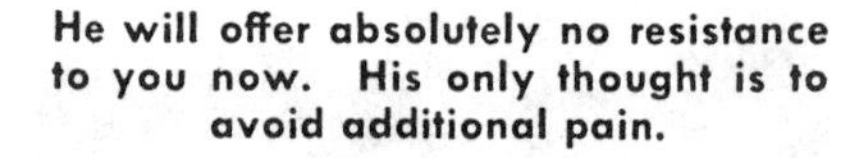

He will offer absolutely no resistance to you now. His only thought is to avoid additional pain.

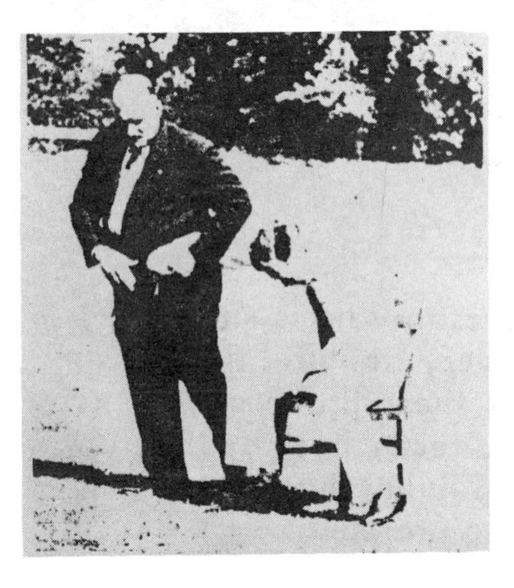

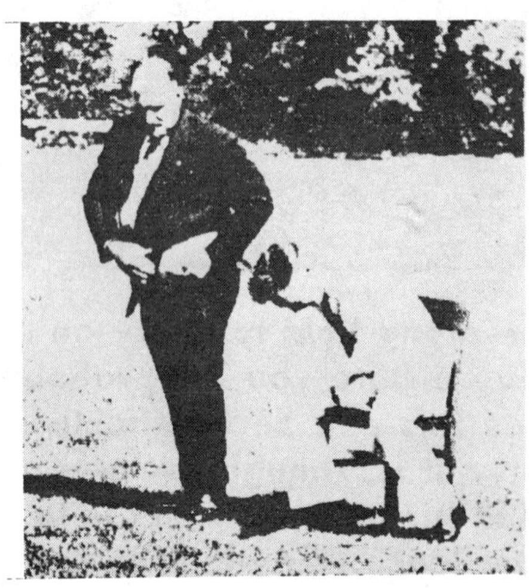

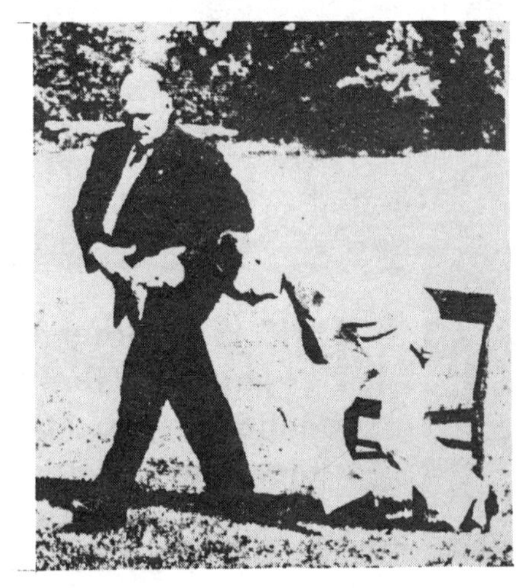

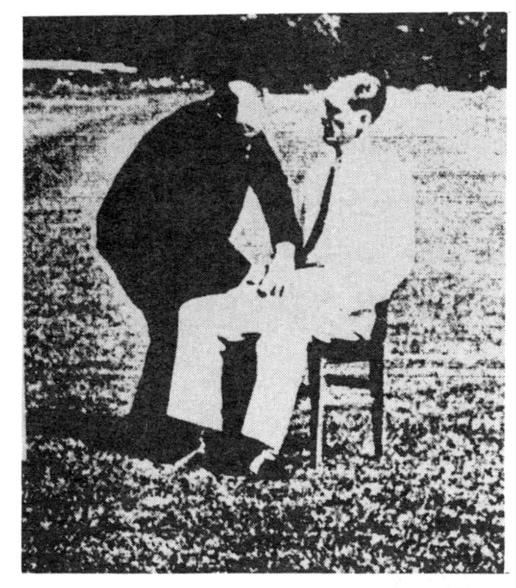

If you are going to operate on his right side grasp his right wrist quickly just above his hand, then,

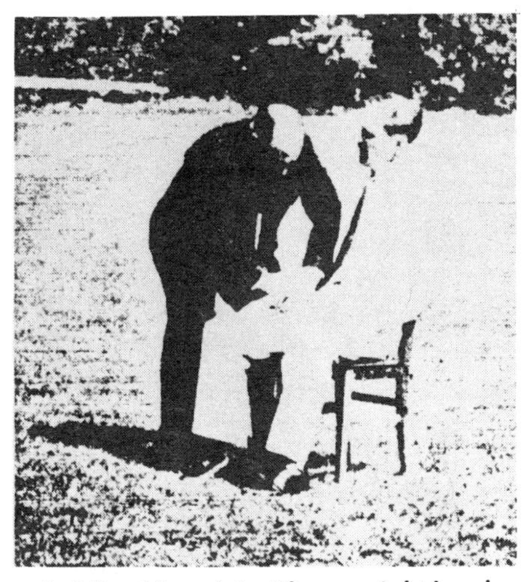

holding his wrist with your right hand, take hold of his thumb with the fingers of your left hand.

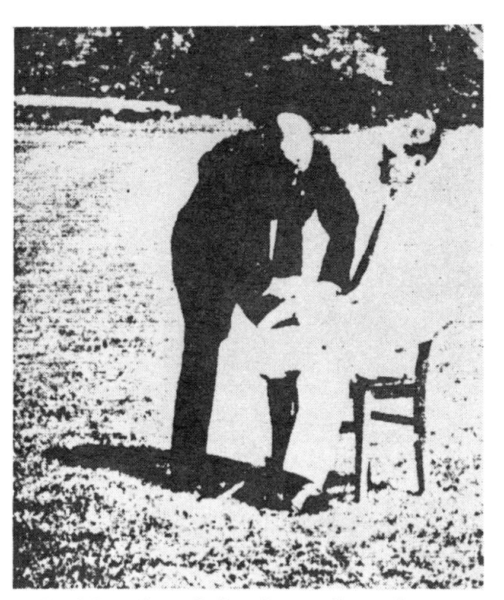

Pull his thumb backward, at the same time keeping it pointing downward, not out to the side.

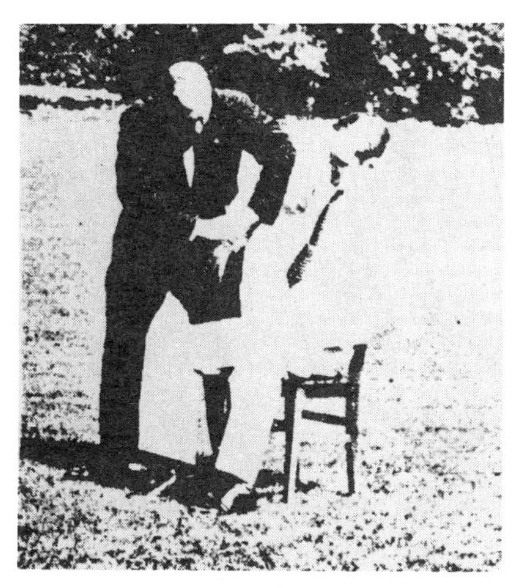

Pull his hand and wrist into close contact with the side of your hip and

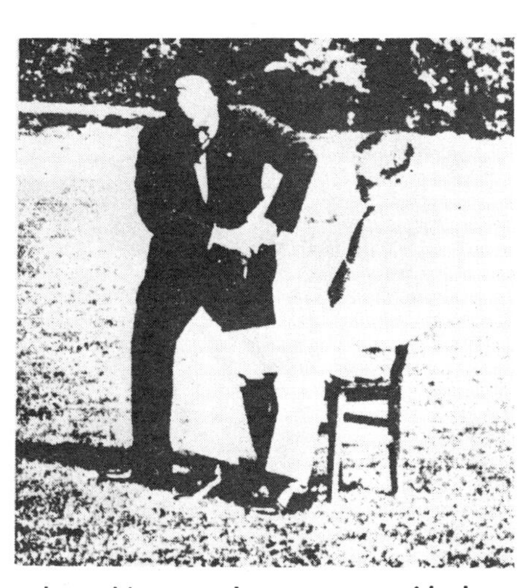

keep his arm close to your side by pressure of your left forearm.

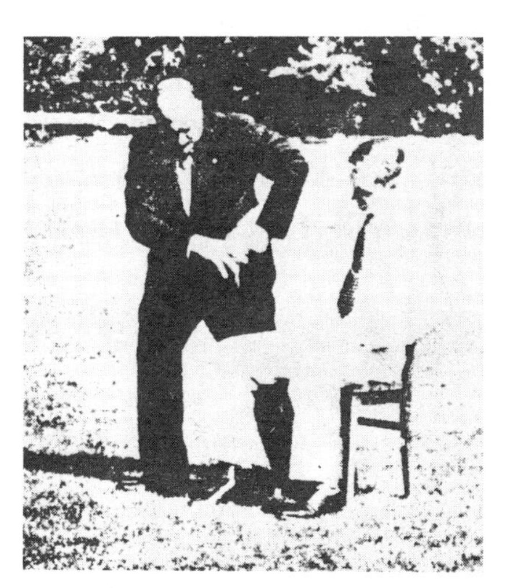

Your left thumb is now on top of his wrist and the fingers of your left hand have drawn his right thumb far back.

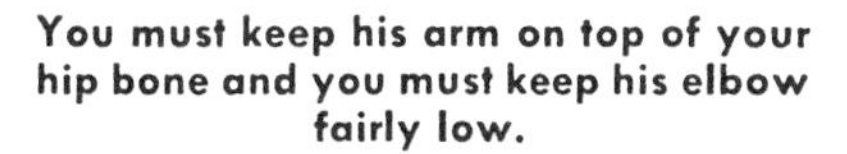

You must keep his arm on top of your hip bone and you must keep his elbow fairly low.

There is practically no pressure on yourself and you can easily keep your man under control for as long as you care to do so.

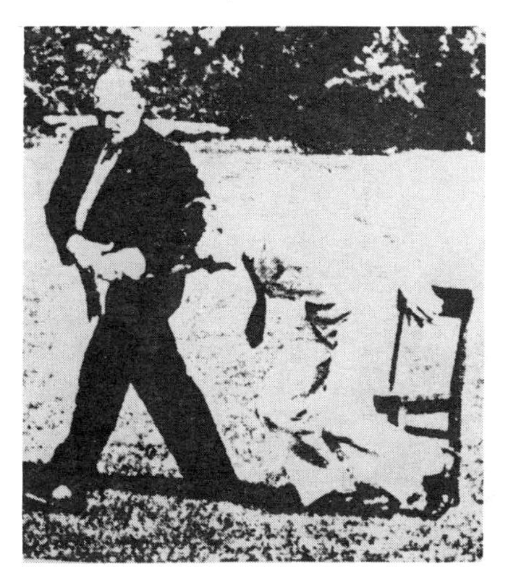

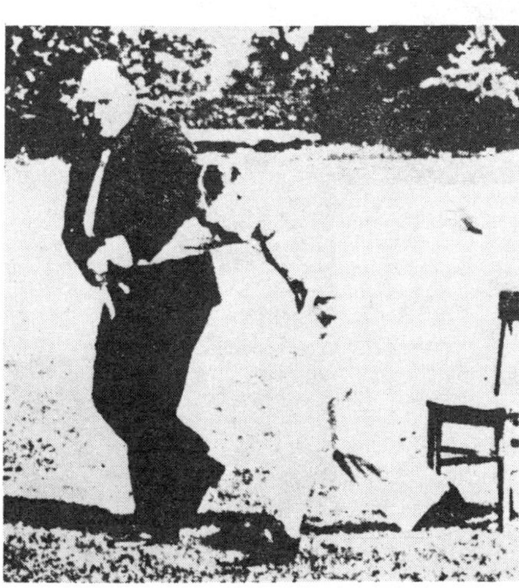

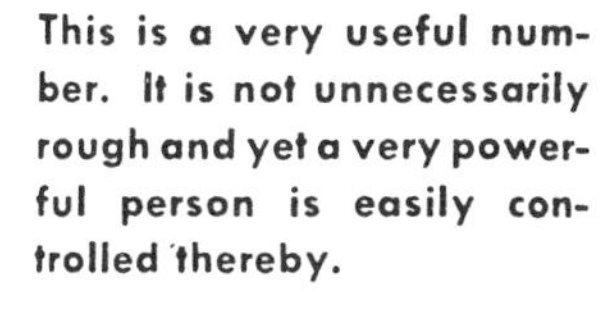

This is a very useful number. It is not unnecessarily rough and yet a very powerful person is easily controlled thereby.

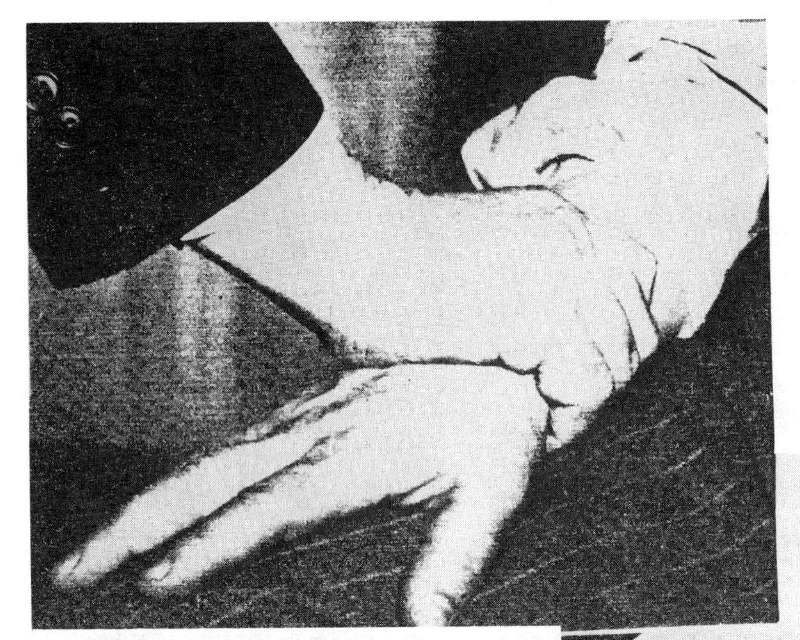

You must remember that this number first required a tight grip on the subject's right wrist by your right hand.

Your left hand reaches across his hand and your fingers pull his thumb backwards. This will force his wrist to bend.

Pull the thumb straight back until your own thumb will go over the back of his wrist while your fingers retain his thumb.

Only your left hand is needed now. Pull his hand up to you and force his wrist to rest on top of your hipbone.

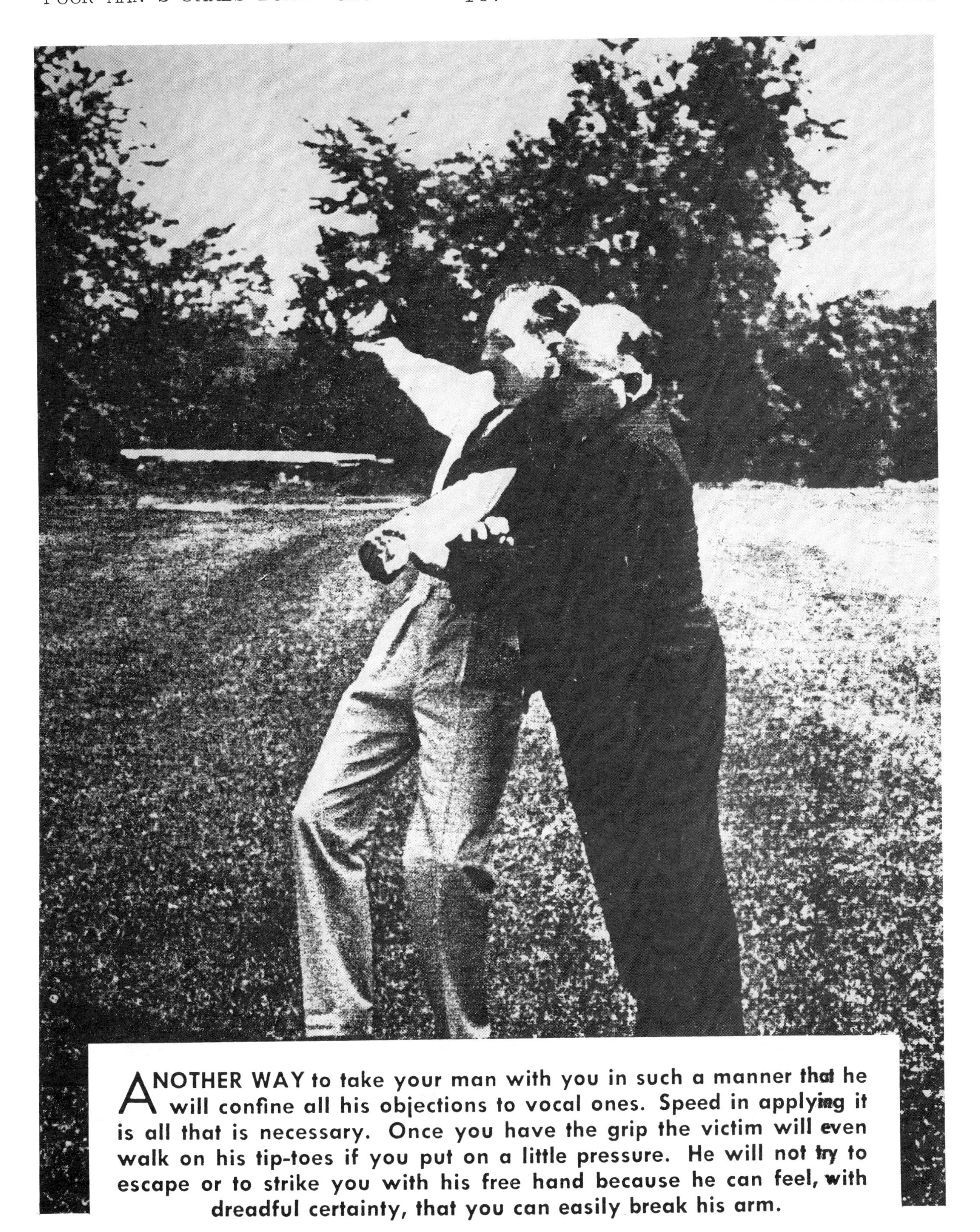

ANOTHER WAY to take your man with you in such a manner that he will confine all his objections to vocal ones. Speed in applying it is all that is necessary. Once you have the grip the victim will even walk on his tip-toes if you put on a little pressure. He will not try to escape or to strike you with his free hand because he can feel, with dreadful certainty, that you can easily break his arm.

This, like most Jiu-Jitsu numbers,—depends largely on quick, proper handling of the very first portion of the action. Get your opponent on the defensive and you're the winner.

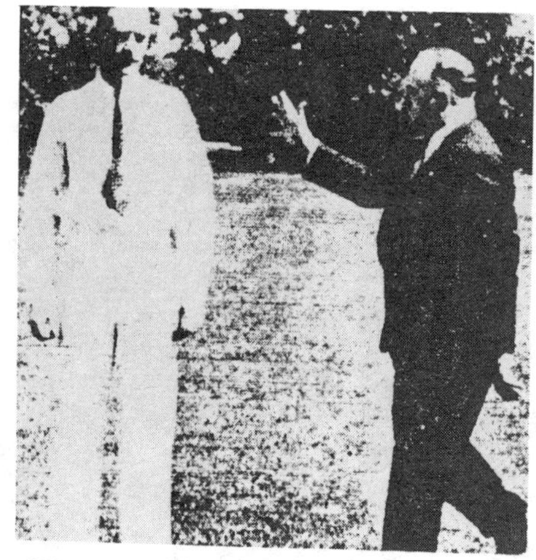

When you grasp his arm don't fumble around; take a real grip.

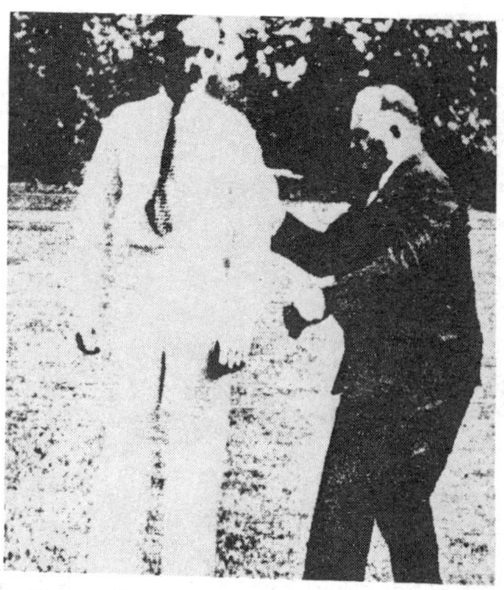

Remember the correct way to hold a person; by the sleeve, not the arm itself.

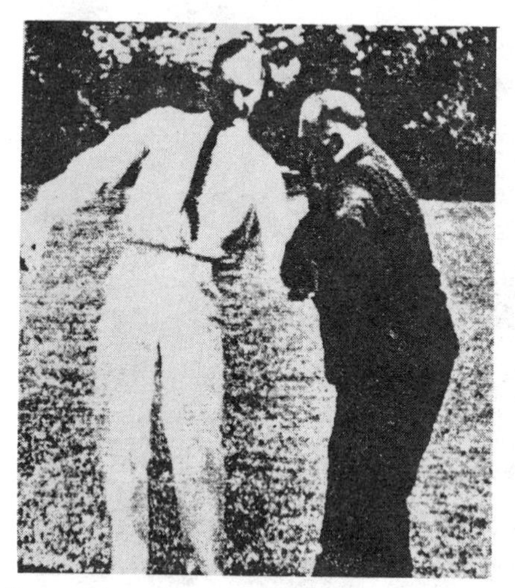

Twist his wrist sharply and at the same time raise his arm.

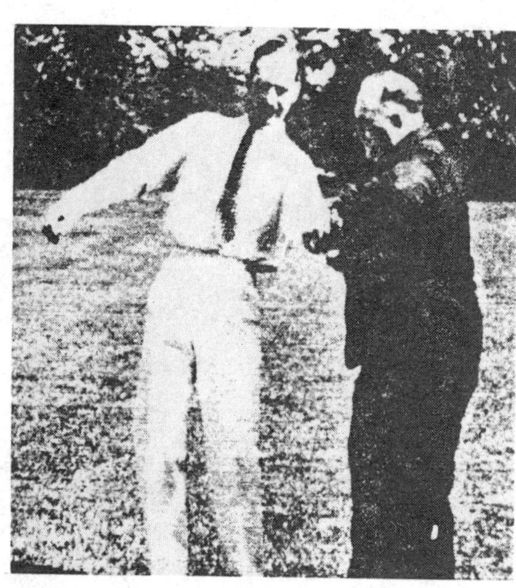

With his wrist twisted until the palm of his hand is pointing upward he'll let himself go off balance slightly.

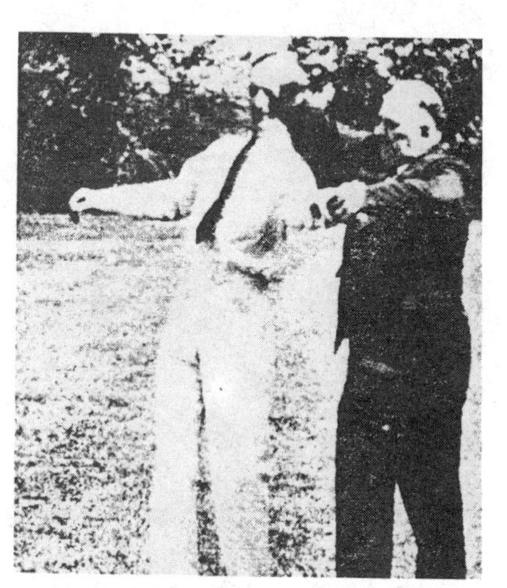

Your right hand has released its grip from his sleeve and your right arm goes over his left arm.

have his arm very snugly tucked under yours. Otherwise you cannot exercise the full force of your position.

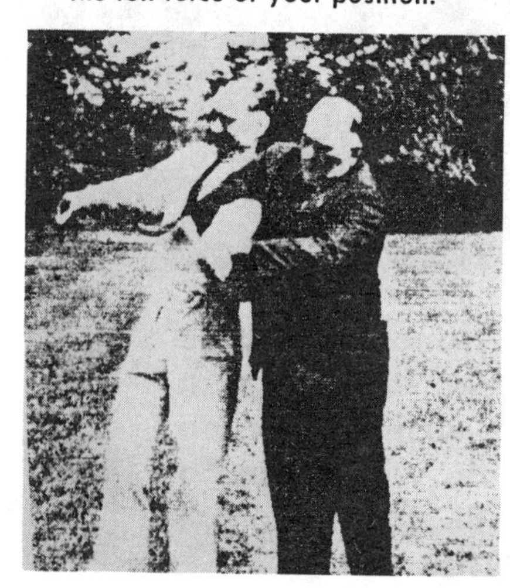

Bring your right hand up and lay it on your left fore arm.

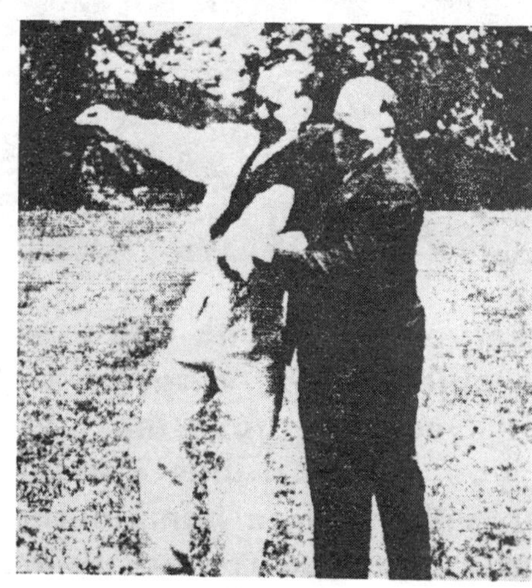

Notice to what an extreme the left arm has been twisted; a full half turn at least.

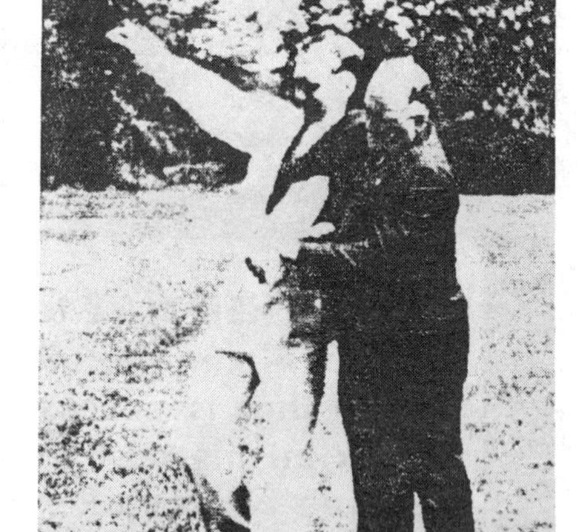

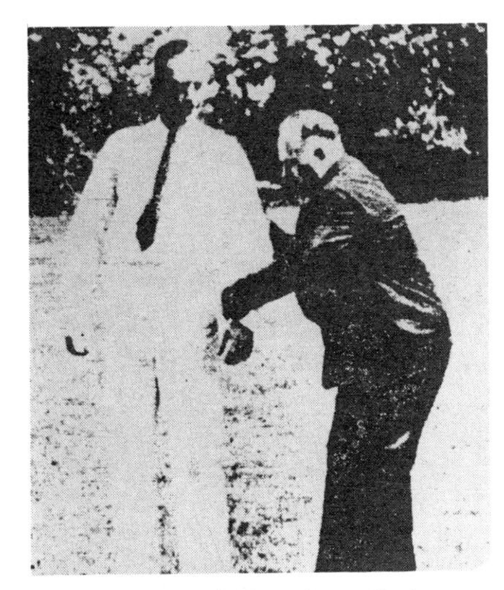

Grasp far around his wrist so that you can give his arm an extreme twist with only one motion. In applying these numbers you should

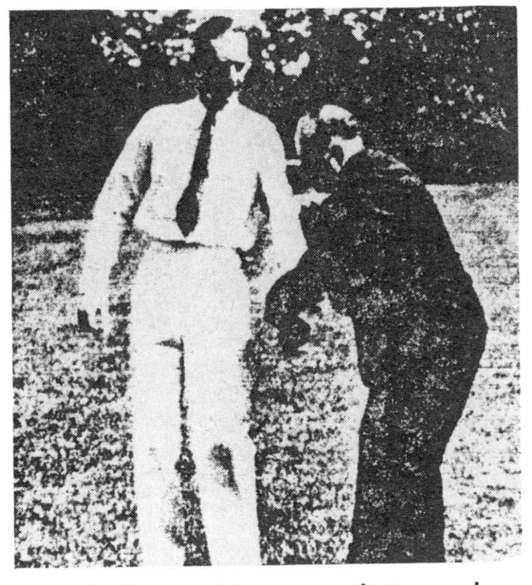

work close to his arm so that you do not have to reach far from your body.

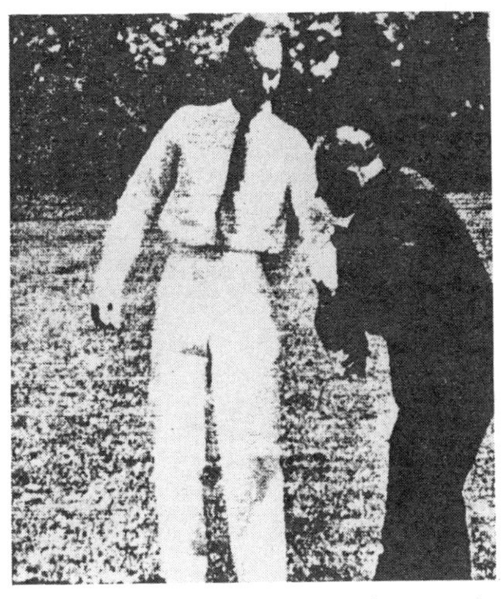

Act very quickly and by the time he has an inkling of your purpose you'll have him off balance.

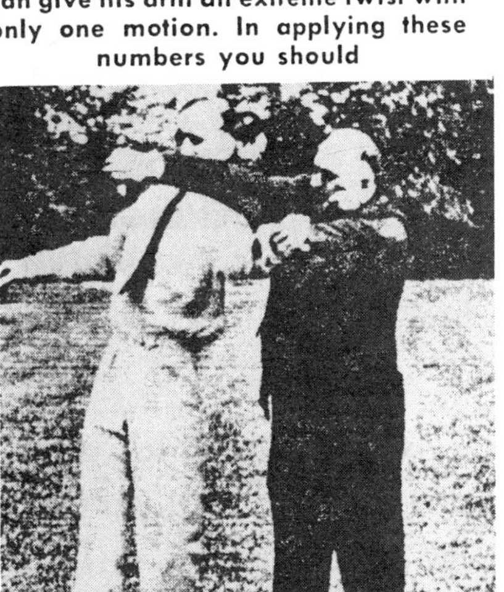

When your opponent's free arm goes straight out from his side—in any Jiu-Jitsu number—it is a sign that he is off balance.

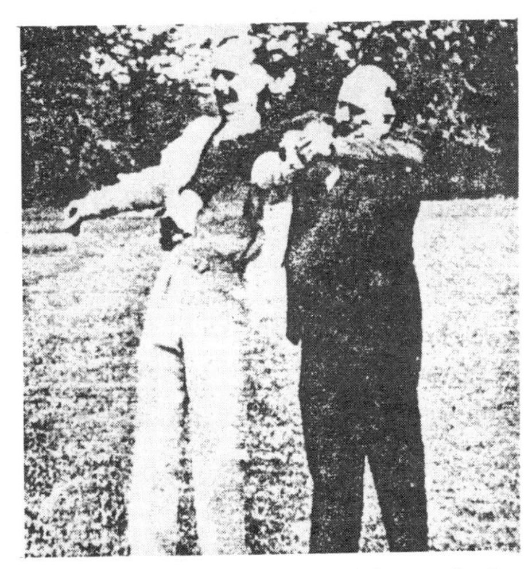

Lay your upper arm over his arm just above his elbow. Don't relax your grip on his wrist.

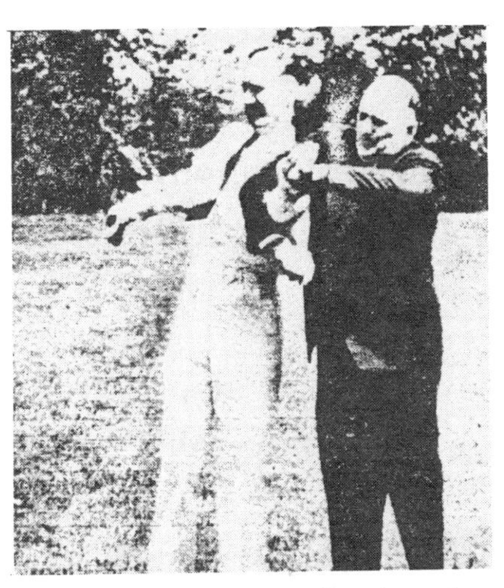

Now bring your arm directly underneath his elbow. Keep him very close to you and

His arm is securely locked now and it is impossible for him to escape.

You are able to exert powerful leverage, enough even, to easily snap his elbow joint.

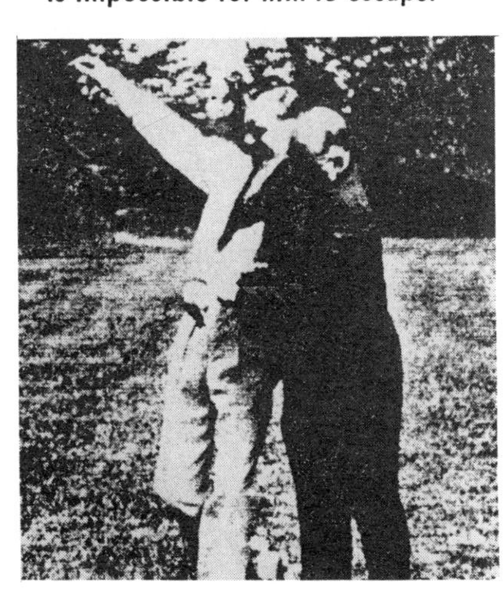

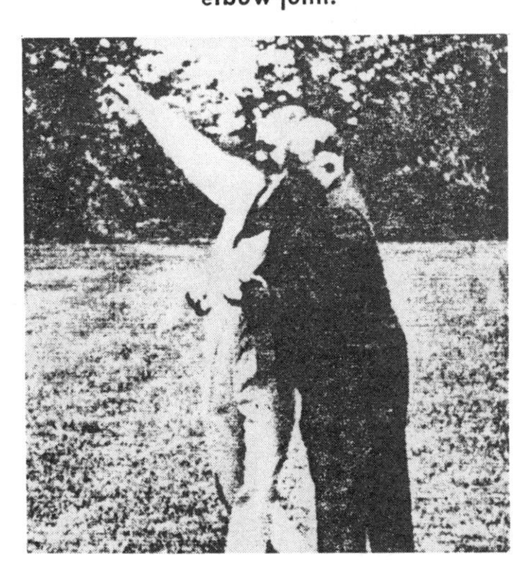

Once you have his arm securely in this lock it requires little effort for you to keep your victim subdued indefinitely.

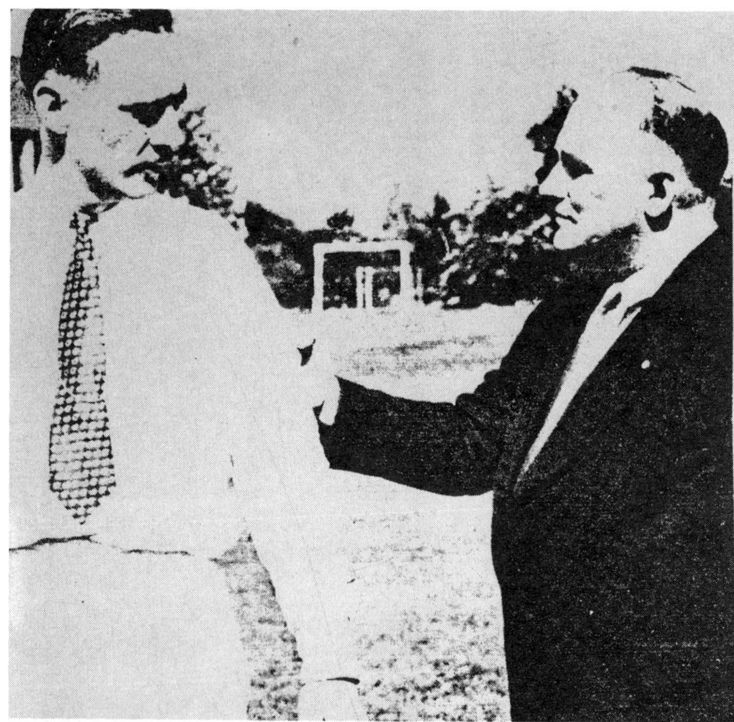

The first important move was to grip the man's sleeve in the approved manner.

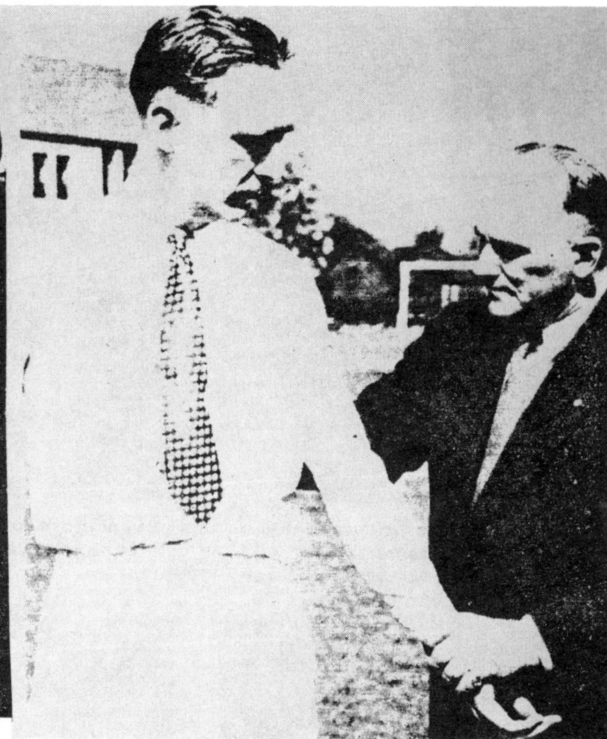

Then you grasped and quickly twisted his wrist.

The next step was to put your right arm just above his elbow.

This was followed by having your forearm go under his arm and putting your right hand on your left wrist.

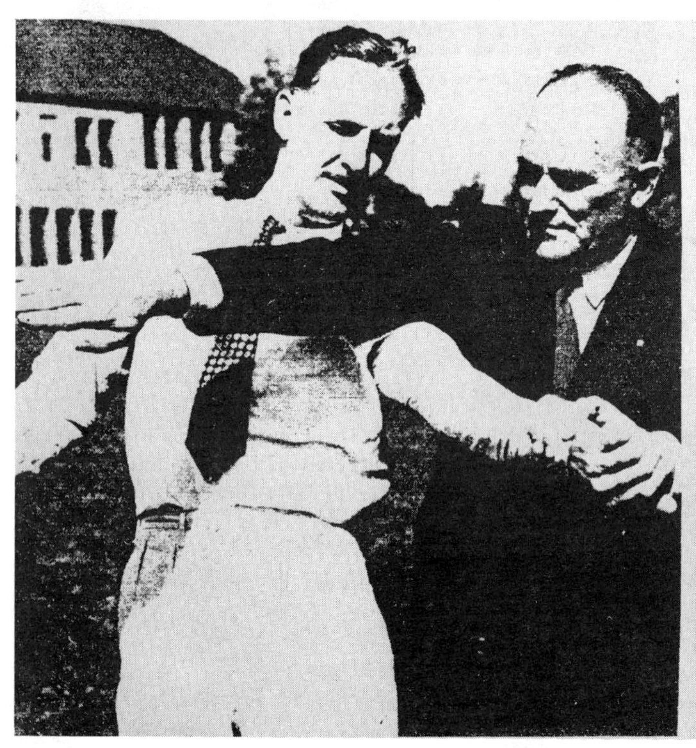

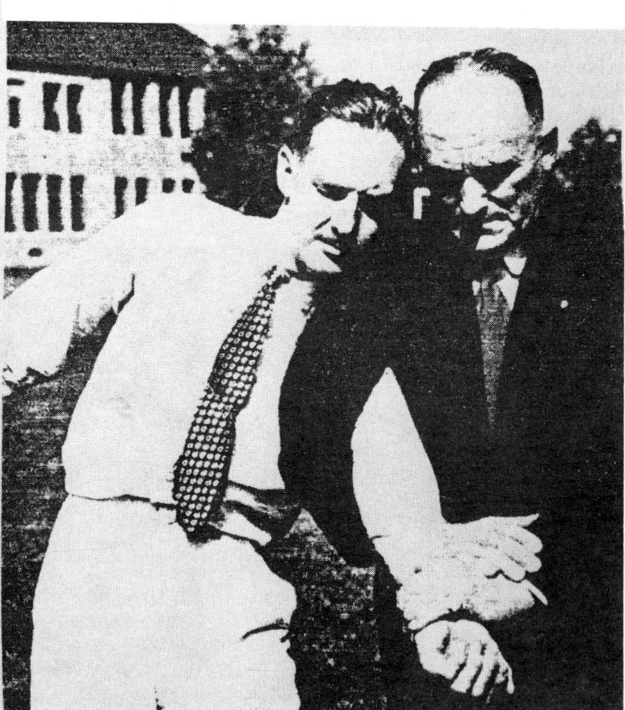

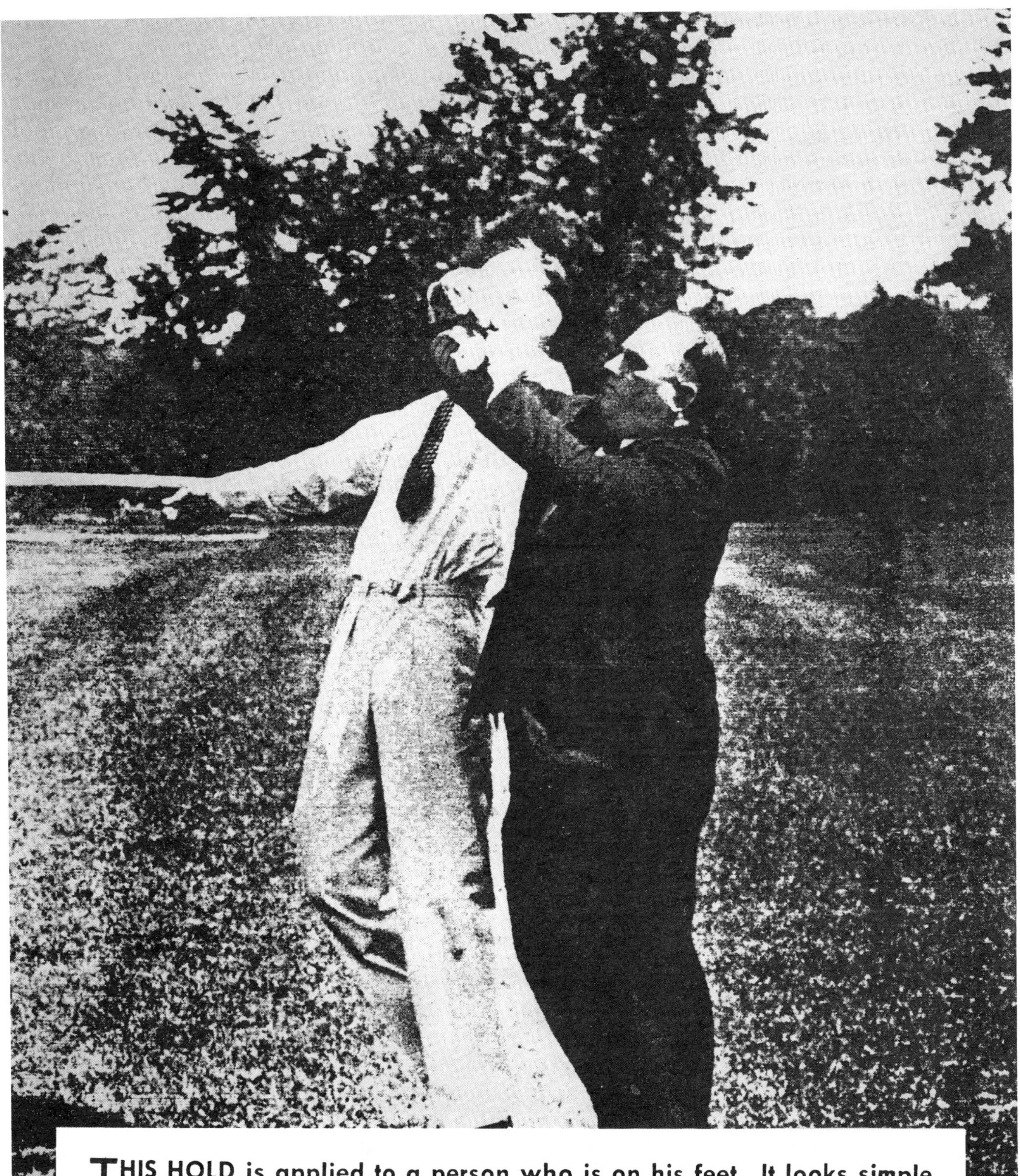

THIS HOLD is applied to a person who is on his feet. It looks simple in the picture. It is simple too, but it does its job. Your upper arm acts as a fulcrum in such a way that you find it easy to hold your victim's arm and hand down leaving him to keep his arm from being broken by stretching up on his toes and hurrying along with you. The exertion on your part is negligible.

The action of this number is somewhat similar to the one preceding. Some people find this routine a little easier to apply.

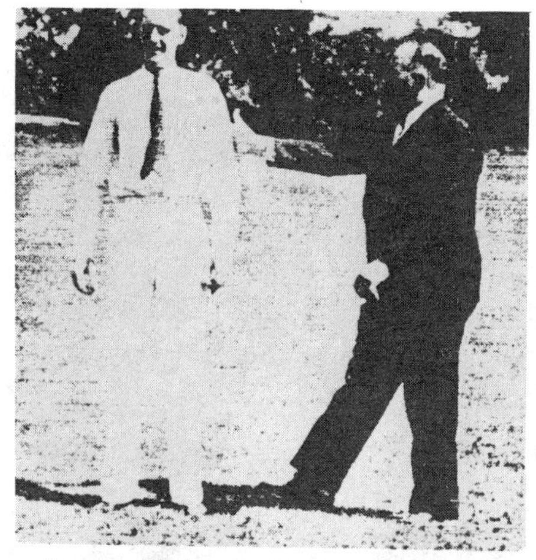

Approach your subject in the same way that you did in the previous number.

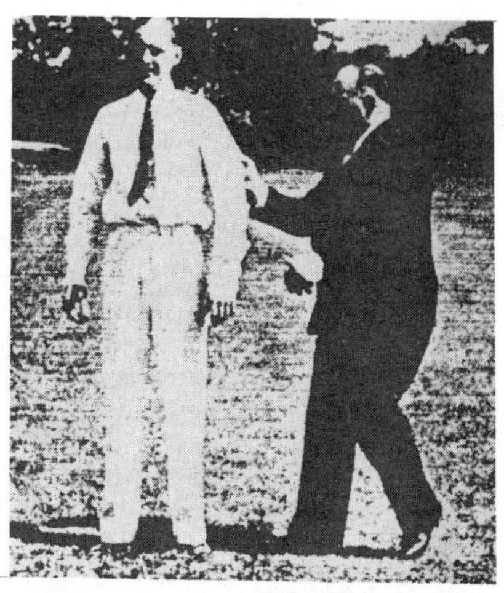

These holds can be worked equally well on either the left or right arm.

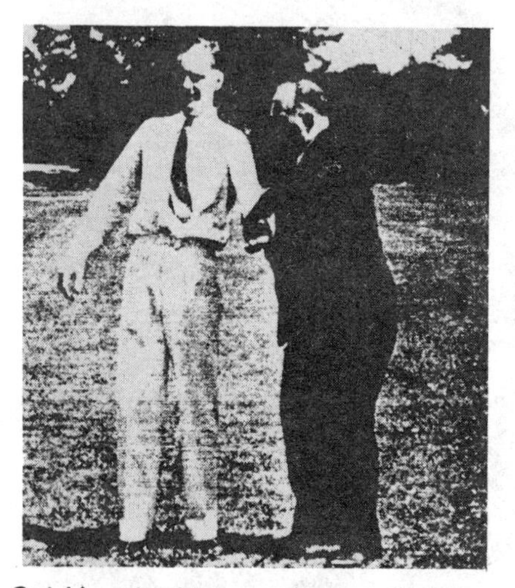

Quickly raise his arm as you twist his wrist. As your left hand brings his hand up

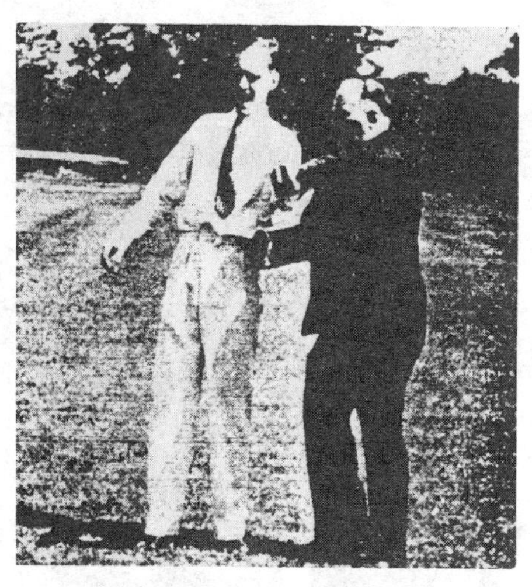

your right arm goes under his left arm exactly at his elbow.

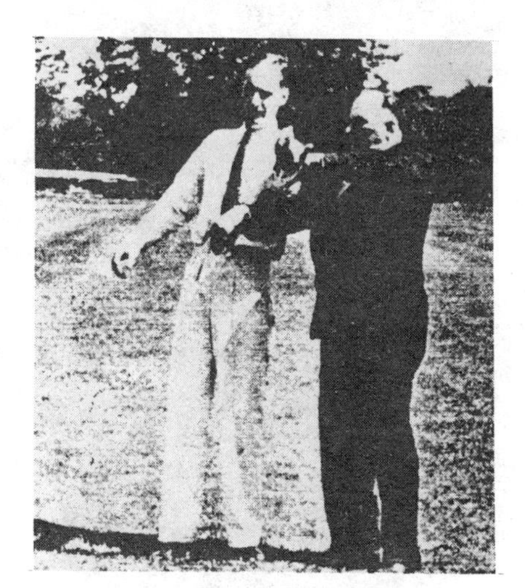

Keep his left arm stretched straight out from his shoulder.

Rest the tips of the fingers of your right hand on your left hand. The leverage you now exert

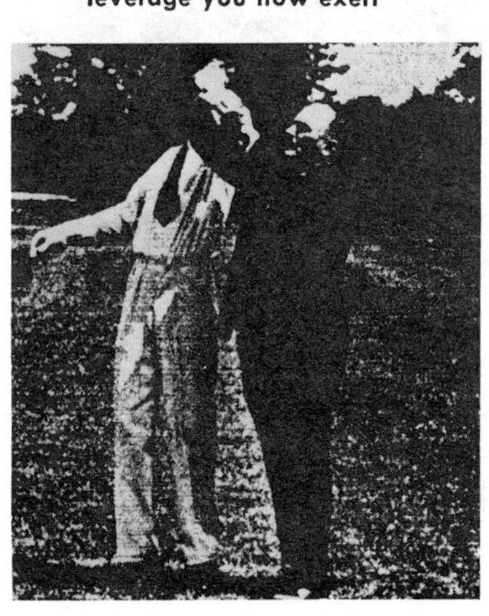

on his arm will bring him right up on his tip toes.

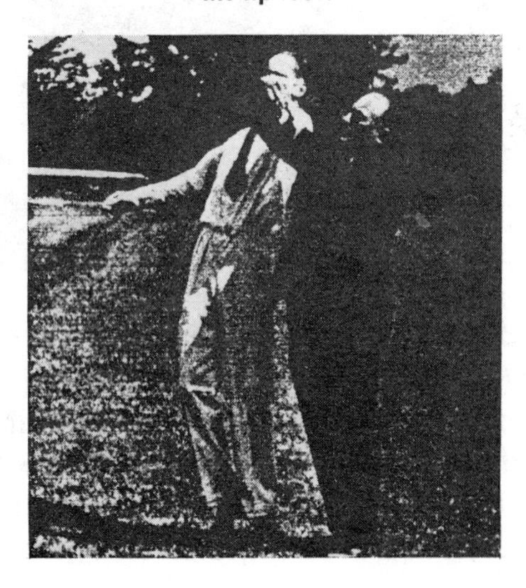

Raising or lowering your right elbow just a fraction of an inch increases or decreases his pain.

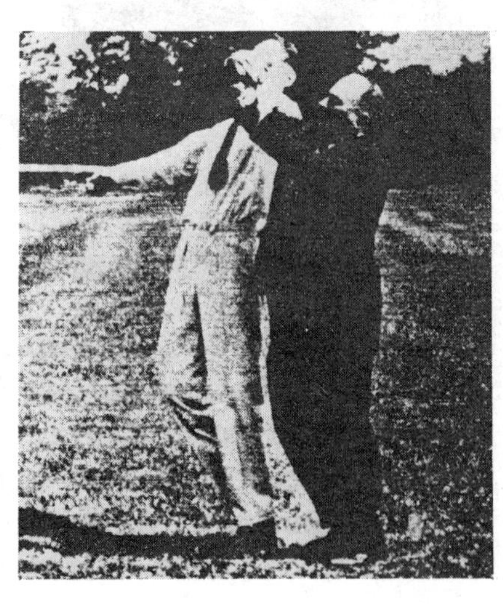

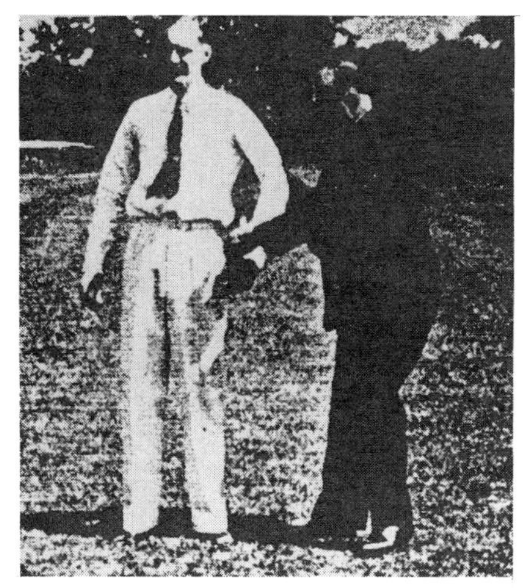

Never hesitate at any point while applying any hold—to do so gives your opponent a chance to retaliate.

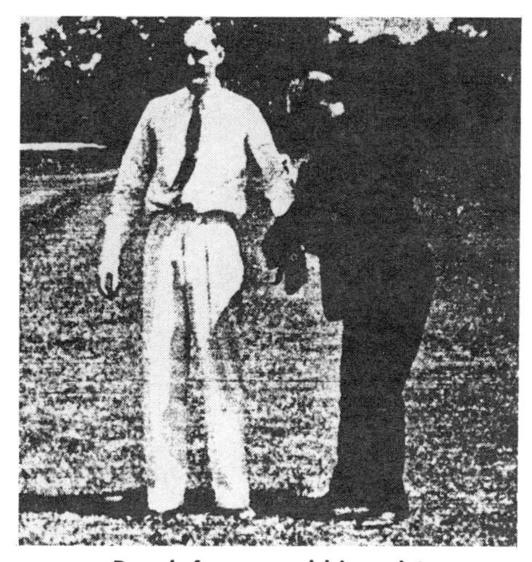

Reach far around his wrist.

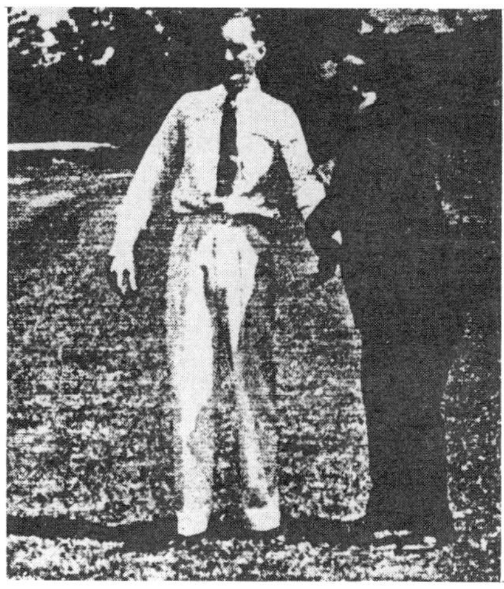

When you have a firm grasp on his wrist your right hand releases his upper arm.

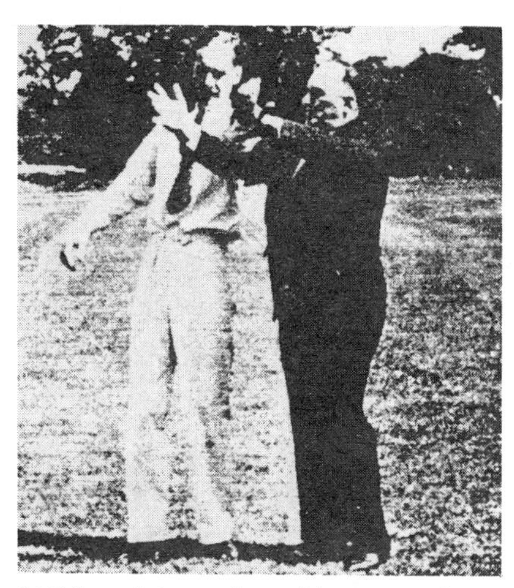

At this point you have him somewhat off balance which makes the finish comparatively easy.

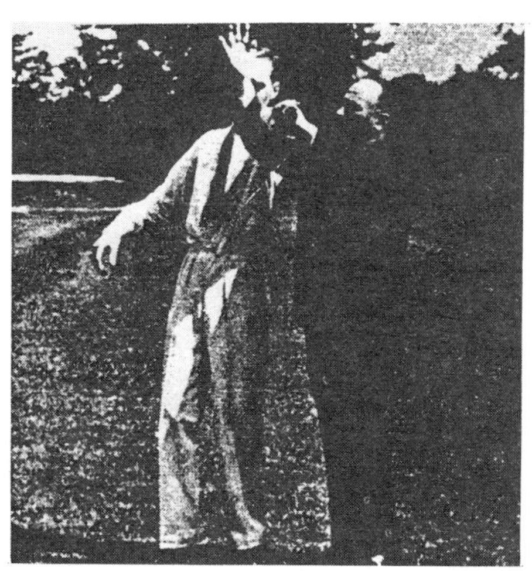

Your man's elbow rests on the inside of your arm just above your own elbow joint.

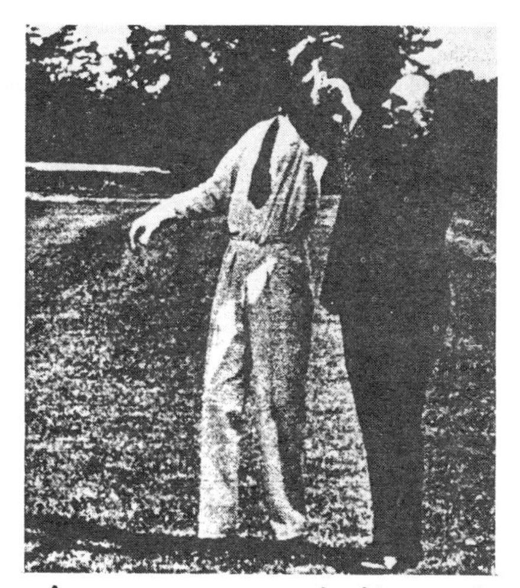

As your arm goes under his arm the practical effect is that your weight is on one end of his arm and his weight is on the other.

You can now keep him in this position by the exertion of a very small amount of pressure.

He cannot possibly escape and he cannot do a single thing to injure you.

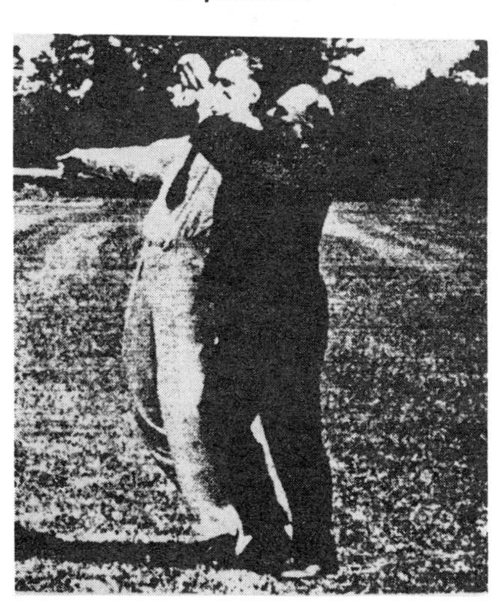

This hold clearly shows how a subject's own weight is put to use against himself.

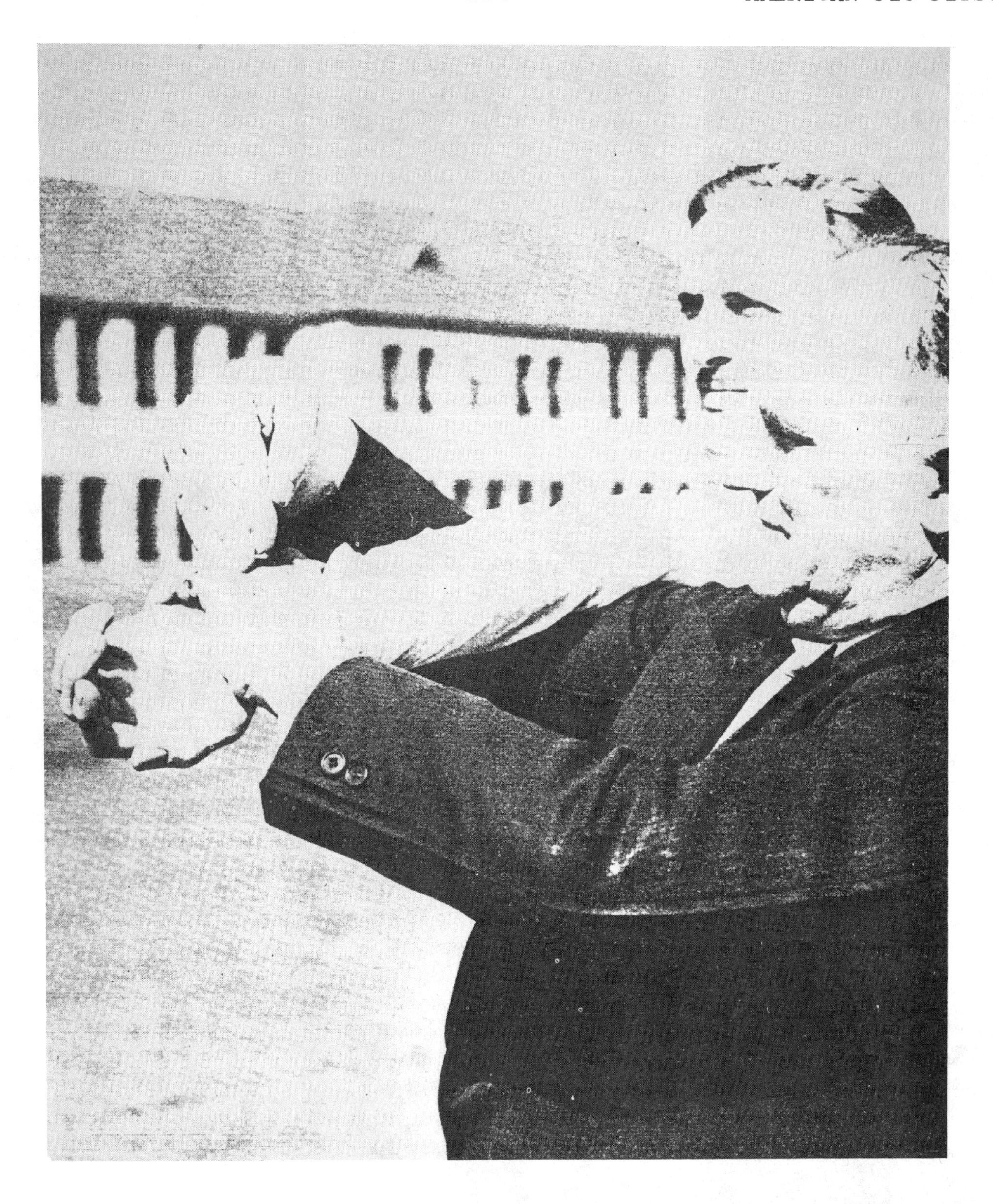

The secret of this "come-along" hold is the manner in which the right hand is held so that only its fingers touch your left hand. Look at the bend in the victim's arm!

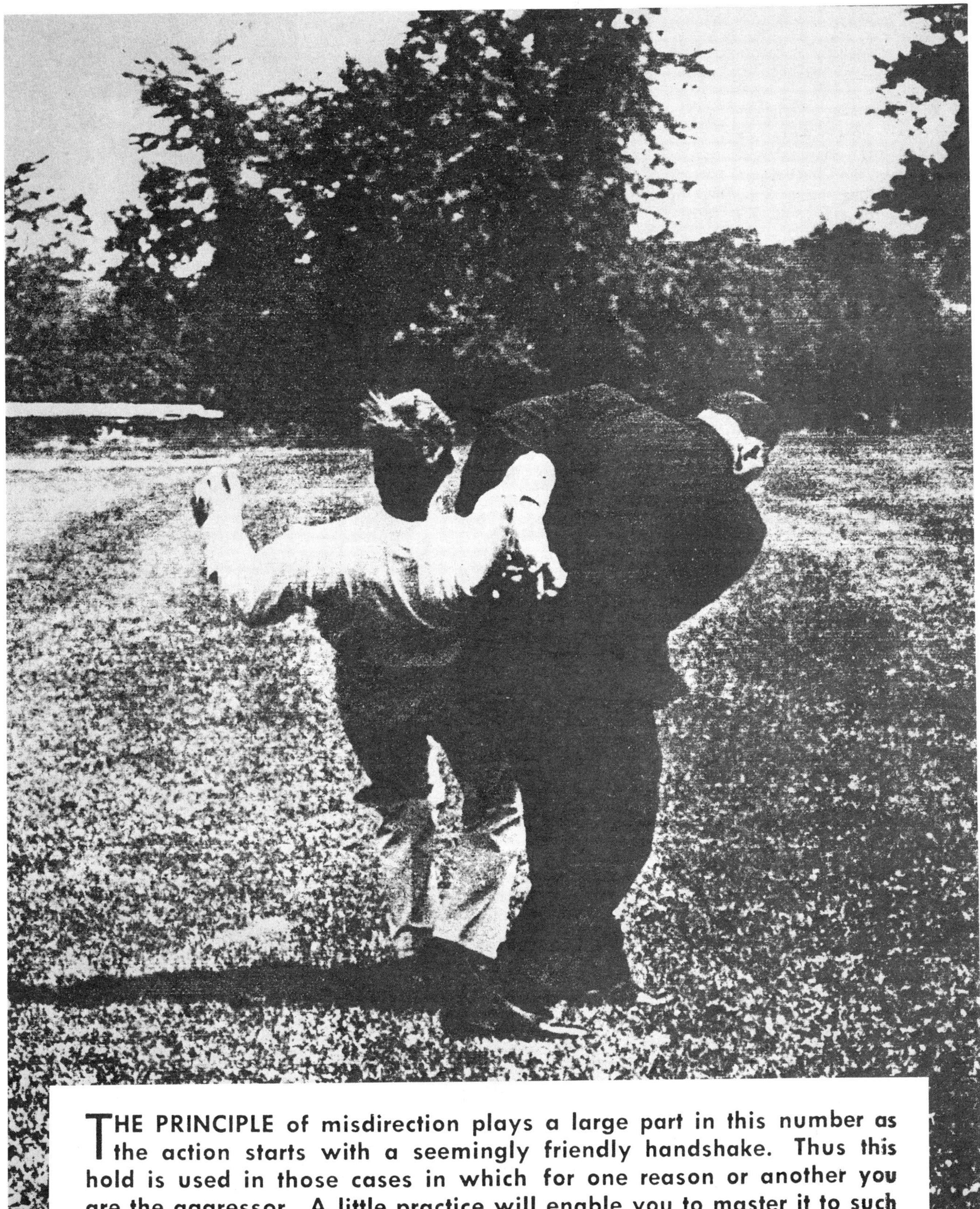

THE PRINCIPLE of misdirection plays a large part in this number as the action starts with a seemingly friendly handshake. Thus this hold is used in those cases in which for one reason or another you are the aggressor. A little practice will enable you to master it to such an extent that you can throw a person to the ground in two seconds. To save his arm he must go down and he'll do it as fast as he can.

A handshake which you convert into a vicious throw is certainly a prime example of misdirection. But because it does take the man by such surprise it is always easy to accomplish.

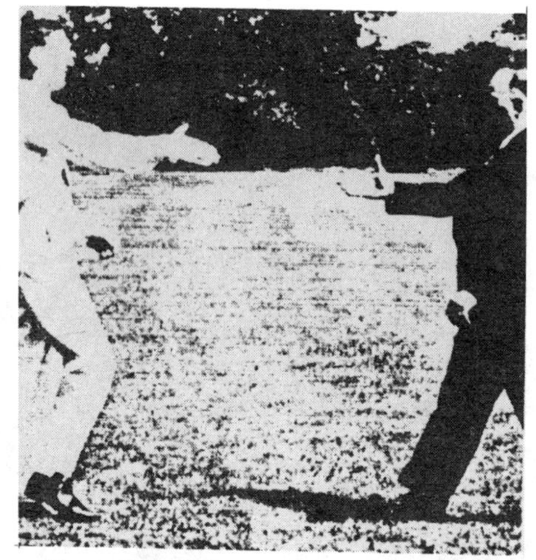

Give a friendly greeting to throw your intended victim off guard.

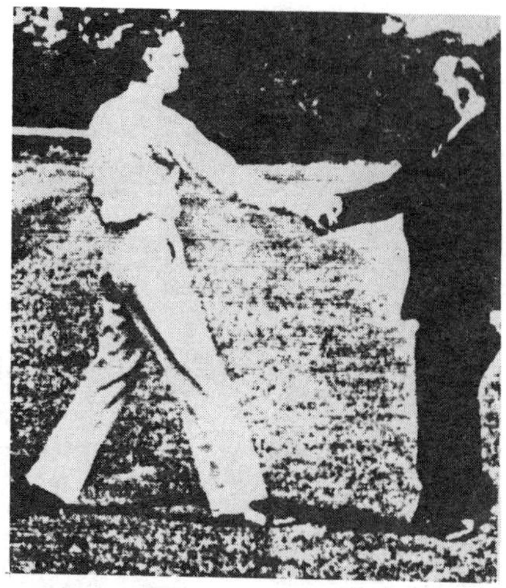

Take a good firm grip on his hand.

The pain in his shoulder and wrist force him around and down.

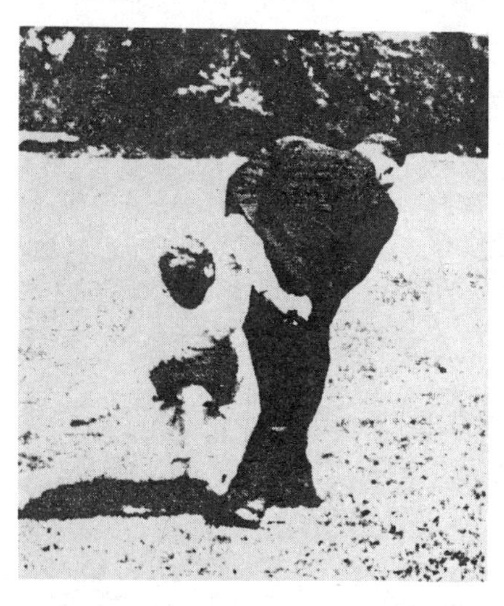

He cannot save himself from falling.

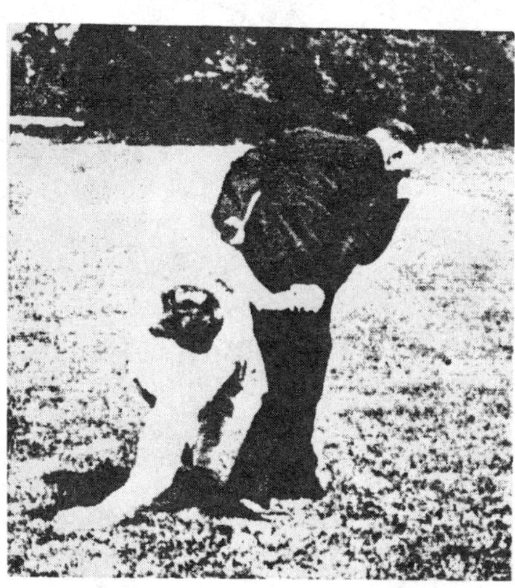

Your left hand has released his elbow.

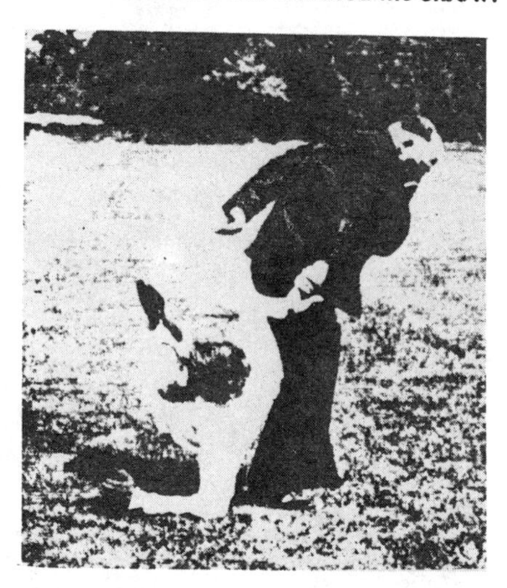

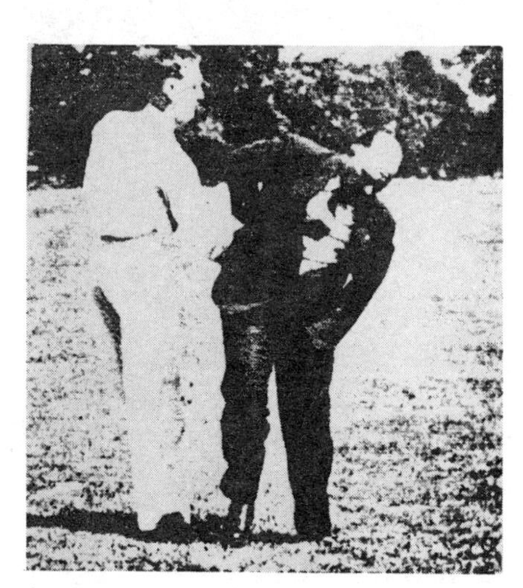

As you turn, the palm of your right hand is facing away from your back.

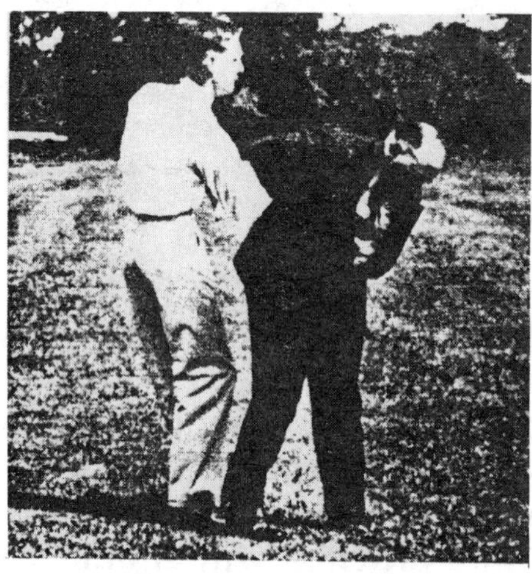

You now have your back squarely turned to your man and

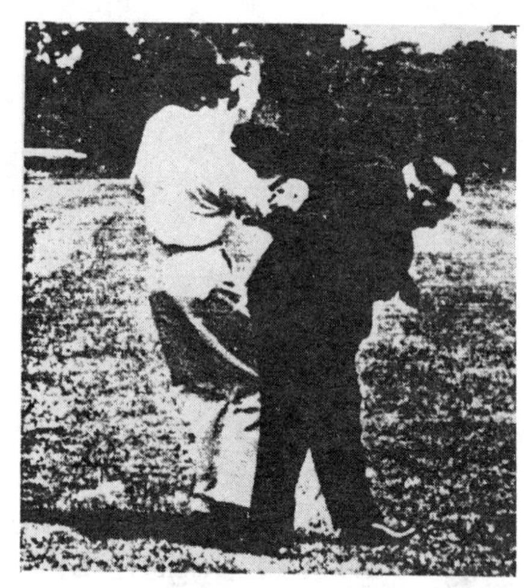

with your left hand you reach behind your back and firmly grasp your opponent's right elbow.

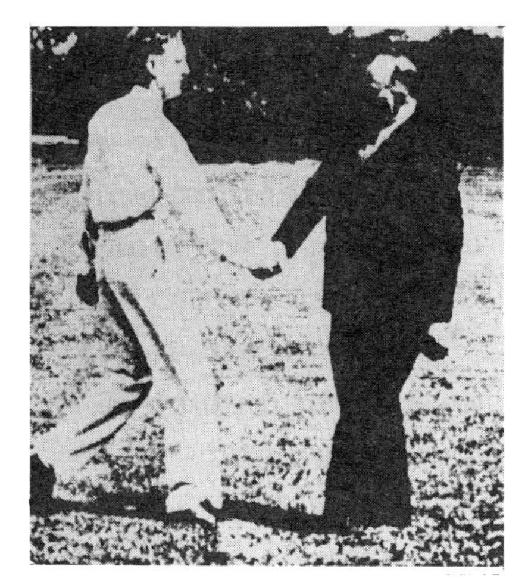

The action is extremely fast from this point to the finish.

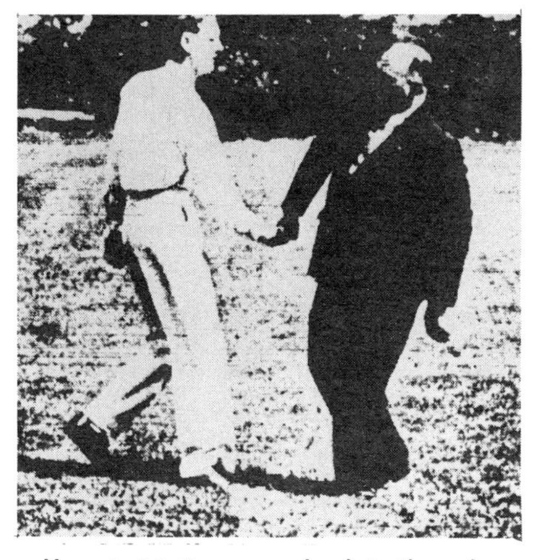

You start to turn your back to the subject all the while

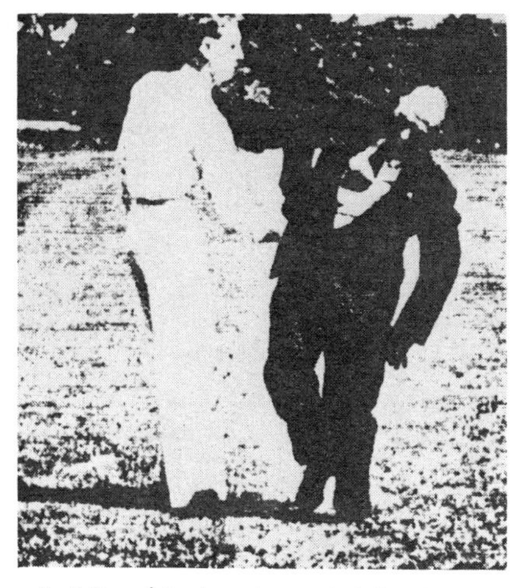

holding his hand so tightly that he cannot withdraw it.

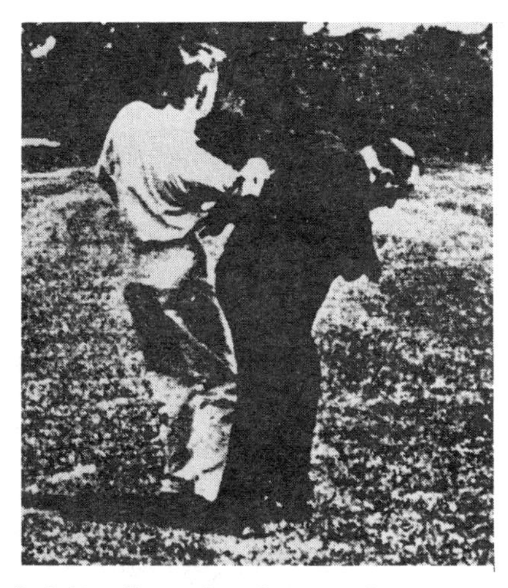

Pull his elbow sharply up and toward your back, while at the same time twisting his hand down.

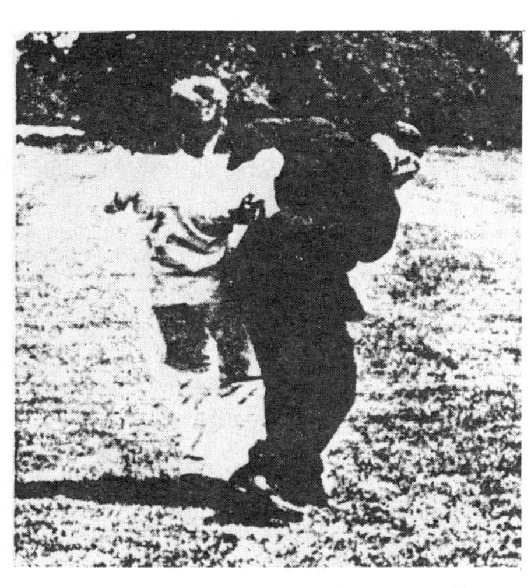

Retention at this point of a very firm grip on his hand is absolutely necessary to insure that

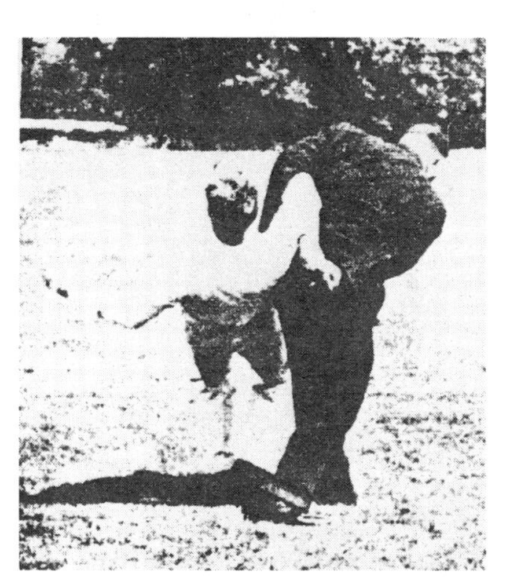

your opponent is not able to retain his balance.

At this point you retain your grip on his hand only if you want to hold him on the ground.

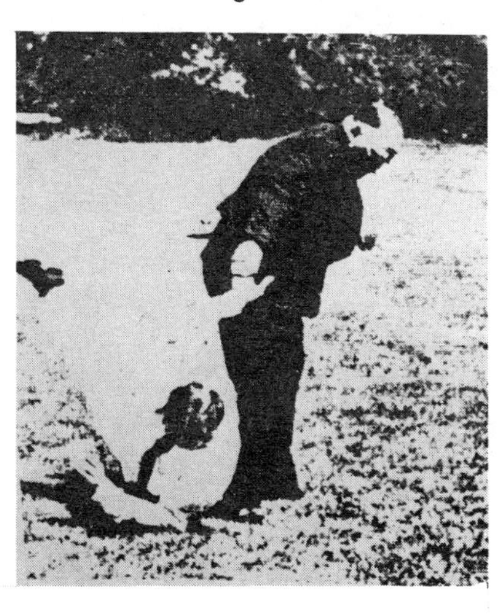

You now can bend his arm backward over your knee if you want him to stay down.

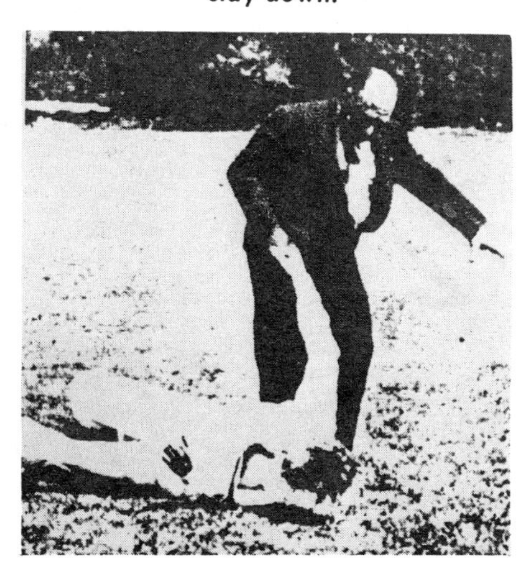

"The hand is quicker than the eye" applies one hundred per cent to Jiu-Jitsu. Before your opponent can SEE what you are doing you should have the hold firmly fixed.

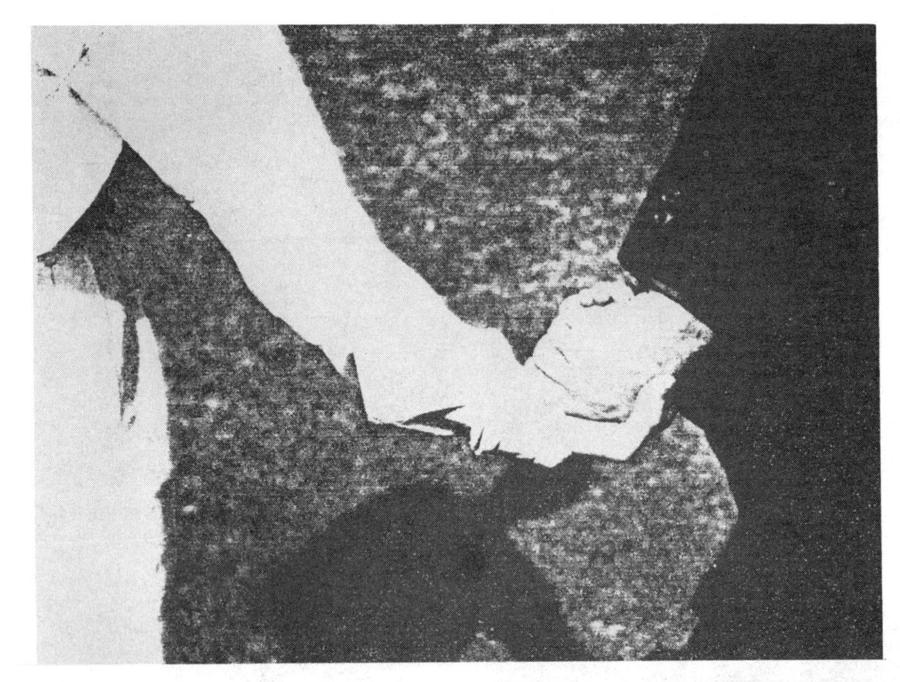

These two pictures re-emphasize the important action of the last hold. As soon as you have your enemy's hand, swing your body very quickly around until you are holding him behind you like this. You are the one who turns; don't try to swing him around you.

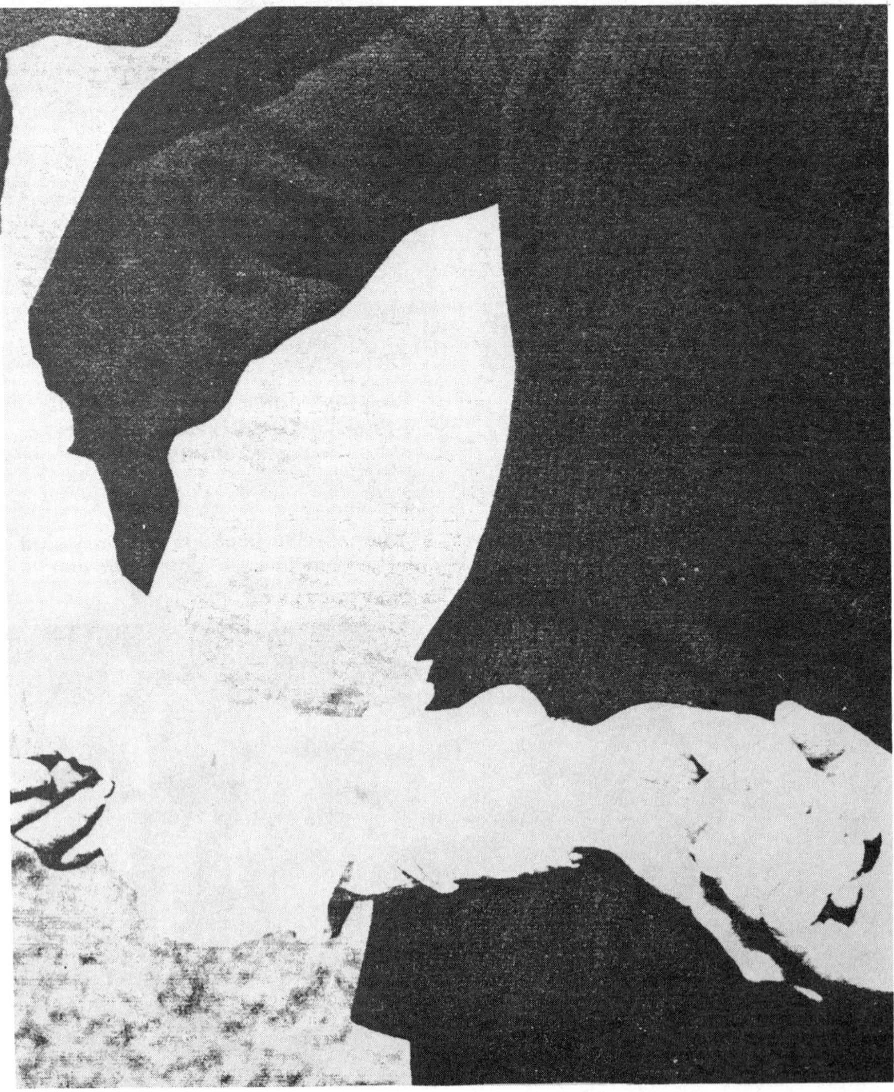

You continue turning until your left hand can, by reaching behind you, grip his right arm just above his elbow. Then by pulling his elbow up and toward you he will be thrown.

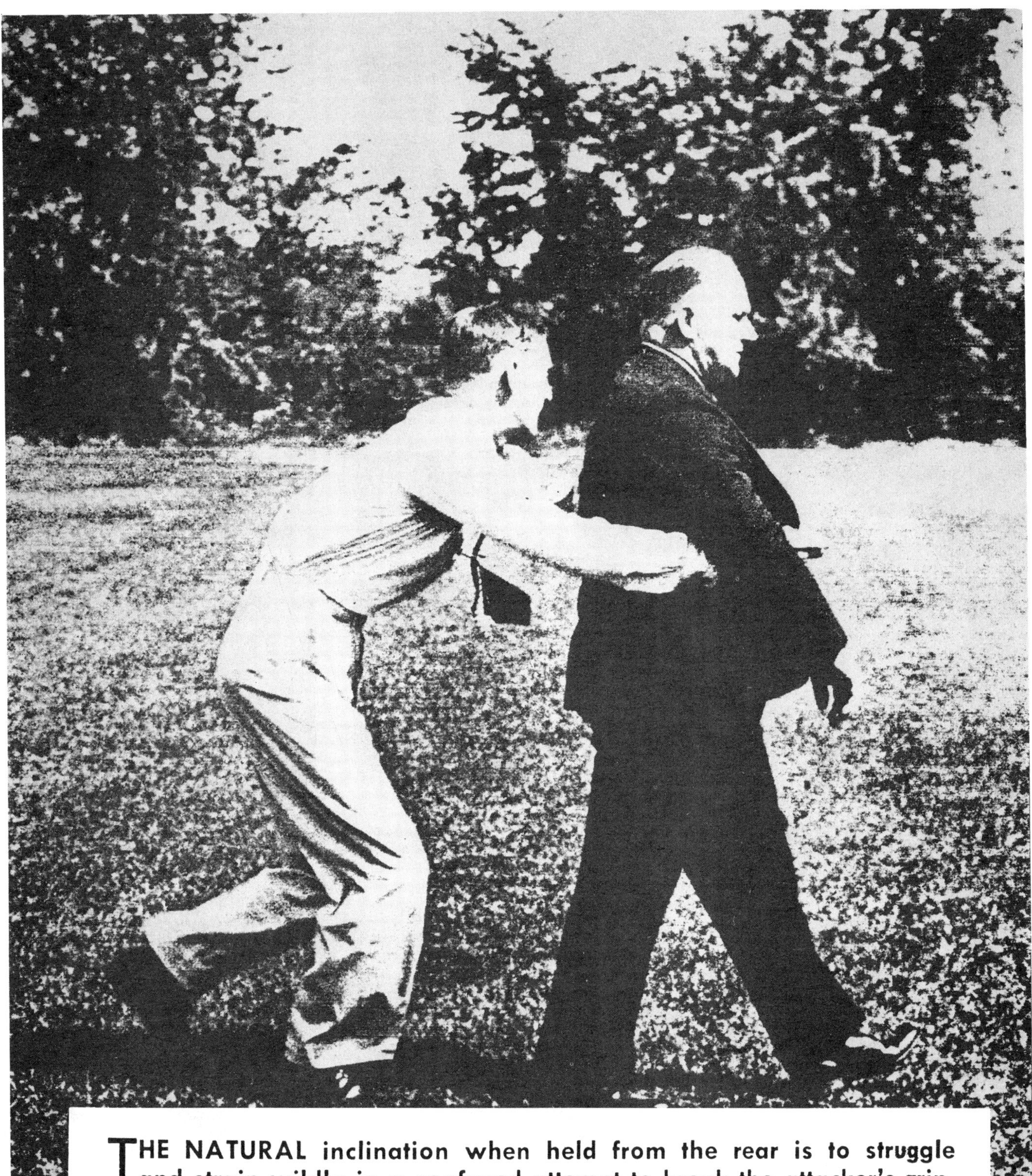

THE NATURAL inclination when held from the rear is to struggle and strain wildly in a confused attempt to break the attacker's grip. The hold can be broken very simply and easily though, by following the directions of this lesson, and at the finish the aggressor ends up on the ground. This is the first number in this book which makes use of the hip throw which is an important part of a great many Jiu-Jitsu operations.

As you can see, this lesson only applies when your arms are not pinned to your side by your assailant. In those cases we use a different Jiu-Jitsu release.

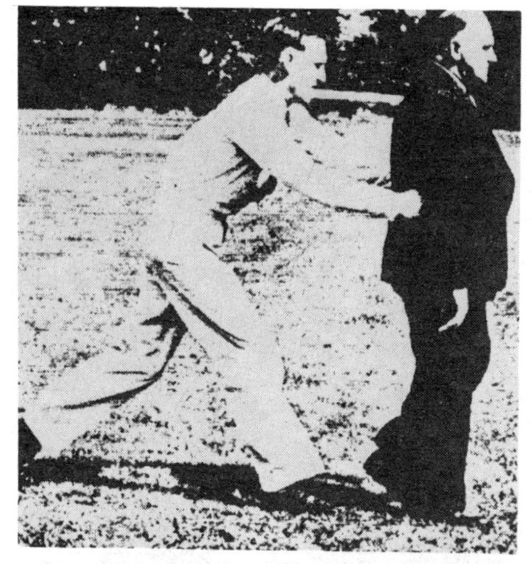

Attackers very frequently try to overpower their victims by seizing them from behind.

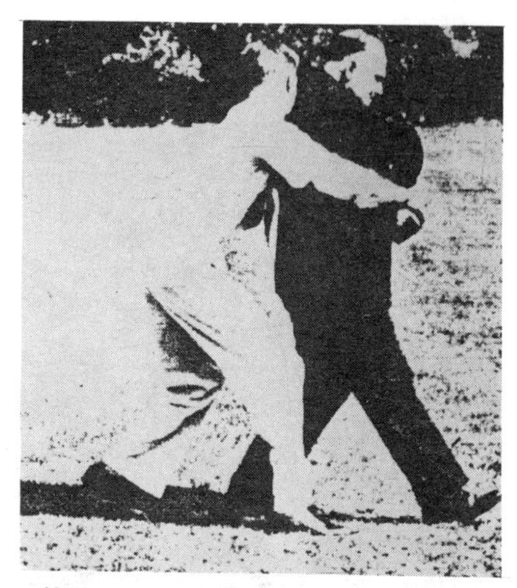

If this should happen to you do not waste your strength or time trying to turn around.

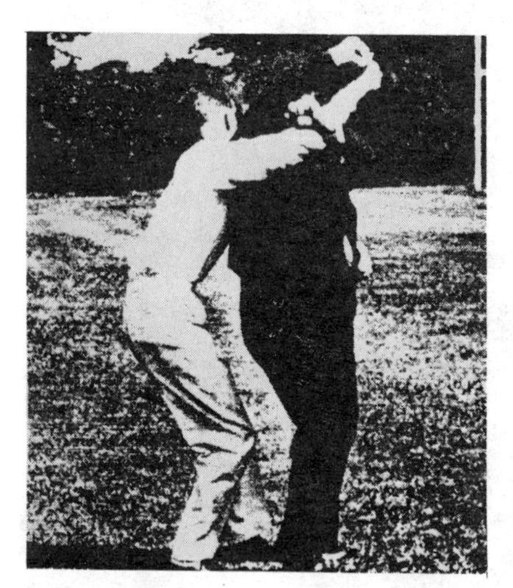

Bring your left arm over underneath his arm right at his elbow and

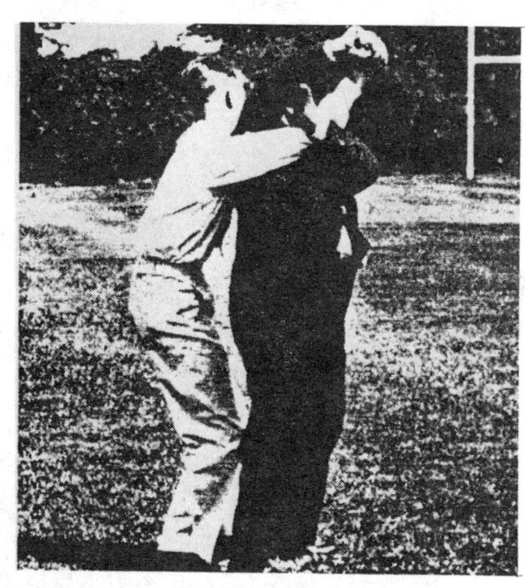

lock his arm in by resting the fingers of your left hand on your right arm just above your elbow.

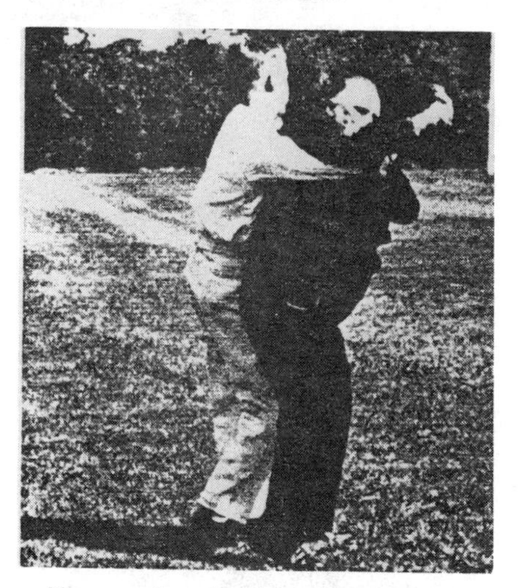

Now, using the hip throw, you are going to throw him fast and hard. To do this you

You have retained your lock on his arm and your grip on his thumb.

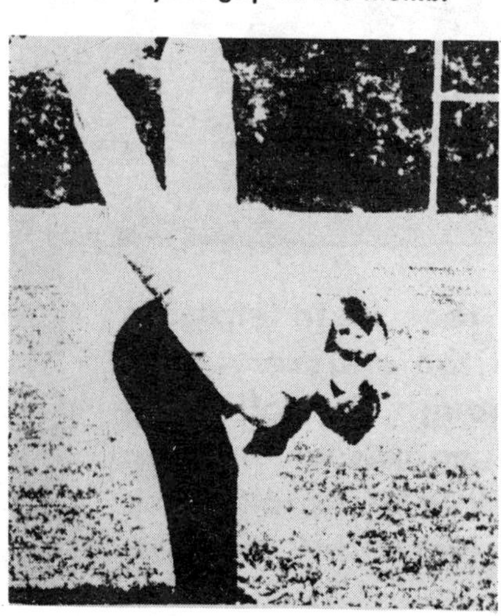

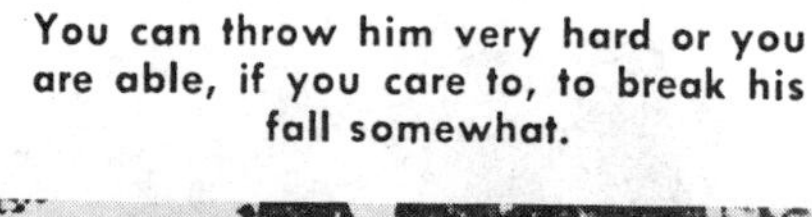

You can throw him very hard or you are able, if you care to, to break his fall somewhat.

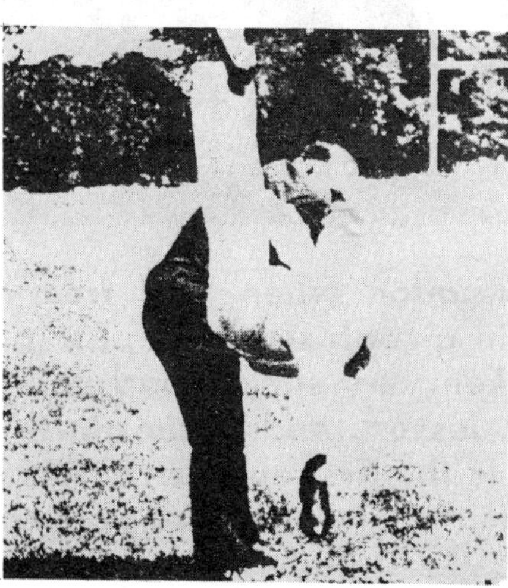

Don't let go of his thumb yet because you're going to want to keep control of anyone who has attacked you from behind.

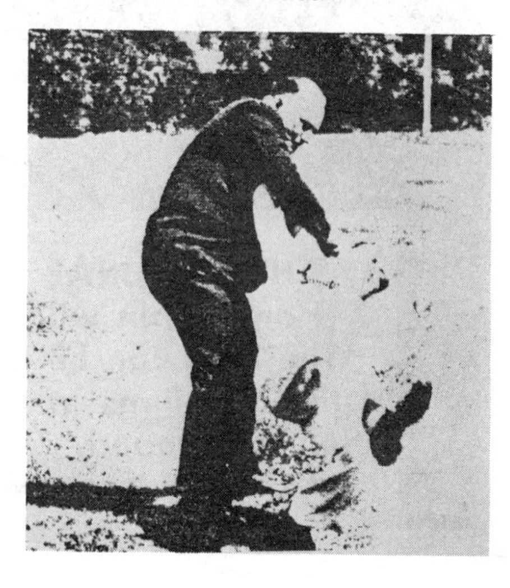

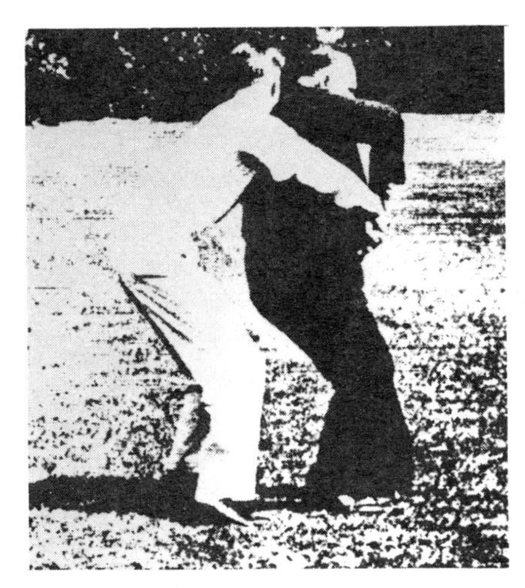

In breaking this hold you must obtain a strong grasp on the attacker's right thumb by

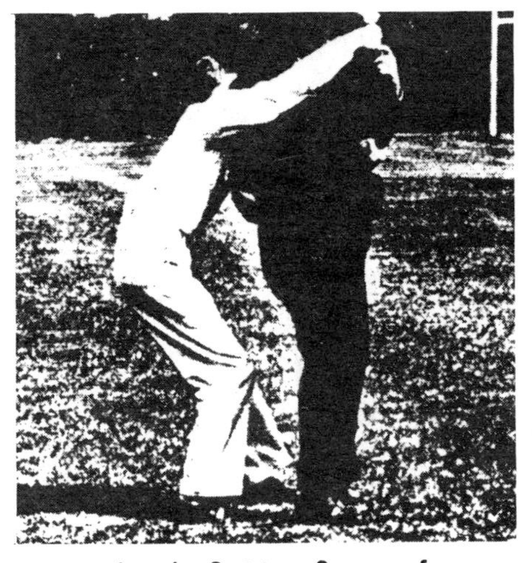

wrapping the first two fingers of your right hand around his thumb with the back of your hand toward you.

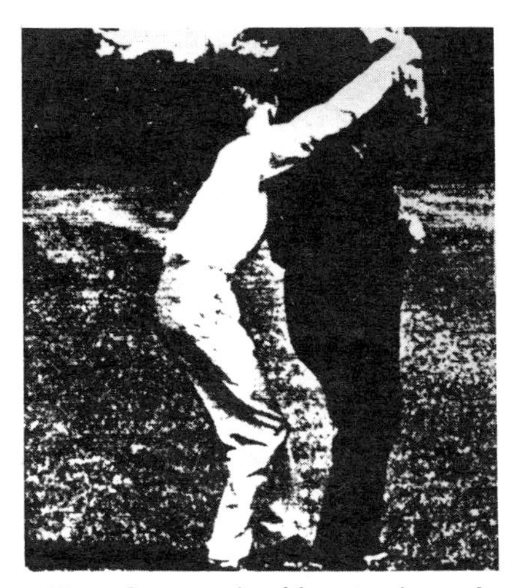

Your fingers should extend as far down the base of his thumb as they will reach. Stretch his arm to the full limit at the same time raising it away up in the air.

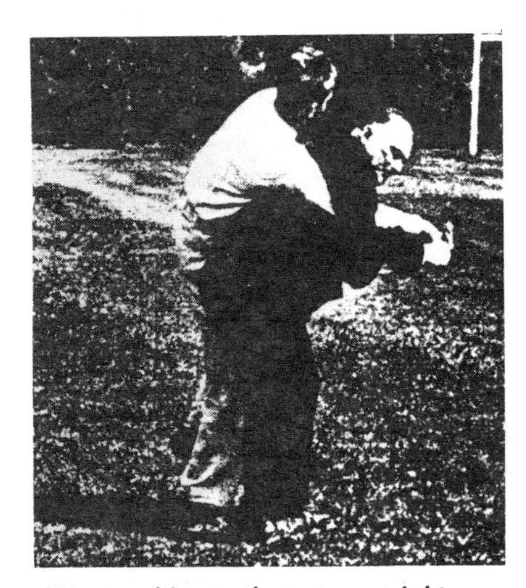

shift your hips to the extreme right as you simultaneously bend over and jerk him forward.

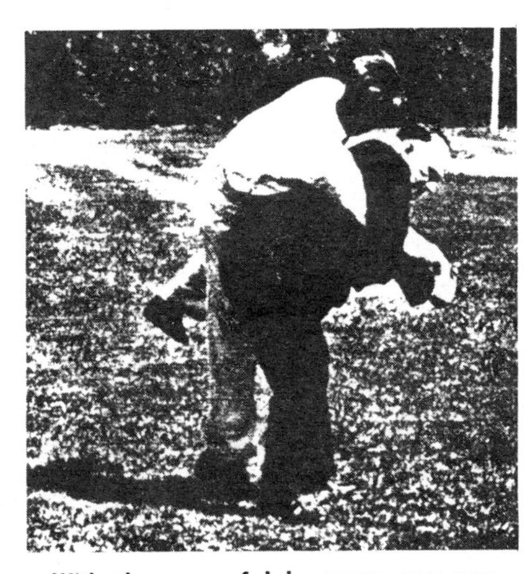

With the powerful leverage you are exerting on his arm he'll leave the ground easily.

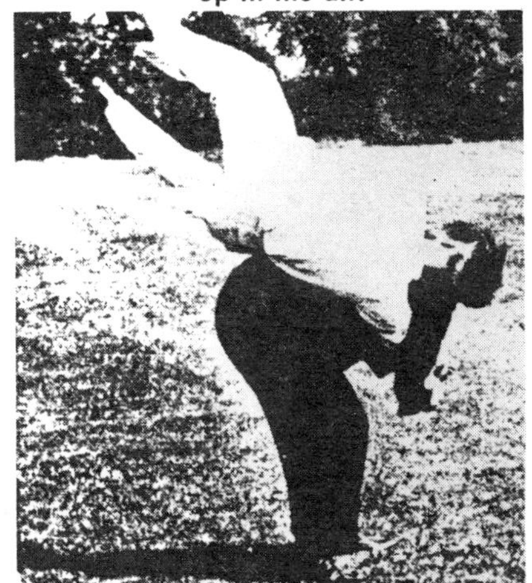

Actually the larger the man the easier it is to throw him over this way.

Once he is on the ground release his thumb and very quickly grasp his first and second fingers in one of your hands. With your other hand

grip his third and fourth fingers. With the palm of his hand bent far back from his wrist spread his fingers apart and bend them back. This will hold him.

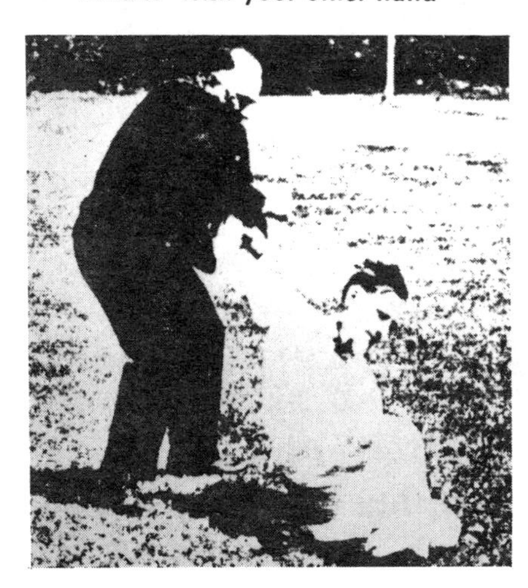

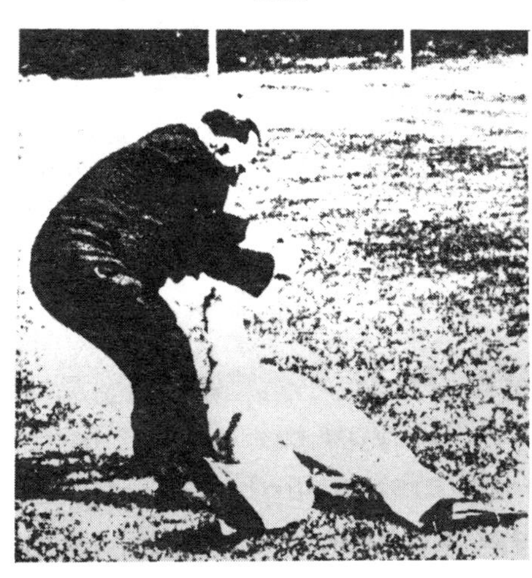

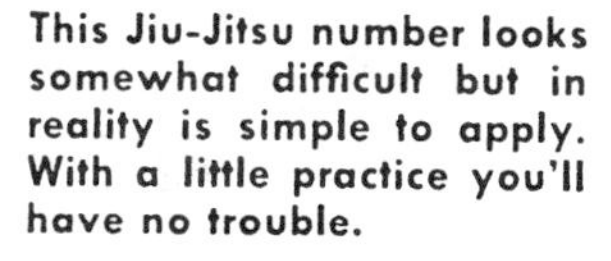

This Jiu-Jitsu number looks somewhat difficult but in reality is simple to apply. With a little practice you'll have no trouble.

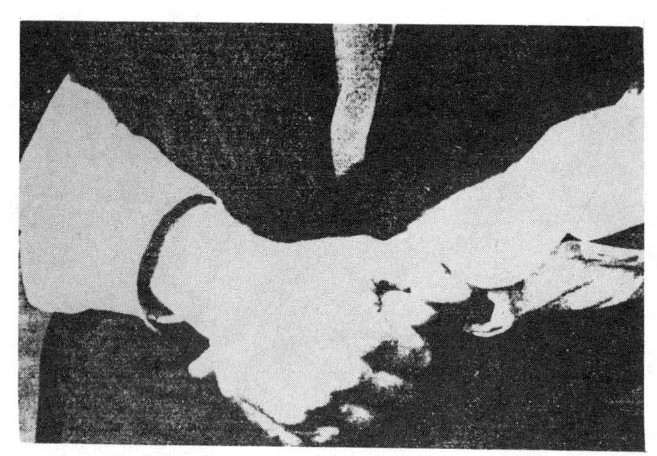

If his hand is so tightly closed that it is difficult to grasp his thumb, close your right hand and use your big knuckle to bore into the nerve on the back of his hand. He'll open his hand, quickly.

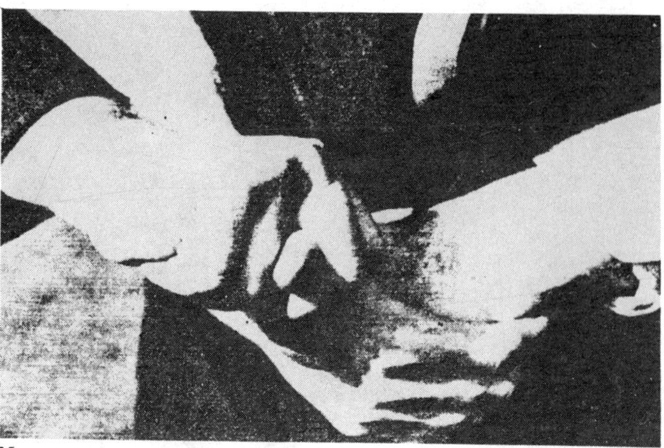

You use only your thumb and first two fingers to grip his thumb. To do this correctly you must hold far down toward the big knuckle of his thumb and at an angle. Your fingers should point down over the large joint of his thumb.

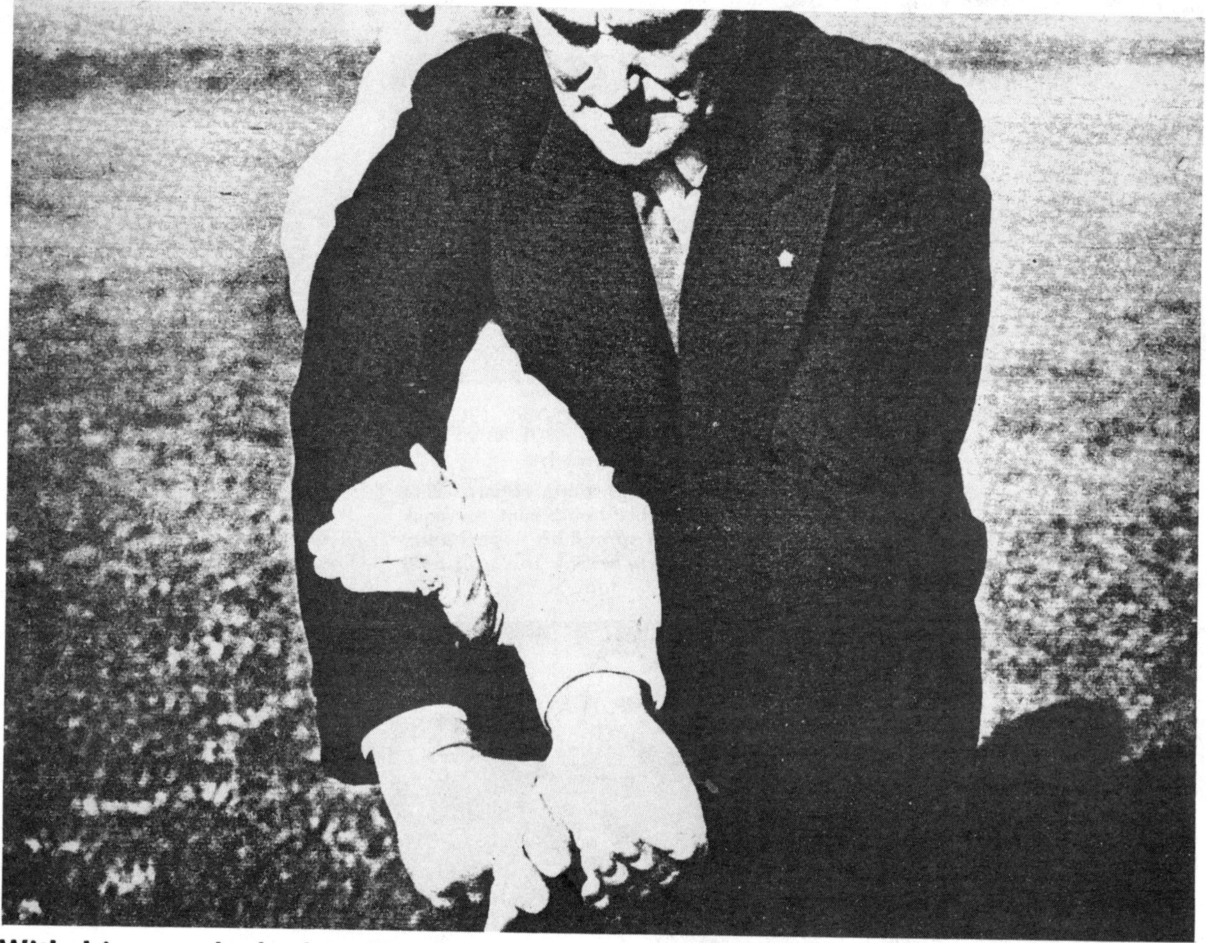

With his arm locked in like this you are all set to throw him over by the hip throw. Keep the pressure severe enough in this position so that he is in pain and will not try to hit you with his free hand.

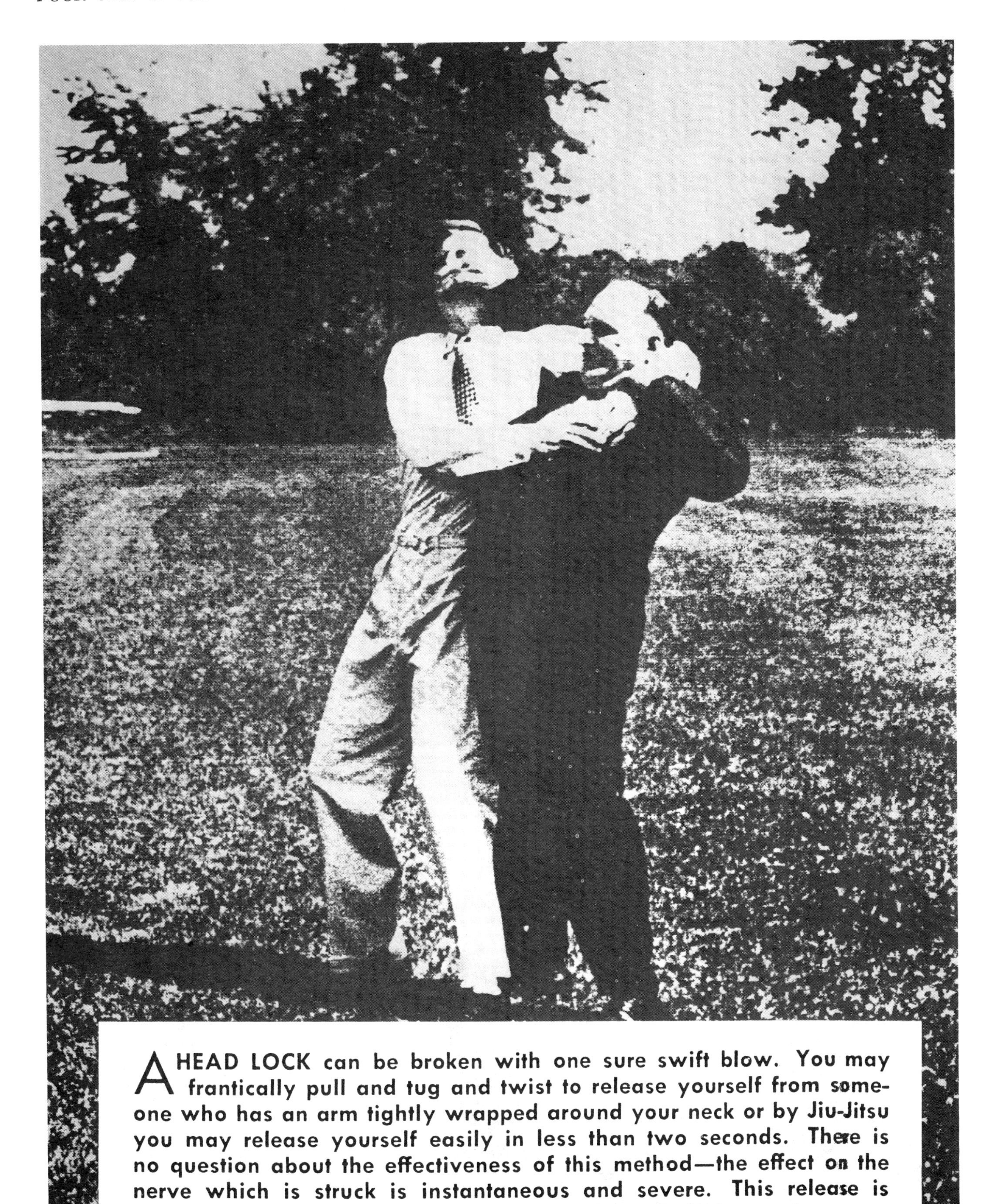

A HEAD LOCK can be broken with one sure swift blow. You may frantically pull and tug and twist to release yourself from someone who has an arm tightly wrapped around your neck or by Jiu-Jitsu you may release yourself easily in less than two seconds. There is no question about the effectiveness of this method—the effect on the nerve which is struck is instantaneous and severe. This release is very easy to apply and needs comparatively little practice.

This is a one hand break for a head lock which you can depend upon whenever you may have an occasion to apply it.

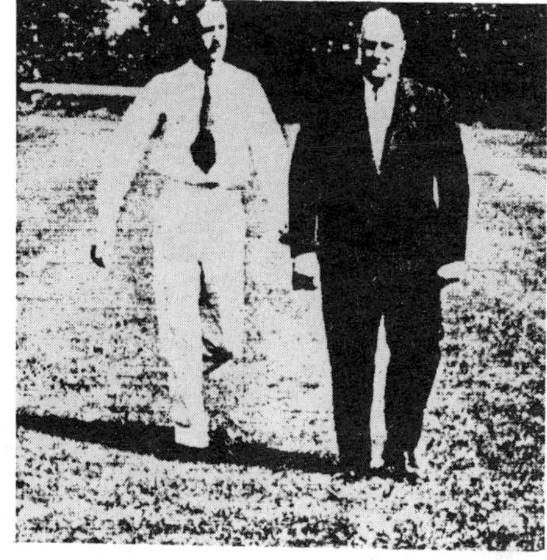

In Jiu-Jitsu there are several ways to release yourself from such a predicament

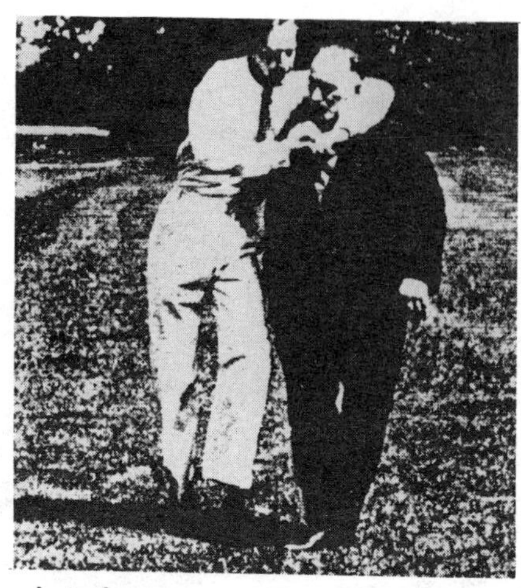

but there are none easier or more simple than this method.

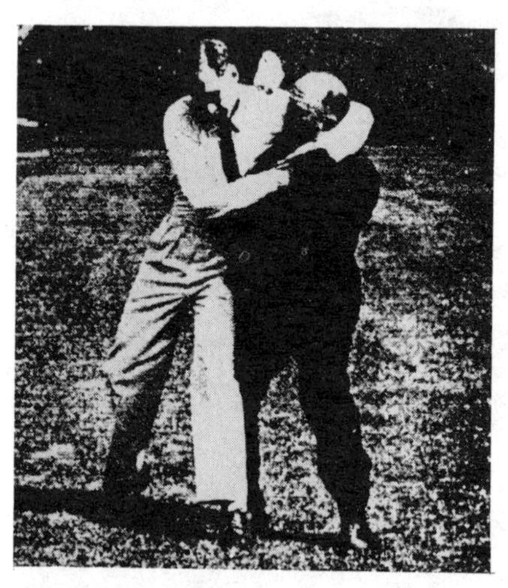

and bring your right arm up behind your opponent's back

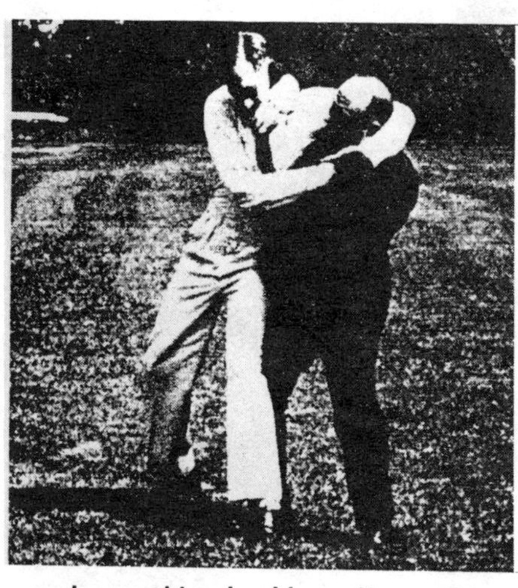

and over his shoulder. Have your right hand in the position recommended for a knife blow.

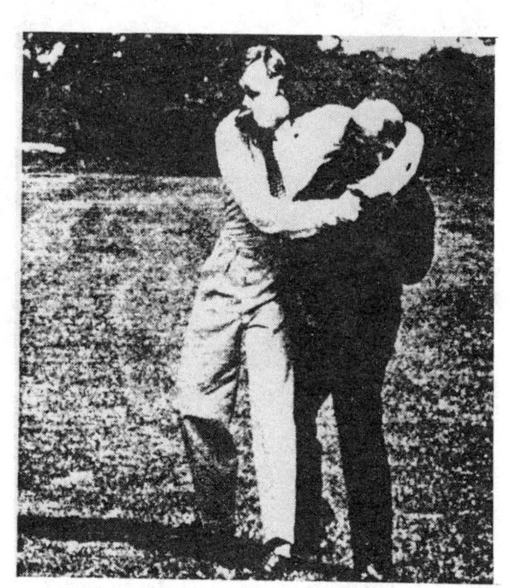

In the meantime waste none of your effort in trying to break the grip of his arms by pulling

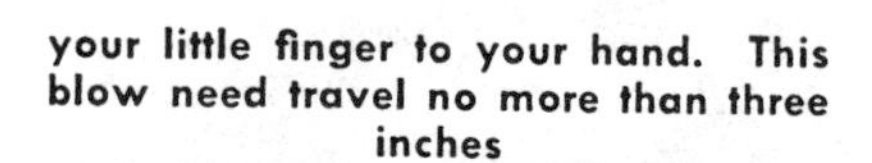

your little finger to your hand. This blow need travel no more than three inches

to completely incapacitate your man for further action for some time.

His grasp around your neck will be broken at once and

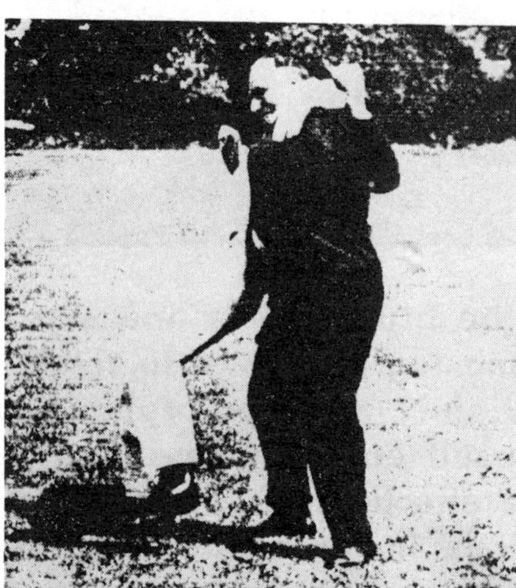

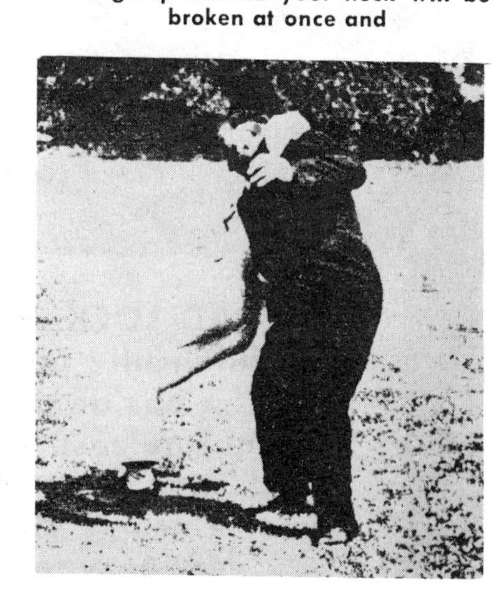

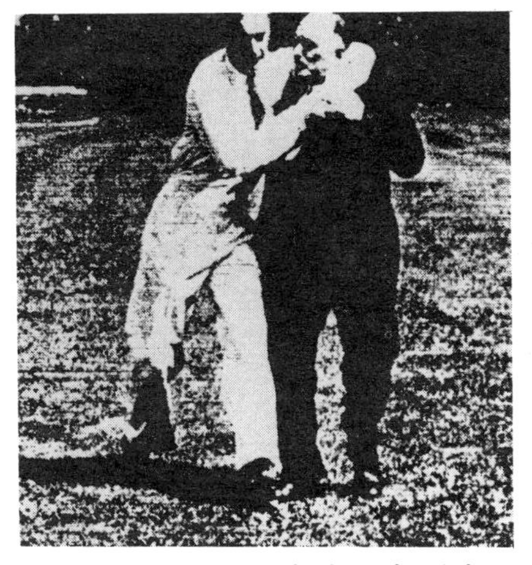

Whether you are attacked on the right or left side makes no difference in the ease of your release.

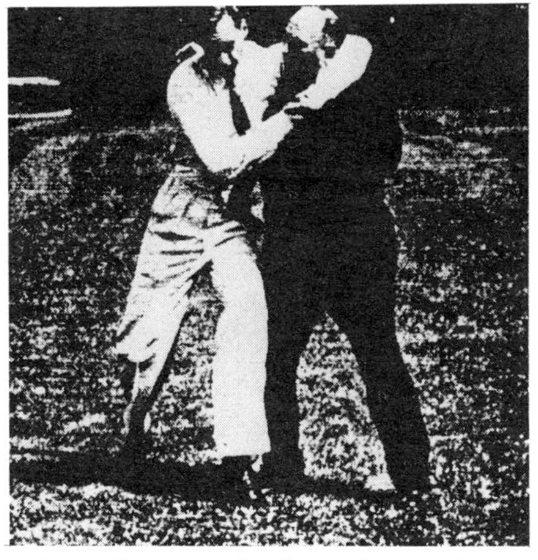

As in the example shown here, when your assailant is on your right side

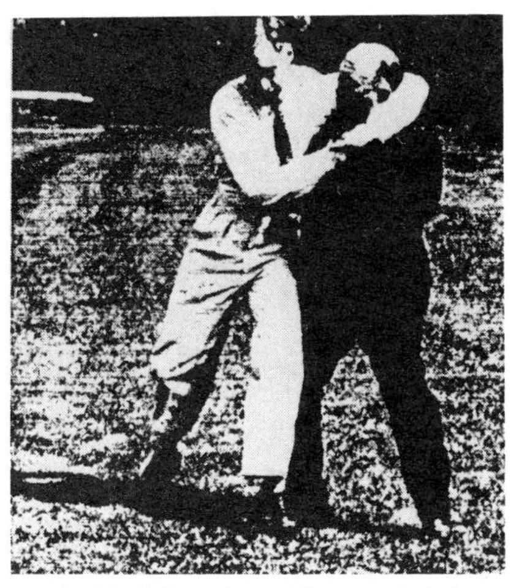

grip his left wrist with your left hand

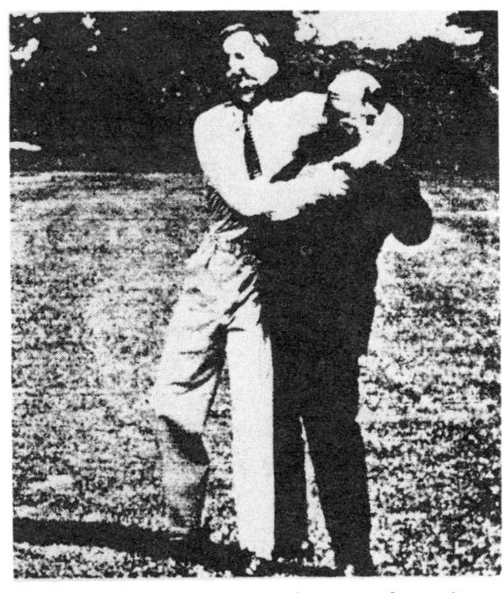

on his arms or trying to loosen the grip of his hands. Strike with the knife edge

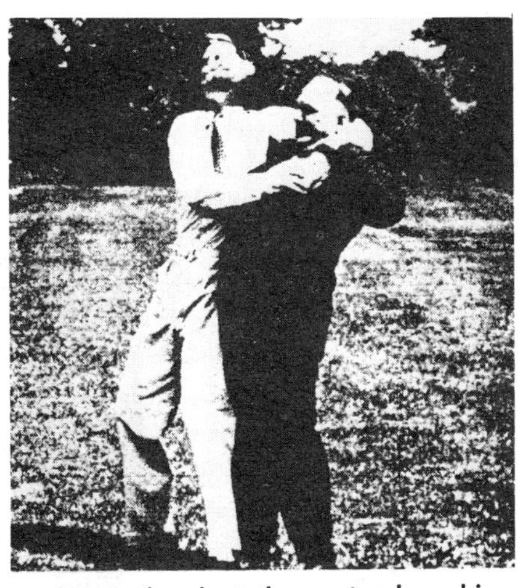

of your hand at the spot where his upper lip meets his nose.

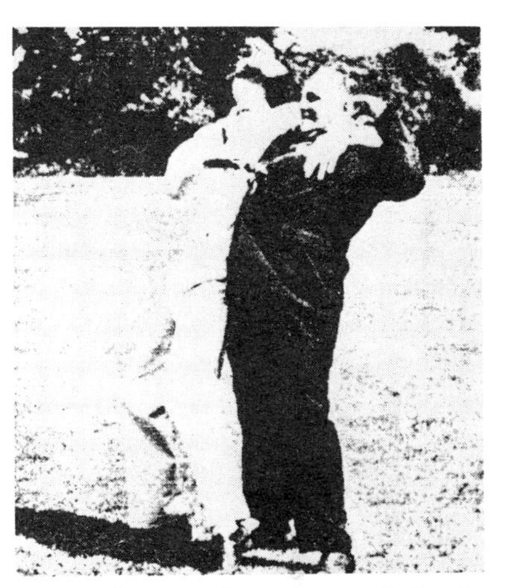

Have the actual contact made by the big knuckle which joins

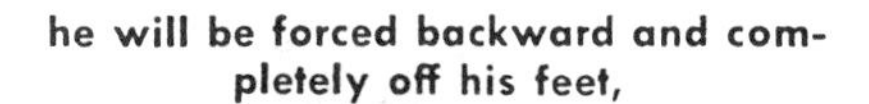

he will be forced backward and completely off his feet,

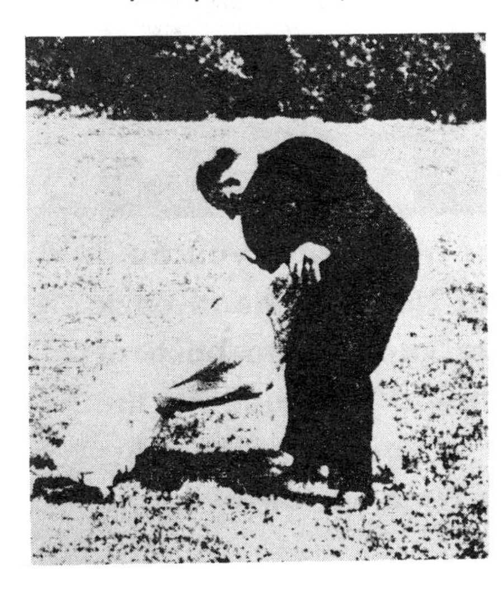

thus giving you a perfect opportunity to take further action should it appear necessary.

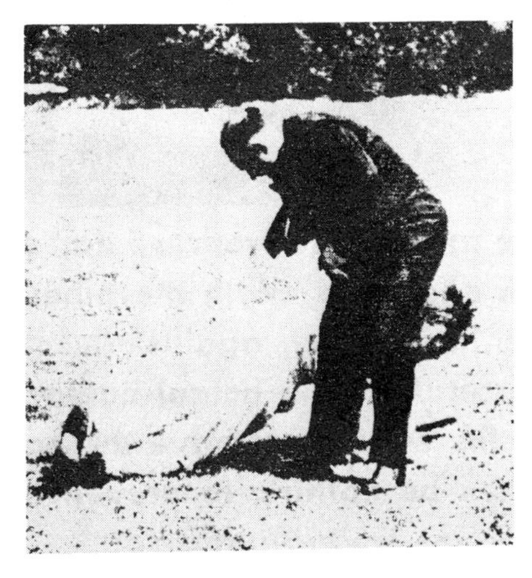

When you are practicing this number just push on the nerve spot below your partner's nose instead of actually giving it a blow.

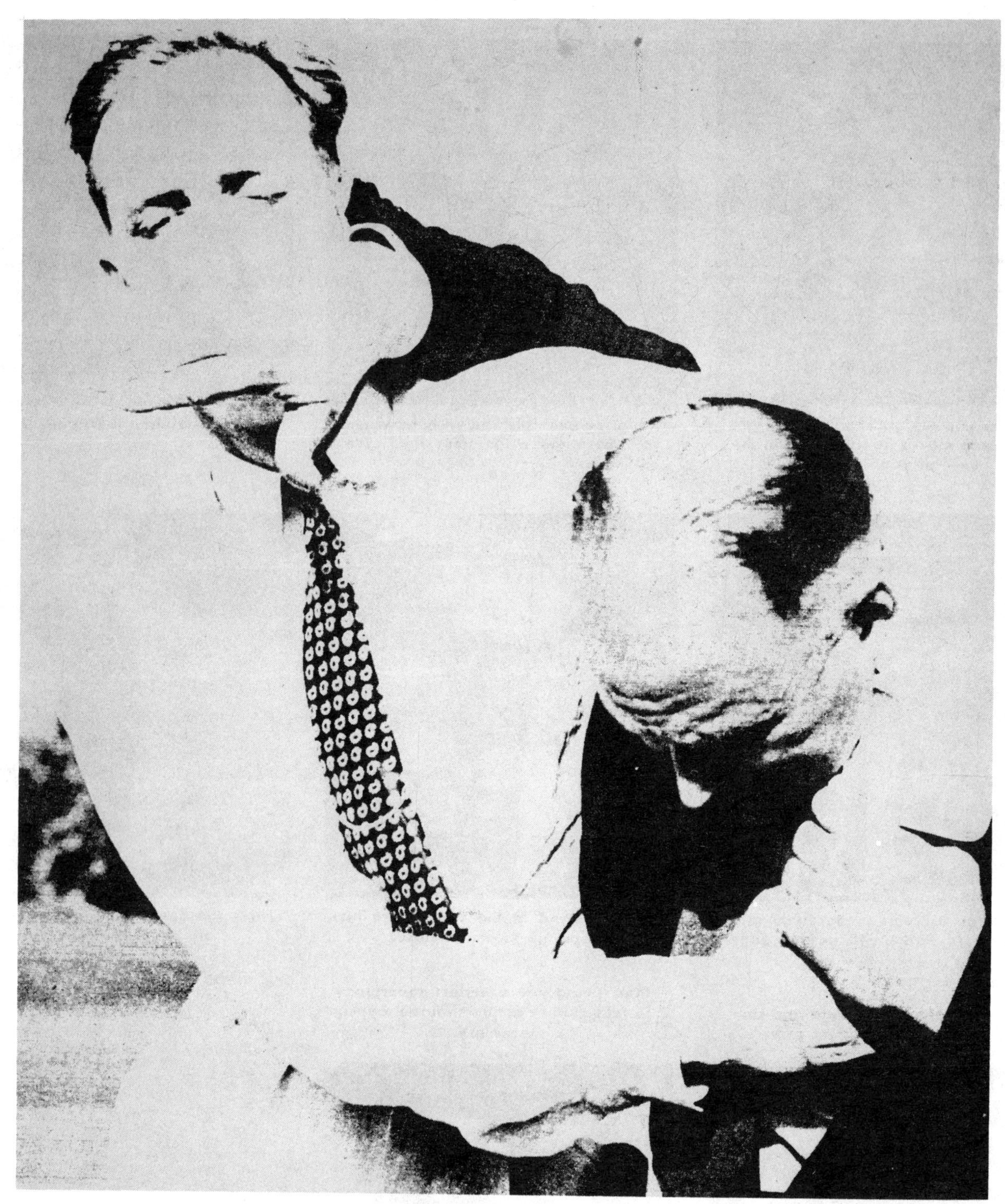

Checking over once more the release from a head lock, notice that you hold the assailant's wrist with one hand. With the other you force his head back by placing your hand, knife fashion, against the nerve spot at the base of his nose and pushing forcefully. The actual contact should be made by the big knuckle of your little finger. Do not have the palm of your hand over his mouth as there would then be nothing to prevent him from viciously biting your hand.

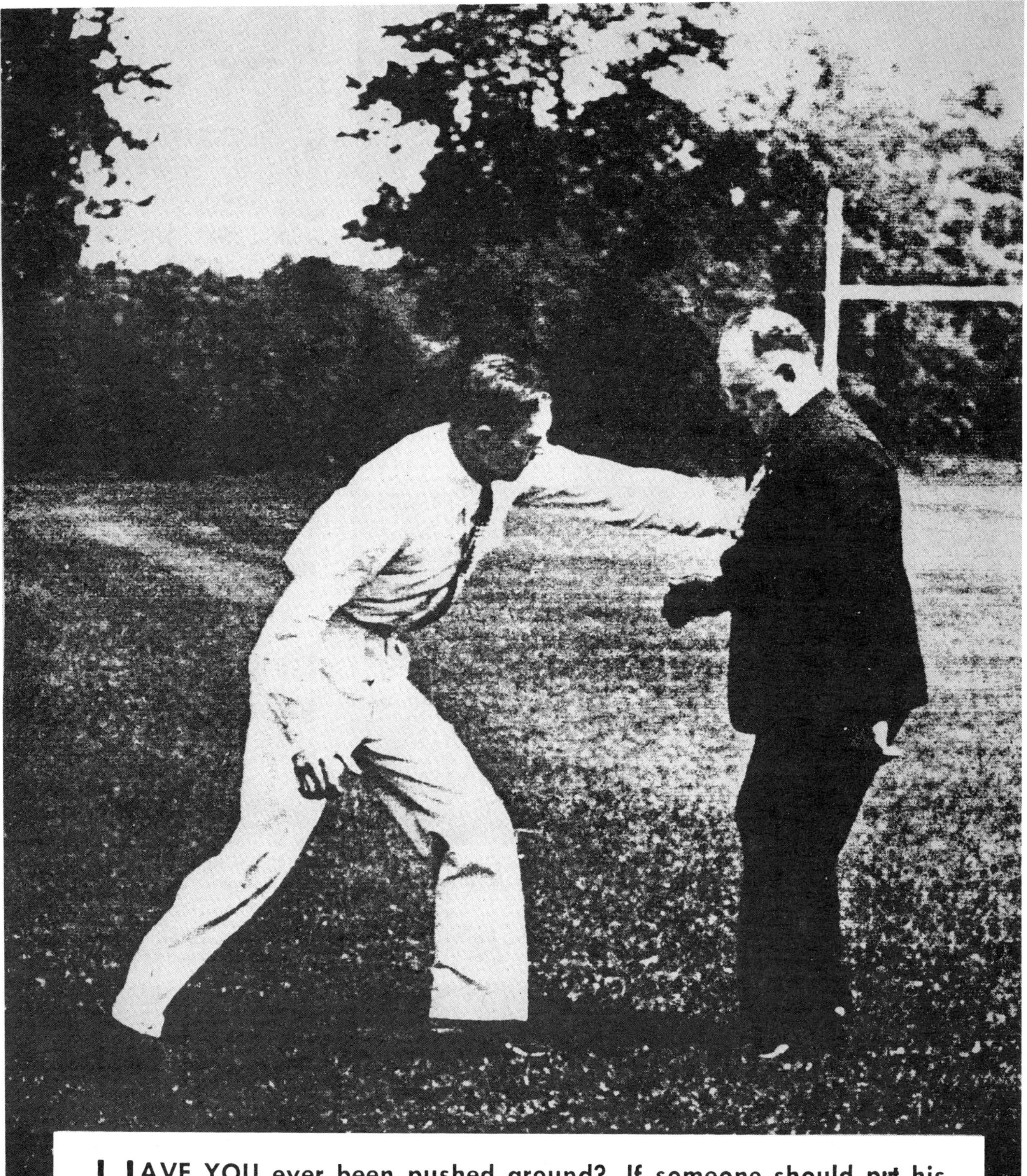

HAVE YOU ever been pushed around? If someone should put his hand on your shoulder or chest and try to push you against your will you can, in less than one second, have your assailant lying at your feet. You don't have to be bigger or stronger than he is, you don't have to engage in a 'fight'. Literally, a simple 'twist of the wrist' and he's lying on the ground or floor, at your mercy.

This number uses the wrist throw which, you will find, is the basis for a great many Jiu-Jitsu holds.

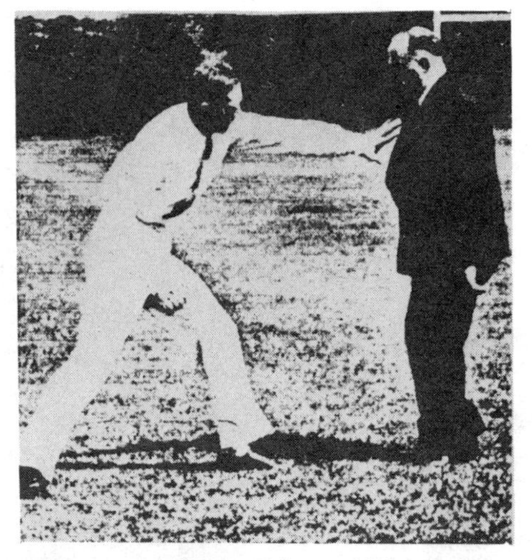

This is another number which works equally well against either a left or a right hand assault.

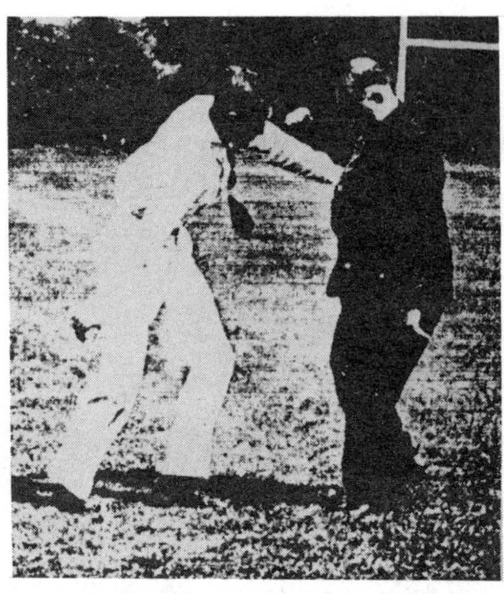

If the opponent attempts to push you, using his left arm,

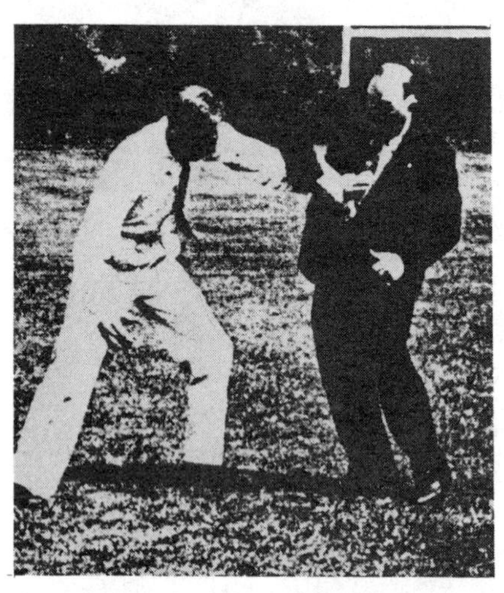

over the first and second finger bones. Press hard with your thumb.

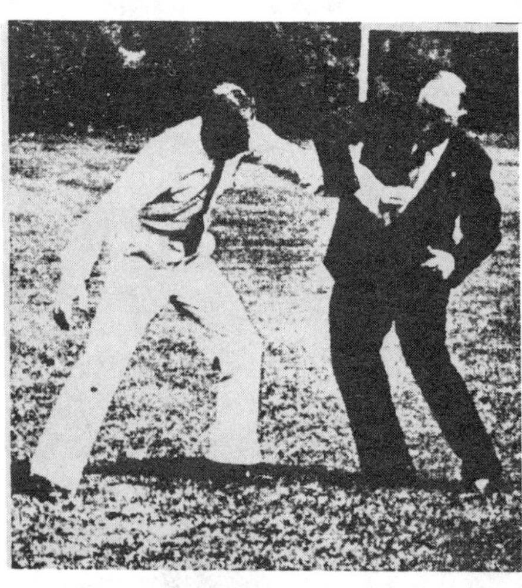

Turn your body somewhat to the left and pull his hand down to the left.

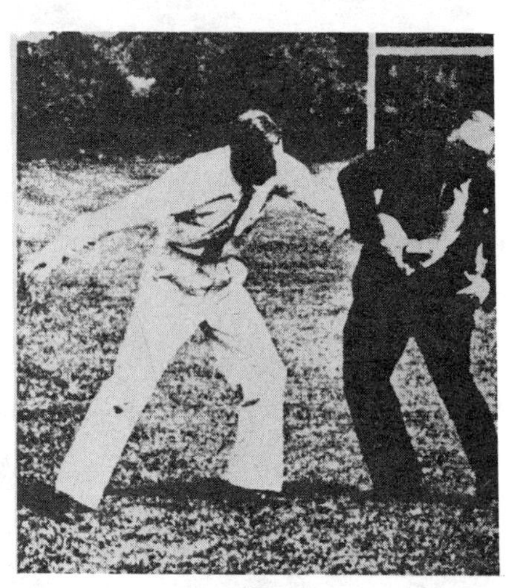

This tends to upset your assailant's balance as you pull him forward.

quickly bring his hand and arm high up in the air with his hand twisted so

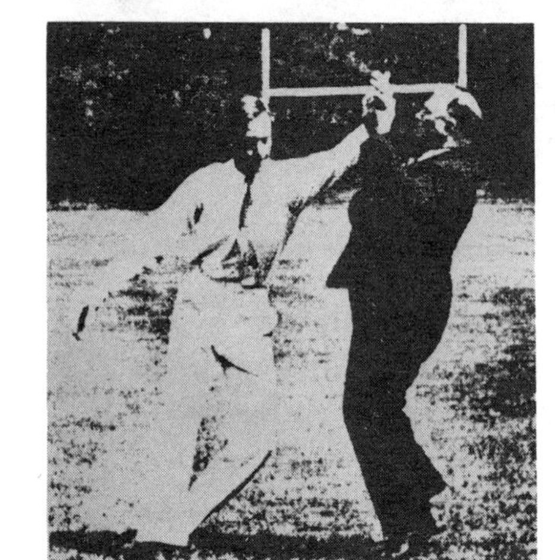

that the palm of his hand is pointing right at his head.

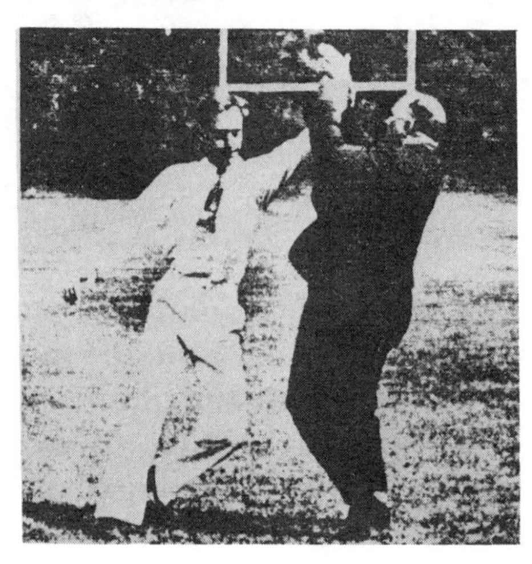

Keep twisting his hand and wrist further to your right and down he goes.

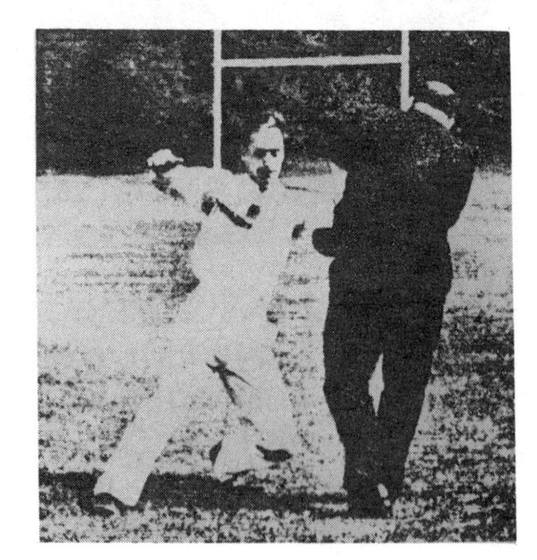

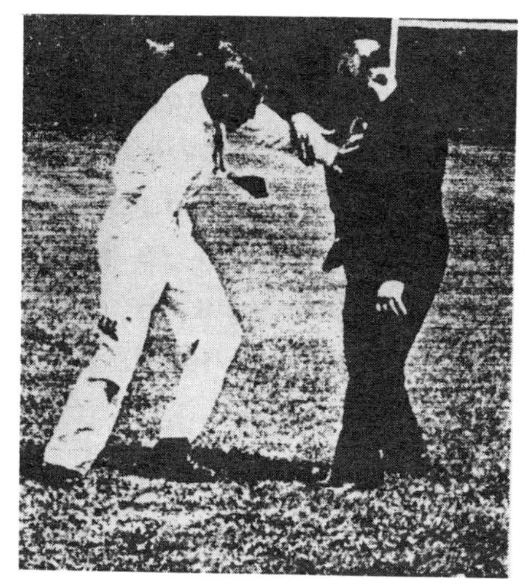

bring your right hand over his wrist

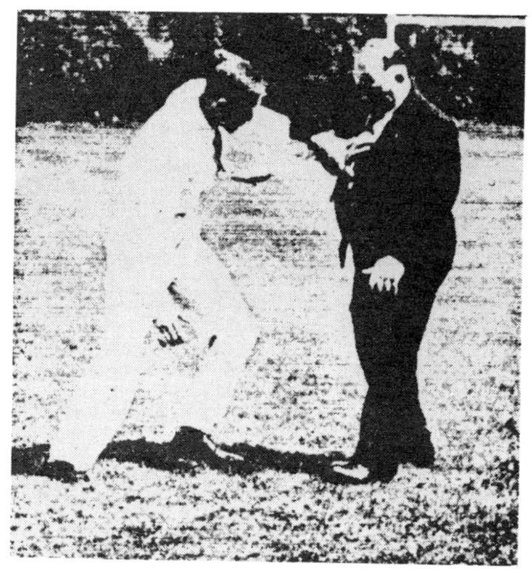

putting your fingers in the palm of his hand

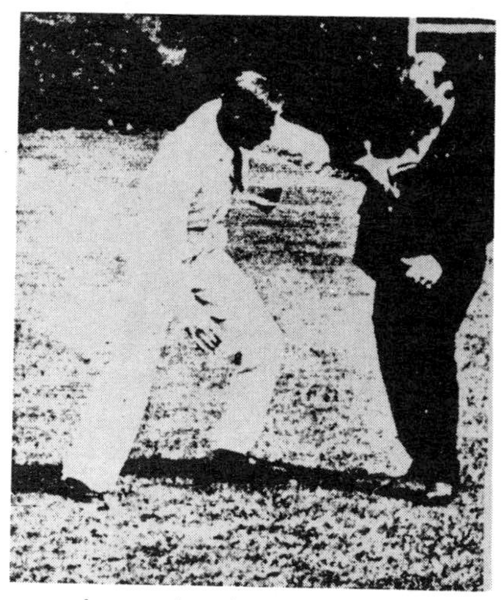

and your thumb on the back of his hand

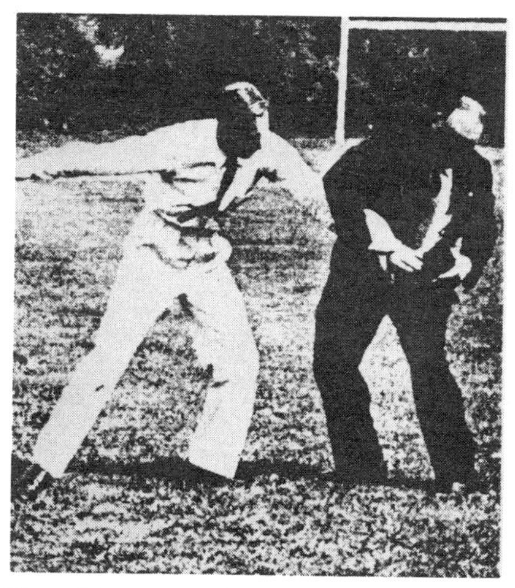

Now bring your left hand up to take a grip on his hand.

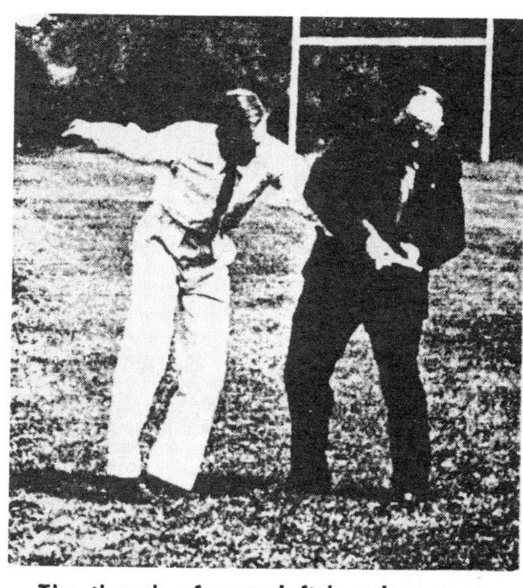

The thumb of your left hand goes on the back of his hand and your fingers across his palm.

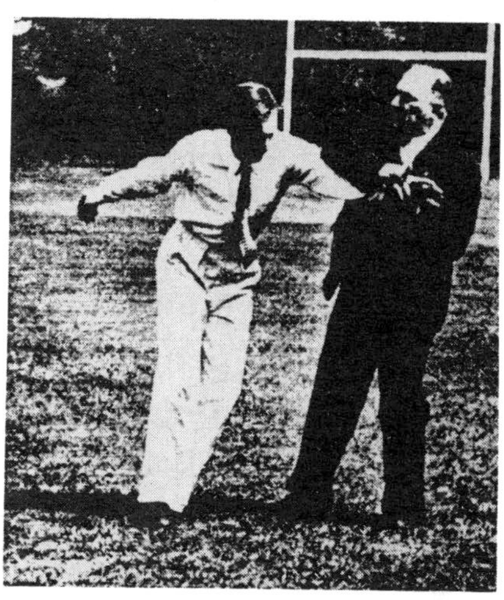

Press hard with your thumbs on nerves in back of his hand, at the same time

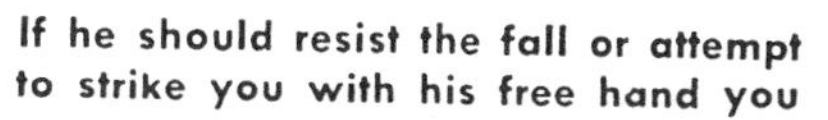

If he should resist the fall or attempt to strike you with his free hand you

will easily and surely severely injure his wrist.

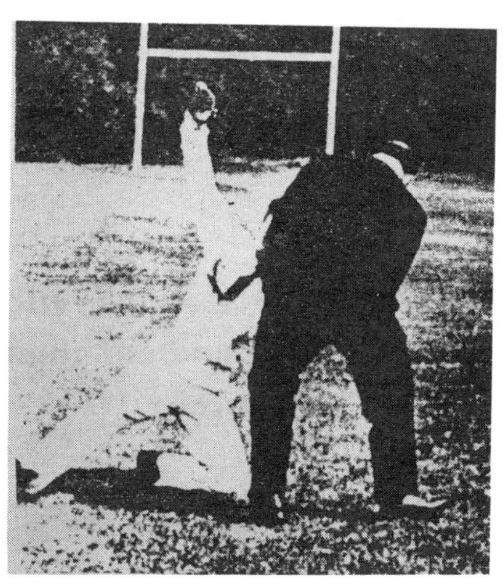

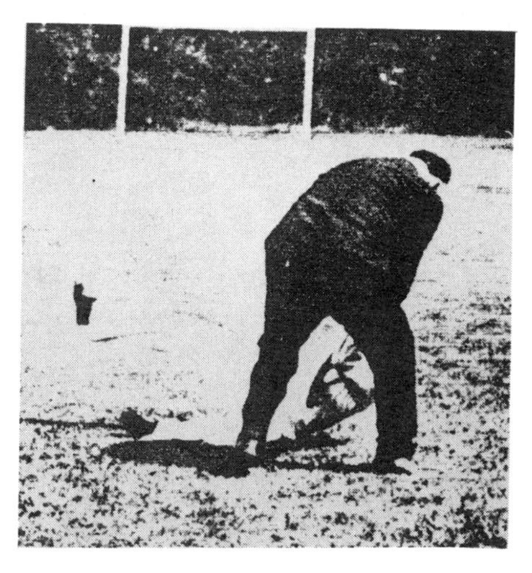

Practice this throw until you are very proficient at it. It is the basis of many other Jiu-Jitsu numbers.

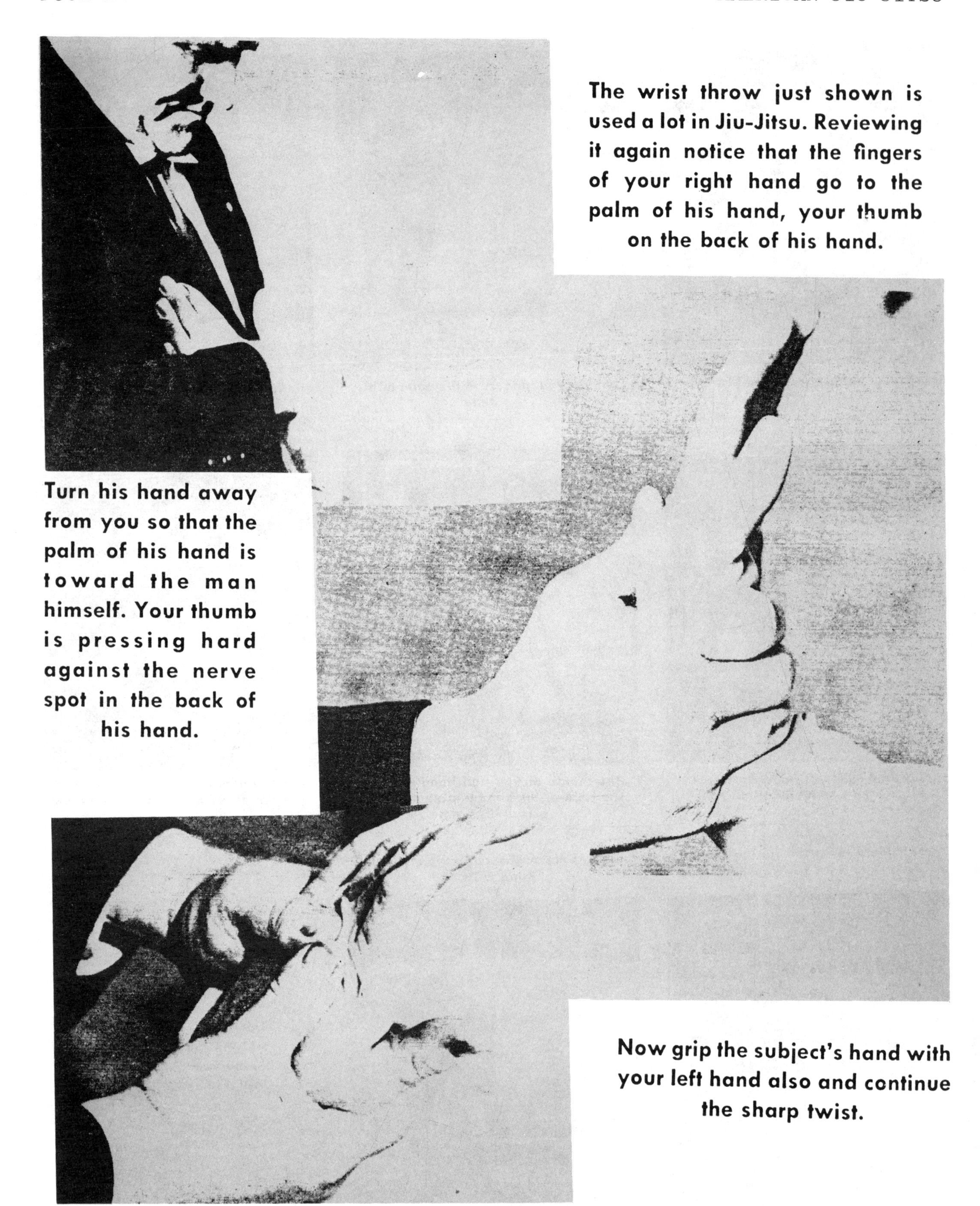

The wrist throw just shown is used a lot in Jiu-Jitsu. Reviewing it again notice that the fingers of your right hand go to the palm of his hand, your thumb on the back of his hand.

Turn his hand away from you so that the palm of his hand is toward the man himself. Your thumb is pressing hard against the nerve spot in the back of his hand.

Now grip the subject's hand with your left hand also and continue the sharp twist.

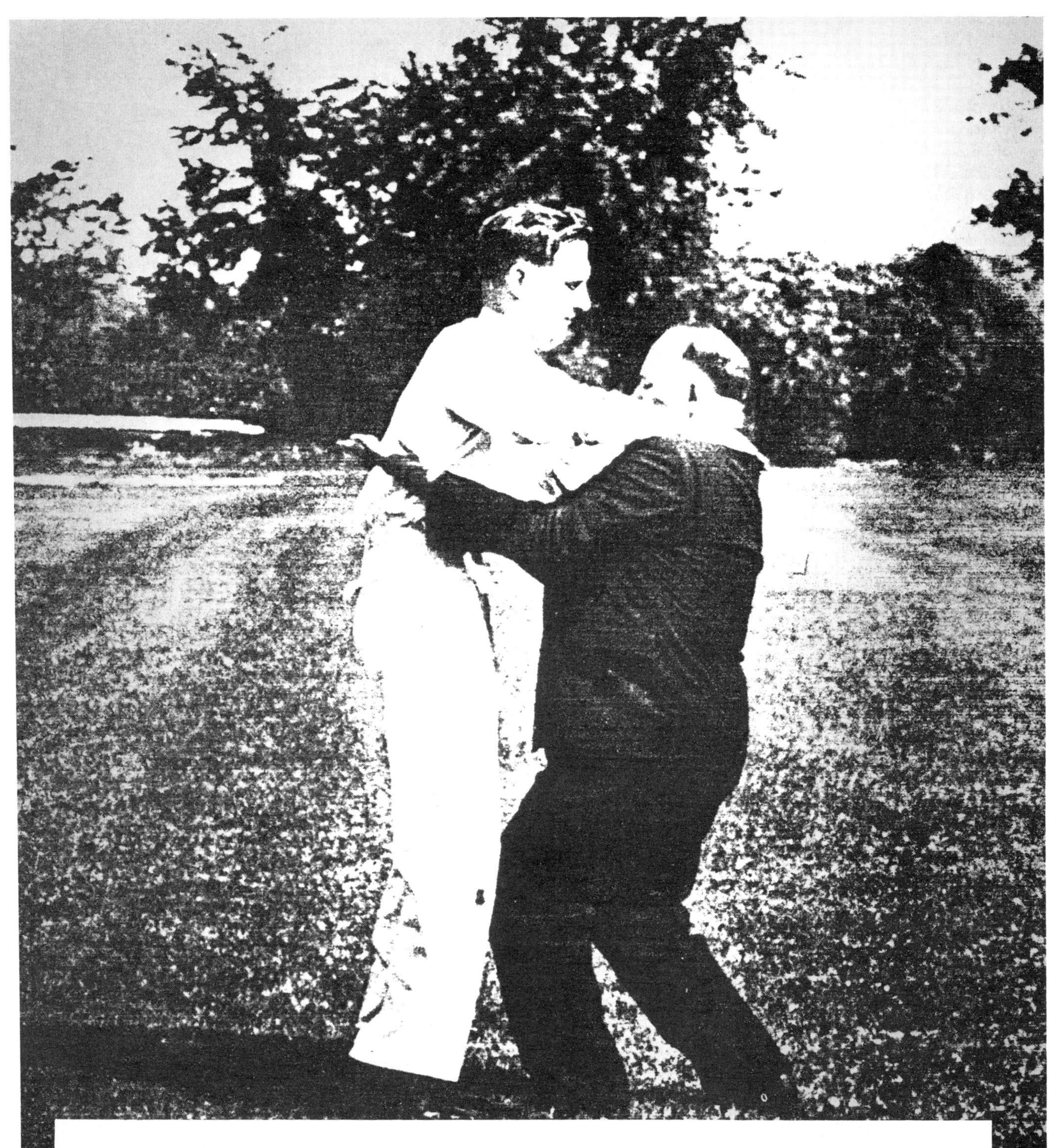

A GREAT MANY instances occur every year in which people are choked, some to death and others painfully but not fatally. There are a number of Jiu-Jitsu defenses or releases from choking, some more complicated than others. This one, involving a single, sharp, accurate blow is easy to accomplish and entirely effective. It has the added advantage, if sharply and correctly administered, of ending the trouble at once as the attacker has little fight left in him.

Use this defense when your attacker is not wearing a lot of heavy clothing. A heavy overcoat, for instance, would soften your blow too much, robbing it of its full effectiveness.

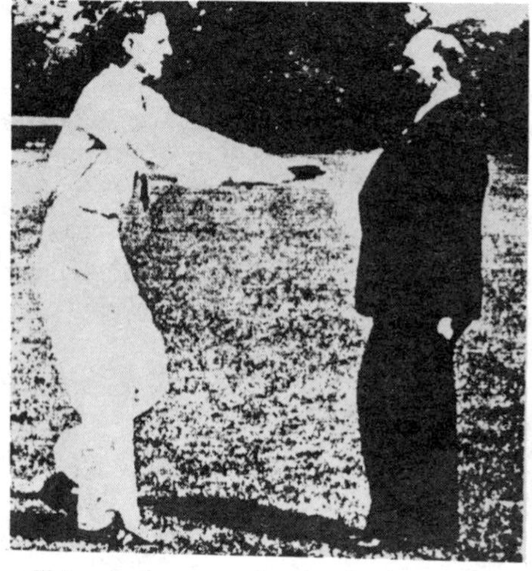

This number may be used when ever your opponent is in front of you.

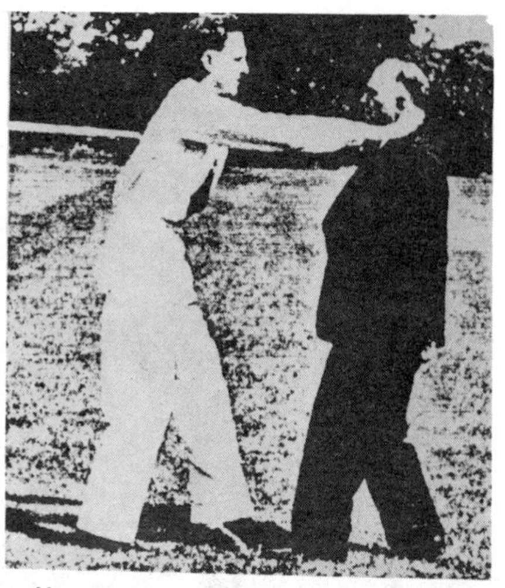

He must be within easy reach of you as, of course, he is if he is attempting to choke you.

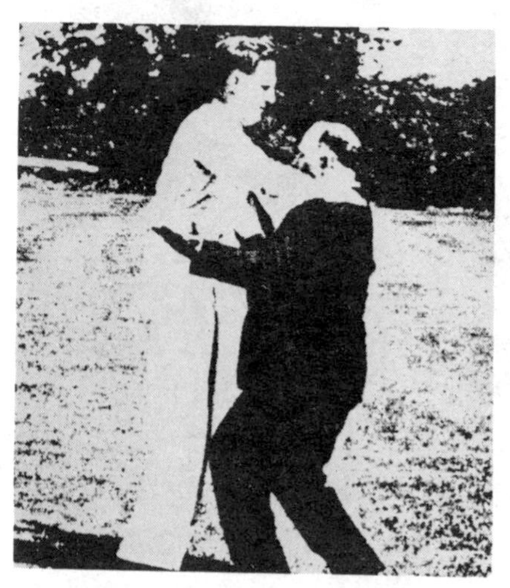

Your hands must be in the "knife blow" position

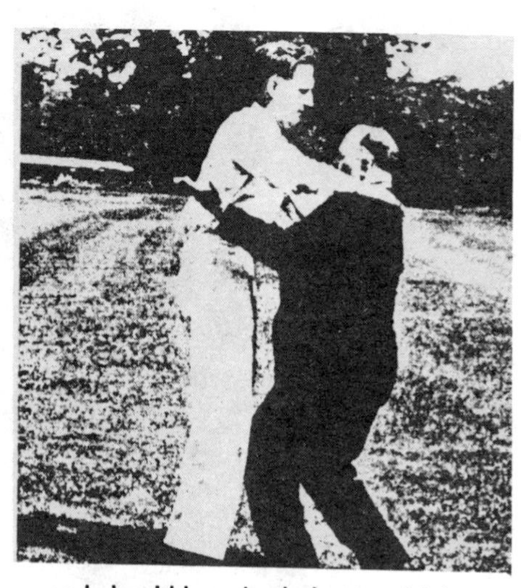

and should be raised about as high as your shoulders.

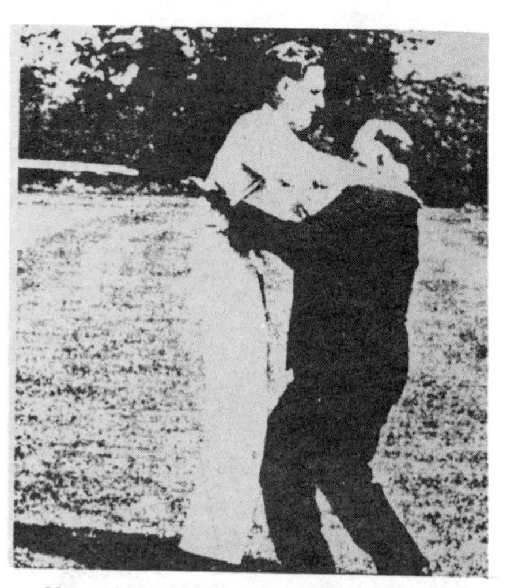

You strike hard against both sides of his body simultaneously, about at his fifth or sixth ribs.

The man will fall to the ground severely injured, gasping for breath.

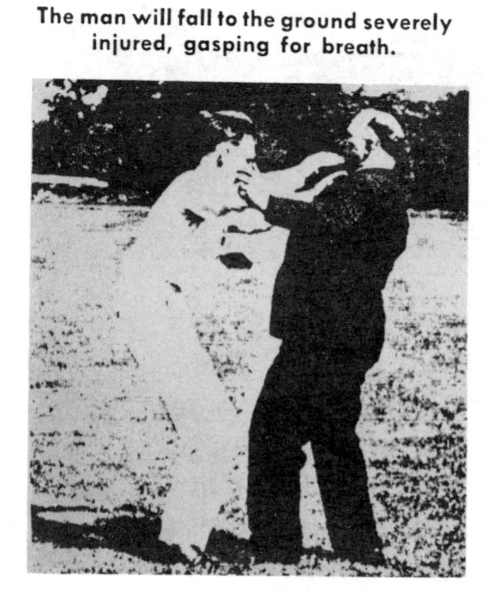

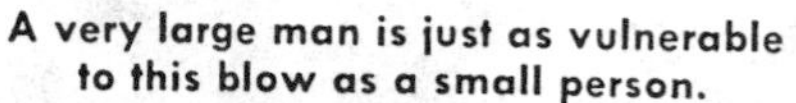

A very large man is just as vulnerable to this blow as a small person.

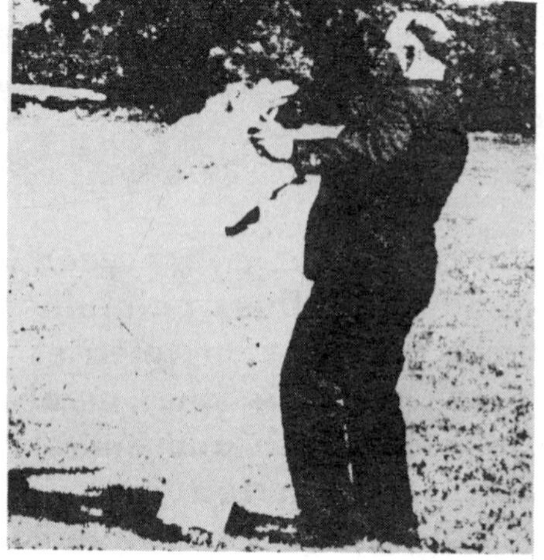

The larger the man the bigger your target and consequently the big man is easy to hit.

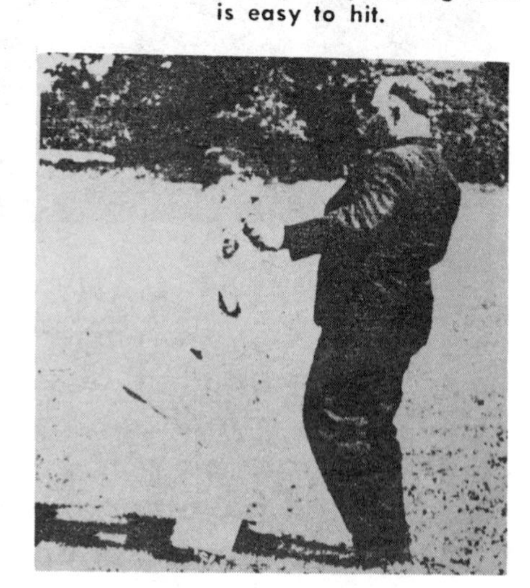

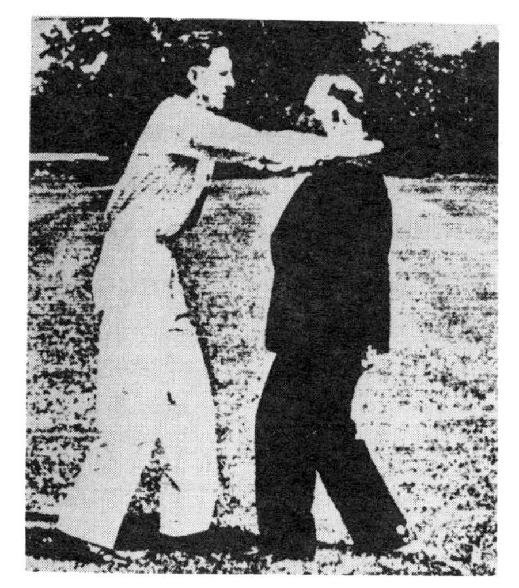

His hands are around your throat. Bend your knees a little.

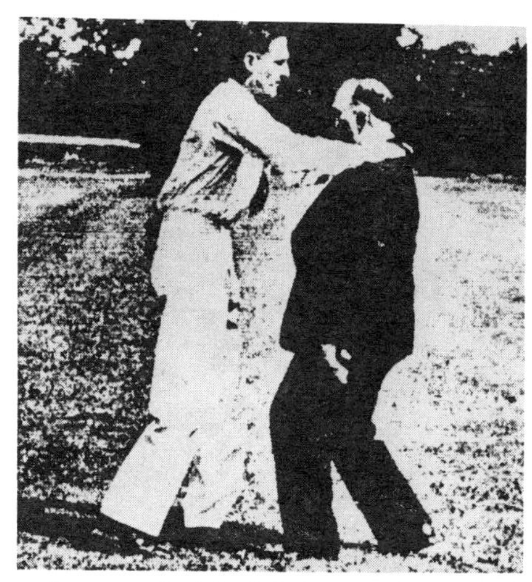

As you start to bring your arms up you should crouch down slightly.

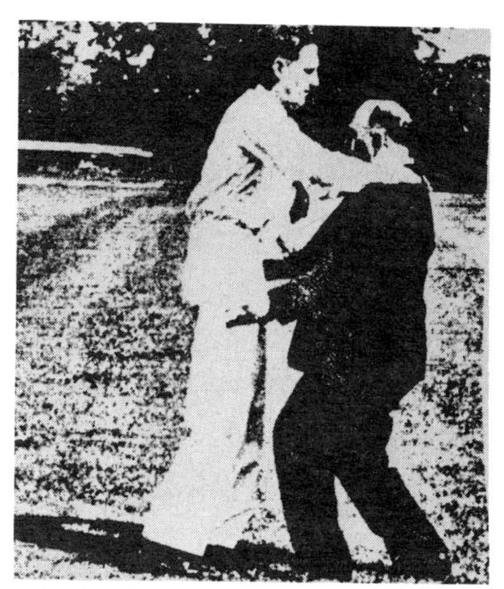

Both of your hands should come up at the same time.

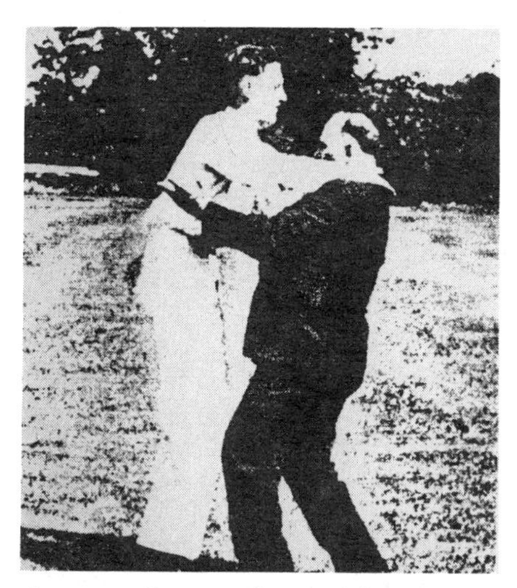

As you strike you also straighten your knees, which tends to give added power to the blow.

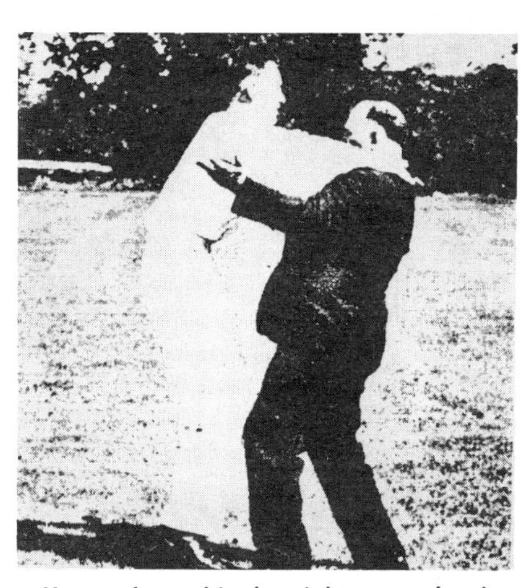

If you have hit the right spots hard enough

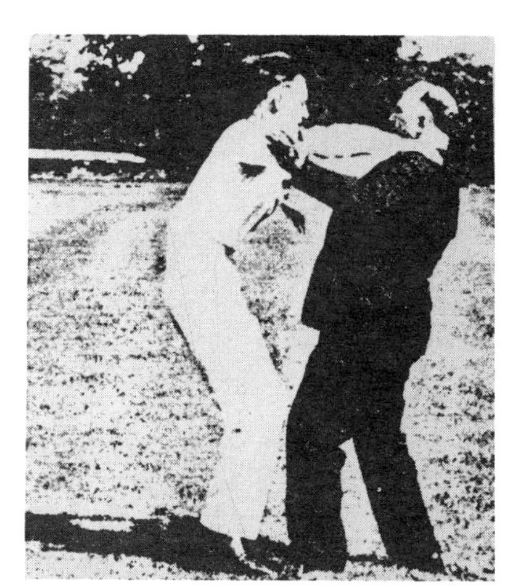

he will release his grasp on your throat at once.

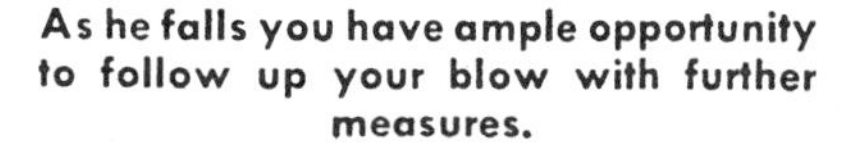

As he falls you have ample opportunity to follow up your blow with further measures.

Remember in executing this number, as well as all Jiu-Jitsu numbers involving a blow, that you use the knife blow, not your fist.

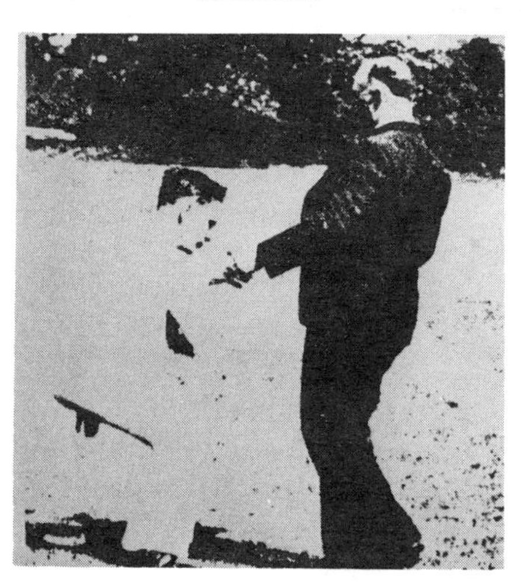

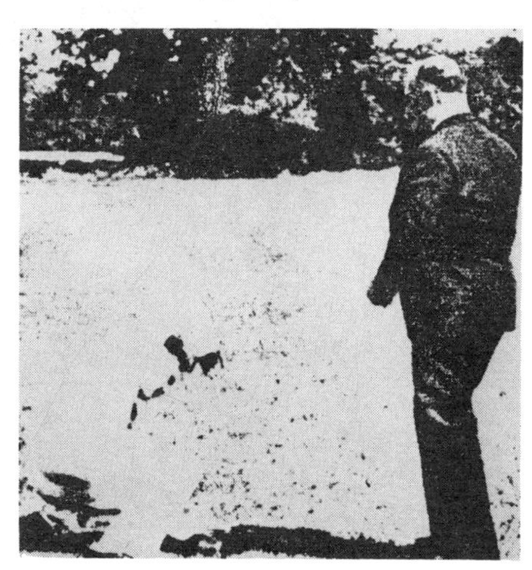

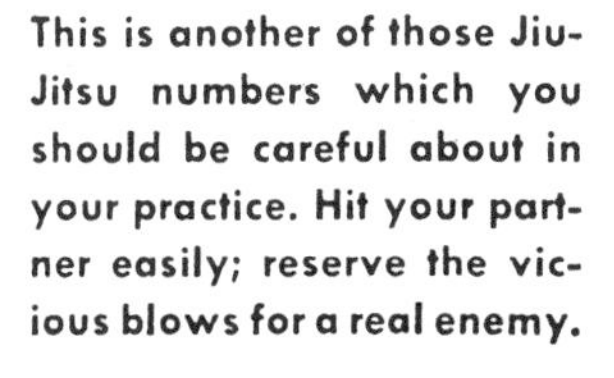

This is another of those Jiu-Jitsu numbers which you should be careful about in your practice. Hit your partner easily; reserve the vicious blows for a real enemy.

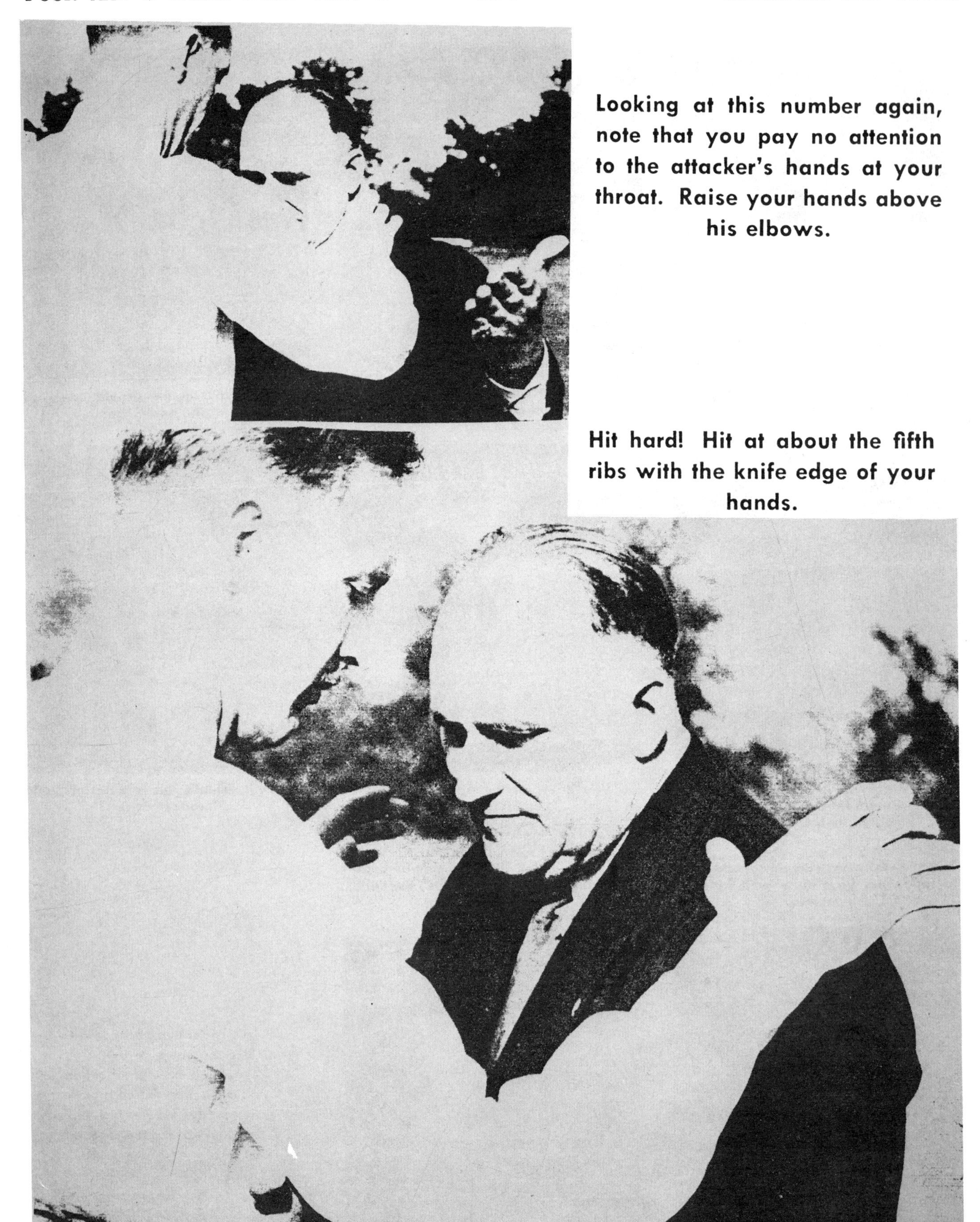

Looking at this number again, note that you pay no attention to the attacker's hands at your throat. Raise your hands above his elbows.

Hit hard! Hit at about the fifth ribs with the knife edge of your hands.

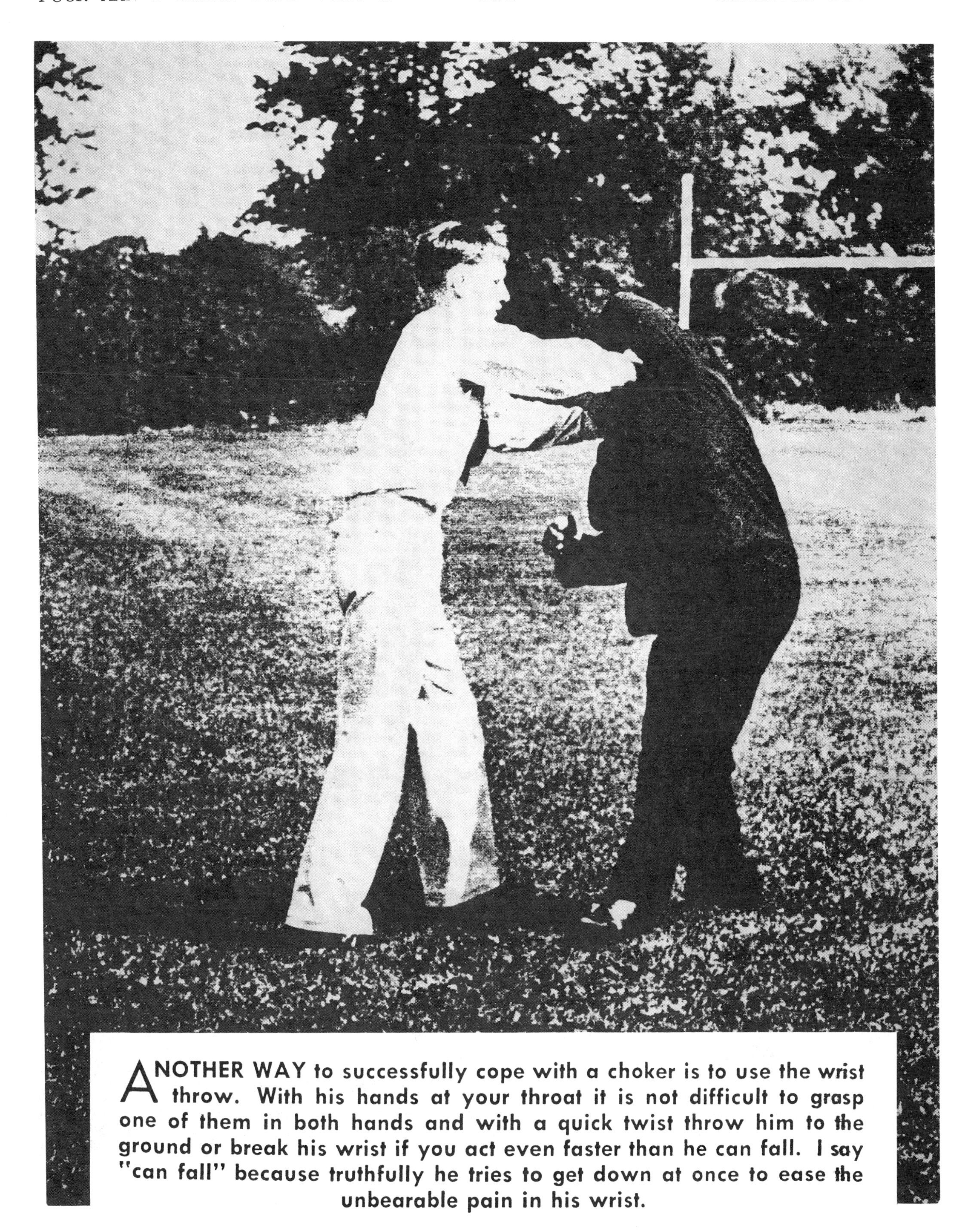

ANOTHER WAY to successfully cope with a choker is to use the wrist throw. With his hands at your throat it is not difficult to grasp one of them in both hands and with a quick twist throw him to the ground or break his wrist if you act even faster than he can fall. I say "can fall" because truthfully he tries to get down at once to ease the unbearable pain in his wrist.

This number shows you another use of the wrist throw which you first encountered in the defense against pushing.

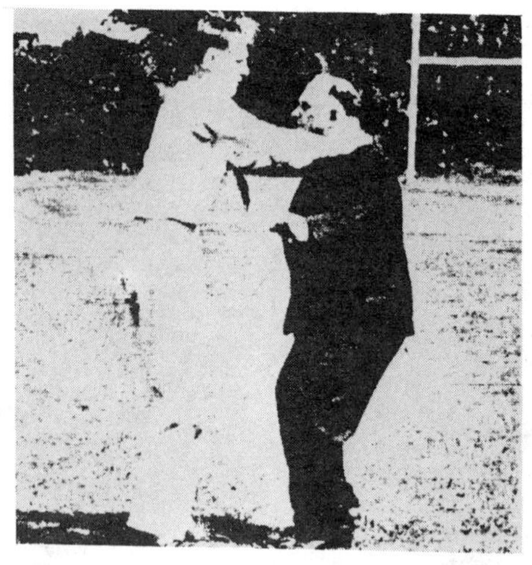

You can work upon your attacker's right or left arm with equal certainty of success.

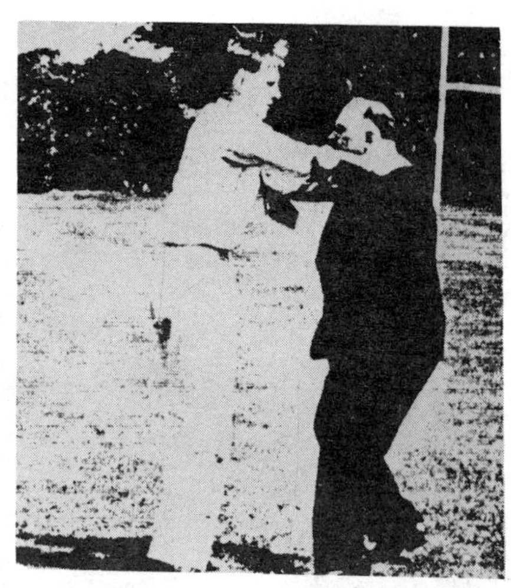

If you choose to throw him to your left, as above,

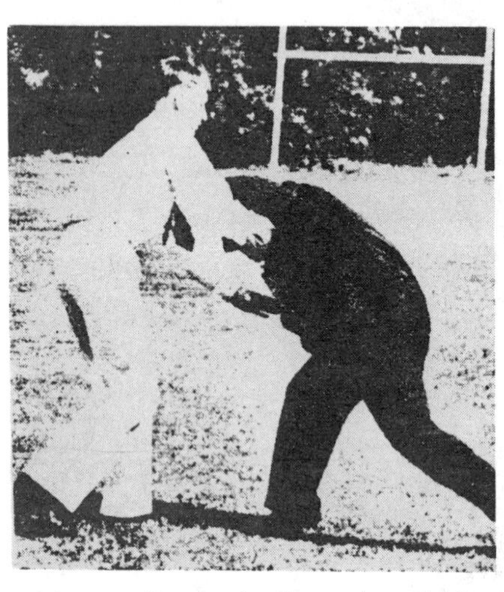

and your fingers in the palm of his hand.

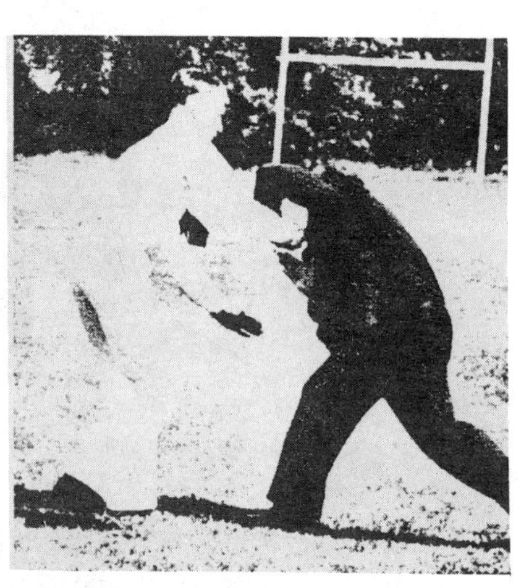

Bend forward and far to the right, helping to throw

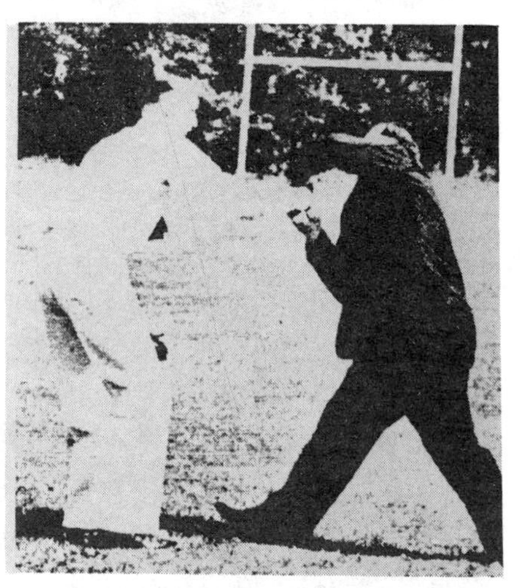

your opponent off balance, and to gain momentum for your next move.

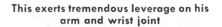

This exerts tremendous leverage on his arm and wrist joint

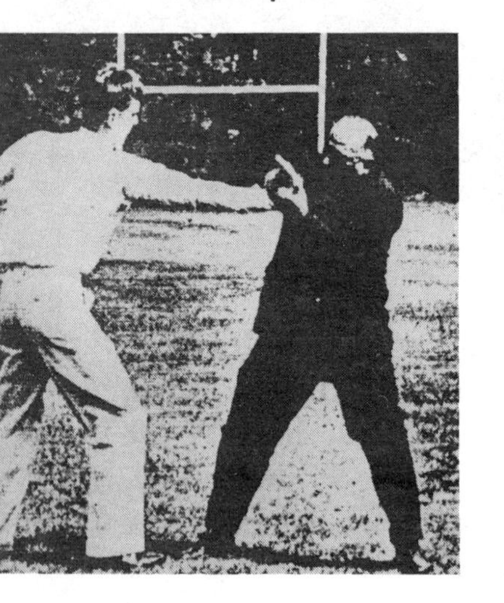

and inflicts so much pain that it cannot be withstood.

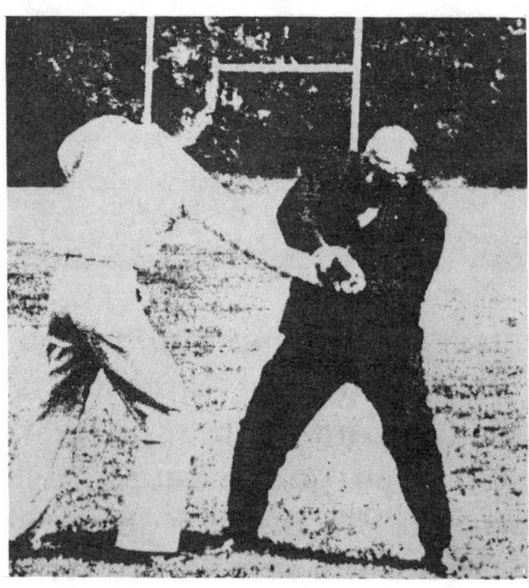

If it could be endured and the man attempted to strike you or break away

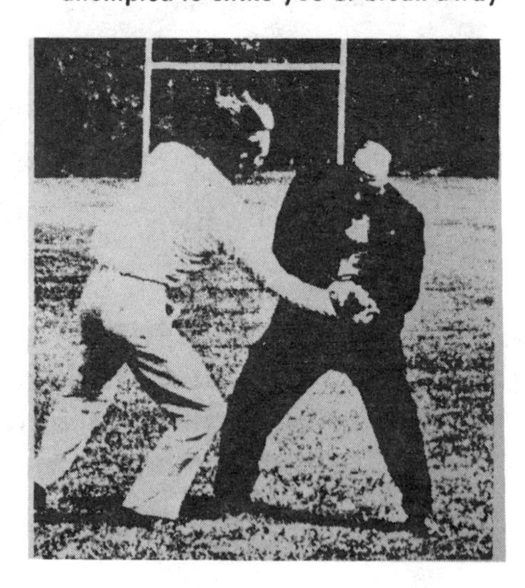

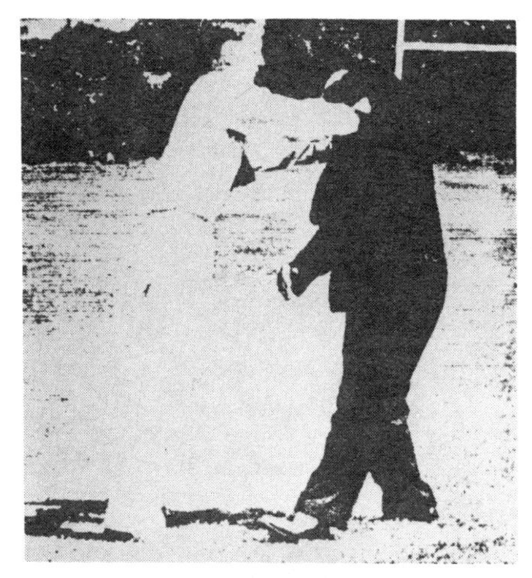

reach with your left hand for his right hand which is for the moment at your throat.

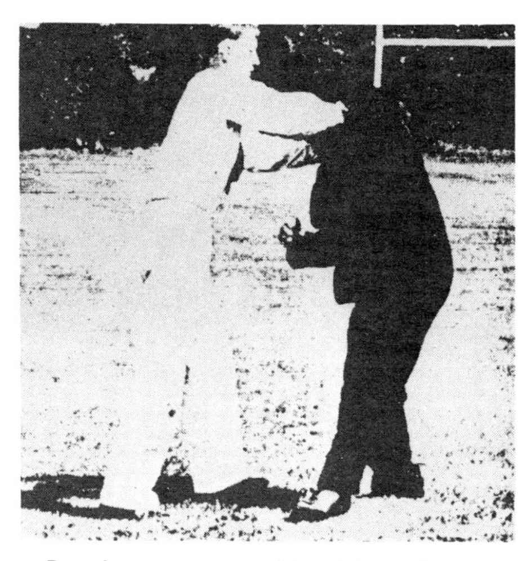

Reach away over his right wrist so that you grasp

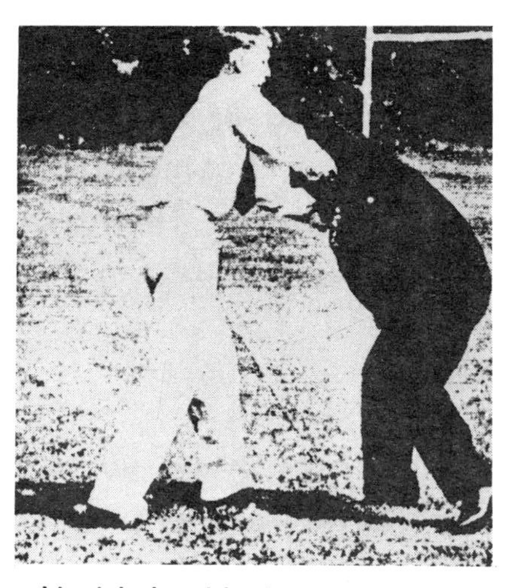

his right hand by having your thumb on the back of his hand

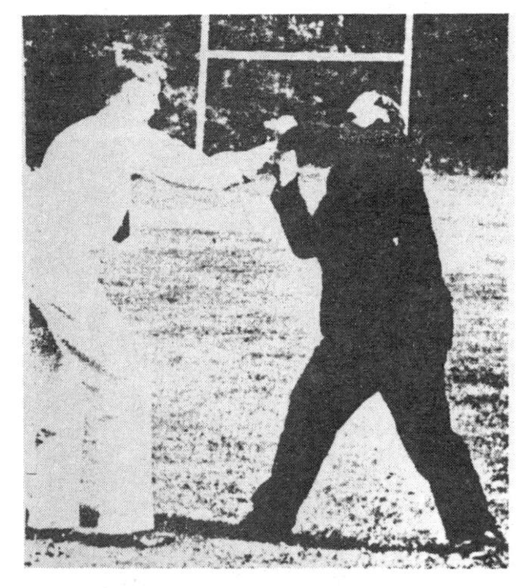

Your right hand has reinforced your left on the victim's hand with fingers in palm, thumb on back.

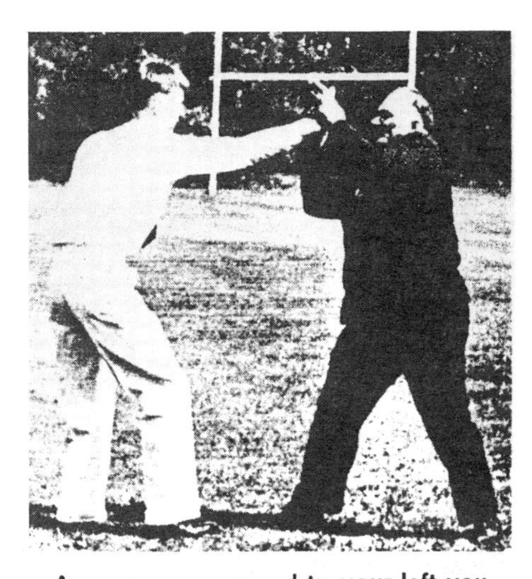

As you come up and to your left you are exerting strong pressure on the nerves in the back of his hand

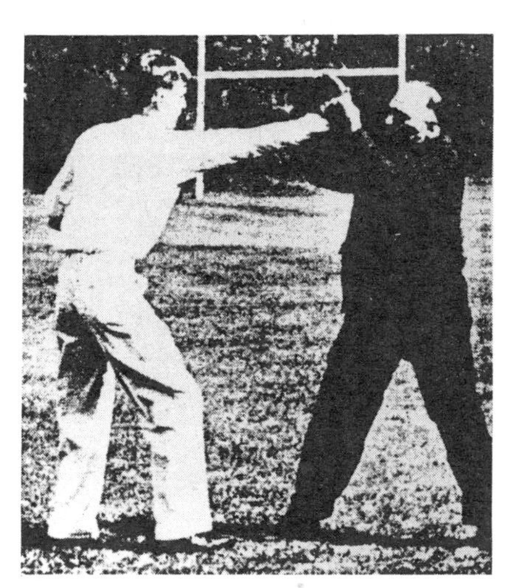

and are bending his hand toward the inside of his wrist.

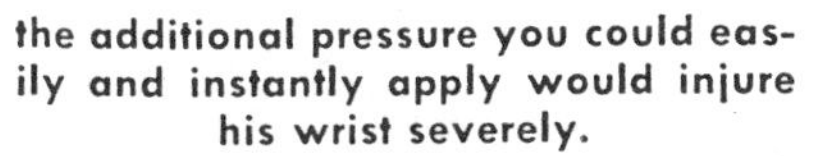

the additional pressure you could easily and instantly apply would injure his wrist severely.

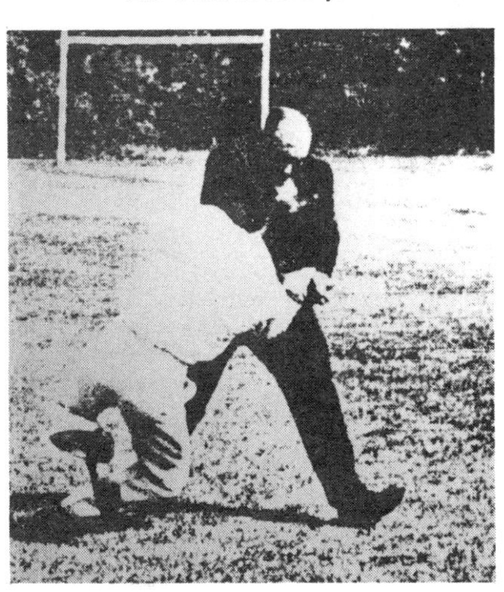

When he falls he will spin around in an attempt to straighten out the twisted arm.

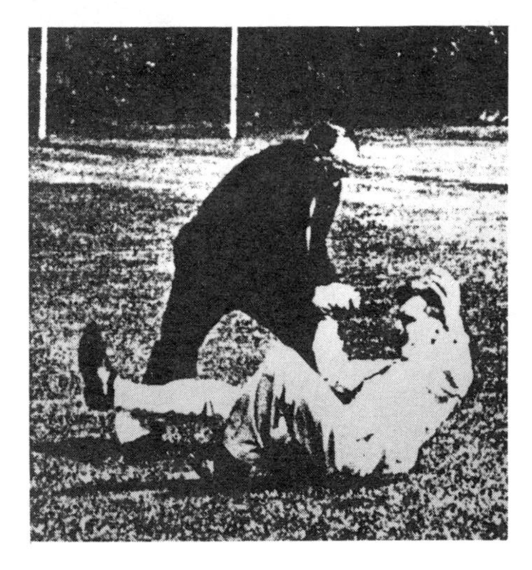

He is, however, at your mercy because you still have control of his wrist and can continue to apply pressure, or change to some other but equally punishing, grip.

This method of releasing yourself from a choking grip utilizes the wrist throw. Thumb on back of hand and fingers to the palm.

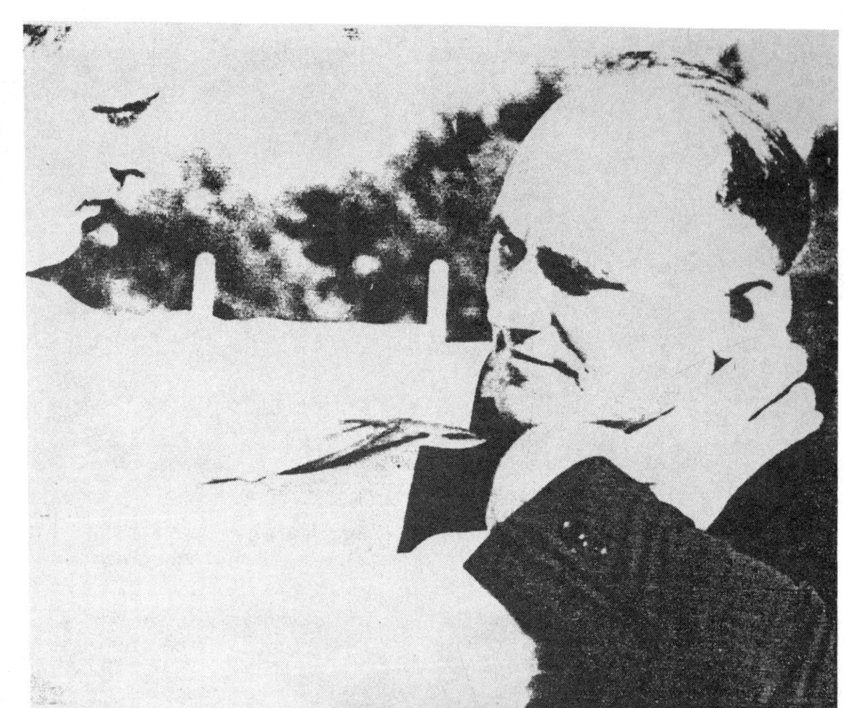

This shows how your fingers should be in the palm of his hand and the thumbs on the back. This picture shows the extreme twist that is given the attacker's arm.

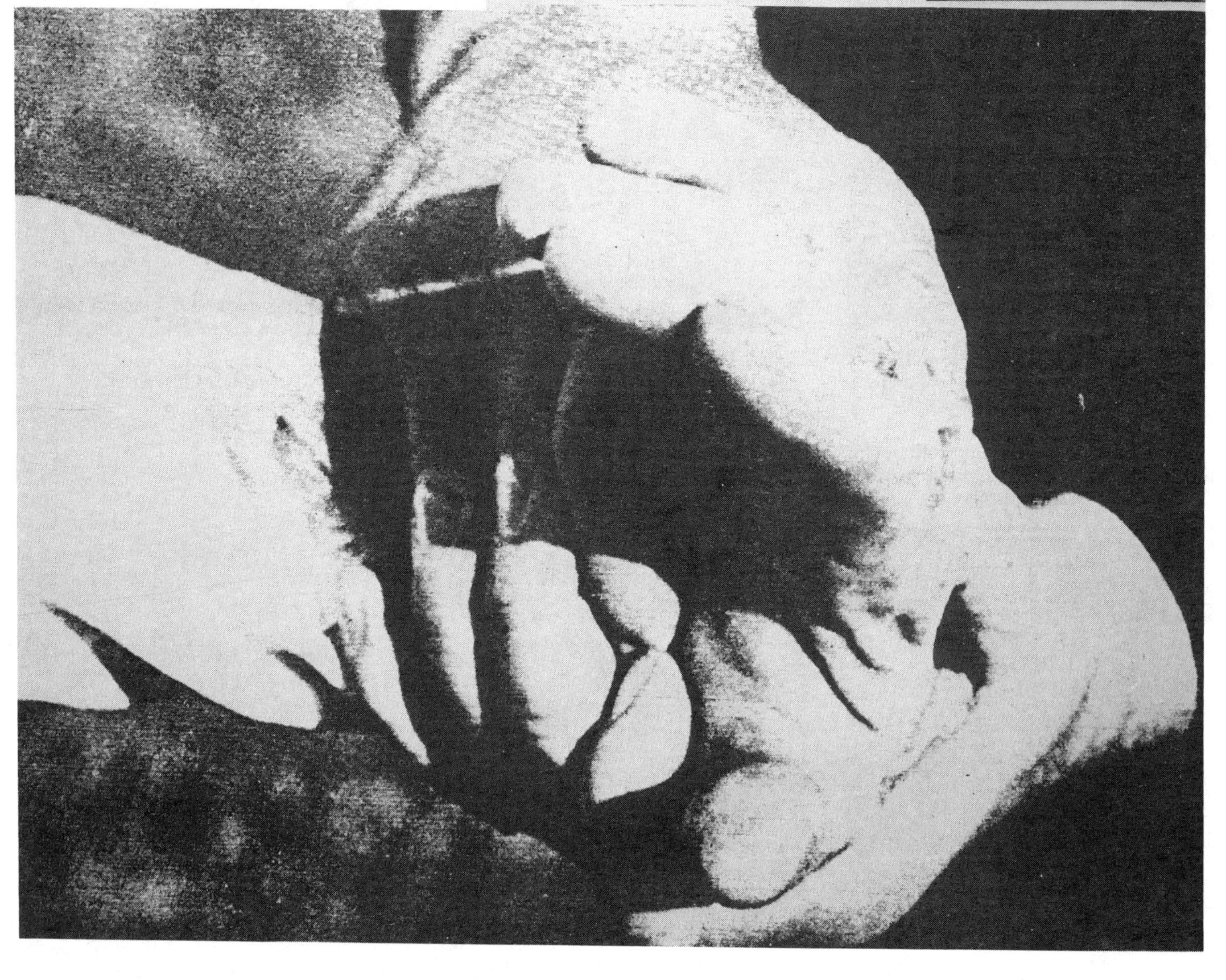

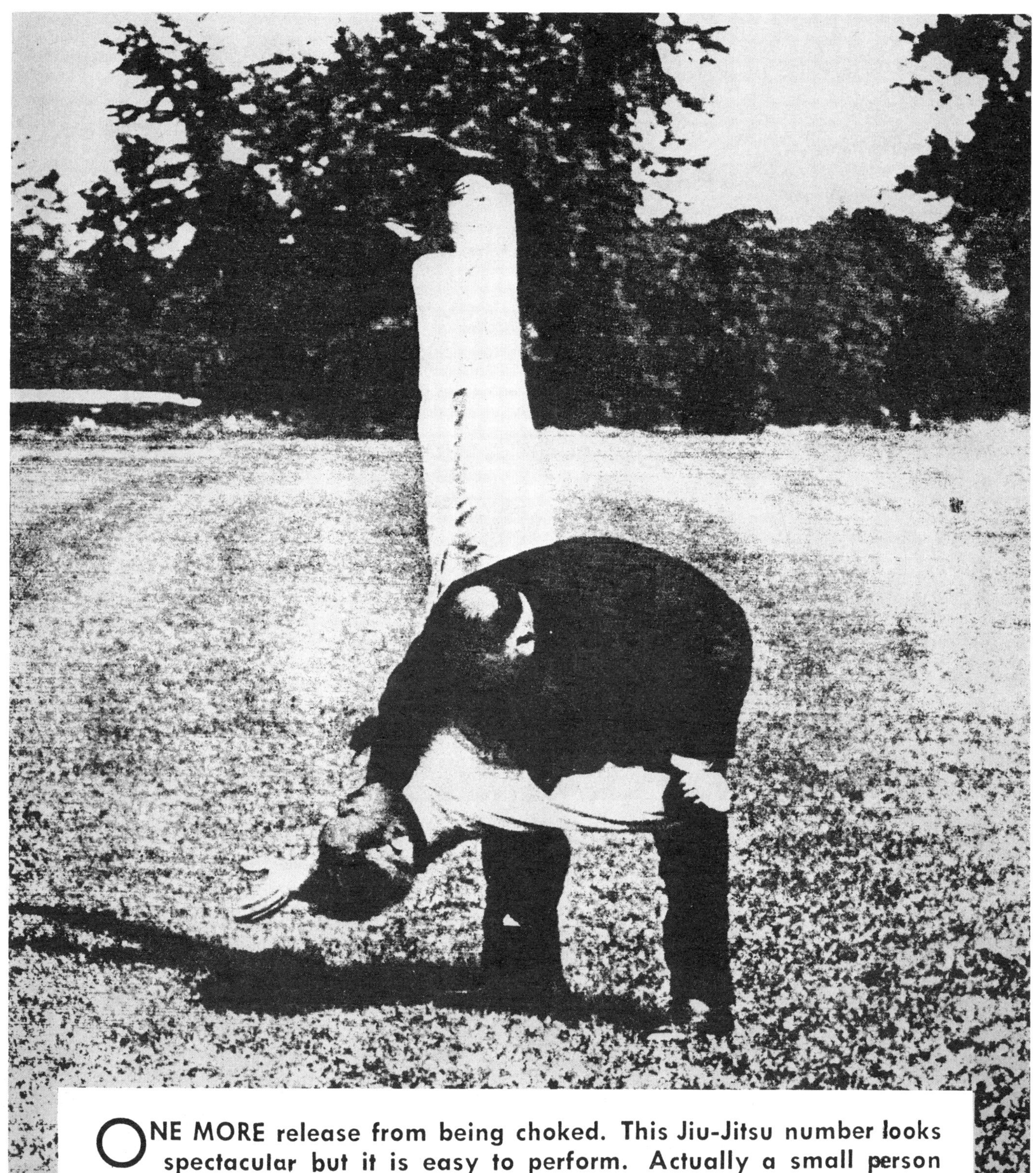

ONE MORE release from being choked. This Jiu-Jitsu number looks spectacular but it is easy to perform. Actually a small person can release himself from, and throw, a much larger and stronger person by this method.

The advantage of having several counter-attacks for any one type of attack lies in the fact that different circumstances will often indicate that use of one certain defense is more likely to succeed than any other.

I repeat that this is an easy number to use—but it cannot be used successfully without adequate practice.

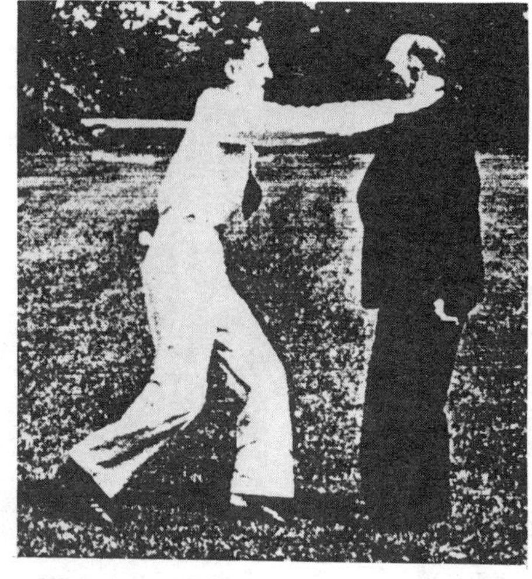

With this number you release yourself from an assailant's clutch

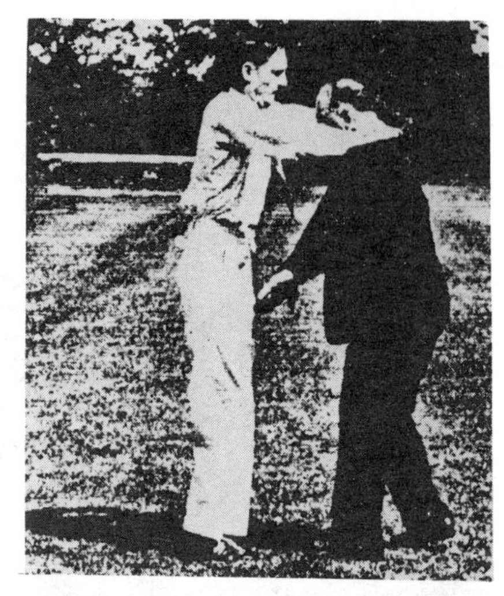

and throw him so hard upon his back that he may be stunned by the fall.

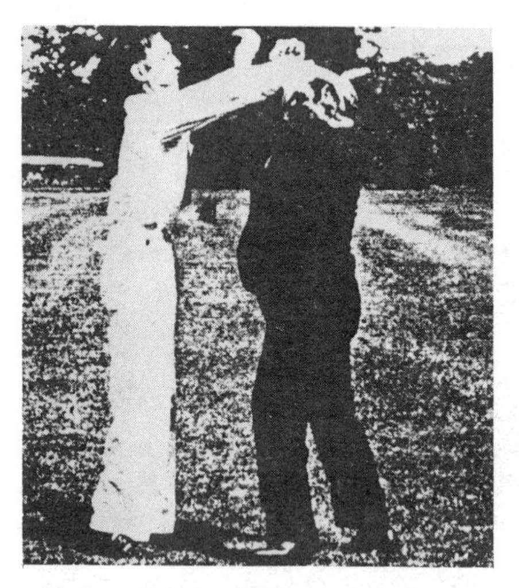

and your force will free your throat from the grip of your enemy.

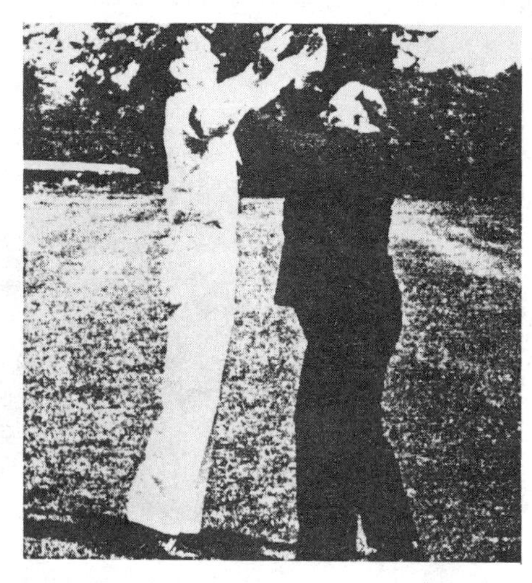

As you knock his hands away get a good firm grip around his upper right arm with your left hand. This will be easy as your arms and hands are still in motion.

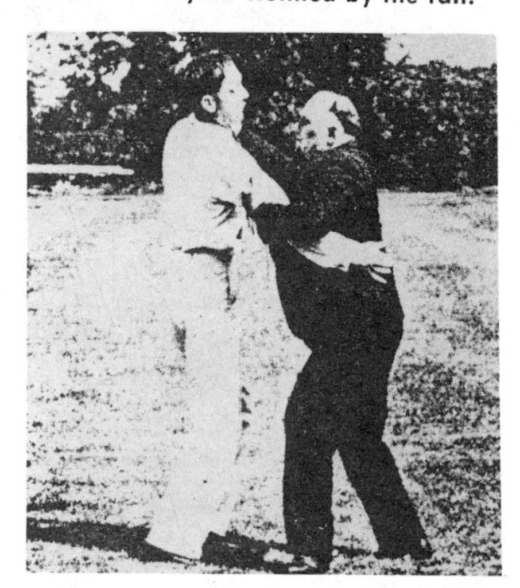

Your right hand now takes a firm hold on his shoulder right up close to his neck. Up to this point you have been standing face to face

If you make your lift with the hip and the pull with your hands simultaneously,

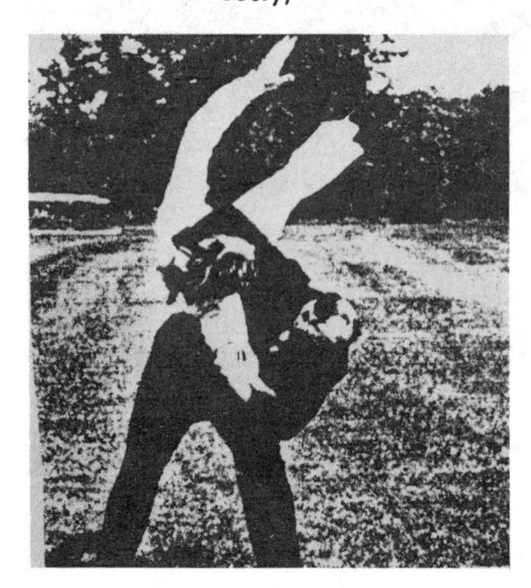

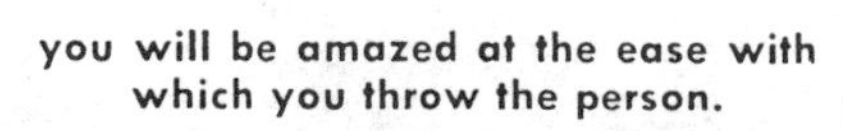

you will be amazed at the ease with which you throw the person.

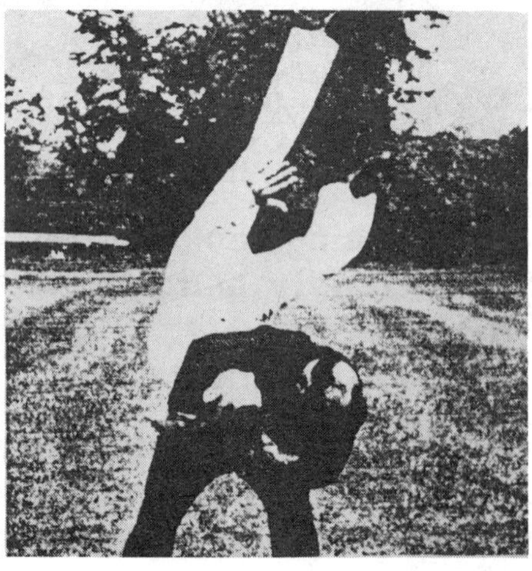

You can throw the subject very heavily or you can ease up a little as he goes over

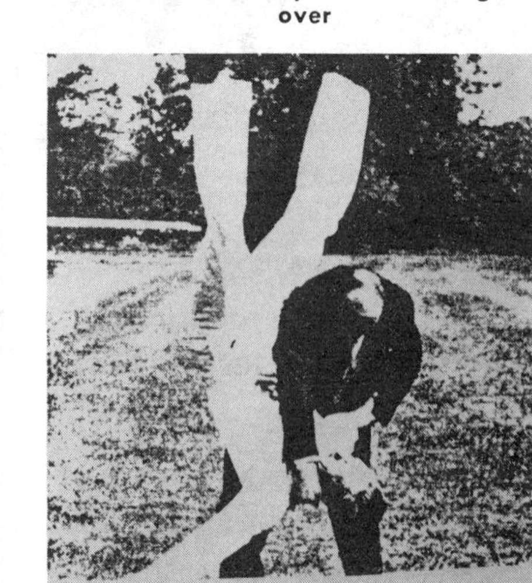

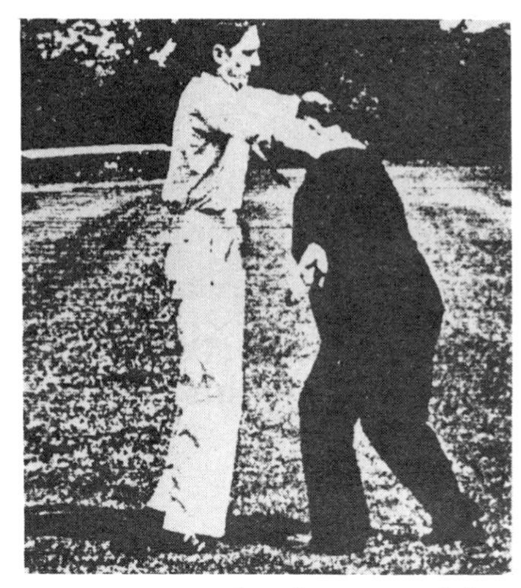

For the first part, the release, you sink down several inches by bending your knees.

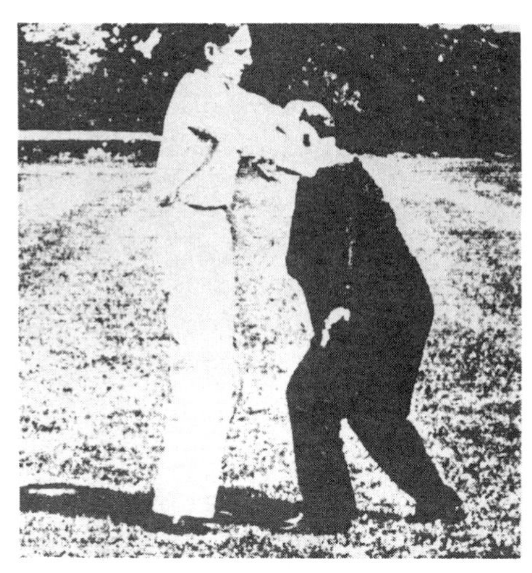

By dipping down thus you gather momentum for your upward push.

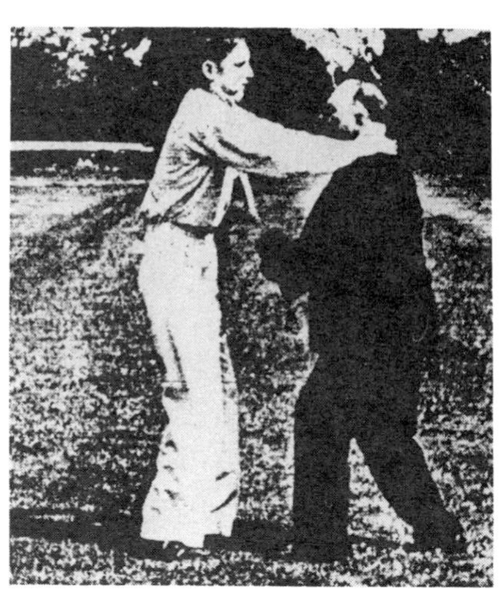

Thrust your arms upward between his arms. Push outward as well as upward

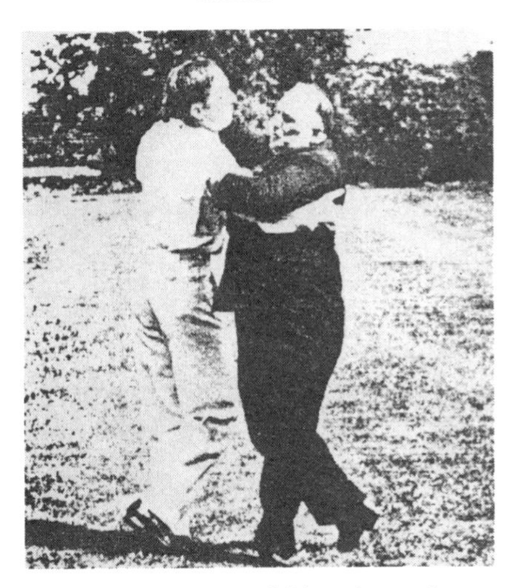

whereas now you quickly take a step directly to your left with your right foot

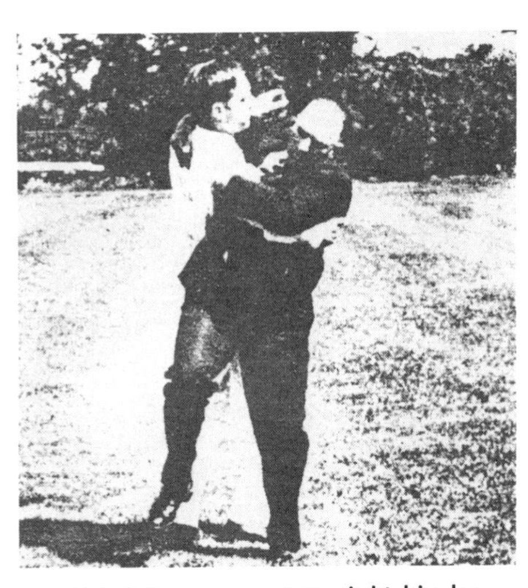

which brings your own right hip behind your opponent's right hip. Now raise your right hip

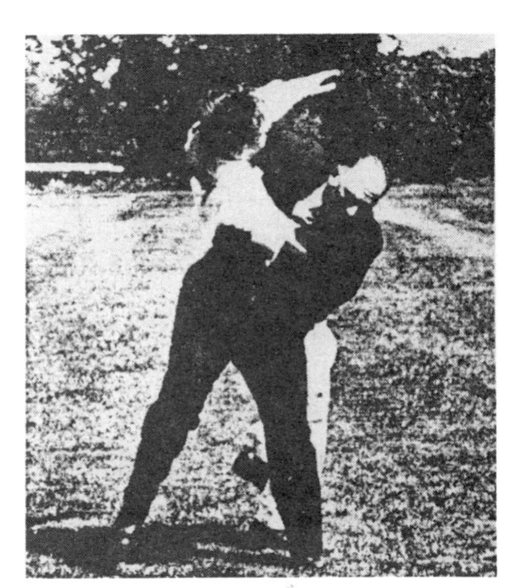

which raises him upon it and at the same time give a strong pull forward on his shoulders. Pull down on his right arm and pull up and over on his left shoulder.

and break his fall somewhat. Of course if someone has attempted to choke you, you

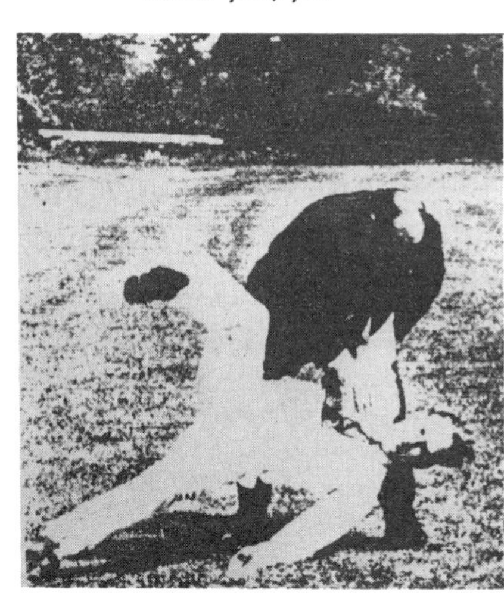

are not going to want to ease his fall too much. Retain his right arm by your left and bend it backward over your forearm to keep him under control.

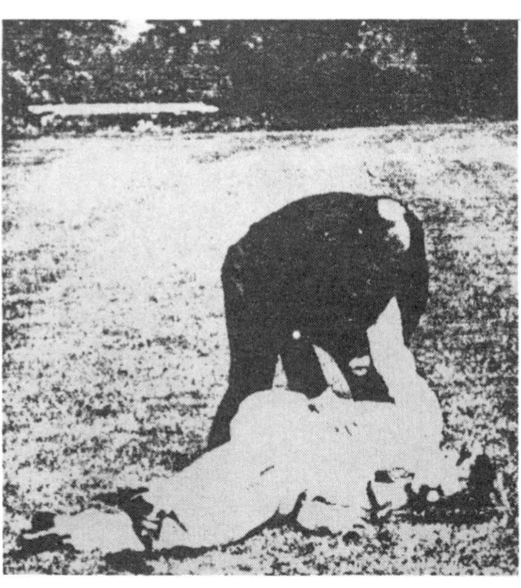

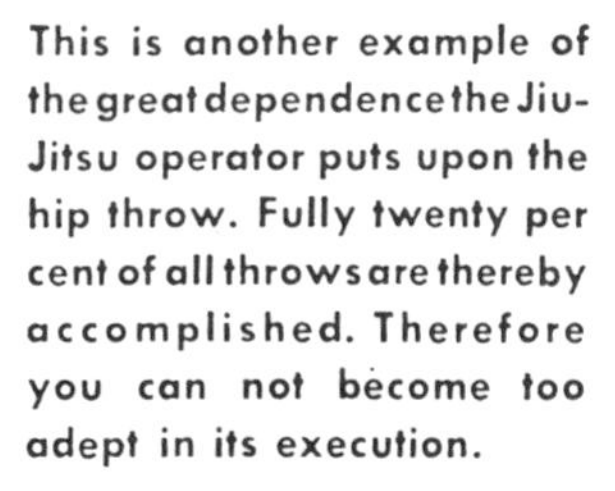

This is another example of the great dependence the Jiu-Jitsu operator puts upon the hip throw. Fully twenty per cent of all throws are thereby accomplished. Therefore you can not become too adept in its execution.

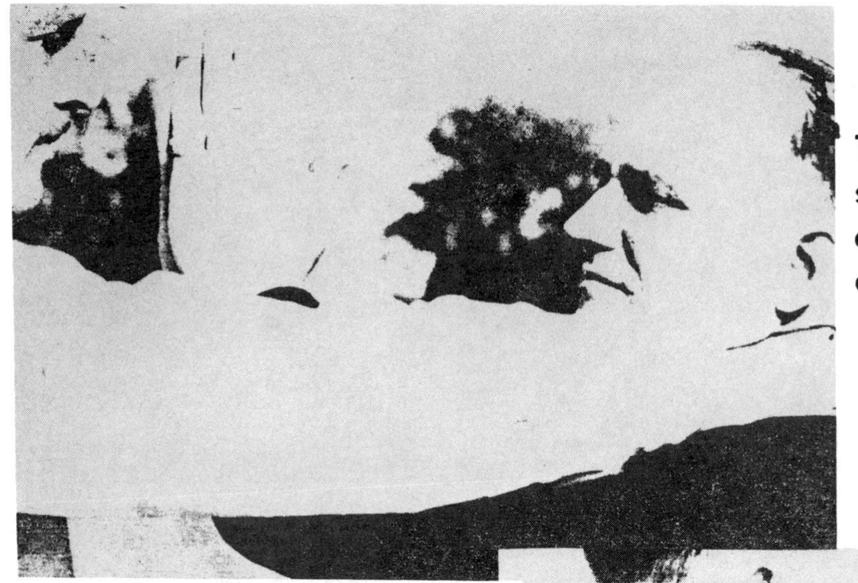

The first part of this number consists of the release. Your hands and arms thrust upward, with considerable force, between his arms and break his grip.

Then you hold his right arm closely under your left arm and your right arm goes to his left shoulder.

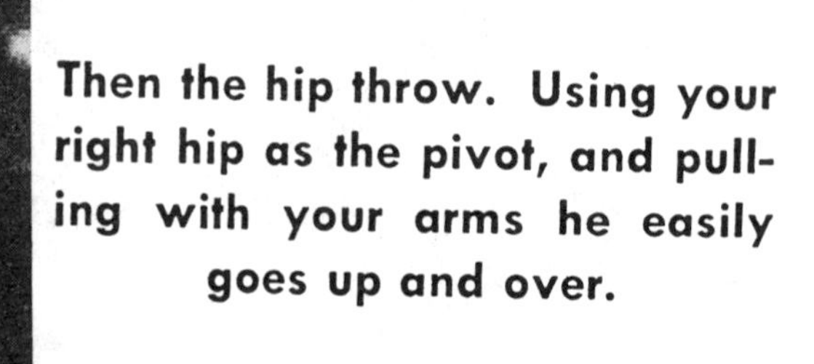

Then the hip throw. Using your right hip as the pivot, and pulling with your arms he easily goes up and over.

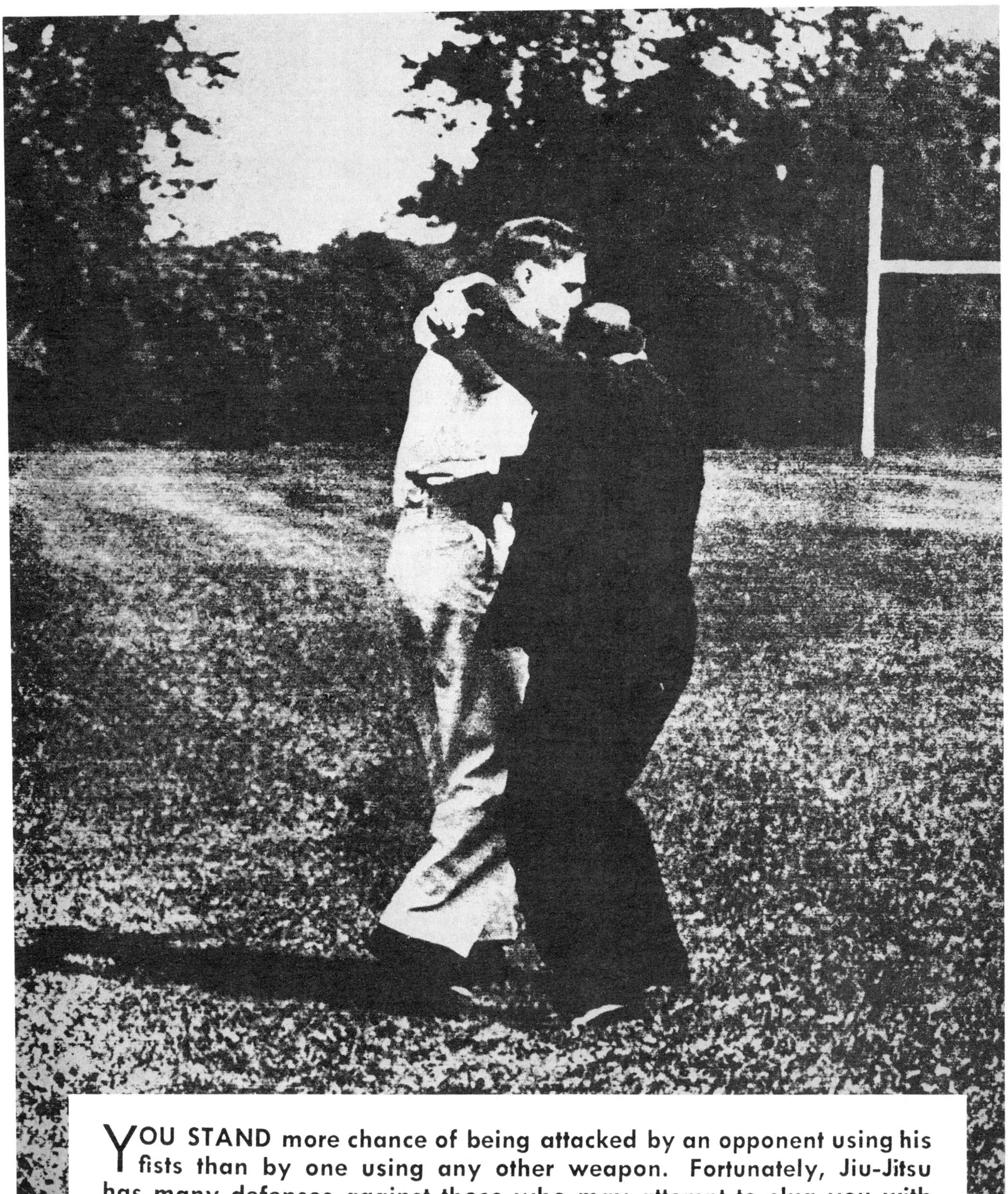

YOU STAND more chance of being attacked by an opponent using his fists than by one using any other weapon. Fortunately, Jiu-Jitsu has many defenses against those who may attempt to slug you with their fists. The one described here is to be used against a right-hand blow. Just two moves to make, one to block your opponent's blow, one to make your counter blow, and if you do it correctly the trouble is over.

This is a very useful number. A person who attempts to hit you with a right hand blow gives you a wide open opportunity to knock him out.

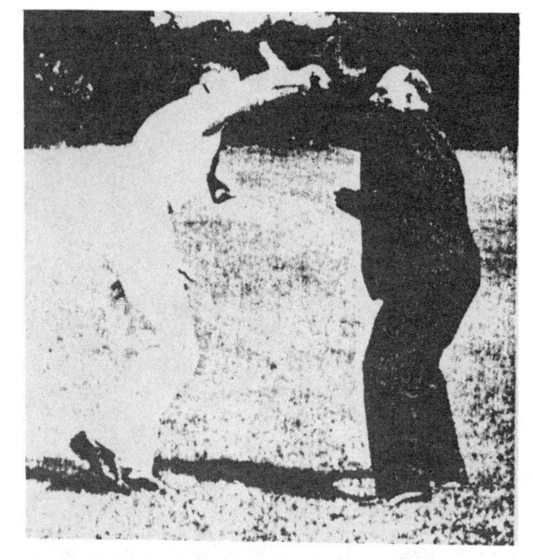

As an attacker's right fist flashes toward you, counter the blow

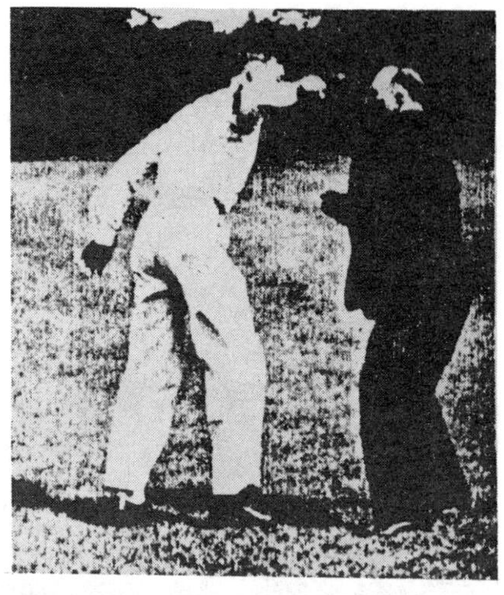

by a hard smash with the knife part of your hand to his forearm

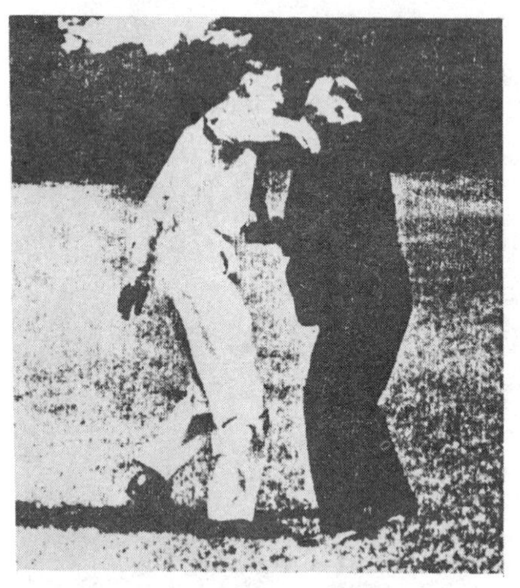

which will momentarily paralize his wrist and hand. As you do this

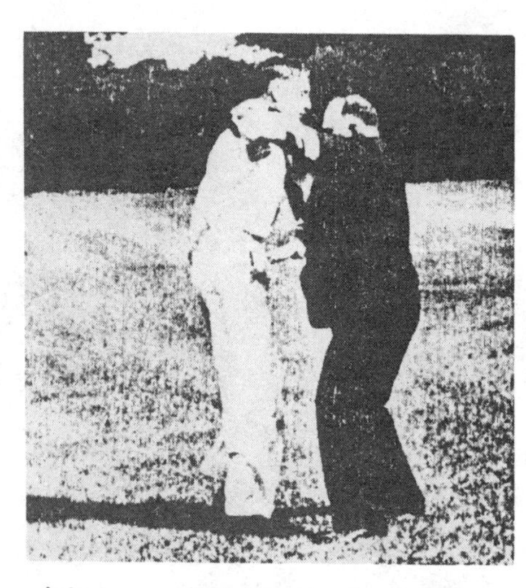

bring your right hand and arm over, across your body, with your hand in knife blow position.

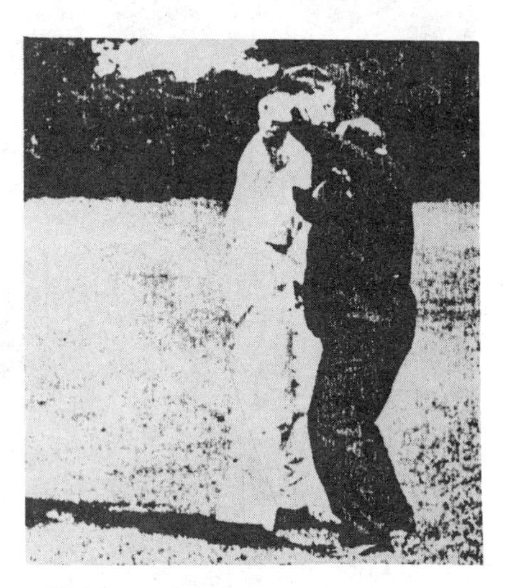

With your left hand hold your opponent's right arm out of the way and bring

your right hand high on your left side. Then hit, very hard, at a spot right over his lowest rib.

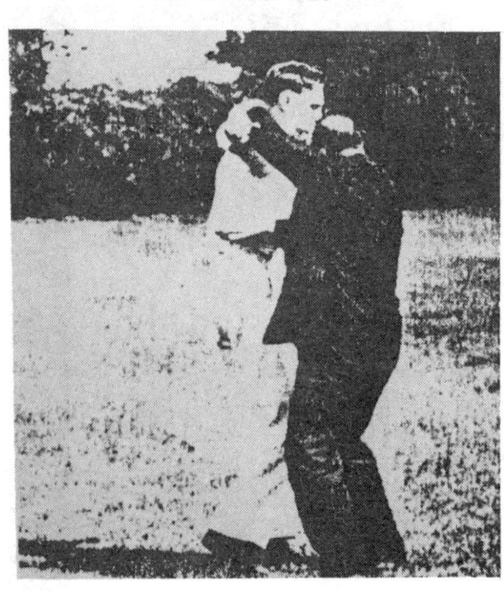

In most cases this will be a knockout blow as few people can stand such a blow to their liver.

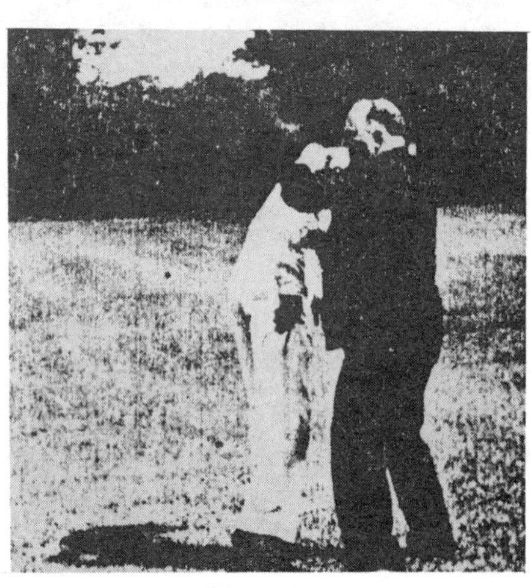

Let me caution you to use this blow very lightly in practice. Do, however, practice hitting the right spot but this can be determined by very light taps.

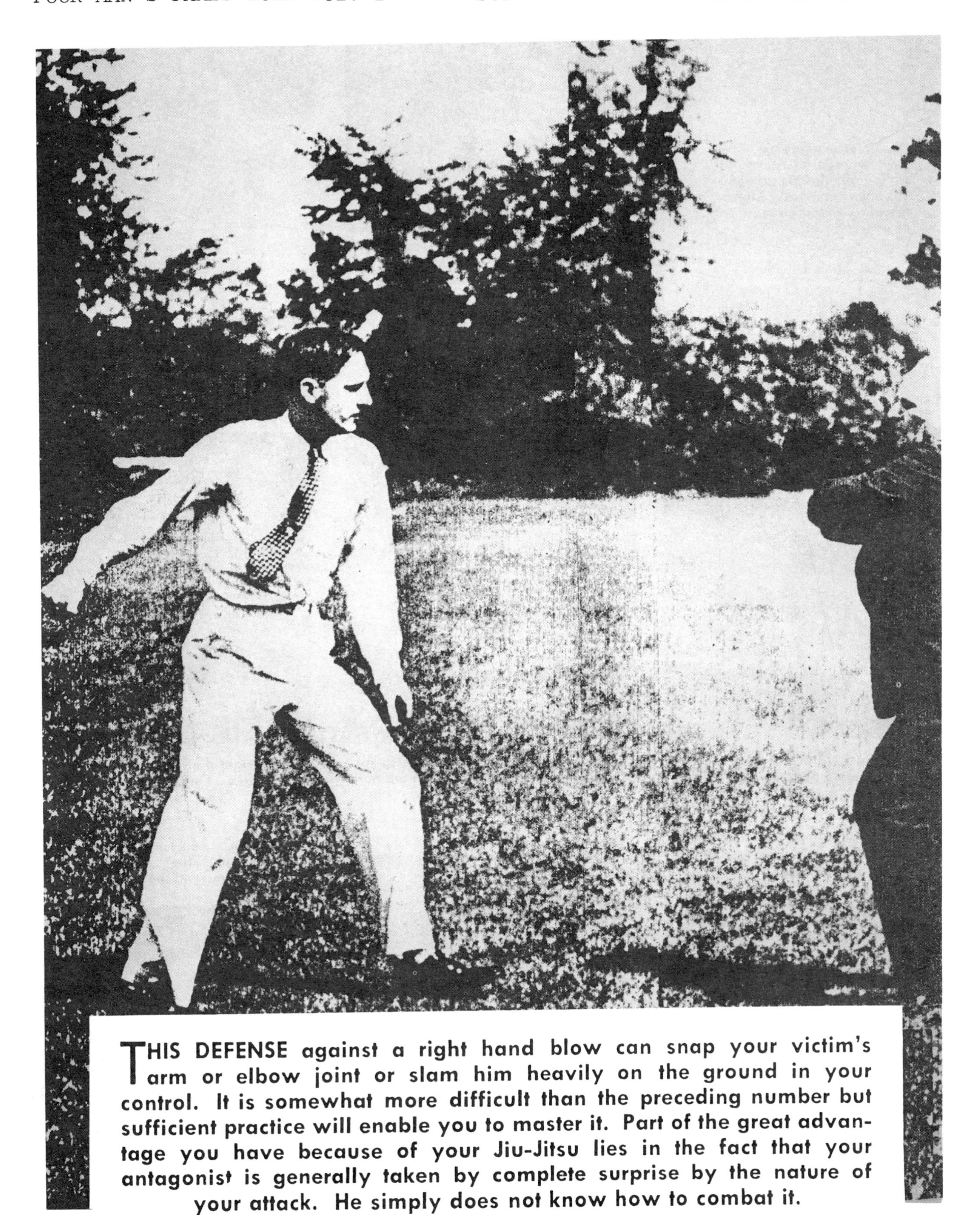

THIS DEFENSE against a right hand blow can snap your victim's arm or elbow joint or slam him heavily on the ground in your control. It is somewhat more difficult than the preceding number but sufficient practice will enable you to master it. Part of the great advantage you have because of your Jiu-Jitsu lies in the fact that your antagonist is generally taken by complete surprise by the nature of your attack. He simply does not know how to combat it.

This defense against a blow by a fist requires speed but comparatively little strength. The leverage involved takes the place of an abundance of power.

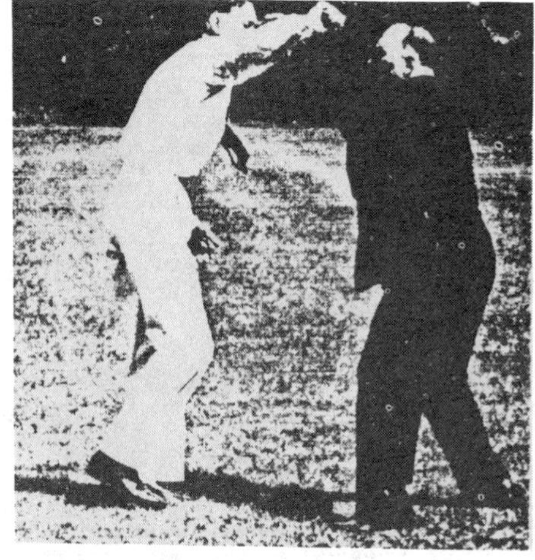

Parry the blow with the knife edge of your hand against attacker's forearm

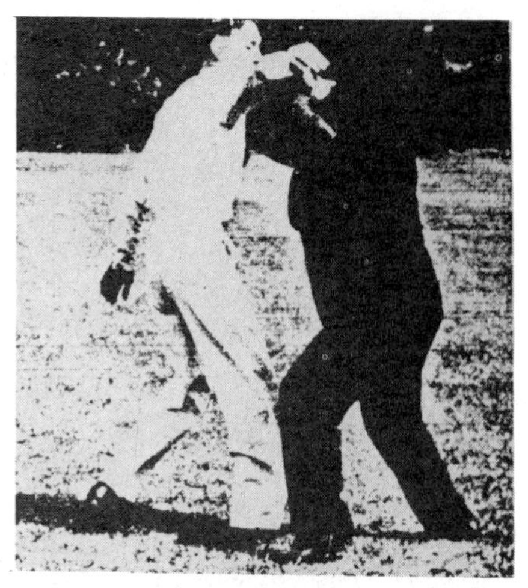

and grasp his wrist and force his arm upward. Grasp his left shoulder close to his neck.

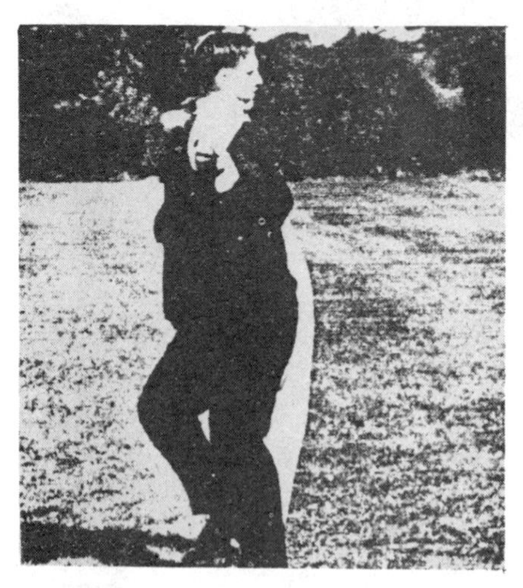

the palm of his hand will be slightly upward. Retain your hold on his left shoulder.

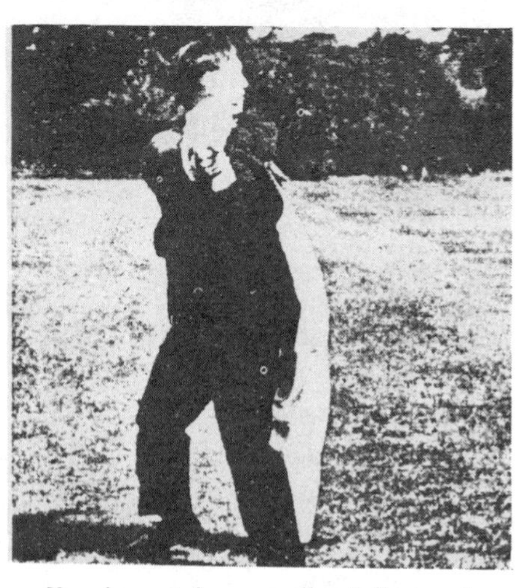

You have taken another full step forward and you and your man are now nearly back to back.

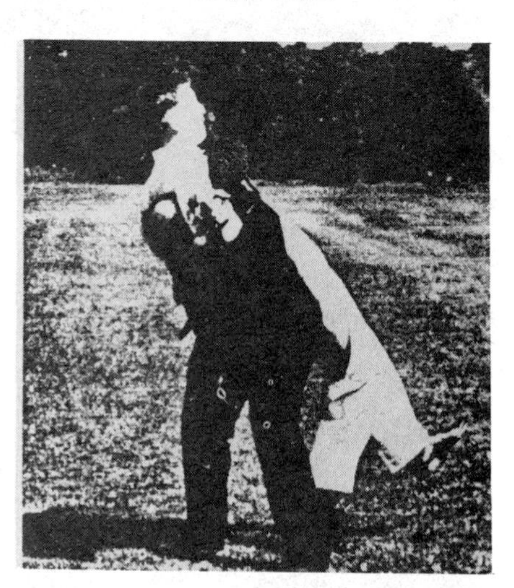

Your right hip is in close contact with the back of his right hip. Now shift your hips suddenly

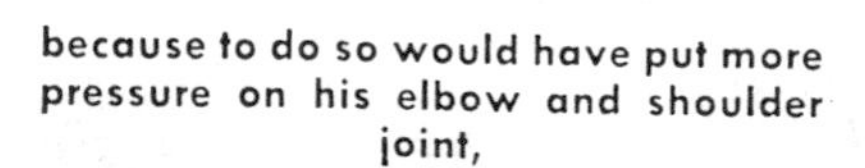

because to do so would have put more pressure on his elbow and shoulder joint,

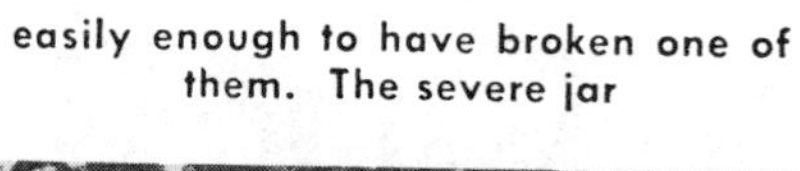

easily enough to have broken one of them. The severe jar

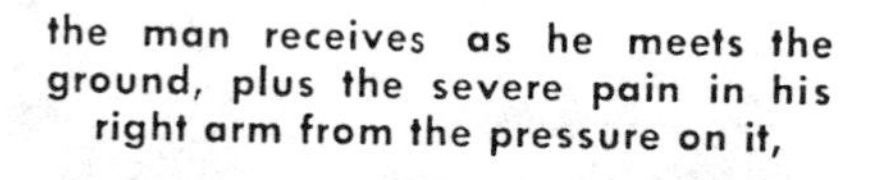

the man receives as he meets the ground, plus the severe pain in his right arm from the pressure on it,

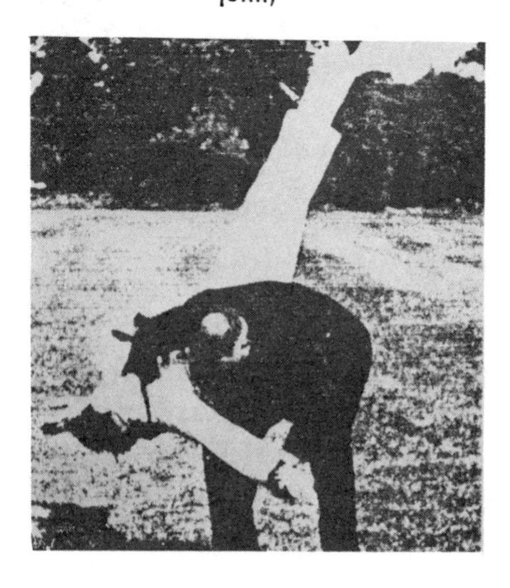

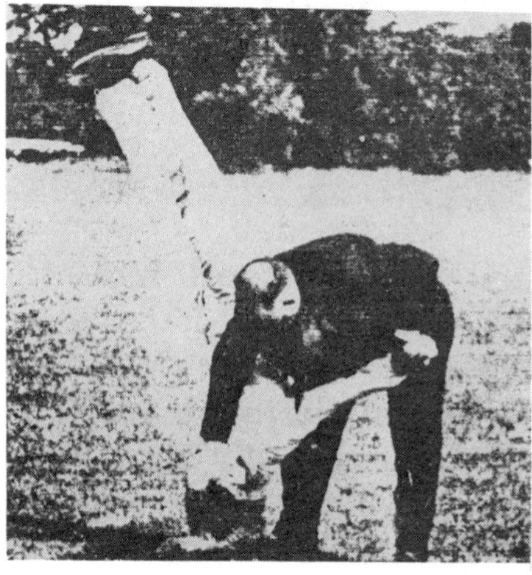

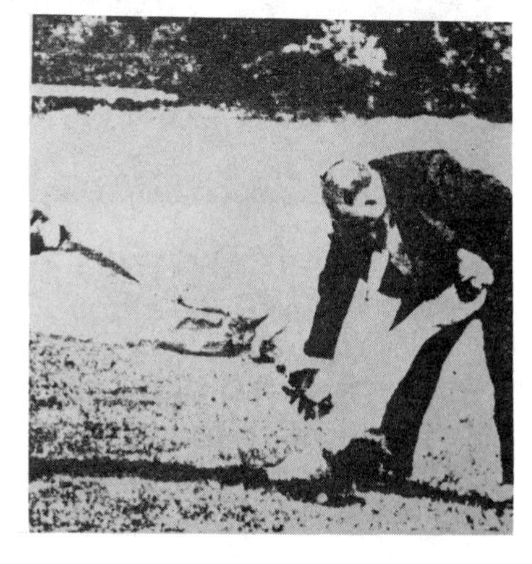

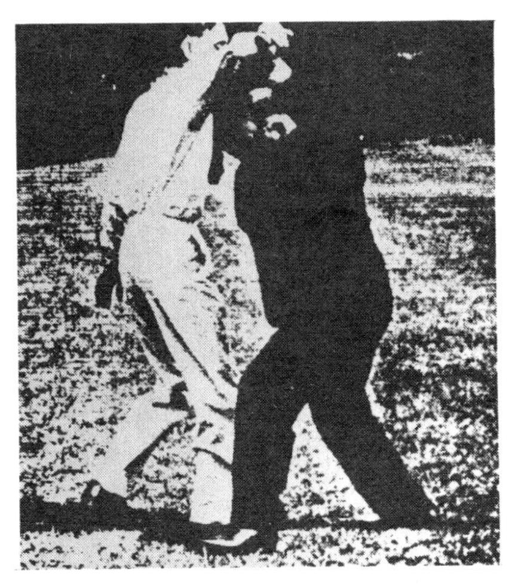

Duck your head, if necessary, to go under his outstretched right arm, stepping forward as you do so.

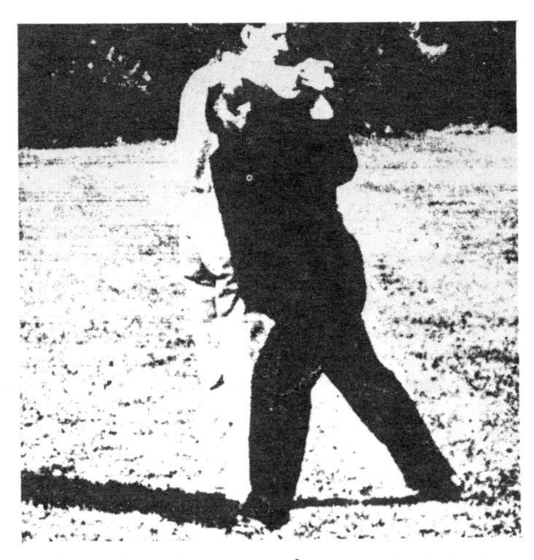

Bring his right arm down across your shoulders. His elbow should rest upon the back of your neck.

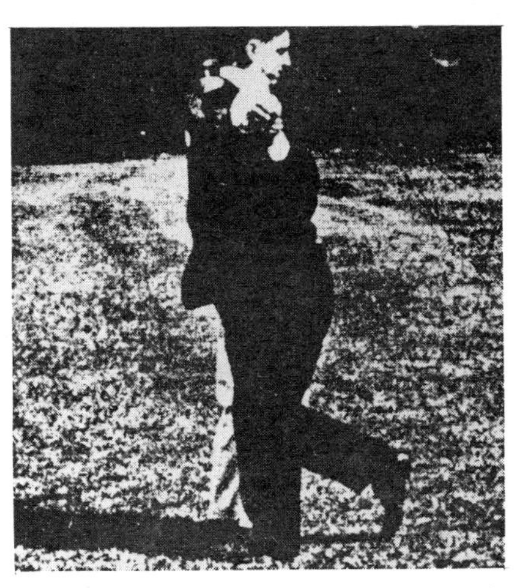

With your left hand, which is firmly grasping your attacker's wrist, rotate his arm so that

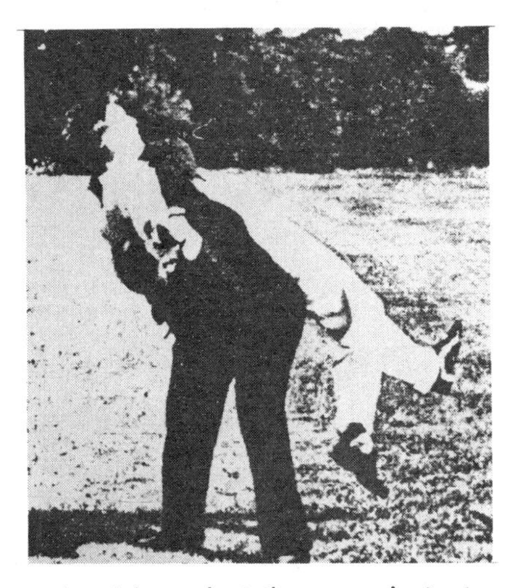

to the right and at the same instant lunge upward and forward with arms and upper body.

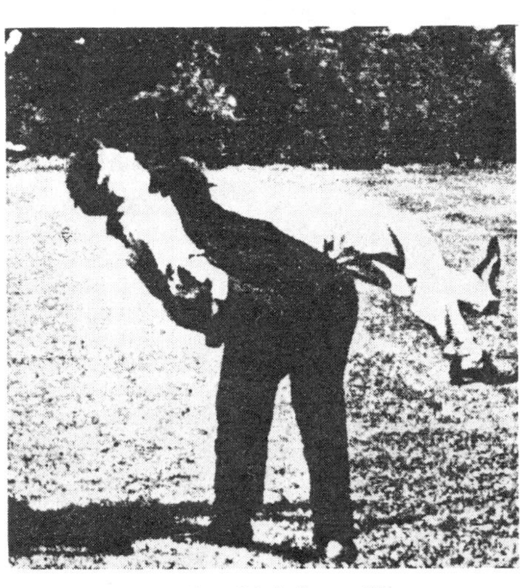

The ease with which he will come up on your back is amazing.

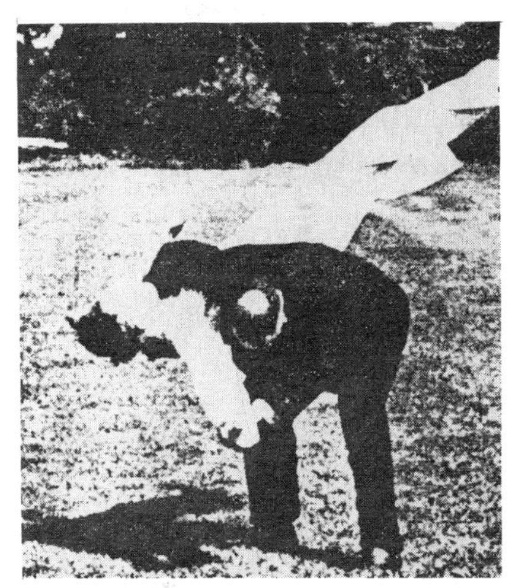

During the moment when you had his arm across your shoulders he could make no resistance

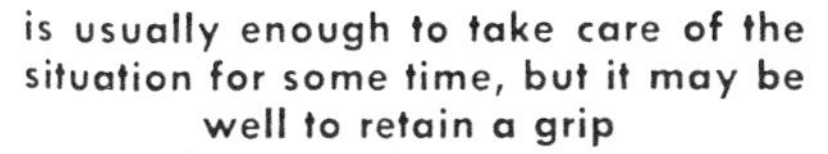

is usually enough to take care of the situation for some time, but it may be well to retain a grip

on his right arm and hold it in a lock until you can see whether he has any fight left in him.

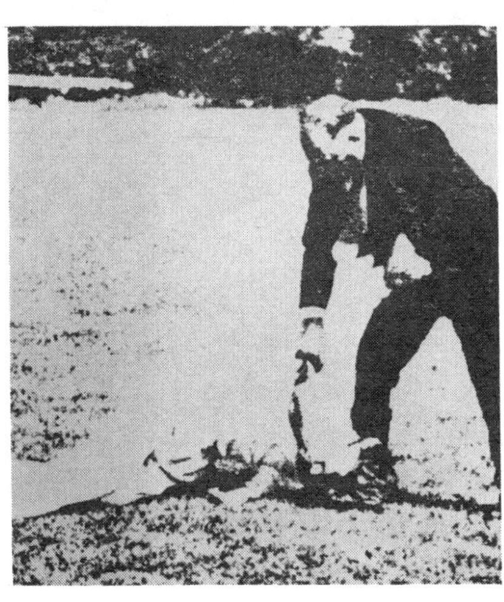

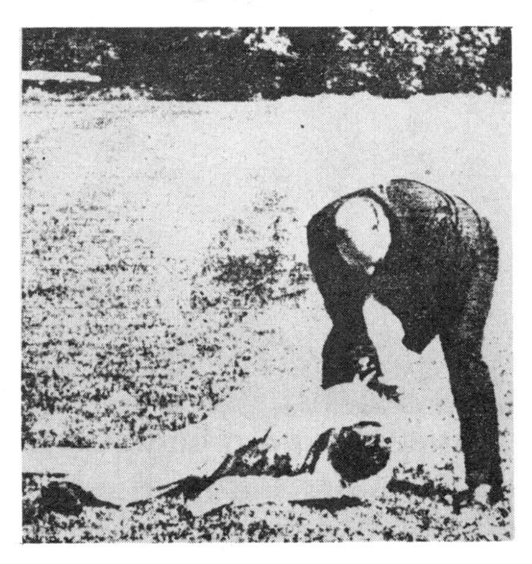

Hold his right hand with your right hand, bend his forearm forward, put your left arm through the V formed by his arm and rest your hand on your right wrist. Then bend his right hand forward until he indicates "enough"!

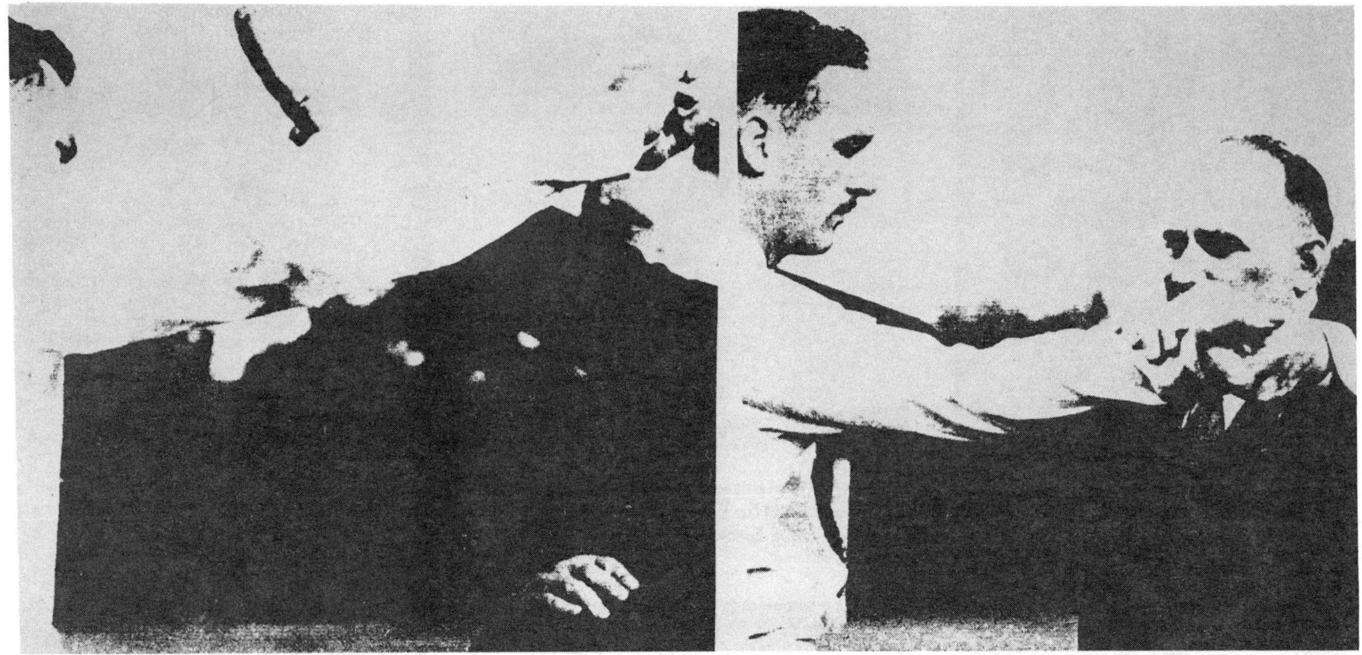

The first part of this number consists of blocking the blow with your left hand.

Next you grasp his right wrist with your left hand and turn his wrist so that the palm of his hand faces upward.

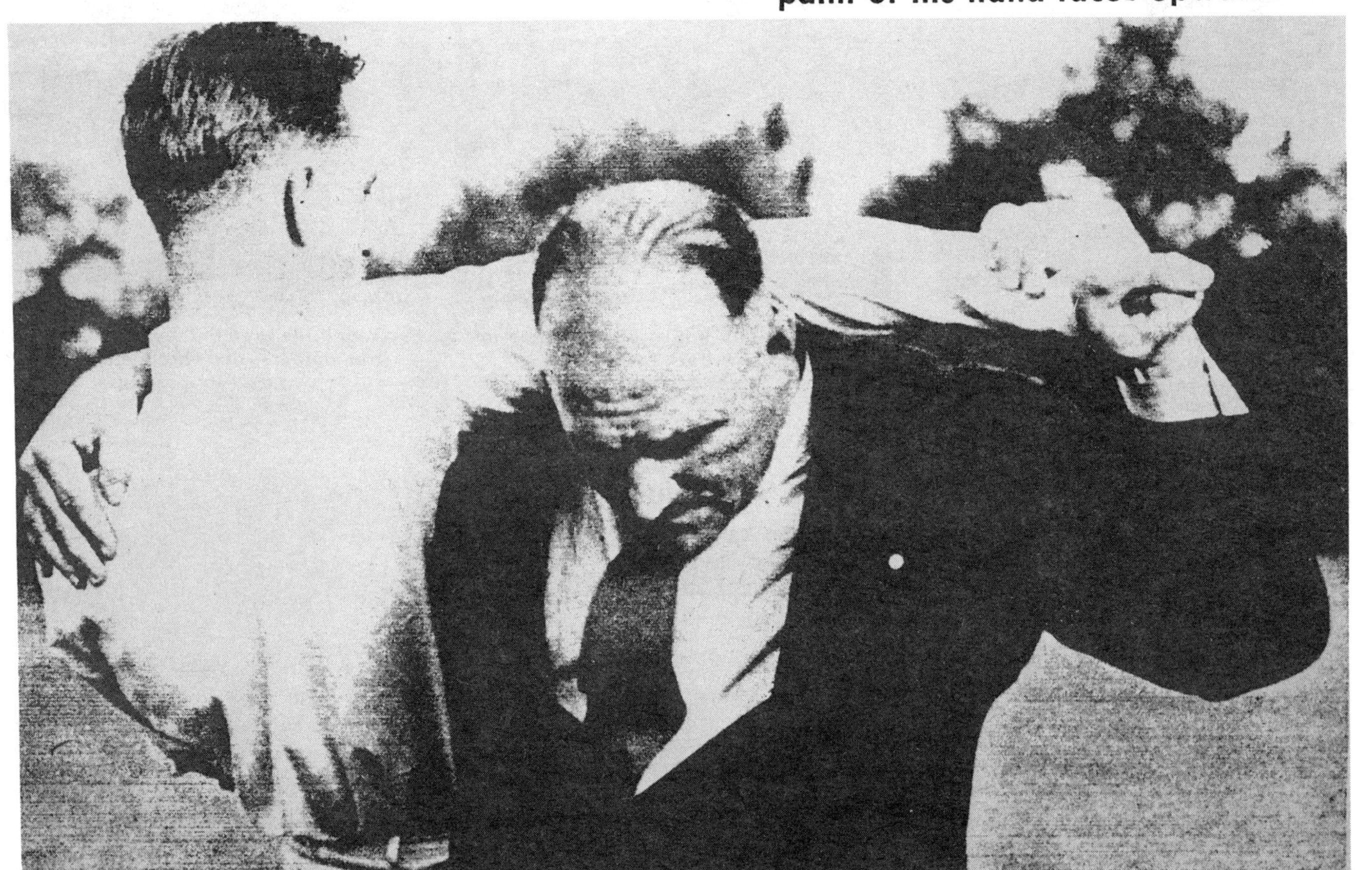

His arm is raised over your head and brought down across the back of your neck. Your hip is close to his back and the next step is to throw him up and over.

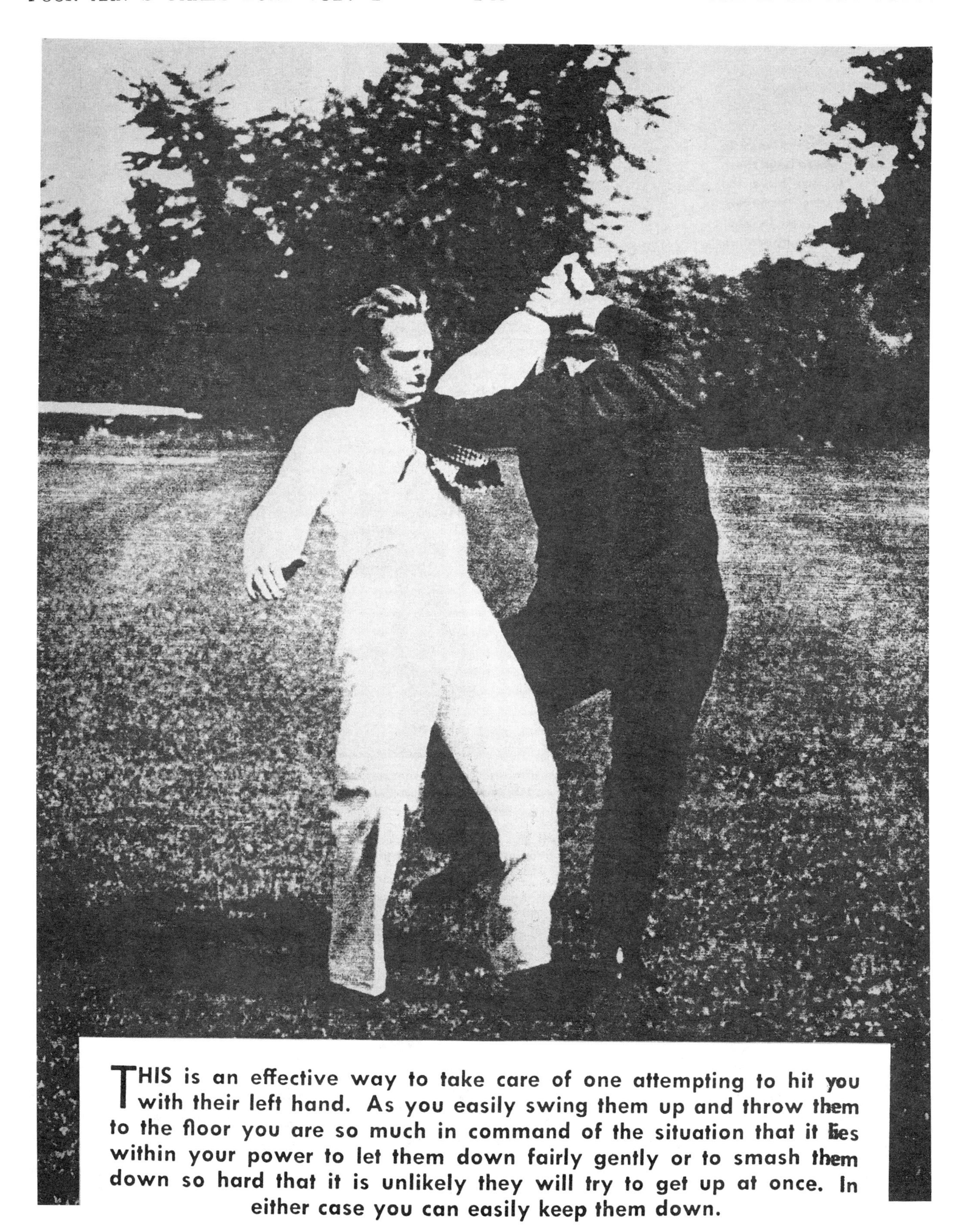

THIS is an effective way to take care of one attempting to hit you with their left hand. As you easily swing them up and throw them to the floor you are so much in command of the situation that it lies within your power to let them down fairly gently or to smash them down so hard that it is unlikely they will try to get up at once. In either case you can easily keep them down.

This number is as easy to use as it looks to be in these pictures. If you have the proper sequence of movements firmly fixed in your mind the actual application is not difficult.

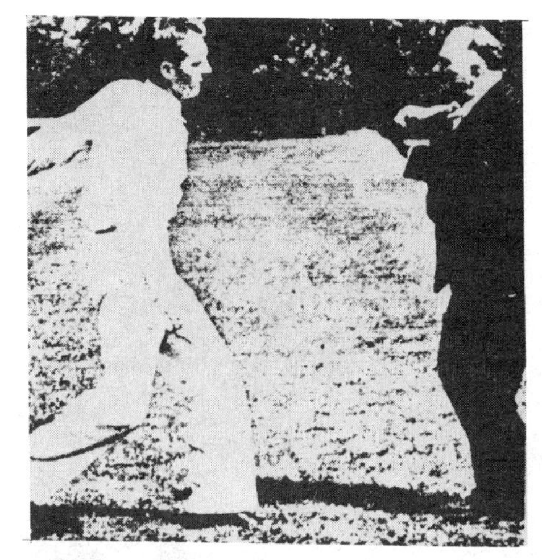

While it is shown here as a defense against a left-hand blow it is equally effective against a right.

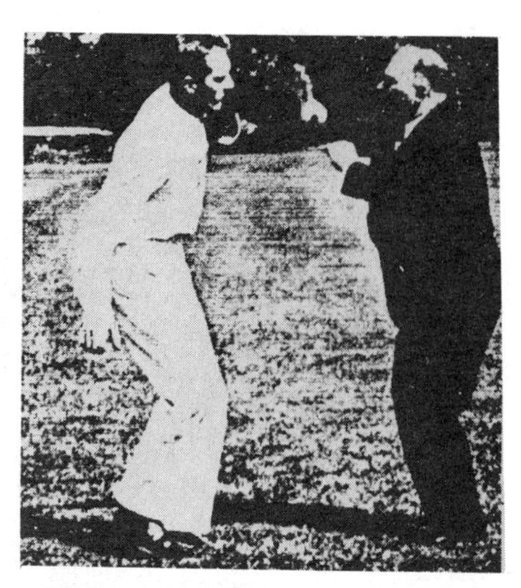

You should always be ready for any type of attack. If you are not, a surprise offensive catching

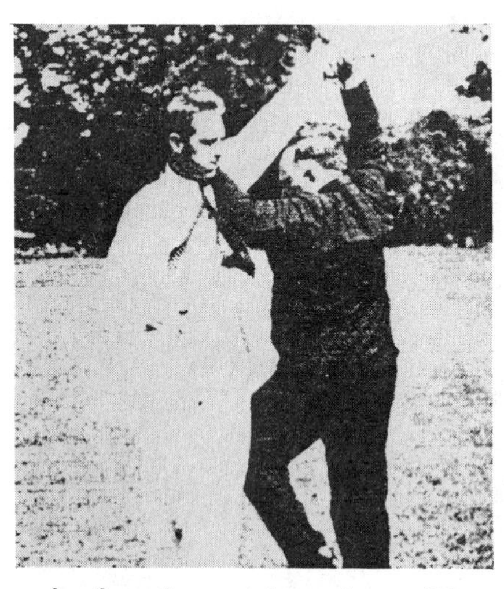

make the grip as tight as is possible for you. Make it as close to his neck as you can.

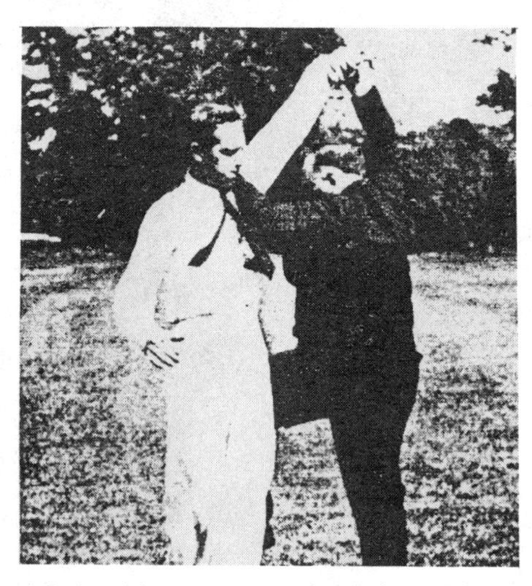

Raise his arm as high in the air as you can reach and also keep it fully extended

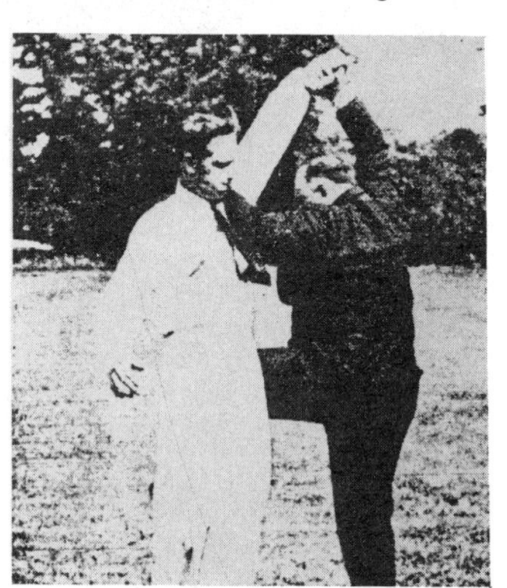

which will keep him off balance and out of position to resist effectively.

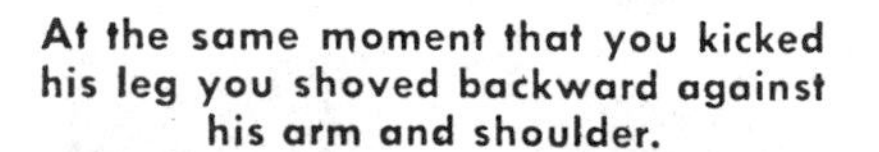

At the same moment that you kicked his leg you shoved backward against his arm and shoulder.

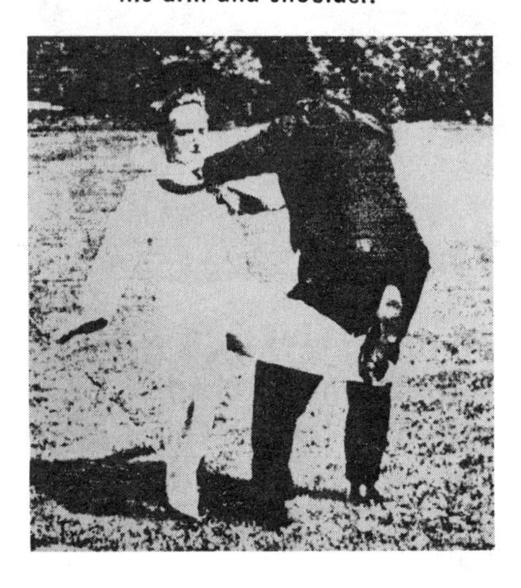

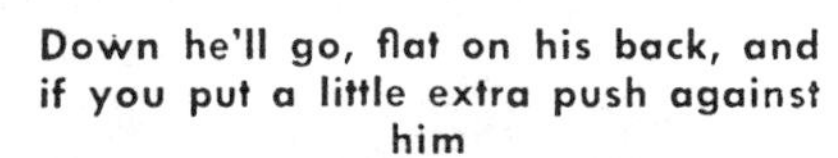

Down he'll go, flat on his back, and if you put a little extra push against him

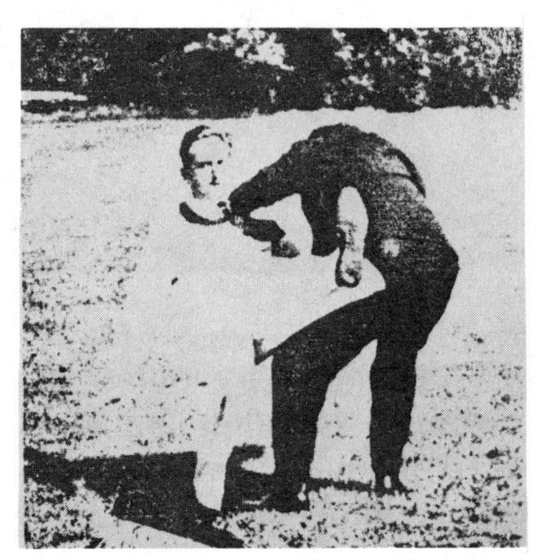

as he is going down he'll land with enough force to be disabled, at least temporarily.

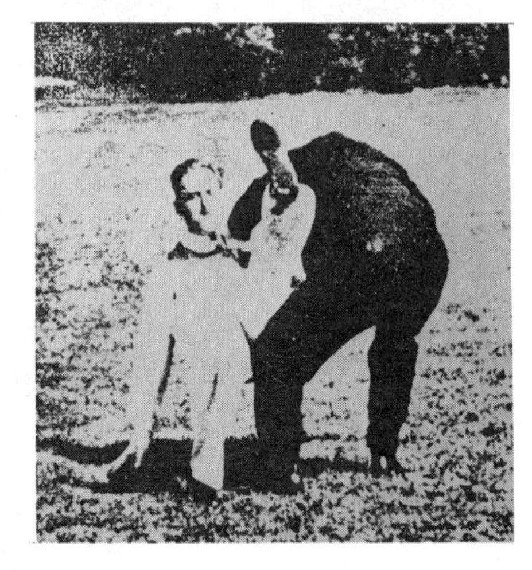

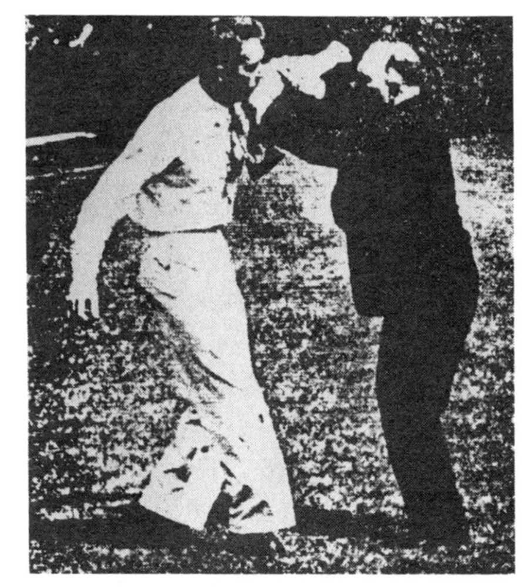

you off guard can be just as disastrous to you as you intend it to be to your opponent.

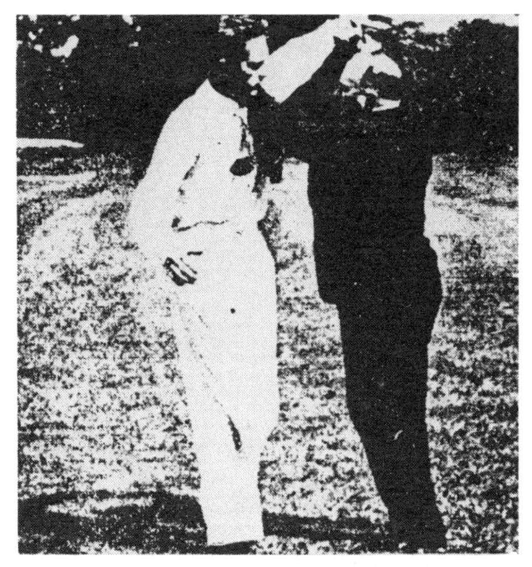

Block the blow with the knife edge of your right hand and then obtain a grip on his left wrist.

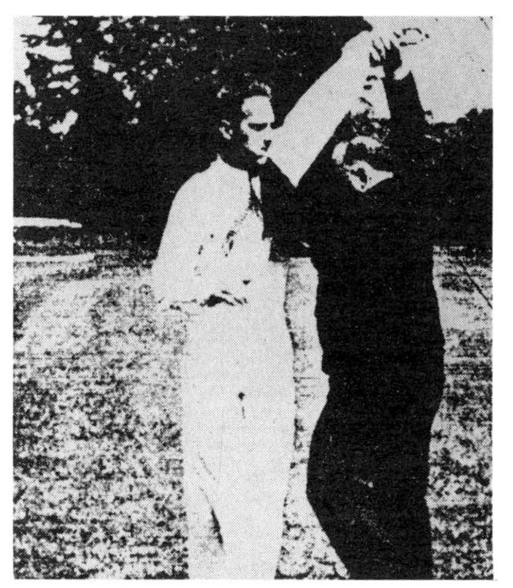

With your left hand hold the attacker's shoulder. Don't merely use his shoulder as a resting place for your hand—

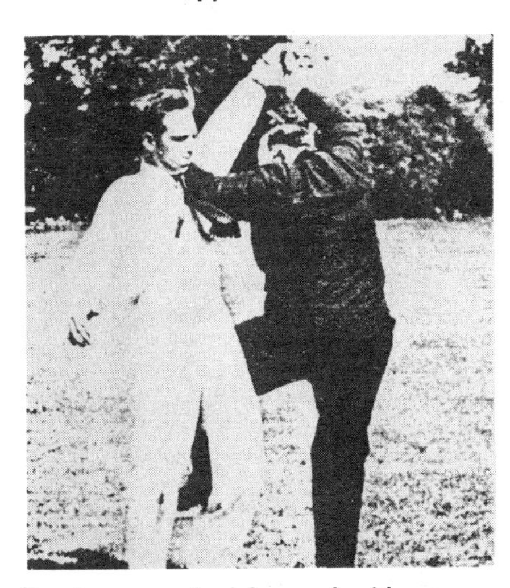

You have reached forward with your left leg until it is well behind his left leg.

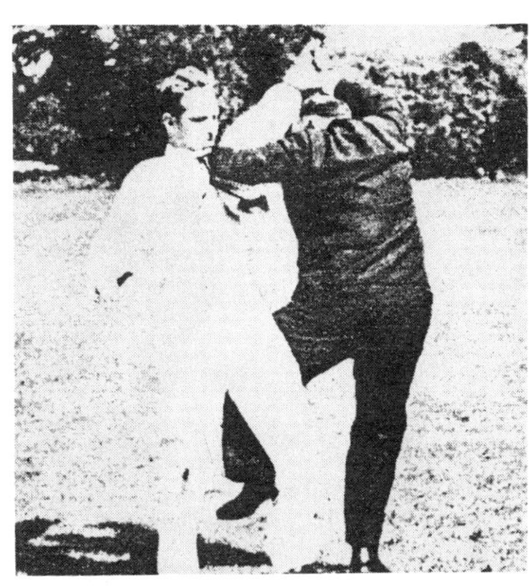

Now with your left heel kick the calf of the assailant's leg. I said "kick" and do it hard!

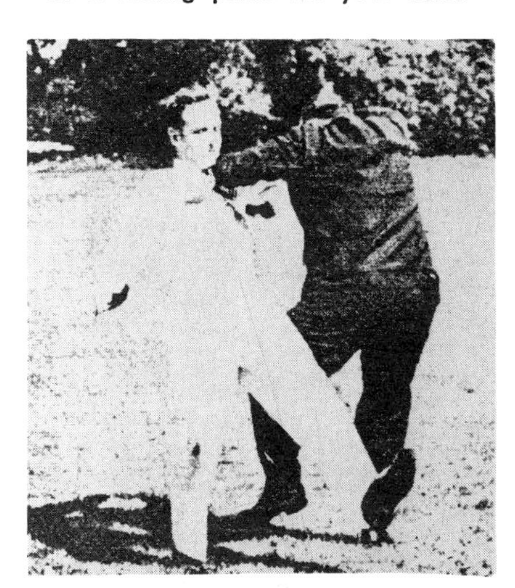

A shove won't do the job, but the kick will really take his legs out from under him as he is already off balance.

Some of the older Jiu-Jitsu numbers included instances in which YOU, intentionally, also fell to the ground.

I definitely will not let my students use numbers which even momentarily place themselves in such dangerous positions.

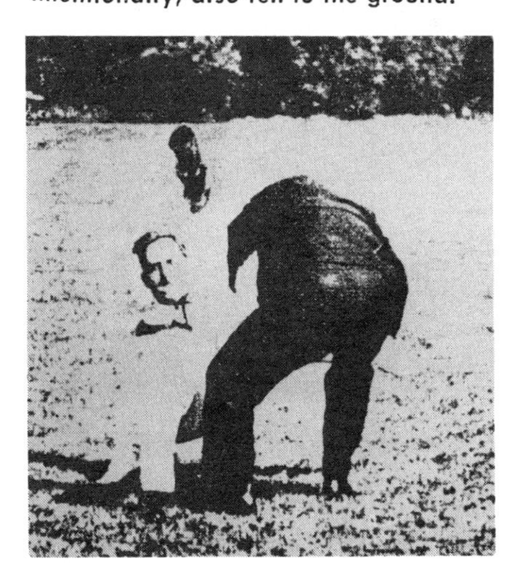

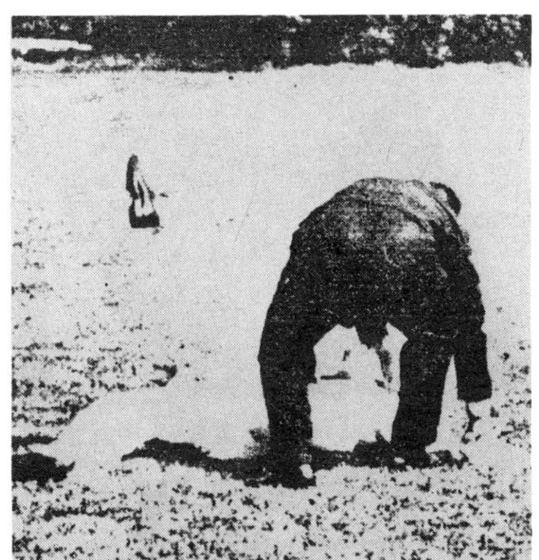

Jiu-Jitsu has successful defenses for every attack and I allow the use of only those which control the various situations with the most speed and least bother to the operator.

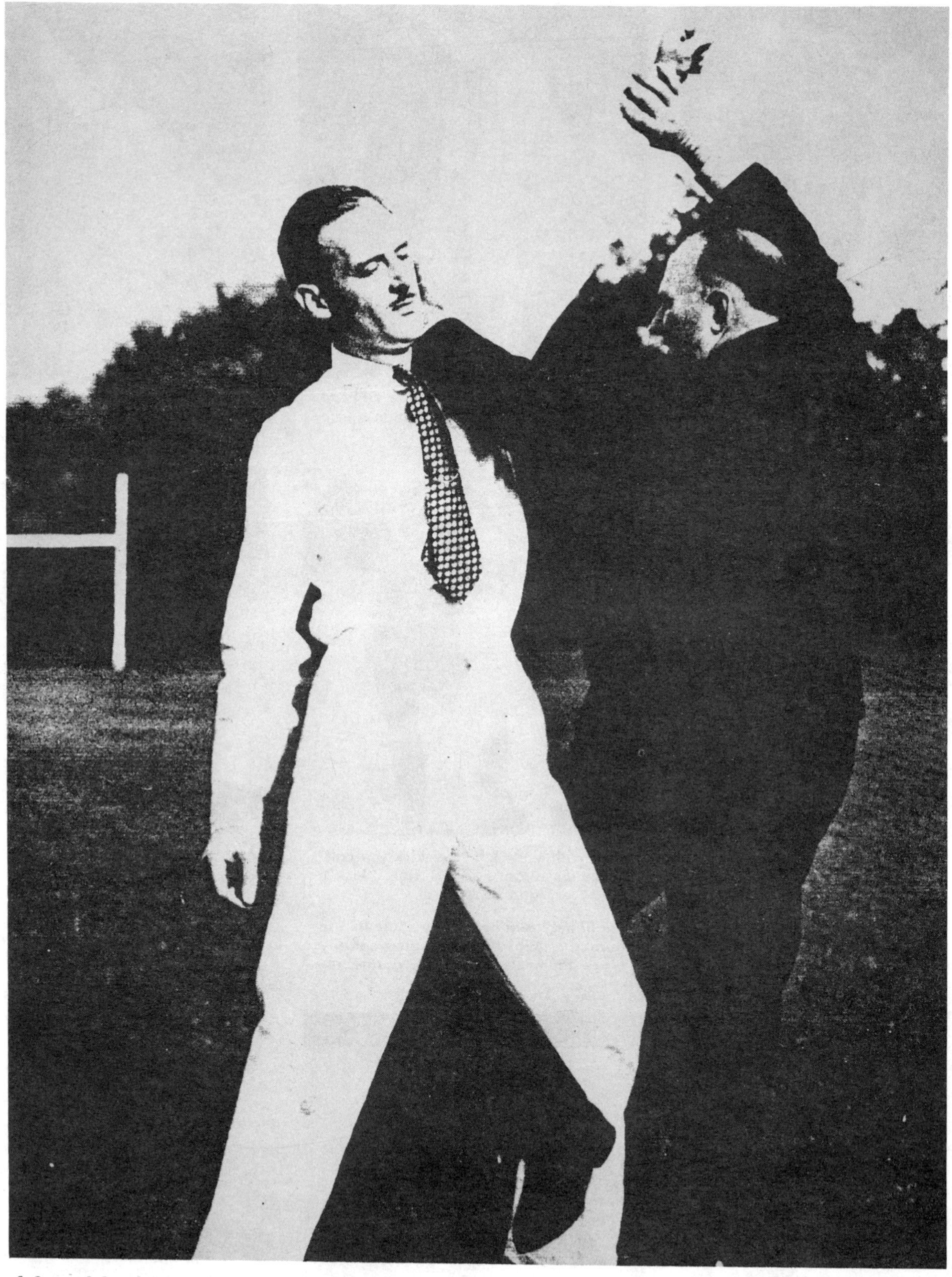

After blocking the left hand blow you hold your man's wrist and shoulder and raise his arm high in the air to throw him off balance. Then a solid kick with your left heel against his left leg and he is thrown to the ground.

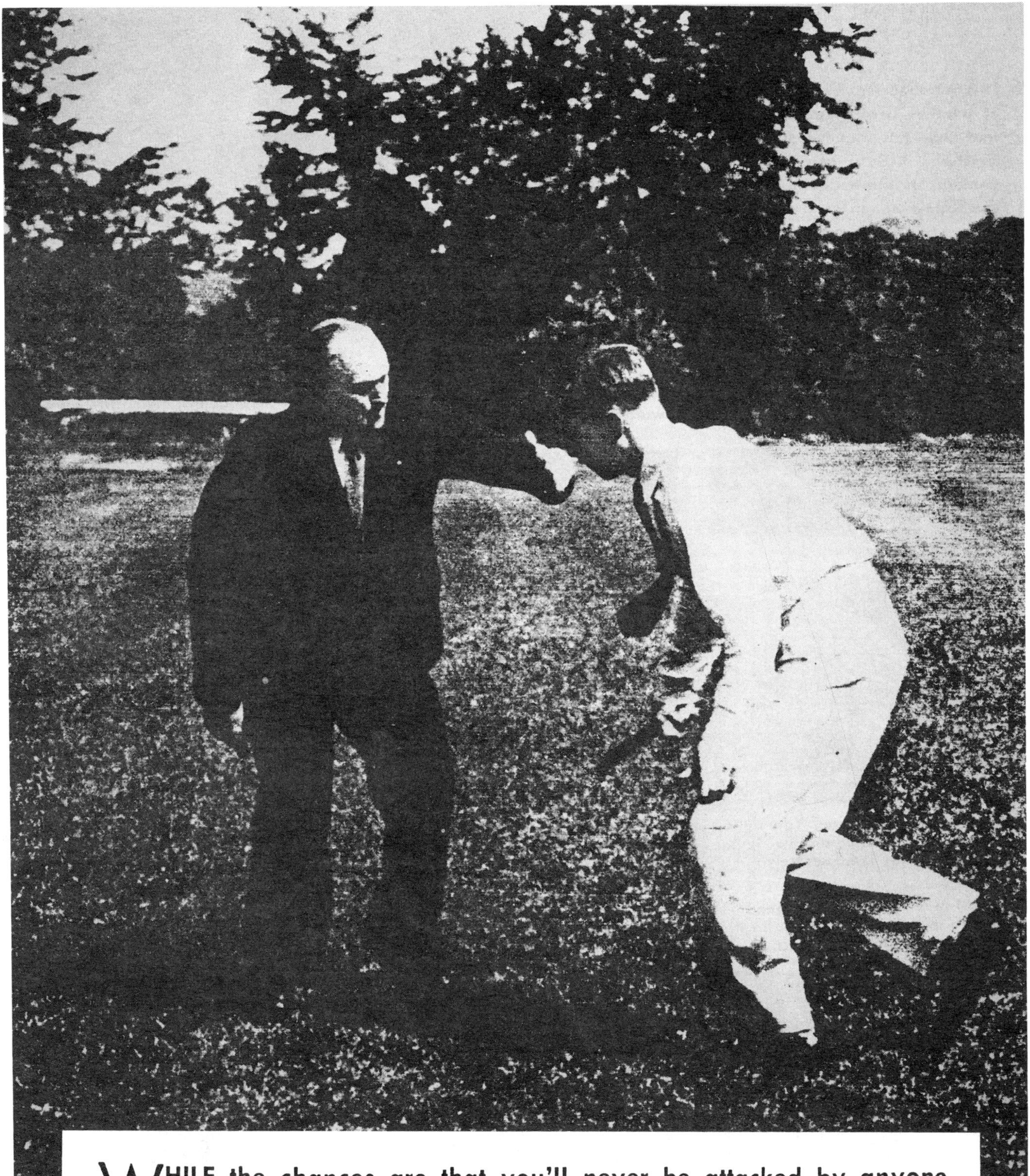

WHILE the chances are that you'll never be attacked by anyone wielding a knife, the Jiu-Jitsu defense against such a person is so easy that you cannot afford to neglect it. When practicing, use a knife of the proper weight and shape, but have the blade covered by some protective sheath so that there is no possibility of anyone being needlessly injured.

This number requires a lot of practice before you can know that you have really mastered it. But when you can apply it as shown in the following pictures you own a real defense against anyone approaching you in this manner with a knife.

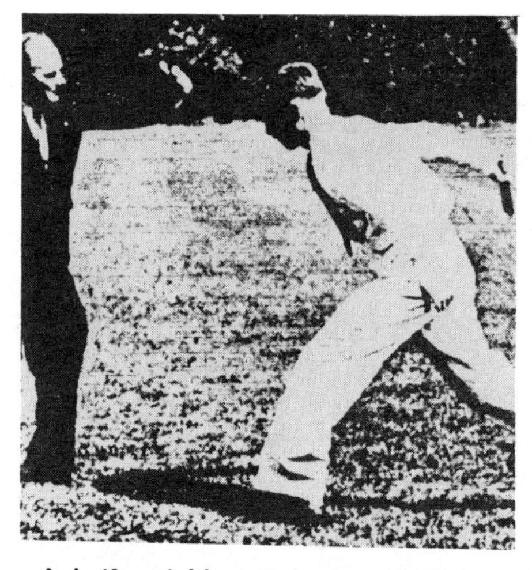

A knife wielder attempts to stab by either a downward lunge or an upward slash of his weapon. This defense is for the latter action.

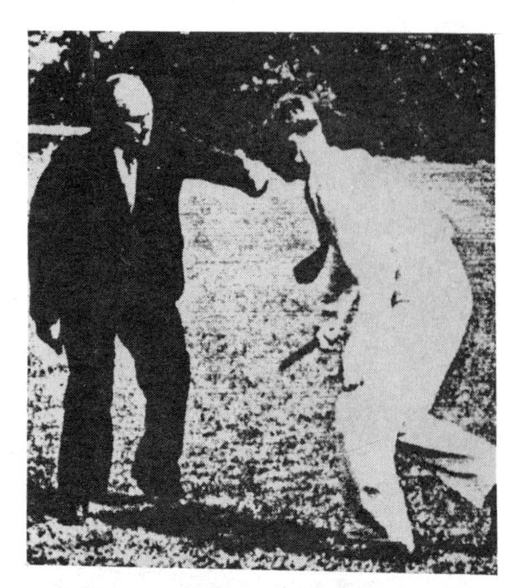

As he comes to you, you must quickly do two things; parry the blow and swing your body to one side out of the way.

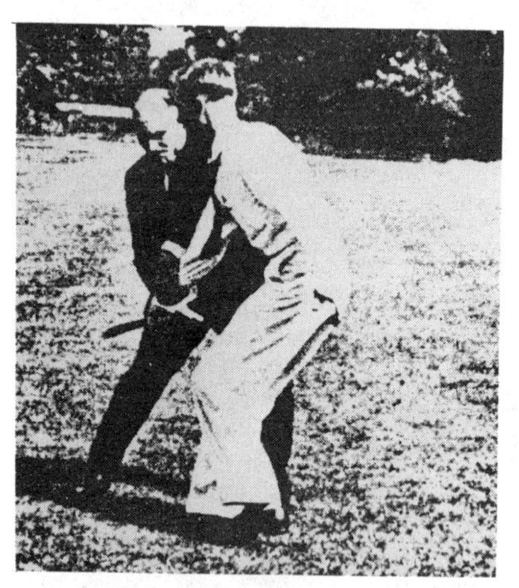

where you take a firm grip. Your right hand joins in this action and you thus hold his knife hand securely

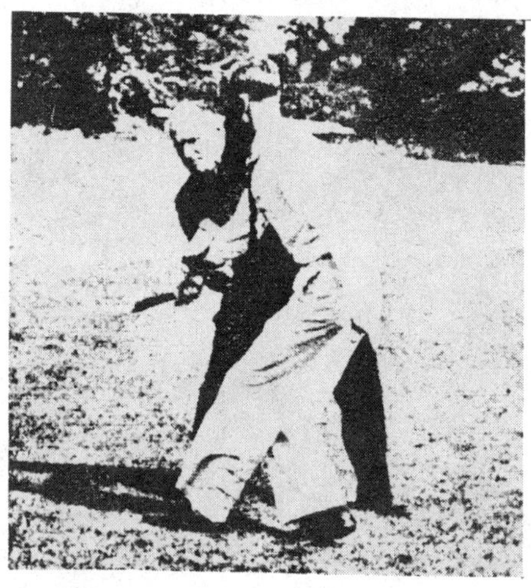

with your thumbs exerting pressure on the nerve center on the back of his hand

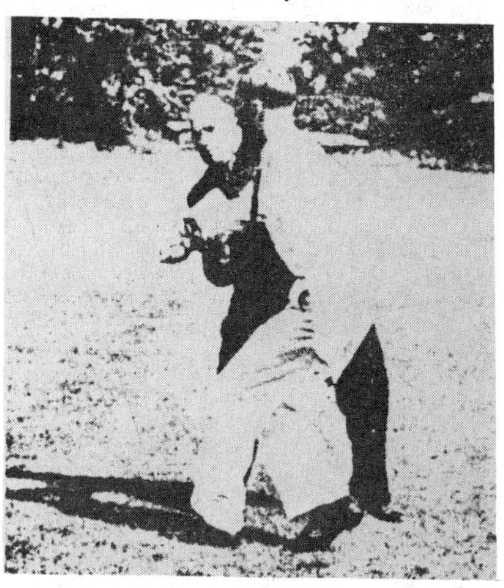

and your fingers to the inside of his wrist. You are now in no danger from the knife

This will make him open his hand—letting go of the knife which will sail through the air out of reach.

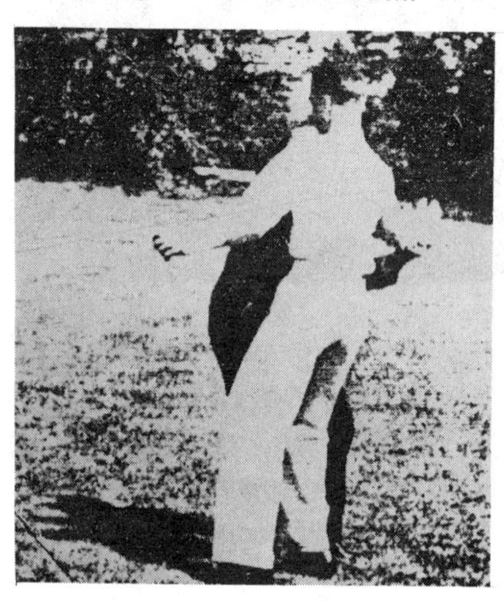

You still have one more objective and that is to throw him to the ground—you are doing that by

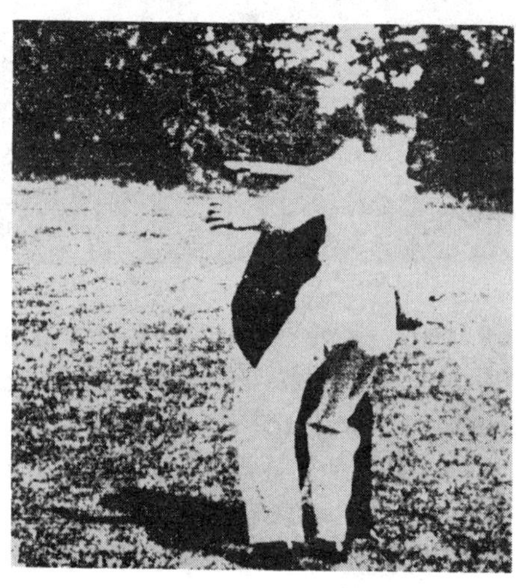

twisting his hand, wrist and arm farther backward all the time until the leverage on his elbow and wrist produces

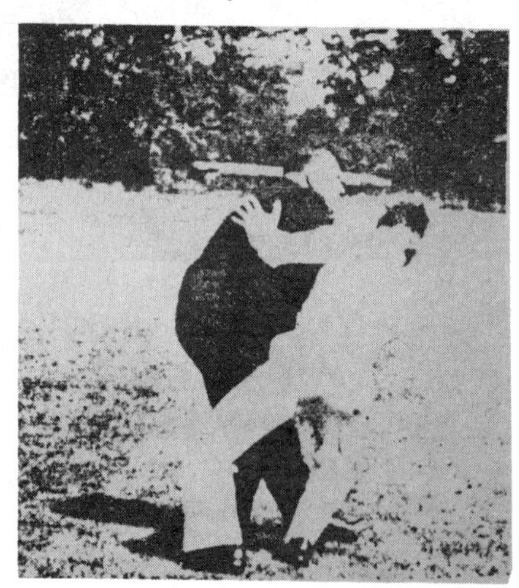

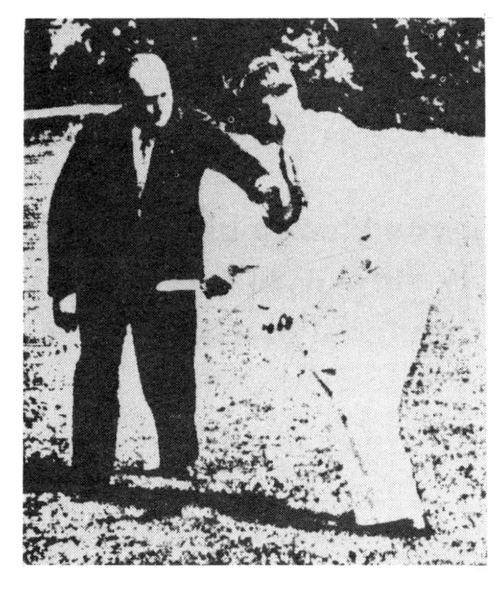

Smash, with the knife blow of your hand, into your enemy's lower right arm breaking the force of his thrust.

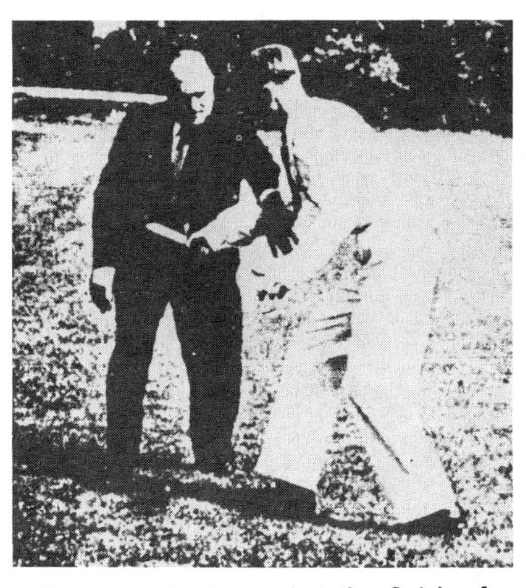

Turn your body so that the finish of his arrested blow will slide harmlessly past you.

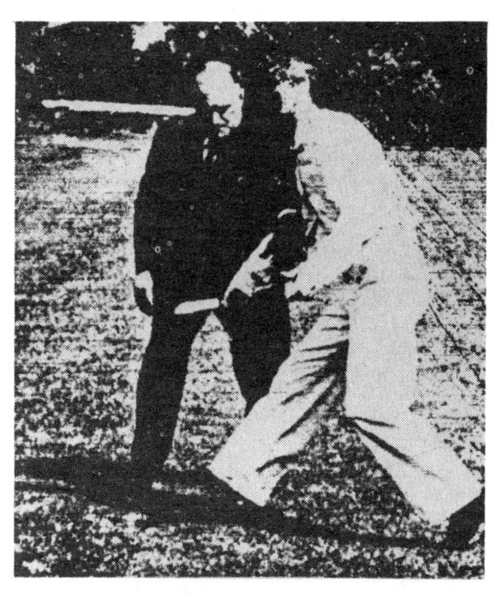

Slide your left hand from the spot you hit down to his wrist

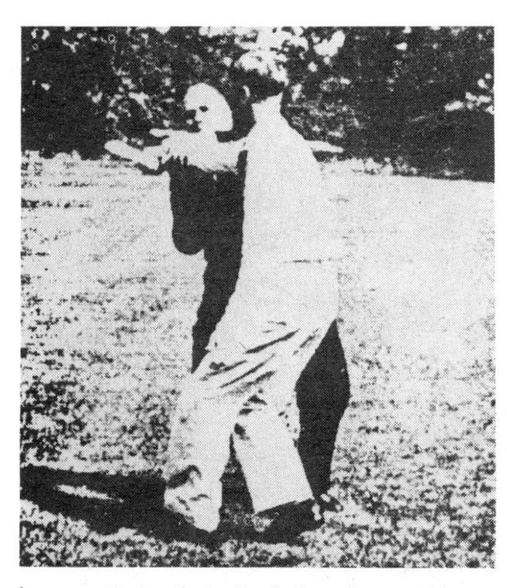

but until the assailant is weaponless and on the ground you cannot relax your grip.

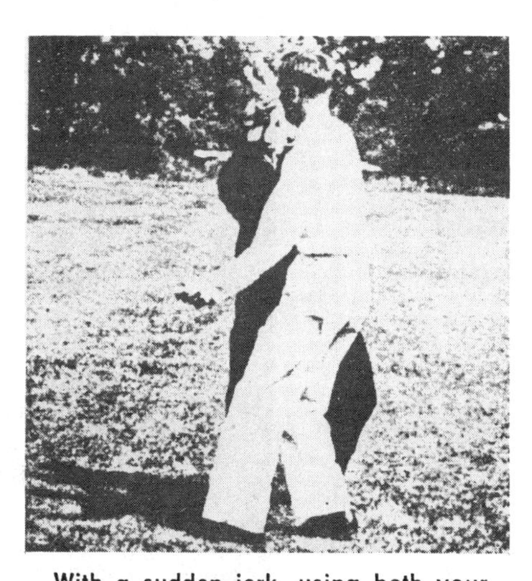

With a sudden jerk, using both your hands, bring his arm up and as you do so exert pressure

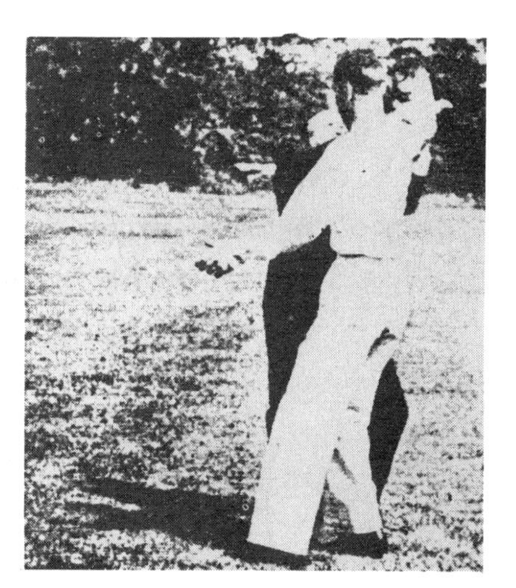

with your thumbs on the nerve spot on the back of his hand between the first and second fingers.

more pain than he can stand. This will bring him to the ground in a hurry. Resistance would result

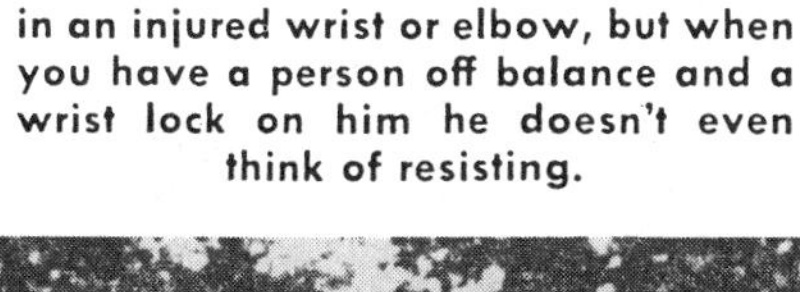

in an injured wrist or elbow, but when you have a person off balance and a wrist lock on him he doesn't even think of resisting.

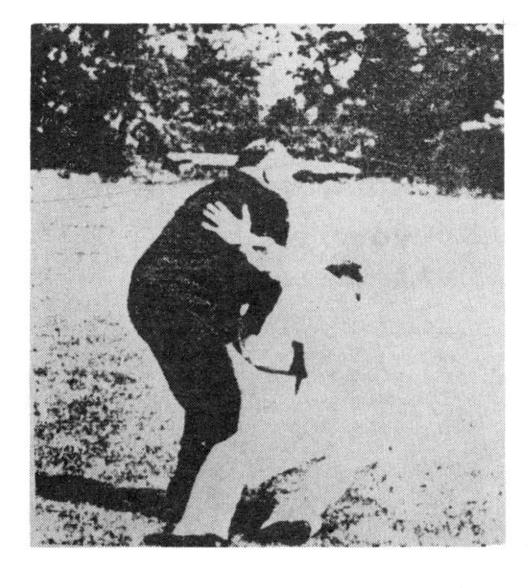

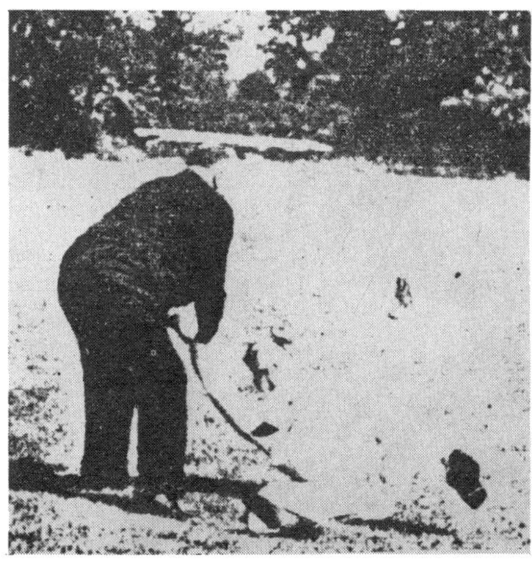

In analyzing this hold I discussed the several steps such as blocking the blow, getting rid of the knife and throwing the man, as if they were separate parts of the number. Of course they are all part of one smooth flowing action which accomplishes the final goal.

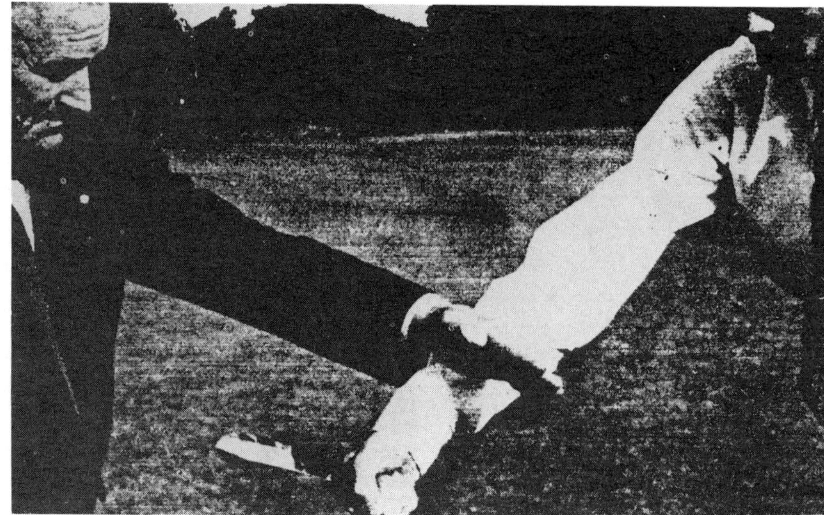

When you block a blow don't merely slow it down. Hit as hard as you can.

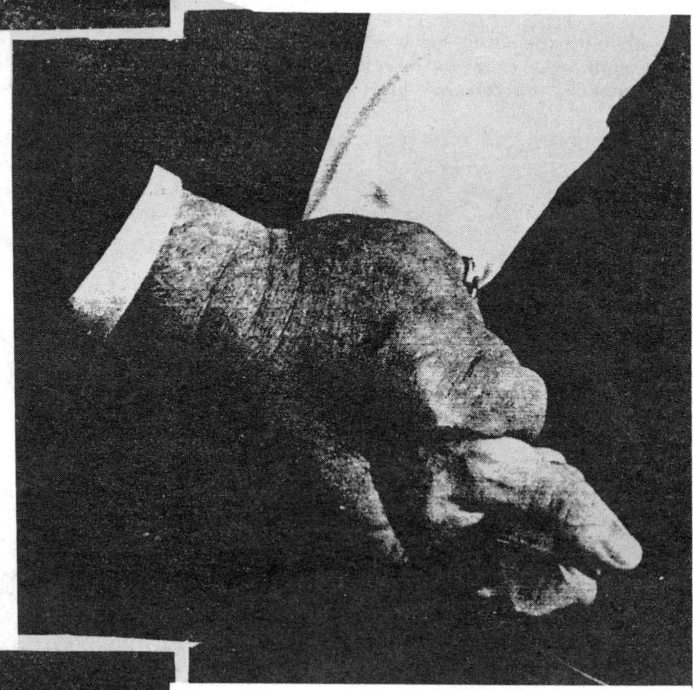

The instant you block this blow your hand moves down and grips his hand with your thumb to the back of his hand.

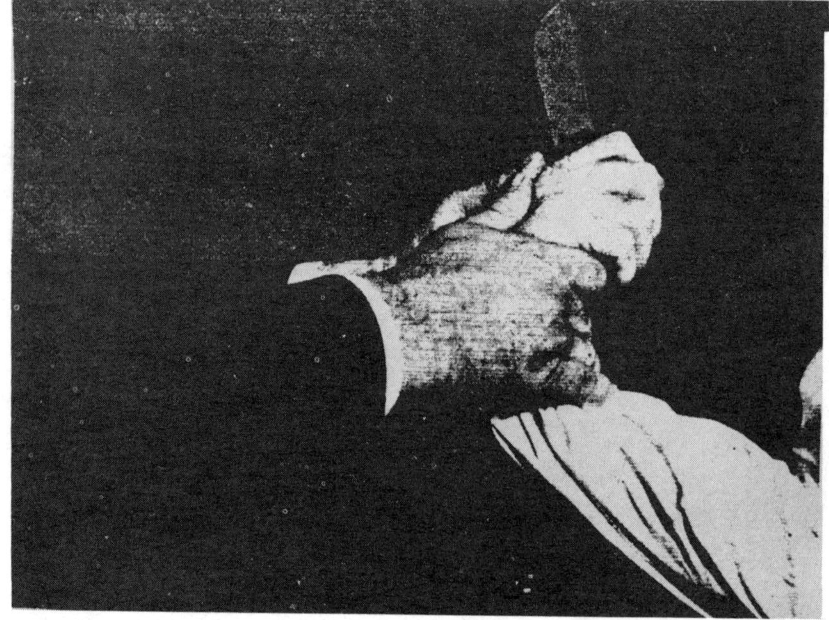

Your left hand then re-inforces your right and you twist his hand back and to your left.

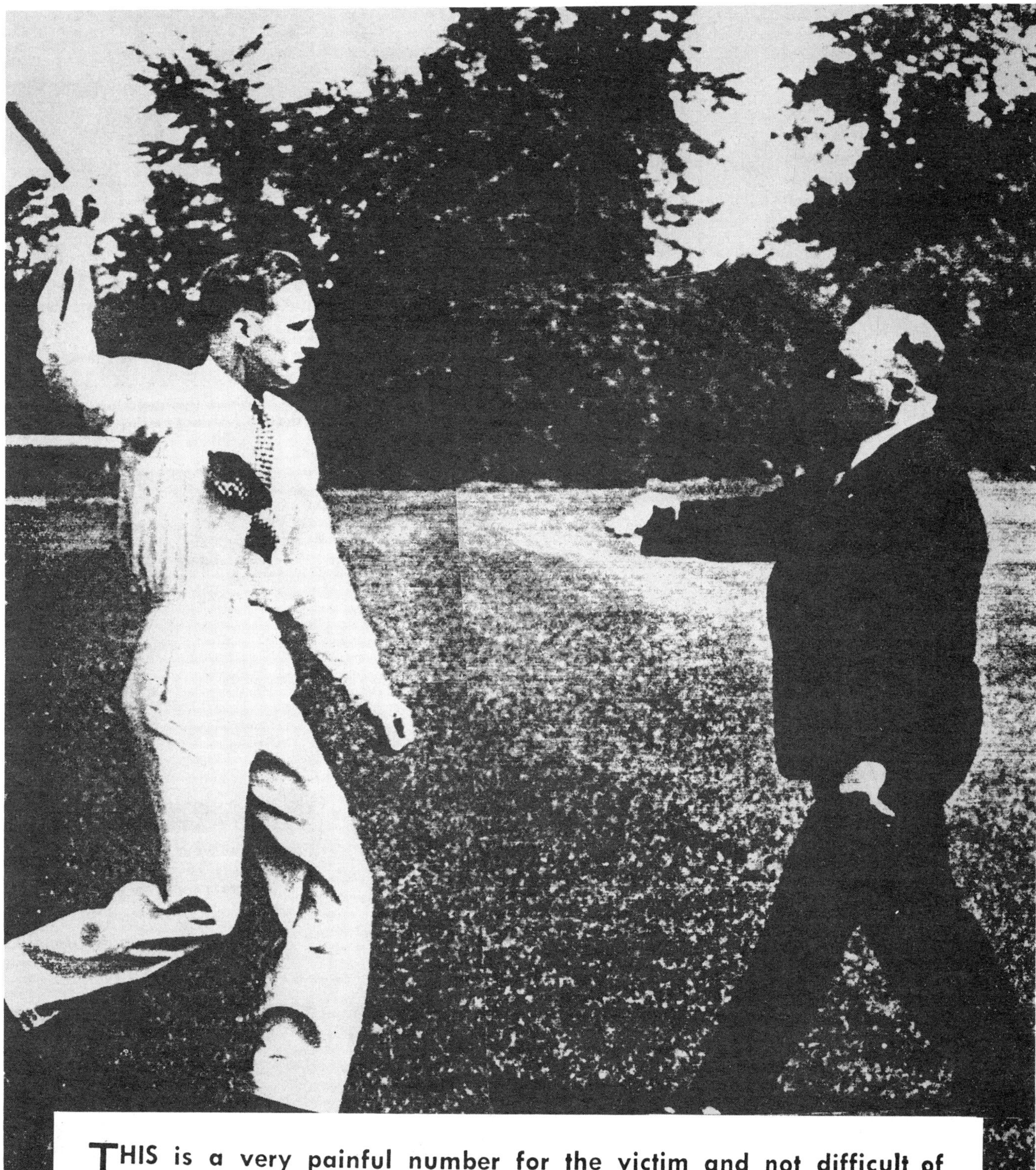

THIS is a very painful number for the victim and not difficult of performance by the operator. I show this defense being used against a person carrying a club but it is equally effective against any other weapon, such as a bottle or knife. Speed and aggressiveness are the important factors and every minute you spend on your Jiu-Jitsu practice helps to make you quicker and more alert. You'll think faster and act faster.

One important way in which Jiu-Jitsu differs from other forms of self defense is that the Jiu-Jitsu expert is anxious for actual close contact with the opponent whereas other defenses endeavor to keep the attacker away.

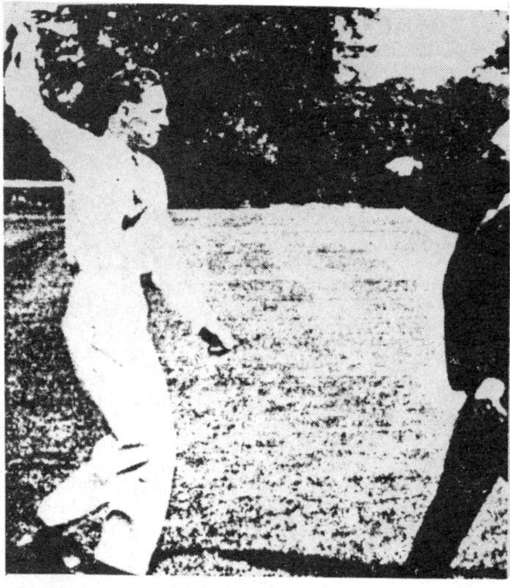

As anyone potentially dangerous to you nears, you must be alert for any type of attack

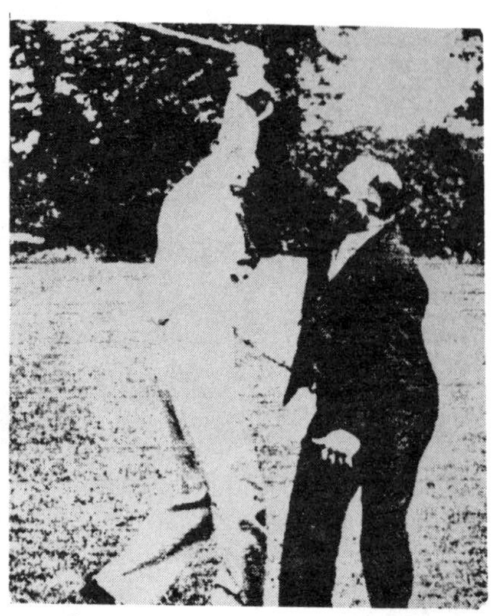

and maintain yourself in such position that you cannot be drawn off balance.

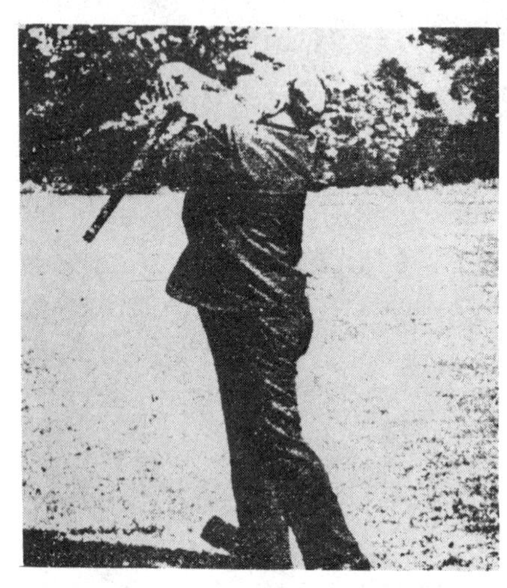

As you blocked the blow your left arm came up under his elbow and then

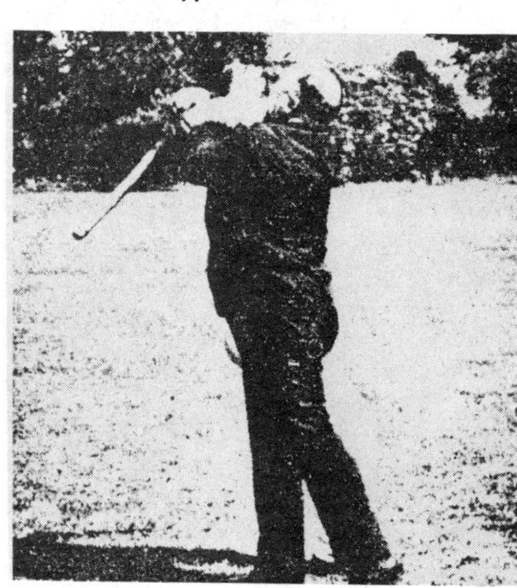

your left forearm goes between the V formed by his arm and your right arm, and your left hand

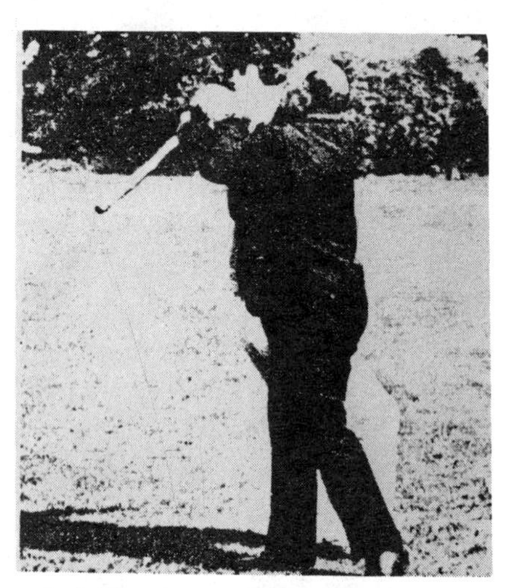

is laid on your right wrist or forearm. This locks your opponent's arm in a very punishing position

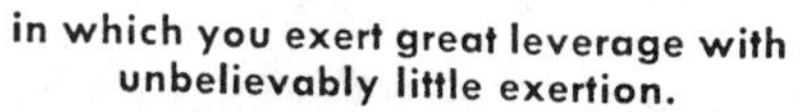

in which you exert great leverage with unbelievably little exertion.

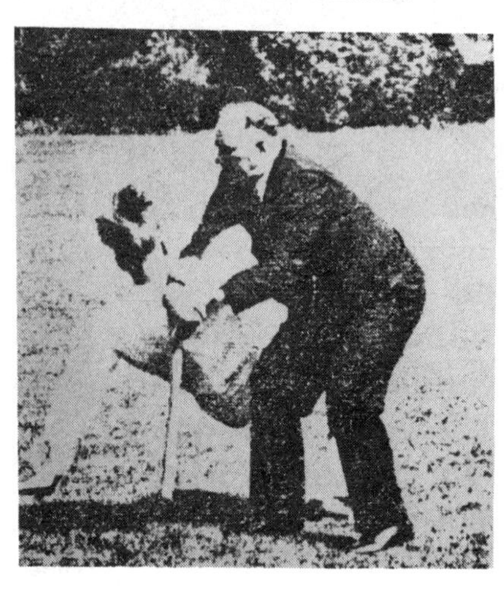

Always maintain your holds as your man falls, for to release him and depend

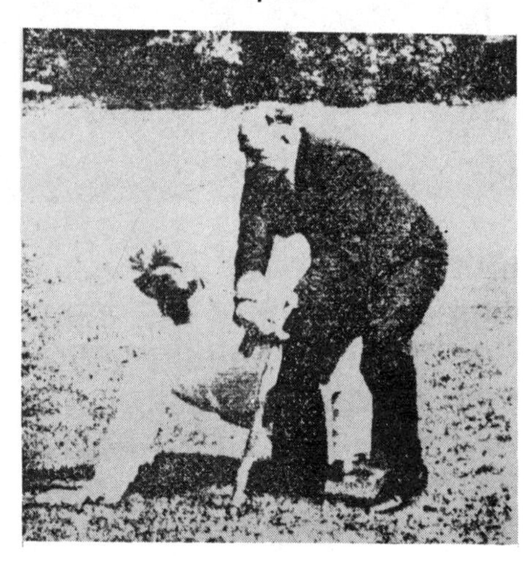

upon the fall alone to incapacitate him is to give up your advantage needlessly.

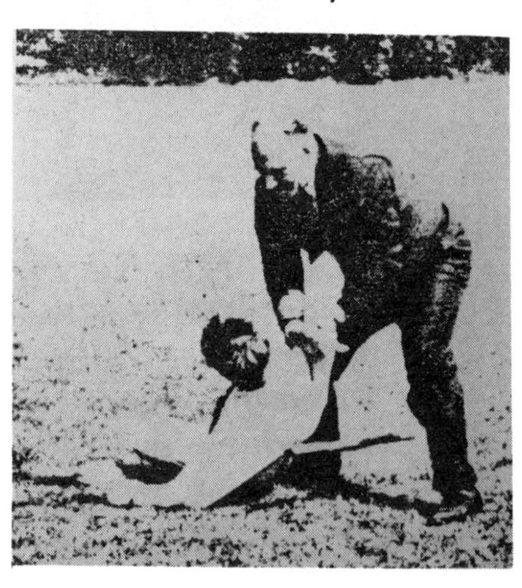

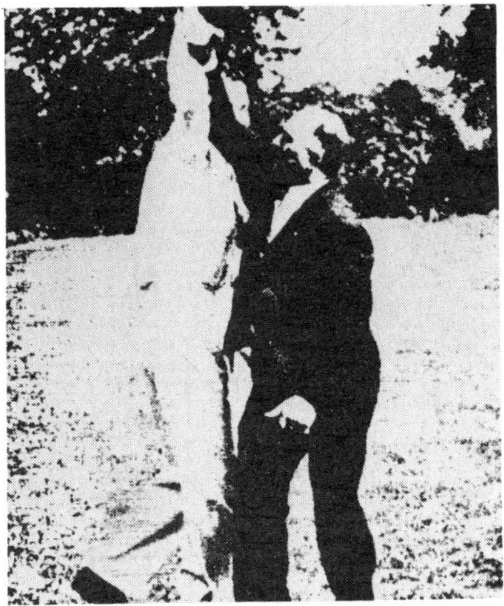

As the weapon is being swung at you your first concern is to block the blow,

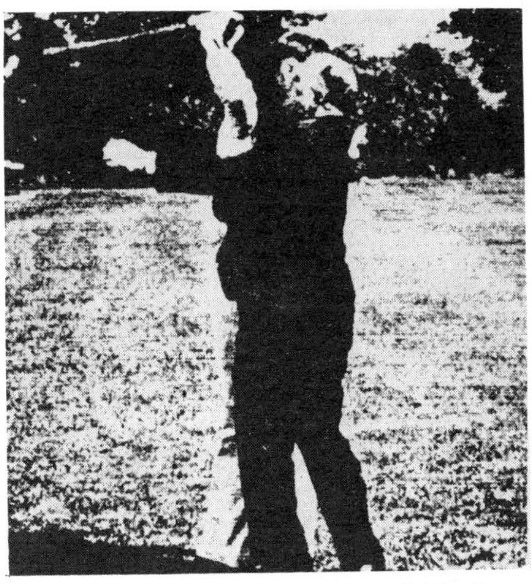

which you do by striking the clubber's forearm with your knife-hand blow.

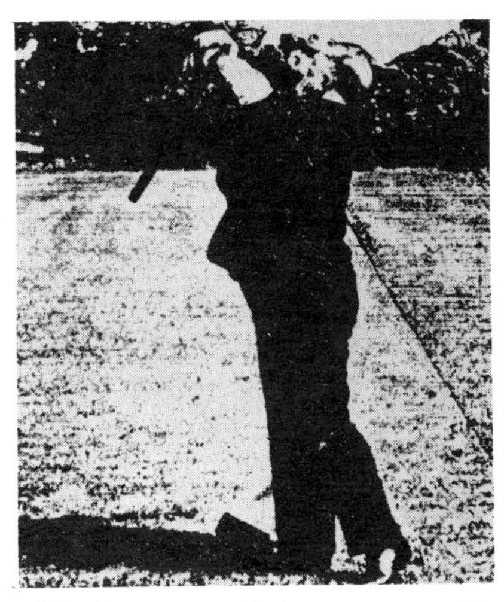

When you are aiming at a specific target such as this keep your eye on the hand or arm, not on his face or elsewhere.

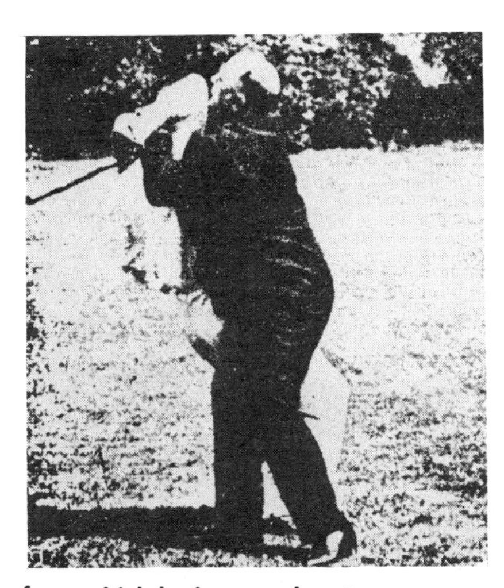

from which he is powerless to escape. Don't bother about the club because he'll drop that himself.

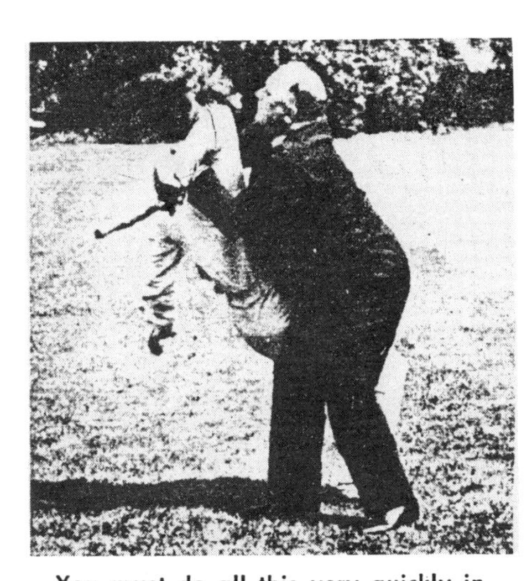

You must do all this very quickly in one fast, smoothly flowing sequence

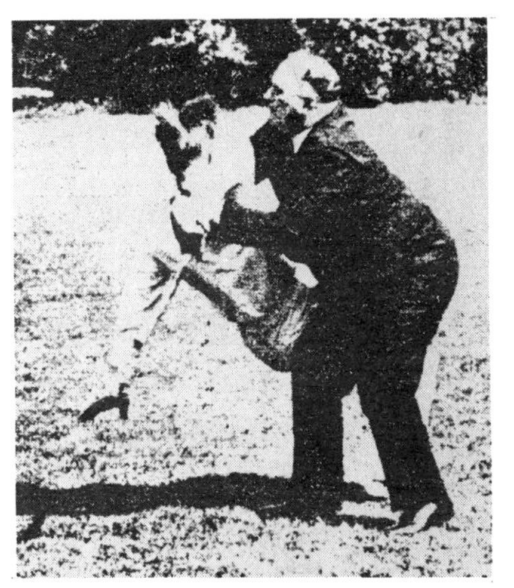

which surprises him, knocks him off balance, and puts his arm in a lock

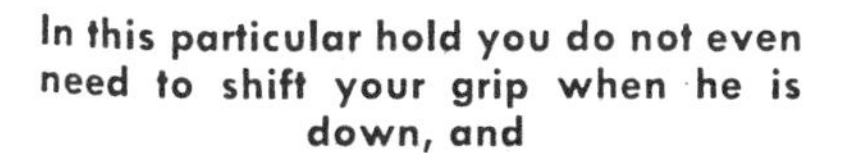

In this particular hold you do not even need to shift your grip when he is down, and

as long as you hold him as shown here he is powerless to make more trouble.

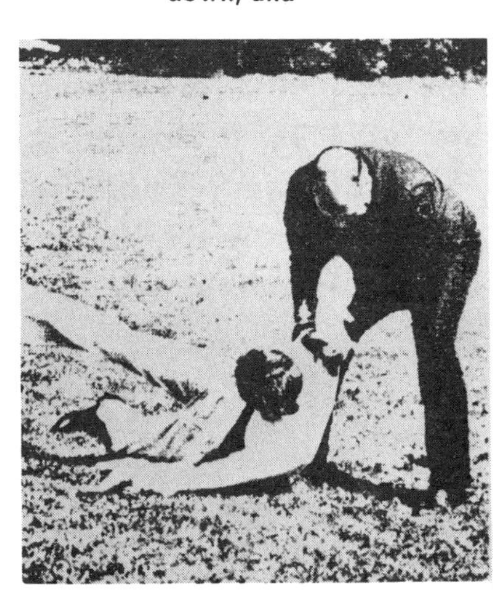

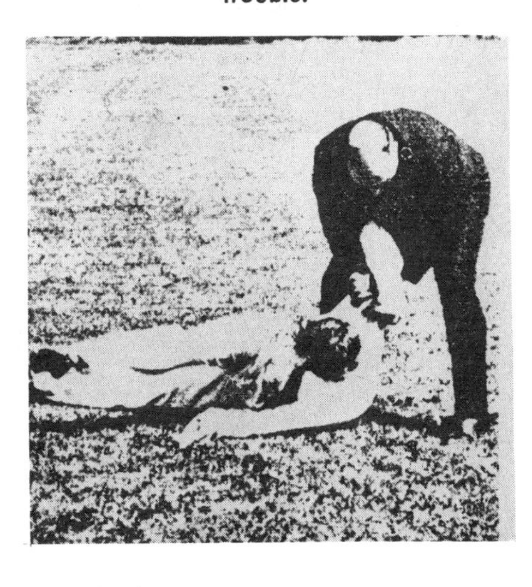

Of course any struggling he did from such a position would only convince him that he was in grave danger of receiving a broken wrist.

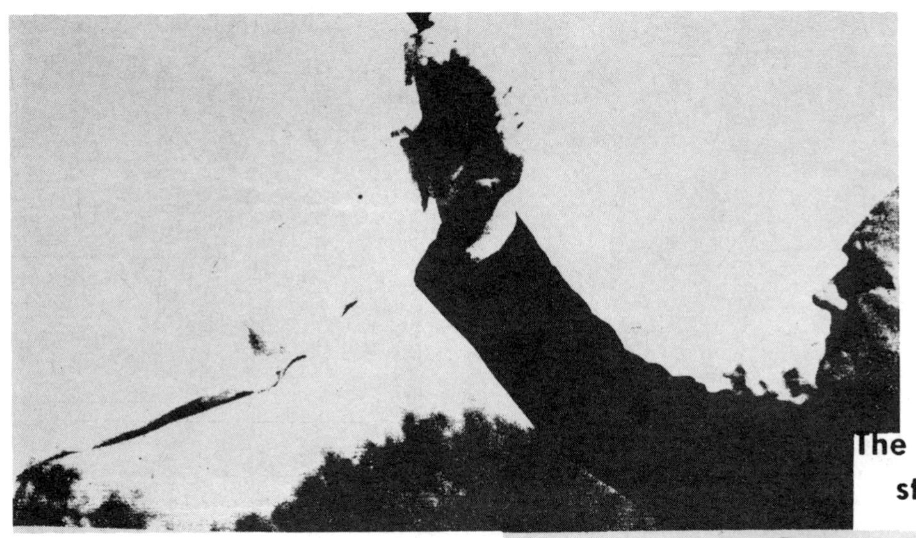

The club hand is blocked in the standard Jiu-Jitsu manner.

Your right hand forces his forearm back. Your left arm goes up through the bend of his arm and your left hand rests on your right wrist.

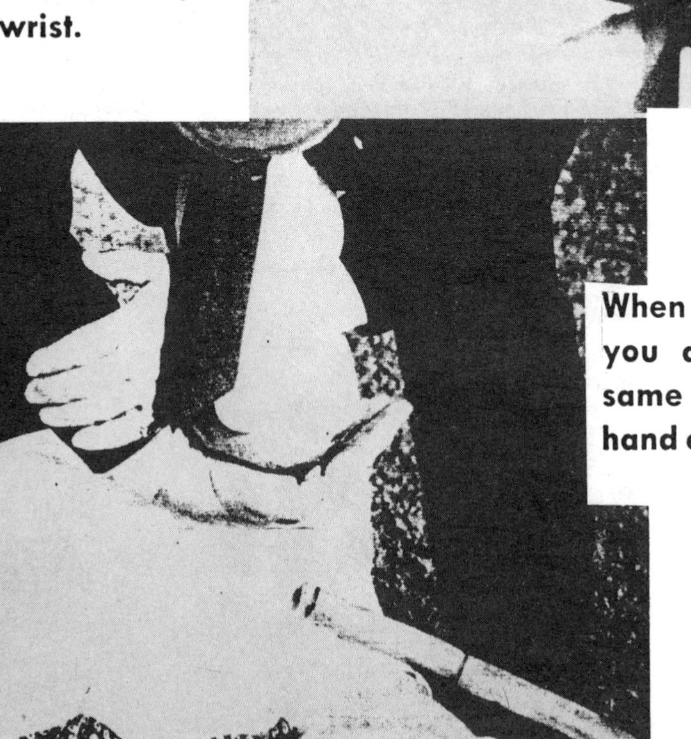

When the clubber is forced down you are able to maintain the same hold on him. Your right hand exerts pressure on the back of the man's hand.

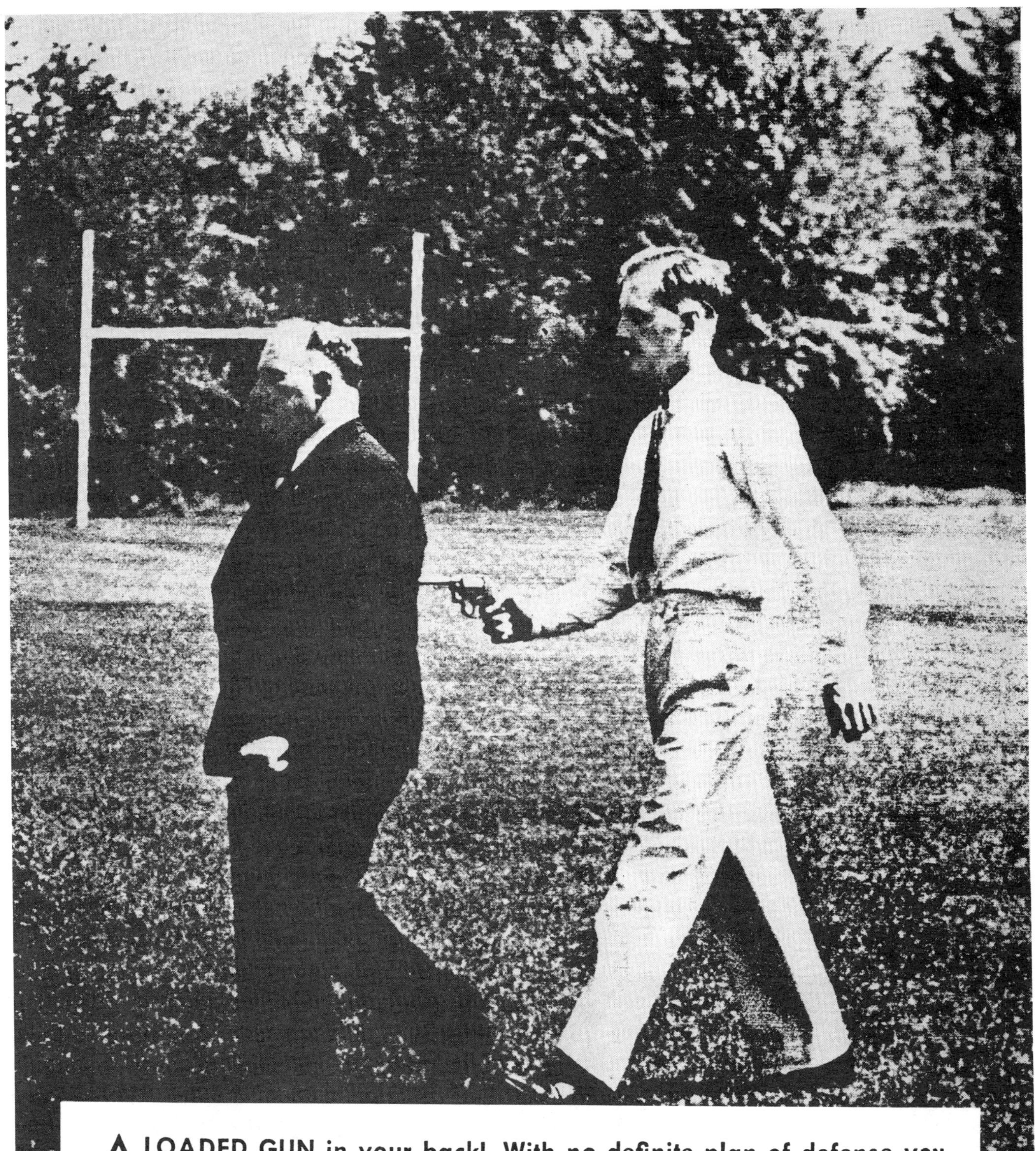

A LOADED GUN in your back! With no definite plan of defense you have no choice other than to surrender meekly and take the consequences. This Jiu-Jitsu number shows you how to avoid being shot and to quickly disarm the gunman. Of course the gun must be in contact with you to enable this defense to succeed. Jiu-Jitsu cannot help you if a person stands six feet away from you and pulls the trigger.

You may never be poked in the back by a gun and told to "stick 'em up" but every day that experience comes to many people. If the gun is right at your back you can capture the gunman as shown here.

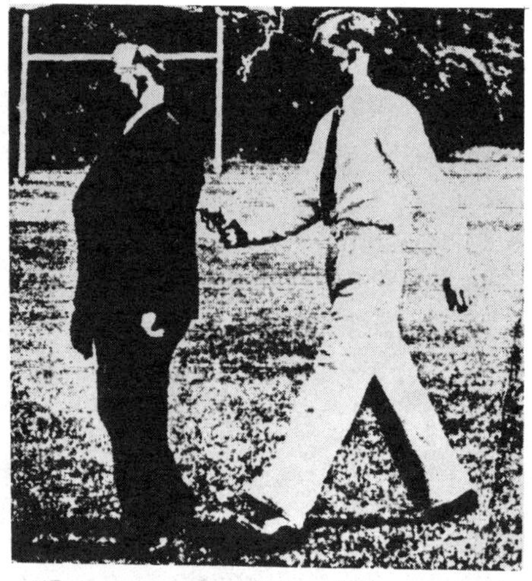

"Put up your hands," calls for action. The man with the gun expects you to do as you are told so that when you say "Yes Sir,"

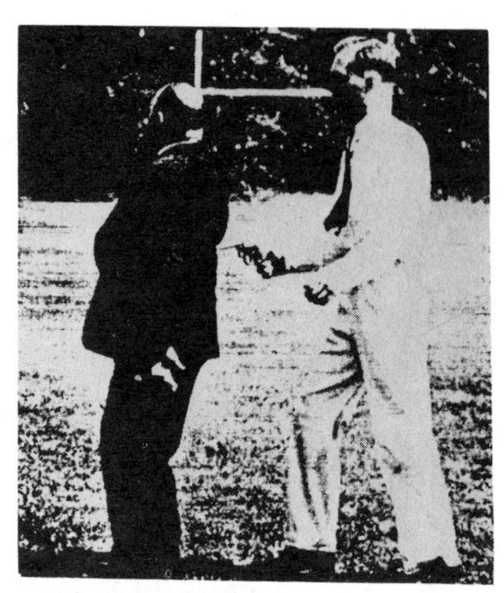

and move, he is not surprised. His surprise, however, is to have you turn, instead of putting your arms up.

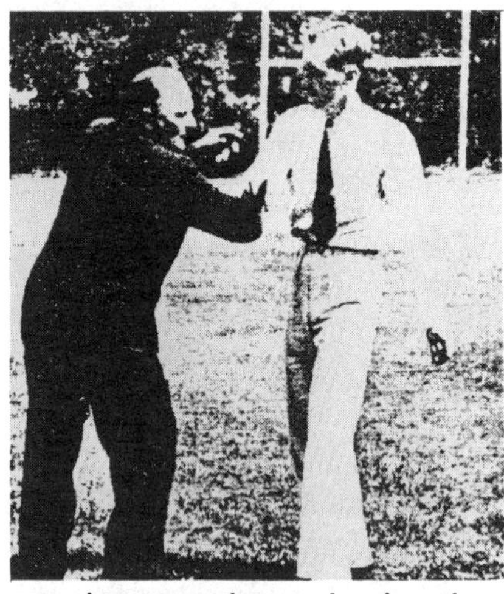

around to grasp the gun hand as the first move to disarm the attacker.

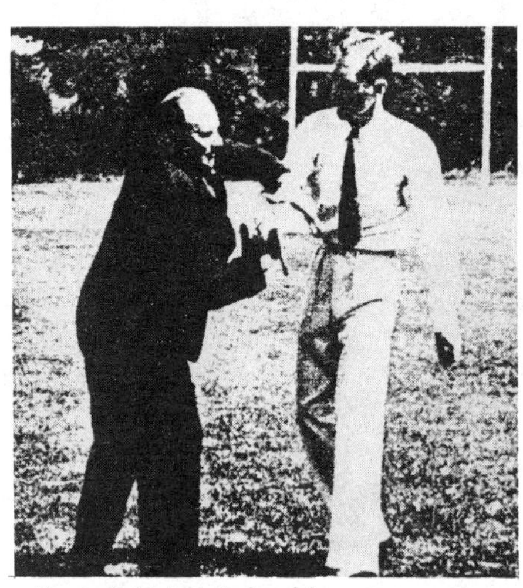

Your right hand should now come up to take the man's wrist as your left hand

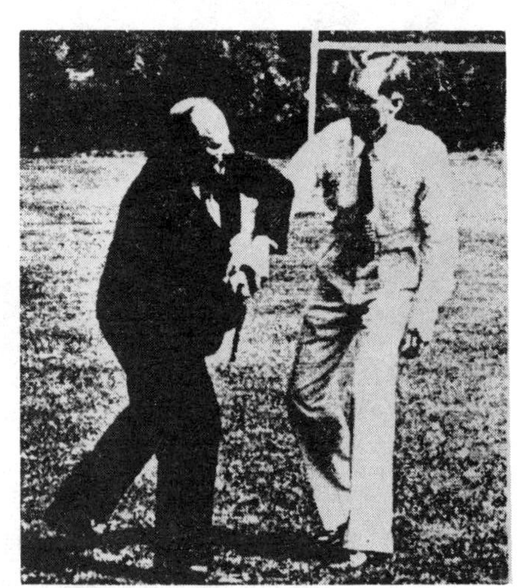

grips his gun hand with your thumb on the back of his hand. Next force

The pressure you have exerted on the back of his hand will have forced his hand open.

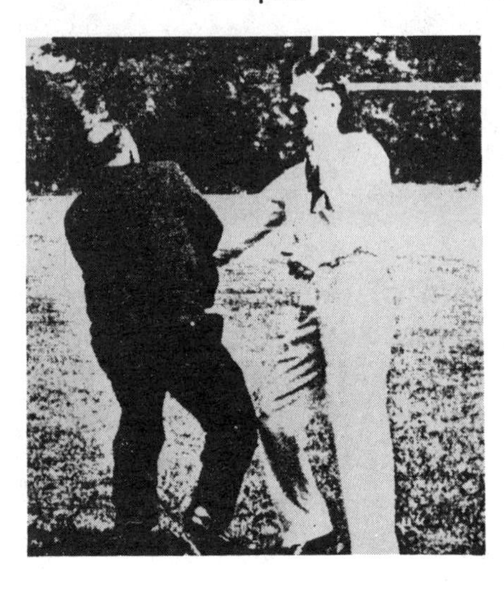

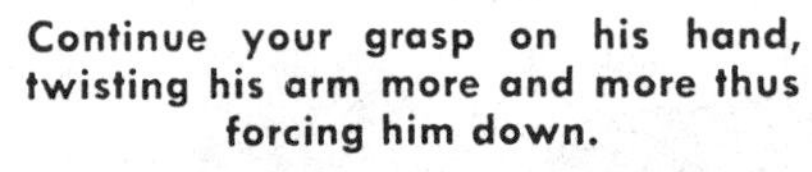

Continue your grasp on his hand, twisting his arm more and more thus forcing him down.

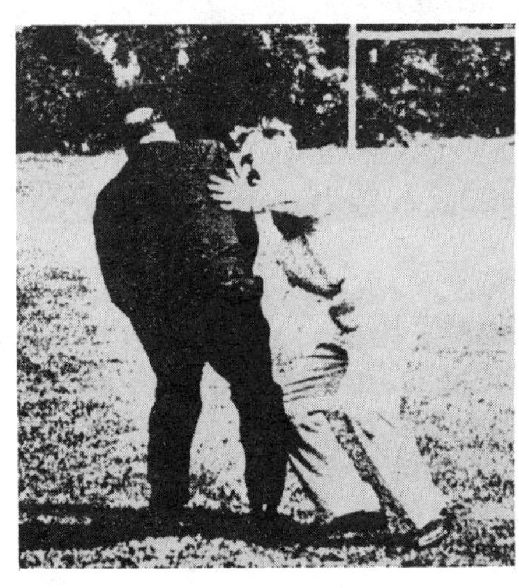

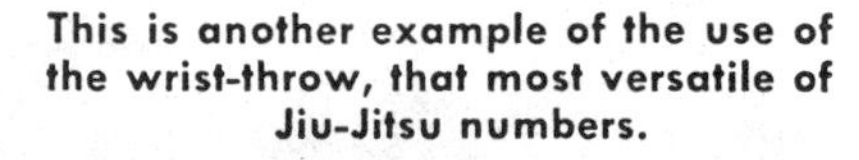

This is another example of the use of the wrist-throw, that most versatile of Jiu-Jitsu numbers.

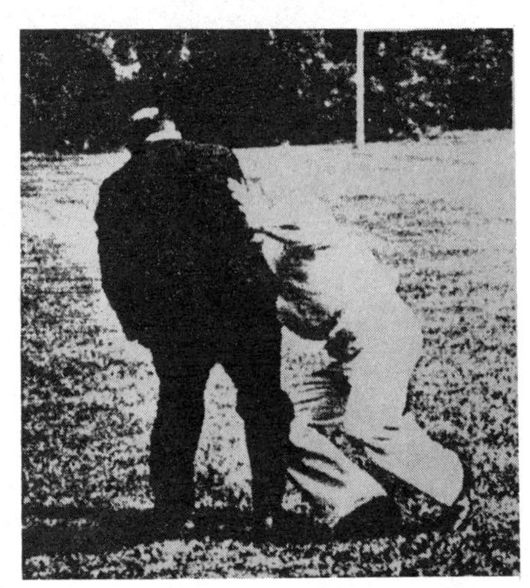

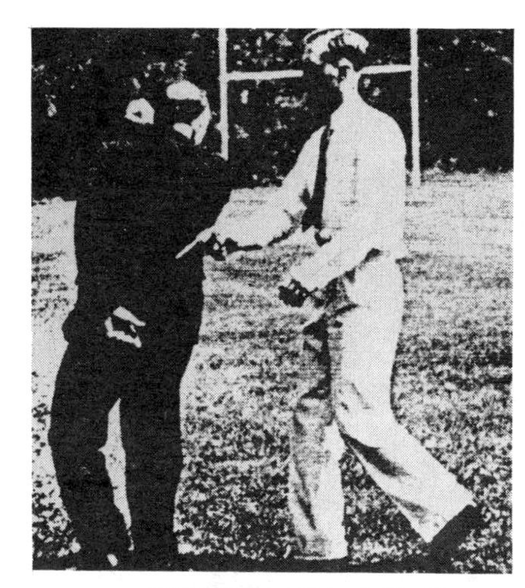

You turn QUICKLY to the right. Even if he should, in this split second, fire his gun you would not be shot

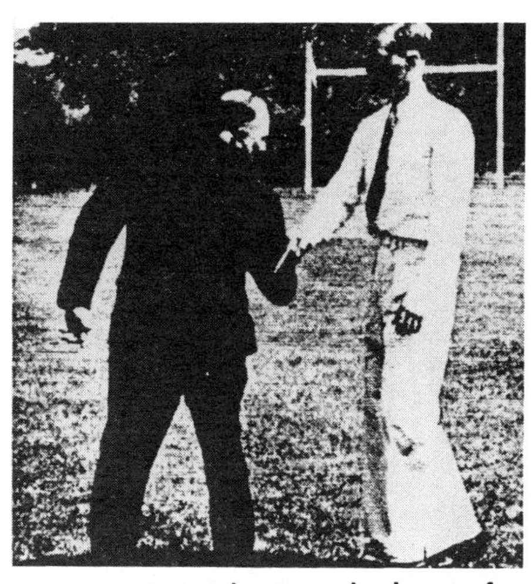

as your turn takes your back out of the possible line of fire. Hit the gun or gun-arm with your right elbow

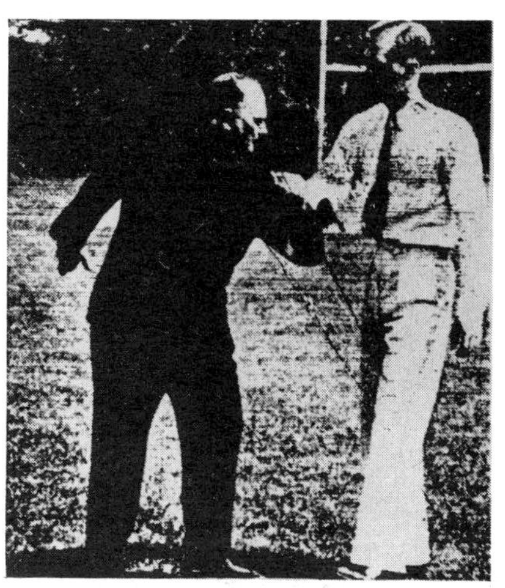

pushing it still further away from a dangerous position. Bring your left hand

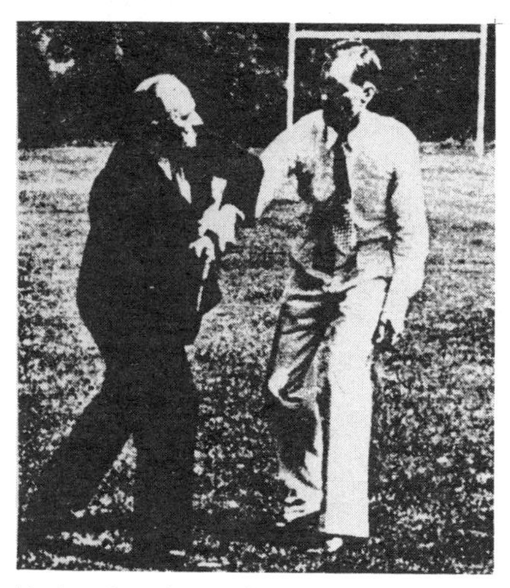

his hand and arm down to get set for a quick, violent upward movement. Now bring his hand up

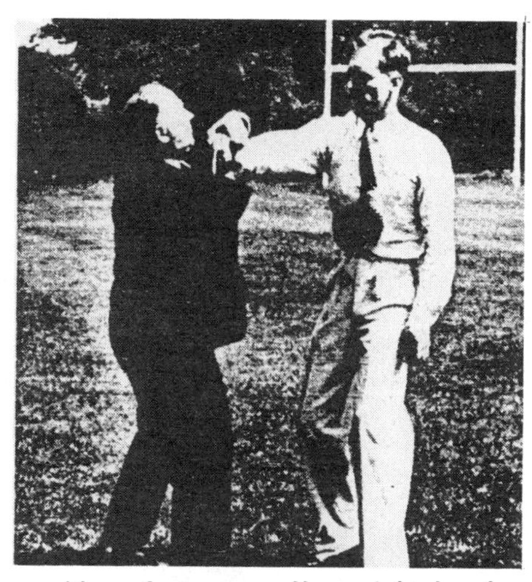

with a fast snap. Your right hand gripping his wrist and your left his hand.

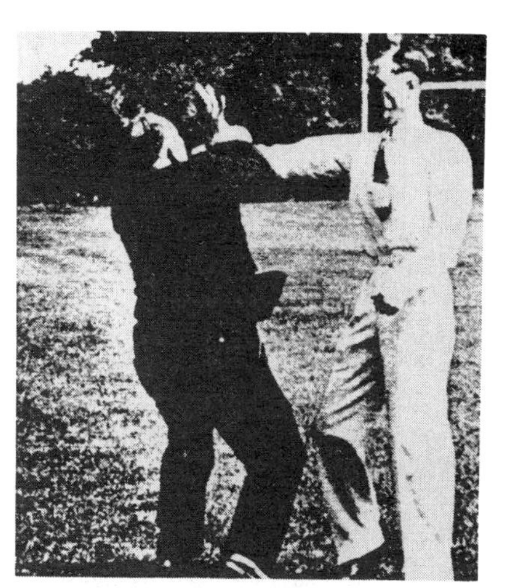

When you reach the top of the swing his hand will open and the gun will be thrown through the air.

The gun has been thrown far away and you have your man on his back on the ground.

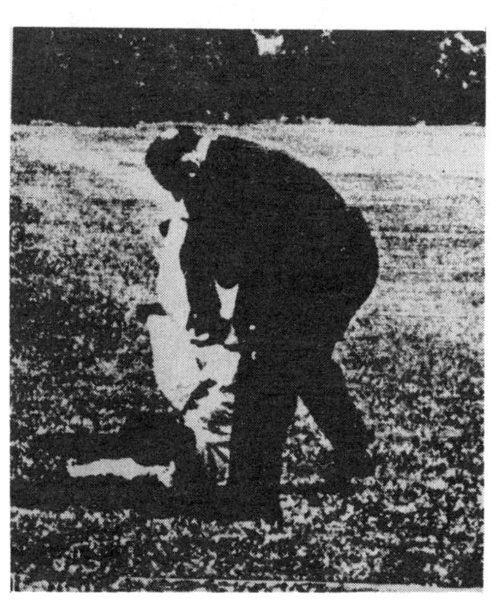

You can easily keep him there by an arm lock such as I have shown you at the finish of the last number or you can use a finger spread as shown here.

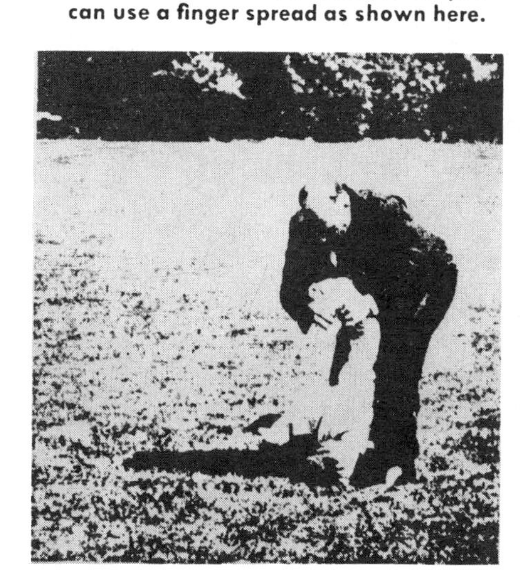

With your left hand grip the victim's fourth and fifth fingers and with your right hand take his first and second fingers then bend his hand far back, and at the same time stretch the fingers apart.

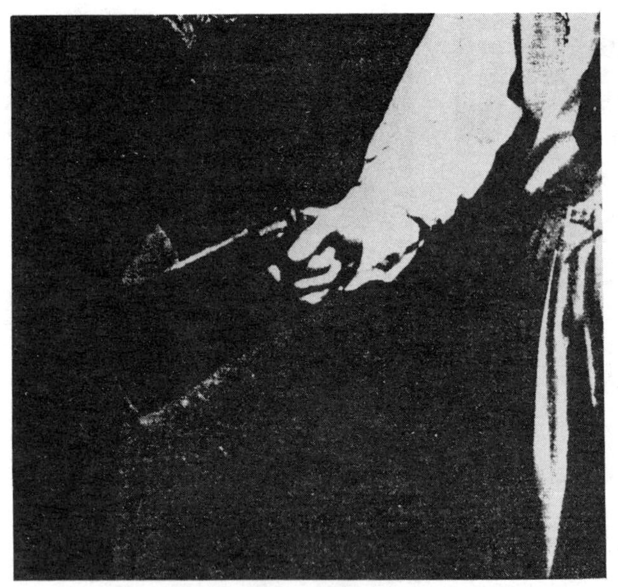

As you turn to face the gunman you swing your right elbow so that it hits the gun, deflecting its aim from your back.

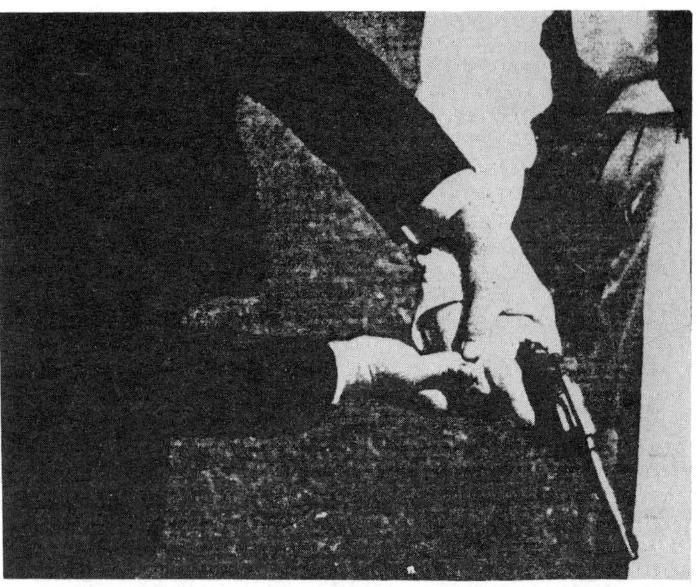

This is a close-up of the proper grip on the man's gun-hand. Notice that it is an adaptation of the wrist throw position so widely used in Jiu-Jitsu.

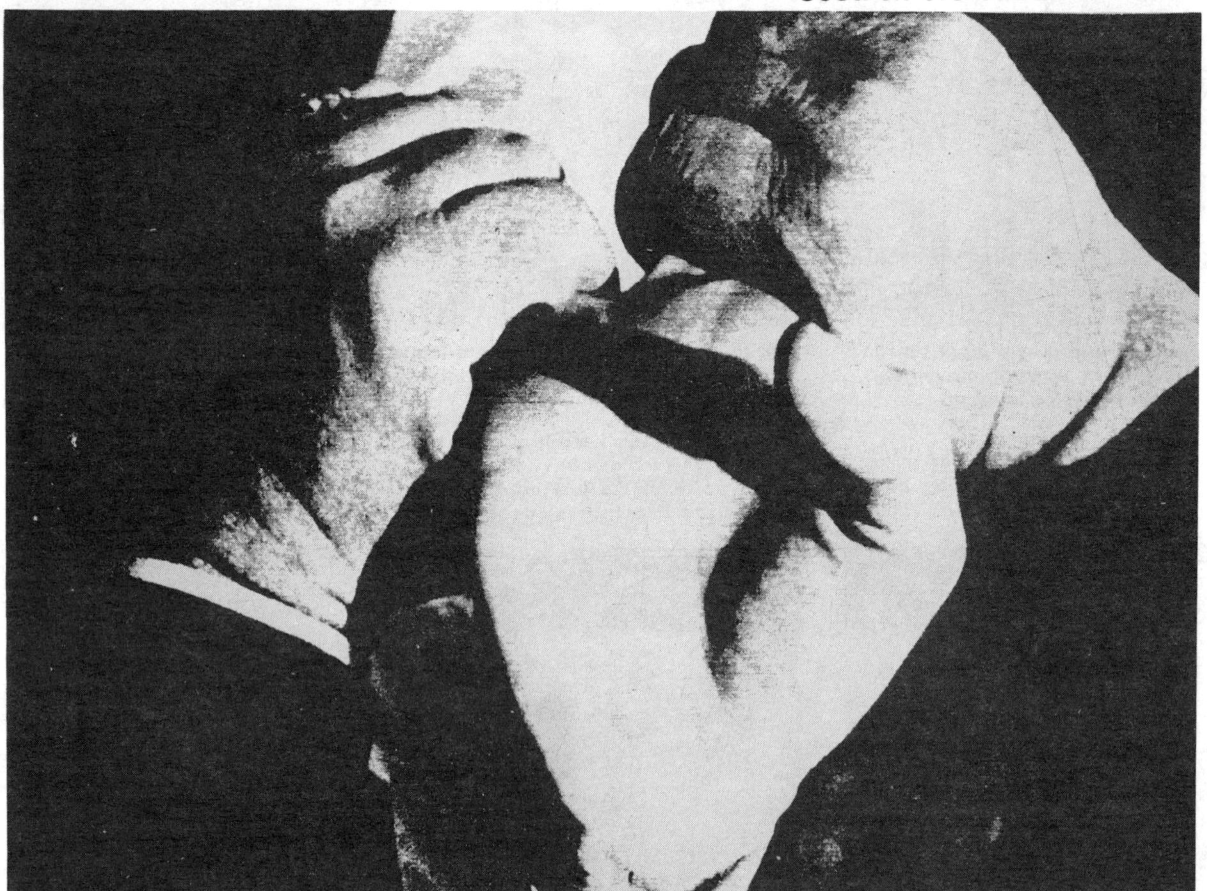

To hold the attacker on the ground you have his hand pointing away from you. Two of his fingers are held by one of your hands and two by the other. Then the fingers are stretched apart.

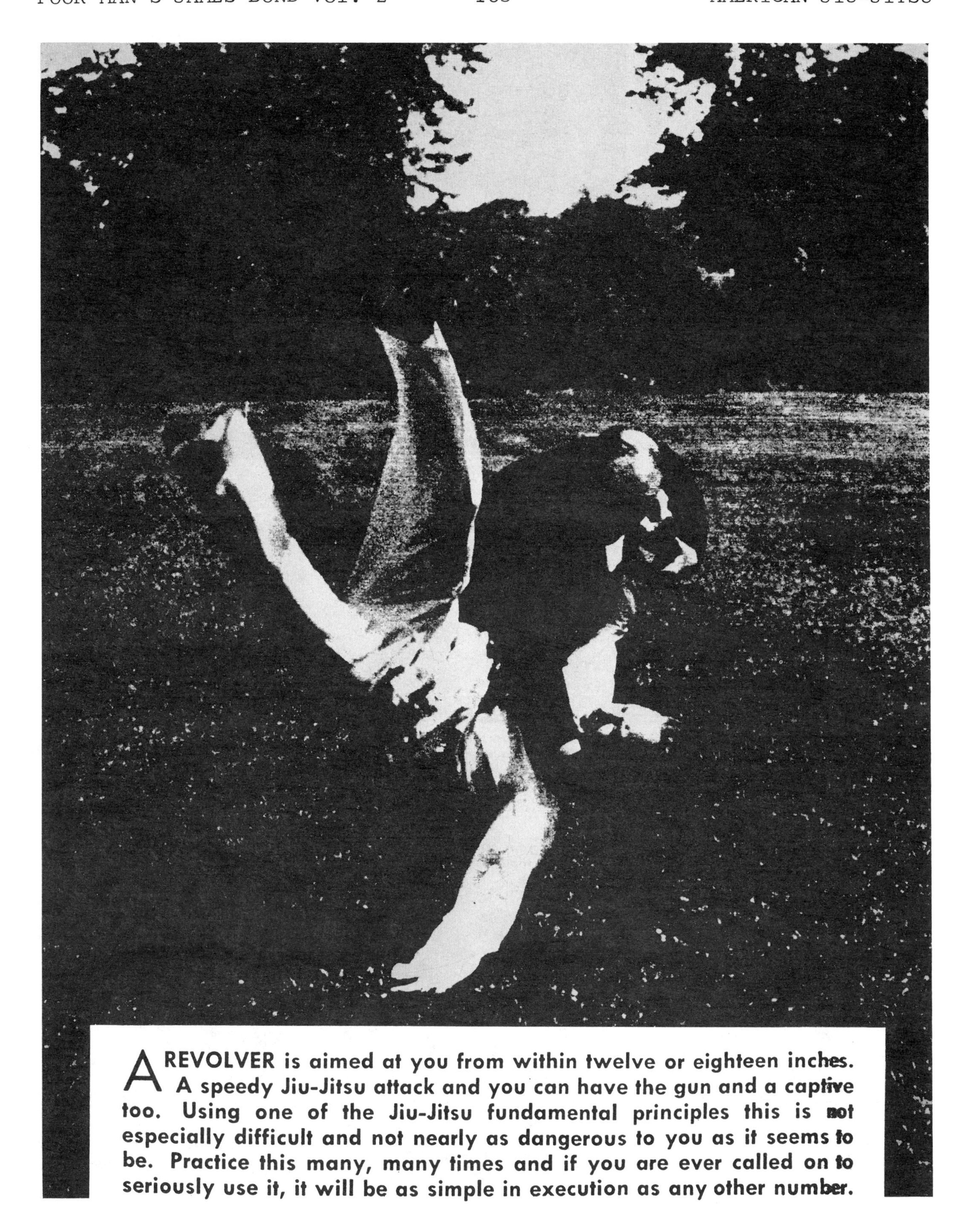

A REVOLVER is aimed at you from within twelve or eighteen inches. A speedy Jiu-Jitsu attack and you can have the gun and a captive too. Using one of the Jiu-Jitsu fundamental principles this is not especially difficult and not nearly as dangerous to you as it seems to be. Practice this many, many times and if you are ever called on to seriously use it, it will be as simple in execution as any other number.

Don't ever attempt to resist a gunman who is standing outside of your easy reach. Eighteen inches is about the outside limit of the possibility of successful application.

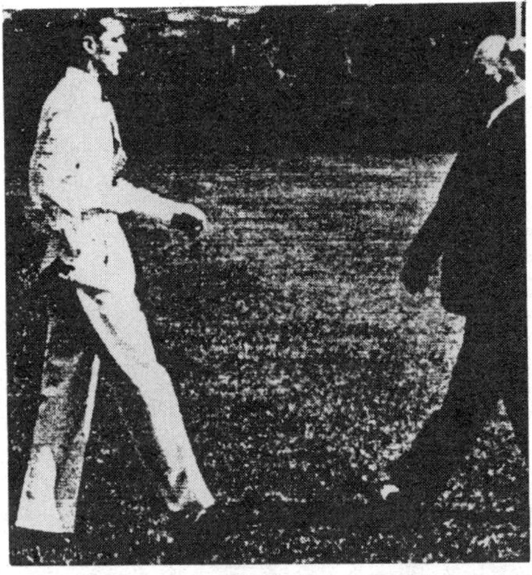

After you have become proficient at Jiu-Jitsu defense it is unlikely that you will ever be caught off your guard.

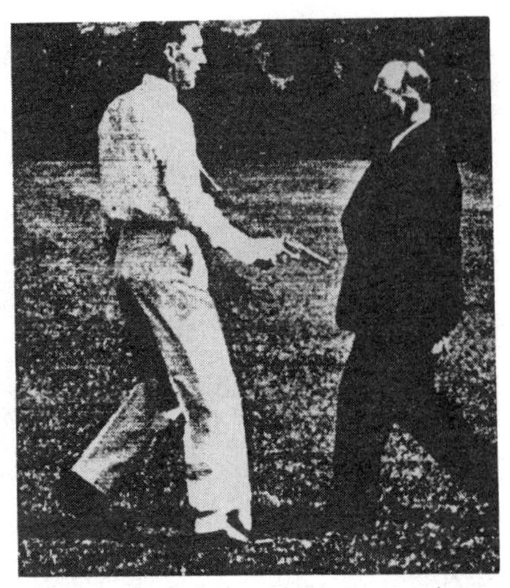

As a revolver is flashed at you with an ugly command to put up your hands

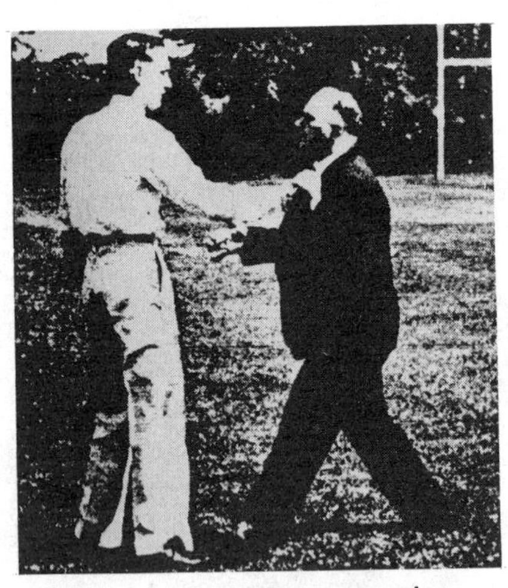

Continue forcing the gun toward your assailant, meanwhile giving him no chance to remove his trigger finger

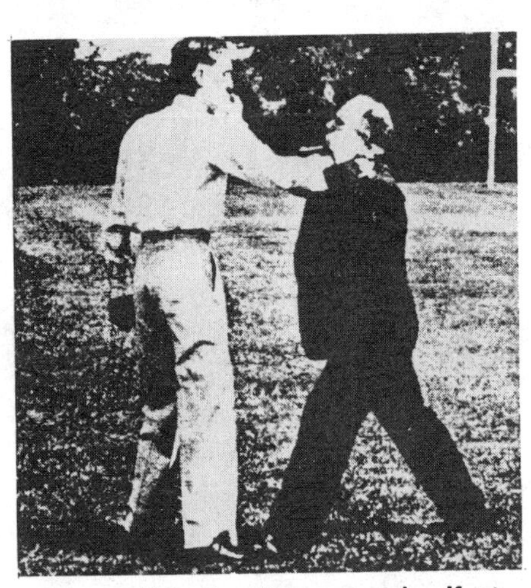

from within the tigger guard. If at this stage the gun should be fired, the gunman himself would be the victim.

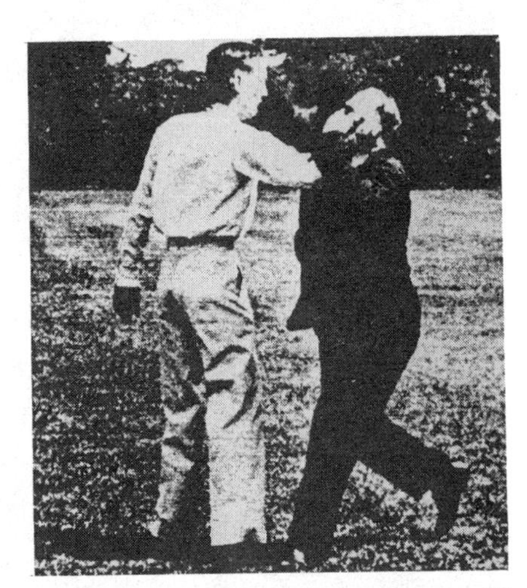

You have stepped forward and with right hand gripped his left shoulder close to his neck. Keep a firm grip on the revolver and with his trigger finger painfully

with your right hand. Lift up suddenly with your right hip and pull him

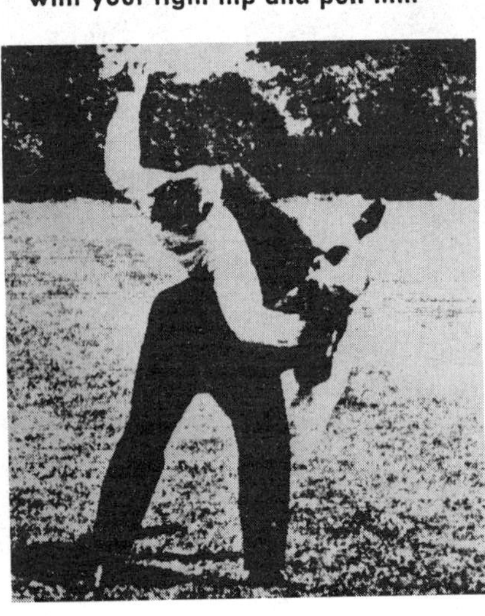

over with your arms. This is easy to do as your hip acts as the fulcrum and

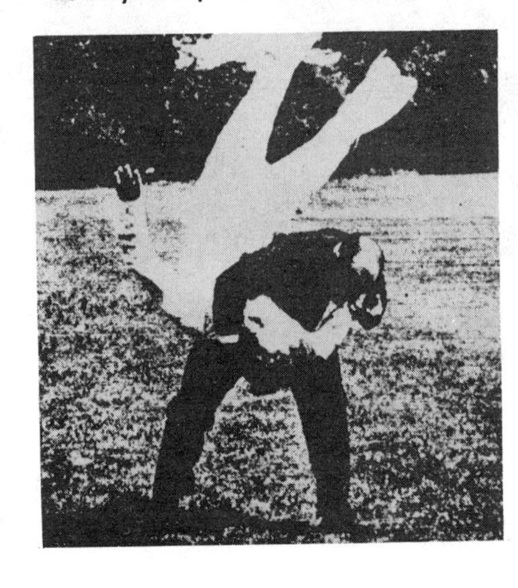

you already have him off balance. When you have him up in the air like this,

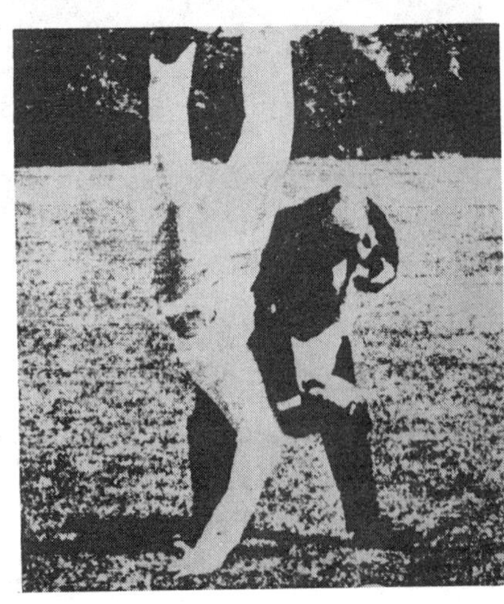

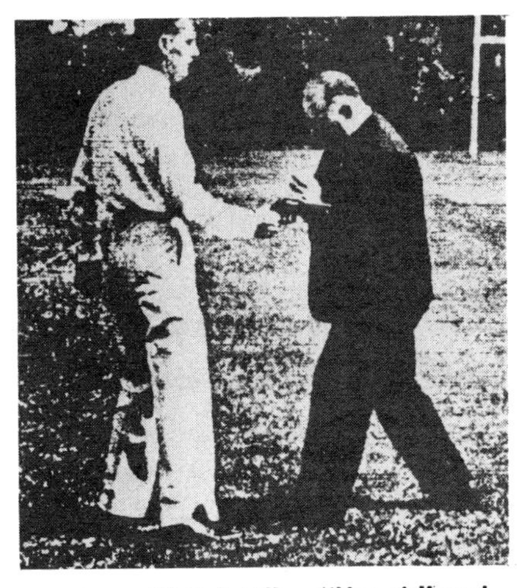

you'll say "All right" or "Yes sir" and start such a motion but as you raise your arms you'll push the barrel of the gun to one side

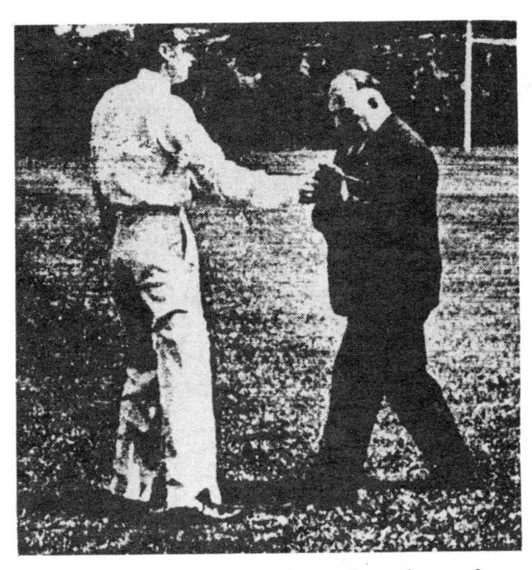

and turn your hand so that the palm of your left hand is against the chamber,

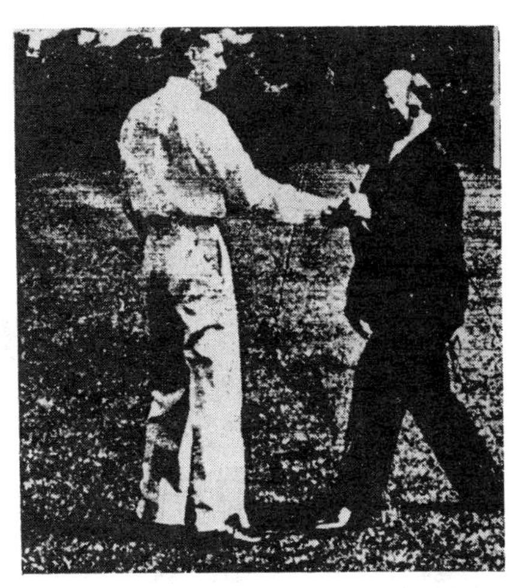

enabling you to close your fingers over it tightly thus preventing the revolver from being fired. As you probably know the chamber must be free to turn, otherwise you cannot pull the trigger of a revolver.

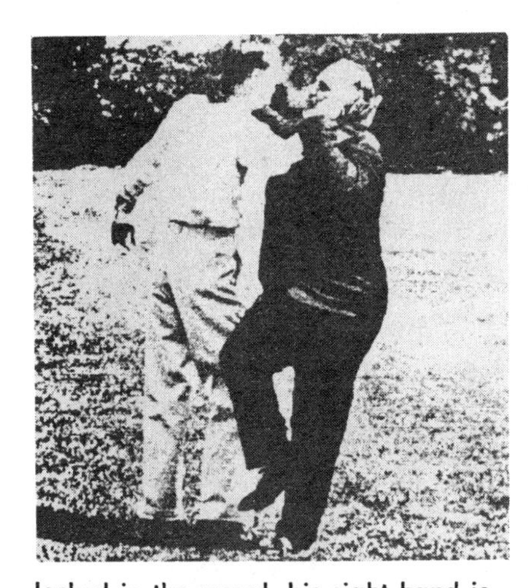

locked in the guard, his right hand is incapable of rendering him any assistance whatever.

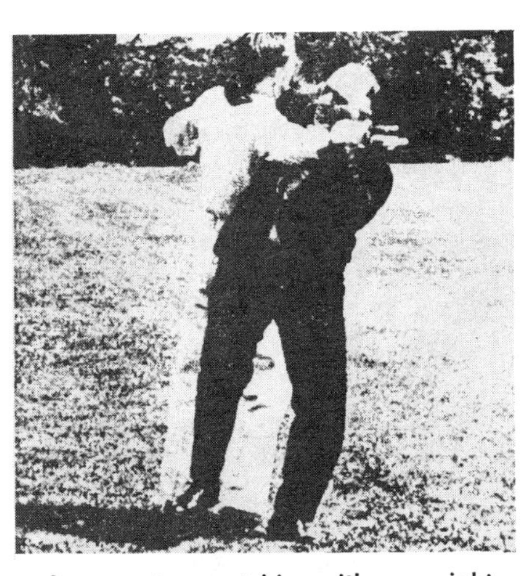

As you step past him with your right leg you prepare to throw him by a hip-throw.

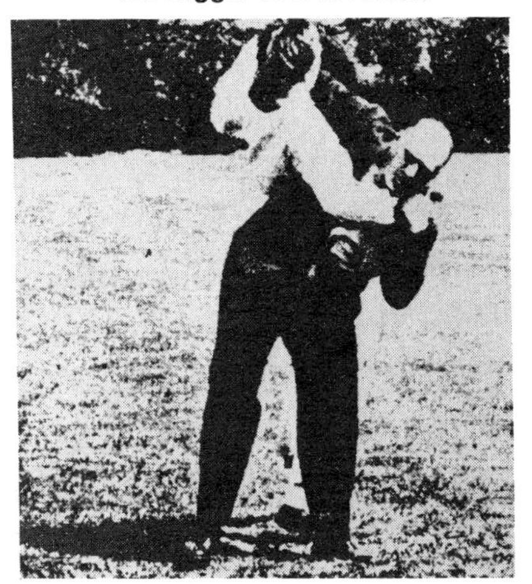

Shift your right hip up and over to the right. Hold his right arm close to you and continue your grip on his left shoulder

exert all your force suddenly to slam him down to the ground.

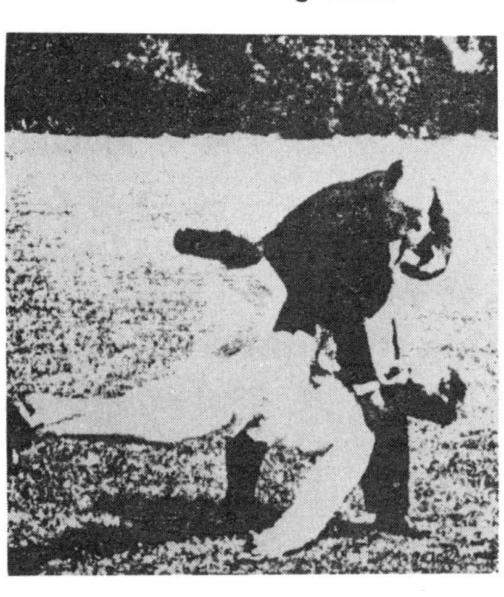

The impact of the hard fall and the fact that you continue to hold his finger in the trigger guard combine to keep him under control.

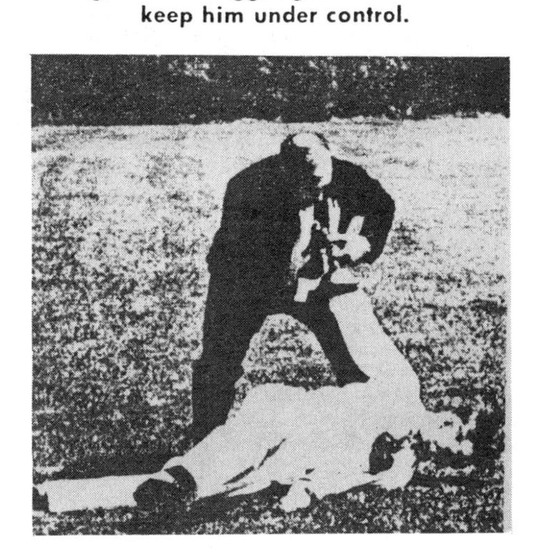

You can easily take the revolver away from him and then hold him by bending his arm backward, with the back of his elbow against your knee.

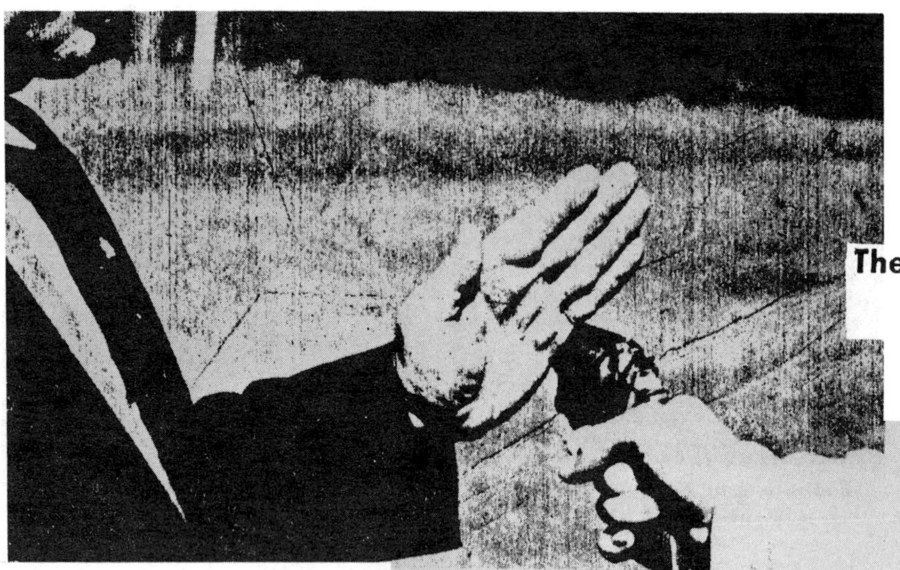

The gun is struck by the left hand and turned away.

The muzzle is forced around until it points at the gunman himself. His finger is imprisoned in the trigger guard.

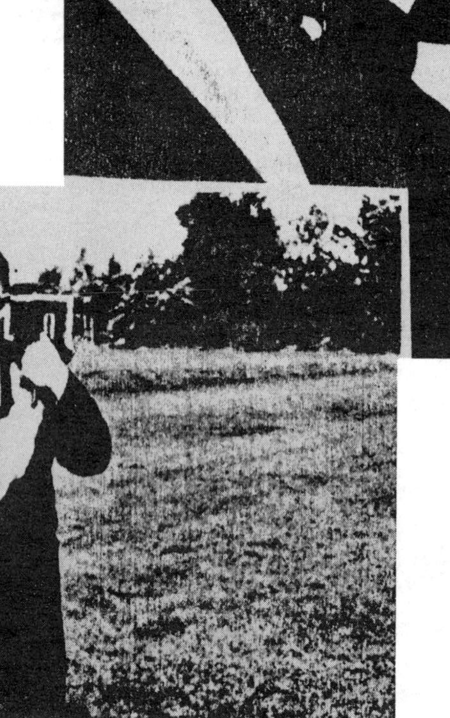

This shows the proper position used in completing the capture by using the hip-throw.

CHEMICALS IN WAR

A Treatise on Chemical Warfare

McGRAW-HILL BOOK COMPANY, Inc.
NEW YORK AND LONDON
1937

BY

AUGUSTIN M. PRENTISS, Ph.D.

Brigadier General, Chemical Warfare Service
United States Army

ABOUT THIS BOOK

This book is complete except for irrelevant chapters such as: Relation of Chemical Industry to Chemical Warfare, International Situation, Chemical Technique and Tactics of Cavalry, Military Organization for Chemical Combat, Chemical Techniques and Tactics of Air Corps, etc.

Also left out was the extensive bibliography and hundreds of footnotes referring to books long out of print and generally unobtainable. For the most part, their subject matter concerned the historical record of the use of toxic substances in World War One and would have been of no use nor of any interest to one contemplating the making and use of chemical warfare substances in our time.

ABOUT TABLE IV.—PROPERTIES OF CHEMICAL AGENTS

The original chart was a large foldout of 14 by 28 inches. This was impractical to reproduce in the present format. However, the 25 substances and their characteristics have have been reproduced on the following six pages. For ease in following the chart, the substances have been numbered. To follow the chart, simply pick the substance of interest and follow its number across the chart, page by page.

PREFACE

The three outstanding developments of the World War were the military airplane, the combat tank, and chemical warfare. Each of these new instruments of war made its appearance on the battlefield at about the same time, each exerted an important influence in shaping the character of modern combat, and each is destined to play an even greater role in future warfare.

Since the World War, all nations have actively pushed the development of these new arms and much has been written concerning the first two—military aviation and mechanization—both in this country and abroad. But, for reasons not altogether clear, the literature of chemical warfare has not kept pace with its development since the war, although much has been done during the past few years in the principal countries of Europe to supply this deficiency. The dearth of publications on chemical warfare in this country is truly remarkable, considering the position of the United States among the industrial nations of the world, and particularly in view of the phenomenal growth of its chemical industry during the past fifteen years.

With the exception of one book by General Fries and Dr. West, which appeared in 1921 and was largely a narrative account of the Chemical Warfare Service in the World War, and one or two books concerning certain phases of gas warfare, no authoritative texts on chemical warfare have appeared in this country, despite the European literary activity in this field in the past few years.

There is perhaps no military subject that is so little understood and so much misrepresented as chemical warfare. During the late war it suffered much vilification and abuse which was not only wholly without

Continued on page 176

Table IV. PROPERTIES OF CHEMICAL AGENTS (See also page 174)

Agent, common name	Chemical name	CWS. symbol	Physiological classification	Tactical classification	Persistency (summer)	Persistency (winter)	Lowest irritant concentration, mg. per liter or oz. per 1,000 cu. ft., 10 min. exposure
Bromacetone (1)	Bromacetone (CH_3COCH_2Br)	BA	Lacrimator	Harrassing agent	1 to 2 hr. in open; 3 hr. in woods	2 days in open; 7 days in woods	0.0015
Brombenzyl cyanide (French: Camite) (2)	Brombenzyl cyanide ($C_6H_5CHBrCN$)	CA	Lacrimator	Harrassing agent	3 days in open; 7 days in woods	Several weeks	0.00015
Chloracetophenone (3)	Phenyl chlormethyl ketone ($C_6H_5COCH_2Cl$)	CN	Lacrimator	Harrassing agent	Solid for days; burning mixture, 10 min.	Several weeks in solid; burning mixture 10 min.	0.0003
Chlorine (4)	Chlorine (Cl_2)	Cl	Lung injurant	Casualty agent	5 min. in open; 20 min. in woods	10 min. in open; 1 hr. in woods	0.029
Phosgene (5)	Carbonyl chloride ($COCl_2$)	CG	Lung injurant	Casualty agent	10 min. in open; 3 min. in woods	20 min. in open; 2 hr. in woods	0.005
Diphosgene (German: Perstoff) (French: Surpolite) (6)	Trichlormethylchloroformate (diphosgene) ($ClCOOCCl_3$)	German Green Cross	Lung injurant	Casualty agent	15 min. in open; 60 min. in woods	30 min. in open; 3 hr. in woods	0.005
Chlorpicrin (vomiting gas) (7)	Trichlornitromethane (Cl_3CNO_2)	PS	Lung injurant and lacrimator	Casualty agent and harrassing agent	1 hr. in open; 4 hr. in woods	12 hr. in open; week in woods	0.009
Ethyldichlorarsine (German: Dick) (8)	Ethyldichlorarsine ($C_2H_5AsCl_2$)	ED	Lung injurant, sternutator, and vesicant	Casualty agent and harrassing agent	1 to 2 hr. in open; 2 to 6 hr. in woods	2 to 4 hr. in open; 12 hr. in woods	0.001
Hydrocyanic acid (9)	Hydrocyanic acid (HCN)	French 4	Systemic toxic	Casualty agent	5 min. in open; 10 min. in woods	10 min. in open; 1 hr. in woods	0.020
Cyanogen chloride (10)	Cyanogen chloride (CNCl)	French 4B	Systemic toxic	Casualty agent	10 min. in open; 20 min. in woods	20 min. in open; 2 hr. in woods	0.0025
Mustard (11)	ββ' Dichlorethyl sulfide ($(ClCH_2CH_2)_2S$)	HS	Vesicant	Casualty agent	24 hr. in open; 1 week in woods	Several weeks both in open and in woods	0.001
Lewisite (12)	β Chlorvinyldichlorarsine ($ClCH{:}CHAsCl_2$)	M-1	Vesicant	Casualty agent	24 hr. in open; 1 week in woods	1 week	0.0008
Methyldichlorarsine (German: Methyldick) (13)	(CH_3AsCl_2)	MD	Vesicant and lung irritant	Casualty agent	1 hr.	2 to 3 hr.	0.002
Diphenylchlorarsine (German: Clark I) (14)	Diphenylchlorarsine ($(C_6H_5)_2AsCl$)	DA	Respiratory irritant (sternutator)	Harrassing agent	5 min. by H.E. detonation; 10 min. by candle dissemination	Same as summer	0.0005
Diphenylcyanarsine (German: Clark II) 15	Diphenylcyanarsine ($(C_6H_5)_2AsCN$)	CDA	Respiratory irritant (sternutator)	Harrassing agent	Same as DA	Same as DA	0.0001
Adamsite (16)	Diphenylaminechlorarsine ($(C_6H_4)_2NHAsCl$)	DM	Respiratory irritant (sternutator)	Harrassing agent	10 min. in open from candles	10 min. in open from candles	0.00038
Crude oil (17)	Mixture of paraffin hydrocarbons	CO	None	Screening agent	While source is operating plus 5 min.	Same as summer	None
White phosphorus (18)	White phosphorus (P_4), yellow phosphorus	WP	None	Screening agent and incendiary agent	Depends upon size of burning particle; usually 10 min. or less in open	Same as summer	Smoke irritation negligible

Intolerable concentration, mg. per liter or oz. per 1,000 cu. ft., 10 min. exposure	Lethal concentration, mg. per liter or oz. per 1,000 cu. ft., 10 min. exposure	Melting point	Boiling point	Volatility, 20°C. (68°F.)	Vapor pressure, 20°C. (68°F.)	Vapor density compared to air	Density of solid, 20°C. (68°F.)	Solvents for
0.010 (1)	3.20	−54°C. (−65°F.)	135°C. (275°F.)	75 oz. 1,000 cu. ft. air	9 mm. Hg	4.7	1.60	Fats and organic solvents
10 min. exposure, 0.0008 (2)	30 min. exposure, 0.9; 10 min. exposure, 3.5	25°C. (77°F.)	225°C. (437°F.)	0.13 oz. 1,000 cu. ft. air	0.0112 mm. Hg	6.6	1.47	Chlorbenzene, chloroform, PS, CG
10 min. exposure, 0.0045 (3)	30 min. exposure, 0.34; 10 min. exposure, 0.85	59°C. (138°F.)	247°C. (476°F.)	0.106 oz. 1,000 cu. ft. air	0.013 mm. Hg	5.2	1.30	Chloroform, PS, ethylenedichloride, monochloracetone
10 min. exposure, 0.10 (4)	30 min. exposure, 2.53; 10 min. exposure, 5.60	−102°C. −(152.5°F.)	−33.6°C. (−28.5°F.)	19,369 oz. 1,000 cu. ft. air*	4,993 mm. Hg	2.5	1.46	CG, PS, CCl_4
10 min. exposure, 0.020 (5)	30 min. exposure, 0.36; 10 min. exposure, 0.50	−118°C. (−190°F.)	8.2°C. (46.7°F.)	6,370 oz. 1,000 cu. ft. air†	1,180 mm. Hg	3.5	1.38	Cl and PS
10 min. exposure, 0.40 (6)	30 min. exposure, 0.36; 10 min. exposure, 0.50 (U.S.); 0.05 (Germany)	−57°C.	127°C. (260.6°F.)	120 oz. 1,000 cu. ft. air	10.3 mm. Hg	6.9	1.65	CG, PS, DA
10 min. exposure, 0.050 (7)	30 min. exposure, 0.80; 10 min. exposure, 2.00	−69.2°C. (−92.4°F.)	112°C. (231.5°F.)	165 oz. 1,000 cu. ft. air	18.3 mm. Hg	5.6	1.66	Chloroform, CG, chlorine, CS_2, C_6H_6 C_2H_5OH
10 min. exposure, 0.01 (causes sneezing) (8)	30 min. exposure, 0.10; 10 min. exposure, 0.50	−30°C. (−22°F.)	156°C. (312°F.)	100 oz. 1,000 cu. ft. air	5.0 mm. Hg	6.5	1.70	Ethyl chloride
10 min. exposure, 0.030 (9)	30 min. exposure, 0.150; 10 min. exposure, 0.200	−15°C. (5°F.)	26°C. (79°F.)	873 oz. 1,000 cu. ft. air	603 mm. Hg	0.93	0.75	$ASCl_3$, $SbCO_2$
10 min. exposure, 0.005 (10)	30 min. exposure, 0,120; 10 min. exposure, 0.40	−6°C. (21°F.)	15°C. (59°F.)	3,300 oz. 1,000 cu. ft. air	1,000 mm. Hg	1.98	1.22 at 0°C.	Organic solvents
Eye-casualty concentration—1 hr. exposure, 0.001 (11)	30 min. exposure, 0.07; 10 min. exposure, 0.15	14°C. (57°F.)	217°C. (422.6°F.)	0.625 oz. 1,000 cu. ft. air	0.065 mm. Hg	5.5	1.27	Oils, PS, alcohol, carbon tetrachloride
Minimum irritating concentration, 0.0008 (12)	30 min. exposure, 0.048; 10 min. exposure, 0.12	−18.2°C. (0°F.)	190°C. (374°F.)	4.5 oz. 1,000 cu. ft. air	0.395 mm. Hg	7.1	1.88	HS-PS, oils, alcohol
1 min. exposure, 0.025 (13)	30 min. exposure, 0.125; 10 min. exposure, 0.75	54.8°C. (−66.6°F.)	132°C. (269.6°F.)	75 oz. 1,000 cu. ft. air	8.5 mm. Hg		1.85	Organic solvents
10 min. exposure, 0.0012 (14)	30 min. exposure, 0.60; 10 min. exposure, 1.50	45°C. (113°F.)	383°C. (720°F.)	0.00068 oz. 1,000 cu. ft. air	0.0005 mm. Hg	Practically no vapor; all solid particles	1.4	Acetone, chloroform, chlorpicrin
10 min. exposure, 0.00025 (15)	10 min. exposure, 1.00	31.5°C. (91°F.)	350°C. (662°F.)	0.0015	0.0001 mm. Hg	8.8	1.45	Organic solvents, chloroform
3 min. exposure, 0.005 (16)	30 min. exposure, 0.65; 10 min. exposure, 3.00	195°C. (387°F.)	410°C. (770°F.) Decomposes below boiling point	Negligible	Negligible	No vapor; disseminated as solid	1.65	Furfural acetone
None (17)	None	−20°C. (−3°F.)	200°C. (392°F.)	Negligible	Negligible		0.8	Benzene, gasoline
Smoke irritation negligible (18)	Smoke harmless	44°C. (111°F.)	287°C. (549°F.)	0.1728 oz. 1,000 cu. ft. air	0.0253 mm. Hg	Vapor negligible; disseminated as a solid	1.83	Carbon disulfide, ether, benzene

Action on metals	Stability on storage	Action with water	Hydrolysis product	Odor in air	Odor detectable at mg. per liter or oz. per 1,000 cu. ft.	Physiological action
Very corrosive to iron (1)	Unstable in heat or light	None	None	Pungent and stifling	0.0005	Vapor, severe lacrimation; liquid, produces blisters; often toxic
Very corrosive to iron; lead or enamel lined shells required (2)	Slowly decomposes	Slowly hydrolyzes	HBr and various compounds	Like sour fruit	Irritates before odor can be detected	Severe lacrimation and nose irritation
Tarnishes steel slightly (3)	Stable	None	Not readily hydrolyzed	In low concentrations like apple blossoms	0.0002	Eye and skin irritation
None if dry; vigorous corrosion if wet (4)	Stable in iron cylinders, if dry	A little dissolves forming HCl, HOCl, and ClO_2	HCl; HOCl; ClO_2	Pungent	0.0100	Burns upper respiratory tracts
None if dry; vigorous corrosion if wet (5)	Stable in dry steel containers	Hydrolyzes rapidly	HCl; CO_2	Like ensilage; fresh-cut hay	0.0044	Burns lower lung surfaces, causing edema
None if dry, corrosion if wet (6)	Stable in dry steel containers	Hydrolyzes slowly	$ClCO_2$; CO_2; HCl	Disagreeable, suffocating	0.0088	Burns lower lung surfaces, causing edema
Produces slight tarnish only (7)	Stable for long periods in steel containers	Very slightly soluble	Hydrolyzes with difficulty	Sweetish, like fly-paper	0.0073	Lacrimates; irritates nose and throat; produces nausea and lung irritation in order as concentration increases
None (8)	Stable	Hydrolyzes slowly	Ethylarseneous oxide and HCl (hydrolysis product is poisonous if swallowed)	Biting, irritant	0.0010	Vesicant, $\frac{1}{8}$ as powerful as HS; powerful sternutator; causes paralysis of fingers
None except on copper, if dry; corrodes all if wet (9)	Stable when mixed with strong acid and dissolved in solvents	Miscible, slowly decomposes	Ammonium cyanide	Like bitter almonds	0.0010	Paralysis of central nervous system
None if dry; corrodes metals if moist (10)	Unstable; stability increased when mixed with $AsCl_3$	Slightly soluble	HCl; cyanuric acid		0.0025	Irritates eyes and lungs
None (11)	Stable in steel containers	Slowly hydrolyzes	HCl and $(HOCH_2CH_2)_2S$; not toxic	Like garlic or horse-radish	0.0013	Dissolves in skin or lung tissue, then produces burns
None (12)	Stable in steel containers	Hydrolyzes readily	HCl; Ml oxide; (ClCH)(CHAsO); very toxic	Like geraniums, then biting	0.014	Dissolves in skin, then burns and liberates Ml oxide which poisons body
None (13)	Very stable	Slightly soluble	None		0.0008	Asthma, dyspnea; lung injurant, skin vesicant
Vigorous corrosion on steel (14)	Slowly decomposes	Slowly hydrolyzes	HCl; Da Oxide (Da oxide is poisonous if swallowed)	Like shoe polish	0.0003	Sneezing; vomiting; headache
Vigorous corrosion on iron and steel (15)	Very stable	None	None	Like garlic and bitter almonds	0.0003	Sneezing; vomiting; headache
Very slight (16)	Stable in steel containers	Insoluble, hydrolyzed with difficulty	HCl; DM oxide $[(C_6H_4)_2NHAs]_2O$; DM oxide is very toxic if swallowed	No pronounced odor	Almost no odor to average man, up to 0.0025	Headache, nausea, violent sneezing, followed by temporary physical debility
None (17)	Very stable	None	None	Slightly suffocating	None	None
None (18)	Stable out of contact with oxygen	None; stored under water in concrete tanks	Smoke in air; phosphoric acid (H_3PO_4) dissolved in water	Like matches		Solid particle burns flesh; vapors very poisonous, cause bone decay; smoke relatively harmless

Protection required	Method of neutralizing	First aid	Munitions suitable for use	American marking on munitions
Gas mask; absorbent only (1)	Alkali	Wash eyes with boric acid; wash skin with warm sodium carbonate solution	Projectiles and grenades	2 green bands BA gas
Gas masks; absorbents in canister only (2)	Alcoholic sodium hydroxide spray	Wash eyes with boric acid solution	75-mm. artillery shell or airplane spray	2 green bands CA gas
Gask masks; both absorbent and effective filter (3)	Strong hot sodium carbonate solution	Wash eyes with boric acid; wash skin with warm sodium carbonate solution	Candles and grenades as burning mixtures; grenades; artillery shell; 4.2-in. CM; 4-in. CM; airplane spray and bombs as solution	Burning type munitions, 1 green band, CN gas
Gask masks; absorbents in canister only (4)	Alkali, solution or solid	Keep patient quiet and warm and treat for bronchial pneumonia	Mixed with CG and PS in cylinders and LP shells	1 green band Cl gas
Gas masks; absorbents in canister only (5)	Steam hydrolyzes; alkalies and amines react with CG	Keep patient quiet; administer heart stimulants; give oxygen in severe cases; treat like pleurisy	LP shells; cylinders; 4.2-in. CM; 4-in. CM; 155-mm. howitzer shell	1 green band CG gas
Gas masks; absorbents in canister only (6)	Steam hydrolyzes alkalies and amines react with CG	Keep patient quiet; administer heart stimulants; give oxygen in severe cases; treat like pleurisy	LP shells; cylinders; 4.2-in. CM; 4-in. CM; 155-mm. howitzer shell	
Gas masks with high-grade absorbents in canisters (7)	Sodium sulfite solution	Wash eyes with boric acid; keep patient warm; protect throat from infection	Mixed with CN in 75-mm. shell; air bombs; 4-in. CM and 4.2-in. CM shell; pure in spray; w/GG in LP and 4.2-in. shell	2 green bands PS gas
Gas masks and protective clothing (8)	Sodium hydroxide solution	Wash skin with warm sodium carbonate solution	Artillery shell; 4.2-in. CM shell; airplane spray	2 green bands ED gas
Gas mask; absorbents only (9)	None necessary	Fresh air; cold water in face; artificial respiration	Artillery shell	
Gas mask; absorbents only (10)	None necessary	Fresh air; cold water in face; artificial respiration	Artillery shell	
Gas masks and protective clothing (11)	Bleaching powder, 3 % sodiumsulfide (Na_2S) in water; steam; gaseous chlorine; or bury under moist earth	Wash affected parts with kerosene or gasoline, then with strong soap and hot water; rub dry; rinse with hot clean water; agent must be removed within 3 min.	Airplane spray; airplane bombs; 75-mm. guns; 155-mm. howitzer; 155-mm. gun; 4.2-in. CM	2 green bands HS gas
Gas masks and best of protective clothing (12)	Alcoholic sodium hydroxide spray	Wash with oils, hot water, and soap; dry; first aid must be applied at once	Airplane spray; airplane bombs; 75-mm. shell; 155-mm. howitzer shell; 4.2-in. CM	2 green bands M-1 gas
Gas masks and best of protective clothing (13)	Sodium hydroxide solution	Wash with soap and water, then with sodium hydroxide (5 %); wash eyes with boric acid	Artillery and mortar shell	2 green bands MD gas
Best type of filter in gas-mask canister. (14)	Caustic gaseous chlorine	Chlorine in low concentrations	Burning-type munitions	1 green band DA gas
Gas masks, best type of filter (15)	Caustic gaseous chlorine	Chlorine in low concentrations	Artillery shell	
Best type of filter in gas-mask canister (16)	Gaseous chlorine bleach liquor	Breathe low concentrations of chlorine from bleaching-powder bottle	Candle; destroyer smoke attack; burning-type air bombs	1 green band DM gas
None (17)	None necessary	None necessary	Incomplete combustion by naval vessels	1 yellow band CO smoke
None needed against smoke; fireproof suits against burning particles (18)	None needed; copper sulfate solution stops burning of particles, as does water	Apply copper sulfate solution; pull out solids; treat burn with picric acid; keep burning part under water until medical aid arrives if no $CuSO_4$ is available	Grenades; artillery shells; 4-in. CM; 4.2-CM; airplane bombs in.	1 yellow band WP smoke

Table IV. **PROPERTIES OF CHEMICAL AGENTS**

Agent, common name	Chemical name	CWS. symbol	Physiological classification	Tactical classification	Persistency (summer)	Persistency (winter)	Lowest irritant concentration, mg. per liter or oz. per 1,000 cu. ft., 10 min. exposure
Sulfur trioxide........ (19)	Sulfur trioxide $(SO)_3$		None	Screening agent	While container is operating	Same as summer	Smoke irritation negligible
Oleum (60 per cent).... (20)	$(SO_3XH_2SO_4)$		None	Screening agent	While container is operating	Same as summer	Smoke irritation negligible
HC Mixture........... (21)	Hexachlorethane (C_2Cl_6)†, zinc and zinc oxide (ZNO)	HC	None	Screening agent	Only while burning	Same as summer	Smoke irritation negligible
Titanium tetrachloride.. (22)	Titanium tetrachloride $(TiCl_4)$	FM	None	Screening agent	10 min. in open	Same as summer	Smoke irritation negligible
Sulfur trioxide solution.. (23)	Sulfur trioxide (SO_3), about 55 per cent; chlorsulfonic acid $(HClSO_3)$, about 45 per cent by weight	FS	None	Screening agent	While container is operating	Same as summer	Smoke irritation negligible
Thermite....... (24)	Thermite $(Al+Fe_3O_4)$	Th	None	Incendiary agent	None	None	None
Solid oil.............. (25)	Mixture of paraffin hydrocarbons	SO	None	Incendiary agent	None	None	None

* This volatility is at 4,993 mm. Hg. At 760 mm. Hg, the volatility of chlorine is 3,708 oz./1,000 cu. ft

† This volatility is at 1,180 mm. Hg. At 760 mm. Hg, the volatility of phosgene is 4,420 oz./1,000 cu ft.

Intolerable concentration, mg. per liter or oz. per 1,000 cu. ft., 10 min. exposure	Lethal concentration, mg. per liter or oz. per 1,000 cu. ft., 10 min. exposure	Melting point	Boiling point	Volatility, 20°C. (68°F.)	Vapor pressure, 20°C. (68°F.)	Vapor density compared to air	Density of solid, 20°C. (68°F.)	Solvents for
Smoke irritation negligible (19)	Smoke harmless	40°F. (104°F.)	45°C. (113°F.)	Negligible	242.27 at 25°C.		1.94	
Smoke irritation negligible (20)	Smoke harmless	5°C.	Decomposes	Negligible	Negligible		1.99	
Smoke irritation negligible (21)	Smoke harmless	Hexachlorethane 184°C. (363°F.)	185°C. (sublimes) (365°F.)	2.85 oz. 1,000 cu. ft. air	0.22 mm. Hg	Vapor negligible; disseminated as a solid	2.0	Alcohol, ether (for hexachlorethane only)
Smoke irritation negligible (22)	Smoke harmless	−23°C. (−9°F.)	136°C. (277°F.)	86.4 oz. 1,000 cu. ft. air	8.32 mm. Hg		1.7	Ethylene dichloride
Smoke irritation negligible (23)	Smoke harmless	Below −30°C. (−22°F.)		About 80°C. (176°F.)			1.91	Strong sulfuric acid
None (24)	None	1,500°C. (2,732°F.)	None	None	None	None	3.3	None
None (25)	None	30°C. (86°F.)	None	None	None	None	0.9	Organic solvents

	Action on metals	Stability on storage	Action with water	Hydrolysis product	Odor in air	Odor detectable at mg. per liter or oz. per 1,000 cu. ft.	Physiological action
(19)	Corrosive unless dry	Stable if dry	Hydrolyzes	H_2SO_3 and H_2SO_4	Acrid suffocating smoke		Hacking cough
(20)	Corrosive unless dry	Stable if dry	Hydrolyzes	H_2SO_3 and H_2SO_4	Acrid suffocating smoke		Like strong acid
(21)	None if dry	Stable	C_2Cl_6 slowly hydrolyzes; mixture ignites	Smoke in air; ($ZnCl_2$) zinc chloride in water solution	Acrid suffocating smoke		None from solid; slightly suffocating action by heavy smoke
(22)	Vigorous corrosion by smoke; none by liquid on steel if dry	Stable in steel containers when dry	Hydrolyzes	Smoke in air; $TiCl_4 \cdot 8H_2O$; then HCl and $Ti(OH)_4$	Acrid		Liquid burns like strong acid; vapors and smoke irritating to throat
(23)	Vigorous corrosion if wet; vigorous corrosion in presence of moisture	Stable in steel containers	Reacts violently like strong sulfuric acid	Smoke in air; hydrochloric acid (HCl) and sulfuric acid (H_2SO_4) mixed in water solution as fog particles	Acid or acrid		Liquid burns like strong acid; smoke causes pricking sensation on skin
(24)	None	Stable	None	None	None		Burns like molten iron
(25)	None	Stable	None	None	None		Burns like oil

	Protection required	Method of neutralizing	First aid	Munitions suitable for use	American marking on munitions
(19)	None	Wash freely with cold water		Artillery and CM shell; airplane spray	
(20)	None	Wash freely with cold water		Smoke grenades; airplane tanks	
(21)	None	None needed	None needed	Burning-type munitions only; grenades; candles; smoke floats; special air bombs	1 yellow band HC smoke
(22)	None for ordinary smoke clouds; gas masks needed for heavy concentration only	Alkali; solid or solution	Wash with sodium bicarbonate solution, then with warm water; treat burn with picric acid	Artillery shell; 4-in. CM; 4.2-in. CM; airplane spray; airplane bombs; special munitions	1 yellow band FM smoke
(23)	None for ordinary smoke; gas masks for high concentrations, only rubber gloves for handling liquid	Any alkali, solid or solution	Like an acid burn	From cylinders under gas pressure; airplane spray tanks; explosive shell	1 yellow band FS smoke
(24)	Fireproof clothes	None	Like ordinary burn	Drop bombs; artillery shell	1 purple band Th incendiary
(25)	Fireproof clothes	None	Like hot-liquid burn	Drop bombs; artillery shell	1 purple band SO incendiary

foundation in fact, but which was deliberately disseminated as propaganda to influence the neutral nations of the world against Germany, just as in the Middle Ages the first use of firearms was similarly excoriated.

Chemical warfare has been the favorite topic of discussion at international conferences because it is a popular subject of condemnation, and one concerning which treaties and conventions can be made without the slightest probability of being lived up to, as was the case in the World War.

Finally, the subject of chemical warfare has been the happy hunting ground for sensational newspaper and magazine writers whose imaginations have furnished lurid pictures of whole populations being wiped out at a single blow with poison gas dropped from airplanes.

In view of the general public interest in this question and its importance to our national defense, it seemed to the author that it was high time for someone to produce an authoritative American text on chemical warfare, and so he reluctantly undertook this task as a patriotic duty.

The purposes of this book are threefold: (1) to trace the development of the art and science of chemical warfare from its beginning in the World War to the present time; (2) to present an American viewpoint on chemical warfare; and (3) to make available to the public an authentic text on a much misrepresented and misunderstood subject of great importance to our future national security.

General acknowledgment is made in the reference notes to the many sources to which the author is indebted for much of his material.

Special acknowledgment is made to Major George J. B. Fisher, Chemical Warfare Service, United States Army, who not only furnished the chapters on the Protection of Civilian Populations from Chemical Attack and the International Situation with respect to chemical warfare, but also rendered much valuable assistance in the general preparation of the text; and to Dr. Arthur B. Ray, who had charge of the development work on incendiaries in this country during the World War, for his kind permission to use material from his work in the chapter on Incendiary Agents.

Many of the illustrations are reproduced by permission of the War Department, and the diagrams of the German gas bombardments in 1918 are reproduced by the kind permission of the British Royal Artillery Institution.

The author is also indebted to Major General C. E. Brigham, Chief of Chemical Warfare Service, whose sympathetic cooperation made this book possible.

AUGUSTIN M. PRENTISS.

WASHINGTON, D. C.,
January, 1937.

TABLE OF CONTENTS

INTRODUCTION

From the dawn of antiquity to the present century men have fought their battles by physical blows, and it was not until the World War that the history of organized conflict recorded a deviation from this fundamental principle of battle.

The blows by which man subdued his opponent were delivered by hand until his ingenuity devised instruments for adding distance to the striking power of the human arm. But the weakness of primitive devices for projecting missiles put on hand-to-hand fighting a premium that persisted down through the Middle Ages. The invention of firearms at last enabled soldiers to fight their battles at a distance, for by superseding brawn with the propulsive power of gunpowder it became possible to penetrate all known forms of protection and to strike fatal blows from a distance. It then became an important aim of tactics to weaken an enemy by means of missiles hurled at a distance before closing with him to accomplish his final defeat.

The attention lavished upon various types of guns made these weapons so tremendously powerful that at last they came to defeat the very purpose they served. Thus, the fire power of modern weapons of impact—machine guns, supported by artillery of various calibers—has grown so great that, when properly located in defensive positions, they are capable of repulsing every assault against them. Soldiers cannot advance under the withering fires of machine guns and artillery barrages without prohibitive losses and any attempt to do so only results in futile slaughter. Modern armies are forced to seek protection in trenches so deep and strong as to defy even the colossal power of modern artillery, and tactical movement is thus eventually paralyzed.

This result was foreshadowed in our own Civil War, to be grimly demonstrated in the World War. In the latter conflict there were, at least on the Western Front, no flanks to be turned. Yet the absence of exposed flanks was here no more than proof that, given sufficient modern rifles and guns, and enough soldiers to man them, a battle front may be extended until it defies outflanking. Linear formations are then reinforced in depth so that substantial penetration becomes prohibitive and the task of subduing a belligerent must be accomplished by economic instead of military force.

In order to counteract the power of modern impact weapons and the resulting deadlock of trench warfare, toxic gas finally was resorted to. It was hoped by this new means to restore movement in battle and thus again permit tactical maneuver and fire power to open the way to victory.

But gas, for reasons which we shall presently discuss, did not immediately fulfill these early expectations, although the ensuing struggle for technical protection led to an examination of practically every compound in the whole catalogue of chemistry that offered any promise of military utility and to the actual trial in battle of scores of chemical agents. The results, *in toto*, was *chemical warfare*, and the opening up of a new field for the implementation of military effort.

History records numerous earlier but abortive attempts to utilize the powers of chemistry for military ends. It is not within the scope of this book to examine in detail such occurrences preceding the World War. With the exception of Greek fire, none of them produced important results and none permanently challenged the supremacy of existing weapons. They are of interest to us here only as indicating man's eagerness to experiment with any means that promises to promote his fortunes in battle and his final dependence upon technical knowledge to produce such means.

The value of chemicals as war weapons had attracted the serious speculation of military minds as early as our Civil War, but no practical progress was made in this field because of the then undeveloped state of the chemical industry. Many chemical substances having powerful physiological effects had already been discovered and classified before the commencement of the World War; a number of these were well known and had been manufactured in quantity before the war. It was only natural then that these substances were utilized as chemical-warfare agents in the war and no new chemical was specially developed for war purposes. Yet there is a wide gulf between laboratory research and the colossal production needed to supply modern armies in the field. The use of chemicals as warfare agents was not practicable, even though the possibilities may have been recognized, until the chemical industry had attained sizeable proportions.

But during the decades preceding the World War the chemical industry, particularly in Europe, had been expanding apace. A remarkable feature of this new major industry was the tremendous development of dye production, which during the early years of the twentieth century largely centered in Germany. In 1913 the world production of dyes reached approximately 150,000 tons, of which Germany controlled three-quarters, producing at the same time something over 85 per cent of the intermediates entering into the finished dyes. When it is remembered that these intermediate products may also be used in compounding

military chemical agents and that the dye factories provide both technical skill and manufacturing equipment needed for the production of these substances, the peculiar military significance of this industry becomes apparent.

The basic chemical industries, producing nitrogen compounds, chlorine, sulfuric and nitric acids, and the alkalies, had attained major proportions before the beginning of the war, especially in Germany. Thus chlorine, which was used on an enormous scale, not only as a war gas itself, but as the basis for the manufacture of nearly all other chemical agents, was being produced in Germany at the rate of tens of thousands of tons annually. The highly developed coal-tar industry, as well as facilities for production of arsenic, bromines, and phosphorus, stood ready to furnish important contributions to war effort.

The immense chemical factories along the Rhine were producing these potentials of chemical warfare on a large scale and, what was equally vital, possessed the technical talent capable of directing the conversion of their products into warfare agents. With the stage thus set, it needed no more than the urge of dire military necessity to insure the advent of chemical warfare.

Not only was the military crisis of the winter of 1914–1915 brought about by the collapse of the classical methods of attack so successful in former wars of movement, but (as far as Germany was concerned) the situation was even more critical because of the serious depletion of supplies of explosive ammunition. Germany entered the World War with plans for but a few months of intensive campaign, for which she believed that her accumulated stocks of ammunition would suffice. As these stocks rapidly dwindled with victory still distant, Germany was obliged quickly to mobilize her national industries behind her armies. That the great German chemical industry should have been immediately utilized to this end was inevitable; the wonder is rather that the first German gas attack was such a surprise to the Allies.

The introduction of chemicals as active agents of war was readily recognized as a portent that in the future, military weapons are to be forged in laboratories as well as in foundries. Thus, even in 1915, few students of military technique failed to discern the dawn of a new era in the long history of warfare. The two decades that have elapsed since the first German gas attack at Ypres have not only confirmed this early appreciation but have added greatly to the comprehension of both soldier and scientist as to the role and power of chemicals in war.

Not only has the introduction of chemicals in war changed the character of modern combat, but it has also vastly accelerated the evolution of military weapons. Thus, more than a century passed after the British first brought cannon into the field at Crécy without witnessing

substantial improvement in the technique of supporting artillery; yet within a few years chemical warfare has advanced from an untried theory to a recognized principle of modern war.

This progress has been marked by two distinct phases. First there was the crucible of war—more than three years of fierce struggle that taxed the chemical resources of the most highly industrialized nations. Then followed the postwar period of evaluation, research, and assimilation. The latter phase has probably contributed no less than the former to the early maturity of this new arm of war.

Notwithstanding the remarkable results achieved with chemicals during the World War, the means and methods employed in that conflict appear as crude and feeble beginnings when viewed in the light of our present knowledge and our cooler conceptions of the future. As we draw away from the late war we apprehend more clearly that the potential power of chemicals was then only dimly foreshadowed. Today we realize that all nations are facing new and powerful instrumentalities involving as profound changes in the art and science of war as were brought about by the invention of gunpowder. In a word, armies have already advanced well into the era of chemical warfare.

CHAPTER I

BASIC PRINCIPLES

COMPARISON OF CHEMICAL AND EXPLOSIVE WEAPONS

An understanding of the true character of chemical warfare can best be approached by a consideration of the action of combat chemicals as compared to that of explosive weapons.

Certain important differences between the effects of chemical and of explosive munitions emphasize the peculiarity and novelty of chemical warfare and suggest some of its potentialities. These differences are particularly noticeable in the mechanism of the action of chemical agents and their effects in terms of time and space.

Chemical substances used in war for their direct physiological or chemical effects are called *chemical agents*. A chemical agent does not exert its effect by direct physical impact upon its target, like a rifle bullet or a shell fragment. On the contrary, chemicals may be liberated in place, depending on wind to move them to their targets; they may be transported to a point of release over or on the target by airplanes or wheeled vehicles; or they may be carried to that point in projectiles. In any case, the container is merely a conveyance for the chemical agent.

The effect of a chemical agent then is derived from the reactions that take place after the agent is freed from its container. Tactical and technical considerations indicate the point of release; natural forces then complete the processes of dispersion and ultimate effect. Herein lies a fundamental difference between chemicals and explosives.

Also, chemicals do not strike a physical target—they pervade the atmosphere over an area. The area may be wide when a volatile gas is dispersed, or it may be restricted to a few acres saturated with slowly evaporating liquids. Yet always the effect is as permeating as the active range of the component molecules.

In contrast to this wide distribution of effect characteristic of chemicals, let us analyze the action of high explosives. As the high-explosive shell detonates, its effect is derived from the concussion of the explosion and from the striking force of flying fragments. This action, however, does not extend beyond a relatively small area surrounding the point of burst. Even within this danger area, of two soldiers standing side by side, one may be killed and the other escape unharmed.

Such uncertain and uncontrollable results are impossible with gas. When gas is released everyone within its compass becomes *equally*

exposed to its effect. The soldier may counter that effect with artificial protection, but otherwise he cannot escape it even though he is some distance from the point of release, for gas saturates the entire atmosphere overlying the target area.

Again, in the matter of *time*, gas offers a striking contrast to weapons of impact. The effect of the rifle bullet is instantaneous; a second after the bullet strikes it is spent and harmless. But even the most fleeting gas clouds are effective for a matter of many minutes, while persistent chemicals may continue to contaminate an area for days.

Another unique characteristic of gas is its searching effect. A hastily dug fox hole affords individual shelter from machine-gun bullets. A copse of trees may well protect a whole company of infantry from artillery fire. But gas follows no narrow trajectory; it permeates the air and overcomes all incidental obstacles of terrain to stalk its quarry relentlessly. These distinctive features combine to enhance the power and utility of chemical agents, particularly in their action against personnel.

Before examining the basic principles underlying the science of chemical warfare, it is important to understand the meaning and usage of certain technical terms.

DEFINITIONS

We have said that chemical substances used in combat are designated as chemical agents. Of these agents, three distinct groups—*gases, smokes,* and *incendiaries*—constitute what is generally understood as the matériel of chemical warfare.

Gases are chemical agents which produce physiological effects. These agents are used in war to incapacitate military personnel. Physically they are often dispersed as liquids and not infrequently as particulate clouds; yet the term *gas* has attained in military parlance a generic meaning that embraces any chemical used for its direct effect upon the human body. A gas which produces death is called a *lethal* agent, while a gas which, under field conditions, does not cause death or serious casualties is an *irritant* agent.

A *smoke* agent, as its name implies, is one capable of obscuring vision in sufficient measure to afford concealment. It may incidentally burn or corrode, yet primarily it screens.

Incendiary agents start destructive fires, igniting even materials that ordinarily are slow to burn.

A *toxic* is any substance which, by its direct chemical action, either internally or externally, on the human or animal organism, is capable of destroying life or seriously impairing normal body functions.

Toxicity is the measure of the inherent poisonous effect of a chemical agent and is the product of its concentration times the period of exposure to its action.

Lacrimators cause intense, though temporary, irritation of the eyes; they are commonly known as *tear gas* (see Chap. VI).

Lung injurants are those gases that particularly attack and injure the bronchial tubes and the lungs. The "injurant" gases are quite distinct from "irritant" gases; the former are highly toxic and frequently lethal in action, whereas the latter are characteristically nonlethal and include generally lacrimators and sneeze gases (see Chap. VII).

Systemic toxics are substances which by systemic action exert a direct paralyzing effect upon the heart and nervous system. They are usually the most deadly of all gases (see Chap. VIII).

Vesicants are agents which exert a blistering (vesicant) effect upon the skin (see Chap. IX).

Irritant gases (sometimes called *sneeze* gases or *sternutators*) attack the nasal passages, causing nausea and headache of a few hours' duration. They are never lethal in concentrations encountered in the field (see Chap. X).

Symbols.—During the World War, code symbols or names were used to designate the various chemical agents employed, without revealing their chemical identity. The symbols were usually two or three letters, arbitrarily chosen, to designate the chemical agent, and the names were generally fanciful and were derived from some place or event incident to the first use of the agent. As most substances used as chemical agents were complex compounds with long chemical names, the short symbols and names proved very convenient in referring to the agent and came into general use even where secrecy was not essential. In the course of a short time, the chemical identity of the agents used on both sides in the war became generally known and the code symbols and names lost their secrecy value. They are, however, still employed as a matter of convenience in preference to the chemical names of the compounds.

Table I shows a list of the principal chemical agents used in the war and their code symbols or names. For convenience, chemical agents will generally be designated throughout this text by their symbols, as indicated in Table I.

Concentration refers to the quantity of chemical vapor present in a given volume of air. It is expressed in four ways, as follows: (1) as parts of gas per million parts of air; (2) as grams of gas per cubic meter of air; (3) as milligrams of gas per liter of air; or (4) as ounces of gas per thousand cubic feet of air.

Numerically, grams per cubic meter is the same as millgrams per liter, and is almost the same as ounces per thousand cubic feet; all these are

6

TABLE I.—NOMENCLATURE OF CHEMICAL AGENTS

Chemical name	Chemical formula	English name	American CWS symbol	French name	German name
Gases					
Acrolein	CH_2CHCHO	—	—	Papite	—
Arsenic trichloride	$AsCl_3$	—	—	Marsite	—
Benzyl bromide	$C_6H_5CH_2Br$	—	—	Cyclite	T-Stoff
Benzyl iodide	$C_6H_5CH_2I$	—	—	Fraissite	—
Bromacetone	CH_3COCH_2Br	BA	BA	Martonite	B-Stoff
Brombenzyl cyanide	$C_6H_5CHBrCN$	—	CA	Camite	—
Bromine	Br_2	—	—	—	Brom
Brommethylethyl ketone	$CH_3COCHBrCH_3$	—	—	Homomartonite	Bn-Stoff
Carbonyl chloride	$COCl_2$	Phosgene	CG	Collongite	D-Stoff
Chloracetone	CH_3COCH_2Cl	—	—	Tonite	A-Stoff
Chloracetophenone	$C_6H_5COCH_2Cl$	—	CN	—	—
Chloracetophenone	$C_6H_5COCH_2Cl$ }				
Chloroform	$CHCl_3$ }	—	CNS	—	—
Chlorpicrin	CCl_3NO_2 }				
Chlorine	Cl_2	Chlorine	Cl	Bertholite	Chlor
Chlorpicrin	CCl_3NO_2	Vomiting gas	PS	Aquinite	Klop
Chlorvinyldichlorarsine	$CHClCHAsCl_2$	Lewisite	M-1	—	—
Cyanogen bromide	CNBr	CB	—	Campellit (Italian)	Ce (Austrian)
Cyanogen chloride	CNCl	—	—	Vitrite	—
Dianisidin	$(NH_2(OCH_3)C_6H_3)_2$	—	—	—	X
Dibromethyl sulfide	$(BrCH_2CH_2)_2S$	—	—	—	Bromlost
Dibrommethyl ether	$(CH_2Br)_2O$	—	—	—	X
Dichlorethyl sulfide	$(ClCH_2CH_2)_2S$	Mustard gas	HS	Yperite	Lost; also Yellow Cross
Dichlormethyl ether	$(CH_2Cl)_2O$	—	—	—	X
Dimethyl sulfate	$(CH_3)_2SO_4$	—	—	Rationite	D-Stoff
Diphenylaminechlorarsine	$(C_6H_4)_2NHAsCl$	Adamsite	DM	—	—
Diphenylchlorarsine	$(C_6H_5)_2AsCl$	—	DA	—	Clark I
Diphenylcyanarsine	$(C_6H_5)_2AsCN$	—	CDA	—	Clark II
Ethylbromacetate	$CH_2BrCOOC_2H_5$	—	—	X	—
Ethylcarbazol	$(C_6H_4)_2NC_2H_5$	—	—	—	Blue Cross-1
Ethyldibromarsine	$C_2H_5AsBr_2$	—	—	—	X
Ethyldichlorarsine	$C_2H_5AsCl_2$	—	ED	—	Dick. also Green Cross-3
Ethyliodoacetate	$CH_2ICOOC_2H_5$	SK	—	—	—
Ethylsulfuryl chloride	$ClSO_2OC_2H_5$	—	—	Sulvanite	—
Hydrocyanic acid	HCN	JL and VN	—	Forestite	—
Iodoacetone	CH_3COCH_2I	—	—	Bretonite	—
Methyldichlorarsine	CH_3AsCl_2	—	MD	—	Methyldick
Methylsulfuryl chloride	$ClSO_2OCH_3$	—	—	—	X
Monochlormethylchloroformate	$ClCOOCH_2Cl$	—	—	Palite	C-Stoff, K-Stoff
Perchlormethylmercaptan	$SCCl_4$	—	—	Carbontetrachlorsulfide	—
Phenylcarbylamine chloride	$C_6H_5CNCl_2$	—	—	—	Green Cross-1

7

Chemical name	Chemical formula	English name	American CWS symbol	French name	German name
Phenyldibromarsine	$C_6H_5AsBr_2$	—	—	—	X
Phenyldichlorarsine	$C_6H_5AsCl_2$	—	—	Sternite	Blue Cross-1
Thiophosgene	$CSCl_2$	Thiophosgene	—	Lacramite	—
Trichlormethylchloroformate	$ClCOOCCl_3$	Diphosgene	—	Surpalite	Perstoff
Xylyl bromide	$CH_3C_6H_4CH_2Br$	—	—	—	T-Stoff
Smokes					
Chlorsulfonic acid	$HClSO_3$	X	X	X	X
Hydrocarbons	—	Crude oil	CO	—	—
Niter, sulfur, pitch, borax, and glue	$KNO_3 + S + C + Na_2B_4O_7$ + glue	Type S mixture	Type S mixture	—	—
Silicon tetrachloride	$SiCl_4$	—	—	—	X
Stannic chloride	$SnCl_4$	KJ	KJ	Opacite	—
Sulfur trioxide	SO_3	—	—	X	N-Stoff
Sulfur trioxide + chlorsulfonic acid	$SO_3 + SO_3HCl$	X	FS	X	X
Sulfuryl chloride	SO_2Cl_2	—	—	X	X
Titanium tetrachloride	$TrCl_4$	—	FM	Fumergerite	F-Stoff
White phosphorus	P_4	WP	WP	X	—
Zinc, carbon tetrachloride ammonium chloride, and magnesium carbonate	$Zn + CCl_4 + NH_4Cl + MgCO_3$	—	BM	—	—
Zinc plus carbon tetrachloride plus zinc oxide plus kieselguhr	$Zn + CCl_4 + ZnO$ + kieselguhr	—	—	Berger Mixture	—
Zinc plus hexachlorethane and zinc oxide	$Zn + C_2Cl_6 + ZnO$	—	HC	—	—
Incendiaries					
Barium nitrate, magnesium, and linseed oil	$BaNO_3 + Mg$ + linseed oil	Incendiary mixture	—	—	—
Barium peroxide plus magnesium	$BaO_4 + Mg$	Incendiary powder	X	—	—
Modified thermite	$3Al + 6BaNO_3 + 8Fe_3O_4$	Modified thermite	X	—	—
Potassium perchlorate and paraffin	$KClO_4 + C_nH_{2n+2}$	Incendiary mixture	—	-	—
Sodium	Na	Sodium	X	X	X
Solidified hydrocarbons	—	Solid oil	—	—	—
Sulfur thermite	$8Al + 3Fe_3O_4 + 9S$	—	—	Daisite	—
Thermite	$8Al + 3Fe_3O_4$	Thermite	Th	X	X
White phosphorus in carbon disulfide		Inflammable liquids	—	X	—

X denotes employment without special name or symbol.
— denotes nonemployment.

8

ratios between *weight* of gas and *volume* of air. On the other hand, parts per million is purely a volumetric ratio and differs essentially from the other three ratios, in that the molecular weight of the gas must be taken into consideration. As all four of these ratios are met with in the literature of pharmacology, toxicology, and other branches of science closely allied to chemical warfare, it is frequently necessary to convert one expression into another. Mathematical formulas for doing so are given in Appendix A.

An *irritating* concentration is one which produces an irritant effect upon a man without injuring his body functions or seriously impairing his working efficiency. The lowest irritant concentration is often called the *threshold of action* or *threshold concentration.*

An *intolerable* concentration is one which cannot be withstood for more than a very limited time without serious derangement of some body function. As applied to lacrimators, it is usually synonymous with the maximum concentration in which a man can maintain his vision without masking.

A *lethal concentration* is one which the average unprotected man cannot survive after a definite brief period of exposure. The numerical value of the lethal concentration decreases as the time of exposure increases.

Volatility refers to the capacity of a liquid to change into vapor in the open air. Quantitatively, the volatility of an agent is the amount held as a vapor in a unit volume of saturated air at any given temperature and pressure. Volatility increases with temperature. If the volatility of a chemical compound is considerably greater than its lethal concentration for a 10-minute exposure, it is possible to set up killing concentrations under field conditions and the substance is a casualty-producing agent. For relation of volatility to vapor pressure, see Appendix A.

Hydrolysis is the reaction of any chemical substance with water whereby new compounds are created. This is a reaction of great importance in chemical warfare, as many chemical agents are rendered harmless after a time by hydrolysis. If the hydrolysis product is itself a poison, as is the case with all agents containing arsenic, considerable effort is required to neutralize the agent effectively.

Vapor Pressure.—Evaporation is constantly taking place from the exposed surfaces of all liquids and volatile solids. The pressure exerted by the escaping vapor is called the *vapor tension* of the liquid or solid. When its vapor tension equals the surrounding atmospheric pressure, a liquid is said to boil and a solid to sublime, for at that temperature its vapor is able to lift the air above it and so freely escape. At all temperatures below the boiling point of a liquid or the subliming point of a solid, the vapor tension of the substance is less than atmospheric pressure,[9] so that the escape of the vapor is opposed by the surrounding air. Much of the vapor is thus forced back into the liquid or solid. Under these conditions the vapor is in equilibrium with the liquid or solid. A vapor in equilibrium is said to be saturated, and the equilibrium pressure is called the *vapor pressure*, which for a given substance depends only on

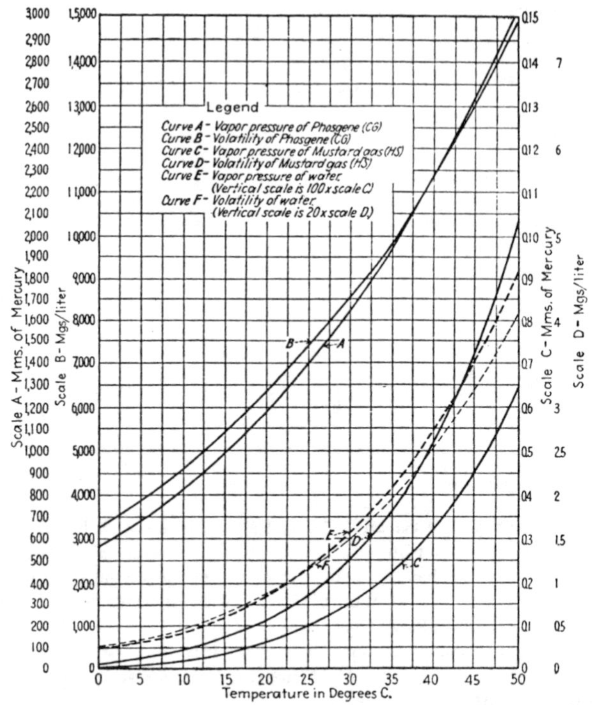

CHART I.—Typical vapor pressure and volatility curves for nonpersistent (CG) and persistent (HS) gases.

the temperature. If the vapor is not allowed to accumulate over the liquid or solid, it will remain unsaturated, equilibrium will not be reached, and the liquid will gradually disappear by evaporation. This is the usual case with chemical-warfare agents that are dispersed over the ground as liquids. No general relation is known connecting the vapor pressure and temperature, but curves showing this relationship have been determined by observation for a great number of chemical substances[10] that are liquids at ordinary temperatures. For purposes of comparison, the vapor-pressure–temperature curves for two of the most typical chemical agents, including the curve of water, are shown in Chart I.

Persistency is the length of time a chemical agent remains effective at the point of its release. If a gas remains in sufficient concentration to require protection of any kind at the end of 10 *minutes*, it is classed as *persistent*. If the concentration at the end of 10 minutes is too weak to require any protection, the gas is classed as *nonpersistent*. This is the American rule, but is not the same in other countries. In some foreign countries three classes of persistency are recognized, as follows:

Nonpersistent.
Moderately persistent.
Very persistent.

In such classifications the nonpersistent class is essentially the same as ours, while the moderately persistent and very persistent classes are in reality subdivisions of our persistent class. The advantage of such subdivision of the persistent class of gases is not apparent, as will be brought out in our further discussion of the subject of persistency.

The most important properties of a casualty-producing gas are toxicity and persistency, for upon the first depends its inherent power to incapacitate, and upon the second depends the extent of time during which the gas is effective in the field. The persistency of a gas also measures the length of time that must elapse before unprotected troops may occupy infected ground; thus it greatly influences the proper tactical use of the gas. As toxicity and persistency are not simple properties, but are functions which involve several other properties of a gas, they will be further considered at this point.

TOXICITY

Chemical agents have a wide range of toxicity, varying from simple local irritation, such as lacrimation, to fatal systemic poisoning, as from hydrocyanic acid. The measure of this toxicity, in terms of physiological reaction, may be determined with considerable scientific accuracy, not only within the laboratory, but also under the widely varying conditions encountered on the field of battle. Toxicities, thus established, furnish a criterion by which the most important agents of chemical warfare are judged and their tactical uses formulated. Since a general knowledge of the toxicity of agents is necessary to any comprehensive study of chemicals in war, a brief survey of the subject is presented at this point.

At the outbreak of the World War, German scientific research had produced, as a by-product of their chemical industry, extensive data on the toxicities of chemical substances.[11] From these data, many chemical compounds were selected and tried out in military operations between 1915 and 1918. The majority of these substances were eventually discarded because the actual results obtained in the field failed to measure up to theoretical expectations. Yet the experience thus gained not only increased knowledge of the absolute toxicities of many chemical compounds, but also permitted the formulation of definite relations between the various factors entering into the problem, so that basic principles could be deduced and the whole subject established on a scientific foundation.

While the study of this field of toxicology has, since the war, engaged the attention of scientists generally, the interest and talent devoted to this subject in Germany continues to command respect. It is, therefore, believed that the German viewpoint on toxicity of war gases deserves consideration and we accordingly follow with some freedom the presentations of German authorities in this field, notably those of Drs. Haber, Flury, Meyer and Buscher.

The effects of chemical agents upon the human organism result either from internal contact, as inhalation, or from external contact with various body surfaces. Chemicals such as dichlordiethyl sulfide (mustard gas) combine both of these types of effect. Yet the two must be approached independently before cumulative toxicity may be quantitatively determined.

Considering first those agents whose vapors when inhaled produce deleterious internal reactions, it is found that a definite relation exists between the concentration of vapor present in the air, the amount of such contaminated air that is admitted into the body, and the toxic effect produced upon the body. This relation has been established by Haber as follows:

Most toxic substances on contact with the body react chemically with the living tissues and destroy them by forming chemical combinations therewith. The degree of intoxication or poisonous effect is proportional to the chemical reaction of the toxic substance on the body tissues. This reaction is a function of three independent variables:

1. The time of exposure to the toxic substance.
2. The concentration of the toxic substance.
3. The concentration of the living material (body tissues).

Let c = the concentration of the vapors or droplets of the toxic substance in the air, expressed in milligrams per cubic meter,
v = volume of air breathed in, per minute,
t = time of exposure to the contaminated atmosphere, in minutes,
G = weight of the body, in kilograms;

then the quantity of poison inhaled and generally retained in the body would be[12]

$$ctv \tag{1}$$

and the degree of intoxication or poisoning, I, is

$$I = \frac{ctv}{G} \tag{2}$$

Death occurs when the degree of intoxication, I, equals a constant critical limit, W, which is specific for each kind of animal and for each toxic substance, *i.e.*, when

$$\frac{ctv}{G} = W \qquad (3)$$

In general, the amount of air inspired per minute is proportional to the body weight of the higher animals, so that the ratio v/G is constant for a given species and may be written as unity for the purposes of comparing the toxicities of gases on the same kind of animals. Then

$$ct = W \qquad (4)$$

The product $ct = W$ is called the *product of mortality* (*Tödlichkeitsprodukt*) or the *lethal index* of the particular toxic substance for the given animal. This product W varies inversely as the toxicity of the toxic substance, *i.e.*, the smaller the value of W, the more toxic is the substance.

By taking a large number of observations on various animals exposed to constant concentrations of toxic gases for definite periods of time under carefully controlled conditions and tabulating the mortality results, it has been found that the relation between the minimum lethal dose and time of exposure follows a definite curve for each toxic gas. Chart II shows this curve for phosgene on dogs and expresses the concentration required for each length of exposure in order to produce death. Such curves are generally known as toxicity curves and the form of curve shown in Chart II is typical of all such curves, and illustrates the tremendous increase in concentration required when the time of exposure is reduced below 10 minutes. For this reason, it is customary to base relative toxicity figures on 10 minutes for short exposures and 30 minutes for long exposures.

Upon examining internal physiological reactions to toxic vapors, it appears that some differentiation must be made between those substances characterized by *local* effects as distinguished from those that induce general *systemic* poisoning. Compounds of the latter category, such as carbon monoxide and hydrocyanic acid, are in part neutralized by certain physiological counterreactions, and their reactions with the body tissues are reversible up to a certain point. To allow for this

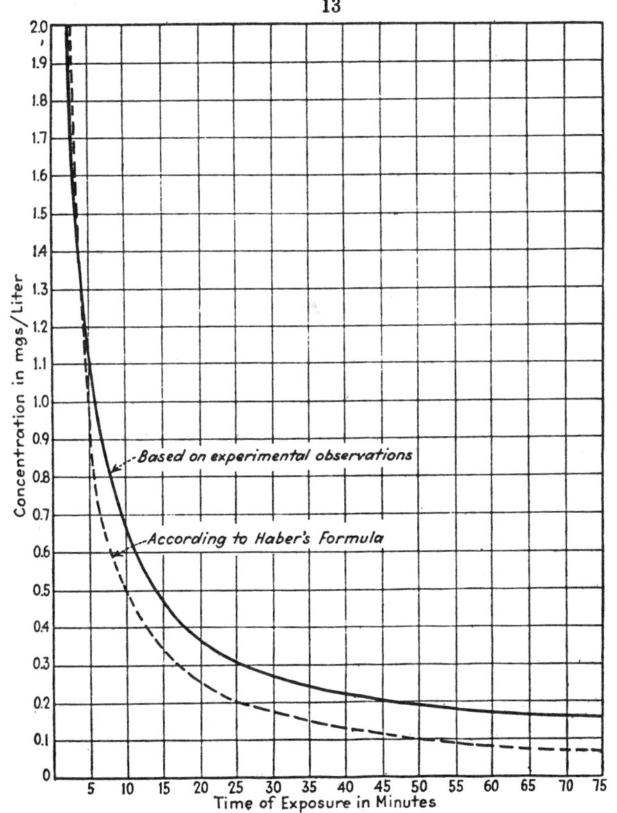

CHART II.—Toxicity curve for phosgene (on dogs).

phenomenon it is necessary to insert an "elimination factor," e, in the Haber formula, which then reads

$$(c - e) \times t = W \qquad (5)$$

Here the relation between c and e demands a critical density of concentration below which systemic poisons are noneffective, and the observed data confirm this result.

In accordance with these formulas, toxicity data are experimentally determined by closely observing the physiological reactions of test

animals under carefully controlled experimental conditions. While the effects on the higher animals are not in all cases absolutely parallel with human reactions, they do furnish valuable relative toxicological data as between various chemical agents. The following table presents lethal indices so computed for certain well-known chemical substances.

RELATIVE TOXICITY FROM INHALATION
(After Haber)

Agent	Lethal Index
Irreversible Reactions	
Phosgene	450
Diphosgene	500
Lewisite	1,500
Mustard gas	1,500
Chlorpicrin	2,000
Ethylsulfuryl chloride	2,000
Ethyldichlorarsine	3,000
Ethylbromacetate	3,000
Phenylcarbylamine chloride	3,000
Chloracetone	3,000
Benzyl iodide	3,000
Methyldichlorarsine	3,000
Acrolein	3,000
Diphenylchlorarsine	4,000
Diphenylcyanarsine	4,000
Bromacetone	4,000
Chloracetophenone	4,000
Benzyl bromide	6,000
Xylyl bromide	6,000
Brombenzyl cyanide	7,500
Chlorine	7,500
Reversible Reactions	
Hydrocyanic acid	1,000–4,000*
Carbon monoxide	70,000*

* The lethal indices of the *systemic* poisons depend upon the degree of concentration c, and the product $c \times t$ for these compounds is therefore not constant.

From the above table it appears that fatalities result from normal inhalation for 1 minute in an atmosphere contaminated with a concentration of 450 mg. of phosgene per cubic meter of air. The deadliness of agents of the phosgene type is further emphasized by the fact that they may be equally effective in smaller quantities when inhaled over longer periods, which does not hold true with the systemic toxics, such as hydrocyanic acid and carbon monoxide. In the case of phosgene, the absolute quantity of vapor required to produce death (toxicity index 450) is about 3.6 mg., based on a normal inspiration of 8 liters of air per minute, or $8 \times {}^{450}\!/_{1000} = 3.6$. Generally speaking this quantity of phosgene vapor introduced into the lungs will, as Flury (5) indicates, cause death even when inspired more slowly in a concentration corre-

spondingly lighter than 450 mg. per cubic meter. The absolute quantity of hydrocyanic acid, according to the foregoing toxicity index, averages 20 mg.; but as dilution increases, the toxicity of gaseous hydrocyanic acid falls off rapidly, until at 0.03 gram per cubic meter the human organism is able finally to counteract wholly its toxicity; thus concentrations below this strength become actually innocuous. Considering the extreme volatility of carbon monoxide and hydrocyanic acid, and the resulting impracticability of creating effective concentrations of their vapors in the field, it is evident that these chemicals, while commonly regarded as highly poisonous, are unsuited to military usage.

The foregoing toxicity figures must be accepted with reservations, as they apply to one set of conditions only, *i.e.*, to one animal (the cat) and to one rate of breathing. While experimental determinations of toxicity on animals yield valuable relative data as to certain classes of toxic agents, these data cannot always be applied to man, because certain animals are more sensitive to certain gases than man and others are less so. Also the rate of breathing is a very important factor. Thus, a man at rest breathes on an average about 8 liters of air per minute, but, if he is exercising moderately, he will breathe 32 liters of air per minute, and with violent exercise he will breathe at a proportionally greater rate. Hence, when exposed to a toxic atmosphere of a certain concentration for the same length of time, he will take in four times as much poison when moderately exercising as when at rest. Body weight is another factor, for, in general, the larger the body, the greater the amount of a toxic substance required to produce the same degree of intoxication. Because of these factors, it is more accurate to state the specific amount of the toxic agent that will cause death when absorbed into the body. But such a criterion is impracticable of application in the field, and so an average constant concentration is assumed over a fixed time of exposure—usually 10 to 30 minutes for nonpersistent gases.

For comparison with the German toxicity data presented in the foregoing tabulation, the American data in the table on page 16, show the quantities of gases required to produce fatal effects on 10 minutes' exposure.

The wide discrepancy between the German and American toxicity data is strikingly shown in this tabulation. This discrepancy has been attributed to various causes, such as that the German data were based on cats, while most of the American data were based on dogs and mice; that cats are peculiarly susceptible to some gases and resistant to others; that the cats used in the German tests during the war were undernourished, and therefore less than normally resistant; that the degree of activity, and therefore the rates of breathing, may have been widely different in the German and American tests. While the subnormal

16

condition of the German test cats would tend to explain partially the generally higher toxic effects obtained in the German experiments (*i.e.*, generally lower lethal indices), none of the reasons advanced are sufficient to explain the great number of widely divergent results.

Lethal Concentrations of Gases
(10 Minutes' Exposure)

Agent	American data		German data
	Mg. per liter	Lethal index	Lethal index
Phosgene	0.50	5,000	450
Diphosgene	0.50	5,000	500
Lewisite	0.12	1,200	1,500
Mustard gas	0.15	1,500	1,500
Chlorpicrin	2.00	20,000	2,000
Ethylsulfuryl chloride	1.00	10,000	2,000
Ethyldichlorarsine	0.50	5,000	3,000
Ethylbromacetate	2.30	23,000	3,000
Phenylcarbylamine chloride	0.50	5,000	3,000
Chloracetone	2.30	23,000	3,000
Benzyl iodide	3.00	30,000	3,000
Methyldichlorarsine	0.75	7,500	3,000
Acrolein	0.35	3,500	3,000
Diphenylchlorarsine	1.50	15,000	4,000
Diphenylcyanarsine	1.00	10,000	4,000
Bromacetone	3.20	32,000	4,000
Chloracetophenone	0.85	8,500	4,000
Benzyl bromide	4.50	45,000	6,000
Xylyl bromide	5.60	56,000	6,000
Brombenzyl cyanide	0.35	3,500	7,500
Chlorine	5.60	56,000	7,500
Hydrocyanic acid	0.20	2,000	1,000–4,000
Carbon monoxide	5.00	50,000	70,000

One of the difficulties is to be found in the form of the observed toxicity curve shown in Chart II. By selecting various times of exposure, finding the corresponding minimum lethal doses from the curve, and multiplying these figures by each other, we obtain the variations in the lethal index for phosgene as shown in the table on page 17.

Thus, by increasing the time of exposure from 2 to 75 minutes, we find that the lethal index increases threefold, whereas, according to Haber's formula, the lethal index should remain constant, irrespective of the time of exposure. The theoretical toxicity curve for phosgene,

17

according to Haber's Formula, is shown in dotted lines on Chart II, based on American data (*i.e.*, 0.5 mg. per liter on 10 minutes' exposure). A comparison of the two curves on Chart II shows that, while the observed data follow in general Haber's Formula, there is not a sufficiently close agreement to maintain a constant lethal index.

Time of exposure, minutes	Minimum lethal dose, Mg. per liter	Lethal index
2	2.00	4,000
5	1.10	5,500
10	0.65	6,500
15	0.46	6,900
20	0.37	7,400
25	0.30	7,500
30	0.27	8,100
45	0.20	9,000
60	0.17	10,200
75	0.16	12,000

While the difficulty mentioned in the foregoing paragraphs would account for such differences in the lethal index as are shown for certain agents, such as ethyldichlorarsine, phenylcarbylamine chloride, and methyldichlorarsine, it is altogether inadequate to explain the other large discrepancies shown above, which in many cases are as much as tenfold.

Many chemical-warfare agents are not fatal in concentrations encountered in the field and their combat value is due to their irritant action on the body. One group of irritant substances act primarily on the eyes and are commonly known as *lacrimators;* others attack the nose and throat and are generally termed *respiratory irritants,* or *sternutators:* a few have special selective effects against other organs such as the ears (termed *labyrinthic agents* by the French). Also many lethal agents have an irritant effect far below their lethal concentrations.

All irritant agents, regardless of their special physiological action, have an *intolerable limit,* which means the maximum concentration that an *unprotected* man can endure without physical incapacitation, for the period of time considered. Usually this period is 1 minute.

The intolerable limits for the majority of irritant agents as determined by investigators in different countries are in much closer agreement than toxicity determinations, most of the differences being well within experimental error.

The following tabulation shows the intolerable limits of the principal irritant agents and agents of other classes having an irritant effect:

18

Limits of Human Tolerance for Irritants

Agent	CWS symbol	Mg. per liter
Diphenylcyanarsine	CDA	0.00025
Diphenylaminechlorarsine	DM	0.0004
Lewisite	MI	0.0008
Mustard gas	HS	0.0010
Diphenylchlorarsine	DA	0.0012
Chloracetophenone	CN	0.0045
Bromacetone	BA	0.0100
Ethyldichlorarsine	ED	0.0100
Ethyliodoacetate	.....	0.0150
Xylyl bromide	.....	0.0150
Phosgene	CG	0.0200
Methyldichlorarsine	MD	0.0250
Phenylcarbylamine chloride	.....	0.0250
Brombenzyl cyanide	CA	0.0300
Benzyl iodide	.....	0.0300
Ethylbromacetate	.....	0.0400
Methylsulfuryl chloride	.....	0.0400
Dichlormethyl ether	.....	0.0400
Diphosgene	.....	0.0400
Ethylsulfuryl chloride	.....	0.0500
Chlorpicrin	PS	0.0500
Acrolein	.....	0.0500
Dibrommethyl ether	.....	0.0500
Benzyl bromide	.....	0.0600

Cyanogen bromide	.....	0.0600
Cyanogen chloride	.....	0.0610
Perchlormethylmercaptan	.....	0.0700
Chlorine	Cl	0.1000
Chloracetone	.....	0.1000

Of these compounds, diphenylcyanarsine appears to exert the greatest irritant effect, since only 0.00025 mg. of this gas per liter of air is intolerable after 1 minute, and 0.00000001 *gram per liter of air* proves decidedly disagreeable.

From what has been said above, it is evident that high toxicity, while an important factor, does not solely determine the utility of warfare gases. An irritant agent of even low intrinsic toxicity becomes extremely effective when not countered by the protection of the gas mask, so that some sacrifice of toxicity value is clearly warranted if this serves to circumvent or increase the burden of protection. Thus, forcing the enemy to mask frequently becomes an end in itself, which is attained positively and most efficiently by the irritant nonlethal gases.

PERSISTENCY

Persistence is, in general, an expression for the length of time during which a chemical agent remains and exerts its effect on the place where it has been released. The physical properties of a substance are nearly always the determining factors in its persistence.

In considering persistence, we distinguish two groups of chemical agents:

1. Pure *gases, e.g.,* Cl and CG and toxic smokes (DA and DM).
2. *Liquids* and *solids, e.g.,* HS and M-1.

In the case of substances of the *first* group, the entire amount of the combat chemical is distributed over the target area and there is none on the ground in liquid or solid form. If it is later deposited on the ground, as is sometimes the case with toxic smokes, it plays no important role. Since these true gases are completely distributed in and float with the air, they have about the same persistency as the air with which they are mixed. They follow completely every current of air and, if a layer of air which has been over the target area moves away, the chemical agents of this group follow its course. There are, however, always small differences in the persistence of these substances.

The pure gases (Cl, CG) are heavier than the air, and so they have a tendency to sink into depressions in the ground and remain for a time in the form of gas pockets in the deep spots where the air currents cannot easily penetrate and carry them further away. But, even in a complete calm, they diffuse from these sheltered places and gradually become harmless through dilution with air.

The toxic smokes (DA, DM) sink finally to the ground, as does every smoke, with a speed which is proportionate to the size of the smoke particles. Once on the ground, they can no longer rise and, like ordinary dust, they are carried away by the atmospheric precipitations.

But both the diffusion of the pure gases and the fall of the smoke particles proceed so comparatively slowly that these factors play no essential part as compared with the diffusing and dividing effect of the vertical and horizontal air currents. The persistence of the chemical agent of this group depends, therefore, chiefly on the conditions of wind and, so far as the wind is affected by the lay of the land and its covering, on these factors also. It is thus easily seen that deep depressions in the ground or thick high-standing forests may considerably increase the persistence of the materials.

In the case of the materials of the *second* group (HS, M-1), the persistence is considerably greater than it is with the first group, yet it varies greatly according to the specific properties of each substance. Most of the materials of this kind are liquids, which on the explosion

of the shell in which they are placed are sprayed out over the terrain in large or small drops, whence they evaporate into the air layers above the ground. As long as there is liquid chemical material on the ground, it is a constant source of replacement for the evaporated portion of the material, which has been thinned down or carried away by the air currents. The air is constantly contaminated anew with toxic or irritant gases. Similar to the liquid chemical agents are some agents which in the open air evaporate without first becoming liquid (*e.g.,* CA).

For tactical considerations, it is of decisive importance to know how long this process continues on a target area that has been covered with gas. If we leave out of consideration, at first, the ordinary external influences, then it appears that, above all else, the air temperature is the determining factor.

Chemical agents volatilize with a rapidity proportional to the temperature of the air, but in this they show great differences among themselves. For example, HS volatilizes in the cold so slowly that the air above the contaminated ground often does not contain enough of the vapor to endanger respiration. In summer it always vaporizes fast enough, yet so economically that it may persist on the contaminated ground under favorable conditions for three weeks or longer. On the other hand, CG volatilizes so quickly that an open country treated with it may be entered without danger a quarter of an hour to half an hour later.

The physical reasons for the great differences in the persistence of chemical agents are to be found in the fact that these substances have very different vapor pressures and in the degree to which these pressures vary on change of temperature. The higher the vapor pressure at a given temperature of the air, the less persistence at that temperature. But the rapidity of volatilization of a chemical, which alone gives an objective measure for its persistence, is not simply proportionate to the vapor pressure, but has a complicated dependence on other decisive factors.

A more satisfactory basis for gauging the persistence of the combat materials is a table of the reciprocal values of rapidity of volatilization which serves as a table of the relative persistence of the chemical agents. For purposes of comparison, the rapidity of volatilization of water at 15°C., is assumed to be 1.

The reciprocal values of the rapidity of volatilization are taken because the persistency of a combat material is greater in proportion as its rapidity of volatilization is small; water was selected as the material for comparison because the rapidity of its volatilization, by observation, has come within the experience of everyone. Computing the rapidity of the volatilization from the vapor pressure was accomplished by the

inversion of a process which, in principle, was first applied by the American physicist Langmuir (*Phys. J.,* vol. 14, p. 1273) in the formula

$$S = \frac{c_1}{c} = \frac{p_1}{p}\sqrt{\frac{M_1 T}{M T_1}}$$

In this formula S signifies the persistency of the chemical agent, c_1 the rapidity of volatilization of water at 15°C., c the rapidity of volatilization of the chemical at the absolute temperature T, p_1 the vapor pressure of water at 15°C., p the vapor pressure of the substance at the temperature T, M_1 the molecular weight of the water, M that of the substance, T the absolute temperature of the air, T_1 the absolute temperature corresponding to the Celcius temperature of 15°.

Persistency of Some Typical Chemical Agents
(That of Water at 15° Assumed as 1)

Chemical agent	Physical state	Temperature, °C.								
		−10	−5	0	5	10	15	20	25	30
CA	Solid	6,930	4,110	2,490	1,530	960	610	395	260	173
	Liquid	(2,720)	(1,830)	(1,250)	(860)	(600)	(427)	(307)	(222)	(163)
HS	Solid	2,400	1,210	630	333	181	Melts at 13.9°C.			
	Liquid	(1,162)	(690)	(418)	(258)	(162)	103	67	44	29
M-1	Liquid	96.0	63.1	42.1	28.5	19.6	13.6	9.6	6.9	5.0
Diphosgene	Liquid	2.7	1.9	1.4	1.0	0.7	0.5	0.4	0.3	0.2
PS	Liquid	1.36	0.98	0.72	0.54	0.4	0.3	0.23	0.18	0.14
CG	Liquid	0.014	0.012	0.010	0.008	Boils at 8.02°C.				

In the case of CA and HS, under the normal melting point, are given in brackets the persistency of the liquid phases. These materials, especially the first, are obstinately inclined to remain liquid when cooled below the freezing point. Moreover, the freezing point of the commercial product, on account of the unavoidable impurities contained therein, is of itself lower than that of the chemically pure compound.

The use of the table is shown by the following examples. Liquid HS has, at 15°C., a persistence of 103; liquid CA has a persistence of 427. This means that the first material under otherwise similar conditions (similar average size of drops, similar wind conditions, etc.), takes 103 times as long to disappear from the ground by evaporation as an equal mass of water, and CA is $^{427}/_{103}$, or about four times, as persistent as HS.

Diphosgene and phosgene are also two materials which are chemically closely related. But the difference in persistence between them is an important factor in their tactical use. This can be compared directly, as a rule, only under 8°C. (the boiling point of phosgene). Above this

22

temperature, phosgene no longer exists as a liquid under atmospheric pressure, but changes into a heavy gas which seeks a way through uneven lands, partly following its own weight, partly the air currents. In level country, it moves only with the wind. Under 8°, phosgene can exist as a liquid in the open, but even at 10° the persistence of diphosgene is 100 times greater than that of phosgene.

HS and M-1 are likewise two materials of very similar physiological effect, distinguished by the vesicant effect on the skin which they produce, especially when they are in liquid condition. But their persistence is quite different. In summer HS has a persistence seven to eight times greater than that of M-1. This is a well-known disadvantage of M-1 in most of the tactical uses for these materials, and it is still further emphasized by the fact that M-1 easily undergoes chemical decomposition in warm weather if moisture is present, which is often the case at this season. But in winter M-1 is superior to HS, as we shall see. The difference of the persistence of the two materials is greater then than it is in summer, for HS freezes; as a solid body, it does not moisten the uniforms, clings to them less, and cannot work through them to the skin. M-1, however, remains fluid even in winter and, moreover, its persistence increases to the degree possessed by HS in summer. So HS may be called a summer gas and M-1 a winter gas.

CA, a lacrimator, is, so far as concerns persistence, the king of all the combat materials. The great persistence which it attains in low temperatures has a limited value, however, as its rapidity of evaporation is then so small that the air, in movement, does not become sufficiently charged with the vapor of the material and so cannot exert a satisfactory physiological effect. Even in summer, the persistence of CA is so great that it is frequently too long for most of the tactical uses of an irritant agent. For this reason, the Americans prefer CN, another irritant that has other advantages also, such as simple preparation and compounding with explosive materials. On the explosion of the shell, it vaporizes. The vapor exercises intense physiological irritation, but it disappears quickly from the air of the combat terrain for, on its further attenuation (on account of the negative specific heat of the saturated vapor), it precipitates and falls to the ground where, owing to very slow evaporation, it exercises no effect worthy of note.

In the above tabulation all data are based on the rapidity of evaporation of water at 15°C., without making any assumption as to the absolute time of evaporation. Different influences play a weighty role on the length of time that passes before a chemical agent, placed on a terrain, is completely volatilized.

First, the average size of the surface of the drops of the chemical, which are sprinkled over the terrain, is of some significance. The

23

greater this surface is, the quicker, as a rule, volatilization will take place. But in this regard it appears that the difference between most of the liquid chemical agents is not considerable. This is due to the fact that their surface tensions, as measured in the laboratory, are about equal. But the chemical agents can be scattered in very different sized drops by varying the amount of explosive material in the shells. Very large drops will be divided up into very small drops in their flight through the air and when they strike the ground. On the other hand, small drops unite and form large ones through constant contacts which take place among their great number. So there results a fairly constant average size for the drops, which makes it possible to disregard the influence exerted by the size of the drops in rough estimates.

But it is different with the influence of the weather, of the ground formation, and of the covering. These factors can naturally affect greatly the rapidity of volatilization. We can estimate their effect approximately only by empirical rules.

If we compare the data that may be deduced from war experience, which in general agree fairly well with the figures in the above tabulation, the following conclusion may be drawn:

The persistence of a chemical agent in dry weather and on open even ground, for the duration of 1 hour, is taken as the unit of persistence in the figures of the above tabulation. In greatly cut up land, double value is to be assigned; in heavy forest, three times the value.

It must be noticed that heavy or continuous rain brings a premature end of the persistence of the chemical agents that are clinging to the ground, by washing them away; a heavy snow fall makes them ineffective by covering them over with a thick layer of snow. Where precipitation is frequent, persistencies of more than two or three weeks are seldom realized, if we except house ruins and similar places which are protected from the weather.

Summary.—The method developed above for determining the persistence of chemical agents makes it possible:

1. To form a dependable judgment in regard to the persistence of even those chemicals, concerning which no war or other practical experiences are available;
2. To take into consideration, as accurately as desired, the temperature of the air, which, next to air currents, exerts the most important tactical influence of the day on the persistence of the chemical agents.

EFFECT OF WEATHER ON CHEMICAL WARFARE

While chemical agents are influenced by weather conditions more than any other weapons, this does not mean that the occasions on which chemicals may be used in battle are limited to favorable weather. Cloud gas released from cylinders is the only form of chemical attack that cannot

24

be launched with some degree of effectiveness in almost any weather in which combat takes place. However, weather conditions do largely influence the form and technique of chemical attack and are frequently the deciding factor in the success or failure of the undertaking. Hence, a thorough understanding of the effect of weather conditions on the employment of chemicals is essential to a successful use of chemicals in war.

The Six Weather Elements.—The weather at any particular time and place is completely determined by the following:

Wind.
Precipitation.
Temperature.
Pressure.
Clouds.
Humidity.

Since weather is the condition of the atmosphere at any time and place, it is best described by giving numerical values for its elements. These six elements will be taken up and considered separately. Chemical-warfare operations are more or less concerned with all of them. For example, the factors influencing gas or smoke clouds are, in order of importance: (1) wind, under which should be considered the direction, steadiness, and velocity of the wind, and eddy currents due to the proximity of woods, uneven terrain, etc.; (2) precipitation; (3) temperature; (4) pressure; (5) clouds; (6) humidity. The effectiveness of all smokes is greatly increased by high humidity; on the other hand, high humidity tends to destroy some of the irritant agents by hydrolysis. Cloudiness has a very marked effect on the rise of smoke clouds. The persistency of agents is largely dependent upon temperature and wind velocity. So it will be seen that no chemical-warfare operation can be considered without reference to the weather elements.

The numerical values of the weather elements are by no means constant, but are always undergoing change or variations.

WIND

Air in motion near the earth's surface and nearly parallel to it is called *wind*. All other motions of masses of air should be spoken of as air currents. In connection with wind there are three things to be determined or measured, *viz.*, the direction, the velocity, and the gustiness.

Direction.—The wind is named for the direction from which it comes; thus, if the air moves from the north toward the south, it is called a *north* wind.

25

In noting wind direction, eight points of the compass are used, *viz.*, the cardinal points, north, south, east, and west, and the four intermediary points, northwest, southwest, northeast, and southeast. The magnetic azimuth of winds is sometimes used in chemical-warfare operations.

Wind direction can be determined in the field by measuring with a compass the direction of drift of smoke or of dust thrown into the air and adding 180 degrees. It can also be determined by means of a portable wind vane previously oriented by compass, or by taking the magnetic azimuth from the wind vane to a point indicated by its arrow.

Velocity.—Wind velocity can be estimated by using the following table:

Titles	Description	Meters per second	Miles per hour
Calm	Calm, smoke rises vertically	Less than 0.3	Less than 1
Light air	Direction of wind shown by smoke drift but not by wind vanes	0.3–1.5	1–3
Slight breeze	Wind felt on face; leaves rustle; ordinary vane moved by wind	1.6–3.3	4–7
Gentle breeze	Leaves and small twigs in constant motion; wind extends light flag	3.4–5.4	8–12
Moderate breeze	Sways branches of trees, blows up dust from the ground, and drives leaves and paper rapidly before it	5.5–9.8	12–22
Fresh breeze	This sways whole trees, blows twigs and small branches along the ground, raises clouds of dust, and hinders walking somewhat	9.9–14.3	23–32
High wind	This breaks branches, loosens bricks from chimneys, etc., litters the ground with twigs and branches of trees, and hinders walking decidedly	14.4–32.2	33–72
Hurricane	Complete destruction of almost everything in its path	32.2 on	72 on

Wind velocity can be measured by means of an anemometer and a watch. The anemometer measures the distance in meters traveled by the wind in the space of time measured by the watch. Thus, if in 1 minute the anemometer registers 606 meters, the wind has traveled 606 meters in 60 seconds or

$$606 \div 60 = 10.1 \text{ meters per second}$$

$$\text{Meters per second} \times 2.237 = \text{miles per hour}$$

$$\text{Miles per hour} \times 0.447 = \text{meters per second}$$

26

Wind velocity increases markedly with altitude. This will often be noted in observing the travel of smoke clouds. The higher velocity above the ground sometimes causes a rolling movement of the top of the cloud and the top is carried forward faster than the body of the cloud. The increase in velocity with altitude is very rapid in the first 100 to 200 ft., particularly over land.

The effects of surroundings on wind should be carefully considered in any local observation of direction and velocity.

Gustiness.—Wind, both as regards direction and velocity, is probably more affected by the immediate surroundings of the place at which observations are made than any other of the meteorological elements. There are four things to be especially considered: valleys, buildings, nature of the surface, and altitude. Valleys influence wind direction markedly and velocity to a slight extent. Valleys have a tendency to cause the wind to blow along their length. Buildings increase the wind velocity near them and also make the wind gusty. In fact, one result of all unevennesses in the surface over which air passes is to cause gusts. The nature of the surface also has a marked influence on wind velocity. On land the wind velocity is very much reduced near the earth's surface. This is brought about not only by friction but also by the intermingling of air masses and by the formation of eddies that result from the uneven surface. *Turbulence* may be defined as the sum of all the local air currents. It causes a complete mixing of the atmosphere and consequently the dilution of a gas or smoke cloud. *Steadiness* is the opposite of gustiness.

Effect of Wind on Chemical Warfare.—*Persistent agents* are used to saturate the surface of the ground and the vegetation and hence are not easily blown away. Winds have little effect on their use. Evaporation will be slightly increased by high winds, but the high winds blow the vapors away so rapidly that their effectiveness is not greatly increased.

Nonpersistent Agents.—With this class of agents the wind is of primary importance, especially if the method of propagation is by the use of cylinders. The three characteristics of the wind which are especially important are the *direction*, the *velocity*, and the *steadiness*.

1. *Direction.*—When cylinders or irritant candles are used, the direction of the wind must be such that it will carry the agent from our emplacement to the enemy's position without carrying it into any portion of our own position. When our own lines and the target for projectors or mortars are in close proximity, the wind direction is similarly of importance. When we are using chemicals from artillery shells, bombs, or airplanes, the direction may not be so important unless the action is long sustained with a wind toward our own troops. Then the fumes may be carried to our position and cause trouble.

27

2. *Velocity.*—When cylinders and irritant candles are used, the velocity should not be less than 3 miles per hour because winds having a lower velocity than this are likely to be gusty and variable. They may die down or even reverse and blow the agent back on our own troops. However, when the agent is delivered by artillery, mortars, projectors, or bombs, this lower limit of wind velocity need not be considered.

The velocity should not be over 12 miles per hour because winds having higher velocities than this tear the cloud apart and, immediately after the agent is released, mix it with large quantities of air (through turbulence) and cause the concentration to be lowered.

The higher the wind velocity, the faster a given wave or cloud will pass over the enemy's position, the shorter the time he will be exposed to it, and the less effective it will be. If a certain result is desired and if a high wind is blowing, more agent must be used.

It is clear from the foregoing that, in general, a low rather than a high wind velocity is to be desired in order that the cloud may stay over the enemy as long as possible and in order that economy in the use of agents may be practiced.

The higher wind velocities also tend to cause turbulence and eddies over trenches and valleys, causing the agent to rise and preventing it from penetrating into trenches and dugouts.

With high wind velocities the cloud may also be so torn apart that groups of the enemy will be left in gas-free "islands" and so escape its effect.

The upper limit of 12 miles per hour is just as important with artillery and projector shoots as it is with cylinder attacks, owing to the tendency of high winds to tear the clouds apart and disperse them before they have existed long enough to be effective.

The technical limit of 12 miles per hour is sufficiently high to prevent the enemy from running out of the cloud to safety. This becomes evident when we consider that a man at a brisk walk covers only 4 miles per hour, that a horse at a trot covers 8 miles per hour and at a gallop 12 miles per hour.

3. *Steadiness* is important both as to direction and velocity. The wind should maintain its direction and velocity over a wide front for at least as long as the chemical attack is to last. Otherwise, conditions will be gusty and squally and the gas cloud will be broken, whirled up into the air, and rarefied. For obvious reasons, the nearer the cloud approaches any portion of our own trenches, the steadier the wind should be.

Irritant Smoke Clouds and Screening Smokes.—Irritant smoke clouds may be generated from candles or from shells or bombs. In the first case, the same principles apply as were discussed under nonpersistent

28

clouds. Again in the two latter cases, only the upper wind-velocity limit need be considered, when the cloud might be dispersed or blown over the enemy too rapidly for sufficient effect.

Screening smokes may also be generated from candles, shells, bombs, or airplanes. When a smoke screen is generated from candles, the wind must be in the proper direction to accomplish the desired result. It must usually blow toward the enemy. Here again, and for the same reasons as stated above, the upper velocity limit should not be exceeded. The lower limit is not so important since, even if the wind did reverse itself, the screening smokes are harmless to personnel. Steadiness of the wind is important with screening smokes so the smoke cloud or screen will not be torn asunder, leaving gaps through which the enemy may see. Generally, variations in wind velocity are accompanied by variations in the wind direction, even as much as 180 degrees. Large wind-direction changes, occurring at rapid intervals, often produce turbulent conditions, especially if accompanied by large velocity changes.

The effect of varying winds makes successful screening difficult because of the breaks in the screen and the rapid dissipation of the smoke.

Convection currents, due to bright sunshine, lift the cloud high in the air and often prevent satisfactory screening.

Convection currents are not so strong in presence of high winds as in the cases of light winds because high winds rapidly mix the warm surface-heated air with the superimposed and surrounding cooler air and tend to prevent their development.

Wind and Safety Limits.—Since the successful use of nonpersistent agents is largely dependent on wind conditions, it is essential to establish rules governing the relation of the wind direction and velocity to the use of nonpersistent agents. Wind-direction limits are prescribed primarily in the interest of safety to friendly troops, while wind-velocity limits insure a reasonable chance of success in the operation. Safety precautions require wind limits for the portable cylinder, the irritant candle, the Livens projector, and the 4-in. chemical mortar.
They are not required for artillery weapons or for the 4.2-in. chemical mortar unless the range is less than 1,200 yd.

A general rule for the use of mustard gas and other highly persistent vesicants is as follows:

Let X = safe distance from our lines to near edge of target area,
A = depth of target area in direction of fire,
B = width of target area.

Then

$$X = \frac{A + B}{2} \text{ (but never less than 1,000 yd.)}$$

29

TEMPERATURE AND CLOUDS

Effect of Temperature on Chemical Warfare.—*Persistent agents* are much more effective when used in hot weather. Under these conditions there is sufficient vapor generated to cause skin and lung casualties. Hot weather without rising air currents gives the ideal temperature condition. Under cold-weather conditions the blister effect from the vapor is not obtained, although the agents will still cause casualties if personnel comes in actual contact with the chemical, as by walking through vegetation on which the agent has been sprayed.

Nonpersistent Agents.—In contrast to the effect on the persistent agents, high temperatures are a serious handicap to the use of nonpersistent agents. High temperatures cause the atmosphere near the ground to become heated, and thus lighter than the overlying and surrounding air. It then has a tendency to rise or be displaced by the cooler, heavier air, and rising or convection currents may be set up. These will cause the cloud or agent to rise rapidly over the heads of the enemy and to mix with large quantities of air, thus lowering both the persistency and the concentration. Convection currents are especially prevalent in the afternoon over dry or plowed ground or ground free from vegetation. On the other hand, on days when the temperature is low, the lower layers of the air will remain cool and there will be no tendency for an overturning of the atmosphere. The length of time that a definite amount of agent will give an effective cloud of a desired persistency and concentration is thus increased.

It may be said, then, that high temperatures which usually occur on bright sunny days usually produce conditions unfavorable to the success of nonpersistent gas attacks, and that the cooler parts of the day, such as from midnight to dawn, are the most favorable periods for gas attacks. Normally, the coldest part of the 24 hours occurs at approximately sunrise.

Irritant Smokes and Screening Smokes.—The smokes are comparatively free from the influence of atmospheric temperature insofar as the formation of the original cloud is concerned. The cloud once formed is affected in the same way as clouds of nonpersistent agents.

Temperature Effects at Night.—During the daytime the temperature over a limited area, say a square mile, is about the same unless there are marked changes in topography or soil. On days with much sunshine and a low wind velocity, the lower points, particularly those in narrow valleys, may be a few tenths of a degree warmer than the upper parts of the area. At night, the layer of air next to the ground grows colder and denser and drains like water into the valleys and places of low elevation. If the wind is unable to remove these pockets of cold air, a

30

marked variation in temperature over a limited area will be found. For every limited area, there will be a critical value of wind velocity, which for most areas is probably not far from 3 miles per hour. As long as the wind velocity remains higher than 3 miles per hour, these pockets of air will be removed and mixed with air at other points and no variation in temperature will be found. Since the question of variation in temperature depends upon the interplay between the drainage of colder air and the ability of the wind to remove these pockets of cold air, the variation will depend not only upon the elevation but also upon the openness of the valleys, their direction, the roughness of the surface, and the direction from which the wind comes.

Because of the tendency of surface air to cool and drain into valleys and depressions, such places in the vicinity of gassed areas will, on calm nights particularly, be likely to contain dangerous concentrations of toxic agents. This is a matter which should receive careful consideration in the disposition of troops near a gassed area.

Effects of Clouds on Chemical Warfare.—Clouds as meteorological formations have no direct effect on any chemical agent. It is through their effects upon other meteorological elements that they become important to the chemical-warfare officer. Clouds attain their effects through their control over temperature. They shut off the sun's rays and thus shield the surface of the earth from some of the heat of the sun. A clear hot sunshiny day has been described as one favorable to convection currents and to a rapid rise of the agent from the ground. An overcast or cloudy day is less favorable for the development of rising air currents, and hence the agent will stay near the surface of the earth for a longer period of time. A sunshiny day, then, is unfavorable to the success of chemical attacks and a cloudy day is favorable.

PRECIPITATION

Effects of Precipitation on Chemical Warfare. *Persistent Agents.*—Heavy rain is unfavorable to the successful use of any chemical agent. Under this weather condition the cloud of any agent will be washed from the air and beaten to the ground. Even the liquid agent, such as mustard, will be washed away, hydrolized, and destroyed.

Nonpersistent Agents.—The concentration of clouds of other agents such as phosgene and chlorine is immediately lowered by rain. Snow and hail, to a lesser extent, act in the same way.

Irritant Smokes.—These agents not being hydrolized, light rains and mists are not especially unfavorable and may even be of assistance in hiding the characteristic color of the cloud. Heavy precipitation, however, is unfavorable in the case of irritant smokes. Heavy rains wash the agent from the air in the same way that they clear the air of

31

other dust particles. Heavy snow will also remove toxic smokes from the air by coming in contact with the smoke particles and carrying them to the ground.

Screening Smokes.—For the same reasons that a high humidity is favorable for the use of the screening smokes, so also are light precipitation, fogs, and mists. These furnish the necessary water for the hydrolysis reaction. Also under conditions of fog, light rain, or mist, visibility will be very much restricted and hence the amount of screening smokes necessary to obtain a desired end will be reduced. This is due both to the obscuring power of the mist and to the increased efficiency of the smoke in the damp air. On the other hand, here again heavy precipitation tends to beat the smoke cloud down and wash it from the atmosphere.

Humidity

Humidity is defined as the state of the atmosphere as regards moisture. If the air were absolutely dry, its humidity would be spoken of as zero. It is the humidity, as much as the temperature, which makes one uncomfortable on a hot sultry day. A moist hot day in summer is much more oppressive than a dry hot day because the moisture in the atmosphere prevents that free evaporation of the perspiration from the human body which cools it. The cold is also more penetrating on a damp day than on a dry day. The reason is that the moisture makes the clothing a better conductor of heat and hence the body is cooled faster. *Absolute humidity* is defined as the actual quantity of moisture present in a given quantity of air. It may be expressed in grains per cubic foot or grams per cubic meter. By *relative humidity* is meant the ratio of the actual amount of water vapor present in the atmosphere to the maximum quantity it could hold without precipitation. Relative humidity is always expressed in percentage.

Effect of Humidity on Chemical Warfare. *Persistent Agents.*—The humidity of the air will have no appreciable effect on the persistent agents regardless of how they may be released.

Nonpersistent Agents.—The nonpersistent agents are very slightly hydrolized by water vapor in the air. Phosgene shows the greatest effect in this, but even it is not greatly attacked. Thus the first part of a phosgene cloud moving through an extremely damp atmosphere will have a slightly lower content of phosgene than the following portions of the cloud, but still the cloud as a whole will be effective.

Irritant Smokes.—These agents are not affected by the amount of water vapor in the air, since the agents hydrolize very slowly.

32

Screening Smokes.—These agents are made much more effective by a high absolute humidity in the surrounding air. Since the initial chemical reaction generally produces a compound which is readily hydrolized and which in being hydrolized is broken into still smaller particles, the cloud becomes more effective on damp days. It is not necessary in the field, however, to make measurements of the humidity because the other weather conditions favorable to smoke screens are usually accompanied by a sufficiently high humidity. If humidity is low and other conditions are favorable, a satisfactory screen may be maintained by firing a somewhat greater quantity of agent.

Atmospheric Pressure

The pressure of the atmosphere is simply the weight of the column of air above the station in question, extending to the limits of the atmosphere. Atmospheric pressure thus diminishes with elevation above the earth's surface because there is a smaller quantity of air to exert a downward pressure. We are probably less conscious of atmospheric pressure and its changes than of any of the other weather elements. In meteorological work the pressure of the atmosphere is usually expressed in terms of inches of mercury. Thus a pressure of 30 in. means that the pressure of the atmosphere is the same as the pressure exerted by a column of mercury 30 in. long.

Effects of Pressure on Chemical Warfare.—Pressure has no appreciable effect upon any of the chemical agents except insofar as it controls vertical air currents and winds. The winds tend to move from highs toward lows, and the greater the change in pressure, the stronger the winds which may be expected.

Rising air currents are unfavorable since they cause the cloud of agent to be carried upward, in spite of its weight, and to rise over the heads of the enemy and be carried away. Rising air currents are often formed when the pressure is low, and they tend to follow the center of the low area.

Descending air currents are to be desired. These are often found when the pressure is high, and they tend to accompany high areas in their movements. In the presence of these currents the air tends to carry the agent downward and thus holds the cloud close to the surface of the earth where it is most effective.

MILITARY APPLICATION

Now that the basic principles of chemical action have been broadly outlined, there remains to be considered the manner in which chemical agents are employed in battle.

33

Viewing the typical modern battlefield in panoramic plan, each military arm may be regarded as responsible for definite areas which are largely delimited by the ranges of the weapons of that arm. Infantry, for example, is directly concerned to a distance of say 1,000 yd. to its front, which is about as far as infantry rifles are practically effective. Chemical troops operate in the next zone out to about 2,500 yd. from the front lines. Light artillery can reach well beyond this limit and therefore is concerned with areas up to about 8,500 yd. beyond its own front lines. Beyond this zone the longer ranges of corps and army artillery come into play, extending the depth of attack to 15,000 yd. Attack aircraft employing chemicals usually cover the enemy's combat zone to a depth of about 15 miles. Bombardment aircraft are seldom utilized within the effective range limits of artillery, but beyond this may be employed so far as cruising radii permit (about 1,150 miles). Flanks are usually given over to mechanized cavalry, which may be expected to penetrate for considerable distances within enemy territory (see Diagram I, Chap. III). Weapons appropriate for the dispersion of chemical agents are characteristically employed in each of these distinct areas of military action.

Within their range (2,500 yd.), the special weapons of the chemical troops afford most effective and efficient means of laying down chemical concentrations. For this reason, chemical troops are attached to the front-line infantry units in the attack and render close support by accompanying them in the advance and treating the vital zone directly in front of the attack with concentrations of gas and smoke upon targets most threatening to the advancing infantry.

The zone next beyond that covered by chemical troops' weapons is treated by the divisional artillery with chemicals as well as high explosives. Medium and heavy artillery of the corps and army are then called upon to disperse gas and incendiary agents at longer ranges; aircraft utilize the same agents in operations which in most cases may be termed *self-completing, i.e.*, they are not dependent upon ground force for consolidation and exploitation. To support and supplement the action of mechanized cavalry, special chemical troops are attached and act as components of these units, dispersing smoke and both persistent and nonpersistent gases.

Means for employing of chemical agents in military operations are therefore characterized by considerable flexibility, and properly so, because the successful use of the chemicals in battle often hinges on natural and tactical circumstances not predictable long in advance. The infantry and cavalry are thus not encumbered by chemical weapons, but are supported within their immediate zones by the attachment of chemical units from higher tactical reserves when the need for them

34

arises; the supporting arms—artillery, air and chemical—are habitually provided with suitable chemical munitions which permit the establishment of appropriate concentrations of chemical agents in the areas with which they are particularly concerned.

So the chemical arm has been assimilated into the organic structure of modern armies without necessitating material changes in their basic organization. But the use of chemicals in combat has brought about the extension of military action into the fourth dimension, thus completing a cycle of evolution that has witnessed battles successively waged with fists, clubs, arrows, bullets, and molecules.

By means of molecular "bullets," man has finally learned the secret of waging war in such manner as to temper the blows of battle with something of the nicety of a skilled anesthetist. For, among chemical agents, it is actually practicable to select those that vary in effect all the way from simple lacrimation to quick death; it is thus within the range of possibility to conduct a virtually deathless war with chemicals—a result entirely beyond the scope of explosive munitions or any other military agents heretofore devised.

As to those gases that are potentially lethal, we know with certainty what the expectancy of fatalities per hundred casualties will be under any given conditions, while complete recoveries from nonfatal gas casualties are surprisingly high. In fact, the military value of chemicals derives not from their deadliness per se, but from their direct influence upon tactical situations, from their effect upon military units rather than on individuals.

The gradations with which this effect may be exerted are wide, thus affording a flexibility never previously attainable in weapons of warfare. The laws of diffusion and dilution of gases, and of the travel of gas clouds in the field, have been carefully determined and have been found to be as definite and exact as the laws of ballistics, so that, while effective concentrations of gases may be extended over wide areas, such concentrations may also be carefully delimited so as never to extend beyond the areas intended to be gassed. Moreover, within a specific area concentrations may be strengthened or reduced according to the nature of the task at hand. *Controlled effect*, resulting from technically correct application, is therefore a novel and outstanding characteristic of chemical warfare.

From this it follows as an underlying principle of chemical action that any sizable gas attack, delivered with due regard to tactical and technical considerations, may be depended upon to produce predictable military results. In subsequent chapters is to be found an elucidation of the corollary principle that the number of outright casualties so inflicted upon an opponent will be increasingly high in proportion to his deficiencies in gas discipline.

35

CHAPTER II

TECHNICAL AND TACTICAL REQUIREMENTS OF CHEMICAL AGENTS

The total number of compounds known to chemical science has been variously estimated at from 300,000 to 500,000. Of these, some 200,000 have been studied to the extent that their principal properties are of record (8). As nearly all chemical compounds exert some toxic effects (either local or general) upon the body, it is not possible to estimate with accuracy the total number of toxic substances. However, several thousands of compounds have such pronounced toxic properties as to bring them distinctly within the field of toxicology, and their toxic powers are well known.

From this vast field, over 3,000 chemical compounds were selected and investigated for use as chemical agents during the World War, but only about 30 were found suitable for actual use in the field. From this group, about a dozen were finally adopted and used extensively as war agents, and of these not more than half were notably successful. This may seem remarkable when it is recalled that the combined efforts of the world's leading chemists were intensively concentrated for nearly four years on the problem of finding and producing the most effective chemical agents. The reason for this apparent meager return for the effort expended is found in the many exacting requirements which a chemical substance must meet before it can qualify as a successful chemical-warfare agent.

These requirements may be logically considered in two groups—(1) technical and (2) tactical. The technical requirements are those concerned with the problems of quantity production and utilization in the various forms of chemical munitions; the tactical requirements are those involved in the effects produced on the field of battle.

TECHNICAL REQUIREMENTS

Since the technical requirements for chemical agents are common to all the classes, *i.e.*, gases, smokes, and incendiaries, these requirements will be considered without distinction as to class of agent.

Raw Materials.—To be effective in war, chemical agents must be used in enormous quantities, and hence the raw materials from which these agents are made must receive first consideration. It is obvious

36

that before a chemical substance is adopted for use in war, the raw materials from which it is manufactured must be available in the quantities required for, no matter how militarily effective a substance may be, it should not be adopted as a chemical agent unless it can be made in sufficient quantities from materials that are available under war conditions. Thus, if a chemical compound requires for its manufacture one or more ingredients which cannot be produced in quantities from domestic materials, dependence must be placed on importation from some foreign country. Such a source of supply may be cut off in war, for even neutral sources of supply will be unavailable if control of the sea or intervening land areas is lost.

For certain critical materials which are not required in prohibitive quantities and are stable in long storage, it is possible for a government to acquire in time of peace a sufficient stock to last through the duration of a war. Such cases will be exceptional, and we may therefore lay down as a first requirement that the raw materials for a chemical agent should be available from domestic sources. This requirement at once rules out a vast field of possible compounds depending upon the extent of the domestic resources of a country.

Ease of Manufacture.—Of hardly less importance than availability of raw materials is the next general consideration—ease of manufacture. No matter how effective a compound may be on the field of battle, if it is difficult to make, there is always the serious threat of failure of supply under war conditions. Complicated chemical processes require highly skilled personnel to carry them out successfully, and such personnel is difficult to make available when the whole industrial machinery is in high gear to meet mobilization demands. Moreover, special apparatus and equipment are frequently needed in the more complex chemical processes, often limiting production.

A classic example of the difficulties and delays, encountered in attempting to produce a chemical agent that involves a complicated process of manufacture, is mustard gas. Notwithstanding that a process of making mustard gas had been worked out by Victor Meyer years before the war, France was unable to manufacture mustard and use it in retaliation against the Germans for nearly a year while England did not use it until after 15 months of intensive effort. Even when the Allies did produce mustard gas they had to make it by a much simpler process than that used by the Germans.

Simplicity in production not only makes far less demands on the chemical industry but immensely simplifies the supply problem in war. Simple processes can easily be completely performed in one plant, thus avoiding unnecessary transfer of intermediates from one plant to another with the attendant confusion and difficulty of coordinating production.

37

Chemical Stability.—The next most important general requirement is perhaps chemical stability under all conditions of storage. Many compounds otherwise suitable for chemical warfare react with iron and therefore cannot be stored either in bulk in steel tanks, or in ordinary shells, bombs and other projectiles. This seriously detracts from the value of the compound for war purposes since it necessitates special linings of lead, porcelain, etc., in all containers and munitions into which the chemical is filled.

The most effective lacrimators used in the war were bromine compounds, and these were not stable in contact with iron and steel containers. Much time and effort was therefore expended in developing and producing special linings for all receptacles for these gases.

The production of satisfactory linings in this country proved to be such a formidable task that immediately after the war the United States Army developed a new tear gas (CN) which did not contain bromine and was stable in long storage under all conditions.

Hydrolysis.—Closely associated with chemical stability is the matter of hydrolysis. If a compound hydrolyzes in contact with water it not only greatly reduces its effectiveness in the field but seriously complicates its storage and loading into munitions. Since water vapor is always present in the atmosphere, compounds that hydrolize must be completely protected from contact with the air in storage and also special precautions must be taken in loading such chemicals into shells and other projectiles.

Thus, phosgene slowly hydrolyzes in contact with water; hence, when filling phosgene into shell, great care must be exercised that the cavity of the shell is absolutely dry before filling. Even water vapor from the air condensing on the inside walls of the shell may be sufficient to hydrolize the phosgene and break it down into hydrochloric acid which at once attacks the steel walls of the shell body.

Polymerization.—Another form of chemical instability which is frequently fatal to the use of a compound as a chemical agent is polymerization. When a chemical compound polymerizes, it usually changes into a substance which has radically different physical and physiological properties. Thus a chemical compound may be a very active lacrimator in one form while its polymer will have no lacrimatory power at all, so that, if polymerization occurs after filling into munitions, such a compound will be useless in the field. This was the difficulty with the French tear gas "Papite" used in the war. Chemically, "Papite" is acrolein (CH_2:-CHCHO) and is a rather powerful lacrimator in its primary form. In storage, however, it polymerizes into a secondary form which has little or no lacrimatory power. Hence this substance was subsequently abandoned as a chemical agent.

38

Dissociation.—An important requirement of a chemical agent, when used in projectiles, is capacity to withstand the heat and pressure of dispersion from strong thick-walled containers (such as artillery shell) without decomposition or dissociation.

In order properly to open an artillery shell and effectively release its chemical contents, a high-explosive charge is used. Upon explosion, temperatures as high as 3,000°C. are created while pressures as great as 80,000 lb. per square inch are generated in the shell. Many compounds that are perfectly stable at ordinary temperatures and pressures will break down and decompose under the high temperatures and pressures generated upon explosion of the bursting charge.

In some cases, the decomposition upon explosion may be complete, as when chlorpicrin is used with a large bursting charge. Here the loss is complete, and such compounds cannot be employed in projectiles which require heavy bursting charges to open them.

In other cases, only a partial destruction of the chemical filling results, as when too large a bursting charge is used with volatile gases, such as phosgene. But to the extent of the decomposition involved, the efficiency of the shell is lowered. To avoid such losses, a shell of lower tensile strength and a low-temperature type of explosive charge may be used. Such shell of cast iron and semisteel were employed by the British and French during the war. But the capacity of these shell was much less than that of the steel shell so that the net gain was not great. Another solution was the thin-walled steel shell which could be opened with a smaller explosive charge. In any case, however, compounds which tend to break down at elevated temperatures and pressures involve limitations and technical difficulties that make it very desirable to find substances that are unaffected by such conditions.

Another form of decomposition is inflammability. If a chemical filling ignites upon explosion and is consumed in flames, its physiological effect is lost; so it is obvious that a prime requisite of a chemical agent for use in bursting munitions is capacity to withstand the temperatures and pressures of explosion without dissociation through burning.

Physical State.—Chemical compounds may be either solids, liquids, or gases at ordinary temperatures. If gaseous at ordinary temperatures, it is essential that the compound be capable of being held in a liquid state under moderate pressures, since the quantity of a *gaseous* substance that can be contained in an ordinary projectile is negligible. Chlorine and phosgene are examples of substances that are gaseous at ordinary temperatures under atmospheric pressure, but these gases may be held in the liquid state under moderate pressures which can be maintained in ordinary projectiles. On the other hand, such compounds as hydrocyanic acid and carbon monoxide, while extremely toxic, cannot be liquefied

39

at ordinary temperatures with moderate pressures, and hence these gases cannot be used successfully in projectiles. Accordingly, we may lay it down as a basic requirement that chemical agents must either be solids or liquids at ordinary temperatures and under moderate pressures.

As between solid and liquid chemical agents, the solids are generally to be preferred as shell fillers since solids have many advantages over liquids in projectiles. If the chemical agent is a solid, the cavity in the projectile may be completely filled, as in the case of high-explosive filling, and there is then no difference in ballistic behavior between such chemical shell and H.E. shell. On the other hand, if the chemical agent is a liquid, the shell cavity cannot be completely filled but a certain percentage of empty space must be left in the shell to permit expansion of the liquid with rise in temperature. The void thus left in the shell affects its ballistic characteristics, and the general experience in the war showed that liquid-filled shell had to be fired with special range tables. But whether or not special range tables are required for liquid-filled shell, it is certain that the behavior in flight of liquid-filled shell differs from solid-filled shell. This difference is bound to be reflected in the dispersion of shots and the impact patterns obtained. This problem will be further considered in a later chapter on artillery shell.

Liquids have one possible advantage over solids as chemical fillings for projectiles in that they are generally more easily dispersed on the opening of the shell. As a rule, solids require a greater bursting charge to disperse them effectively, and the solid particles resulting do not disseminate into the surrounding air so readily as the vapors generated by liquid fillings.

Boiling Point.—Among the liquid chemical agents those with the higher boiling points and lower vapor pressures are preferred. In general, the higher the boiling point, the lower the vapor pressure at ordinary temperatures and the less the pressure generated in the container in storage. Hence, generally, a smaller void may be employed in filling the shell and less leakage is apt to occur in storage and handling. On the other hand, the higher the boiling point, the greater the explosive charge required effectively to disperse the substance, and the less chemical will be contained in the shell.

Another factor of great importance in connection with the boiling point is the difficulty of filling the shell. A chemical whose boiling point is below ordinary summer temperatures, *e.g.*, phosgene (b.p. 47°F.), must be artificially cooled and held below its boiling point during the filling operation. This requires refrigeration facilities for precooling the empty shell and bulk phosgene and greatly complicates the process of filling.

40

Melting Point.—While not so important as boiling point, the melting point of a chemical agent is often of considerable importance if this point occurs within the range of ordinary atmospheric temperatures. Thus, the melting point of pure mustard gas is about 57°F., so that mustard is a liquid in summer when the temperatures are above 57° and a solid in winter when the temperatures are below that point. In order to secure uniformity in ballistic effects and dispersion, it is necessary to keep the chemical filler in one physical state and, since it is impracticable to keep it as a solid above its melting point, it is necessary to keep it as a liquid at ordinary temperatures below its boiling point by the use of solvents. Concerning this use of solvents, Fries, gives the following interesting data from the World War:

> In order that the product (mustard gas) in the shell might be liquid at all temperatures, winter as well as summer, the Germans added from 10 to 30 per cent of chlorbenzene, later using a mixture of chlorbenzene and nitrobenzene and still later pure nitrobenzene. Carbon tetrachloride has also been used as a means of lowering the melting point. Many other mixtures, such as chlorpicrin, hydrocyanic acid, bromacetone, etc., were tested, but were not used. The effect on the melting point of mustard gas is shown in the following table:

MELTING POINT OF MUSTARD-GAS MIXTURES

Per cent added	Chlorpicrin		Chlorbenzene		Carbon tetrachloride	
	°C.	°F.	°C.	°F.	°C.	°F.
0	13.9	57	13.9	57	13.9	57
10	10.0	50	8.3	47	10.0	50
20	6.1	43	6.1	43	6.7	44
30	2.8	37	−1.1	30	3.3	38

While the difficulties of melting points in the range of ordinary temperatures can be solved by the use of solvents, all these additional steps greatly complicate production and reduce the efficiency of chemical agents.

Specific Gravity.—Substances used as chemical agents during the war varied greatly in specific gravity. Some were lighter than water while others were nearly twice as heavy as water. This large variation in weight creates filling difficulties. On the other hand, all the high explosives ordinarily used as shell fillers closely approximate a specific gravity of 1.5 so that different kinds of explosive charges introduce little variation in the weight of loaded H.E. shell. As it is desirable that all shell be brought to the standard weights, for which range tables are calculated, the nearer a chemical filler approaches the mean H.E., specific gravity 1.5, the less variation there is between the chemical and H.E. shell: also the difficulties of filling chemical shell are fewer.

41

Vapor Density.—Regardless of whether the chemical agent is a gas or a smoke, it must have a vapor density greater than that of air for otherwise, as soon as the agent is released from its container, it will immediately rise from the surface of the ground and thus lose its physiological or obscuring effect.

All the principal chemical agents used in the war met this requirement except hydrocyanic acid, the vapor of which was only 0.93 times as heavy as air. In consequence of its light vapor, this substance proved very disappointing in battle, although it is physiologically one of the most deadly gases known to chemists. Carbon monoxide is another very toxic gas which cannot be used in battle chiefly because its vapor density is less than air. Although the various substances used as chemical agents in the war varied only about twofold in specific gravity in their solid or liquid forms, they varied nearly tenfold in vapor density. Thus, the lightest gas used was HCN with a vapor density of 0.93, while one of the heaviest gases used, DA, has a vapor density of 9.0. The average vapor density of the more important agents was about 5.0.

In general, the heavier the vapor, the better it will cling to the ground and roll into depressions, dugouts, and trenches thus exerting a more intensive and lasting effect upon men taking shelter in such places.

As regards vapor density of a substance, we may say that it must at least be heavier than air and the heavier it is, the better its substance is suited for use as a chemical agent.

TACTICAL REQUIREMENTS

Under the heading of Technical Requirements, we have reviewed the essential qualities which chemical agents must possess in order that they may be manufactured and loaded into projectiles in sufficient quantities to meet the vast requirements of modern war. We now come to a consideration of those properties which chemical agents must possess in order to exert the effects required in battle. These we call *tactical requirements*. As the tactical effects of gases are markedly different from smokes and incendiaries, it will be more convenient to consider the tactical requirements of each of these three classes of agents separately.

Gases

We shall begin with the gases and note first those requirements which apply particularly to the gases used on the tactical offensive, as these are the most exacting requirements.

Toxicity.—In general, it may be said that, for the lethal and casualty-producing gases, toxicity is probably the most important requisite. Since the casualty effects of most gases are in direct proportion to their toxicities, it follows that the more toxic the gas, the more effective and 42 efficient it is as a chemical agent. Or, stated in another way, the same casualty results can be produced with decreasing quantities of the agent and with shorter periods of exposure, in proportion as its toxicity increases. This follows from Haber's generalization that toxic effect is proportional to toxicity times exposure time (see page 12). Perhaps the only exception to this toxicity requirement is in the case of the lacrimators, where toxic effects are not desired but where temporary incapacitation over the widest area with the minimum expenditure of chemicals is the prime consideration. Such a result, however, is hardly a war requirement but belongs more properly to the class of agents suitable for quelling domestic disturbances. Indeed, with far more effective agents available for general harassment of troops in war, it is difficult to foresee the future use of lacrimators in battle, although they undoubtedly will continue to be widely used in war for the training of troops behind the lines.

With the exception of lacrimators, we may say that toxicity is a fundamental requirement of all battle gases. High toxicity alone, however, does not necessarily make an effective casualty agent on the field of battle, as many other factors enter into the final effect. This fact was not sufficiently appreciable in the early years of the war and many very costly mistakes were made. Thus, the French were deceived into adopting HCN as a toxic shell filler by the extremely high toxicity of this gas in laboratory tests. However, owing to the fact that it is extremely volatile in the open air and that its vapor is lighter than air, it proved to be almost impossible to set up effective concentrations in artillery shoots with these shell. Another peculiarity of HCN is that, unless its concentration exceeds a certain critical figure, it is almost harmless. These two peculiarities made the French Vincennite (HCN) shells one of the most outstanding failures in chemical warfare during the war.

Multiple Effects.—Next to toxicity, the manner in which a gas exerts its action upon the body is the most important tactical consideration. Many gases have more than one mode of action. Thus, chlorpicrin is both a lacrimator and a lung-injurant gas so that both the eyes and lungs must be protected from this agent. Dimethyl sulfate (German D-Stoff) is both a lacrimator and a vesicant, and the eyes as well as the body must be protected; mustard gas has a triple effect, being a vesicant, lung injurant, and lacrimator combined. Hence mustard is the most difficult gas to protect against and for this reason it is one of the most valuable tactical agents.

In general, the more extensive the mode of action of a gas, *i.e.*, the greater the number of physiological effects it produces, the more valuable it is from a tactical viewpoint.

43

Persistency.—Since the toxic effect of a gas is a product of its toxicity and time of exposure, the next most important requirement for a casualty-producing gas is its persistency. By persistency is meant the duration of time an agent will remain around its point of release in an effective concentration. It is obvious that, no matter how toxic a gas may be, if it is so volatile that it lasts only a few seconds after being released, it cannot produce worth while casualty effects. Persistency is a function of the boiling point of a substance. That is, the higher the boiling point, the slower the liquid will evaporate and the longer it will persist in the field. Also, since volatility is a measure of the rate at which a liquid evaporates, persistency is an inverse function of volatility, and the more volatile a liquid is, the less persistent it will be.

Duration of Effects.—Assuming that the primary object of battle is to defeat the enemy by inflicting upon him, not fatalities, but rather non-fatal casualties of as long duration as possible, those chemical agents which produce the most lasting casualty effects are the most efficient. In this requirement, mustard is the most efficient chemical agent that was used in the war, as it produced slow-healing wounds but was fatal in only a small percentage of casualties.

Speed of Action.—The next most important tactical requirement is rapidity of action. Some substances act with remarkable speed in producing effects upon the body while others act very slowly, and their effects are not noticeable until many hours after exposure. Thus, HCN acts with almost lightning rapidity when present in lethal concentrations. One or two full breaths of this gas are sufficient to cause instant collapse and death within a few minutes. On the other hand, mustard gas is very slow acting and, in usual field concentrations, does not produce noticeable symptoms until several hours after exposure.

Regardless of the type of gas, it is obvious that the quicker it produces its effects, the sooner it secures the desired tactical results. Gases that are intended for casualty effects on the offensive must obviously be quick-acting and bring about incapacitation during the attack which may last only a few minutes. For this reason, mustard gas, which does not incapacitate for several hours after exposure, is unsuitable as an offensive gas and would be of more general value as a war gas if its speed of effect were greater.

Insidiousness.—If a gas produces uncomfortable or painful physiological effects upon first exposure to it, men will at once be aware of its presence and take measures to protect themselves and thus render ineffective the power of the gas. On the other hand, if a gas is insidious in action and produces no warning discomfort during the necessary period of exposure, it will exert its full casualty effect before countermeasures can be taken. Obviously, therefore, the more insidious the action of a 44 gas, the greater its surprise effect and tactical value. Moreover, the slower the action of a gas in producing its physiological effects, the greater the need for insidiousness in action. Thus, mustard-gas vapor is effective in low concentrations only after several hours' exposure, so that, if it were not insidious in its action and difficult to detect in low concentrations, troops would not remain exposed to it for a sufficient time to become casualties. But because mustard-gas vapor is both insidious in action and almost impossible to detect in low concentrations,.

it has a high casualty power, although it is slow in action and although its effects do not manifest themselves for several hours after exposure.

Volatility is also an important property of a casualty gas since it determines the maximum concentration which can exist in the open air at any given temperature. In general, liquids of low boiling points and high vapor pressures build up much heavier concentrations in a given volume of air than liquids with high boiling points and low vapor pressures. In fact the maximum concentration that can be held in the air (saturation point) is a direct function of the volatility of a substance (see definition on page 8). The mathematical relations between persistency, volatility, and vapor pressure are shown by the formulas in Appendix A.

The foregoing remarks concerning volatility apply particularly to the lethal or casualty-producing gases. With the neutralizing gases, such as mustard, and the harassing gases, such as DA, where immediate casualty effects are not primarily sought, the best tactical results are secured by maintaining a low concentration on the target area for a maximum period of time, and persistency then becomes of paramount importance. The principal requirements for the neutralizing and harassing gases are, first, great persistency and, second, effectiveness in low concentrations over long periods of time.

Penetrability.—Other things being equal, the greater the power of a gas to penetrate the enemy's masks, protective clothing, and other means of chemical defense, the greater will be the offensive power and tactical value of the gas. It has been estimated that the mere wearing of a mask (even of the latest improved type) reduces the physical vigor of troops about one-fourth. The addition of protective clothing still further reduces the physical activity and stamina of troops and thus greatly impairs their fighting ability. The greater the penetrating power of a gas, the more elaborate must be the protective equipment of the enemy with a corresponding reduction in this combat power. Hence, the penetrability of a gas is an important factor in its tactical value.

Invisibility.—Regardless of the type or kind of gas, it is generally agreed that it is most effective in the field when used as a surprise. The more difficult a gas is to detect by the senses, the more readily men are taken unawares—hence the importance of invisibility, which prevents

45

troops from seeing the approach of a gas cloud and perceiving the extent and limits of its concentration.

Odorlessness.—Next to visibility, gas concentrations are most usually detected in the field, especially at night, by the characteristic odor of the agent. The more nearly odorless the substance is, the more deadly is its surprise effect.

SMOKES*

* The smokes here considered are the nontoxic screening smokes. Toxic smokes are tactically the same as casualty gases except with regard to visibility.

Total Obscuring Power.—Passing now to a consideration of the second class of chemical agents—the smokes—we find quite different tactical requirements. Since the purpose of a smoke is to obscure vision, conceal terrain, and not to cause casualties, there is no necessity for a smoke to be odorless, while visibility or rather obscuring power is a fundamental requirement. Smokes are generally rated on the basis of their total obscuring power (T.O.P.). Total obscuring power is a function of the opacity of the smoke particle and its density per cubic foot of air. More specifically, the total obscuring power of a smoke is the product of the volume of smoke produced per unit weight of material and the density of the smoke. Chemical agents vary greatly in obscuring power and only those with high total obscuring powers are suitable as screening smokes.

Persistency.—Next to total obscuring power, persistency is the most important requirement for a smoke agent. The more persistent a smoke is, the less material is required to maintain a screen for a given time, and hence the more effective and economical the agent is.

Capacity.—The third requirement for a smoke agent is its smoke-producing capacity per pound of agent. Smoke-producing chemical compounds vary greatly in their output per unit of material and the compound which produces the greatest quantity of smoke per pound of material is the most efficient.

Density.—The next most desirable property for a smoke is density, or specific weight relative to air. It is obvious that the heavier the smoke is, the less it will rise from the ground and the better it will cling to and cover the areas to be screened, so that density or heaviness is an important requirement.

Harmlessness.—Another important requirement for a screening smoke is that it should exert no deleterious effect upon personnel, since smoke is frequently used to envelop friendly troops for their protection. If a smoke is irritating, the time during which troops can be blanketed is reduced and the effect upon the morale of the troops is adverse, even if no undesirable physiological effects are produced.

46

Temperature.—Other things being equal, a cold smoke is preferable to a hot one, for the hotter a smoke is, the more it will tend to ascend in the air, and the less its screening value will be. For this reason, smokes which are the products of chemical action, such as hydrolysis (*e.g.*, FM) possess certain advantages over smokes which are the result of combustion, as burning-oil smoke.

Color.—White smoke in most terrains blends better with the horizon line and is preferred to black or colored smokes for general concealment.

INCENDIARIES

The purpose of incendiary agents is to destroy enemy material by conflagration. Accordingly, the fundamental requirement of an incendiary agent is that it have the capacity to set fire, under the most adverse conditions encountered in the field, to whatever targets it is employed against.

Temperature.—The first tactical requirement of an incendiary agent is that it generate within its own substance an extremely hot fire, preferably one emitting flames. The higher the temperature generated by the incendiary substance, the greater its capacity to set fire to target material of low inflammability.

Time of Burning.—The next requirement is one of time of burning. The longer an incendiary agent burns, per pound of material, the longer it will sustain initiating fires and the greater will be the chances of igniting the material against which it is employed.

Unquenchability.—A military incendiary agent should also preferably be unquenchable by water, as water is generally the only means available in the field for putting out fires.

Spontaneous Combustion.—From a tactical viewpoint, spontaneous combustion is a distinct advantage in an incendiary material, since all that is necessary to use this material for initiating fires is to spread it over the target area and spontaneous combustion will create the desired results. From a technical viewpoint, spontaneous combustion is advantageous in that such a material does not require a fuse and special igniting charge with the resulting complications that these elements involve. On the other hand, technical difficulties in storage, handling, and filling into projectiles are created when an incendiary agent is spontaneously combustible, and these must be carefully weighed against the above advantages.

Extinguishment in Flight.—If an incendiary agent is to be used in a scatter-type projectile, *i.e.*, where the incendiary charge is to be scattered over a large target area, an additional requirement is demanded of the incendiary material, *viz.*, the burning particles must not be extinguished in flight after burst of the projectile. This is a very difficult requirement

47

to meet unless the incendiary material is spontaneously combustible for the reason that there is always a critical velocity above which a burning particle cannot be projected through the air without extinguishing its flames. This was the principal reason for the failure of the early types of incendiary bombs which were dropped from the German Zeppelins on London and Paris. These bombs were made of nonspontaneously combustible materials and were ignited, either on release from the bomb rack or by a time fuse after a short period of flight. The bombs would then burst into flames while high in the air. The increasing velocity acquired during the remainder of their fall would exceed the critical flame velocity and extinguish the flames from the bombs before they reached the ground.

The same difficulty occurred with the early types of incendiary artillery shell which were constructed on the shrapnel principle. It was found that when these shell burst they expelled their contents (as lumps of burning incendiary materials) at such high velocities as to extinguish the flames from the lumps. Consequently, if an incendiary material is not spontaneously combustible, it must be able to maintain its fire when expelled from the projectile by the bursting charge so that the incendiary particles will be brought in contact with the target material in a burning condition.

REQUIREMENTS FOR IDEAL AGENTS

Since we have now reviewed the requirements for chemical agents at some length, we may summarize this subject by stating the qualities and characteristics of an ideal chemical agent of each type.

Offensive Gas.—The ideal combat gas for use on the tactical *offensive* should meet the following requirements:

Tactical	Technical
1. High toxicity.	1. Availability of raw materials.
2. Multiple effectiveness.	2. Ease of manufacture.
3. Nonpersistency.	3. Chemical stability.
4. Effects of maximum duration.	4 Nonhydrolyzable.
5. Immediate effectiveness.	5. Withstands explosion without decomposition.
6. Insidiousness in action.	6. A solid at ordinary temperature.
7. Volatility (maximum field concentration).	7. Melting point above maximum atmospheric temperature.
8. Penetrability.	8. Boiling point as low as possible.
9. Invisibility.	9. High vapor pressure.
10. Odorlessness.	10. Specific gravity approximately 1.5.
	11. Vapor density greater than air (the heavier the better).

Phosgene, which is described in detail in Chap. VII, came closer to meeting the above requirements than any other substance. It fell short

48

of the ideal requirements chiefly in respect to the following: it lacked multiple effectiveness, being a lung injurant only; except in high concentrations, it was not immediately effective; it was not odorless and, in contact with water vapor in the air, it formed a white steamlike cloud and was thus not invisible; it hydrolyzed slowly with water and hence was not effective on very wet days; being a gas at ordinary temperatures, it had to be artificially cooled to be filled into projectiles. But even with these limitations, phosgene was the best all-round *offensive* gas used in the war.

Defensive Gas.—The ideal combat gas for use on the tactical *defensive* should also meet the above requirements except that it should be persistent rather than nonpersistent and it should be effective in low concentrations.

Mustard gas came close to the ideal defensive gas, being deficient only in the following particulars: it was not immediately effective; it had a faint odor; it was not easy to manufacture; it slowly hydrolyzed in contact with water vapor in the air and with water on the ground; it was a liquid at summer temperatures and a solid at winter temperatures; it had a rather low vapor pressure. But, even with these limitations, mustard gas proved to be not only the best defensive gas but the best all-round casualty agent used in the war.

Harassing Gas.—The ideal harassing gas should have the same requirements as defensive gas but should also be effective in very much lower concentrations in order that it may cover a large area with minimum expenditure of ammunition, and thus justify its use despite low toxicity.

DA was the most effective harassing gas used in the war and fell short of ideal requirements only as to the following: it had only one physiological effect—sternutatory; it was not very persistent; its effects were of short duration, generally a few hours; it was not volatile; it had a detectable odor; it was extremely difficult to make; it had high melting and boiling points and low vapor pressure; it was difficult to disperse in an effective form. Notwithstanding these deficiencies, however, this compound is a very effective harassing agent when used under proper conditions.

The ideal smoke agent should meet the following requirements:

Tactical	Technical
1. High total obscuring power.	Same as for gases.
2. High persistency.	
3. Large smoke-producing capacity.	
4. High specific weight relative to air.	
5. Low temperature of generation.	
6. No harmful physiological effect.	

White phosphorus was the most successful smoke agent used during the war, although it failed to meet the ideal requirements in the following

49

particulars: unless used on the progressive burning principle, it was low in persistency; the smoke generated, being lighter than air, tended to rise rapidly from the ground and, also being a product of combustion, the smoke was hotter than the surrounding air, which still further accelerated its upward movement. While the smoke itself was relatively harmless, the vapors generated by the burning particles of phosphorus were very poisonous, although the effects were not manifest until long after exposure. Also the burning particles of phosphorus caused painful wounds when brought in contact with the body so that phosphorus had a very decided casualty power in addition to its obscuring power.

As to technical requirements for smoke shell, phosphorus was very satisfactory, the only difficulties involved with its use in projectiles being those encountered in any spontaneously combustible material. It had to be stored and loaded under water so as to exclude all contact with air, and any leakage in storage and handling immediately caused fires.

However, notwithstanding its limitations, phosphorus was the best World War smoke agent and in many respects remains among the best smoke producers today although many new cold smokes, generated by noncombustible chemical reaction, have been developed since the war to compete with phosphorus as a smoke agent and are better adapted for erecting smoke screens from airplanes.

The ideal incendiary agent should meet the following requirements:

Tactical	Technical
1. High combustibility.	Same as for gases.
2. High temperature of combustion.	
3. Fire unquenchable with water.	
4. Fire not extinguishable in flight.	
5. Spontaneously combustible.	
6. Sustained fire generation.	
7. Combustion with flames.	

The incendiaries used during the war were chiefly of two kinds: (1) the *scatter type* consisting mainly of mixtures of inflammable oils, resins, tar, etc., primed with phosphorus, sodium, and the like; and (2) the *intensive type*, consisting chiefly of thermite and similar metallic chemically reactive mixtures producing intense though highly concentrated fires.

None of the World War incendiaries proved to be outstandingly successful, and much room for improvement remained in this field at the close of the war.

Although primarily a smoke producer, white phosphorus was about as satisfactory an incendiary agent as any material used in the war, although it lacked many desirable qualities.

50

In the light of what has been said above as to the many exacting requirements which chemical compounds must meet in order to qualify as chemical agents, it is not difficult to understand why, with many thousands of compounds from which to choose, so few met with success in the World War and why so many of the early chemical agents were failures.

This does not mean, however, that there will not be greatly superior chemical agents in the future. On the contrary, the progress that has been made in chemical-warfare research and development during the few years since the war completely negatives such an idea. Future developments will undoubtedly be along two general lines of effort (1) to find more effective ways and means of using known chemical agents and (2) to find more powerful compounds.

The progress since the war has been mainly in the first field, *i.e.*, improving the ways and means of using known chemical agents. The reason for this is that the full power of successful World War chemical agents was by no means developed by the military technique under which they were employed. There is consequently little advantage in finding more powerful agents while the full possibilities of those already known remain unexploited. For example, it has been determined that 20 mg. (about two-thirds of a teaspoonful) of mustard vapor quickly absorbed into the lungs of a man will cause his death. At this rate, there is enough potential poison in 1 ton of mustard gas to kill 45,000,000 men. Yet, during the last war 12,000 tons of mustard caused only 400,000 casualties, or an average of 33 casualties to every ton of mustard used in battle. With this great discrepancy between the potential and actual casualty-producing power of mustard gas, there is little reason to look for still more powerful compounds. On the contrary, if sufficient effort is expended in finding more efficient ways of using it, mustard will undoubtedly yield far greater results. Already two means of using mustard gas have been developed which greatly increase its effectiveness in the field, *viz.*, sprinkling from ground vehicles and spraying from airplanes, of which more will be said in a later chapter.

However, while military effort is being principally devoted to improving field technique in the use of chemical agents, industrial research is constantly discovering and studying new compounds, some of which will undoubtedly prove more powerful than any chemical agents heretofore employed. In fact, so vast is the field of chemistry and so far-reaching are its potential powers that no man will presume to predict its ultimate possibilities in either peace or war. The only certainty in the future is that of *progress;* no government worthy of the name will risk the security of its people by failure to take military advantage of the unremitting progress that has been and will continue to be made in the ever-widening fields of science.

51

CHAPTER III

DISSEMINATION OF CHEMICAL AGENTS

To be effective in battle, chemical agents must be properly disseminated over a suitable target area. Dissemination comprises two processes—the delivering of the chemicals to the target (accomplished by *projection*), and the spreading of the chemicals over the target in an effective state (accomplished by *dispersion*). Dissemination of chemicals, therefore, consists broadly of their projection and dispersion.

The various methods and processes of dissemination are considered in this chapter, while the weapons and material utilized for this purpose are treated in Chaps. XIV to XVIII, in connection with the arms to which they pertain.

MEANS OF PROJECTION

During the World War, chemicals were disseminated by every military arm, although the air corps did not use toxic gases. When chemical warfare made its appearance in 1915, there was already a large variety of high-explosive weapons in use. As chemical warfare was born during the war and there was no prewar development of its matériel, the first chemical munitions were hasty adaptations of high-explosive weapons, although subsequent experience showed that some of these weapons were not suitable for chemical dissemination and were every inefficient for this purpose.

The first use of gas in the World War was from hand grenades, which could be thrown about 25 or 30 yd. Owing to their limited range, they could be used only in hand-to-hand combat and frequently exposed the using troops to the chemicals employed almost to the same extent as the enemy. They were, therefore, of advantage only when employed by masked troops against an unmasked enemy. When masks were available to both sides, their general combat effectiveness largely disappeared.

The next step was to put chemicals into rifle grenades which could be projected from 200 to 250 yd. This was still too close to permit the troops using them to employ them without masks and, as masks furnished complete protection against the gases in these grenades, they were not much more effective than the hand grenades. However, when used with smoke fillings, especially white phosphorus, they did afford

52

considerable protection to small bodies of infantry in the attack and continued to be used for this purpose throughout the war.

Although chronologically the next use of gas was in artillery shell (in January, 1915, by the Germans on the Russian Front), these shell were a failure and the successful use of gas in artillery shell was not accomplished until the summer of 1915 after the great cloud-gas attacks from cylinders in the spring of 1915. We may, therefore, say that the next development in chemical warfare was the cylinder method of dispersion. The effective range of gas released from cylinders varied greatly with the weather and other local conditions and the numbers of cylinders employed. As a general rule, it may be said that gas clouds were effective to a depth approximately equal to the front from which they were projected, although in several notable instances the effective depth was much greater. As the diffusion and dilution of the gas released from cylinders increase roughly as the cube of the distance downwind from the point of release, very large quantities of gas are required to project effective concentrations for distances greater than 2,500 yd., and we may, therefore, delimit the effective zone of cylinder attacks by this range, except for unusually large operations.

Beginning in the summer of 1915, chemicals were loaded into artillery shell, first of the light calibers, and then of heavier calibers, as the war progressed. By 1917, artillery of all calibers were firing chemical shell although many of the heavier shell were unsuitable for chemical dissemination.

Following the artillery shell, the use of chemicals next extended to the trench mortars, though here again the slow rate of fire and immobility of heavier calibers were altogether unsuitable for chemicals; the lighter calibers did not have shells of sufficient capacity for this purpose.

It was soon found that artillery was not adapted to disseminate chemicals within the zone of infantry combat because of the flat trajectory of the guns, the low chemical capacity of the shell, and the difficulty of placing effective concentrations relatively close to our own front lines, without danger to friendly infantry. Since existing types of trench mortars which normally covered this zone with high-explosive fires were unsuitable for establishing and maintaining gas and smoke concentrations, and since cylinder operations were too limited by adverse winds and weather conditions, the problem of how to cover the infantry combat zone with effective chemical concentrations at all times became very acute.

This problem was finally solved by the British, who first devised special (Livens) projectors which were adapted to fire in one salvo a large number of high-capacity bombs for a maximum distance of 1,800 yd., and thus create extremely heavy gas concentrations within the enemy's

53

defensive positions. The chemicals released from Livens bombs were already on the target area and hence did not have to travel across unoccupied terrain with resulting loss of strength, as in the case of gas released from cylinders. The Livens projector was a very effective means of chemical projection and was extensively employed on both sides during the remainder of the war. However, it required much labor and time to install and was adapted for use only in very stabilized situations.

To supplement the Livens projector and to provide a more mobile device which could be used in open warfare, the British also developed a special chemical (4-in. Stokes) mortar, which was a compromise in mobility and capacity between the 3-in. and the 6-in. H.E. mortars. The 4-in. chemical mortar had the same range and rate of fire (20 rounds per minute) and almost the same mobility as the 3-in. mortar and, at the same time, a shell holding nearly three times the amount of chemical. The 4-in. chemical mortar thus had a gas-projecting capacity nearly three times that of the 3-in. mortar and proved to be one of the most valuable means of projecting chemicals devised in the war. Because of its mobility and the fact that it could be used in small and large groups equally well, it was a very flexible weapon well adapted for a wide variety of tactical situations.

The cylinder, projector, and chemical mortar were all used to lay down chemical concentrations in the infantry combat zone. Each was necessary to supplement the other in order to fully cover this important field with chemicals in all tactical situations, and these devices were, therefore, grouped together as special chemical weapons. Because of the skill and special training required to place effective concentrations of gas and smoke in the infantry combat zone, close to friendly troops, it was early found necessary to organize special troops to man these special chemical weapons. These troops were particularly trained in the use of these special weapons and thoroughly understood the capabilities and limitations of each. They were known in the war as *special gas troops* and, while originally organized as engineer units, they devoted their full time to chemical operations and were in fact chemical troops.

Although gas was not disseminated from airplanes during the late war, incendiary and smoke agents were employed in drop bombs early in the war. Since the war, many nations have developed means for employing chemicals from airplanes.

Numerous special chemical devices such as land mines, toxic smoke candles, smoke generators on tanks, etc., have also been developed during the postwar period by many of the principal world powers.

We may summarize the possible means for projecting chemical agents by operating arms as follows:

54

Munition	Operating Arm
Smoke generators on tanks Hand and rifle grenades Smoke candles	Infantry and cavalry
Smoke generators, portable Accompanying mortar (81-mm.) smoke	Infantry
Toxic gas cylinders Livens projectors Chemical mortars Chemical sprinklers (mechanized) Toxic smoke candles Flame projectors	Special chemical troops
Artillery shell (Light and medium calibers)	Field artillery
Drop bombs Chemical sprinklers and sprayers	Air corps

With the addition of the postwar chemical armament, there now exists means for disseminating chemicals, not only to all parts of the battlefield, but even to the areas behind the front and as far into the interior of the enemy's country as the cruising radius of bombardment planes will permit.

In order to coordinate all the various means for disseminating chemicals and to insure that each is used to supplement the others in the most efficient manner, the Theater of Operations is divided into zones progressively increasing in depth from the battle front. Diagram I (page 55) shows in schematic form such a zoning of the Theater of Operations.

METHODS OF PROJECTION

Regardless of the technical means employed, there are but three basic methods of placing chemicals on a target area. First, by releasing the chemical from containers installed in one's own front lines, and depending upon the wind to carry it to and over the target area. This may be called the method of release *at origin*. Second, by releasing from containers projected *on the target area* by some physical means, such as firing from a gun (chemical shell), dropping from an airplane (chemical bomb), or placing in position by retreating troops (chemical mines). This is the method of release *on target*. Third, by releasing the chemical from containers carried by airplanes over the target area and depending upon gravity to carry it down to the target area. This is the method of release *over target*.

From what has been said above, we may now summarize the possible methods of projecting chemicals as shown on page 56.

55

A discussion of the technical means and matériel used for projecting chemicals will be found in subsequent chapters pertaining to the several arms which employ chemicals.

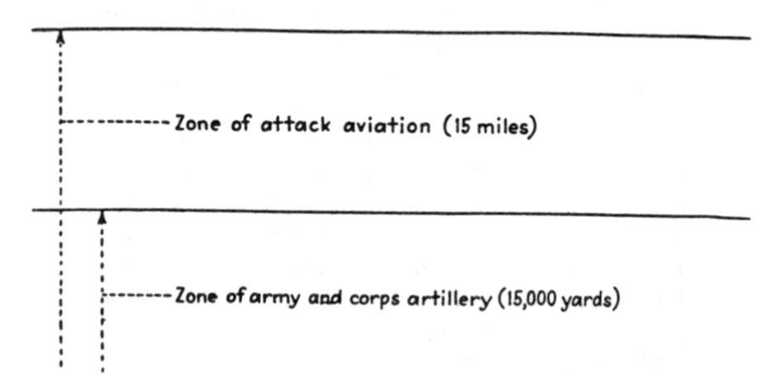

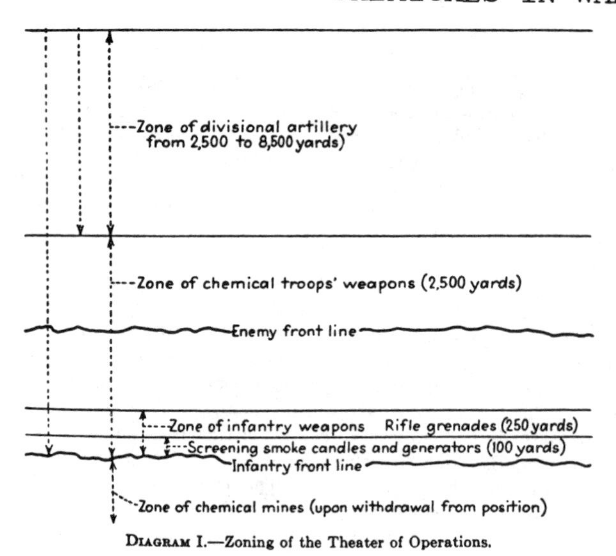

DIAGRAM I.—Zoning of the Theater of Operations.

METHODS OF DISPERSION

In previous chapters we have seen that chemicals to be tactically effective must be brought into contact with the body or the body must be surrounded by a toxic atmosphere in which the concentration of the chemical is at least equal to the minimum effective strength for a given time of exposure. Since troops in battle normally take advantage of all available sheltering cover, it is not ordinarily possible to bring a combat chemical (in its original physical state) directly in contact with the body. This being the case, it is necessary to distribute the chemical as uniformly as possible, in a finely divided form, throughout the atmosphere covering the target area, so as to create a toxic concentration which envelops the unprotected body and penetrates it through the lungs or skin. This is the problem of dispersion.

56

METHODS OF PROJECTING CHEMICALS

Basic method of projection	Technical means utilized	Operating arm of service	Type of chemicals employed	Depth of normal zone covered
Release at origin....	Toxic gas cylinders	Chemical troops	Nonpersistent toxic gases	2,500 yd.
	Toxic smoke candles	Chemical troops	Respiratory irritant gases	1,500 yd.
	Screening smoke Candles and generators	Infantry and cavalry	Screening smokes	100 yd.
Release on target....	Artillery shell	Artillery	All kinds of toxic gases, screening smokes, and incendiaries	2,500 to 15,000 yd.
	Chemical mortar shell	Chemical troops	All kinds of toxic gases, screening smokes, and incendiaries	2,500 yd.
	Chemical sprinklers (mechanized)			
	Livens projectors	Chemical troops	Toxic gas and incendiaries	1,800 yd.
	81-mm. mortar shell	Infantry	Smoke	3,000 yd.
	Hand and rifle grenades	Infantry and cavalry	Toxic gas, smoke, and incendiaries	25 to 250 yd.
	Chemical mines	Chemical troops	Toxic gas	Area evacuated
Release over target....	Drop bombs	Air corps	Toxic gas, smoke, and incendiaries	1,150 miles
	Airplane sprinklers	Air corps	Persistent gases	15 miles
	Airplane sprayers	Air corps	Persistent gases	15 miles

Physical States.—Under ordinary field conditions, combat chemicals may originally be either solids, liquids, or gases; only a very few (Cl and CG) are true gases; a few (DA, DM, and CN) are solids; the majority are liquids.

Dispersion as a Gas.—If the chemical is a gas at ordinary temperatures [say +20°C. (68°F.)] and atmospheric pressure, its dispersion is easily accomplished. It has only to be released from its container, when it will escape into the air and rapidly permeate it by expansion and diffusion, until a fairly homogeneous mixture is obtained. The problem of dispersion of a gaseous chemical is, therefore, very simple; it being necessary only to release a sufficient amount of the chemical to insure an effective concentration by the time the toxic cloud covers the target area.

57

Dispersion as an Aerosol.—The dispersion of liquid and solid chemicals is much more difficult. All liquids and many solids give off some vapor at ordinary temperatures even though their boiling points are far above maximum atmospheric temperatures. These vapors act like true gases and, from a chemical-warfare viewpoint, may be regarded as such.* But the percentage of vapors given off by most liquid and solid combat chemicals under ordinary field conditions is so small as to be practically negligible unless the substance is heated, in which case the larger part, if not all, of the substance may be vaporized and pass off into the air in vapor form. Excepting the few chemicals that are true gases in the field and those that can be readily vaporized at ordinary field temperatures, chemical agents are usually dispersed in the form of exceedingly small solid or liquid particles.

* In physics, a vapor is a gas at a temperature below the boiling point of the corresponding liquid.

As each molecule in a vapor is free to move according to the gas laws, vapors, *in general*, obey the laws of gases and yield with air *homogeneous* mixtures. In smokes, however, the molecules are not free to move individually, but are clustered together in bunches, so that smokes do not rigidly obey the laws of gases, but yield with the air *heterogeneous* mixtures. Such mixtures are *dispersed systems*, comprising a gaseous phase —the air—and a solid or liquid phase—the toxic substance—in very finely divided particles. The most common forms of dispersed systems are those in which a solid or a liquid is dispersed in a liquid. These are called *colloidal solutions*, or *sols*. If the dispersing medium is water, the system is a hydrosol and, if the dispersing medium is air, the system is an *aerosol*. As a colloidal solution is intermediate between a true solution and a suspension of large particles in a liquid, an aerosol is intermediate between a true gaseous mixture and a suspension of large particles in the air. Accordingly, aerosols, although elastic fluids, do not rigidly obey the laws of gases, but closely approximate the properties of colloidal solutions. As chemical smokes are aerosols, they also in general follow the laws governing colloidal solutions.

Regardless of whether the aerosol is a toxic or simple obscuring smoke, the *method* of dispersion is the same and consists basically of the condensation in the air, by a physical or chemical process, of a substance emitted in the state of molecular dispersion. The structure and stability of the aerosols thus obtained are subsequently modified by secondary phenomena, such as: condensation of water on the surface of the minute solid particles or drops, oxydation on contact with the air, or hydration.

Processes of Dispersion.—The *primary dispersion* of the substance may be effected by either a physical or a chemical process.

58

Physical Means of Dispersion.—In the *physical* process, three general means are employed: (1) mechanical force, as when a very fine dust is sprayed from an airplane; (2) heat, as when a substance is distilled in the air (from smoke candles); and (3) a combination of force and heat, as when the contents of a chemical shell are scattered by the explosion of a bursting charge.

When *mechanical force* alone is employed for primary dispersion, the substance must be first reduced to an impalpable powder and must also have, when thus finely divided a sufficient vapor pressure to be vaporized on contact with the air.

When *heat* is the means employed for primary dispersion, the solid or liquid chemical is heated and distills into the atmosphere in a gaseous state and then condenses to a dispersed or aerosol state. Certain smoke producers, such as phosphorus, oleum, and chlorsulfuric acid, for example, are dispersed in this manner. The vapors of these substances act as fog producers, for their anhydrides have a strong affinity for water and by hydration form acids which are themselves very hygroscopic. Thus, the sulfuric anhydride (SO_3) in oleum and chlorsulfuric acid reacts with water to form sulfuric acid (H_2SO_4), which in turn absorbs large quantities of water. A smoke composed of liquid droplets, *i.e.*, fog, is in reality a dispersed solution of acid in water.

When *mechanical force and heat* are both employed for primary dispersion, the former scatters the substance in very finely divided form, while the latter volatilizes it and reduces it to the vapor phase.

Chemical Means of Dispersion.—When the primary dispersion is effected by a *chemical* process, two substances in a gaseous state are simultaneously emitted and, by chemical reaction on each other, yield a liquid or solid compound in the dispersed state. Thus, gaseous hydrochloric acid and ammonia yield ammonium chloride in the form of a dense white fume. Similarly, sulfuric acid fumes formed by the hydration of sulfuric anhydride form, on contact with ammonia, ammonium sulfate, another dense white smoke, thus:

$$H_2SO_4 + 2NH_3 = (NH_4)_2SO_4$$

If the products of decomposition are volatile, as in these cases, the reactions are reversible, and we have the general equation

$$\text{Salt} \rightleftarrows \text{Acid} + \text{Base.}$$

The direction and intensity of all reversible reactions [according to Gibbs' Phase Rule (10)] depends upon the factors of temperature, pressure, and concentration of reacting bodies. Thus the reaction

$$NH_4Cl \rightleftarrows HCl + NH_3$$

59

depends for its direction primarily on the amount of moisture present, for gaseous hydrochloric acid and ammonia mixed together in the air form ammonium chloride up to a certain point, when further formation of the same is inhibited by the reverse reaction.

Of all the factors affecting the formation of fogs and smoke, water plays the most important role. It not only converts anhydrides (P_2O_3, SO_3) to corresponding acids and precipitates them in the dispersed state, but also assures the dissociation of hydrolyzable salts and their reprecipitation in colloidal dimensions. The water vapor in the air can also adhere to the surfaces of minute solid particles floating in the air, and convert them to liquid droplets, as is the case when natural fogs form over smoky cities.

In the chemical process of dispersion, salts that are both volatile and easily hydrolyzable produce the best smokes. Hence oxides with feeble bases or feeble acids, because readily hydrolyzable, are most generally employed.

Summary.—Chemicals then are dispersed in two forms, one, in which a vapor (or gas) is mixed with air (gas clouds) and the other, a suspension of solid or liquid particles in the air (smoke clouds). As the behavior in the field of these two forms of chemical dispersion are somewhat different, the principal characteristics of each will be briefly summarized.

Gas Clouds

Density.—As a liquid changing into a gas absorbs heat from the air during vaporization, the air in contact with the vapor is cooled. The magnitude of this cooling effect depends upon the material used and its concentration and, while usually small, it is sufficient to cause an appreciable increase in the density of the air mixed with the vapor. Also, war gases themselves are heavier than air. The result of these two phenomena is to cause gas clouds to hug the ground and flow into all depressions and low places.

Lateral Spread.—When a gas is released in the open air, it immediately expands and diffuses into the atmosphere. This causes the cloud to spread laterally and vertically. Shifting wind and air currents also increase lateral spread as the cloud moves downwind. Under average conditions, the lateral spread is about 20 per cent of the distance traveled, while for favorable conditions it is about 15 per cent, and for unfavorable conditions it will amount to as much as 50 per cent.

Vertical Rise.—The expansion and diffusion of a gas upon its release in the open air also cause the cloud to rise as it travels with the wind, notwithstanding that the gas itself may be heavier than the air and that it cools the air when expanding. The vertical rise of a gas cloud depends

60

upon several factors, chief among which are convection currents. These currents are strongest when the ground is dry and warmer than the air and when the sun is shining brightly. On the other hand, at night and in the early morning, the ground surface is usually cooler than the surrounding air, and there are no convection currents, so that gas clouds have much less vertical rise under such conditions. This rise will vary

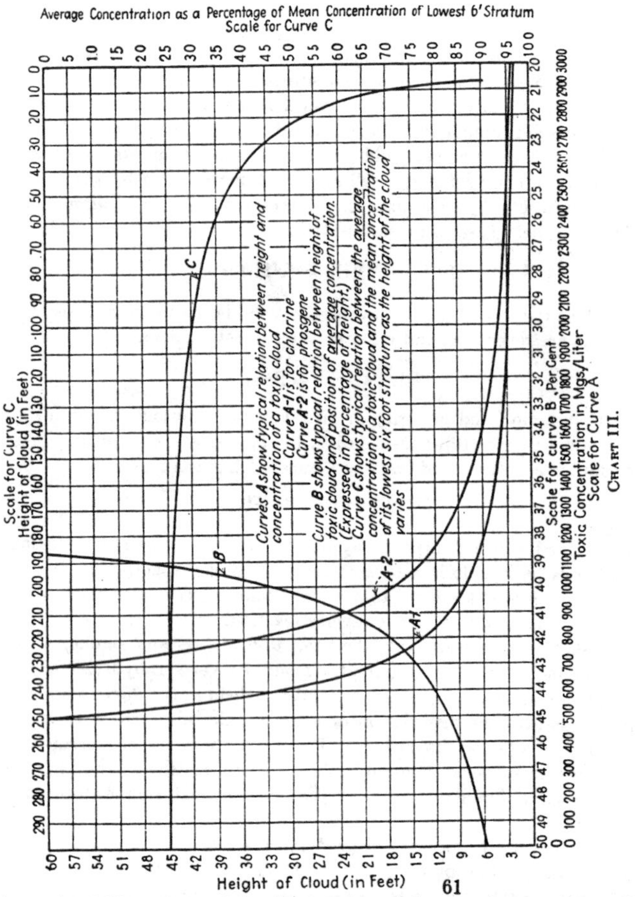

61

from about 10 per cent of the distance traveled under the most favorable conditions to as much as 35 per cent under adverse conditions.

Drag Effect.—Since the wind velocity along the ground is practically zero, but increases rapidly upward, gas clouds are carried over the ground with a sort of rolling motion, which causes the cloud to incline forward and stretch out in length more at the top than the bottom. This increase in the length of the cloud is called the *drag effect* and, for clouds released on the ground, amounts to from 10 to 30 per cent of the distance traveled, depending upon the nature of the terrain. For gas released from airplanes, up to 100 ft. above ground, the drag effect is equal to 100 per cent of the distance traveled, owing principally to the high velocity of the airplane.

Variation of Concentration.—The concentration of vapor in a gas cloud varies inversely as the logarithm of the height above ground. Thus, if C_1 is the concentration at a height H_1 and C_2 the concentration at a higher point H_2, then

$$C_2 = C_1 \times \frac{\log H_1}{\log H_2} \qquad (1)$$

This causes the lower layers of the gas cloud to be more dense and more toxic than the upper layers, as is clearly shown in Chart III, in which curve *A* shows the general relation between heights above ground (ordinates) and the concentrations at these heights (abscissas) and indicates the form of the relation between height and concentration.

Average Concentration.—In a gas cloud, the average concentration is not in the geometrical center of the cloud, but varies therefrom as the height of the cloud increases. In Chart III, curve *B* shows the change in the position of the *average* concentration, as the height varies.

If the concentration at any height in a toxic cloud is known, the concentration at any other height may be computed from Eq. (1). If the concentration is not known for any given height, then the total height and the average concentration of the toxic cloud may be computed from a given quantity of chemical as shown on pages 64–66. The position of the average concentration is then located from curve B in Chart III. With the average concentration and its position thus determined, the concentration at any other height in the cloud can be computed from Eq. (1). Also the effective concentration in the lowest 6-ft. layer of the cloud may be determined from curve *C* in Chart III.

Smoke Clouds

Density.—When chemicals create a smoke they either burn or hydrolyze in the air, thus generating heat which warms the air imme-

62

diately downwind from the source of smoke. Smoke clouds thus rise more than gas clouds, since air containing hot smoke particles, being less dense, tends to rise above the surrounding cooler air. Again, unlike gas clouds, smoke clouds have an *even* concentration at *all* elevations above ground.

Lateral Spread and Drag Effect.—The *lateral* spread and *drag effect* of smoke clouds are substantially the same as for gas clouds.

Vertical Rise.—The rate of *vertical rise* of smoke is much greater than that of gas because the smoke particles absorb heat waves from the sun and are warmed up thereby. The transfer of heat to and from smoke particles by radiation is also very important, especially in bright sunshine. Since each smoke particle has a diameter of 10^{-3} to 10^{-6} cm. and is surrounded by a tightly held air film about 10^{-3} cm. thick, it acts like a tiny air-filled balloon, rising when heated and falling when cooled below the surrounding air. Thus, while convection currents tend to give the same rise to both gas and smoke, radiation primarily affects the smoke particles only. In addition, smoke particles in the air are heated by radiation from the ground surface as well as from the sun and, when the ground is cooler than the air, the smoke particles actually lose their heat by radiation to the ground. Hence smoke clouds are more influenced by ground temperature and time of day than gas clouds.

RELATION BETWEEN QUANTITY AND RANGE

The amount of chemical required to establish an effective concentration on a target is determined by the general relation between a quantity of chemical and its effective range.

Let W = weight of chemical released from one point, in pounds,
D = density of chemical released (air = 1),
V = original volume of chemical released from one point, at atmospheric temperature and pressure, in cubic feet,
V_s = volume of chemical after it has traveled a distance S, in cubic feet,
S = distance traveled from point of release at any time T, in feet,
T = time of travel, in minutes,
C_a = *average* concentration of the toxic cloud,
C_1 = ground concentration of the toxic cloud (*i.e.*, mean concentration of lowest 6-ft. stratum),
C = minimum effective concentration expressed as a volumetric ratio of chemical to air, in parts per thousand,
H_a = height of C_a above ground, and
H_1 = height of C_1 above ground.

63

Experience shows that the dimensions of a chemical cloud generated from one point of emission can be expressed in terms of the distance traveled under various field conditions as follows:

Let S = distance traveled by top of cloud,
F_s = width of cloud at any distance, S,
H_s = height of cloud at any distance, S,
R_s = drag effect of cloud at any distance, S.

The values of F_s, H_s, and R_s, as functions of S, for various field conditions, are shown in the following tabulation:

Values of Width, Height, and Drag of Chemical Clouds*

Field conditions	Sky	Time of day	Terrain	Ground temperature	Winds, m.p.h.	Value of F_s		Value of H_s		Value of R_s	
						Gas	Smoke	Gas	Smoke	Gas	Smoke
Favorable..	Heavily overcast	Night or early morning	Level fields or water	Colder than air	Steady 0–4	0.15S	0.15S	0.03S	0.10S	0.10S	0.10S
Average...	Partly	Mid-	Moder-		Slightly	0.20S	0.20S	0.10S	0.20S	0.20S	0.20S

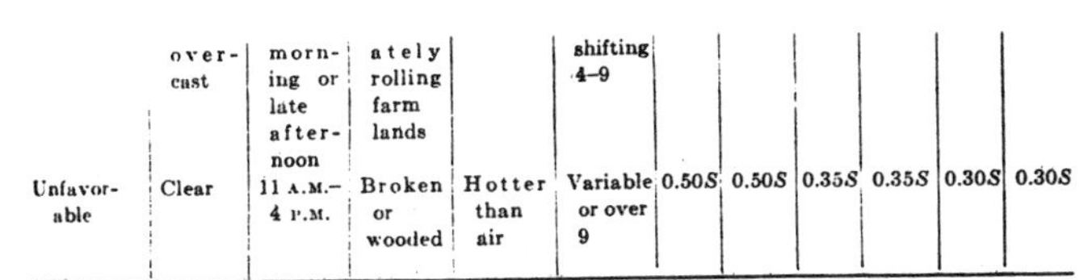

	over-cast	morning or late afternoon	ately rolling farm lands		shifting 4–9						
Unfavorable	Clear	11 A.M.–4 P.M.	Broken or wooded	Hotter than air	Variable or over 9	0.50S	0.50S	0.35S	0.35S	0.30S	0.30S

* NOTE: The values given for *smoke* in the above table apply only to a *range* smoke, *i.e.*, one blowing directly toward the target area. For data pertaining to *lateral* smoke clouds, see Chap. XIII.

In the above table, it is shown that, under *average* field conditions, a *gas* cloud will have a vertical rise of 10 per cent and a drag and lateral spread of 20 per cent of the distance traveled. After the gas has traveled a distance S, we have a toxic cloud of the following dimensions:

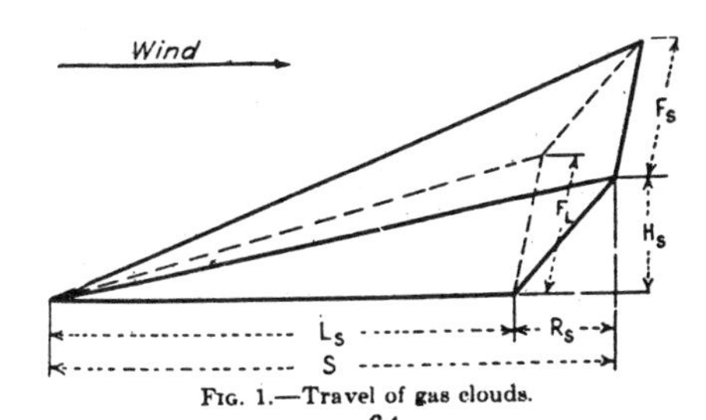

FIG. 1.—Travel of gas clouds.

64

Top length of cloud at distance S $= S$
Bottom length of cloud at distance S $= L_s$
Drag of cloud at distance S $= R_s$
Bottom width of cloud at distance S $= F_l$
Height of cloud at distance S $= H_s$

Hence
$$V_s = \frac{L_s F_l H_s}{6} \quad (2)$$

But
$$L_s = S - R_s \quad (3)$$

And, for *average* field conditions,

$$R_s = 0.2S$$

Hence
$$L_s = 0.8S$$
$$F_l = 0.2 \times 0.8S = 0.16S$$
$$H_s = 0.1S$$

Therefore
$$V_s = \frac{0.8S \times 0.16S \times 0.1S}{6} = 0.00213S^3 \quad (4)$$

If we denote the coefficient of S by the symbol K, Eq. (4) takes the form

$$V_s = KS^3 \quad (5)$$

When the toxic cloud reaches a length S,

$$V_s = \frac{V}{C_a} \quad (6)$$

where C_a is the average concentration at the distance, S. Substituting value of V_s from (6) in Eq. (5), we have

$$\frac{V}{C_a} = KS^3 \quad (7)$$

Hence
$$V = KC_aS^3 \quad (8)$$

or
$$S = \sqrt[3]{\frac{V}{KC_a}} \quad (9)$$

Since
$$V = \frac{W}{D}$$
$$W = KC_aDS^3 \quad (10)$$

and
$$S = \sqrt[3]{\frac{W}{KC_aD}} \quad (11)$$

From Eq. (1), page 61, we have

$$C_a = \frac{C_1 \log H_1}{\log H_a} \quad (12)$$

65

Since C_1 is the mean concentration of lowest 6-ft. stratum of the toxic cloud,

$$H_1 = 3 \text{ ft. (curve } B\text{, Chart III)}$$

and
$$\log H_1 = 0.4771$$

Also, when the cloud reaches its maximum *effective* length,

$$C_1 = C \quad (13)$$

C is a definite quantity for each gas according to the physiological effect desired and the time of exposure to the gas.

Hence, when the cloud reaches its maximum *effective* length:

$$C_a = \frac{0.4771}{\log H_a} \times C \quad (14)$$

Substituting the value of C_a from Eq. (14) in Eqs. (10) and (11), we have

$$W = \frac{0.4771KCDS^3}{\log H_a} \quad (15)$$

$$S = \sqrt[3]{\frac{W \log H_a}{0.4771CKD}} \quad (16)$$

Since the ground distance, or range, L in any given case is a definite percentage of the distance S [Eq. (3) and table on page 63], we see from Eq. (15) that the quantity of chemical required to set up an effective concentration on a distant target increases as the cube of the distance to the target and, from Eq. (16), the effective range of a given quantity of chemical varies directly as the cube root of the weight of chemical released and inversely with the cube root of its density and effective concentration.

Since the values of K in the foregoing equations depend upon the corresponding values of F_s, H_s, and R_s, which in turn vary with the distance S, as shown in the table on page 63, the values of K for gases and smokes, under varying field conditions, may be summarized as follows:

Field conditions	Values of K	
	Gas	Smoke
Favorable	0.000608	0.002025
Average	0.002133	0.004267
Unfavorable	0.014292	0.014292

66

As H_a, the height above ground of the *average* concentration, also varies with the distance S, we might express H_a as a function of S and so convert Eqs. (15) and (16) to functions of S and the quantities K, C, D, which are definite constants for any given case. Such a procedure, however, leads to very complicated formulas for W and S, which would be cumbersome to apply in practice.

A shorter and simpler method is to plot a curve for Eq. (14) from which the value of C_a in terms of C_1 may be read directly for any given case and then inserted in Eqs. (10) and (11). Curve C on Chart III is such a curve and expresses the value of C_a as a percentage of C_1 for any rise up to 300 ft. Above a rise of 300 ft., which corresponds to a gas range of 3,000 ft. under average field conditions, the value of C_a is obtained from Eq. (14).

In order to illustrate the time and space factors involved in dissemination of a gaseous chemical, from a single point of emission, let us take the simplest case of a cylinder discharging chlorine. We shall assume that the cylinder holds 30 lb. of liquid phosgene. A cubic foot of air at 20°C. (68°F.) and atmospheric pressure weighs 0.075 lb. and, as the density of gaseous chlorine is 3.5 times the density of air at this temperature and pressure, it weighs 3.5 × 0.075 = 0.2625 lb. per cubic foot. Using Eq. (11) above, and a lethal concentration of 1:10,000, we have for *average field* conditions

$$S = \sqrt[3]{\frac{30}{\frac{0.002133 \times 0.2625}{10{,}000}}} = 812.2 \text{ ft.}$$

for an *average* concentration of 1:10,000. But at this range the ground concentration equals approximately three times average concentration. Substituting this value for C_a in Eq. (11), we have

$$S = 1{,}172 \text{ ft.}$$
$$L_e = 0.8S = 942 \text{ ft.}$$

Thus, 30 lb. of phosgene under *average* field conditions will have a range of 942 ft., with ground concentration of 1:10,000 (0.434 mg. per liter), which is lethal on 15 minutes' exposure. With *favorable* field conditions, the same amount of chlorine will have an equally effective range of 1,233 ft., while with *unfavorable* field conditions this effective range will be reduced to 430 ft. In this case, favorable conditions increase it to 53 per cent of the range under average conditions.

If the wind is blowing steadily toward the target at a rate of 5.4 miles per hour (475 ft. per minute), the cloud will, under average field con-

67

ditions, reach its full development (in the form shown in Fig. 1) in $^{942}/_{475} = 1.98$, or approximately 2 minutes. To maintain an average concentration of 1:10,000, our cylinder should be emptied in that time, requiring a discharge rate of approximately 15 lb. per minute. If a slower rate of discharge is used, the gas cloud will be attenuated and its concentration will be correspondingly lowered. Also, if there is an increase in the wind velocity, there should be a corresponding increase in the discharge rate in order to maintain the same concentration.

On the other hand, with a 5.4-mile wind and a discharge rate greater than 15 lb. per minute, the initial concentration of the cloud will be raised above the strength of 1:10,000 (0.434 mg. per liter). After the cloud has traveled the same ground distance (942 ft.), its concentration will fall off, as indicated above, but will still be higher than 1:10,000 by the time the cloud reaches the target. There is, therefore, a theoretical advantage in increasing the discharge rate, but there are practical difficulties involved in so doing. In the first place, much higher pressures are required for greater velocities of discharge, the pressure increasing as the square of the velocity. Also, if the emission is too rapid, there is insufficient time for the ejected liquid to change into vapor and the liquid chemical falls to the ground where part of it is lost by absorption. Moreover, the liquid on the ground produces a very high local concentration immediately adjacent to the operating troops and may endanger them if there is any unsteadiness in the wind.

Size of Target.—Another very important factor in the cloud or wave method of disseminating gas is the size of the target area to be covered.

Width.—The width of the target area should be approximately equal, but should not exceed the width of the gas cloud at the front edge of the target, *i.e.*, the value of F_l as shown in the following table:

Field conditions	Values of F_s		Values of F_l		Per cent of range L_e	
	Gas	Smoke	Gas	Smoke	Gas	Smoke
Favorable	0.15S	0.15S	0.135S	0.135S	0.90	0.90
Average	0.20S	0.20S	0.160S	0.160S	0.80	0.80
Unfavorable	0.50S	0.50S	0.350S	0.350S	0.70	0.70

For chemicals emitted from a single point, with a range of 1,000 ft., the width of target should be: for favorable conditions, 90 ft.; for average conditions, 80 ft.; and for unfavorable conditions, 70 ft.

Depth.—If the target area is of material depth as compared to its distance from the point of emission of the gas, it should always be *included as a part of the range.* Otherwise, by the time the gas cloud reaches the

68

rear boundary of the target, its concentration will have fallen below the required effective strength. As an illustration of this point, let us assume that the discharge from the cylinder mentioned above travels over a target 200 ft. deep whose front edge is at the distance $L = 1{,}050$ ft. from the cylinder emplacement. We shall also assume that the cylinder is emptied in 2 minutes, so that, by the time the first chlorine discharged reaches the front edge of the target, the last chlorine will have just been released from the cylinder. Traveling at the rate of 6 miles per hour (528 ft. per minute) it will require 0.40 minute for the cloud to pass over the target area. During this time, the cloud will expand to the larger

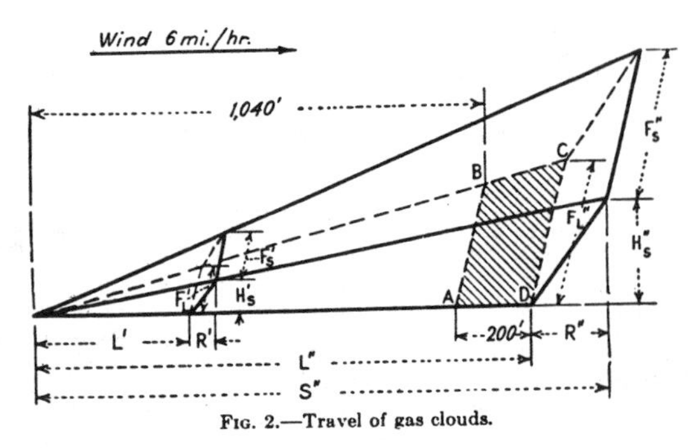

Fig. 2.—Travel of gas clouds.

dimensions indicated by ('') letters in Fig. 2. At the same time, the rear part of this volume, following the expiration of the cylinder discharge and indicated by (') letters, will be uncontaminated air.

$$ABCD = \text{target area: } AD = 200'$$

Assuming *average* field conditions,

$$S'' = S' + \frac{200}{0.8} = 1{,}563'$$
$$R'' = 0.2S'' = 312.6'$$
$$L'' = S'' - R'' = 1{,}250'$$
$$F_l'' = 0.16S'' = 250'$$
$$H_s'' = 0.1S'' = 156.3'$$
$$V_s'' = \frac{L''F_l''H_s''}{6} = \frac{1{,}250 \times 250 \times 156.3}{6} = 8{,}140{,}625 \text{ cu. ft.}$$
$$V_s' = \frac{L'F_l'H'}{6} = \frac{200 \times 40 \times 25}{6} = 33{,}300 \text{ cu. ft.}$$

The volume of the expanded toxic cloud is $V_s'' - V_s' = 8{,}107{,}325$ cu. ft., while its *average* concentration is

69

$$8{,}107{,}325 \div \frac{30}{0.1865} = 1:50{,}000$$

and its ground concentration is 1:15,000 which is only one-fifteenth of the lethal concentration.

Time of Emission.—Again referring to the example given on page 66, we see that 30 lb. of chlorine will produce a lethal concentration of 1:1,000 over a target area 168 ft. wide at a distance of 1,050 ft. from the point of emission if discharged at the rate of 15 lb. per minute. This concentration is, however, lethal only after 30 minutes' exposure, so that 450 lb. of chlorine would be required to produce *deaths* per 168 ft. of enemy front, or almost 3 lb. per foot of front. Of course, *nonfatal* casualties will be produced over a much wider front, since chlorine causes such casualties in concentrations of 1:10,000, or approximately one-tenth the lethal concentration. In this case, nonfatal casualties could be secured with the same amount of chlorine over a target area 361 ft. wide at a distance of 1,806 ft.

Comparison with Smoke.—If instead of a gas we used the same quantity (30 lb.) of a toxic smoke of the same density, under the same conditions, in a concentration of 1:10,000, we should have

$$S = \sqrt[3]{\frac{\dfrac{30}{0.004267 \times 0.1865}}{10{,}000}} = 1{,}556 \text{ ft.}$$
$$L_e = 0.8 \times 1{,}556 = 1{,}245 \text{ ft.}$$
$$F_l = 0.2L_e = 249 \text{ ft.}$$

from which we see that our effective range is 1,245 ft. and our width of target 249 ft.

When a gas concentration is increased tenfold and all other factors remain the same, the effective range is increased by the cube root of 10, or 2.154 times. The *smoke* cloud in our example does not realize such an increase over the gas cloud because the vertical rise of smoke is twice as great as that of gas, *i.e.*, K smoke $= 2K$ gas (table, page 63).

Multiple Points of Emission.—In the foregoing discussion concerning the relation between a quantity of chemical and its effective range, we have considered only emissions from a single point. In actual practice, however, the gas-cloud method of chemical attack is always carried out on a large scale over a considerable portion of the enemy's front. To cover such an area the chemical must be discharged from a sector of one's own front bearing relation to the size of the target to be covered, *i.e.*, the chemical is discharged from a large number of cylinders uniformly distributed along a line substantially parallel to the enemy's front and of a length in proportion to the target area.

70

In order to determine the relation between the amount of chemical and its effective range when discharged from multiple points of emission and the optimum arrangement of these points with reference to the target

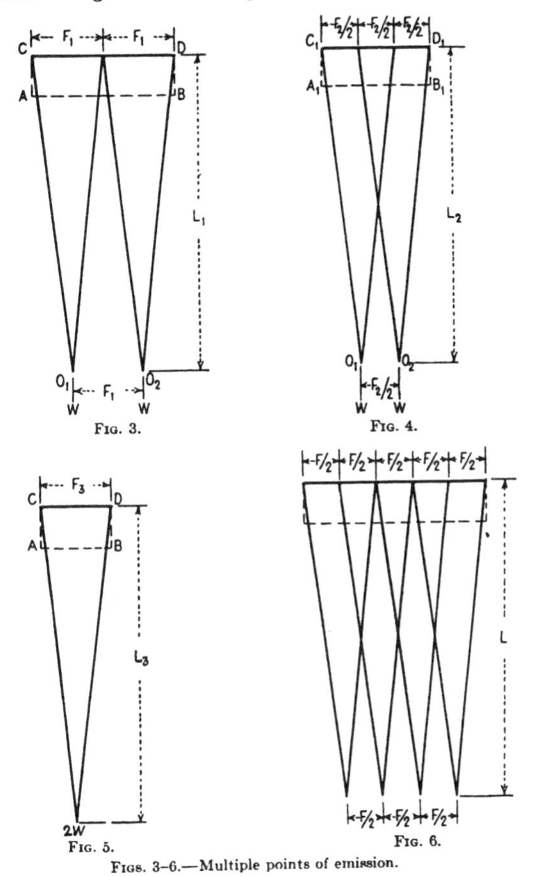

FIGS. 3–6.—Multiple points of emission.

area, we shall first consider some fundamental elements of the problem As the vertical rise of a gas or smoke cloud bears a constant ratio to its length in any case, it will somewhat simplify our discussion if we confine our attention to the *plan* views of the chemical clouds considered.

71

Accordingly, in Figs. 3, 4, and 5 we have plan views of three possible arrangements of *two* cylinders, or points of chemical emission. In Fig. 3, the cylinders, each containing a quantity of chemical W, are placed at points O_1 and O_2, F_1 distance apart, along a line parallel to the front of the target area $ABCD$ and at a distance $L_1 = 1{,}000$ ft. therefrom. Thus arranged, the contents of the two cylinders cover a target $2F_1$ in width with a concentration C. In Fig. 4, the same cylinders are placed at points O_1 and O_2, half the distance apart, shown in Fig. 3, $F_1/2$, so that their clouds overlap a distance $F_2/2$ at the target line A_1B_1. Thus arranged, the cylinders cover a target $1.5F_2$ in width with a concentration C.

In Fig. 5, both cylinders are placed at the same point O so that their clouds coincide and cover a target F_3 in width with a concentration C. Our first inquiry is as to the relative ranges obtained by these three arrangements, *i.e.*, the relations of L_2 and L_3 to L_1.

It is apparent from inspection that Figs. 3 and 5 show the extreme cases and Fig. 4 shows the mean case of all the ways in which two cylinders or points of chemical emission could be arranged in practice, and that the range L_1 in Fig. 3, is equal to that of a single cylinder. Considering Fig. 5 next, we see that this is really the case of a single cylinder of $2W$ capacity, so that from Eqs. (3) and (11), page 64.

$$L_3 = \sqrt[3]{2} \times L_1 = 1.26L_1 \quad \text{and} \quad F_3 = 1.26F_1$$

Comparing these two extreme arrangements, we find that the range in Fig. 5 is 26 per cent larger than that in Fig. 3, while the front covered is only 63 per cent as large.

Now considering Fig. 4, we see that the ground area covered by the two clouds is

$$2F_2\frac{L_2}{2} - F_2\frac{L_2}{8} = \frac{7}{8}F_2L_2$$

while their volume is

$$\frac{7}{8}F_2L_2 \times \frac{H_2}{3} = \frac{7F_2L_2H_2}{24}$$

Since the ground length of a gas cloud is eight-tenths, the spread two-tenths, and the rise one-tenth, of the distance traveled, S, the volumes of the two clouds in Figs. 3, 4, and 5 are, respectively,

$$V_1 = 2\left(\frac{F_1L_1H_1}{6}\right) = \frac{1}{3}\left(\frac{L_1}{4} \times \frac{L_1}{1} \times \frac{L_1}{8}\right) = \frac{L_1^3}{96}$$

$$V_2 = 7\left(\frac{F_2L_2H_2}{24}\right) = \frac{7}{24}\left(\frac{L_2}{4} \times \frac{L_2}{1} \times \frac{L_2}{8}\right) = \frac{7L_2^3}{768}$$

$$V_3 = \frac{F_3L_3H_3}{6} = \frac{1}{6}\left(\frac{L_3}{4} \times \frac{L_3}{1} \times \frac{L_3}{8}\right) = \frac{L_3^3}{192}$$

72

But

$$V_1 = 2\frac{W}{DC}$$

$$V_2 = 2\frac{W}{DC}$$

$$V_3 = 2\frac{W}{DC}$$

where D is the density and C the concentration of the gas.

Hence $$V_1 = V_2 = V_3$$

And

$$\frac{7L_2^3}{768} = \frac{L_1^3}{96}$$

$$L_2 = L_1\sqrt[3]{\frac{768}{672}} = 1.045L_1$$

And

$$\frac{L_3^3}{192} = \frac{L_1^3}{96}$$

$$L_3 = L_1\sqrt[3]{\frac{192}{96}} = 1.260L_1$$

From the foregoing we see that, if the range L_1 in Fig. 3 is 100 per cent, the range in Fig. 4 is 4.5 per cent greater, while the range in Fig. 5 is 26 per cent greater.

From the above we conclude that with a given quantity of chemical the maximum *range* is obtained by discharging the whole quantity from one point, while the maximum *width* of target is obtained by discharging half the quantity from each of two points spaced apart a distance equal to half the target width. If the points of emission are further apart than half the target width, then there will be gaps between the clouds over the target area and, if the points are closer together than half the target width, there will not be a uniform concentration C over the target, but an increase above C where the clouds overlap.

When more than two points of emission are used, optimum results are obtained when the points are spaced a distance apart equal to half the width of target covered by one cylinder. With this arrangement, as indicated in Fig. 6, it may be shown that the distance S traveled by the composite cloud emitted from a number of points, N, varies in accordance with the following general equation:

$$S = \sqrt[3]{\frac{W}{N/(N-1)KC_oD}} \tag{17}$$

73

and since $L = 0.8S$ for *average* field conditions

$$L = 0.8\sqrt[3]{\frac{W}{N/(N-1)KC_aD}} \qquad (18)$$

If the range L for one point of emission is given a value of unity, we have the following relation between the range from one point of emission and the successive ranges from multiple points of emission:

Points of Emission	Range to Target
1	1.000
2	1.045
3	1.063
4	1.072
5	1.077
6	1.081
7	1.084
8	1.086
9	1.087
10	1.089
N	1.100

From the foregoing table, it is seen that the range slowly increases with the number of points of emission and approaches a limit of 1.1 times the range from a single point of emission, as the number of points of emission is indefinitely increased. Also, the optimum arrangement of cylinders, as indicated in Fig. 6, gives a front of emission practically equal to the width of the target to be covered.

From what has been shown above, the number of cylinders needed to cover a given target may be determined as follows: Let the target be 1,000 ft. wide by 500 ft. deep and at a distance of 2,000 ft. from the nearest section of front from which the cylinders can be installed. It is desired to set up and maintain a lethal concentration (1:10,000) of phosgene on the target, under average field conditions and with a range wind of 6 miles per hour. Each cylinder holds 30 lb. of phosgene. Required: the number of cylinders and their distribution.

At 20°C. (68°F.), the density of phosgene is 0.2654 lb. per cubic foot.

From Eq. (2):

$$2{,}500 \text{ ft.} = S - 0.2S \qquad \text{or} \qquad S = 3{,}125 \text{ ft.}$$

$$F_s = 500 \text{ ft.} \qquad H_s = 312.5 \text{ ft. (table, page 63)}$$

From curve B, Chart III,

$$H_e = \frac{312.5}{3} = 104.17 \text{ ft.}$$

74

From Eq. (14)

$$C_a = \frac{0.4771}{2.1271} \times \frac{1}{10{,}000} = 0.00002243$$

Since here F_s equals half the target width and the optimum arrangement of cylinders is at intervals of $F_s/2$, four groups of cylinders, spaced 250 ft. apart, are required to cover the target area.

From Eq. (18),

$$2{,}500 \text{ ft.} = 0.8\sqrt[3]{\frac{W}{(4/3)0.002133 \times 0.00002243 \times 0.2654}}$$

from which

$$W = 560 \text{ lb.}$$

and the total phosgene required is $4 \times 560 = 2{,}240$ lb.

As the wind is blowing at the rate of 528 ft. per minute, it will require 5 minutes for the cloud to reach the rear boundary of the target and an equal time to move over the target. As the phosgene concentration of 1:10,000 is lethal only after 10 minutes' exposure, it takes twice 2,240 or 4,480 lb. to maintain this concentration on the target area for the necessary time to produce fatal casualties. This is equivalent to a total of 150 cylinders divided into four groups spaced 250 ft. apart.

In the preceding example, it was shown that 2,240 lb. of phosgene are required to establish a concentration of 1:10,000 on a target 500 by 1,000 ft. at a distance of 2,000 ft. (667 yd.) from the line of emission. If the phosgene could be released *on* the target and dispersed uniformly thereover, it would require only

$$\frac{500 \times 1{,}000 \times 6 \times 0.2654}{10{,}000} = 80 \text{ lb.}$$

to set up a lethal blanket of gas 6 ft. high over the target area. Thus, at a distance of only 2,000 ft. (667 yd.), it takes 28 lb. of chemical to disseminate 1 lb. in an effective form on the target area by the cloud-gas method of projection. Moreover, as the quantity of chemical required to establish an effective concentration varies as the cube of the range, the cloud-gas method of attack becomes very wasteful of chemical agents when the range exceeds 1,000 yd., since so large a portion of the chemical is dissipated before it reaches the target or is disseminated in the upper parts of the cloud where it serves no useful purpose. For this reason various forms of projectiles were early employed to carry the chemicals to the target and to release them *on* the target area. The first projectiles used for this purpose were artillery shell. These were soon supplemented by trench-mortar shell and later by special (Livens) gas-projector bombs which were fired in only one salvo and thus released the entire chemical

75

concentration at one instant, thereby greatly increasing the surprise effect and the initial toxic concentration. Finally, special (4-in. Stokes) rapid-fire mortars were developed for projecting chemicals in mobile situations and were used very effectively throughout the war.

DISSEMINATION BY PROJECTILES

While the theoretical economy of releasing chemicals on the target area is very large, as indicated above, the practical advantage is not nearly so great, for several deterrant factors enter into the projection and dispersion of chemicals from projectiles.

In the first place, projectiles are not very efficient as carriers of chemicals, for their walls must be made thick enough to withstand the shock of discharge, and this greatly limits their chemical capacity. The efficiency of a chemical projectile may be defined as the ratio of the weight of chemical filling to the gross weight of the projectile. On this basis, the best artillery shell have an efficiency of about 12 per cent. The short-range trench and chemical mortars, having to withstand far less violent shocks of discharge, may have thinner walled projectiles with correspondingly greater chemical capacity. Thus, chemical-mortar shell have an efficiency of about 30 per cent. Livens projector bombs, having a still shorter range, have 50 per cent chemical capacity. Finally, chemical drop bombs and land mines, which are merely dropped or placed in position and thus have no shock of discharge to sustain, have an efficiency of 60 to 70 per cent.

Another factor which greatly reduces the efficiency of artillery for chemical projection is the large increase in dispersion of the projectiles as the range increases. The standard target unit for artillery fire is a square 100 yd. on a side, generally called the *artillery square*. At 3,000 yd., the dispersion of shots from a 75-mm. gun is so small that approximately 91 per cent of the projectiles fired fall within an artillery square. At 8,000 yd., however, owing to greatly increased dispersion of shots, only 41 per cent of the shell fall within an artillery square. Thus, about 2.2 times as many shell and chemical must be expended to produce an effective concentration on a 75-mm. artillery square at 8,000 yd. as at 3,000 yd. The same is true of all other calibers of artillery and, while a greater percentage of shell will fall within a large target area than a small one, a greater amount of chemical is also required for the larger target, although not quite in the same proportion. It thus arises that the efficiency of the artillery as a means for projecting chemicals falls off very rapidly as the range increases.

A third factor limiting the efficiency of artillery shell as chemical vehicles is the loss of chemical on the burst of the shell. On account of its rugged construction, an artillery shell requires a considerable force

76

to open it and, when this force is applied from the bursting charge in the shell, it drives a portion of the chemical charge into the ground; also, it throws a portion into the air above the 6-ft. effective stratum, where it is largely lost insofar as any useful effect is concerned. It is variously estimated that from 25 to 50 per cent of the chemical contents of an artillery shell is thus lost on the burst of the shell if the gas is nonpersistent. For persistent gases this loss is much less. Also, the loss is much less if the shell is burst in the air just above the target, as air-burst chemical shell release from 80 to 90 per cent of their contents in an effective form.

What has been said of artillery shell applies also, but to a far less extent, to short-range projectiles such as Livens bombs and chemical-mortar shell and, to a still less extent, to aviation drop bombs and land mines. Not only are all these latter projectiles of greater efficiency, but they also have much less dispersion than artillery shell at the longer ranges and do not require such large bursting charges to open them.

Because of the great variation in efficiency of the several classes of chemical projectiles, it is obvious that only the most efficient types should be used in the zones they can reach. Thus, the special chemical-projecting devices, such as gas-cloud cylinders, Livens projectors, and chemical mortars, which cover the vital infantry combat zone out to a distance of 2,500 yd. from the front lines, are far more efficient and effective for chemical projection than artillery with its shells of relatively low capacity and efficiency. For the same reasons, aviation drop bombs are more efficient than long-range artillery for dissemination of chemicals beyond a distance of 10,000 yd. (about 6 miles) from the infantry front lines. It is principally on the basis of the relative efficiencies of the several chemical-projecting means that the normal zones for their employment, indicated on page 54, were arrived at.

Regardless of the type of projectile employed to carry the chemical to the target, the dispersion of the chemical after release from the projectile is essentially the same as when released from cylinders. That is to say, the chemical, when released from projectiles, volatilizes, expands, and diffuses into the air, and thus forms a toxic cloud which then moves with the wind exactly as the clouds formed by cylinder discharges.

The same relation between quantity of chemical and the effective range of the chemical obtains when the chemical is released from projectiles as when it is released from cylinders, except, of course, that there is no loss from expansion and diffusion before the toxic cloud reaches the target area.

In addition to obviating this loss, projectiles have two very important advantages over cylinders as a means for disseminating chemicals. First, all kinds of chemicals may be employed in projectiles regardless of their physical state, whereas only chemicals which are relatively volatile liquids

77

may be employed in cylinders. Secondly, chemicals can be used in projectiles regardless of the direction of the wind, whereas cylinders can only be used when the wind is blowing toward the enemy's lines. Even when the wind is blowing directly toward one's own lines, chemicals may be put over in projectiles without danger to friendly troops if the dosage is adjusted to the distance between the target and one's own lines in accordance with the quantity-range relation discussed above.

This relation is thus one of the most important in chemical warfare, for it not only enables one to determine the quantity of chemical required to establish and maintain an effective concentration on a given target at a given range, but, what is equally important, it also enables one to determine how much of a chemical can be safely placed at a given distance from one's own troops under the most adverse conditions. Except for cloud-gas emission from one's own front lines, for which favorable winds are required, it is possible by these determinations to use chemicals at all times and under all conditions with perfect safety to one's own troops. It is at once apparent that, if it requires W pounds of chemical to establish an effective concentration on an enemy position X distance from one's own front lines, any amount of this chemical less than W, released within the enemy position, will not produce an effective concentration on friendly troops, even in an adverse wind, since the relation between a quantity of chemical and its effective range applies alike to both situations

CONTROL OF CHEMICAL WARFARE

Because of this definite relationship between chemical quantities and effective ranges, chemical warfare is susceptible of much closer control than is possible with bullets and H.E. shell. When a bullet or shell once leaves the gun, the gunner cannot tell what its effect will be. It may ricochet or be deflected from its path by striking some intervening obstacle, and its ultimate point of impact may be far removed from the intended target. Even if it strikes within the target area, no one can predict where its fragments will strike or what their ultimate effect will be. On the contrary, a given quantity of chemical will have a definite and predictable effect when intelligently used by properly trained troops who thoroughly understand the behavior of chemical concentrations in the field and know how to employ them, for chemical concentrations follow closely the laws of gases and these laws are just as certain and definite as the law of gravity.

This fact cannot be too strongly emphasized, as there is much misapprehension concerning it, not only on the part of the public in general, but even on the part of military men of high rank and position. One of the main arguments advanced against chemical warfare at peace conferences and in other public discussions in the years immediately following

78

the late war was the mistaken notion that chemicals employed in military operations cannot be controlled and confined to the battlefield, but will unavoidably extend their deleterious effects to areas far behind the combat zone and thus kill or injure noncombatants and civilian populations.

A typical illustration of this erroneous idea is contained in General March's book on the World War. He says:

> We had had the use of gas forced on us in the war by the action of Germany, and in self-protection had to organize the Chemical Warfare Service. And no soldier can say that he prefers to be killed by being torn to pieces by a shell rather than to be gassed. But the use of poison gas, carried wherever the wind listeth, kills the birds of the air, and may kill women and children in rear of the firing line. When I first reached France I found in Paris an American organization, headed by Miss Lothrop, which had a hospital in which, when I inspected it, were over 100 French women and children who had been living in their homes in rear of and *near the front*, and who were gassed. The sufferings of these children, particularly, were horrible and produced a profound impression on me. War is cruel at best, but the use of an instrument of death which, once launched, cannot be controlled, and which may decimate non-combatants—women and children—reduces civilization to savagery.

The instances in which women and children were gassed in the war were very few and in every such case they were gassed because they were living (as in this case) in areas so close to the battle front that they might easily have become victims of bullets, shells, or any of the other weapons of war, as were many thousands of others who risked their lives by remaining in the combat zone.

As a matter of fact, the largest gas attacks in the war did not extend beyond 10 or 12 kilometers behind the firing lines. Moreover, the concentrations beyond 2 to 3 kilometers from the front were so weak as to require prolonged exposure to produce even light casualties whereas deaths from such concentrations were unheard of. Since the normal range of medium and heavy artillery is from 12 to 15 kilometers behind the front lines, it is obvious that any civilians remaining in this zone do so at their own risk and are in daily jeopardy of their lives. Yet no one advocates the abolishment of artillery as a weapon of warfare. The case is even worse against high-explosive long-range artillery shell and aviation drop bombs, for these two weapons were extensively used throughout the war on Paris and other cities far behind the combat zone where noncombatant civilians had every right to pursue their peaceful occupations without jeopardy of life and limb. Nothing is said of the thousands of women and children who were killed and maimed by long-range artillery and aviation bombs in areas far behind the battlefields. It is apparently considered legitimate for a combatant to fire H.E. shell at random into a large city some 70 kilometers behind the front, as when the Germans fired long-range guns on Paris and with a single shell killed or maimed 80 people worshiping in a church. Instances of this kind could be cited by the score,

79

yet the advocates of humanity in warfare are apparently prepared to accept such wholesale destruction when carried out by means of the older and more familiar methods of warfare.

The record of gas in the World War as affecting noncombatants is singularly free from the charge of indiscriminate and uncontrolled injury, for gas was not used in long-range artillery shell or aviation bombs, or in any way beyond a distance of 10 or 12 kilometers behind the firing lines, which zone is universally regarded as the field of battle in modern warfare.

Whatever objections might be logically advanced against the use of chemicals in war, the lack of control of their effect is not one, for chemicals can be far more accurately controlled and their effects more carefully adjusted to the purpose sought than any other weapon heretofore devised by man.

107

CHAPTER V

CLASSIFICATION OF CHEMICAL AGENTS

Chemical agents may be classified in several ways depending upon the point of view and the purpose of the classification. Broadly speaking, we may divide the several classifications into two general groups—theoretical and practical. In the theoretical group are included classifications according to: (1) chemical composition, (2) physical state, and (3) physiological effect, whereas the practical group comprises classifications according to: (1) persistency, (2) degree of action, and (3) tactical employment. In this chapter we shall discuss briefly these several classifications, both during and since the World War, including the system of marking to denote the various classes of chemical agents used by the principal nations, and we shall conclude with some general observations on the subject of classification.

Unfortunately, many of the classifications heretofore in use were based upon classes that were not mutually exclusive but tended in many instances to overlap. This was unavoidable from the properties of the agents themselves, as will be more particularly brought out in discussing the various classes of agents, and there is probably no system that can be devised which is absolutely free from this defect. Nevertheless, classifications serve many useful purposes and, for use in the field, should be made as simple and as clear-cut as possible.

CHEMICAL CLASSIFICATION

Although a vast amount of effort has been expended during and since the late war in an attempt to establish some general laws governing the relation between chemical structure and physiological action on the living body, there is, strictly speaking, today no simple classification of toxic substances in accordance with chemical composition. We have mentioned in Chap. II the tremendous number of chemical compounds among which physiologically active substances may be found. With this vast reservoir from which to draw, it is obvious that much research effort would be saved if the field of search could be delimited by the establishment of the general relation between chemical composition and physiological action. Consequently chemists and toxicologists have worked hand in hand on this complex problem for many years and, while they

108

have not yet solved it, they have succeeded in throwing much light upon the subject and enabled investigators to confine their research to certain families of compounds where desired physiological properties are most apt to be found.

We cannot go very deeply into this subject here; to attempt to do so would lead us far into the field of biochemistry and pharmacology and space does not permit; but we shall state briefly certain limited generalizations which have been established and found useful. The clearest simple statement of this complex subject known to the author is that of Hederer and Istin (15), of which the following is a condensed extract.

It has long been known that certain metals and metalloids possess well-defined toxic properties and that they often confer upon the compounds in which they are present marked physiological activity. Such metals are arsenic, antimony, tin, mercury, lead, and bismuth. Other elements, themselves of indifferent toxicological action, are capable of combining to form groups or radicals which, although they do not always have an actual existence, have the power of giving to their compounds special physiological properties. For example: (1) the ions H^+ and OH^- which form, respectively, the acids and the bases; (2) the oxidizing groups —SO_3, SO_4, NO_3, and P_2O_5; and (3) the reducing groups—SO_2, SH, P_2O_3, and CO.

These materials being known, we can distinguish, without attempting to formulate a law of general application, three different classes in accordance with the organization of toxic molecules; each of them is characterized by particularities of molecular structure and common physiological properties.

In the *first class*, the atom or the toxic group is combined, according to its valence, either with one or several halogens (F, Cl, Br, I) or with one or several radicals (SO_3—, SO_4—, NO_2—, NO_3—, CN—) but never with an atom of carbon. The substances constructed on this model are *mineral compounds*, and their schematic formula can be written

$$X—M—X$$

where the symbol X represents either a halogen or a reducing group, and M, the toxic atom or group.

The substance mercuric chloride ($HgCl_2$), the formula of which may be written

$$Cl—Hg—Cl$$

is an example of compounds of the first class. Other toxic compounds of military importance in this class are:

109

Sulfur monochloride	S_2Cl_2
Arsenic trichloride	Cl—As<(Cl)(Cl)
Sulfuric chlorhydrin	O_2S<(Cl)(Cl)

In the *second class*, the toxic elements (M) are combined with one or several organic radicals (such as CH_3—, C_2H_5—, C_2H_3—, C_6H_5—) and are found linked by carbon, or by one or several atoms of hydrogen—the most simple organic radical. There are thus obtained the *organic compounds*, many of which (to indicate the presence of the characteristic element) merit the name *organo-minerals*. They respond to the general formula

$$R—M—R$$

in which the symbol M is the same as before and in which the R represents an organic radical. The substance cacodyl ($((CH_3)_4.As_2)$), the formula of which may be written:

$$(CH_3)_2>As—As<(CH_3)_2$$

is an example of compounds of the second class. Other toxic compounds of military importance belonging to this class are:

Methylmercaptan	$H—S—CH_3$
Methylarsine	$CH_3—As=H_2$
Lewisite (III)	$As\equiv(CH=CHCl)_3$
Methylformate	O=C<(H)(OCH_3)
Acrolein	O=C<(H)($CH=CH_2$)
Hydrocyanic acid	H—C—N
Phenylcarbylamine	$C\equiv N—C_6H_5$

In the *third class*, the basic materials can combine, in one or several valences, with halogens or with ionizable mineral radicals, as bodies of the first class and thus, or by the remaining free valences, either with carbon or organic radicals or with hydrogen, as bodies of the second class. In order to realize similar compounds, called *organic* or *organo-mineral halogens*, the primary elements should be at least bivalent. The formula for compounds of this class is

$$R—M—X$$

in which all the symbols are the same as above.

110

Ethyl mercuric chloride, the formula of which may be written

$$C_2H_5—Hg—Cl$$

is an example of compounds of the third class. Other important military toxic compounds belonging to this class are

Mustard gas	S<($CH_2—CH_2—Cl$)($CH_2—CH_2—Cl$)
Dichlormethylarsine	$CH_3—As=Cl_2$
Lewisite (II)	$(ClCH—CH)_2=As$
Phosgene	$O=C=Cl_2$
Chloroformate of methyl chloride	O—C<(Cl)($OCCl_3$)
Iodoacetone	O=C<(CHI)(CH_3)

Cyanogen chloride	$Cl{-}C{\equiv}N$
Phenylcarbylamine chloride	$Cl_2{=}C{=}N{-}C_6H_5$
Methylchlorsulfate	$SO_2{-}H{<}^{Cl}_{OCH_3}$
Chlorpicrin	$Cl_3C{-}N{<}^{O}_{O}$

While it appears from the foregoing that many of the World War chemical agents may be classified in accordance with the scheme outlined, it does not follow that all such agents are so classifiable, as there are many known exceptions, and undoubtedly many more exceptions will be found as new chemical agents are discovered.

Another chemical classification of combat toxics is indicated by Hederer and Istin as follows:

1. Oxydizers, *e.g.*, chlorine, chlorpicrin, or
2. Reducers, *e.g.*, acrolein, ketones.
3. Ionizable, *e.g.*, hydrocyanic acid, arsines, or
4. Nonionizable, *e.g.*, carbon monoxide.

However, there are not clear-cut lines of demarcation between these classes, nor do they in any way help to associate chemical composition with physiological action so that little seems to be gained by efforts to classify toxic compounds along these lines.

Our conclusion, then, as regards the chemical classification of toxic compounds is that at present only very sketchy approximations can be made. Moreover, among compounds of military importance there are

111

so many exceptions to any general chemical classification that the whole subject abounds in technical difficulties. Fortunately, however, chemical classification is not of any great importance in chemical warfare, other than as an aid to research. Perhaps the most important point to be emphasized here is the fact that many of the most formidable toxic agents known today belong to two well-defined families of compounds—the cyanides and the organic arsenicals—and it is from these fields that most of the future chemical agents seem likely to be drawn.

PHYSICAL CLASSIFICATION

The physical classification is very simple and is based upon physical state or form of the substance *under ordinary conditions, i.e.*, temperature 68°F. (20°C.) and atmospheric pressure (760 mm. Hg). Thus, an agent is a true *gas*, if its boiling point is below ordinary atmospheric temperature, as is the case with chlorine (b.p. – 28°F.). This classification as a *true gas* is not to be confused with the broad generic term *gas*, used to refer generally to toxic chemical agents, but means that the substance is in a gaseous state under ordinary temperatures and pressures.

CLASSIFICATION OF CHEMICAL AGENTS ACCORDING TO PHYSICAL STATE

Gases	Boiling point, °F.	Liquids	Boiling point, °F.	Solids	Melting point, °F.
Carbon monoxide	–310	Brombenzyl cyanide	+77*	Dichlorethyl sulfide	+57
Chlorine	– 28.3	Hydrocyanic acid	79.7	Brombenzyl cyanide	77
Phosgene	+ 46.7	Acrolein	126.3	Diphenylcyanarsine	91
Hydrocyanic acid	+ 79.7	Monochlormethylchloroformate	228.2	White phosphorus	111
		Chlorpicrin	231.5	Diphenylchlorarsine	113
		Chloracetone	246.2	Ethylcarbazol	154
		Trichlormethylchloroformate	260.6	Diphenylaminechlorarsine	387
		Methylsulfuryl chloride	269.6		
		Brommethylethyl ketone	271.4		
		Bromacetone	275		
		Perchlormethylmercaptan	300.2		
		Ethyldichlorarsine	312.8		
		Ethylbromacetate	318.2		
		Dimethyl sulfate	370.4		
		Lewisite	374		
		Benzyl bromide	393.8		
		Phenylcarbylamine chloride	406.4		
		Xylyl bromide	420.8		
		Dichlorethyl sulfide	57*		
		Phenyldichlorarsine	484.7		

* Melting point.

An agent is a *liquid* if its melting point is below ordinary temperatures and its boiling point is above such temperatures, *i.e.*, when the

112

range of atmospheric temperatures lie between the melting and boiling points of an agent, *e.g.*, chlorpicrin (m.p. – 92.4°F., b.p. 235.4°F.).

Similarly, an agent is a *solid* when its melting point is above ordinary atmospheric temperatures, *e.g.*, white phosphorus (m.p. 111°F.).

The tabulation on page 111 shows the principal World War chemical agents classified according to physical state.

PHYSIOLOGICAL CLASSIFICATION

This classification arranges chemical agents according to the effects they produce upon the living body. Both during and since the late war, the physiological classification systems of the principal countries has differed considerably; in order to compare these systems, we shall review briefly the salient points of each.

American Classification (World War) —In this system, the toxic substances are classified according to the predominant effects which they exert, with the understanding, however, that the action of any substance is not limited to a single tissue or group of tissues. Thus, a substance, the vapor of which causes injury to the respiratory passages, may, when applied to the skin, cause blistering. If the sole or chief usefulness of a substance in warfare depends upon its effect on the respiratory tract, it is classed as a *respiratory irritant.* If its power to produce casualties is due to its action on the skin, it is classed as a *skin irritant.* If both actions are useful, it is placed in both groups.

1. *Respiratory Irritants.*—By far the greatest number of substances thus far used injure the respiratory apparatus. Three groups may be differentiated:

a. Those which exert their chief effects on the delicate membranes in the lungs through which oxygen passes from the air into the blood. The main result of this injury is to cause fluid to pass from the blood into the minute air sacs and thus to obstruct the oxygen supplied to the blood. Death from one of these substances may be compared to death by drowning, the water in which the victim drowns being drawn into his lungs from his own blood vessels, *e.g.*, phosgene, chlorine, chlorpicrin, diphosgene.

b. Substances which injure the membranes which line the air passages. During normal life these membranes insure protection to the lungs against mechanical injury by particles which may be taken in with the air and against bacterial infection. As a result of the action of substances of this group, their protective power is lost. Portions of the membrane may become swollen and detached and may plug up the smaller passages leading to the lung tissue, or the damaged tissue may become the seat of bacterial infection, thus setting up bronchitis and pneumonia, *e.g.*, mustard gas, ethyldichlorarsine.

113

c. Substances which affect chiefly the upper air passages, *i.e.*, the nose and throat. These substances cause intense pain and discomfort, but are not dangerous to life. They cause sneezing, painful smarting of the nose and throat, intense headache, a feeling of severe constriction of the chest, and vomiting. For varying periods after exposure, they may cause general muscular weakness and dizziness, loss of sensation in parts of the body or any transitory unconsciousness, *e.g.*, diphenylchlorarsine, diphenylcyanarsine.

2. *Tear Producers* (*Lacrimators*).—Certain substances have a powerful effect upon the eyes, causing copious flowing of tears, followed by reddening and swelling of the eyes, producing thereby effective temporary blindness. These effects are often produced by extremely minute quantities of tear-producing substances. Large quantities of the same substances usually act as lung irritants as well, *e.g.*, brombenzyl cyanide, bromacetone, ethyliodoacetate, chlorpicrin.

3. *Skin Blisterers* (*Vesicants*).—Certain substances have a powerful irritating effect upon the skin, very much like that produced by poison ivy. The same effect is produced upon all the surfaces of the body with which the substance may come in contact, such as the eyes and the breathing passages. Accordingly, a substance producing skin blistering will, if inhaled, also act as a powerful irritant of the air passages, *e.g.*, mustard gas.

American Classification (Postwar).—Agents are classified physiologically according to their most pronounced effect. The following are the terms usually employed:

1. *Lung Irritants.**—Agents which, when breathed, cause inflammation and injury to the interior cavity of the bronchial tubes and the lungs, *e.g.*, phosgene, diphosgene, chlorpicrin.
2. *Irritants (Sternutators).*—Those substances which produce violent sneezing and coughing followed by temporary physical disability. Sternutators are usually in the form of irritant smokes and the two are regarded as synonymous, *e.g.*, diphenylchlorarsine, diphenylaminechlorarsine, diphenylcyanarsine.
3. *Lacrimators.*—Agents which cause a copious flow of tears and intense, though temporary, eye pains, *e.g.*, bromacetone, brombenzyl cyanide, chloracetophenone.
4. *Vesicants.*—Agents which, when absorbed or dissolved in any part of the human body, produce inflammation and burns with destruction of tissues.

* The author has substituted the term *lung injurants* for this class of gases to distinguish them from the nose and throat irritants (sternutators).

British Classification (World War).—During the early part of the war, the British employed four classes, as follows:

1. Gases of permanent effect, roughly corresponding to our class of vesicants, *e.g.*, dichlorethyl sulfide.
2. Gases of temporary effect, roughly corresponding to our class of lung injurants, *e.g.*, phosgene.

3. Gases having a nonfatal effect, corresponding to our irritants, *e.g.*, ethyliodoacetate.
4. Gases having a fatal effect, corresponding to our class of systemic poisons, *e.g.*, hydrocyanic acid gas.

Later on in the war, the British reduced their physiological classification to only two classes:

1. Lacrimatory agents (ethyliodoacetate).
2. Lethal agents (phosgene, chlorpicrin, mustard gas).

British Classification (Postwar).—Since the war, the British have adopted the following classification:

a. Vesicants, *e.g.*, mustard gas and lewisite.
b. Lung irritants, *e.g.*, phosgene, chlorine, chlorpicrin.
c. Sensory irritants, *e.g.*, diphenylchlorarsine, diphenylcyanarsine.
d. Lacrimators, *e.g.*, brombenzyl cyanide, xylyl bromide, etc.
e. Direct poisons of the nervous system, or paralysants, *e.g.*, hydrocyanic acid gas.
f. Gases which interfere with the respiratory function of the blood, *e.g.*, carbon monoxide.

"Broadly speaking, the gases in groups (*b*) and (*e*) may be regarded as lethal agents, and those in groups (*c*) and (*d*) as irritants, capable of putting a man out of action immediately, though only temporarily; whilst those of group (*a*), though intensely poisonous, have, when used against troops who are well disciplined in defence against gas, a casualty-producing power enormously in excess of their killing power".

French Classification (World War).—The French classification recognized seven classes as follows:

1. Highly toxic gases, *e.g.*, hydrocyanic acid.
2. Suffocating or asphyxiating gases, *e.g.*, chlorine, phosgene, diphosgene, chlorpicrin.
3. Lacrimators, *e.g.*, chloracetone, acrolein.
4. Vesicants, *e.g.*, mustard gas, dimethyl sulfate.
5. Sternutators, *e.g.*, diphenylchlorarsine, diphenylcyanarsine.
6. Labyrinthic, which affect the ear, *e.g.*, dichlormethyl ether.
7. Carbon monoxide.

French Classification (Postwar).—Since the war, the French have simplified their physiological classification to the following:

1. Irritant toxics comprising:
   a. Lacrimators, *e.g.*, benzyl bromide and xylyl bromide.
   b. Respiratory irritants or sternutators, *e.g.*, diphenylchlorarsine, diphenylcyanarsine.
2. Caustic toxics comprising:
   a. Lung caustics or suffocants, *e.g.*, chlorine and phosgene.
   b. Skin caustics or vesicants, *e.g.*, mustard gas, lewisite.
3. General toxics, *e.g.*, hydrocyanic acid type, comprising no actual well-differentiated subdivisions.

German Classification (World War).—The early German classification distinguished three classes as follows:

1. Irritant gases (*Reizstoffe*) which cause only temporary injuries, comprising:
   a. Lacrimators, e.g., T-Stoff.
   b. Irritants, e.g., B-Stoff, Bn-Stoff, D-Stoff.
2. *Combat gases (Kampfstoff)* which cause more permanent injuries, *e.g.*, C-Stoff and K-Stoff.
3. Toxic gases (*Giftstoff*) which cause death or serious incapacitation, *e.g.*, hydrocyanic acid, diphosgene, chlorpicrin.

Later on in the war the middle-class (2) gases gradually dropped out and the Germans came to recognize only two great classes: (1) the nonfatal irritants, and (2) the fatal toxic gases.

German Classification (Postwar).—Since the war the Germans have adopted the following classification :

1. Lacrimators (*tränenerregende Kampfstoffe*), *e.g.*, bromacetone, xylyl bromide, brombenzyl cyanide, chloracetophenone.
2. Sternutators (*niesenerregende Kampfstoffe*), *e.g.*, diphenylchlorarsine, diphenylcyanarsine.
3. Lung irritants (*lungenreizende Kampfstoffe*), *e.g.*, chlorine, phosgene, diphosgene, chlorpicrin, lewisite B.
4. Vesicants (*blasenziehende Kampfstoffe*), *e.g.*, chlorovinyldichlorarsine, dichlorethyl sulfide.
5. Nerve poisons (*Nervengifte*), *e.g.*, hydrocyanic acid.

On comparing the several World War physiological classifications with those of the postwar period, we find that there was much greater divergence among the various systems during the war than since then.

Thus it is noted that the German World War classification differed in principle from those of the Allies, the German classification being based solely upon the *degree* of physiological effect, while all the Allies' systems were based upon the *nature* of the effect.

Since the war there has been a gradual rapprochement of viewpoint in the matter of physiological classification so that now we find the principal nations in substantial agreement upon the following physiological classification of chemical agents:

1. *Lung injurants*—compounds which attack the pulmonary passages and lungs and generally prove fatal in a few hours if the gas is present in the usual field concentration.

2. *Irritants* (often called *sternutators*)—compounds which produce a strong local irritation of the nose and throat, causing violent sneezing and coughing. This irritation often extends to the stomach through the swallowing of saliva containing the irritant substance and causes severe headache, nausea, and vomiting. Exposure to strong concentrations of irritant compounds generally results in marked physical debility. How-

ever, these effects are only temporary and are limited to the period of exposure and a few hours thereafter.

3. *Lacrimators*—compounds which act almost exclusively upon the eyes, producing a copious flow of tears and rendering vision impossible during the period of exposure and for from half an hour to an hour thereafter. Lacrimatory gases seldom have any other physiological effects in the concentrations employed in the field.

4. *Vesicants*—compounds which attack all body surfaces with which they came in contact (both internal and external), producing blisters and a general destruction of tissue similar to burns from fire. In addition to this surface action, most of the vesicants were also toxic if inhaled into the lungs in the form of vapor. Because of their multiple effects upon the body, the vesicants were by long odds the most prolific casualty producers of any military agents used in the late war.

5. *Systemic poisons*—compounds which usually attack the blood (as carbon monoxide) or the nerve centers (as hydrocyanic acid) and produce almost instant death by arresting the vital processes of the body at their motor centers. These agents are the most virulent poisons with respect to the quantity required to produce death but they are not the most fatal gases on the battlefield owing to their extreme volatility, light vapor density, and other peculiar properties which detract from their effectiveness in the field.

In addition to the above classes of gases, there are also the smoke and incendiary agents but, as they produce only slight or incidental physiological effects, they are usually omitted from the physiological classifications.

CLASSIFICATION ACCORDING TO PERSISTENCY

As the persistency of an agent in the field measures the length of time its effective concentration can be maintained and hence the duration of its action in battle, the classification of chemical agents according to persistency of great practical importance.

For the purpose of comparison, we shall note briefly the practice of the principal nations with regard to this classification during and since the World War.

American Classification (World War).—The classification shown in the table on page 117 was employed by the American Army during the War:

American Classification (Postwar).—Since the World War, the American classification has been reduced to two classes by the elimination of the intermediate (moderately persistent) class, so that now agents which persist for more than 10 minutes in the open field are classed as *persistent*, while agents which persist less than 10 minutes are

117

classsed as *nonpersistent*. In accordance with this scheme, only the following important chemical agents are nonpersistent: Cl, CG, HCN, CN, DM, DA, DC, WP, FM. All other agents are persistent.

AMERICAN WORLD WAR CLASSIFICATION ACCORDING TO PERSISTENCY

Class	Agents	Persistency		Remarks
		In open	In woods	
I. Nonpersistent....	VN Cl CG CNL DA DC	10 min.	3 hr.	These gases are very volatile, vaporizing entirely at the moment of explosion. They form a cloud, capable of giving deadly effects, but which loses, more or less rapidly, its effectiveness by dilution and dispersion into the atmosphere.
II. Moderately persistent.	NC PS PG PCC DG	3 hr.	12 hr.	These gases, having moderately high boiling points, are only partially vaporized at the moment of explosion. The cloud formed upon explosion is generally not deadly, but it immediately gives penetrative lacrimatory or irritant effects. The majority of the gas contents of the shell is pulverized and projected in the form of a spray of fog, which slowly settles on the ground and continues to give off vapors that prolong the action of the initial cloud.
III. Highly persistent.	HS CA BA	3 days	7 days	These gases, having a very high boiling point, are but little vaporized at the moment of explosion. A small portion of the contents of the shell is atomized and gives immediate effect, but by far the greater part is projected on the ground in the form of droplets which slowly vaporize and continue the action of the initial cloud.

Other Classifications.—The British, French, and Germans, neither during nor since the war, adopted any sharply defined classification of

118

chemical agents in accordance with persistency. On the contrary, all three, while recognizing generally the two main classes—nonpersistent and persistent—failed to specify any definite time units to distinguish these classes.

Thus, from the British point of view,

. . . gases are generally divided into two main categories:

Nonpersistent.
Persistent.

Nonpersistent substances when liberated are rapidly converted into gas or smoke; clouds of gas so produced continue to be effective until dissipated by the wind and the sun.

Persistent substances used in gas warfare are generally liquids, which contaminate the area on which they are released and continue to give off vapor for a considerable period. Mustard gas and most tear gases are typical examples. Whilst evaporation is going on the immediate neighborhood to leeward of the contamination is dangerous. In the case of gases such as mustard gas, which attack the skin, actual contact with contaminated ground or objects must be avoided.

The French view of this subject is clearly expressed by Hederer and Istin as follows:

The military employment of the chemical arm leads to the distinction, on the basis of total particular toxic effect, between two categories of aggressive substances; the volatile substances and the persistent substances. The volatile substances are either gases, such as chlorine, or liquids of low boiling point and high vapor pressure, such as phosgene and hydrocyanic acid, which boil, respectively, at 46°F. and 79°F., or solids dispersed as ultramicroscopic particles, such as the chloride or cyanide of diphenylarsine.

The first constitute the gaseous "clouds" and the second smokes which diffuse and rapidly vanish in open country.

The persistent substances are, on the contrary, liquids of high boiling point and low vapor pressure, such as chlorpicrin and mustard gas, which boil, respectively, at 224°F. and 423°F. Their clouds condense upon the soil in the form of minute liquid droplets and evaporate slowly. These substances are generally endowed with great stability. They do not oxydize readily in contact with air and they hydrolyze only with difficulty.

As to German practice, Hanslian says:

By persistence we understand the period of time during which a combat substance remains on the spot where it was liberated for tactical purposes, and exerts its effects there. This persistence is dependent first of all upon the volatility of the substance in question; it is greater the lower the volatility, and vice versa.

. . . .

From a tactical viewpoint, persistency is a matter of vital importance since it is this property which mainly determines whether or not a chemical agent is suitable for use on the offensive. Since attacking troops must traverse the ground between their

119

own position and that of the enemy, and, if their attack is successful, they must occupy the enemy's position, it is manifest that chemical agents employed in support of the attack must be of very low persistency so as to leave the terrain treated with such agents safe for occupancy by the attacking troops when they reach the enemy lines. Under normal battle conditions, it has been found that gases which persist for more than ten minutes after release upon open ground are dangerous to attacking troops when they traverse or occupy such treated areas and hence only nonpersistent gases are suitable for offensive operations, except when the attack is made on such a broad front that certain strong defensive areas can be avoided in the attack, in which case such areas may be treated with persistent gases.

For general harrassing and for defensive operations, where the ground treated with chemical agents is not to be occupied by friendly troops, persistent agents are more effective and are generally employed for these purposes.

For use of troops in the field, no military classification of chemical agents can ignore persistency and the more clear cut and definite the classification according to persistency, the more useful it is.

He then gives a tabulation of the persistencies of several of the more important chemical agents, calculated according to the Leitner formula (see page 21) and arranged in inverse order of persistence, but no segregation into classes according to persistency is made.

CLASSIFICATION ACCORDING TO DEGREE OF ACTION

By degree of action is meant the seriousness of the casualties inflicted by chemical agents and, as chemical agents vary all the way from simple lacrimation to almost instant death, there is a wide range in their degree of action.

From the viewpoint of military operations in the field, chemical agents are generally divided into three classes:

1. *Light-casualty* agents which produce simple lacrimation or temporary irritation of some part of the body, as the nose and throat, *e.g.*, sternutators.
2. *Moderate-casualty* agents which incapacitate for a period of from a few days to several weeks, but seldom cause permanent injuries or death, *e.g.*, the vesicant agents (mustard gas).
3. *Serious-casualty* agents which cause prolonged or permanent casualties and a high percentage of deaths, *e.g.*, lung injurants such as phosgene.

Closely associated with, and really forming a logical part of, the classification according to degree of action, is the further consideration as to the speed of action of chemical agents, *i.e.*, whether they produce immediate or delayed effects. In general, agents of the light-casualty class (1) and serious-casualty class (3) produce immediate effects, whereas those of the moderate-casualty class (2) produce delayed effects, but this rule is variable and there are notable exceptions both ways.

120

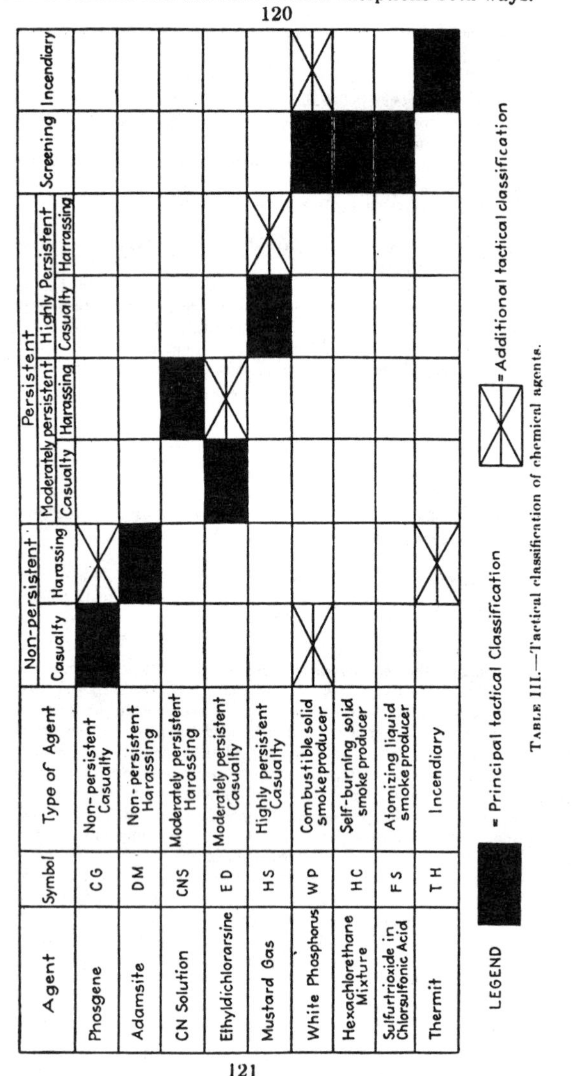

Agent	Symbol	Type of Agent	Non-persistent: Casualty	Non-persistent: Harassing	Persistent, Moderately persistent: Casualty	Persistent, Moderately persistent: Harassing	Persistent, Highly Persistent: Casualty	Persistent, Highly Persistent: Harrassing	Screening	Incendiary
Phosgene	CG	Non-persistent Casualty	■	X						
Adamsite	DM	Non-persistent Harassing		■						
CN Solution	CNS	Moderately persistent Harassing				■				
Ethyldichlorarsine	ED	Moderately persistent Casualty			■	X				
Mustard Gas	HS	Highly persistent Casualty					■	X		
White Phosphorus	WP	Combustible solid smoke producer	X						■	X
Hexachlorethane Mixture	HC	Self-burning solid smoke producer							■	
Sulfurtrioxide in Chlorsulfonic Acid	FS	Atomizing liquid smoke producer							■	
Thermit	TH	Incendiary		X						■

LEGEND: ■ = Principal tactical Classification; X = Additional tactical classification

TABLE III.—Tactical classification of chemical agents.

121

TACTICAL CLASSIFICATION

This classification is according to tactical use and logically embraces the following classes (see Table III):

1. Casualty agents, which include:
   - *a.* Lung injurants.
   - *b.* Vesicants.
   - *c.* White phosphorus.
2. Harassing agents, which include:
   - *a.* Lacrimators.
   - *b.* Irritants (sternutators and irritant smokes).
3. Screening agents (obscuring smokes).
4. Incendiary agents.

MILITARY CLASSIFICATION

From the six classifications described above may be worked out a single mixed classification which is useful in military operations. This mixed or *military* classification groups all chemical agents into categories most useful to the using troops.

As the two things which are of paramount importance to commanders in the field are (1) *persistency* and (2) *nature of effects* produced upon the enemy, the most logical military classification is as follows:

MILITARY CLASSIFICATION OF COMBAT GASES

I. *Nonpersistent agents*

A. *Lung injurants*

1. Simple
   - Chlorine .... (Cl_2)
   - Methylsulfuryl chloride .... ($ClSO_3CH_3$)
   - Ethylsulfuryl chloride .... ($ClSO_3C_2H_5$)
   - Chlormethylchloroformate .... ($ClCOOCH_2Cl$)
   - Phosgene .... ($COCl_2$)
   - Dimethyl sulfate .... ($(CH_3)_2SO_4$)
   - Perchlormethylmercaptan .... ($SCCL_4$)
   - Trichlormethylchloroformate .... ($ClCOOCCl_3$)
   - Chlorpicrin .... (NO_2CCl_3)
   - Phenylcarbylamine chloride .... ($C_6H_5CNCl_2$)
   - Dichlormethyl ether .... ($(CH_2Cl)_2O$)
   - Dibrommethyl ether .... ($(CH_2Br)_2O$)
2. Toxic
   - Phenyldichlorarsine .... ($C_6H_5AsCl_2$)
   - Ethyldichlorarsine .... ($C_2H_5AsCl_2$)
   - Phenyldibromarsine .... ($C_6H_5AsBr_2$)

B. *Respiratory irritants* (sternutators)

1. Simple
   - Diphenylchlorarsine .... ($(C_6H_5)_2AsCl$)
   - Diphenylcyanarsine .... ($(C_6H_5)_2AsCN$)
   - Ethylcarbazol .... ($((C_6H_4)_2NC_2H_5)$)
   - Diphenylaminechlorarsine .... ($NH(C_6H_4)_2AsCl$)
2. Toxic
   - Phenyldichlorarsine* .... ($C_6H_5AsCl_2$)
   - Ethyldichlorarsine* .... ($C_2H_5AsCl_2$)
   - Ethyldibromarsine* .... ($C_2H_5AsBr_2$)

* Primarily toxic lung injurants.

122

C. *Systemic toxics*
   - Hydrocyanic acid .... (HCN)
   - Cyanogen bromide .... ($CNBr$)
   - Cyanogen chloride .... ($CNCl$)
   - Phenylcarbylamine chloride* .... ($C_6H_5HCCl_2$)

II. *Persistent agents*

A. *Immediate effect*

1. Pure lacrimators
   - Ethylbromacetate .... ($CH_2BrCOOC_2H_5$)
   - Xylyl bromide .... ($CH_3C_6H_4CH_2Br$)
   - Benzyl bromide .... ($C_6H_5CH_2Br$)
   - Ethyliodoacetate .... ($CH_2ICOOC_2H_5$)
   - Benzyl iodide .... ($C_6H_5CH_2I$)
   - Brombenzyl cyanide .... ($C_6H_5CHBrCN$)
   - Chloracetophenone .... ($C_6H_5COCH_2Cl$)
2. Toxic lacrimators
   - Chloracetone .... (CH_3COCH_2Cl)
   - Bromacetone .... (CH_3COCH_2Br)
   - Iodoacetone .... (CH_3COCH_2I)
   - Acrolein .... (CH_2CHCHO)
   - Brommethylethyl ketone .... ($CH_3COCHBrCH_3$)
   - Chlorpicrin† .... (CCl_3NO_2)
   - Phenylcarbylamine chloride† .... ($C_6H_5CHCl_2$)

B. *Delayed effect*

1. Pure vesicants ..... Dimethyl sulfate† .... ($(CH_3)_2SO_4$)
2. Toxic vesicants
   - Methyldichlorarsine .... (CH_3AsCl_2)
   - Dichlorethyl sulfide .... ($S(C_2H_4Cl)_2$)
   - Phenyldichlorarsine† .... ($C_6H_5AsCl_2$)
   - Phenyldibromarsine† .... ($C_6H_5AsBr_2$)
   - Ethyldichlorarsine† .... ($C_2H_5AsCl_2$)
   - Chlorvinyldichlorarsine .... ($ClCHCHAsCl_2$)

* Primarily toxic lung injurants.
† Primarily lung injurants.

While the above classification is a logical and useful arrangement to combat gases in accordance with properties of primary importance to troops in the field, it is more fortuitous than rigid in its application. Thus, while all vesicant gases heretofore in use have been persistent and have had delayed effects on men and animals, it does not follow that all future vesicants will necessarily have these properties, for there is no known connection between vesication and persistency, or between vesication and delayed effects. On the contrary, it is entirely possible that a nonpersistent vesicant, or one that is immediately effective, will be discovered. There is an urgent tactical demand for such a type of gas and there is no reason why it cannot be found. Similarly, there is no inherent reason why lung-injurant or respiratory-irritant gases should be nonpersistent and it is readily conceivable that persistent gases of these two classes may exist.

Accordingly, all we can say for the military classification indicated above is that it accords with the known facts today and is a logical and useful arrangement. If and when exceptions to this classification appear,

123

as is not at all unlikely, we shall then have to amend our arrangement and formulate a new classification in accordance with the new facts.

MARKING SYSTEMS

In order to indicate to troops in the field essential information concerning the type and character of the fillings contained in chemical projectiles, each nation adopted a special system of marking such projectiles. As the basic theory of the several marking systems used in the war was quite different, the principal features of each will be noted here.

German System.—We have said that the German World War classification of combat gases differed in principle from the classifications of the Allies, in that the German system was based primarily upon the *degree* of effect exerted by the gas, whereas the Allies' systems were predicated upon the *nature* of the effect, *i.e.* whether *lung* injurant or vesicant, etc. Based upon the fundamental idea of degree of effect, the German system grouped all gases into four major classes, with distinguishing marks, as follows:

Class	Physiological action	Marking
1. Harmless gases	Lacrimators (*Augenreizstoff*)	White Cross (*Weisskreuzkampfstoffe*)
T-Stoff	Xylyl bromide	
B-Stoff	Bromacetone	
Bn-Stoff	Brommethylethylketone	
2. Slightly harmful gases	Irritants (*Reizstoffe*)	Blue Cross (*Blaukreuzkampfstoffe*)
Clark I	Diphenylchlorarsine	
Clark II	Diphenylcyanarsine	
Dick	Ethyldichlorarsine	
3. Moderately harmful gases	Vesicants (*blasenziehende Kampfstoffe*)	Yellow Cross (*Gelbkreuzkampfstoffe*)
Lost	Dichlorethyl sulfide	
D-Stoff	Dimethyl sulfate	
	Dichlormethyl ether	
4. Severely harmful	Lung injurants (*lungenreizende Kampfstoffe*)	Green Cross (*Grünkreuzkampfstoffe*)
Chlor	Chlorine	
Phosgen (D-Stoff)	Carbonyl chloride	
Perstoff (diphosgene)	Trichlormethylchloroformate	
Klop (chlorpicrin)	Nitrochloroform	
K-Stoff	Monochlormethylchloroformate	

All projectiles containing gases belonging to any one of the above groups were marked with a corresponding colored cross, as indicated.
124
To identify further particular gases within a group, additional marks were used. Thus, if a shell contained diphosgene, it was marked with a green cross; if it contained diphosgene mixed with chlorpicrin, it was marked with a green cross and the figure 1; if it contained phosgene, diphosgene, and diphenylchlorarsine, it was marked with a green cross and the figure 2. Similarly, diphenylchlorarsine was marked with a blue cross and the figure 1, while diphenylcyanarsine was marked with a blue cross and the figure 2. Also ethyldichlorarsine was distinguished from mustard gas (yellow cross) by adding the figure 1 to denote the former filling.

The earlier type shell containing lacrimators and simple irritants were marked with large white letters thus, "B" for B-Stoff, "C" for C-Stoff, and "D" for D-Stoff, etc. There was no uniform body color to denote gas shell as a whole; the earlier types of gas shell were painted gray, whereas the later types were painted blue with a yellow ogive. Smoke shell were painted gray with a black letter "N" (*Nebel*, fog) to distinguish them from gas shell.

Incendiary shell were painted red all over with the word "Brand-Gr" on the side in black letters to distinguish from certain types of HE shell which were also painted red.

The principal defects in the German marking system were: (1) the lack of a distinctive uniform body color to distinguish chemical shell from other types; and (2) the absence of means for indicating the relative persistency of the various chemical fillings, which is of great importance to tactical operations in the field. This second defect was somewhat mitigated by the circumstances that, as a whole, the Green and Blue Cross shell were nonpersistent, while the Yellow Cross were persistent. But this was more fortuitous than deliberate, and the lines of demarcation were not clear cut. Shell containing ethyldichlorarsine were at first marked as Yellow Cross 1, but were later changed to Green Cross 3, when it was found that this gas was sufficiently nonpersistent to be used on the offensive.

French System.—French chemical shell were distinguished from other types by a body color of dark green, and the incendiary shell were distinguished from the gas shell by a red ogive. There were no French smoke shell, distinguished as such. Certain gas shell had a sufficient amount of smoke-producing material to make a visible cloud on burst, but they were regarded as gas shell.

Chemical fillings, regardless of whether they were gas, gas with smoke, or incendiary, were denoted by certain code numbers, sometimes in combination with colored bands or stripes on the shell. The code numbers were purely arbitrary and were not arranged in any way to indicate persistency or even the type of chemical filling. On the contrary, the
125
numbers seem to have been chronologically assigned to each filling as it was adopted.

The following table gives the principal French chemical shell with their markings:

Shell	Charge	Markings
75 mm. incendiary	Carbon disulfide; white phosphorus; cylinder of incendiary in celluloid	Green ogive, red body, No. 2 on top of ogive and also on bottom
75 mm. incendiary	White phosphorus; neutral liquid	Green ogive, red body, No. 3 on top and bottom
75 mm. gas	Vincennite quarternaire (V4)	Green, 2 white rings, No. 4 on top and bottom
75 mm. gas	Vitrite; manganite; marsite	White Bands, "4B" on ogive, base and shell case
75 mm. gas and smoke	Collongite, ⅔; opacite, ⅓	Green, 1 white ring, No. 5 on top and bottom
75 mm. gas and smoke	Aquinite, ¾; opacite, ¼	Green, 1 orange-yellow ring, No. 7 on top and bottom
75 mm. gas and smoke	Martonite; opacite	Green, 1 orange-yellow ring, No. 9 on top and bottom
75 mm. gas	Yperite with solvent	2 orange-yellow bands, "20"
75 mm. gas	Camite, 13; aquinite, 100	1 orange-yellow band, "21"
155 mm. gas and smoke	Collongite, ⅔; opacite, ⅓	Green body, 1 white ring, No. 5 on top ogive
155 mm. gas	Aquinite, ¾; opacite, ¼	Green body, 1 white ring, No. 7 on top of the ogive
155 mm. gas	Yperite with solvent	2 orange-yellow bands, "20" on top of ogive
155 mm. F.A. gas	Camite, 13; aquinite, 100	1 orange-yellow band, "21" on top of the ogive
15 mm. F.A. incendiary, Naud.	Carbon disulfide and tar; phosphorus 1; kilogram cylinder of incendiary matter	Green body, red head, and black ring
155 mm. Naud (steel)	Carbon disulfide and tar; white phosphorus; cylinder of incendiary	Green body, red head, and black ring

The French system of marking, being purely arbitrary, had little to recommend it. The information denoted by the code numbers applied only to the filling and, unless troop commanders were very familiar with the properties of these fillings (which was seldom the case), they had little or no guidance in the use of chemical shell in the field. Moreover, the numbers painted on the shell frequently became more or less obliterated, and when they were illegible, the different kinds of gas shell frequently could not be distinguished.
126
British System.—The three classes of British chemical shell were distinguished from each other and from all other types of shell by distinctive body colors, as follows: gas shell were painted gray; smoke shell, light green; and incendiary shell, red. In addition, for gas shell, the kind of *gas* filling was indicated by a system of colored stripes encircling the body of the shell as follows:

Filling	Marking bands
SK (ethyliodoacetate)	No bands

KSK	No bands, letters HVV
PS (chlorpicrin)	1 white
PG (50 per cent chlorpicrin)	2 white
NC (80 per cent chlorpicrin; 20 per cent stannic chloride)	1 white, 1 red, 1 white
VN (vincennite)	1 white, 1 red
CG (phosgene)	1 red, 1 white, 1 red
CBR	1 red
BB (mustard gas)	4 red

The smoke shell were also distinguished by having a red ring painted around the ogive, close to the nose of the shell, and the letters "PHOS" stenciled in black on the side of the shell to denote phosphorus filling.

The incendiary shell were without distinguishing marks, except all over red color.

From the foregoing, it is apparent that the British system was an improvement of the French, in that each class of chemical shell was distinguished from all other types and the kind of filling was indicated by bands that were more readily identified than the French code numbers. However, the British system also failed to denote the persistency of the gas fillings as a guide to use in the field; in this respect it was open to the same objections as the French system.

American System (World War).—In the war, American chemical shell were distinguished from all other types by a gray body color and black letters reading "Special Gas," "Special Smoke," or "Special Incendiary." The three classes of chemical shell were further distinguished by distinctive color stripes encircling the body of the shell, as follows: gas shell—white and/or red stripes; smoke shell—yellow stripes; incendiary shell—purple stripe.

Among gas shell, those filled with nonpersistent gases were distinguished by white stripes; those with persistent fillings by red stripes; and those with semipersistent fillings with combination white and red stripes. Furthermore, within each group of gases the number of stripes denoted the relative persistency. That is, the least persistent gas of the nonpersistent group was denoted by one white stripe, the next least persistent gas by two white stripes, etc. Similarly, among the persistent

127

group, the least persistent gas was denoted by one red stripe, the next least persistent by two red stripes, etc.

The following tabulation shows the chemical fillings used in the war and the markings employed to denote them:

Filling	Marking stripes
Nonpersistent Gases	
DA (diphenylchlorarsine)	1 white
CG (phosgene)	2 white
PD (CG and DA)	3 white
Semipersistent Gases	
PS (chlorpicrin)	1 red, 1 white
NC (chlorpicrin and stannic chloride)	*1 yellow, 1 red, 1 white
PG (PS and CG)	1 white, 1 red, 1 white
Persistent Gases	
BA (bromacetone)	1 red
CA (brombenzyl cyanide)	2 red
HS (mustard gas)	3 red
Smokes	
WP (white phosphorus)	1 yellow
FM (titanium tetrachloride)	2 yellow
Incendiary	
Incendiary mixture	1 purple

* Stannic chloride is a smoke producer, hence the yellow stripe to denote this fact.

From the foregoing, it will be seen that the American marking system was by far the most logical and informative scheme of identifying chemical fillings of any of the marking systems used in the war. It not only distinguished chemical shell from other types, and the three classes of chemical fillings from each other, but it also identified each gas by a mark which indicated to what persistency group the gas belonged and its relative persistency therein. The American system had the further advantage that if a more effective gas of any group were substituted for a less effective gas, no change in the marking of the shell would be necessary. Thus, suppose a more effective lacrimator were substituted for BA. If this new gas were less persistent than CA the shell containing it would continue to be marked with one red stripe. If, however, the new gas were more persistent than CA, but less than HS, the new gas shell would be marked with two red stripes and the shell thereafter filled with CA would be marked with one red stripe to denote the fact that CA was now the least persistent gas of the persistent group.

American System (Post War).—The only disadvantage of the American World War marking system was the number and variety of markings used to denote gas shell, but this was due to the large number of gases which had to be distinguished. Since the war the effort has been to reduce the number of standard chemical fillings to the minimum. To this end, only one chemical filling of each type is now approved as stand-

128

ard, *i.e.*, one nonpersistent, one persistent gas, one irritant gas, one smoke and one incendiary filling. When a new filling is developed to a point where it is found to be more effective than any of the existing standard types, it is adopted as the standard for its type and the former standard gas then becomes a substitute standard if it is desired to retain it for possible substitute use, or if not, it is declared obsolete and dropped.

A comparison of the present classification and marking system with the American World War practice shows a marked simplification. While the system of stripes to denote type of chemical agent is retained, these stripes no longer distinguish degree of persistency as between gases of the same type. This is not serious, however, so long as there is but one gas of any one type in use, as is now contemplated.

129

CHAPTER VI

LACRIMATORY AGENTS

The first toxic gases employed in the World War were the lacrimators, *i.e.*, substances having a specific action on the eyes and producing a copious flow of tears and temporary blindness. In the concentrations used in battle, neither the eyeball nor the optic nerve was injured and only in rare cases (as when a soldier was so near a shell burst as to have the liquid chemical splashed in his eyes) was any corneal injury experienced. In fact, so transitory was the effect of these early lacrimatory gases that no one, at the time of their introduction, appeared to regard them as *toxic* gases coming within the prohibitions of the Hague Conventions of 1899 and 1907. As a matter of fact, however, most of the World War lacrimators were equally as toxic as many of the lethal gases used. For a comparison of the relative toxicities of the lacrimatory and lethal gases see the tables on pages 14 and 16.

Perhaps the reason why no protest was made over the initial use of lacrimatory gases was that, in the low concentrations ordinarily encountered in the open, temporary lacrimation was the only effect produced, and no one regarded these substances as militarily effective. However, when these gases were employed against enclosed places, such as field fortifications, deep trenches, dugouts, etc., where their vapors could accumulate, toxic concentrations could be built up and serious casualties result. Since toxic concentrations could thus be produced in battle, it is clear that most of the World War lacrimators were in fact *toxic* gases and did come within the prohibitions of the Hague Conventions.

The principal lacrimators employed in the late war, in the order of their introduction are shown in the table on page 130.

As will be noted in the table, the lacrimators fall naturally into two groups: (1) *simple* lacrimators, which in ordinary field concentrations affect the eyes only; and (2) *toxic* lacrimators, which in ordinary field concentrations not only affect the eyes but also exert certain toxic effects against other parts of the body. All the toxic lacrimators, in addition to their lacrimatory action, are also lung injurants. In the cases of chlorpicrin and phenylcarbylamine chloride, their lung-injurant effects are so much more pronounced than their lacrimatory effects that they are usually classed as lung-injurant agents (see Chap. VII).

130

Agent	Introduced by	Date
Simple lacrimators		
Ethylbromacetate	French	August, 1914
Xylyl bromide	Germans	January, 1915
Benzyl bromide	Germans	March, 1915

Brommethylethyl ketone	Germans	July, 1915
Ethyliodoacetate	British	September, 1915
Benzyl iodide	French	November, 1915
Brombenzyl cyanide	French	July, 1918
Chloracetophenone	Americans	Postwar
Toxic lacrimators		
Chloracetone	French	November, 1914
Bromacetone	Germans	July, 1915
Iodoacetone	French	August, 1915
Acrolein	French	January, 1916
Chlorpicrin*	Russians	August, 1916
Phenylcarbylamine chloride*	Germans	May, 1917

* Primarily lung injurants.

GROUP CHARACTERISTICS

The lacrimators, as a group, have certain well-defined properties in common, the most important of which are the following:

1. They all have the power to irritate certain tissues only, *i.e.*, the eyes, and without producing noticeable lesions; their action is thus both elective and reversible since they affect only one organ, and the irritation produced quickly disappears.
2. Their threshold of action is low, *i.e.*, they are effective in extremely low concentrations, such as a few thousandths of a milligram per liter, and can produce an intolerable atmosphere in concentrations as low as one-thousandth of that required for the most effective lethal agents.
3. They are quick acting, producing almost instantaneous physiological effects (in less than 1 minute) in the form of a muscular reaction of the eyelids, closing the eyes, and a glandular reaction from the lacrimatory glands, producing a copious flow of tears.
4. Chemically they are very closely related, being formed by a central atom of carbon, carrying a halogen and one or several negative groups in which the hydrogen atoms are readily displaced. Hederer and Istin (15), quoting Professor Job, give the following type formulas which explain the chemical relationships of the lacrimators to each other:

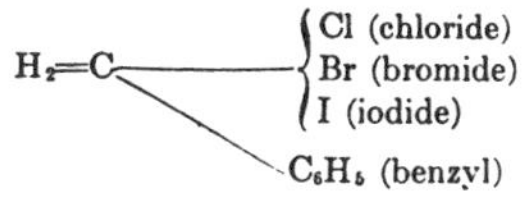

$H_2{=}C$ — {Cl (chloride), Br (bromide), I (iodide)} and C_6H_5 (benzyl)

131

$H_2{=}C$ — {Cl (chlor-), Br (brom-), I (iod-)} and $CO{-}CH_3$ (acetone)

$H_2{=}C$ — Cl (chlor-) and $CO{-}C_6H_5$ (acetophenone)

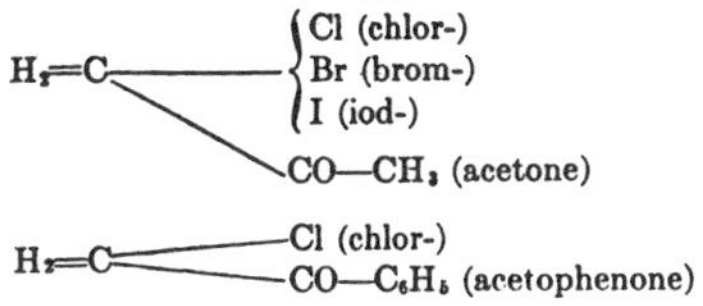

5. Physically, the lacrimators are, in general, liquids of relatively high boiling points and low vapor pressures. They are, therefore, essentially nonvolatile substances that form persistent gases.

Since all the lacrimators are practically insoluble in water, although readily soluble in fats and organic solvents, on coming in contact with the moist surfaces of the eyeball and conjunctiva, they are not diluted by the moisture encountered but are rapidly absorbed by the epithelial surfaces. The effect upon the sensitive nerves at once produces an irritation that passes rapidly from a slight tingling sensation to an intolerable smarting and terminates in a muscular reaction, closure of the eyelids, and a secretion of tears. The reflex action of closing the eyelids and the profuse secretion of tears produces a suspension of vision which, however, usually persists but a few minutes after termination of the exposure to the lacrimatory atmosphere, and rarely produces any pathological lesion or injurious aftereffects.

A marked peculiarity of the lacrimators as a group is their relative ineffectiveness against animals. Thus it was noted early in the war that concentrations which caused profuse lacrimation in men produced no visible effect upon horses and mules. From careful tests, using brombenzyl cyanide as the agent, it was found that it was necessary to use a solution 100 times as strong to lacrimate a dog and 1,000 times as strong to lacrimate a horse to the same degree as a man. The reason for this great difference in the sensitiveness to lacrimation between men and animals has never been satisfactorily explained, though the fact is well established by tests and war experience.

Although lacrimators were used throughout the World War, their employment was more and more limited as other more powerful gases were introduced. During the whole period of the war, about 6,000 tons of lacrimators were used in battle. This was less than 5 per cent of the total tonnage of toxic gases used. However, owing to their effectiveness in extremely low concentrations, forcing troops to mask, with its attendant disadvantages, lacrimators served a useful purpose in the war. Also, owing to their total lack of permanent injury, lacrimators are well adapted for controlling mobs and suppressing domestic disturbances; they have been used in increasing amounts for this purpose since the World War.

132

As the later lacrimators are far more powerful than their earlier predecessors, they are of the greatest interest, particularly, as to the future. However, in order to trace the development of the lacrimators as a group and to compare the properties of each with the others, a brief description will be given of each in the chronological order of its introduction.

Ethylbromacetate ($CH_2BrCOOC_2H_5$)

The first combat gas used in the war was *ethylbromacetate*, which was employed by the French in rifle grenades as early as August, 1914. In November, 1914, owing to a shortage of bromine from which brominated compounds could be made, chloracetone was substituted as a filling in the French gas grenades (1).

Ethylbromacetate was first prepared by Perkin and Duppa in 1858 by heating bromacetic acid and alcohol in sealed tubes. The compound was thus known long before the World War and was used in many ways in industry in the manufacture of other chemical substances. Its highly irritant effect upon the eyes was also well known to chemists. This property and the fact that it is easily manufactured and handled were perhaps the reasons for its employment in 1912 as a filling for hand bombs by the Paris police for temporarily disabling criminals and facilitating their arrest. The success attained by the French police in suppressing lawless gangs with this gas undoubtedly led to adoption by the French Army as a filling for 26-mm. rifle grenades.

According to German authors, the French had actually manufactured a quantity of these gas-rifle grenades before the outbreak of the World War, and 30,000 were taken into the field by the French Army in August, 1914, and used during that summer. The French deny this and assert that the hand bombs filled with ethylbromacetate were used for police purposes only. However, regardless of whether or not the French actually manufactured rifle gas grenades prior to the World War, they certainly appear to have been employed by the French Army during the first months of the war, and the chemical filling used was ethylbromacetate.

According to Mueller, ethylbromacetate is prepared by the bromination of acetic acid in the presence of red phosphorus and the subsequent esterification with alcohol of the bromacetic acid obtained.

It is a transparent liquid of 1.5 specific gravity, which boils without decomposition at 168°C. (334.4°F.), and does not react with iron. It is almost insoluble in water and is only slowly hydrolyzed thereby.

Ethylbromacetate is very irritating to the eyes and nasal passages, causing lacrimation in concentrations as low as 0.003 mg. per liter. At 0.04 mg. per liter, the concentration becomes intolerable to the eyes, and

133

a concentration of 2.30 mg. per liter is lethal on 10 minutes' exposure. Its toxicity is, therefore, over twice that of chlorine. Its volatility is 21.00 mg. per liter at 20°C. (68°F.), so that field concentrations of nearly ten times the lethal dose are practicable.

On account of the scarcity of bromine, ethylbromacetate was displaced by chloracetone in November, 1914, and was not used thereafter. Its use was, therefore, very limited and, aside from the fact that it was the first combat gas used in the World War, this compound was not important.

Chloracetone (CH_3COCH_2Cl)

French: "Tonite"

Chloracetone was introduced by the French in November, 1914, as a substitute for ethylbromacetate in hand and rifle gas grenades. It is obtained by the direct chlorination of acetone and is a clear liquid, of 1.16 specific gravity, which boils at 119°C. (246.2°F.), yielding a vapor 3.7 times heavier than air. Chloracetone is only slightly soluble in water and is not decomposed thereby. It tends, however, to polymerize into a relatively inert form on long storage.

It has a pungent odor like that of hydrochloric acid and lacrimates the eyes (conjunctiva) in concentrations as low as 0.018 mg. per liter. A concentration of 0.10 mg. per liter is intolerable after 1 minute of exposure, and a concentration of 2.30 mg. per liter is lethal on 10 minutes' exposure. It is, therefore, about as toxic as ethylbromacetate. However, it is much more volatile so that its ordinary field concentrations are much higher than those of ethylbromacetate.

Because charcoal readily absorbs chloracetone and therefore even the early gas masks afforded adequate protection against it and because bromacetone proved to be a better tear gas, chloracetone was displaced in 1915 by bromacetone and other more powerful lacrimators then introduced. A relatively small amount of chloracetone was used in the war, and it played but a minor role in the early stages of gas warfare.

Xylyl Bromide ($C_6H_4CH_3CH_2BR$)

German: "T-Stoff"

In the early experiments with various chemical compounds, in an effort to produce more powerful lacrimators, the Germans found that, in general, the bromine derivatives were far more effective than the corresponding chlorine compounds; as there was then no shortage of bromine in Germany (as in France and England), the German chemists proceeded to develop for chemical warfare a series of bromine compounds of which

134

xylyl bromide was the first. The first use of this gas in battle was in artillery shells fired against the Russians at Bolimow on Jan. 31, 1915, and its first employment on the Western Front was against the British at Nieuport in March, 1915. The firing of these shells against the Russians not only constituted the first use of gas in artillery shell* but was also the first use of gas in a major operation in the World War, antedating, as it does, the celebrated cloud-gas attack at Ypres in April, 1915, by three months.

* Strictly speaking, the first German gas used in the World War was chlorsulfate of ortho-dianisidin, a powder which was filled between the lead balls of the 10.5-mm. shrapnel. However, only one trial lot of these shell was used on Oct. 27, 1914, at Neuve-Chapelle and, as the success obtained was not sufficient to warrant further use of this material, it was abandoned.

Xylyl bromide is prepared by the direct bromination of xylene and consists of a mixture of the three isomeric substitution products of the ortho-, meta-, and para-xylene present. When pure, the xylyl bromides are light yellow slightly viscous liquids, while the xylylene bromides are solids. Crude xylyl bromide consisted of a mixture of xylyl and xylylene bromides and, as used in gas warfare, was a black liquid, of 1.4 specific gravity, which boils at from 210° to 220°C. (410° to 428°F.), yielding a pungent aromatic vapor, 8.5 times heavier than air, with an odor resembling lilacs. As it corrodes iron and steel very rapidly, xylyl bromide had to be loaded into lead containers which were in turn placed in the shell. Later in the war, lead and enamel linings were developed which successfully protected the shell from corrosion and made the inner lead containers unnecessary.

Xylyl bromide is an extraordinarily powerful irritant to the eyes (conjunctiva). It can be detected by sensitive individuals in concentrations as low as 0.00027 mg. per liter, whereas its lacrimatory concentration is 0.0018 mg. per liter. A concentration of 0.015 mg. per liter is intolerable after 1 minute, and a concentration of 5.60 mg. per liter is lethal on 10 minutes' exposure. Hence while xylyl bromide is a much stronger lacrimator, its toxicity is only half that of ethylbromacetate.

On account of its low volatility (0.60 mg. per liter at 68°F.), xylyl bromide was not very effective at low temperatures, and it was also very readily absorbed by the charcoal in gas-mask canisters, so that masks furnished adequate protection against it. Owing to these facts and its corrosive properties, it was replaced in 1917 by more volatile and powerful substances. However, xylyl bromide played an important role in the history of gas warfare. About 500 tons of T-Stoff were fired by the Germans and, while no serious casualties were produced thereby, this gas first showed the tactical importance of gas shell and paved the way for the more effective gas shell which followed.

135

Benzyl Bromide ($C_6H_5CH_2Br$)

German: T-Stoff; French: "Cyclite"

The second bromine compound introduced by the Germans was benzyl bromide. It was first used by them at Verdun in March, 1915, in an effort to obtain a more volatile substance than xylyl bromide, but the improvement was not marked for, while benzyl bromide is somewhat more volatile, it is less irritating than xylyl bromide. The French also later used this compound under the name of "Cyclite."

Benzyl bromide is prepared by the direct bromination of toluene in the same way as xylyl bromide is obtained from xylene. In its pure state, benzyl bromide is a transparent liquid, with a specific gravity of 1.44, which boils at 201°C. (393.8°F.), yielding vapor 6.0 times heavier than air and with a pleasant aromatic odor resembling water cress. It is insoluble in water and is only very slowly decomposed thereby. Its great chemical stability, low vapor pressure, 2.0 mm. Hg at 20°C. (68°F.), and low volatility, 2.4 mg. per liter at 20°C. (68°F.), assures its persistence on the terrain.

While benzyl bromide is a decided eye irritant, its effect is not nearly so great as that of xylyl bromide. Thus, a concentration of 0.004 mg. per liter is required to produce any irritation at all, and the concentration does not become intolerable until it attains 0.06 mg. per liter. In higher concentrations, it also produces much irritation of the nose, throat, and air passages with salivation and nausea. Its lethal concentration for 10 minutes' exposure is 4.50 mg. per liter, as compared to 5.60 mg. per liter for xylyl bromide.

Like other bromide compounds, benzyl bromide corrodes iron and steel and must, therefore, be kept in lead- or enamel-lined containers. It was used in battle in small quantities for a short time because its irritant power was much less than that of other compounds, and its basic component—toluene—was more urgently needed for the manufacture of high explosives. For these reasons, and the fact that charcoal thoroughly absorbs its vapors, it is unlikely that benzyl bromide will ever be used again as a chemical agent.

Bromacetone (CH_3COCH_2Br)

German: "B-Stoff"; French: "Martonite"; British and American: "BA"

Not satisfied with the slight improvement of benzyl bromide over xylyl bromide, the Germans soon brought out a third bromine compound —bromacetone—in an effort to solve the problem of a more easily volatilized irritant. It was also used by the French, mixed with 20 per cent chloracetone, under the name "Martonite," and by the British and Americans under the symbol "BA." This compound was the most

136

widely employed of any of the pure lacrimators, more than 1,000 tons being fired in projectiles alone, not to mention use in other weapons such as hand and rifle grenades. Bromacetone is the bromine compound which corresponds to chloracetone and is produced in a similar manner, *i.e.*, by the direct bromination of acetone. It is a colorless liquid, of 1.6 specific gravity, which boils at 135°C. (275°F.), yielding a vapor 4.7 times heavier than air. On long standing, bromacetone decomposes, gradually changing to a black resinous mass, during which process hydrobromic acid is released. Although bromacetone is not soluble in and is not decomposed by water, it is nevertheless a rather unstable compound, as it decomposes even in its purest form, particularly under the influence of heat and light.

Bromacetone was one of the most effective lacrimators used in the war. It produces an irritating effect upon the eyes in concentrations as low as 0.0015 mg. per liter while, a concentration of 0.010 mg. per liter is intolerable, and a concentration of 3.20 mg. per liter is lethal on 10 minutes' exposure. The toxicity of bromacetone is thus intermediate, between that of ethylbromacetate (2.30 mg. per liter) and xylyl bromide

(5.60 mg. per liter).

At 20°C. (68°F.), the vapor pressure of bromacetone is 9 mm. Hg and its volatility 75.0 mg. per liter. Owing to its relatively high volatility, toxic concentrations of bromacetone were often encountered in the field, so that, in addition to its lacrimatory power, this compound is classed as a toxic lacrimator. Moreover, *liquid* bromacetone, on contact with skin, produces blisters which, although they heal rapidly, are extremely painful on the sensitive parts of the body.

In the late war, bromacetone was used by the Germans in artillery (Green T) shells and trench-mortar bombs (B-Minen) for only a short time, owing largely to the ever-increasing demand for acetone for other purposes. The British also used it for a short time until it was replaced by more effective iodine compounds. In the mixture Martonite (80 per cent bromacetone and 20 per cent chloracetone), it was used by the French and Americans throughout the war, although it was rapidly being displaced toward the end of the war by the more powerful compound, brombenzylcyanide, introduced by the French in the summer of 1918.

Brommethylethyl Ketone ($CH_3CO.CH.Br.CH_3$)

German: "Bn-Stoff"; French: "Homomartonite"

By the summer of 1915, the demand for acetone as a solvent for nitrocellulose in the manufacture of powder and dopes for airplane fabrics became so great that both sides began to look for substitutes for bromacetone, with the result that in July, 1915, the Germans introduced brom-

137

methylethyl ketone (Bn-Stoff), while the French followed with a mixture of brommethylethyl ketone and chlormethylethyl ketone, under the name "Homomartonite," so called because of its great similarity to Martonite (80 per cent bromacetone and 20 per cent chloracetone) in chemical composition and physiological action.

Methylethyl ketone is present in large quantities in the "acetone oils," which are by-products in the manufacture of acetone from wood, and, if this compound is brominated in a way similar to acetone, brommethylethyl ketone is obtained. When freshly distilled, it is a faintly yellow liquid, insoluble in water, of 1.43 specific gravity, and boils with some decomposition at 145°C. (293°F.), yielding a vapor 5.2 times heavier than air.

The vapor pressure of brommethylethyl ketone is 15.0 mm. Hg at 14°C. (57.2°F.), while its volatility at 20°C. (68°F.) is 34.0 mg. per liter. It is thus less persistent than xylyl bromide. Like all bromine compounds, it corrodes iron and steel and requires lead- or enamel-lined receptacles for storage.

Brommethylethyl ketone is a powerful lacrimator, being more powerful than benzyl bromide and only slightly less powerful than bromacetone, which it resembles to an extraordinary degree in its other properties. Thus, its minimum lacrimatory concentration is 0.0126 mg. per liter, while a concentration of 0.016 mg. per liter is intolerable and a concentration of 2.00 mg. per liter is lethal on 10 minutes' exposure. Owing to its high toxicity and volatility, toxic concentrations of brommethylethyl ketone may readily be produced in the field; for this reason this compound is classed as a toxic lacrimator.

On the whole, brommethylethyl ketone was not so effective a war gas as bromacetone, and its substitution for bromacetone was solely for economic reasons relating to the shortage of acetone.

Iodoacetone (CH_3COCH_2I)

French: "Bretonite"

The scarcity of bromine caused the French and British to turn to the iodine compounds corresponding to the bromine compounds in use by the Germans, with the result that during the latter part of 1915 three such iodine compounds—iodoacetone, ethyliodoacetate, and benzyl iodide—made their appearance in the war. These substances were, on the whole, somewhat superior in irritant and toxic effects, but less stable than the corresponding bromine compounds.

The first of the iodine compounds to make its appearance was iodoacetone which was introduced by the French in August, 1915, as a filling for artillery shell.

138

Iodoacetone is prepared by treating chloracetone with sodium or potassium iodide in alcoholic solution. When first prepared, it is a clear faintly yellow liquid, with a specific gravity of 1.8, which boils at 102°C. (215.6°F.) and turns brown on contact with the air. Iodoacetone decomposes on heating more easily than bromacetone and is converted on standing about one week into symmetrical diiodoacetone. Its vapor possesses a very pronounced pungency and is of about the same lacrimatory strength as brommethylethyl ketone (0.120 mg. per liter), but is more toxic than any of the halogenated ketones.

Iodoacetone was used only a short time by the French, being superseded toward the end of 1915 by benzyl iodide. The British manufactured some iodoacetone but do not appear to have used it in the field, preferring the more powerful ethyliodoacetate.

Ethyliodoacetate ($CH_2ICOOC_2H_5$)

British: "SK"

This compound was introduced by the British at the battle of Loos, Sept. 24, 1915, as a filling for 4.2-in. howitzer shell. It was later also used in 4-in. Stokes-mortar bombs and gas grenades and was the British standard lacrimator throughout the war.

Like iodoacetone, ethyliodoacetate is obtained by the double decomposition of the corresponding chlorine compound (ethylchloracetate) with potassium iodide in alcoholic solution. It is a colorless oily liquid, of specific gravity 1.8, which boils at 180°C. (356°F.) and quickly turns brown in the air, liberating iodine. At 20°C. (68°F.), its vapor pressure is 0.54 mm. Hg, and its volatility is 3.1 mg. per liter. It is somewhat more stable than iodoacetone, but is still quite easily decomposed. Unlike the bromine compounds, it does not attack iron and may, therefore, be loaded into projectiles without any protective lining.

Ethyliodoacetate is extremely irritant and lacrimatory and is moderately toxic as well. Its lowest lacrimatory concentration is 0.0014 mg. per liter; the intolerable concentration is 0.015 mg. per liter; a concentration of 1.5 mg. per liter is toxic on 10 minutes' exposure. It is, therefore, more irritant, lacrimatory, and toxic than any of the lacrimators previously employed in the war. While its toxicity is about one-third that of phosgene, its volatility is very low, and for that reason lethal concentrations were not encountered in the field. To increase its volatility, it was usually diluted with alcohol before filling into projectiles.

While ethyliodoacetate was one of the most powerful lacrimators used in the war, the British were forced to adopt it because of a shortage of bromine and the fact that they then had access to large supplies of iodine from South America. At the present time, the price and scarcity of iodine make the future use of this compound as a chemical agent undesir-

139

able, particularly since other even more powerful lacrimators are now available.

Benzyl Iodide ($C_6H_5CH_2I$)

French: "Fraissite"

This substance was the last of the three iodine compounds used as chemical agents in the war. It was introduced by the French in November, 1915, to replace iodoacetone, on account of the shortage of acetone, and was intended to serve the same purpose as benzyl bromide used by the Germans.

Benzyl iodide is obtained by the double decomposition of benzyl chloride with potassium iodide in alcoholic solution. It is a white crystalline solid which melts at 24°C. (75°F.) and boils with complete decomposition at 226°C. (438°F.). Its specific gravity is 1.7; it is insoluble in water and has a marked ability to undergo double decomposition on storage.

As a lacrimator, benzyl iodide has about twice the power of benzyl bromide. Thus, its lowest irritant concentration is 0.002 mg. per liter; its intolerable concentration is 0.03 mg. per liter; its lethal concentration is 3.00 mg. per liter on 10 minutes' exposure. However, its volatility (1.2 mg. per liter at 20°C.) is only half that of benzyl bromide, and for that reason it was usually employed in the field in the form of a 50-50 mixture with benzyl chloride under the name "Fraissite."

While benzyl iodide was an improvement over iodoacetone, it was used for only a short time and was displaced early in 1916 by acrolein. Except for ethyliodoacetate, the iodine compounds were used only in very small quantities and for a short time by the Allies as a temporary measure, owing to the scarcity of bromine, and were soon displaced by other more effective substances.

Acrolein (CH_2CHCHO)

French: "Papite"

Acrolein was introduced by the French in January, 1916, as a filling for gas grenades and artillery shell, in an effort to obtain an effective lacrimator which did not require bromine or acetone for its manufacture. Acrolein is obtained by the dehydration of glycerine, by distilling it in the presence of potassium bisulfate or crystallized magnesium sulfate as a catalyst.

When freshly prepared, acrolein is a clear liquid of greenish yellow color and pungent odor, with a specific gravity of 0.84 at 15°C. It boils at 52°C. (125.6°F.), yielding a light vapor only 1.9 times heavier than air, is very unstable, and is easily oxidized into acrylic acid. Even when

140

protected from the air, acrolein gradually polymerizes into disacryl or acrolein gum, an inactive gelatinous substance which has none of the physiological powers of acrolein.

In order to prevent polymerization, the French added about 5 per cent amyl nitrate as a stabilizer. While this tended to prevent polymerization into disacryl, it did not prevent the formation of acrolein gum, so that it was not very effective.

Acrolein is a fairly powerful lacrimator and respiratory irritant, the effects on the eyes and throat occurring simultaneously. In higher concentrations, it is also a lung-injurant toxic gas. In concentrations as low as 0.007 mg. per liter, acrolein lacrimates and greatly irritates the conjunctiva and the mucous membranes of the respiratory organs. At 0.05 mg. per liter, it becomes intolerable, while a concentration of 0.35 mg. per liter is lethal on 10 minutes' exposure. Because of its toxic properties, acrolein is classed as a toxic lacrimator. On account of its great lack of chemical stability, acrolein was not a successful chemical agent in the World War and can never play an important role in chemical warfare.

Chlorpicrin (CCl_3NO_2)

French: "Aquinite"; German: "Klop"; British and American: "PS" and "NC"

Chlorpicrin lacrimates in concentrations as low as 0.002 mg. per liter. A concentration of 0.05 mg. per liter is intolerable, and 2.00 mg. per liter is lethal on 10 minutes' exposure. Chlorpicrin is thus both a lacrimatory and lung-injurant toxic gas, but, as its lung-injurant effects are so much more pronounced than its lacrimatory effects, it is usually considered as a lung-injurant gas and is so regarded here (see Chap. VII).

Phenylcarbylamine Chloride ($C_6H_5CNCl_2$)

This compound is both a lacrimator and a lung injurant. Its minimum lacrimatory concentration is 0.003 mg. per liter, which makes it intermediate between benzyl bromide (0.004 mg. per liter) and benzyl iodide (0.002 mg. per liter). At 0.025 mg. per liter it is intolerable for more than 1 minute, while 0.05 mg. per liter is lethal on 10 minutes' exposure. As its toxic properties are so much more important than its lacrimatory power, it is generally regarded as a lung-injurant agent and is so treated in Chap. VII.

Brombenzyl Cyanide ($C_6H_5CHBrCN$)

French: "Camite"; American: "CA"

Brombenzyl cyanide was the last and most powerful lacrimator used in the World War. It was introduced by the French in July, 1918, as the

141

culmination of their efforts to produce more powerful and effective lacrimators. It was also simultaneously adopted by the Americans as their standard lacrimator and manufactured in the United States in the fall of 1918.

Brombenzyl cyanide was first prepared by Riener in 1881 by brominating phenyl cyanide, and its manufacture in industry was commenced in 1914. Industrially, brombenzyl cyanide is prepared in three steps, as follows: (1) chlorination of toluene to form benzyl chloride; (2) the conversion of benzyl chloride to benzyl cyanide by the action of sodium cyanide in alcoholic solution; (3) the bromination of the benzyl cyanide with bromine vapor in the presence of sunlight.

In its pure state, brombenzyl cyanide is a yellow-white crystalline solid which melts at 25°C. (77°F.) into a brownish oily liquid of 1.47 specific gravity, and boils at 225°C. (437°F.). After a slight initial decomposition upon exposure to air, the compound is chemically fairly stable at ordinary temperatures, although it slowly decomposes in storage. When heated above 150°C. (302°F.) it decomposes very rapidly. It is soluble in water, which decomposes it only very gradually. It is also very soluble in phosgene, chlorpicrin, and benzyl cyanide. Its vapor pressure is 0.012 mm. Hg at 20°C. (68°F.), and its volatility is 0.13 mg. per liter at the same temperature. Its persistency in the open is three days; in woods, seven days; and in the ground, from 15 to 30 days. Like most compounds containing bromine, brombenzyl cyanide corrodes iron and steel and can be kept only in glass-, porcelain-, or enamel-lined containers.

This substance has an odor like soured fruit and produces a burning sensation of the mucous membranes and severe irritation and lacrimation of the eyes with acute pain in the forehead. As a lacrimator it is seven times as powerful as bromacetone. Thus, brombenzyl cyanide can be detected in concentrations as low as 1:100,000,000 (0.000087 mg. per liter); it has an irritating effect on the eyes in concentrations of 0.00015 mg. per liter and it produces lacrimation in concentrations of 0.0003 mg. per liter. A concentration of 0.0008 mg. per liter produces an intolerable irritation, and a concentration of 0.90 mg. per liter is lethal on 30 minutes' exposure. It is thus less toxic than phosgene and, owing to its low volatility, toxic concentration cannot be realized in the field.

While brombenzyl cyanide was by far the most powerful lacrimator used in the war, it has three very serious defects: (1) it corrodes iron and steel, requiring specially lined containers; (2), it is not chemically stable, but slowly decomposes in storage; (3), its great sensitiveness to heat makes its use in artillery shell very difficult. If the bursting charge is not kept very small, it causes loss of the chemical filling through decomposition on explosion. An additional disadvantage might also be found in its rather extreme persistency in the soil.

142

From a tactical standpoint, therefore, brombenzyl cyanide seems quite limited in its possibilities in the future.

Chloracetophenone ($C_6H_5COCH_2Cl$)

American: "CN"

Because of the difficulties attending the use of brombenzyl cyanide, the Americans toward the end of the war began to investigate the properties of chloracetophenone as a combat gas. This compound was discovered in 1869 by the German chemist, Graebe, who described the powerful effects of its vapors upon the eyes. Owing to the short time it was under study in the war and the difficulty of its manufacture, no chloracetophenone was used in the World War. Shortly after the war, however, American investigators became convinced of its superiority as a tear gas and worked out a satisfactory process of manufacture. This process consists of the following steps:

1. Chlorination of acetic acid to obtain monochloracetic acid, according to the equation

$$CH_3COOH + Cl_2 \rightarrow CH_2ClCOOH + HCl$$

2. The chlorination of this compound with sulfur monochloride and chlorine to obtain chloracetyl chloride according to the equation

$$4CH_2ClCOOH + S_2Cl_2 + 3Cl_2 \rightarrow 4CH_2ClCOCl + 2SO_2 + 4HCl$$

3. Treatment of chloracetyl chloride with benzene in the presence of anhydrous aluminum chloride, according to the equation

$$CH_2ClCOCl + C_6H_6 \rightarrow C_6H_5COCH_2Cl + HCl$$

See Chart VIII.

Unlike the lacrimators used in the late war, chloracetophenone is a solid, and remarkably resistant to heat and moisture. It does not corrode metals, including iron and steel, so it may be loaded direct into shell, either by casting or pressing, without danger to the workmen handling it.

When pure, it consists of colorless crystals, of 1.3 specific gravity, which melt at 59°C. (138°F.) and boil at 247°C. (476°F.), yielding a vapor which in low concentrations has an odor resembling apple blossoms. At 20°C. (68°F.) its vapor pressure is very low (0.013 mm. Hg) and its volatility is 0.106 mg. per liter.

Chloracetophenone is only slightly soluble in water and is not decomposed thereby. It is not decomposed by boiling and may therefore be distilled and poured into shells in the molten state, which greatly facili-

143

tates loading into munitions. It is not affected by explosion of high explosives and may even be mixed with same in shell.

In lacrimatory power, chloracetophenone is about equal to brombenzyl cyanide. Thus, it produces lacrimation in concentrations as low as 0.0003 mg. per liter while a concentration of 0.0045 mg. per liter is intolerable and a concentration of 0.85 mg. per liter is lethal on 10 minutes' exposure.

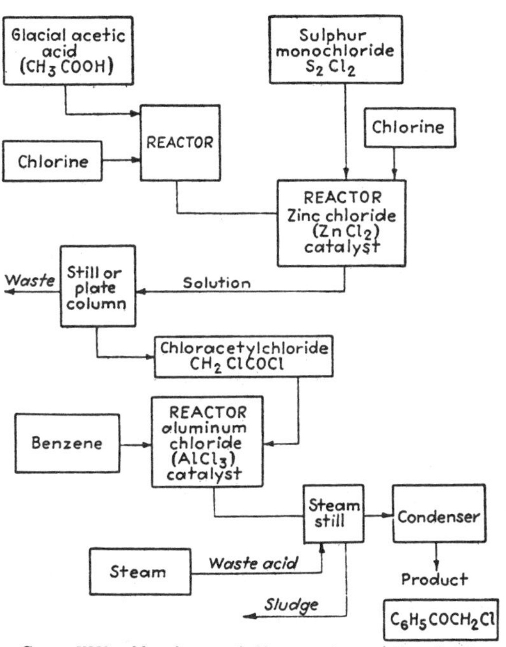

CHART VIII.—Manufacture of chloracetophenone (flow sheet).

In addition to its lacrimatory effect, chloracetophenone is a decided irritant to the upper respiratory passages; in higher concentrations, it is irritating to the skin, producing a burning and itching sensation, especially on moist parts of the body. These effects are very similar to sunburn, are entirely harmless, and disappear in a few hours.

Although chloracetophenone can be effectively dispersed by explosion, it is very much more effective when it is distilled into the air by the heat of a burning composition. A very efficient dispersion results when one part of chloracetophenone is intimately mixed with three parts of small-

144

grained smokeless powder and the mixture burned without explosion. Such a progressive burning mixture can be successfully employed in hand and rifle grenades, trench-mortar bombs, and even artillery shell. This mixture is quite stable in storage and has the advantage of being practically inert on exposure to air until actually ignited.

Chloracetophenone is readily soluble in organic solvents and is thus frequently filled into grenades and shells as a liquid solution. Three such solutions have been used as follows: (1) CNB, consisting of CN, benzol, and carbon tetrachloride; (2) CND, consisting of CN and ethylene dichloride; and (3) CNS, consisting of CN, chloroform, and chlorpicrin.

On account of its low volatility, chloracetophenone usually exists in a gaseous form, but in high concentrations at low temperatures it may exist in the form of smoke (solid particules). In this form, it does not react with the charcoal in the gas-mask canister and for that reason canisters must be provided with a mechanical smoke filter in order to insure adequate protection against it.

Aside from its combat use, this substance is excellently suited for use as a training gas for training troops in chemical warfare. It is also of great value in suppressing mobs and internal disorders, as it is safely and easily handled and is not likely to prove injurious to persons who come in contact with it.

COMPARATIVE STRENGTH OF LACRIMATORS

The aggressive power of a lacrimator is a function of its specific lacrimatory power, expressed as the minimum concentration required to produce lacrimation, and its volatility at ordinary temperatures (68°F.). On this basis, the lacrimators described above are arranged below in the descending order of their aggressive powers.

Agent	Minimum lacrimatory concentration (threshold of action), mg. per liter	Volatility, 20°C. (68°F.), mg. per liter
Brombenzyl cyanide	0.00015	0.1300
Chloracetophenone	0.0003	0.1060
Ethyliodoacetate	0.0014	3.1000
Bromacetone	0.0015	75.0000
Xylyl bromide	0.0018	0.6000
Chlorpicrin	0.0020	165.0000
Benzyl iodide	0.0020	0.0012
Ethylbromacetate	0.0030	21.0000
Phenylcarbylamine chloride	0.0030	2.1000
Benzyl bromide	0.0040	0.0024
Acrolein	0.0070	20.0000
Brommethylethyl ketone	0.0126	34.0000
Chloracetone	0.0180	0.1200
Iodacetone	0.0120	0.0031

145

TOXICITY OF LACRIMATORS

The toxicity of the World War lacrimators has been previously mentioned in Chap. I. The following table shows their relative toxicity on the basis of 10 minutes' exposure:

Agent	Minimum Lethal Concentration, Mg. per Liter
Acrolein	0.35*
Brombenzyl cyanide	0.35
Phenylcarbylamine chloride	0.50*
Chloracetophenone	0.85
Ethyliodoacetate	1.50*
Iodoacetone	1.90
Chlorpicrin	2.00*
Brommethylethyl ketone	2.00*
Ethylbromacetate	2.30*
Chloracetone	2.30
Benzyl iodide	3.00
Bromacetone	3.20*
Benzyl bromide	4.50
Xylyl bromide	5.60

In the cases of those compounds marked with an asterisk (*), their volatilities at 20°C. (68°F.) exceed their minimum lethal doses, so that fatal concentrations of these compounds may be encountered in the field at ordinary temperatures. Moreover, it must be remembered that, even in the cases of those compounds whose volatilities are below their minimum lethal doses, as shown above (unmarked), a smaller concentration over a correspondingly longer time is equally fatal, so that if these compounds are released in protected places, such as trenches, dugouts, woods, etc., where they may persist for a longer period than 10 minutes, they may also prove fatal.

It is also to be noted that all the above lacrimators are much more toxic than chlorine, and that acrolein and brombenzyl cyanide are more toxic than phosgene, although the volatility of the latter is too low to permit fatal concentrations in the field.

FUTURE OF LACRIMATORS

The future role of the lacrimators in war is uncertain. Their great advantage is the extremely small amounts required to force men to mask with the attendant impairment of their fighting vigor. On the other hand, they produce no real casualties and protection is easily obtained. For these reasons, it seems fairly certain that lacrimators will not be used in any future war between first-class powers, as their armies will be equipped with masks affording adequate protection. At the same time, tear gas is very effective against troops having no protection, and

146

for that reason, will probably be used in minor warfare against poorly organized and semicivilized peoples. Also, tear gas will undoubtedly continue to be used to suppress riots and civil disturbances for which purpose it is eminently fitted.

For a summary of the properties of the principal lacrimatory agents, see Table IV.

147

CHAPTER VII

LUNG-INJURANT AGENTS

GROUP CHARACTERISTICS

The lung injurants were the second group of agents to make their appearance in the World War. They form a well-defined group, having many properties in common, and for that reason they were designated by the Germans under a single generic class—*Green Cross substances.* In general, they were all liquids of relatively low boiling points and high vapor pressures. They, therefore, were volatile substances that formed nonpersistent gases upon release from their containers. Their principal physiological action was injury of the pulmonary system of the body. The main result of this injury was to cause fluid to pass from the blood into the minute air sacs of the lungs and thus obstruct the supply of oxygen to the blood. Death from one of these substances may be compared to death by drowning, the water in which the victim drowns being drawn into his lungs from his own blood vessels.

As a rule, the lung-injurant agents are lethal (deadly) in concentrations ordinarily employed in battle and have the following properties in common:

1. Their threshold of useful action is relatively high, varying between 1 and 10 mg. per liter of air.
2. They are effective on very short exposure, usually only a few minutes are required to produce death or serious casualties in the concentrations generally employed in battle.
3. They exert a similar physiological action comprising the following factors:
   a. Irritant effect on the mucous membranes of the respiratory system (nose, throat, and trachea).
   b. Special changes (injury) in the lung tissue.
   c. Secondary sequelae of these changes in the lung tissues, chiefly in the circulatory system and in the composition of the blood gases.
4. Their physiological effect is not immediate, but generally produces death or serious casualties in from 1 to 2 hours after exposure.

From both a chemical and physiological viewpoint, the lung-injurant agents may be divided into two distinct groups: (1) the simple lung injurants, derived from chlorine; and (2) the toxic lung injurants, derived from arsenic. The first group acts only locally on the pulmonary system, while the second group exerts an additional systemic poisoning effect by virtue of the arsenic which they contain.

148

Chlorine (Cl_2)

French: "Bertholite"

Chlorine was the first gas used on an effective scale in war. It was employed by the Germans against British and French Colonial troops at Ypres, Belgium, on Apr. 22, 1915, when 168 tons of chlorine were released from 5,730 cylinders on the front of 6 kilometers. It was effective to a distance of 5 kilometers downwind and caused 15,000 casualties, of which 5,000 were fatal.

During the war chlorine was the principal gas used for cloud-gas attacks. At first, when the Allies had little or no means of protection, it was a very effective weapon and caused many thousands of casualties.

WORLD WAR LUNG INJURANTS

The principal lung-injurant agents in order of their chronological appearance in the World War, are:

Agent	Introduced by	Date
Simple lung injurants		
Chlorine	Germans	April 22, 1915
Methylsulfuryl chloride	Germans	June, 1915
Ethylsulfuryl chloride	French	June, 1915
Monochlormethylchloroformate	Germans	June 18, 1915
Dimethyl sulfate	Germans	August, 1915
Perchlormethylmercaptan	French	September, 1915
Phosgene	Germans	Dec. 19, 1915
Trichlormethylchloroformate	Germans	May 19, 1916
Chlorpicrin	Russians	August, 1916
Phenylcarbylamine chloride	Germans	May, 1917
Dichlordimethyl ether	Germans	January, 1918
Dibromidimethyl ether	Germans	
Toxic lung injurants		
Phenyldichlorarsine	Germans	September, 1917
Ethyldichlorarsine	Germans	March, 1918
Phenyldibromarsine	Germans	September, 1918

Later in the war, when troops were protected with masks, the effectiveness of chlorine was greatly reduced. However, in mixtures with other gases, such as phosgene and chlorpicrin, it continued to be used throughout the war.

At ordinary temperatures and pressures, chlorine is a greenish yellow volatile gas with a pungent odor and caustic poisonous characteristics.

149

It is readily liquefied by moderate pressure (6 atmospheres) at ordinary temperatures (70°F.). When liquid, it has a specific gravity of 1.46 and, when a gas, it is 2.5 times heavier than air, so that when released as a cloud it clings well to the ground as it travels downwind. One liter of liquid chlorine at 25°C. will yield 434 liters of chlorine gas. Since

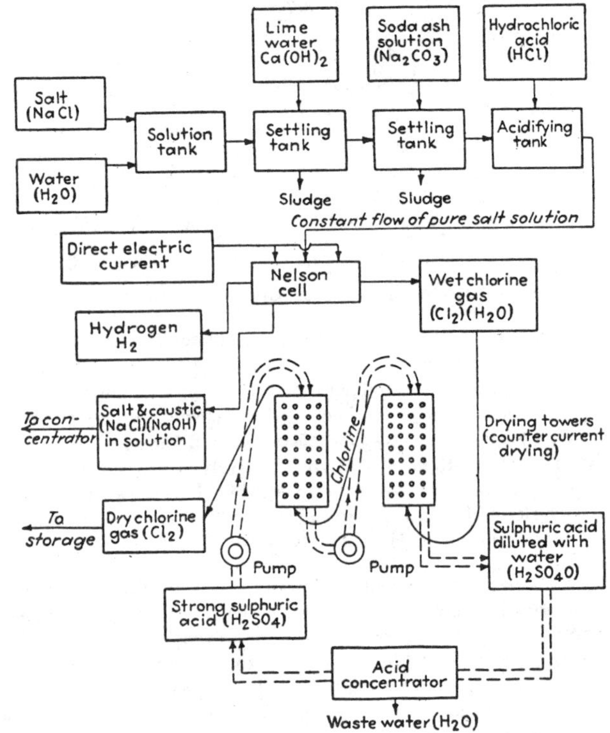

CHART IX.—Electrolytic manufacture of chlorine (flow sheet).

chlorine boils at −33.6°C. (−28.5°F.), it readily vaporizes at ordinary

temperatures and escapes with vigor from its container, so that it is well adapted for cloud-gas operations from cylinders, and this was its principal mode of employment during the war.

Chlorine is manufactured by the electrolysis of common salt (NaCl), as indicated on Chart IX, and is widely used in enormous quantities in industry. In the presence of moisture it is extraordinarily reactive.

150

attacking almost all metals and organic substances. This is its principal disadvantage as a chemical agent, as it is very easily neutralized. Although extremely soluble in water, chlorine does not hydrolyze readily and, when strictly anhydrous, it does not attack iron and steel so that it may be kept in such containers indefinitely.

Physiologically, chlorine is classified as a lung-injurant agent. It also causes a marked irritation of the conjunctiva and the mucous membranes of the nose, larynx, and pharynx.

Concerning the physiological effects of chlorine upon the human body, Gilchrist says:

> The progressive physiological action of chlorine in man as well as in animals may be summarized as follows:
>
> 1. It stimulates the sensory nerves and produces severe pain and spasm of the muscular walls of the bronchi, thus narrowing their lumen and causing a gasping for breath. The muscular spasm soon relaxes and breathing becomes easier.
> 2. Obstruction of the bronchial tubes by an inflammatory exudate, due to the irritation of the gas.
> 3. A flooding of the pulmonary air sacs by serous effusion, with resulting edema and interference with gaseous exchange of respiration.
> 4. A disruptive emphysema of the lungs and of the subcutaneous tissues, due to continuous coughing, and the rupturing of many of the alveolar cells, resulting in the passage of the air into the tissues of the lungs and into the tissues of the neck. Such a condition interferes with normal respiration and leads to a certain degree of asphyxia.

The lethal concentration of chlorine for 30 minutes' exposure is 2.53 mg. per liter; and for 10 minutes' exposure, 5.6 mg. per liter.

Chlorine possesses many of the tactical and technical requirements of an offensive battle gas, as discussed in Chap. II, page 47. Thus it is:

1. Fairly toxic (5.60 mg. per liter is lethal after 10 minutes).
2. Nonpersistent (5 to 10 minutes in the open).
3. Immediately effective (few minutes of exposure).
4. Extremely volatile (19,369 mg. per liter).
5. Raw materials available in unlimited quantities.
6. Easy to manufacture.
7. Chemically stable (when completely anhydrous).
8. Nonhydrolyzable.
9. Not decomposed under shock of explosion.
10. Of low boiling point (−34.6°C.) (−30.3°F.).
11. Of high vapor pressure.
12. Of specific gravity 1.4.
13. Of high vapor density (2.5).

The chief disadvantage of chlorine is its great chemical activity which makes it easy to protect against.

As chlorine is the basis for the manufacture of nearly all chemical agents and is readily available in enormous quantites in industry, it will always be a potential chemical-warfare threat against any nation whose

151

armed forces are not protected against it. However, since present-day gas masks afford complete protection against chlorine and since there are so many more effective combat gases now available, there is little likelihood that chlorine will figure as a chemical agent in any future war between first-class powers.

Methylsulfuryl Chloride ($ClSO_3CH_3$)

Methyl Chlorsulfonate

The great success obtained by the German cloud-gas attacks in April and May, 1915, at once suggested the use of gas in other ways, such as in grenades, trench-mortar bombs, and artillery shell. Since chlorine was too volatile to be loaded into projectiles, a search for a suitable gas for this purpose was begun on both sides.

The first compound to be successfully used in projectiles* was methylsulfuryl chloride, introduced by the Germans in June, 1915. This compound was filled into trench-mortar bombs and hand grenades, but was never employed in artillery shell.

Methylsulfuryl chloride is obtained by the action of sulfuryl chloride on methyl alcohol and is a transparent viscid liquid, of 1.51 specific gravity, which boils at 133°C. (232.4°F.), yielding a vapor 4.5 times as heavy as air, which lacrimates in concentrations as low as 1:750,000 (0.008 mg. per liter). It has a very irritating effect on the conjunctiva and respiratory organs which becomes intolerable when the concentration rises to 0.050 mg. per liter. A concentration of 2.00 mg. per liter is fatal on 10 minutes' exposure, death being caused by lung edema as in the case of chlorine and phosgene poisoning. Its volatility at 20°C. is 60.00 mg. per liter.

Methylsulfuryl chloride was used only a short time, being replaced in the summer of 1915 with K-Stoff.

Ethylsulfuryl Chloride ($ClSO_3C_2H_5$)

French: "Sulvanite"

About the same time that the Germans brought out methylsulfuryl chloride, the French countered with the ethyl compound, as a filling for artillery shell, under the name "Sulvanite."

Ethylsulfuryl chloride is similarly obtained by acting on ethyl alcohol with sulfuryl chloride and is a colorless liquid, of 1.44 specific gravity, which boils with some decomposition at 135°C. (275°F.), yielding a vapor which lacrimates in concentrations as low as 1:1,000,000. A concentration of 0.050 mg. per liter is intolerable and a concentration of 1.00 mg. per liter is toxic.

* The earlier use of xylyl bromide (T-Stoff) in artillery shell on the Russian Front in January, 1915, was unsuccessful.

152

Compared to methylsulfuryl chloride, the ethyl compound is more lacrimatory and toxic, but is less volatile, so that the combat values of the two are probably about the same.

Neither of these compounds played a role of any importance in the war; they mark a milestone in the race for a more effective lung-injurant agent and are of historical interest only.

Chlormethylchloroformate ($ClCOOCH_2Cl$)

French: "Palite"; German: "K-Stoff," "C-Stoff"

This substance, known as "K-Stoff" when used in shells and "C-Stoff" when used in trench mortars and projector bombs, was first used by the Germans in June, 1915, in an effort to find a chemical agent more effective than chlorine.

K-Stoff is a mixture of the incompletely chlorinated methyl esters of formic acid (70 per cent $ClCOOCH_2Cl$ and 30 per cent $ClCOOCHCl_2$) and is a clear liquid, of 1.48 specific gravity, which boils at 1.09°C. (228.2°F.), yielding a vapor 4.5 times heavier than air. It has an ethereal odor, is somewhat lacrimatory, and hydrolyzes easily when warm and even when cold in the presence of alkalies, yielding formaldehyde, carbonic acid, and hydrochloric acid. Its vapor pressure at 20°C. (68°F.) is 5.6 mm. Hg.

Chlormethylchloroformate is prepared by first acting on phosgene with methyl alcohol to obtain methylchloroformate as follows:

$$COCl_2 + CH_3(OH) = ClCOOCH_3 + HCl$$

and then chlorinating this ester in the presence of strong light, so that chlorine progressively replaces the hydrogen atoms of the methyl group, yielding monochlormethylchloroformate ($ClCOOCH_2Cl$) and dichlormethylchloroformate ($ClCOOCHCl_2$).

In concentrations of 1:100,000 (0.0528 mg. per liter), K-Stoff causes slight lacrimation, while a concentration of 1.00 mg. per liter is lethal on 30 minutes' exposure.

It is, therefore, about five times more toxic than chlorine, but only about half as toxic as phosgene and diphosgene, so that, while it was a great improvement over chlorine when first used, it was soon displaced by diphosgene and chlorpicrin when these more powerful compounds were introduced.

Dimethyl Sulfate ($(CH_3)_2SO_4$)

German: "D-Stoff"; French: "Rationite"

The question of who first used this compound as a chemical agent in

the late war is somewhat uncertain. Thus, Dr. Hanslian
153
says this substance was introduced by the Germans as a filling for artillery shell in August, 1915, under the name of "D-Stoff"; the reports of the Allies' laboratories which analyzed the contents of these early German D shells show that dimethyl sulfate was an ingredient of their chemical contents. On the other hand, Dr. Mueller (21, page 96) emphatically denies the German use of this compound and explains the situation thus:

> The oft-repeated statement to the effect that dimethyl sulfate had been used experimentally by the Germans as early as in 1915 is not true. It is to be explained by the fact that methylsulfuryl chloride used at that time temporarily was slightly polluted with a few per cent of dimethyl sulfate, and the impurities still clung to the commercial product after its manufacture. Under no circumstances was dimethyl sulfate purposely added. Those concerned with such matters would never have agreed to its use.

Whether or not the early German use of dimethyl sulfate was deliberate or accidental, it is clear that no one at that time really realized the true combat value of this substance. Thus, it is not only a good lacrimator and very toxic, but is also a fairly powerful vesicant. These properties were later discovered by the French and dimethyl sulfate was adopted by them as a filling for artillery shell and hand grenades in September, 1918, under the name of "Rationite."

Dimethyl sulfate is produced by acting on fuming sulfuric acid with methyl alcohol and distilling in vacuo. Before the war it was used in industry as a methylating agent for amines and phenols and as a reagent for detecting coal-tar oils.

It is a colorless oily liquid, of 1.35 specific gravity, which boils at 188°C. (370.4°F.), yielding a vapor 4.4 times heavier than air with a faint odor of onions.

At ordinary temperatures (68°F.), its volatility is only 3.3 mg. per liter, which is low for a lung injurant but high for a vesicant. Dimethyl sulfate is very readily decomposed by water so that its vapors quickly combine with moisture in the air to form sulfuric acid. This is one of the chief defects of this substance as a chemical agent.

Dimethyl sulfate is a powerful irritant to the mucous membranes, especially the conjunctiva and respiratory system. Its direct toxic action is exerted against the lungs in a manner very similar to that of chlorine, resulting in bronchitis, pneumonia, and lung edema. A concentration of 0.50 mg. per liter is fatal on 10 minutes' exposure. It is, therefore, about as toxic as phosgene. In lower concentrations it exerts a corrosive action on the skin, resulting in a peculiar analgesia of the skin which is said to last for six months after exposure. For this reason, it may also be regarded as a vesicant agent.

154
The limited use of this compound during the war did not definitely establish its combat value. However, the high degree to which it is decomposed by water, and even by the moisture in the air, would require that any tactical effects produced be secured by the vapors directly upon the bursting of the shells before these vapors are decomposed by the moisture in the air. This so greatly limits the combat effectiveness of this substance as to raise a serious question regarding its future value as a chemical agent, particularly since other more toxic and more vesicant compounds have been discovered.

Perchlormethylmercaptan ($SCCl_4$)

Carbon Tetrachlorsulfide

During the summer of 1915, while the Germans were experimenting with halogenated esters, the French conceived the idea of utilizing perchlormethylmercaptan as a chemical-warfare gas, and this substance, which was introduced by the French in the battle of the Champagne in September, 1915, constituted the first use of gas shell by the French Army.

Perchlormethylmercaptan may be obtained by the direct chlorination of methylmercaptan (CH_3SH) or by passing chlorine into carbon disulfide in the presence of a small quantity of iodine as a chlorine carrier. The resulting product is a light yellow liquid, of 1.71 specific gravity, which boils at 149°C. (300.2°F.), yielding a vapor 6.5 times heavier than air. It lacrimates in concentrations as low as 0.010 mg. per liter and is intolerable at 0.070 mg. per liter. A concentration of 3.00 mg. per liter is lethal on 10 minutes' exposure, which makes it about one-sixth as toxic as phosgene.

Perchlormethylmercaptan has the following disadvantages as a chemical agent:

1. Rather low toxicity.
2. Warning odor which betrays its presence before toxic effects are produced.
3. Decomposes in the presence of iron and steel.
4. Charcoal easily fixes its vapors and furnished complete protection against it.

For these reasons, this compound was soon abandoned in favor of other more effective substances and is not likely to be used again as a chemical agent. Commenting on this gas, Izard (23) says, "Its utilization had no other object than to realize a provisional solution."

Phosgene (Carbonyl Chloride) ($COCl_2$)

French: "Collongite"; German: "D-Stoff"; British and American: CG

Phosgene was the second toxic gas to be used in large quantities during the war. It was first employed by the Germans, mixed with
155
chlorine, in a cloud-gas attack against the British at Nieltje, in Flanders, on Dec. 19, 1915, when 88 tons of gas were released from 4,000 cylinders and produced 1,069 casualties, of which 120 were fatal.

In February, 1916, phosgene was adopted as an artillery-shell filler by the French in retaliation for the German K-Stoff shell. Throughout the remainder of the war, this gas was the principal offensive battle gas of the Allies, being used in enormous quantities in cylinders, artillery shell, trench mortars, bombs, and projector drums. More than 80 per cent of gas fatalities in the World War were caused by phosgene. Concerning the use of phosgene in the World War, see Table XVII, pages 663 *ff*.

Phosgene was known to chemists for over a hundred years before the World War, being first made by the British chemist John Davy in 1812 by the reaction of carbon monoxide and chlorine in the presence of sunlight. At the beginning of the present century, phosgene was used extensively as an intermediate in the dye industry and had been manufactured on a considerable scale for many years in Germany. With its well-known toxic properties and its ready availability in large quantities, phosgene was a logical choice of the German chemists for a more powerful substitute for chlorine when the Allies had equipped themselves with masks that afforded adequate protection against chlorine.

At ordinary temperatures and pressures, phosgene is a colorless gas which condenses at 46.7°F. to a colorless liquid of 1.38 specific gravity. Above 46.7°F., phosgene immediately evaporates, although at a slower rate than chlorine, and gives off a transparent vapor, 3.5 times heavier than air, with a stifling, but not unpleasant, odor resembling new-mown hay.

Aside from its characteristic odor, phosgene may also be detected in the field by its so-called *tobacco reaction*, by which is meant that men who have breathed only very slight amounts of phosgene experience a peculiar flat metallic taste when smoking tobacco. Certain other gases, such as HCN and sulfur dioxide, however, also have this effect and must be distinguished from phosgene by their very different odors.

Chemically much more inert than chlorine, phosgene is a very stable compound and is not dissociated by explosion of even strong bursting charges. When dry, phosgene does not attack iron and may, therefore, be kept indefinitely in iron and steel containers. It is, however, extremely sensitive to water, in contact with which it quickly breaks down into hydrochloric acid and carbon dioxide, according to the equation

$$COCl_2 + H_2O = CO_2 + 2HCl$$

Hence, even if slight traces of water are present in loading phosgene into shell, the hydrochloric acid formed will attack the shell walls and gen-
156
erate dangerous pressure in the shell; if sufficient hydrochloric acid is formed, it will eventually destroy the shell. Because of its rapid hydrolysis in the presence of water, phosgene cannot be efficiently employed in

very wet weather.

While phosgene boils at 46.7°F., which is considerably below ordinary summer temperatures, its rate of evaporation is so slow that it has to be mixed with equal quantities of chlorine in order to set up satisfactory cloud-gas concentrations in the field. This was the manner in which phosgene was employed in cloud-gas attacks throughout the war.

The toxicity of phosgene is over ten times that of chlorine, a concentration of 0.50 mg. per liter being fatal after 10 minutes' exposure. In higher concentrations, which are often met in battle, one or two breaths may be fatal in a few hours.

Phosgene appears to exert its physiological and toxic effects chiefly through the medium of its hydrolysis products—hydrochloric acid and carbon dioxide. Its effects upon the upper air passages of the body, where moisture is relatively small, is therefore comparatively slight. With prolonged breathing, however, sufficient phosgene is decomposed in the bronchi and trachea to produce marked inflammation and corrosion. These effects reach their maximum in the alveoli where the air is saturated with water.

Unlike chlorine, phosgene produces but a slight irritation of the sensory nerves in the upper air passages, so that men exposed to this gas are likely to inhale it more deeply than they would equivalent concentrations of chlorine or other directly irritant vapors. For this reason, phosgene is very insidious in its action and men gassed with it often have little or no warning symptoms until too late to avoid serious poisoning. Generally, the victim first experiences a temporary weak spell, but otherwise feels well and has a good appetite. Suddenly he grows worse, and death frequently follows in a few days.

Concerning the physiological action of phosgene, which is typical of the lung-injurant agents, General Gilchrist says:

After gassing with phosgene there is irritation of the trachea or bronchi; coughing is not a prominent symptom, and disruptive emphysema is practically never seen. After moderate gassing, a man may feel able to carry on his work for an hour or two with slight symptoms, but he may become suddenly worse, may show evidence of extreme cyanosis, and subsequently may pass into collapse. There are records of men who have undergone a phosgene-gas attack and who seem to have suffered slightly, but have died suddenly some hours later upon attempting physical effort.

Pulmonary edema appears very early. This edema is at first noncellular but, after about five hours, leucocytes are found, and later the exudate is rich in cells. After inhalation of phosgene, red blood cells are seldom found in the exudate; later fibrin appears. Physical examination at this time reveals focal patches of bronchopneumonia. At the height of illness edema is the outstanding condition. After the

157

second or third day, if death does not occur, the edema fluid is resorbed and recovery follows, barring complication of the bronchopneumonic process.

The important immediate effects of phosgene are practically limited to the lungs. These changes consist of damage to the capillaries. This damage may be noted a half hour after gassing. The capillaries in the walls of the alveoli are markedly constricted and appear collapsed. Later they become dilated and engorged with blood, and blood stasis is the rule. Frequently thrombi form and block the capillaries for some distance, which increases the blood stasis. This dilation and blood stasis in the capillaries is the main cause of pulmonary edema; the latter progresses rapidly from this time on.

A number of theories have been advanced to explain the production of edema. The preponderance of evidence as to the cause of the edema following phosgene gassing is that it is due to local injury of the endothelial cells which results in an increased capillary permeability; the other changes in the blood and in the circulation are secondary to the trauma sustained by the capillary wall.

The injurious effects of phosgene are materially increased by physical exertion. Frequently those parts of the lungs which have not been damaged by the gas would be sufficient for breathing purposes if the body were at rest, but they are not sufficient while the body is in motion, particularly in view of the excess carbonic acid which is formed in the body by the decomposition of the phosgene.

Phosgene is manufactured in industry by the original process of direct synthesis of chlorine and carbon monoxide, as indicated in Chart X. The only change from the original process of making it is the substitution of a catalyst (animal charcoal) for the action of sunlight.

Compared to chlorine, phosgene has the following advantages as a chemical agent. It is:

1. Far more toxic (0.50 mg. per liter at 10 minutes).
2. A little less volatile and more persistent.
3. Greater vapor density (3.5).
4. More insidious in action.
5. Chemically more inert and, therefore, more difficult to neutralize and protect against.

The principal disadvantages of phosgene are its slower physiological action on the body and its inability to discharge itself from cylinders at a sufficient rate for cloud-gas attacks.

In addition to the foregoing, phosgene is relatively easy to protect against and for that reason would probably be displaced in the future by gases of greater toxicity and more difficult to neutralize.

Trichlormethylchloroformate ($ClCOOCCl_3$)

German: "Perstoff"; French: "Surpalite"; British: "Diphosgene"

This gas was first used in the World War by the Germans at Verdun in May, 1916, in retaliation for the French phosgene shell which were introduced in February, 1916.

158

Trichlormethylchloroformate is the completely chlorinated methyl ester of formic acid and is obtained by completing the chlorination of the monochlormethylchloroformate (K-Stoff). In studying the chlorinated methyl esters of formic acid, the German chemists found that their toxic properties increased, while their lacrimatory powers decreased, with

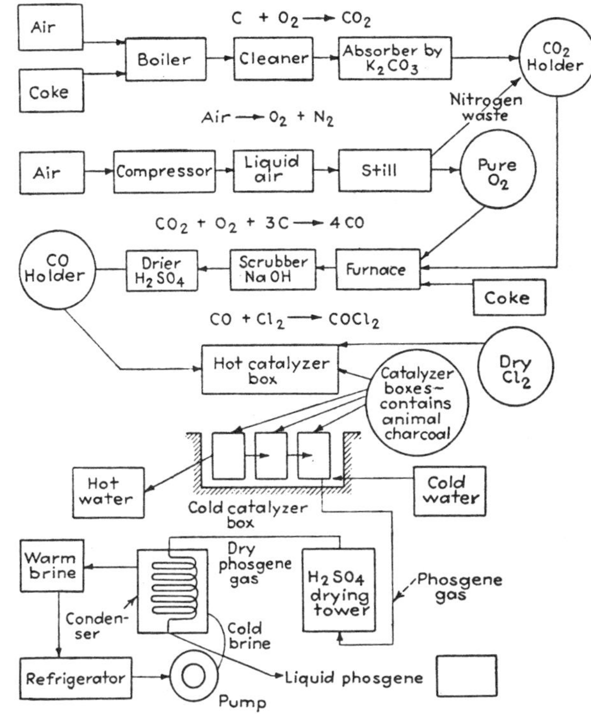

CHART X.—Catalytic manufacture of phosgene (flow sheet).

the addition of chlorine atoms in the methyl group of their molecular structures. Thus, diphosgene, which contains the maximum chlorine atoms, was found to be the least lacrimatory but the most toxic of these compounds and was for that reason substituted for K-Stoff as the standard German nonpersistent lethal gas for shells. An analysis of the gas casualties of the late war indicates that, on the basis of the total

159

number of fatalities, diphosgene was the principal *killing* gas used *in shells* during the war.

Trichlormethylchloroformate is an oily liquid of specific gravity 1.65 and a disagreeable suffocating odor. It boils at 127°C. (260.6°F.), giving off a dense whitish vapor 6.9 times heavier than air, which persists on open ground about 30 minutes. At 20°C. (68°F.), its volatility is 26.00 mg. per liter. When heated to about 350°C. (662°F.) or upon contact with moisture, as in the tissues of the body, trichlormethylchloroformate breaks down, yielding two molecules of phosgene, thus: $ClCOOCCl_3$ =

$2COCl_2$, from which it received its English name—diphosgene. Under ordinary conditions of temperature and pressure, it hydrolyzes slowly, ultimately yielding carbonic acid and hydrochloric acid, according to the following equation:

$$ClCOOCCl_3 + 2H_2O = 2CO_2 + 4HCl$$

Because of its high boiling point and the fact that in its primary form it is relatively inactive physiologically, diphosgene is peculiarly adapted for shell filling. Unlike phosgene, which requires artificial refrigeration to keep it below its boiling point during filling operations, diphosgene can be filled into shells in the field, the workmen requiring no other protection than gas masks. This was of great advantage to the Germans during the war as it enabled them to fill shell close behind the front lines, and the filled shell thus required the minimum transportation, handling, and storage. Because of this fact, the Germans were able to use all sorts of H.E. shell for gas by the simple expedient of cementing the joints in the shells, while the Allies, whose shell were filled far from the front and had to withstand much rough handling and long storage, could not successfully use cemented gas shell, because of leakage difficulties.

The toxicity of diphosgene is about the same as that of phosgene. In fact, it is probable that the toxicity of diphosgene is not a specific property of that compound, but is derived from the phosgene molecules into which it decomposes in the tissues of the body.

The German chemist, Haber , quoting the work of Flury, gives the toxicity index of diphosgene as 500, as compared to 450 for phosgene. For a 10-minute exposure, this is equivalent to a concentration of 0.050 mg. per liter of diphosgene and 0.045 mg. per liter of phosgene. American determinations, however, show that the minimum lethal concentrations of phosgene for a 10-minute exposure is 0.50 mg. per liter which is over ten times the German figure. Many reasons have been advanced to account for the large discrepancy in these figures, such as that Flury's determinations were on cats which were subsequently found to be peculiarly sensitive to phosgene and diphosgene concentrations. The cats were also said to be undernourished, which still further increased

160

their susceptibility. However, regardless of the differences in *specific* toxicity of phosgene and diphosgene, as between the different nations, all agree that there are no perceptible differences in the physiological effects of these two compounds and that they are substantially equal in toxicity.

As phosgene was the choice of the Allies for a standard nonpersistent lethal gas, while the Germans used diphosgene, it is interesting to compare relative merits of these two compounds as chemical agents.

Both have about the same toxicity and physiological effects on men and animals. Diphosgene is about three times as persistent as phosgene, having an open-ground persistency of 30 minutes against 10 minutes for phosgene, so that diphosgene would not be classed as a nonpersistent gas under our present system of classification, which regards all agents having an open-ground persistency greater than 10 minutes as persistent. However, the present limit of 10 minutes for nonpersistent gases is somewhat arbitrary and, from a tactical standpoint, it is believed that a persistency of 30 minutes is not too great for a nonpersistent gas. The main consideration governing the length of time a nonpersistent gas can be allowed to remain on the target area is the time required for the attacking infantry to traverse the ground between their jump-off lines and the enemy's front line. Under the most favorable conditions, with the jump-off line only 800 yd. from the enemy's front line and maximum rate of advance under fire (100 yd. in 4 minutes), this will not be less than 32 minutes, so that a gas which would not persist for over 30 minutes would be suitable for use in offensive operations.

Within the limits of permissible persistency, the nearer this limit is approached by an agent, the easier it is to maintain effective concentrations in the field; therefore a persistency of 30 minutes is an advantage over a persistency of 10 minutes, so that diphosgene has the advantage in this respect. On the other hand, phosgene is more volatile than diphosgene and higher field concentrations can be effected with phosgene.

The speed and duration of the casualty effects of both phosgene and diphosgene are about the same, but phosgene has the advantage of being more insidious in action, as diphosgene is somewhat lacrimatory and gives a noticeable warning in concentrations of 1:200,000, as compared to 1:100,000 for phosgene. The odor and visibility of phosgene and diphosgene are very similar and almost equal, the latter being somewhat more pungent and visible in cloud formation than the former.

Phosgene is made by the direct synthesis of CO + Cl, whereas diphosgene requires the following additional steps:

1. Formation of methylchloroformate from phosgene and methyl alcohol by reaction with calcium carbonate.
2. Formation of diphosgene from methylchloroformate by the reaction of chlorine by the action of electricity (ultraviolet rays).

161

Special title-lined reaction vessels are also required for the manufacture of diphosgene which considerably complicates its production in large quantities. Phosgene is thus far easier to manufacture than diphosgene, and it was primarily on this account that the Allies chose phosgene as their standard lethal agent.

Phosgene is chemically more stable than diphosgene and withstands explosion without decomposition, although diphosgene is first resolved into phosgene by dissociation. Owing to its higher boiling point and relatively inert physiological action in its primary form, diphosgene is far easier to fill into shell, but, on the other hand, it cannot be used for cloud-gas attacks as can phosgene. Finally, diphosgene vapor is more than twice as heavy as phosgene, which gives it greater ground-clinging and searching values in the field.

Chlorpicrin (Nitrochloroform) (CCl_3NO_2)

British: "Vomiting gas"; French: "Aquinite"; German: "Klop"

The next lung-injurant gas to make its appearance in the World War was chlorpicrin. This gas was first used in battle by the Russians in August, 1916, and was subsequently employed by both Germany and the Allies, alone or mixed with other combat substances, in artillery shells, trench-mortar bombs, and in cylinders for cloud-gas attacks. Indeed, chlorpicrin appears to have been the most widely used combat gas in the war, although the total amount used was probably less than that of phosgene and diphosgene.

Like chlorine and phosgene, chlorpicrin was a well-known chemical substance before the World War. It was discovered by the English chemist, Stenhouse, in 1848, and its chemical and physiological properties had been carefully studied many years during the nineteenth century.

Chlorpicrin is a colorless oily liquid, of 1.66 specific gravity, which boils at 112°C. (231.5°F.), giving off a pungent irritating vapor, 5.6 times heavier than air, and having a sweetish odor resembling that of flypaper. Even at ordinary temperatures chlorpicrin evaporates very rapidly, and its vapor pressure is quite high, *e.g.*, at 20°C. (68°F.) it amounts to 18.3 mm. Hg. Its volatility at 20°C. (68°F.) is 165.0 mg. per liter. Chlorpicrin may therefore be used in cylinders for cloud-gas attacks if mixed with chlorine. Mixed with 70 per cent chlorine, chlorpicrin was used in a large number of British gas attacks under the name of "Yellow Star gas."

Chemically, chlorpicrin is quite a stable compound. It is almost insoluble in, and is not decomposed by, water; it does not combine readily with either acids or alkalies. Owing to its chemical inertness, chlorpicrin does not react with any of the chemicals in the gas-mask

162

canister and is removed from the air passing through the canister by the charcoal alone. It is therefore one of the most difficult of the war gases to protect against. Owing to this fact, the protection afforded by gas-mask canisters is usually rated in accordance with the number of hours it will protect against ordinary field concentrations of chlorpicrin.

Chlorpicrin is rather easily manufactured by the direct chlorination of picric acid. In practice, the reaction is carried out by injecting live steam into an aqueous solution of bleaching powder and picric acid, as shown on Chart XI. The yield is 114 per cent of the volume of picric acid employed. Since large amounts of picric acid are used in industry and for high explosives and, since bleaching powder is easily obtainable everywhere, the raw materials necessary in the manufacture of chlorpicrin are readily available. This fact and the ease of manufacture undoubtedly

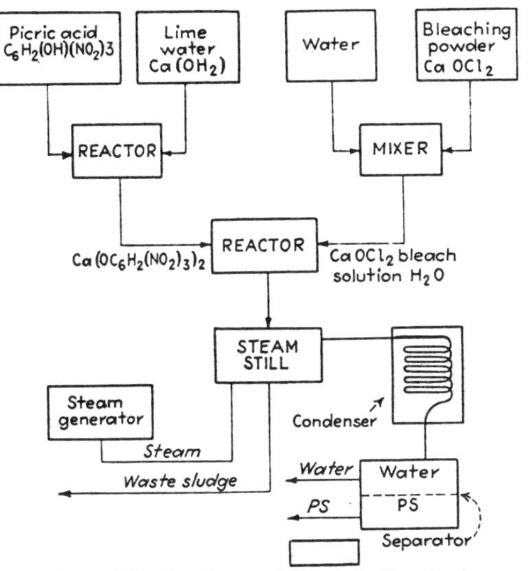

CHART XI.—Manufacture of chlorpicrin (flow sheet).

account for the widespread use of chlorpicrin during the late war.

As a war gas, chlorpicrin has a number of desirable offensive properties. Like chlorine and phosgene, it is a lethal compound which acts primarily as a lung injurant. In toxicity, it is intermediate between chlorine and phosgene, as indicated by the following comparative figures:

163

LETHAL CONCENTRATIONS

Exposure, minutes	Chlorine, mg. per liter	Chlorpicrin, mg. per liter	Phosgene, mg. per liter
10	5.60	2.00	0.50
30	2.53	0.80	0.36

In addition to its lethal (lung-injurant) effects, chlorpicrin is also a strong lacrimator, and has the additional advantage of being capable of penetrating gas-mask canisters that are resistant to ordinary acid gases, such as chlorine and phosgene. The injurious effects of chlorpicrin also extend to the stomach and intestines, causing nausea, vomiting, colic, and diarrhea. These conditions are difficult to combat in the field and often persist for weeks so that even slight cases of chlorpicrin gassing frequently involve large casualty losses.

The main tactical idea in using chlorpicrin, aside from its toxic effect, was to penetrate the mask and produce an intolerable irritation of the eyes, as well as coughing and vomiting from nausea. These effects are sufficient to cause masked troops to remove their masks and thus expose themselves to even more lethal gases, such as phosgene, which would be put over with the chlorpicrin.

The principal disadvantages of chlorpicrin are its relatively low toxicity, as compared to some of the later war gases, and the fact that it decomposes upon heating and when subjected to too high an explosive shock. Notwithstanding this latter peculiarity, the results of the late war showed that chlorpicrin could be successfully used in artillery shells if the bursting charges were properly adjusted to this filling. Another factor limiting the general usefulness of chlorpicrin is its rather high persistency. On open ground chlorpicrin has a persistency of about 3 hours, which would preclude its use on the tactical offensive in ordinary situations.

Owing to the foregoing disadvantages and limitations, the fact that modern gas masks generally furnish adequate protection against chlorpicrin, and the further fact that much more powerful and effective lethal agents were used in the late war and would be in all probability used in any future war, the future role of chlorpicrin as a war gas is at least uncertain, with the probabilities rather against its future use.

Phenylcarbylamine Chloride ($C_6H_5CNCl_2$)

Phenylisocyanide Chloride

This compound, introduced by the Germans in May, 1917, was the last of the simple lung-injurant agents to be employed by them in the

164

World War. Two months later they brought out two entirely new and radically different types of agents—the vesicants (Yellow Cross), of which mustard gas was the prototype, and the sternutators (Blue Cross), of which diphenylchlorarsine was the prototype—and thus changed the whole character of gas warfare.

Phenylcarbylamine chloride was the culmination of an attempt to produce a more persistent and enduring lung-injurant agent, so as to enable concentrations to be maintained in the field for such a length of time as to exhaust the current types of gas-mask canisters. Later it was used in shoots with mustard gas to mask the presence of the latter.

Phenylcarbylamine chloride is produced by chlorinating phenyl mustard oil (C_6H_5NCS), derived from the action of carbon disulfide on aniline. The product is a transparent liquid, of 1.35 specific gravity, which boils at 210°C. (410°F.), yielding a vapor 6.0 times heavier than air. Its volatility at 20°C. (68°F.) is 2.10 mg. per liter. Its lowest irritant concentration is 0.003 mg. per liter; it lacrimates at 1:1,000,000 (0.0072 mg. per liter); it is intolerable at 0.025 mg. per liter; and a concentration of 0.50 mg. per liter is lethal on 10 minutes' exposure.

Phenylcarbylamine chloride was used chiefly in shells for the 10.5-cm. light field howitzer (without a mark) and 15.0-cm. heavy field howitzer (marked 1 Green Cross – variation). Owing to its low volatility, it was very persistent, and for that reason could not be used on the tactical offensive. Moreover, its low vapor pressure often prevented effective concentrations from being realized in the field. Altogether, about 700 tons of this gas were fired by the Germans from the middle of 1917 to the end of the war and, while this gas was a fair lacrimator and was moderately toxic, it failed to achieve any noteworthy success. It was not considered of much value by the British and the reason for its use by the Germans is not apparent, since they already had far more effective lung-injurant agents (*e.g.*, diphosgene and chlorpicrin).

Dichlordimethyl Ether ($(CH_2Cl)_2O$)
Dibromdimethyl Ether ($(CH_2BR)_2O$)

Dichlormethyl ether is one of the lesser combat substances used by the Germans, usually in mixture with ethyldichlorarsine. It was introduced in January, 1918, and was utilized to increase the volatility of ethyldichlorarsine, which was brought into use about the same time.

Dichlordimethyl ether is a colorless liquid, of 1.37 specific gravity, which boils at 105°C. (221°F.) and has a volatility of 0.180 mg. per liter at 20°C. Its lowest effective concentration is 0.015 mg. per liter; it is intolerable at 0.040 mg. per liter and lethal at 0.470 mg. per liter on 10 minutes' exposure.

165

The bromine analogue, dibromdimethyl ether, was also used by the Germans in the same way as dichlordimethyl ether and, as compared to the latter, has the following properties: it has a higher boiling point, 155°C. (311°F.), and a lower volatility (0.022 mg. per liter). It is also less irritant, a concentration of 0.020 mg. per liter being required to produce an irritating effect, while the concentration does not become intolerable until it reaches 0.050 mg. per liter. On the other hand, it is more toxic since a concentration of 0.040 mg. per liter is lethal on 10 minutes' exposure. It is also denser, having a specific gravity of 2.20.

In addition to their typical lung-injurant effects, these two compounds also exert a peculiar selective action on the organs of equilibrium of the body, *i.e.*, the labyrinth of the ear, so that the victim staggers and reels and is unable to maintain his body balance. For this reason the French classified these compounds in a separate class and called them *labyrinthic substances.*

Both dichlormethyl ether and dibrommethyl ether are more toxic than phosgene, and this fact, together with their favorable volatilities and the fact that they are both insidious in action, make them noteworthy combat substances. As they do not appear to have been used to any great extent, except in mixture with ethyldichlorarsine, their individual values as toxic agents were not established in the war. However, their properties and characteristics are such as to make them of considerable potential value, notwithstanding the fact that they are both rather easily decomposed by water.

Phenyldichlorarsine ($C_6H_5AsCl_2$)

French: "Sternite"

The first of the *toxic* lung-injurant agents to appear in the World War was phenyldichlorarsine. This gas was first used by the Germans in September, 1917, with, and as a solvent for, diphenylcyanarsine (Clark 2) in Blue Cross 1 artillery shell, and later by the French in a mixture with 40 per cent diphenylchlorarsine, known as "Sternite."

Phenyldichlorarsine is a clear somewhat viscid liquid, of 1.64 specific gravity, which boils at 252°C. (485.6°F.) giving off dense vapors 7.75 times heavier than air. It is insoluble in water but dissolves readily in the usual organic solvents. It hydrolyzes readily in contact with water and the oxydants destroy it.

Owing to its high boiling point, phenyldichlorarsine has a very low vapor pressure at ordinary temperatures, being equal to only 0.0146 mm. Hg at 15°C. (59°F.).

While the primary physiological effect of phenyldichlorarsine on men and animals is injury to the lungs and death is usually caused by pulmonary edema, phenyldichlorarsine also has a marked vesicant as well

166

as a sternutatory effect on the upper respiratory passages. Its toxicity exceeds that of phosgene, a concentration of 0.26 mg. per liter being fatal in 10 minutes; its vesicant action is somewhat slower than that of mustard gas and the resulting wounds as a rule heal more rapidly.

On the whole, phenyldichlorarsine was not used in the war to any great extent. The principal idea underlying its use was as a solvent for diphenylchlorarsine and to assist in the penetration of the gas-mask canister. A mixture of these two compounds in the proportion of 60 per cent phenyldichlorarsine and 40 per cent diphenylchlorarsine was used by the French under the name of "Sternite." It was claimed that this mixture would readily penetrate the masks then in use and, being a liquid, did not present the difficulties in shell filling that attended the filling with a solid diphenylchlorarsine.

The limited use of phenyldichlorarsine in the late war did not clearly demonstrate any marked superiority for this compound over other organic arsenicals simultaneously employed, but it would seem from a consideration of its properties that it is an agent of considerable promise.

Ethyldichlorarsine ($C_2H_5AsCl_2$)

German: "Dick"

This compound was introduced by the Germans in March, 1918, in an attempt to produce a volatile nonpersistent gas that would be quicker acting than diphosgene or mustard gas and would be more lasting in its effects than "Clark" (see Chap. X). Such a gas was particularly desired for use in the immediate preparation for and in support of infantry attacks in the grand offensive operation planned for the spring of 1918, and ethyldichlorarsine was the answer of the German chemists to this demand.

The German process of manufacturing this compound was complicated and comprised the following principal steps: (1) the conversion of ethyl chloride into ethyl sodium arsenate by treatment with sodium arsenate under pressure; (2) reduction to ethyl arsenious oxide by the action of sulfurous acid; (3) conversion of the ethyl arsenious oxide to ethyl dichlorarsine by treatment with hydrochloric acid.

The final product, when pure, is a clear somewhat oily liquid, of 1.7 specific gravity, which boils at 156°C. (312°F.), yielding a vapor 6.5 times denser than air with a piquant fruity odor. At 20°C. (68°F.), its volatility is 100.0 mg. per liter. Although the liquid ethyldichlorarsine is slowly hydrolyzed by water, the vapor seems sufficiently stable to endure for its ordinary period of persistency in the field. The hydrolysis product, ethylarsenious oxide, is also poisonous when swallowed. Although ethyldichlorarsine is but little soluble in water, it is soluble in

167

alcohol, ether, benzene, or ethyl chloride and is destroyed by oxydants, such as chloride of lime and potassium permanganate. Although ethyldichlorarsine is a fairly powerful sternutator and vesicant agent, its primary action on the body is as a lung injurant. Its first effect in low concentrations is a respiratory irritation which occurs in concentrations as low as 0.001 mg. per liter after 5 minutes' exposure. A concentration of 0.010 mg. per liter is intolerable for more than 1 minute because of the great irritation of the nose and throat. The lethal concentration of ethyldichlorarsine is 0.50 mg. per liter for 10 minutes' exposure and 0.10 mg. per liter for 30 minutes' exposure. Its toxicity is, therefore, the same as phosgene for short exposures (10 minutes), but is over three times the toxicity of phosgene for long exposures (30 minutes). In concentrations as low as 0.005 mg. per liter, this gas causes marked local irritation of the eyes and respiratory tract. The effect upon the eyes and upper respiratory tract is evanescent, while that upon the lower respiratory tract leads to membranous tracheitis and pulmonary congestion, edema, and pneumonia. Arsenic is absorbed rapidly and leads to systemic arsenical poisoning, characterized by lowered temperature, atoxic symptoms, anesthesia, and depression.

On short exposures (*i.e.*, less than 5 minutes), ethyldichlorarsine is not a particularly efficient irritant for the human skin. On exposures greater than 5 minutes, however, positive burns appear which increase in severity with length of exposure. On the basis of rapidity of action, extent of rubefaction, swelling and edema, and time of healing, ethyldichlorarsine is about two-thirds as effective as mustard gas, but for vesication it is only about one-sixth as effective.

Ethyldichlorarsine and its bromic analogue, ethyldibromarsine, were used in mixtures with the equally toxic dichlormethyl ether (21, pages 93 and 95) as fillings for the German Yellow Cross 1 or Green Cross 3 artillery shell. Ethyldibromarsine has the same physiological effects as ethyldichlorarsine, but is less irritant and toxic than the latter and the reason for its use by the Germans is not apparent.

Concerning the use of ethyldichlorarsine in the war, Hanslian says:

> Like the Yellow Cross substance, this combat substance was usually not noticed at all when it was breathed in. It was distinguished from the Yellow Cross substance when used in the field by the fact that in the first place there was no effect on the skin, and in the second place, the injuries to the nose, throat, and chest did not delay for hours but appeared at the end of a few minutes. When small quantities are inhaled, about 5 cc. for 1 minute, the victim is rendered incapable of fighting for as much as 24 hours as the result of dyspnea and pains in the chest, and if large quantities are inhaled the result is fatal. In case small amounts of the substance have already been inhaled before the gas mask is put on, it is impossible to keep the mask on because of the irritation. The substance of the Yellow Cross 1 shell was not nearly
>
> 168
>
> so persistent on the terrain as that of the regular Yellow Cross. These shells were therefore suitable for gassing operations to be followed by infantry assaults. In summer, terrain could be entered 1 hour after the gas cloud had disappeared, and, in winter, 2 hours after. The Yellow Cross substance No. 1 behaved, accordingly, almost in all respects like the Green Cross substance and not like the Yellow Cross substance.

There is no record of the casualties produced by ethyldichlorarsine, nor any reliable record by which its battle efficacy may be judged. However, it possesses many valuable properties and characteristics, chief among which are its quick action and low persistency which makes it suitable as an offensive chemical agent. There is a great tactical need for a quick-acting nonpersistent vesicant and, while the vesicant action of ethyldichlorarsine is secondary to its lung-injurant action, it is, nevertheless, not inconsiderable. We may, therefore, expect to find this compound given careful consideration in any estimate of chemical warfare in the future.

Phenyldibromarsine ($C_6H_5AsBr_2$)

This was the last type of lung-injurant gases of the toxic variety used in the World War. It was introduced by the Germans in September, 1918, and there is very little information as to its effectiveness.

The compound is a colorless or faintly yellow liquid, boiling with slight decomposition at 285°C. (545°F.), and having a density of 2.1 at 15°C. (59°F.). When dispersed by heat, the fumes are slightly lacrimatory and somewhat sternutatory, although this latter effect is very much less than diphenylchlorarsine. A concentration of 0.020 mg. per liter is fatal on 10 minutes' exposure; hence its toxicity exceeds that of any of the lung-injurant agents used in the war.

It was the opinion of the Allies that phenyldibromarsine had very little value during the war. This was no doubt due chiefly to its high boiling point, low vapor pressure, and the relative ease with which it was decomposed in the field. However, definitive data as to the value of this compound are lacking, so that no definite conclusions can be drawn.

COMPARATIVE TOXICITIES OF LUNG INJURANTS

As the lung injurants are compounds of relatively low boiling points and high vapor pressures, their volatilities are well above their lethal concentrations, and therefore the casualty and fatality powers of these agents are in proportion to their minimum lethal concentrations. On this basis, the foregoing lung injurants are arranged in the descending order of their fatal concentrations as shown on page 169.

USE OF LUNG INJURANTS IN WORLD WAR

As a group, the lung injurants were used to a larger extent than any other type of gas and secured the bulk of the gas fatalities in the war.

169

Agent	Minimum Lethal Concentration on 10 Minutes' Exposure, Mg. per Liter
Phenyldibromarsine	0.200
Phenyldichlorarsine	0.260
Dibromethyl ether	0.400
Dichlormethyl ether	0.470
Ethyldichlorarsine	0.500
Phosgene	0.500
Trichlormethylchloroformate	0.500
Dimethylsulfate	0.500
Phenylcarbylamine chloride	0.500
Monochlormethylchloroformate	1.000
Ethylsulfuryl chloride	1.000
Methylsulfuryl chloride	2.000
Chlorpicrin	2.000
Perchlormethylmercaptan	3.000
Chlorine	5.600

Thus it is estimated that, altogether a total of 100,500 tons of these gases were used in battle during the late war and caused 876,853 casualties, or an average of one casualty per 230 lb. of gas. While the ratio of casualties to pounds of gas employed is much lower than in the case of the vesicant gases, it must be remembered that the latter, on account of high persistency, cannot be used on the tactical offensive, whereas the lung-injurant agents are generally nonpersistent and may be employed in any situation.

FUTURE OF LUNG INJURANTS

As the lung injurants were the principal nonpersistent casualty gases of the war and are the only casualty gases suitable for use in the tactical offense when friendly troops are required to occupy terrain within a few minutes after gassing, the lung-injurant agents will continue to play a major role in gas warfare of the future.

The *toxic* lung injurants were but little used during the late war, and their possibilities were not extensively explored. Their high toxicities, dual physiological effects, and other properties are very favorable to offensive chemical warfare, and this field is one from which new and more effective chemical agents may be expected to be drawn in the future.

For a summary of the properties of the principal lung-injurant agents, see Table IV.

170

CHAPTER VIII

SYSTEMIC TOXIC AGENTS

The systemic toxic agents are those compounds which, instead of confining their dominant action to some particular organ or part of the body, usually near the point of impact, have the power to penetrate the epithelial lining of the lungs without causing local damage. They then pass into the blood stream, whence they are diffused throughout the whole interior economy of the body and exercise a general systemic poisoning action which finally results in death from paralysis of the central nervous system. The systemic toxics were the third type of compounds to appear in the World War, the first member of the group being introduced July 1, 1916. The group is very small, consisting of the following compounds used in the war:

Agent	Introduced by	Date
Hydrocyanic acid	French	July 1, 1916
Cyanogen bromide	Austrians	September, 1916
Cyanogen chloride	French	October, 1916
(Phenylcarbylamine chloride)*	Germans	May, 1917

* Primarily a lung injurant.

The systemic toxics are nonpersistent and were used tactically in the same way and for the same purposes as the lung-injurant agents. Their appearance and use in the war was also concomitant in point of time with the lung injurants, and they may, therefore, be tactically regarded as supplementing the lung-injurant group rather than as a separate and distinct group of agents. On the other hand, their physiological effect is quite different from that of the lung injurants and, since our classification is based primarily on physiological effect, with the systemic toxics assigned as a separate subclass under the nonpersistent agents, it is logical to treat them as a separate group.

GROUP CHARACTERISTICS

Chemically, the systemic toxics are closely related. They are all derivatives of the compound cyanogen (C_2N_2) and are divided into two classes: (1) those containing the radical (—C≡N), called ***nitriles;*** and

171

(2) those containing the radical (—N≡C), called ***isonitriles*** or ***carbylamines.*** All are commonly known as *cyanides.*

Physically, the systemic toxics are all light liquids with relatively low boiling points, high vapor pressures, and high volatilities. They are the least persistent of all of the combat agents.

Physiologically, they are, in general:

1. Specialized in their action on the body for, while they pervade the entire circulatory system, they act primarily on the nerve centers and cause death by paralysis of the central nervous system.
2. Extremely quick acting when present in lethal concentrations. A few breaths are sufficient to cause death, which occurs within a few minutes.
3. Reversible in action below a certain critical concentration (about 0.030 mg. per liter), for below this concentration the body appears to have the power to neutralize and eliminate the poison. Hence with the systemic poisons, Haber's simple generalization, that the degree of intoxication equals the toxic concentration times the time of exposure, does not hold true, and an additional factor enters the equation. This is known as the elimination factor* and is specific for each compound, being the quantity which the body can constantly eliminate by reversing the toxic action. Below the critical concentration no lesions are formed by the poison in the body. Even after acute poisoning, few organic lesions are found, for above the critical concentration asphyxiation is so rapid that they do not have time to form.

* See p. 13.

4. Of relatively low threshold of action. Thus, hydrocyanic acid is effective down to the critical concentration of 0.030 mg. per liter.
5. Exceedingly toxic, a concentration of 0.012 mg. per liter of hydrocyanic acid being fatal in from 30 to 60 minutes.
6. Insidious in action, causing practically no premonitory symptoms until after serious poisoning has ensued.

Hydrocyanic Acid (HCN)

French: "Vincennite" and "Manganite"

For over a hundred years before the World War, hydrocyanic acid was known in industry as one of the most virulent of all poisons. During the latter part of 1915, in the race to produce more deadly chemical-warfare gases, it was inevitable that attention would be turned to this compound because of its high toxicity. The French were the first to consider it and were in fact its only exponent during the war. Since the practical difficulties encountered in its use in the field soon convinced the other belligerents that this gas was not suitable for war use, it was never used by them.

Dr. Hanslian, citing a French authority, says that as early as the end of 1915 the French had filled great quantities of gas shells with hydrocyanic acid (Special Shell 4) and phosgene (Special Shell 5), but hesitated to authorize their use at the front because of their high degree of toxicity and lack of splinter effect. In this connection, it will be recalled that the signatories to the Hague Conventions of 1899 [172] and 1907 had agreed not to use *shell*, the sole purpose of which was to diffuse asphyxiating gases, and had laid down the rule that a shell in which the toxic-gas effect was greater than the splinter effect came within the prohibited category. It is, however, difficult to understand the hesitancy of the French to make use of gas shells containing hydrocyanic acid and phosgene in view of their earlier use of gas shell filled with such compounds as ethylsulfuryl chloride and perchlormethylmercaptan, and the prior German use of gas shells filled with bromacetone. To be sure, these earlier compounds were sufficiently lacrimatory to be regarded as such, but they were also toxic enough to cause serious casualties and deaths in ordinary field concentrations and hence could not properly be excluded from the class of asphyxiating shell prohibited by the Hague Conventions.

Regardless of whatever scruples the French may have had against the use of hydrocyanic acid and phosgene shells, they commenced their use in 1916. The phosgene shells were first employed at the front at Verdun on Feb. 21, 1916, and the hydrocyanic acid (Vincennite) shells in the battle of the Somme, July 1, 1916. In view of the superior combat properties of phosgene, which antedated the introduction of hydrocyanic acid, it is not clear why the French ever decided to use the latter. Perhaps the only valid reason is to be found in the fact that the German masks of early 1916 afforded adequate protection against phosgene, but very little protection against hydrocyanic acid. Even this advantage, however, was short-lived for the Germans learned of the contemplated French use of hydrocyanic acid a week before its introduction at the front and soon equipped their troops with mask filters capable of holding back this gas. These filters contained 1 gram of pulverized silver oxide scattered through the potash layers and afforded adequate protection against hydrocyanic acid.

Hydrocyanic acid is derived by distilling a concentrated solution of potassium cyanide with dilute sulfuric acid and absorption of the vapors in water. The anhydrous form used in battle was obtained by subsequent fractional distillation from the aqueous solution. When pure, hydrocyanic acid is a colorless liquid, of 0.7 specific gravity, which boils at 26°C. (79°F.), yielding a light vapor, only 0.93 as heavy as air, with a faint odor resembling bitter almonds. The vapor is exceedingly volatile (873 mg. per liter at 20°C.) and persists in the open only a few minutes after release. In order to prevent the too rapid diffusion of its vapors in the air, hydrocyanic acid was not used in pure form but was mixed with stannic chloride, with the addition of chloroform as a stabilizer to counteract a tendency to polymerize. This mixture was known as "Vincennite," and was used on a large scale in artillery shell by the French. Later, hydrocyanic acid was also mixed with arsenic trichloride, [173] and known as "Manganite." Hydrocyanic acid is miscible with water in all proportions, but is slowly decomposed thereby with the formation of ammonium cyanide. Anhydrous hydrocyanic acid is extremely unstable and is quickly decomposed with the formation of a black resinous mass. However, it can be stabilized by the addition of small percentages of strong acids and by dissolving it in arsenic trichloride or stannic chloride.

According to Hederer and Istin, the toxic action of hydrocyanic acid is typical of the protoplasmic poisons. It suspends certain functions of the living cells, notably oxidation. By inhibiting the action of the respiratory ferments, it brings about a true internal asphyxiation. Under its influence, the tissues become incapable of utilizing the oxygen of the blood and an analysis of the venous blood shows that in oxygen and carbonic acid contents it is very close to the arterial blood. With the higher animals and above all with man, it strikes the central nervous system. After a short period of excitation, the pneumogastric nerve centers, as well as the vasomotor and respiratory centers, are paralyzed. Then the poison, following its general action, gradually arrests cytoplasmic oxidation, and all the tissues suffer from an acute lack of oxygen. But, as the nerve cells are more sensitive than the others, they pay first tribute to the increasing asphyxiation. Their functional death is then shown by noisy symptoms which dominate the scene and mask the divers accompanying troubles.

Hydrocyanic acid is one of the most virulent poisons known. When injected under the skin 0.05 gram is lethal and Vedder (25, page 186) says: "The lethal dose by respiration is usually believed to be less than the above and our figures confirm this view."

However, unlike most toxics, the poisoning effect of hydrocyanic acid is not cumulative, so that Haber's simple generalization does not apply. On the contrary, the body seems to be able to neutralize the effects of this gas up to a critical concentration of about 0.030 mg. per liter. Below this level, the poison is eliminated from the body as rapidly as it is absorbed and no serious toxic effects are produced. Above the critical concentration, however, there is a very rapid poisoning effect and death ensues in a few minutes when the concentration reaches 0.300 mg. per liter. The lethal concentration for 10 minutes' exposure is 0.200 mg. per liter and for 30 minutes' exposure, 0.150 mg. per liter.

Because of its extreme volatility and the fact that its vapors are lighter than air, it is almost impossible to establish a lethal concentration of hydrocyanic acid in the field, and this is particularly true when the gas is put over in artillery shells. This difficulty, coupled with the peculiar action of hydrocyanic acid wherein it produces no casualties until a lethal concentration is established, made the use of this gas in artillery [174] shell a tragic mistake on the part of the French. Despite the vociferous controversies among the Allies as to the effectiveness of hydrocyanic acid on the field of battle, the evidence from all sources is now convincing that extremely few casualties were caused by the French artillery shell containing hydrocyanic acid, although the French used over 4,000 tons of this gas in the war.

Cyanogen Bromide (CNBr)

Austrians: "Ce"; British: "CB"; Italian: "Campillit"

The Austrians introduced cyanogen bromide in September, 1916, shortly after the French brought out hydrocyanic acid. Cyanogen bromide was first employed in a mixture with bromacetone and benzene (25 per cent CNBr to 25 per cent CH_3COCH_2Br and 50 per cent C_6H_6). Later, as a result of poor storing qualities and a resulting decrease in toxic effect, cyanogen bromide and bromacetone were loaded separately into shells. Cyanogen bromide was also used on the Western Front by the British (CB shell).

Cyanogen bromide is made by treating a concentrated solution of potassium cyanide with bromine at 0°C. When freshly sublimed, it is a white crystalline solid, of 2.02 specific gravity, which melts at 52°C. (125.6°F.), and boils at 61.3°C. (142°F.), yielding a vapor 3.4 times heavier than air with a piquant odor and bitter taste. It is soluble in alcohol and in water, but hydrolizes in the latter, yielding a nontoxic hydrate. At 20°C. (68°F.) its vapor pressure is 92.00 mm. Hg and its volatility is 200.00 mg. per liter. Thus, as compared to nonpersistent gases, generally it is highly volatile, yet it is only about one-fourth as volatile as hydrocyanic acid.

The effect of cyanogen bromide on the body is similar to that of hydrocyanic acid. It is, however, less toxic, but has, in addition, a lacrimatory and strong irritant effect. A concentration as low as 0.006 mg. per liter greatly irritates the conjunctiva and the mucous membranes of the respiratory system, while 0.035 mg. per liter is unbearable. Its lethal concentration for 10 minutes' exposure is 0.400 mg. per liter, which makes it somewhat more toxic than phosgene, but only about one-third as toxic as hydrocyanic acid. Moreover, it corrodes metals and suffers decomposition thereby; it also is unstable in storage and gradually polymerizes into a physiologically inert substance. In view of the above, cyanogen bromide is rather unsuitable for use as a chemical agent and the success obtained from its employment in the World War was so slight that the Austrians abandoned it in favor of the German Green Cross (diphosgene) ammunition. [175]

Cyanogen Chloride (CNCl)

French: "Mauguinite" and "Vitrite"

Almost at the same time that the Austrians introduced cyanogen bromide, the French brought out cyanogen chloride, in an attempt to secure a systemic toxic gas that did not have the disadvantages of hydrocyanic acid, *i.e.*, a heavier and less volatile gas with cumulative toxic effects in low concentrations.

Like its bromine analogue, cyanogen chloride is produced by the direct chlorination of a saturation solution of potassium cyanide at 0°C. It is a colorless liquid, of 1.22 specific gravity, which boils at 15°C. (59°F.), yielding a volatile irritant vapor 1.98 times heavier than air. At 20°C. (68°F.) the vapor pressure of cyanogen chloride is 1,000 mm. Hg and its volatility is 3,300 mg. per liter, so that it is more volatile than hydrocyanic acid.

Although cyanogen chloride is but slightly soluble in water, it dissolves readily in the organic solvents. It is chemically unstable and on storage polymerizes into cyanogen trichloride $(CNCl)_3$, which is physiologically far less active. When mixed with arsenic trichloride, which increases the density of its vapors, cyanogen chloride is far more stable, and for that reason it was used in this mixture by the French under the name of "Vitrite."

The toxic action of cyanogen chloride is similar to that of hydrocyanic acid, but it is much more effective in low concentrations on prolonged exposure. Like hydrocyanic acid, in high concentrations it kills by rapid paralysis of the nerve centers, especially those controlling the respiratory system, but, unlike hydrocyanic acid, in low concentrations (0.010 to 0.050 mg. per liter) it is also irritant to the eyes and lungs and has a retarded toxic effect somewhat resembling that of the lung-injurant compounds. Its lethal concentration for 10 minutes' exposure is 0.40 mg. per liter the same as that of cyanogen bromide. Cyanogen chloride is also a moderate lacrimator, 0.0025 mg. per liter producing copious lacrimation in a few minutes.

Phenylcarbylamine Chloride ($C_6H_5CNCl_2$)

This compound has already been considered under the lung-injurant group, as its predominant action is against the pulmonary system. It does, however, have a subsidiary effect resembling that of the systemic toxics, which is attributable to the fact that it is chemically an isonitrile and, therefore, belongs to the family of cyanides. Its systemic toxic effect is not important and it is mentioned here in order to complete its classification.

176

FUTURE OF SYSTEMIC TOXICS

The systemic toxics are as a class the most virulent poisons known. They are, however, extremely volatile and their vapors are very light and diffuse into the atmosphere with extraordinary rapidity. They are also practically noneffective until a certain critical concentration is reached and then they strike with great speed and vigor. Hence, in order to use them effectively in the field, it is necessary to establish the concentration with a high density in a minimum of time and under favorable meteorological conditions, so that the enemy will receive a lethal dose in a few breaths before the concentration falls below its critical effective strength. Because of these requirements concerning its use, the systemic toxics are neither economical nor certain of results on the field of battle. At the same time, their toxicities and rapid actions make them very effective against small well-defined targets, especially where men are sheltered in dugouts, deep trenches, woods, etc., where high concentrations may be established and maintained for several minutes.

177

CHAPTER IX

VESICANT AGENTS

By the term *vesicant agents* we denote those compounds which vesicate (blister) the human and animal body on any surface, either exterior or interior, with which they come in contact. This type of compound constitutes the fourth class of combat gases used in the World War. Most of them are highly toxic substances and nearly all produce multiple physiological effects. Thus, some are fairly lacrimatory, others exert marked lung-injurant effects, while still others are systemic poisons. However, in all compounds classed as *vesicants*, the vesicant effect is so much more pronounced than their other effects as to constitute their dominant characteristic. Where the vesicant effect of a compound is subordinate to its other physiological effects, the compound is classified in some other class, *e.g.*, ethyldichlorarsine is somewhat vesicant, but its primary physiological action is on the pulmonary system of the body, and it is, therefore, considered a lung-injurant agent (see Chap. VII).

At the outbreak of the World War, over 70 vesicant compounds were known to science, yet only five were identified with the war. Of these, but two—dichlorethyl sulfide (mustard gas) and ethyldichlorarsine—were actually used, while the other three—chlorovinyldichlorarsine (lewisite), methyldichlorarsine, and dibromethyl sulfide—were in process of investigation or manufacture at the end of the war and were not actually used in battle. Of the first two, ethyldichlorarsine was primarily a lung injurant and was used only to a limited extent as a vesicant agent. While it proved to be quite effective, it did not play a very important role in the war. On the other hand, mustard gas was widely used by both sides and proved to be so effective that it became the principal battle gas of the last year of the war. In fact, so completely did mustard gas dominate the field of vesicant agents that the story of mustard is practically the story of vesicants in the World War.

GROUP CHARACTERISTICS

While the vesicant agents, in addition to vesication, exert divers complex physiological effects, their physical, chemical, and toxic properties are such that they form a well-defined group with many characteristics in common, and for this reason they were grouped by the Germans under the general name of "Yellow Cross" substances.

Thus, the vesicants, although very soluble in the substance of animal tissues, have weaker chemical affinities for living matter than the lung-

178

injurant agents. They, therefore, disintegrate more slowly and penetrate further into the tissues of the body, thus greatly enlarging their field of action.

Vesicants, in general, are:

1. Nonspecialized in their action on the body, as they destroy the cellular structure of the tissues wherever they come in contact with them.
2. Slow acting, in producing physiological effects on the body. Thus, their toxic effects do not commence to manifest themselves until from 6 to 24 hours after exposure. They are seldom fatal (less than 2 per cent deaths).
3. Nonreversible in action, for their injury to the cellular structure of the tissues is permanent. The lesions produced heal in time, depending upon the depth of penetration of the vesicant agent, but the reaction upon the original cells is irreversible.
4. Low in threshold of action. Thus, mustard gas produces definite incapacitating effects in concentrations as low as 1:100,000 (0.0065 mg. per liter) with 60 minutes' exposure, and on longer exposure equal results are obtained with proportionately lower concentrations.
5. High in boiling point.
6. Low in vapor pressure and volatility.
7. High in persistency.
8. Insidious in action, giving little or no warning of their presence until injury is sustained.

CLASSIFICATION OF VESICANTS

The vesicants may be divided into two classes: (1) simple vesicants which exert a local action only; and (2) toxic vesicants which, in addition to local action, also exert a systemic poisoning effect. The distinction is not of great practical importance since all the simple vesicants of which there is any record of use in the war exert their vesicant effect in a subordinate manner only. That is to say, the known simple vesicants are predominantly compounds of other classes. Thus, dimethyl sulfate, the only simple vesicant used in battle during the war, is a much more powerful lung injurant than a vesicant agent, and for that reason it is generally regarded as a lung-injurant compound (see Chap. VII). On the other hand, mustard gas and the postwar vesicants are all of the toxic variety, so that from a practical-use viewpoint, we may regard the vesicant agents generally as toxic compounds. We do not mean to say, however, that this will always be the case, for it is entirely possible that some new compound will be discovered, the vesicant action of which is simple yet so predominant as clearly to entitle the compound to be classed as a simple vesicant agent.

Dichlorethyl Sulfide ($S(CH_2CH_2)_2Cl_2$)

German: "Lost"; French: "Yperite"; British and American: "Mustard Gas"

The introduction of mustard gas by the Germans on the night of July 12, 1917, in the form of an artillery bombardment against the

179

British front near Ypres in Flanders, marked the beginning of a new phase of gas warfare. It came as a complete surprise to the Allies and caused thousands of casualties before any form of defense could be devised against it. Its tremendous effectiveness perfectly illustrates the ever-threatening potential power of chemical warfare.

During 1916 and the first half of 1917, the principal battle gases used were of the lung-injurant type, and these were based on the principle of attacking the respiratory organs, for which purpose they must necessarily be inhaled. But by the summer of 1917 the gas mask had been so improved that it furnished full protection against all the known lung-injurant gases, so that the only casualties produced by these gases were those where men were caught by surprise and were gassed before they could adjust their masks. In other words, gas defense had caught up with the offense. To break this deadlock, one of two things was necessary—either to find a lung-injurant type of gas that would penetrate the mask or to discover an entirely new type of gas that would go around the mask and incapacitate by attacking some other part of the body. The German chemists solved both of these problems simultaneously by bringing out diphenylchlorarsine (Blue Cross), which, when properly dispersed, would penetrate any of the masks as they were constructed in 1917, (see Chap. X), and mustard gas, which would go through clothing and even rubber and leather boots and produce incapacitating burns on any part of the body with which its vapors came in contact. In addition to its vesicant properties, mustard gas was exceedingly toxic, so that it also caused serious casualties when breathed, even in very minute concentrations. It was, therefore, an almost perfect battle gas, particularly in view of the total absence of any means of protecting the body against it, even though the mask furnished adequate protection for the lungs. There is small wonder, therefore, that mustard gas was soon recognized as the "king of battle gases," and maintained this superior position throughout the remainder of the war.

The gas shells used in bombardment at Ypres on the 12th and 13th of July, 1917, were of 77- and 105-mm. caliber and were marked on the base or side with a yellow cross. The vapors arising from these bursting shells had no immediate irritating action on the eyes or chest, and so at first the troops in the bombardment suffered no discomfort from the gas, except irritation of the nose which caused sneezing. In the course of an hour or two, however, the signs of mustard poisoning began to appear in the form of inflammation of the eyes and vomiting, followed by erythema of the skin and blistering. The conjunctivitis was marked and, by the time the gassed cases reached the casualty clearing stations, the men were virtually blind and had to be led about.

The Ypres area was shelled with mustard gas each night beginning July 12, 1917, until the end of the month. On the nights of the July 21

180

and 22 a particularly heavy bombardment with Yellow Cross shells was directed on Nieuport, which resulted in a heavy toll of casualties of a more serious character than the casualties from the first mustard-gas bombardment at Ypres.

Armentières was shelled with mustard gas on the night of July 20–21, 1917, and on the night of July 28–29 a heavy Yellow Cross bombardment was directed on both Armentières and Nieuport. From then on, Yellow Cross shells were used by the Germans extensively. It was not until July, 1918, that mustard-gas shelling of this type showed any marked diminution, and this was undoubtedly caused by a shortage of Yellow Cross shells.

During the first three weeks of the mustard-gas period (July 12 to Aug. 1, 1917) 14,276 cases of gas-shell poisoning were admitted to the British casualty clearing stations and about 500 deaths occurred among these cases. In this brief period, therefore, the Yellow Cross shelling had accounted for more casualties and practically as many deaths as the entire previous shelling with lung injurants. The total gas-shell casualties admitted to British clearing stations from July 21, 1917, to Nov. 23, 1918, were 160,970, of which number 1,859 died. Seventy-seven per cent of these casualties were due to mustard-gas poisoning, 10 per cent were due to Blue Cross (dichlorethylarsine) gas poisoning, and 10 per cent to Green Cross gas poisoning (phosgene, diphosgene, chlorpicrin).

Concerning the important role played by mustard gas in the war, Dr. Mueller says:

> The German Front would never have succeeded in withstanding the powerful onslaught of the concentrated forces and war materials of almost the whole world if German chemists had not at that moment held the protecting shield of the "Yellow Cross Substance" (mustard gas) before the German soldiers and at the same time thrust into their hands a new sharp sword in the form of the "Blue Cross Substance."

Altogether about 12,000 tons of mustard gas were used in the war and this caused a total of 400,000 casualties, from which it is seen that one casualty was produced for every 60 lb. of mustard used, as compared to one casualty for every 230 lb. of lung injurants used in the war.

Like the other World War gases, mustard was not a new or unknown compound. On the contrary, it was discovered sixty years before the outbreak of the war, and its chemical and physiological properties had been studied and were known to science for many years. Mustard gas was first obtained (in an impure form) by Richie in 1854 (15, page 235). In 1860 it was independently prepared by Guthrie and Niemann by passing ethylene into sulfur chloride; both of these chemists accurately and almost prophetically describing its high toxic and vesicant properties. Thus Guthrie says: "Even the vapors of this substance when in contact with the more delicate parts of the skin of

181

the body cause the most serious destruction." In 1886 the German chemist, Victor Meyer, prepared mustard gas by the action of hydrochloric acid on thiodiglycol and described the terrible effects of the product. Finally, in 1891 the opthalmologist, Theodore Leber, made a summary study of the toxicity of mustard gas.

In searching for a more effective combat gas, therefore, the Germans had available many data in the literature concerning mustard and had only to make it in quantity production and test it in the field. This they did quite secretly in the spring of 1917 and were so well satisfied with the results obtained that they adopted it as an artillery-shell filling and accumulated a large quantity of these (Yellow Cross) shell before the Allies were aware of this development.

In its pure state, dichlorethyl sulfide is a transparent amber oily liquid, of 1.27 specific gravity, which boils with slight decomposition at 217°C. (422.6°F.), yielding a vapor 5.5 times heavier than air. It is almost odorless in ordinary field concentrations and in strong concentrations resembles horse-radish or mustard. Hence the origin of the English name—"mustard gas"—although this substance has no relation chemically to the true mustard oils. It solidifies at 14°C. (57°F.) to form white crystals, and for this reason was used by the Germans diluted with a solvent to lower its freezing point and maintain it in a uniform (liquid) state under all ordinary temperatures.

The vapor pressure and volatility of mustard gas are low, as shown by the following tabulation:

Temperature		Vapor pressure, mm. Hg	Volatility, mg. per liter
°C.	°F.		
0	32	0.0260	0.250
5	41	0.0300	0.278
10	50	0.0350	0.315
15	59	0.0417	0.401
20	68	0.0650	0.625
25	77	0.0996	0.958
30	86	0.1500	1.443
35	95	0.2220	2.135
40	104	0.4500	3.660

Because of its low volatility, mustard gas is very persistent in the field, varying from one day in the open and one week in the woods in summer to several weeks both in the open and in the woods in winter. Its great persistency is the principal limitation on its use, as it cannot be used on the tactical offensive where friendly troops have to traverse or

182

occupy the infected ground. However, by the same token, mustard is peculiarly adapted for use in the tactical defensive, particularly to prevent the occupation by hostile troops of ground evacuated on a withdrawal.

Dichlorethyl sulfide (mustard gas) was made by two radically different processes during the war. The Germans used the more complicated process of Victor Meyer because they had already available facilities for manufacturing the principal components and had only to erect facilities for the final step in the process. The German process was briefly as follows:

1. Ethylene chlorhydrin was converted into thiodiglycol by sodium sulfide according to the equation

$$2(ClCH_2CH_2(OH)) + Na_2S = S\begin{cases}CH_2CH_2(OH)\\CH_2CH_2(OH)\end{cases} + 2NaCl$$

2. The thiodiglycol was chlorinated by treatment with gaseous hydrochloric acid, according to the equation

$$S\begin{cases}CH_2CH_2(OH)\\CH_2CH_2(OH)\end{cases} + 2HCl = S\begin{cases}CH_2CH_2Cl\\CH_2CH_2Cl\end{cases} + 2H_2O$$

The German process had two outstanding advantages, *viz.:* (1) the intermediate products possessed no dangerous properties, and hence there was no danger to personnel working in the plants on any of the intermediate steps. The only danger involved in the whole process was in the last step of chlorinating the thiodiglycol to form mustard gas. This was a relatively simple reaction that was easy to control, and hence the danger to personnel was far less than in many of the steps of the other process. (2) The yield was high and the product pure, since the only other end product was water, which was easily separated by distillation.

On the other hand, the German method had the formidable objection of being a very complicated process, particularly in the method of making the chlorhydrin. To make this intermediate, three steps requiring careful control were necessary: (1) alcohol was split into ethylene by passing its vapors over aluminum oxide at 300°C.; (2) the ethylene gas was pumped into large reactors containing chloride of lime paste which was carefully cooled during the process; (3) the resulting ethylene chlorhydrin was forced out of the lime paste by steam.

While the foregoing steps in the German process of making mustard gas seem simple, in reality they were very difficult and only a chemical technique excellently organized and backed by a wealth of experience could successfully cope with the technical difficulties encountered.

Lacking the facilities and experience in making the intermediates required in the German process, the Allies turned to the older process of

183

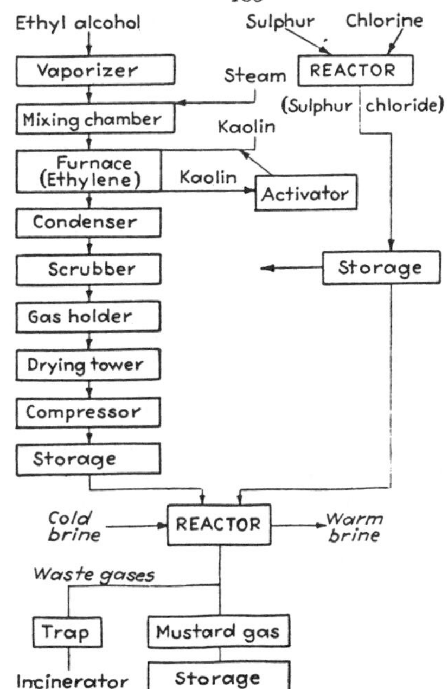

CHART XII.—Manufacture of mustard gas. Levenstein process (flow sheet).

Guthrie and Niemann, in which dichlorethyl sulfide is formed by the direct action of ethylene gas on sulfur monochloride (see Chart XII), according to the equation:

$$2C_2H_4 + S_2Cl_2 = S\begin{cases}CH_2CH_2Cl\\CH_2CH_2Cl\end{cases} + S$$

While this reaction under proper conditions proceeds smoothly, there are actually encountered in quantity-production operations several very formidable difficulties. Thus, the reaction occurs spontaneously with the evolution of much heat. Sulfur is set free, and the temperature must be carefully controlled in order to keep the sulfur in colloidal suspension and thus prevent its precipitation in solid form in the reaction vessels and connecting pipes. There is also considerable difficulty in separating the mustard gas from the colloidal sulfur, so that the resulting

184

product was not so pure as that from the German process, although it seemed to be equally as effective in the field.

It is difficult to emphasize sufficiently the extreme danger that is involved in working with mustard gas even under the best of conditions. The workmen must be equipped with masks and the most efficient protective clothing, and everything coming in contact with even the vapors of mustard gas must be decontaminated at once with chloride of lime or other neutralizing agents. Notwithstanding all these precautions, casualties will occur owing to carelessness, and only the most rigid discipline can keep them within reasonable bounds.

While mustard gas is only slightly soluble in water, it is slowly decomposed thereby. When it is cold, the rate of decomposition is approximately 1 gram of mustard per liter of water in 30 minutes. When it is warm, the decomposition proceeds more rapidly with saponification and the formation of thiodiglycol and hydrochloric acid, according to the reaction:

$$S\begin{cases}CH_2CH_2Cl\\CH_2CH_2Cl\end{cases} + 2H_2O = S\begin{cases}CH_2CH_2(OH)\\CH_2CH_2(OH)\end{cases} + 2HCl$$

This hydrolysis takes place on contact with moisture in the air or with water on the ground and thus mustard gas is slowly destroyed wherever these conditions are encountered; the rate of destruction depends upon the amount of water and the temperature. The hydrolysis of mustard gas is also accelerated in the presence of alkalies, alkaline carbonates, and the solvents of mustard that are miscible with water, such as alcohol. It is rapidly dissolved by the organic solvents, such as ether, chloroform, and acetone, by the light paraffin hydrocarbons, and by all of the organic fats, both animal and vegetable. It is, however, soluble only with difficulty in the mineral oils and in vaseline and paraffin.

Mustard gas is also progressively soluble in gums, such as caoutchouc and rubber; it easily goes through leather and fabrics of cotton and linen. Hence mustard readily penetrates leather and rubber boots and gloves and all articles of clothing, especially if these are brought in direct contact with liquid mustard. It is because of these remarkable powers of solubility and penetration that mustard gas is so difficult to protect against. In fact, the only reliable protection is the destruction of the mustard-gas molecule by decomposing it into its relatively harmless constituents.

In striking contrast to its marked physical activity in solution and penetration, the chemical activity of mustard gas is rather limited, *e.g.*, its slow hydrolysis in contact with water. Its great chemical stability increases the difficulty of decontaminating infected materials with hypochlorites. However, mustard reacts violently with the evolution

185

of great heat, the resulting products being mustard sulfoxide and calcium chloride, in accordance with the equation:

$$CaOCl_2 + S\begin{cases}CH_2CH_2Cl\\CH_2CH_2Cl\end{cases} = SO\begin{cases}CH_2CH_2Cl\\CH_2CH_2Cl\end{cases} + CaCl_2$$

As the sulfoxide is nontoxic, calcium chloride has been widely used to destroy mustard. On the other hand, when very strong oxidizing agents are used, two atoms of oxygen are fixed to the sulfur atom and the resulting product, called *mustard sulfone*, is very toxic. This curious phenomenon adds further difficulties to the problem of decontaminating material infected with mustard.

Chlorine also attacks mustard vigorously and converts it into harmless higher chlorides, according to the equation:

$$Cl_2 + S\begin{matrix} CH_2CH_2Cl \\ CH_2CH_2Cl \end{matrix} = S\begin{matrix} CH_2ClCHCl \\ CH_2ClCHCl \end{matrix}$$

The danger of dissociating mustard into toxic products is, therefore, avoided by the use of chlorine or chlorinating agents, such as dichloramine T and sulfur dichloride.

Mustard gas is lethal in concentrations varying from 0.006 to 0.200 mg. per liter, depending upon the time of exposure. Generally speaking, when inhaled, 0.15 mg. per liter is fatal on 10 minutes' exposure and 0.07 mg. per liter on 30 minutes' exposure. Concentrations as low as 0.001 mg. per liter on 1 hour's exposure, will attack the eyes and render the victim a casualty from conjunctivitis. Mustard is thus five times more toxic than phosgene, which adds greatly to its effectiveness as a combat agent.

Concerning the complex physiological action of mustard gas, we cannot do better than to quote General Gilchrist as follows:

> Mustard is classified as a vesicant gas. . . . At first it acts as a cell irritant, and finally as a cell poison. The first symptoms of mustard-gas poisoning appear in from 4 to 6 hours, but a latent period up to 24 hours may occur. The length of this latent period depends upon the concentration of the gas. The higher the concentration the shorter the interval of time between the exposure to the gas and the first symptoms arising as a result of mustard-gas poisoning.
>
> The physiological action of mustard gas may be classified as local and general. The local action results in conjunctivitis or inflammation of the eyes; erythema of the skin, which may be followed by blistering or ulceration and inflammatory reaction of the nose, throat, trachea, and bronchi. . . .
>
> It is of interest that racial susceptibility to the toxic action of mustard gas exists; whites are more susceptible than negroes. There is also an individual susceptibility to the toxic action of mustard gas, particularly of the skin, and also of the respiratory tract.

186

A great deal of time has been devoted to a study of the mechanism of action of vesicants in general and mustard gas in particular, and a number of theories have been propounded to explain the toxic action of mustard on the living organism. Space does not permit a detailed account of these theories here. Suffice it to say that the simplest and most generally accepted theory is that the toxic effects of mustard are caused by the protoplasmic hydrolysis of the dichlorethyl sulfide molecule and the liberation of free hydrochloric acid in the living cell. Concerning this theory Vedder says:

> Dichlorethyl sulphide is very slightly soluble in water and freely soluble in organic solvents, that is, has a high liquid solubility or partition coefficient. It would, therefore, be expected to penetrate cells very rapidly. Its rapid powers of penetration are practically proved by its effects upon the skin. Having penetrated within the living cell, hydrolysis might occur. The liberation of free hydrochloric acid within the cell would produce serious effects and might account for the actions of dichlorethyl sulphide. The mechanism of the action of dichlorethyl sulphide according to this theory appears to be as follows:
>
> *a.* Rapid penetration of the substance into the cell by virtue of its high lipoid solubility.
>
> *b.* Hydrolysis by the water within the cell, to form hydrochloric acid and dihydroxyethyl sulphide.
>
> *c.* The destructive effects of hydrochloric acid upon some part of the mechanism of the cell.
>
> This theory is very simple, and has been very generally accepted.
>
> Whatever the theory of action, mustard is a cell poison, exerting its necrotizing action on all cells with which it comes directly in contact, including the skin and mucous membranes, with all their structures. The capillaries and other organs that mustard reaches become paralyzed.
>
> It is well known that the injuries produced by mustard heal much more slowly than burns of similar intensity produced by physical or other chemical agencies. This characteristic is explained by this action of mustard on the blood vessels which are rendered incapable of carrying out their functions of repair; and by the fact that necrotic tissue acts as a good culture medium. Hence the great liability to infection of mustard burns.

One of the greatest dangers from mustard gas is the lack of any positive means of identifying it in low concentrations in the field. While it has a characteristic odor resembling mustard or horse-radish in strong concentrations, this odor is very faint in concentrations which are still dangerous on exposures of more than 1 hour. Thus, the odor is said to be detectable at 0.0013 mg. per liter, but a concentration of 0.0010 mg. per liter will cause casualties from conjunctivitis on 1 hour's exposure, and such a concentration cannot be detected even by the keenest perception. Moreover, the sense of smell for mustard gas is quickly dulled after initial exposure, so that much stronger concentrations go unnoticed.

187

Also, many odors, such as those produced by the stronger lacrimators, mask the odor of mustard gas so that it became a common practice to use lacrimators with mustard for this purpose.

The impossibility of detecting mustard gas in the field and the insidious action of this gas, which causes no noticeable symptoms until several hours after exposure, resulted in thousands of casualties in the war which might have been prevented had there been any positive means of detecting mustard and warning troops of its presence. The great importance of this problem caused much effort to be expended in attempts to devise a reliable chemical detector which was practicable for use at the front, but these efforts proved fruitless and the problem still remains unsolved.

Since mustard freezes at 14°C. (57°F.), it is desirable to add to it a small percentage of solvent to keep it in a liquid state at all temperatures ordinarily encountered in the field. If a solvent is not used and the mustard-gas filling in artillery shell changes from a liquid to a solid, with change in temperature, the ballistic behavior of the shells is seriously affected. For this reason, both the Germans and French added from 10 to 25 per cent of some easily volatile solvent such as carbon tetrachloride, chlorbenzene, or nitrobenzene. The Americans found that chlorpicrin could also be used as a solvent with equally satisfactory results and with the additional advantage that the solvent was toxic.

Not only does the addition of a solvent facilitate the ballistic behavior of mustard-gas shells, but it also increases the volatility of the mustard charge in winter weather and renders it more effective on the terrain. Depending upon the solvent used and the force of explosion of the bursting charge in the shell, the mustard-gas solution is scattered in the form of gas clouds, or a finely divided spray composed of liquid particles varying in size from an atomized mist to droplets resembling fine rain. These liquid particles are very stable against humidity and cling firmly to the ground and vegetation. The clouds of mustard vapor formed by the explosion of shells are not at all visible in dry weather and only slightly visible in damp weather. They are effective for about 6 hours on open terrain and for 12 to 24 hours in places protected by vegetation from the wind and sun.

The mustard-gas drops penetrate with great speed and facility any objects with which they come in contact. They easily penetrate leather and rubber boots, uniforms, and other articles of equipment worn by soldiers. The mustard liquid is thus easily carried about by soldiers and spread and evaporated in other previously uninfected places. Frequently in the late war all the occupants of a dugout were contaminated and made ill by the mustard adhering to the clothing of a single soldier who was not even aware of its presence.

188

Not only is mustard gas spread over the battlefield and surrounding areas by the transfer of droplets and the carrying of the liquid substance in clothing, etc., but also by the wind blowing across infected areas and saturating the air more or less with the evaporating mustard fumes. Practical field tests have shown that winds not exceeding 12 miles per hour, blowing over a normally saturated terrain, may transfer concentrations of mustard vapor sufficiently strong (0.070 mg. per liter) to cause death within 30 minutes, for from 500 to 1,000 yd. downwind. Consequently, every mustard-gas bombardment has a direct or immediate effect produced by the liquid spray and the resulting gaseous cloud. as well as an indirect or continued effect produced by the evaporation of the liquid substance from the infected area. The latter may be transferred by the wind in effective concentrations to a distance of from 500 to 1,000 yd. downwind or by men who come in contact with the liquid droplets scattered over the infected area and carry them to other places on clothing and other material.

With its far-reaching diffusion over the battlefields, its insidious action, and its manifold physiological effects, it is no wonder that mustard gas became the "king of battle gases" and, pound for pound, produced nearly eight times the number of casualties produced by all the other battle gases combined.

Compared with the properties of the ideal battle gas, as set forth in pages 47 and 48 of Chap. II, mustard gas meets the following requirements:

1. Very high toxicity (0.15 mg. per liter is fatal in 10 minutes).
2. Extreme multiple effectiveness.
3. Very persistent, which greatly limits its use in the tactical offensive but increases its value on the defensive.
4. Effects of long duration, but not permanent.
5. Effect is delayed for from 6 to 24 hours, which reduces its offensive battle power.
6. Extremely insidious in action. No warning properties or symptoms.
7. Volatility is low. The maximum field concentration is 3.66 mg. per liter on a hot day. This is sufficient for from 10 to 50 times a fatal dose.
8. Extremely penetrative to all forms of organic matter.
9. Vapor is invisible in dry weather and only faintly visible in damp weather.
10. Practically odorless in ordinary field concentrations.
11. Ready availability of raw materials (alcohol, sulfur, and chlorine).
12. Difficult to manufacture, but process is now well worked out in all principal countries.
13. Chemical stability is very high.
14. Hydrolyzes only very slowly at ordinary temperatures.
15. Withstands explosion without decomposition.
16. Not a solid at temperatures above 57°F.
17. Melting point is not above maximum atmospheric temperatures. Hence, use of solvent is advisable.
18. Boiling point, 217°C. (422.6°F.) is very high.

189

19. Vapor pressure is low but sufficient to establish lethal concentrations at ordinary temperatures.
20. Specific gravity (1.27) is below 1.50.
21. Vapor density is 5.5 times that of air.

From the foregoing summary, it may be seen how close mustard gas approaches the ideal battle gas in most of the important requirements. For this reason and the fact that it is extraordinarily difficult to protect against, mustard gas is assured of a secure position in the future, and it is safe to predict that mustard gas will play a dominant role in future chemical warfare until replaced by a more effective agent which has not as yet made its appearance.

Ethyldichlorarsine ($C_2H_5AsCl_2$)

German: "Dick"

Ethyldichlorarsine is a difficult gas to classify according to physiological action as its effects fall in three different classes. It acts as a lung-injurant agent with a toxicity about the same as that of phosgene; it is also a powerful sternutator with about one-fifth the irritant effect of diphenylchlorarsine; and, finally, it is a moderately powerful vesicant, with about two-thirds the skin-irritant power and one-sixth the vesicant power of mustard gas. However, since its casualty power is chiefly by reason of its lung-injurant effect, it is logical to regard this compound as primarily a lung-injurant agent with secondary sternutatory and vesicant effects, and it is accordingly grouped with the lung injurants in Chap. VII. Ethyldichlorarsine is again referred to here, not only because it is fairly vesicant, but also because its origin and early history are associated with the vesicant agents.

The experience of the Germans with the use of mustard gas during the latter half of 1917 showed that a vesicant type of gas was the most effective casualty producer yet devised but, on account of the great persistency of mustard gas, it could not be used on the tactical offensive, where the infected ground had to be immediately traversed or occupied by friendly troops, without prohibitive losses. Mustard also had the further disadvantage that its effects were delayed several hours and therefore it did not immediately incapacitate men so as to make it of any great assistance in local attacks. Having in mind the grand offensive planned for the spring of 1918, Germany called upon her chemists to produce a quick-acting nonpersistent vesicant agent that could be used to better advantage in offensive tactical operations. Ethyldichlorarsine was the answer to this demand and was introduced by the Germans in March, 1918, at the beginning of their great spring offensive on the Western Front.

190

To distinguish it from mustard gas, ethyldichlorarsine was first called "Yellow Cross 1," and it was intended to be used as a typical offensive combat agent along with the "Green Cross" (phosgene type) shells. Somewhat later it was found that the effects of ethyldichlorarsine were not primarily vesicant, but rather lung-injurant, and the vast majority of the casualties produced were from the latter effect. Accordingly, the classification designation of this gas was changed from "Yellow Cross 1" to "Green Cross 3," and it was used as a lung-injurant type of gas during the remainder of the war.

For further information concerning ethyldichlorarsine, see pages 166 *et seq.*

Chlorvinyldichlorarsine ($CHClCHAsCl_2$)

American: "Lewisite"

Chlorvinyldichlorarsine is America's principal contribution to the *materia chemica* of the World War. It was first prepared in 1917 by Dr. W. Lee Lewis (from whom it takes its name), in an effort to create a compound that would combine the vesicant action of mustard gas with the systemic poisoning effect of arsenic. Lewisite is a typical example of the evolution of chemical agents. It will be recalled that in the summer of 1917 the Germans had introduced two radically different types of agents: (1) a vesicant gas (mustard), which penetrated the clothing and burned the body wherever it came in contact and thus produced casualties without having to penetrate the mask; (2) a sternutatory gas (diphenylchlorarsine), which contained arsenic and, when properly dispersed, easily penetrated all existing masks.

Mustard gas was tremendously effective as a casualty producer but had two serious defects from a tactical viewpoint. It was too persistent to be used on the offensive, and its physiological effects were not manifest for several hours after exposure, so that it could not be counted upon to produce casualties during the progress of the attack. On the other hand, diphenylchlorarsine was very disappointing. Owing chiefly to technical errors in the method of its dispersion, it was surprisingly ineffective on the battlefield, although it was highly toxic, was nonpersistent, and readily penetrated the mask.

The year 1917 then closed with the Germans in possession of the most effective defensive chemical agent yet devised (mustard gas), but with no satisfactory offensive agent, since the masks of 1917 afforded adequate protection against all the lung-injurant gases in use. During the winter of 1917–1918, the German High Command was planning the great spring offensive to commence in March, 1918, and must have been much impressed with the vast number of casualties produced by mustard gas during the stabilized warfare in 1917. It was therefore only natural

191

for it to call upon the German chemists for a *nonpersistent* vesicant that would produce immediate casualties. Ethyldichlorarsine was the result of this demand.

This compound was nonpersistent, quick-acting, highly toxic, and contained arsenic. However, it was only about one-sixth as vesicant as mustard gas, did not penetrate clothing to anything like the same extent, and was completely stopped by the existing gas masks. Ethyldichlorarsine proved to be such a disappointment that, when the spring offensive of March 1918, was launched, the Germans resorted to the use of a combination of Yellow, Green, and Blue Cross shells as their principal offensive weapons. The Yellow Cross (mustard gas) were used on sectors not to be penetrated by the Germans during the attack, and the Green Cross (diphosgene) and Blue Cross (diphenylchlorarsine) were used as the main artillery preparation in sectors where the attacks were to be launched.

Closely watching these developments during the spring of 1918, the Americans became convinced that what was most needed was a more effective gas of the ethyldichlorarsine type, *i.e.*, a highly toxic, nonpersistent, quick-acting, vesicant compound containing arsenic. Lewisite was the result of an intensive effort to produce such a compound. How well they succeeded only time can show, as lewisite was produced too late for use at the front. It was not until October, 1918, that the manifold technical difficulties of mass production were finally overcome and manufacture commenced. The first lot manufactured was ready for shipment in November when the Armistice intervened, and it was destroyed at sea.

Curiously enough, the Germans claim that they not only knew about lewisite before the American discovery, but had actually manufactured it during 1917 and 1918. Thus, Hanslian says:

> It is evident from the publications of the German chemist, H. Wieland, (H. Wieland und A. Bloemer: "Über die Synthese der organischen Arsenderivate" in "Liebigs Annalen der Chemie," vol. 451, page 30) that even before the American discovery chlorvinyldichlorarsine was manufactured during the war in 1917 and 1918 in Germany, according to the Germans' own special methods and independently of Lewis' synthesis.

If this is true, it would seem that Germany made a serious error in not employing lewisite in the offensives of 1918, as comparative tests have shown its superiority, in many respects, over the compounds used in 1918. That this opinion is shared by the French may be inferred from the following paragraph from Hederer and Istin.

> The true vesicant arsines have not yet submitted to the proof of battle. They, nevertheless, merit attention by reason of their strong activity and their multiple effects. One can already consider them as persistents of rapid aggressiveness, capable of playing eventually a military role of the first order.

192

The method of making lewisite was suggested by the analogous method of mustard-gas manufacture used by the Allies. Thus, mustard is formed by the action of ethylene on sulfur monochloride, while lewisite is produced by action of acetylene on arsenic trichloride in the presence of aluminum trichloride acting as a catalyst. The dark brown viscid liquid which results from this latter reaction is decomposed by treatment with hydrochloric acid at 0°C. (32°F.), and an oil is obtained which can be fractionated by distillation in vacuo into three chlorvinyl derivatives of arsenic trichloride. These derivatives, which differ from each other only by the successive addition to the arsenic trichloride of one, two, or three molecules of acetylene, are as follows (see Chart XIII):

$$C_2H_2 + AsCl_3 = ClCH{:}CH.As\begin{cases}Cl\\Cl\end{cases}$$

(β-Chlorvinyldichlorarsine)
(Primary lewisite)

$$2(C_2H_2) + AsCl_3 = \begin{matrix}ClCH{:}CH\\ClCH{:}CH\end{matrix}\Big\rangle AsCl$$

(ββ'-Dichlorvinylchlorarsine)
(Secondary lewisite)

$$3(C_2H_2) + AsCl_3 = \begin{matrix}ClCH{:}CH\\ClCH{:}CH\\ClCH{:}CH\end{matrix}\Big\rangle As$$

(ββ'β''-Trichlorvinylarsine)
(Tertiary lewisite)

During the initial reaction considerable heat is liberated and great care must be taken to keep the temperature from rising by regulating the current of acetylene, as otherwise violent explosions may occur. The reaction products are also explosive, and for that reason it is impossible to separate them by direct distillation. Hence, they must be treated with hydrochloric acid until all the aluminum compounds are dissolved. During the distillation of the resulting oily liquid, the unconverted arsenic trichloride passes over first (up to 60°C.); next follows the primary lewisite (up to 100°C.); finally, the balance passes over above 100°C. as a mixture of secondary and tertiary lewisites. The initial distillation yields only about 18 per cent primary lewisite, which is the most active and the preferred product. However, the secondary and tertiary fractions are subsequently converted into the primary form by heating under pressure to 210°C. with an excess of arsenic trichloride, so that the ultimate loss is small.

All the lewisites are liquids at ordinary temperatures, having boiling points ranging between 190° and 260°C., and all are irritating and

193

poisonous compounds but not to anything like the same extent. Thus, primary and secondary lewisites are both highly toxic vesicants, the primary form being more toxic and less vesicant than the secondary, while the tertiary form is very much less active and is practically of no value as a chemical agent. As the primary form is by far the most active, it is the form into which the mixture was practically all converted. Thus, wherever the term, "lewisite" is used without qualification, it will be understood to refer to primary lewisite (β-chlorvinyldichlorarsine).

Pure lewisite is an oily colorless to light amber liquid, of 1.88 specific gravity, which boils at 190°C. (374°F.), yielding a dense vapor 7.1 times

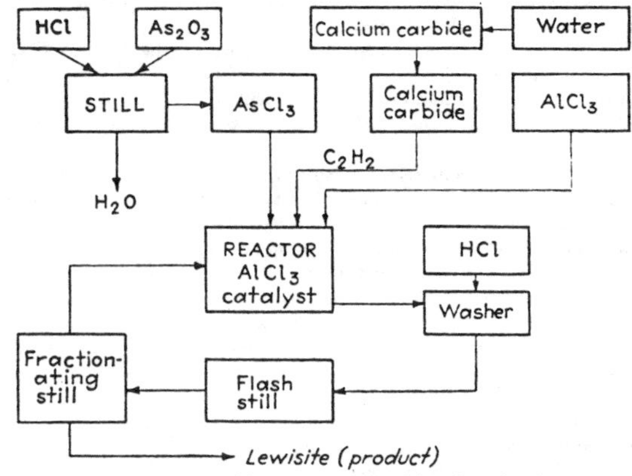

CHART XIII.—Manufacture of lewisite (flow sheet).

heavier than air with a faint odor resembling geraniums. It is readily soluble in the usual organic solvents and petroleum, but is not dissolved by water or weak acids. It is, however, rather easily and quickly decomposed by hydrolysis, yielding hydrochloric acid and an oxide of chlorvinylarsine, according to the equation:

$$ClCH{:}CH.As{:}Cl_2 + H_2O = 2HCl + ClCH{:}CH.As{:}O$$

However, unlike mustard gas, one of the hydrolysis products of lewisite (ClCH:CH.AsO) is a vesicant nonvolatile toxic which is not readily washed away by rains. Hence, while lewisite may be quickly destroyed by hydrolysis in moist air and on watery terrain, its combat value is not lost, since ground which has been contaminated with lewisite will remain dangerous from its oxides for long periods of time. In other words, one should not regard hydrolysis as immediately destructive of the toxic and vesicant powers of lewisite, but as a process in which the compound

194

changes its state, while at the same time retaining its physiological powers in a new form. This view is important in arriving at the true combat value of lewisite, as far too much emphasis has been placed upon its suceptibility to hydrolysis, quite overlooking the fact that, in addition to the combat value of its hydrolysis products, the vast majority of situations in which lewisite would be used would not involve sufficient moisture to destroy it. Most terrains over which armies fight are moderately dry, and the great majority of the days in most parts of the north temperate zone are clear. Also, it must be remembered that in cold frozen countries and hot dry countries hydrolysis is of little importance.

Like mustard gas, lewisite is almost immediately decomposed in the presence of alkalies, such as caustic soda (5 per cent solution) or ammonia, and by active oxydants, such as chloride of lime and the hypochlorites, the reaction being greatly accelerated by heat. Hence terrain and material contaminated with lewisite are decontaminated with the same materials as mustard gas. Also, like mustard, lewisite readily penetrates clothing, leather, rubber, and the tissues of the body, and hence is just as difficult to protect against.

The vapor pressure of lewisite is very much higher than that of mustard. At 0°C. (32°F.) its vapor pressure is 0.087 mm. Hg, as compared to 0.026 mm. Hg for mustard; at 20°C. (68°F.), it is 0.395 mm. Hg, against 0.065 mm. Hg for mustard. The volatility of lewisite at 20°C. (68°F.) is 4.50 mg. per liter, as compared to 0.625 mg. per liter for mustard, and the persistency of lewisite is correspondingly much less than that of mustard. On the basis of Leitner's Formula (see page 21), the persistency of lewisite at 20°C. (68°F.) is 9.6 times that of water, while the persistency of mustard is 67 times that of water.

The freezing point of lewisite is −18°C. (0°F.), which is well below ordinary atmospheric temperatures, so that it is a liquid at all times, except in very cold weather, and hence does not require a solvent as does mustard. Like mustard, lewisite is stable in storage and does not react with iron and steel.

Physiologically, lewisite acts similarly to mustard gas and in addition is a systemic poison when absorbed into the body through the skin or lungs. It may, therefore, be classed as primarily a vesicant, secondarily a toxic lung injurant, and tertiarily a systemic poison when absorbed in the tissues. The mechanism of the physiological action of lewisite is also like that of mustard; both are cell poisons and both undergo endoplasmic hydrolysis within the living cell and release hydrochloric acid in accordance with the following equation (lewisite):

$$ClCH{:}CH.As\begin{matrix}Cl\\Cl\end{matrix} + H_2O \rightarrow ClCH{:}CH.AsO + 2HCl$$

In the case of lewisite, however, the other hydrolysis product—β-chlorvinylarsine oxide—is itself necrosant, and the arsenical residue of this oxide passes into the circulation, fixes itself in various organs, and sets up a general systemic poisoning, typical of arsenal compounds.

Lewisite is then both a local and general toxic of great deadly strength. Thus, a dose of 0.0173 gram per pound of body weight, externally applied, is fatal, so that an average man, weighing 150 lb., would be killed by 2.6 grams (30 drops) applied to his skin. The minimum irritating concentration of lewisite (0.0008 mg. per liter) is far below the minimum concentration at which it can be detected by its odor (0.014 mg. per liter), so that the warning effect of its odor has been greatly exaggerated by some authors. Its blistering (vesicant) concentration (0.334 mg. per liter) is less than 10 per cent of its saturation concentration in the air at 20°C. (68°F.), so that field concentrations ten times that required for vesication are possible. When inhaled, 0.120 mg. per liter is fatal in 10 minutes, and 0.048 mg. per liter is fatal in 30 minutes. Its toxicity thus slightly exceeds that of mustard gas.

Lewisite is quicker acting than mustard gas, as shown by the following comparison, based on experimental tests in which a drop of each agent was placed on the forearm of a man.

Lewisite was completely absorbed in five minutes with a slight burning sensation, while mustard required from twenty to thirty minutes for absorption and produced no noticeable sensation. With lewisite, the skin commences to redden at the end of thirty minutes; then the erythema increases and spreads rapidly and occupies a surface of 12 by 15 centimeters towards the end of the third hour. With mustard, the reaction (salmon colored) does not appear until two hours, and during the third hour covers a surface of only 3.5 by 4 centimeters. The vesiculation of lewisite appears at the end of about thirteen hours and consists of a large blister, the size of a cherry, which soon absorbs all the surrounding small blisters, forming about the twenty-fourth hour, a single, large, bulging, vesicle, surrounded by a reddened fringe which merges with the healthy skin at its outer edge. On the other hand, the first mustard blisters gradually appear in the form of a ring around the infected spot towards the end of the twenty-fourth hour. In the center the lesion is depressed and of a yellowish gray color.

In the absence of a secondary infection, the wounds from lewisite heal more rapidly than those of mustard, but whether these conditions would actually obtain on the field of battle is doubtful, and the probabilities are that in war the wounds of lewisite would be as serious and durable as those of mustard.

The future role of lewisite is uncertain. Under favorable conditions it is undoubtedly superior to any of the other World War gases. The question as to whether or not it would be used in a future war would seem, therefore, to depend primarily upon the meterological conditions to be encountered in the Theater of Operations. In cold countries and in hot

dry countries it would be very effective, but in wet rainy countries much less effective.

Dr. Mueller thinks lewisite would have been a great disappointment to the Americans had it been actually used on the Western Front in the World War. While the climatic conditions in that Theater of Operations were, on the whole, rather unfavorable, it by no means follows that lewisite would have been ineffective if used intelligently, and this is particularly true in view of the highly toxic character of its hydrolysis products which infect contaminated ground for long periods. On the whole, we are inclined to believe that lewisite must be taken into serious consideration in any chemical warfare estimate of the future.

Methyldichlorarsine ($CH_3As.Cl_2$)

This compound is the methyl analogue of ethyldichlorarsine and the properties and characteristics of the two are very similar (see page 166). It was under intensive study by the Americans during the last months of the war, and Flury (28) includes it among the World War toxic gases, although, as a matter of fact, there is no record of its actual use by either side in the war. The preference of the Germans for ethyldichlorarsine, instead of the methyl compound, is difficult to understand in view of the superior properties of the latter, as shown by a comparison of their characteristics. Fries (9, page 181) attributes the German preference for ethyldichlorarsine to the difficulty of manufacturing the methyl compound, but the differences in difficulty of manufacture are so slight as to be no obstacle whatever to the genius of the German chemists who succeeded in solving many more formidable problems.

Like most of the chemical agents used in the war, methyldichlorarsine was not a new compound. It was discovered in 1858 by Baeyer who described its pronounced irritating effects.

The method of manufacture of methyldichlorarsine is complicated and comprises the following principal steps:

1. Sodium arsenite is prepared by dissolving arsenic trioxide in caustic-soda solution, as indicated in the following reaction:

$$6NaOH + As_2O_3 = 2Na_3AsO_3 + 3H_2O$$

The reaction proceeds readily evolving considerable heat.

2. The sodium arsenite solution is next methylated by adding dimethyl sulfate at 85°C

$$Na_3AsO_3 + (CH_3)_2SO_4 = Na_2CH_3AsO_3 + Na.CH_3SO_4$$

3. The disodium methyl arsenite is converted to methyl arsenic oxide by sulfur dioxide, as indicated

$$Na_2CH_3AsO_3 + SO_2 = CH_3AsO + Na_2SO_4$$

4. Methyl arsine oxide is finally converted to methyldichlorarsine by passing hydrogen chloride gas through the mixture, when the following reaction takes place:

$$CH_3AsO + 2HCl = CH_3AsCl_2 + H_2O$$

Methyldichlorarsine is a colorless liquid, of 1.85 specific gravity, which boils at 132°C. (269.6°F.), yielding a vapor with a powerful burning odor. At 20°C., its vapor pressure is 8.50 mm. Hg and its volatility is 75.00 mg. per liter. This compound is chemically very stable, being only slightly soluble in water, though soluble in organic solvents. It does not corrode iron and steel.

Like the ethyl compound, the methyldichlorarsine is a vesicant, toxic lung injurant, and respiratory irritant. A concentration as low as 0.002 mg. per liter causes quite a severe irritation in the nose which produces sneezing and finally extends to the chest where it gives rise to pain. A concentration of 0.009 mg. per liter is distinctly sternutatory; 0.025 mg. per liter is unbearable when inhaled for more than 1 minute, and leads at once to painful attacks of asthma and marked dyspnea which often lasts for 24 hours. Still higher concentrations cause serious injuries to the lungs, 0.56 mg. per liter being fatal on 10 minutes' exposure and 0.12 mg. per liter fatal on 30 minutes' exposure.

Methyldichlorarsine is thus about half as toxic as the ethyl compound and when liquid is less irritant to the skin. On the other hand, its vapors are as irritating to the skin as the vapors of mustard gas and, when liquid it penetrates fabrics much faster than does liquid mustard gas.

The vesicant action of methyldichlorarsine is very similar to mustard, but its lesions are much less severe and heal more rapidly than mustard-gas lesions.

The vapor of methyldichlorarsine is hydrolyzed by moisture, but not rapidly enough to destroy the gas before it can exert its physiological action. Owing to its great volatility, methyldichlorarsine persists in the open for only about 1 hour in warm weather and 2 to 3 hours in cold weather.

Although not proved on the field of battle in the late war, it is believed that, taking everything into consideration, methyldichlorarsine is probably superior to mustard gas and lewisite for producing *rapid* vapor burns of the skin. For this reason, together with its low persistency, it should have a high value for offensive military purposes.

Dibromethyl Sulfide $(S(CH_2CH_2)_2Br_2)$

German: "Bromlost"

The last of the vesicant agents usually identified with the World War, although, strictly speaking, belonging to the postwar period, is the

198

bromine analogue of mustard gas, dibromethyl sulfide, called by the Germans "Bromlost."

This compound was studied by the Germans during the closing days of the war in an effort to find a vesicant compound more persistent than mustard gas, for use on the tactical defensive where it was desired to contaminate ground yielded to the enemy for as long a period as possible.

The three elements which destroy mustard on the ground are humidity, temperature, and wind. A compound less susceptible to hydrolysis and of higher boiling point and lower vapor pressure would, it was thought, persist longer than mustard and be a more effective chemical agent on the tactical defensive. The substitution of bromine for the chlorine atoms in mustard gas was expected to produce such a compound, but dibromethyl sulfide did not measure up to expectations.

Dibromethyl sulfide is a solid at ordinary temperatures, which melts at 21°C. (70°F.) and boils (with decomposition) at 250°C. (464°F.). It has a specific gravity of 2.05 and a volatility of about 0.400 mg. per liter, as compared with 1.27 specific gravity and 0.600 mg. per liter volatility of mustard. It is also far more susceptible to hydrolysis than mustard.

The physiological action of dibromethyl sulfide is very similar to that of mustard gas, but to a far less degree. Its greater density permits about 50 per cent greater amounts to be loaded in the same shell, and this partially offsets its inferior physiological activity. But its sensitiveness to destruction by moisture is a net loss compared with mustard, so that, on the whole, dibromethyl sulfide was not a real advance over mustard gas and would in all probability never be used in war.

COMPARISON OF THE VESICANTS

Considering the factors: (1) rapidity of action; (2) extension of rubefaction, swelling, and edema; and (3) time of healing of lesions, the World War vesicants and those compounds having subsidiary vesicant action may be arranged in descending order of their skin-irritant efficiency as follows:

1. Mustard.
2. Lewisite.
3. Phenyldichlorarsine.
4. Methyldichlorarsine.
5. Ethyldichlorarsine.
6. Phenyldibromarsine.
7. Dibromethyl sulfide.

On the basis of relative toxicity, the above agents would rank as follows:

199

Agent	Minimum Lethal Dose (10 Minutes' Exposure) Mg. per Liter
Lewisite	0.120
Mustard	0.150
Phenyldibromarsine	0.200
Phenyldichlorarsine	0.260
Ethyldichlorarsine	0.500
Methyldichlorarsine	0.560
Dibromethyl sulfide	1.000

USE OF VESICANTS IN THE WORLD WAR

The vesicants rank second in the extent of use in the war, being exceeded in tonnage by the lung injurants only. Altogether, about 12,000 tons of vesicants were used in battle, and of this quantity it is estimated that mustard was fully 95 per cent. No separate records are available as to the exact quantities of the minor vesicants that were used, or as to the casualties produced by them. Mustard gas so nearly completely dominated the vesicant field that all such casualties are generally credited to mustard. The vesicants produced 400,000 casualties, or nearly one-third of the total gas casualties, although the amount of vesicants used in battle was less than 10 per cent of the total gas used. The vesicants secured one casualty per 60 lb. of gas, which was nearly four times the ratio of casualties to gas for the lung injurants.

During the war, the vesicants were used only in artillery and trench-mortar shells, as they were unsuitable for cloud-gas projection, owing to low vapor pressures. By the same token, however, they are well adapted for dispersion by airplane sprays and bombs, and it is accordingly probable that in the future they will be largely employed by the air force, as well as by the artillery.

FUTURE OF THE VESICANTS

The vesicants introduced a new principle in chemical-warfare offense in that they readily penetrated clothing and produced casualties by body burns. Masks, therefore, were wholly inadequate for protection against these agents, and special protective clothing was resorted to. Such clothing is very uncomfortable, especially in hot weather, and greatly lowers the combat ability of troops. It also enormously increases the problem of protection from contamination, not only for men and animals but also for material. Food and water supplies in particular must be specially protected and ready means must be devised to decontaminate enormous quantities of material and large areas of ground.

The introduction of vesicants in the war tilted the scales heavily in favor of the chemical offense, and the war closed leaving the problem

200

of adequate defense against the vesicants largely unsolved. Since the war all nations have expended much time and effort in trying to solve this complex problem. How well they have succeeded only the future can show.

In the meantime, vesicants occupy the center of the stage of chemical armaments and it is a foregone conclusion that they will figure largely in wars of the future. Fortunately for the nations of the world, they exemplify the most humane method of waging war yet devised.

For a summary of the principal properties of the vesicant agents, see Table IV.

201

CHAPTER X

RESPIRATORY IRRITANT AGENTS (Sternutators)

The fifth and last class of toxic agents used in the World War was the respiratory irritants, often called *sternutators* (sneeze producers). They form a small well-defined group having many properties in common and were generally designated by the Germans as "Blue Cross" substances.

By the summer of 1917, the gas masks of all of the belligerents had been developed to a stage where they furnished adequate protection against the lung-injurant gases. Also, the lung-injurant gases theretofore employed were slow acting and did not incapacitate until several hours after exposure. The problem was, therefore, to find a quick-acting nonpersistent gas that would penetrate the mask, and the respiratory irritants were the solution of the German chemists to this problem. While the respiratory irritants produced few serious casualties, by quickly penetrating the mask, nauseating the soldier, and causing frequent vomiting, they usually made it impossible to wear the mask, and upon its removal the soldier soon fell a victim to the lung-injurant agents (Green Cross substances) which were fired simultaneously with the respiratory-irritant agents (Blue Cross substances).

The first large-scale gas attack featuring respiratory-irritant compounds was directed by the Germans against the Russians while crossing the Dvina River at Uexhuell in September, 1917. The Germans employed a combined Green Cross and Blue Cross bombardment against the Russian batteries which commanded the place of crossing. The bombardment lasted for 2 hours and the Russian batteries were silenced with the exception of a few guns which had not been recognized and therefore were not included in the areas shelled.

The great German offensive of Mar. 21, 1918, was based chiefly on the effect of gas. The Allied flanks on the attacking salients were cut off by mustard gas, while the main force was shelled by a mixture of Blue Cross and Green Cross shells. The Allies were at first absolutely defenseless against the respiratory-irritant substances and, had the Germans been able to atomize and disperse their toxic smokes into minute particles, the result would have been disastrous. Toward the end of the war, the Allies incorporated in their gas-mask canisters a mechanical filter, consisting of wadding and layers of felt, and in this way provided adequate protection against these toxic dusts.

202

The Allies claimed that the German Blue Cross shells were not effective, and based their opinion upon the fact that the high explosive in the shell did not sufficiently atomize the toxic chemical to create a dust fine enough to penetrate the mask. There were but 577 casualties and 3 deaths in the American Expeditionary Forces owing to gassing with respiratory-irritant compounds. Deaths from these compounds were very rare.

GROUP CHARACTERISTICS

In general, the respiratory irritants were all solids with high melting points and negligible vapor pressures. They were, therefore, dispersed by heavy explosive charges, in the form of a finely pulverized dust. The particulate clouds thus created lasted only a few minutes in the open, and they were accordingly classed as nonpersistent agents. They were, however, immediately effective and readily penetrated the existing gas masks of the Allies. It was due chiefly to these properties that they were introduced by the Germans on the night of July 11, 1917.

Chemically, all the respiratory irritants belong to the family of arsines (AsH_3) and are compounds consisting of trivalent arsenic in which the arsenic atom is linked by one valence to a halogen atom, or to a monovalent active group, and by two other valences to two atoms of carbon of two carbonyl radicals, thus:

$$(C_6H_5)_2As{-}Cl \text{ (Diphenylchlorarsine)}$$

$$(C_6H_5)_2As{-}CN \text{ (Diphenylcyanarsine)}$$

The respiratory irritants have the power to irritate certain tissues of the body without producing notable lesions, *i.e.*, without injury, at the point of contact when employed in concentrations above their thresholds of action, which are extremely low. They act only on the ends of the sensory nerves, which are anatomically poorly protected against chemical attack, and give rise to more or less acute pains accompanied by muscular reflexes and various secretions, depending upon the nature of the compound and the region infected. The mucous membranes of the respiratory system (nose, larynx, trachea, bronchial tubes, and lungs) are thin and sensitive, and their moist surfaces facilitate the fixation and dissolution of these gases. They, therefore, furnish an excellent field for the action of the respiratory-irritant compounds and are, accordingly, the members chiefly affected by these compounds. Based upon extensive experiments, Flury sums up the physiological action of these compounds, as follows:

203

The intensive cell toxic effect is seen everywhere where the substances come in contact with the living cells in the solid, liquid or gaseous state. They are distinguished from the strong corrosive substances by the fact that even when used in the very lowest concentrations they cause inflammatory phenomena and necrosis in the affected tissues. From the qualitative standpoint, there are no great differences from the effects of the other irritants. The arsenic compounds also act on the respiratory passages and the lungs, the organs of sight and the outer skin, thus causing an acute toxic lung edema, serious injuries to the capillaries, the formation of false membranes in the air passages, inflammation of the conjunctiva and necrosis of the corneal epithelium in the eye, and sometimes also inflammation of the outer skin with the formation of blisters and the deeper destruction of the tissues. The general character of the effect now is more like that of phosgene, again more like that caused by the sulfur-containing irritants such as dichlorethylsulfide. Despite that, there are certain peculiarities to the poisoning caused by the arsenic compounds. The irritation to the sensitive nerves far surpasses in intensity the effect of any chemically accurately defined compounds heretofore known. The irritant action, however, extends not only to the portions of the mucous membranes affected directly by the poison but in a characteristic way also attacks the so-called accessory cavities.

As a rule, the respiratory irritants are nonlethal in concentrations ordinarily employed in battle and have the following properties in common:

1. Their thresholds of action are extremely low; a few thousandths of a milligram per liter produce certain and useful results.
2. They are immediately effective; an exposure of 1 to 2 minutes being sufficient to produce positive effects.
3. Their action is reversible, since the irritation produced disappears rapidly after termination of exposure. They do not destroy the nerve ends and, after the reflexes caused by the irritation, the nerves recuperate their normal functions.
4. Their action is elective, for they affect only the nerve tissues and especially those controlling the respiratory system.

From a physiological viewpoint, the respiratory-irritant agents may be divided into two groups: (1) the simple respiratory irritants, and (2) the toxic respiratory irritants. The first cause only a local irritation of the respiratory system, while the second go further and set up a systemic arsenical poisoning. Only the first group (1) are primarily respiratory irritants, as the compounds in the second group (2) primarily exert other effects and their respiratory-irritant action is only subsidiary. Compounds in the second group, therefore, belong primarily to other groups of agents and are only secondarily regarded as respiratory irritants.

WORLD WAR RESPIRATORY IRRITANTS

The principal respiratory-irritant agents, in order of their chronological appearance in the World War, were:

204

Agent	Introduced by	Date
Simple respiratory irritants		
Diphenylchlorarsine	Germans	July, 1917
Diphenylcyanarsine	Germans	May, 1918
Ethylcarbazol	Germans	July, 1918
Diphenylaminechlorarsine	Americans	Postwar
Toxic respiratory irritants		
Phenyldichlorarsine*	Germans	September, 1917
Ethyldichlorarsine*	Germans	March, 1918
Ethyldibromarsine*	Germans	September, 1918

* Primarily toxic lung injurants.

Diphenylchlorarsine ($(C_6H_5)_2AsCl$)

German: "Clark I"

Diphenylchlorarsine was introduced simultaneously with mustard gas as an offensive companion thereto, since mustard gas was too persistent to be used on the tactical offensive. The purpose of diphenylchlorarsine was to penetrate the Allies' masks, which successfully protected against all the lung-injurant agents. This was accomplished by dispersing the chemical substance in the form of a *dust* which, not being a vapor or gas, was not absorbed by the charcoal and soda lime in the gas-mask canister.

Diphenylchlorarsine was discovered in 1881 by Michaelis and LaCoste. During the war it was manufactured by the Germans in accordance with a complicated process, of which the following were the principal steps:

1. Benzene diazonium chloride was treated with sodium arsenite to form sodium phenylarsenate

$$C_6H_5{-}N_2Cl + Na_3AsO_3 = C_6H_5AsO_3Na_2 + NaCl + N_2$$

2. Sodium phenylarsenate was converted to phenylarsenic acid by treatment with hydrochloric acid

$$C_6H_5AsO_3Na_2 + 2HCl = C_6H_5AsO_3H_2 + 2NaCl$$

3. Phenylarsenic acid was reduced to phenylarsenious acid by treatment with sulfur dioxide and water

$$C_6H_5AsO_3H_2 + SO_2 + H_2O = C_6H_5AsO_2H_2 + H_2SO_4$$

205

4. Phenylarsenious acid was treated with sodium hydroxide to form sodium phenylarsenite

$$C_6H_5AsO_2H_2 + 2HaOH = C_6H_5AsO_2Na_2 + 2H_2O$$

5. Sodium phenylarsenite was converted to sodium diphenylarsenite by treatment with benzene diazonium chloride

$$C_6H_5AsO_2Na_2 + C_6H_5N_2Cl = (C_6H_5)_2AsO_2Na + NaCl + N_2$$

6. Sodium diphenylarsenite was treated with hydrochloric acid to form diphenylarsenic acid

$$(C_6H_5)_2AsO_2Na + HCl = (C_6H_5)_2AsO_2H + NaCl$$

7. This acid was reduced to diphenylarsenious oxide by treatment with sulfur dioxide and water

$$2(C_6H_5)_2AsO_2H + 2SO_2 + H_2O = [(C_6H_5)_2As]_2O + 2H_2SO_4$$

8. Diphenylarsenious oxide was converted to diphenylchlorarsine by chlorination with hydrochloric acid

$$[(C_6H_5)_2As]_2O + 2HCl = 2(C_6H_5)_2AsCl + H_2O$$

Diphenylchlorarsine may also be prepared by a much simpler process, as follows:

1. Triphenylarsine is formed by acting on chlorbenzene and arsenic trichloride with sodium.

2. The triphenylarsine is then heated under pressure with more arsenic trichloride and diphenylchlorarsine is thus obtained.

While the latter was the laboratory method of making diphenylchlorarsine, there appears to be no inherent reason why it could not be used as a basis for a successful commercial method of manufacture and thus greatly simplify the production problem. It was stated that the Germans adopted the more complicated method outlined above because they had previously manufactured several of the intermediates in this process and that the equipment of their chemical plants was peculiarly adapted to this process. Undoubtedly, if diphenylchlorarsine were manufactured in quantity in the future, especially outside of Germany, a simpler and more direct process would be employed.

In the pure state, diphenylchlorarsine is a white crystalline solid, of 1.4 specific gravity, which melts at 45°C. (113°F.), although the somewhat impure commercial substance used during the war melted at 38°C. (100°F.). It boils with decomposition at 383°C. (720°F.). It is insoluble in water, but is readily soluble in organic solvents, including phosgene and chlorpicrin. It decomposes rapidly in contact with water, yielding hydrochloric acid and phenylarsenic oxide which is toxic, but this action is very slow in a merely humid atmosphere. As it is a solid,

206

its vapor pressure (0.0005 mm. Hg at 20°C.) is negligible and its volatility at 20°C. is only 0.00068 mg. per liter.

When diphenylchlorarsine is volatilized by heating, its vapors condense in the air to form very fine liquid droplets or solid particles (depending upon their temperature) which float like particles of smoke or dust in the air; but in order to volatilize and convert this compound into the form of smoke (particulate clouds of solid particles), it is essential that the substance pass through the actual gas or vapor stage. That is to say, a preliminary heating process is necessary. It is impossible to convert this compound by atomization at a low temperature into real smoke, even if it is dissolved in a volatile solvent.

The reason for these peculiarities undoubtedly lies in the size of the particles given off when this substance is distilled by heating, as compared to the smallest sized particle that can be produced by atomization. When volatilized by heat, the particles formed are extremely small, having a diameter of only 10^{-4} to 10^{-5} cm. On the other hand, when dispersed by explosion, the time of detonation is too brief for an appreciable amount of heat to be transmitted to the chemical substance, and the dispersion of the chemical is thus almost entirely due to the physical force of the explosion. The result is that the particles of diphenylchlorarsine dispersed by explosion were many times larger than those resulting from heat distillation. Similarly, when diphenylchlorarsine is dissolved in a liquid solvent and sprayed by a mechanical sprayer, even the best sprayers send out droplets many times larger than the true smoke particles.

These facts were apparently not appreciated by the Germans at the time they adopted diphenylchlorarsine as a filler for their Blue Cross shell, for they first attempted to dissolve this compound in some easily volatilized solvent, such as diphosgene, and disperse it as a liquid spray. When this proved unsatisfactory, they then attempted to disperse it by the use of heavy charges of high explosive which also subsequently proved ineffective on the field of battle. In loading diphenylchlorarsine into the shell, another error was made in placing the explosive charge around, instead of within, the chemical charge. With the explosive surrounding the chemical charge, the force of explosion tended to compress the chemical particles, instead of blowing them apart.

Subsequent experiments by the Allies proved that diphenylchlorarsine was extremely effective in the field when dispersed (by heat distillation) as a true toxic smoke, and they were preparing toxic smoke candles, embodying this principle of dispersion, when the Armistice intervened and prevented their use at the front. The failure to adopt a proper means of dispersing diphenylchlorarsine stands out as one of the few technical mistakes in chemical warfare that the Germans made dur-

207

ing the World War. But it was a costly mistake, as no less than 14,000,000 artillery shells were loaded with this substance (and its analogue, diphenylcyanarsine) and great reliance was placed upon its supposed offensive-combat power in the German drives in the spring of 1918. The evidence of the Allies' casualties from German Blue Cross shell, however, is conclusive that these shell were largely ineffective, notwithstanding the known very powerful physiological properties of these compounds.

When diphenylchlorarsine is pulverized and dispersed by the explosion of a high-explosive charge, and, to a far greater extent, when thermally distilled as a toxic smoke, it is broken up into microscopic particles that float in the air, easily penetrate the ordinary gas-mask canister, and exert their effects directly on the respiratory tract. When used in minimum concentrations, this compound causes great irritation to the upper respiratory tract, the sensitive peripheral nerves, and the eyes; it also irritates the outer skin, but not to so great an extent; when present in stronger concentrations or when inhaled in weaker concentrations for a long time, it attacks the deeper respiratory passages. The irritation begins in the nose, as a tickling sensation, followed by sneezing, with a flow of viscous mucous, similar to that which accompanies a bad cold. The irritation then spreads down into the throat and coughing and choking set in until finally the air passages and the lungs are also affected. Headache, especially in the forehead, increases in intensity until it becomes almost unbearable, and there is a feeling of pressure in the ears and pains in the jaws and teeth. These symptoms are accompanied by an oppressive pain in the chest, shortness of breath, and nausea which soon causes retching and vomiting. The victim has unsteady gait, a feeling of vertigo, weakness in the legs, and a trembling all over the body.

Flury gives the German experience with diphenylchlorarsine:

> In addition to the phenomena of sensory irritation, inhalation of diphenylchlorarsine may lead to serious disturbances of the nervous system from absorption of the poison. These show themselves as motor disturbances, uncertain gait, swaying when standing, and sometimes complete inability to walk. As a rule they are accompanied by severe pain in the joints and limbs. Inhalation of very high concentrations is also often followed by giddiness, attacks of faintness, and loss of consciousness, which may last for many hours. When considerable quantities of diphenylchlorarsine or related organic arsenical compounds are taken through the skin nervous disturbances of various types may arise, and these are to be ascribed not to a local action of the poison but to its general absorption. Hyperesthesia, anesthesia and paresthesia of definite areas of the skin, especially of the lower extremities, could frequently be observed. Twitching of the muscles and convulsions may occur in very severe cases of poisoning by similar substances.

The remarkable part of the effects above described is that they usually set in about 2 or 3 minutes after 1 minute of exposure to the gas

and usually reach their culmination in about 15 minutes after exposure ceases. After 15 minutes in uncontaminated air, the symptoms gradually disappear and in from 1 to 2 hours recovery is complete in the average case. In extreme cases, in enormously high concentrations, sufficient arsenic may be absorbed to produce systemic arsenical poisoning, which then produces the typical aftereffects of such poisoning.

Diphenylchlorarsine is effective in extremely low concentrations. Thus, a concentration as low as 1:25,000,000 (0.0005 mg. per liter) is sufficient to produce marked irritation of the nose and throat, while 0.0012 mg. per liter becomes unbearable after 1 minute. A concentration of 1.50 mg. per liter is lethal after 10 minutes, and 0.60 mg. per liter after 30 minutes' exposure. Since the volatility of diphenylchlorarsine is only 0.00068 mg. per liter, it is impossible to attain even an intolerable concentration in the air in *vapor* form. However, there is theoretically no limit to the concentration which may be built up in the form of *solid* particles suspended in the air, as this is merely a function of the amount of the substance distilled into a given volume of air. Nevertheless, under the actual conditions obtaining on the battlefield, it is very difficult to set up a lethal concentration, and there were few deaths from this gas in the World War.

Diphenylcyanarsine [$(C_6H_5)_2AsCN$]

German: "Clark II"

Diphenylcyanarsine was developed and adopted by the Germans in May, 1918, as an improvement over diphenylchlorarsine to which it is closely related. The main purpose for this development was to correct one of the serious weaknesses of diphenylchlorarsine, *viz.*, its ready decomposition by water. The new compound not only overcame this defect, but also proved to be physiologically more active than its chlorine analogue and was, in fact, the strongest of all the irritant compounds used in the war.

Diphenylcyanarsine was prepared by acting on diphenylchlorarsine with a saturated aqueous solution of sodium or potassium cyanide, during which reaction, the chlorine atom in the latter is replaced by the cyanogen group, thus

$$(C_6H_5)_2AsCl + NaCN = (C_6H_5)_2AsCN + NaCl$$

In a pure state, it is a colorless crystalline solid, of 1.45 specific gravity, which melts at 31.5°C. (91°F.) and boils with decomposition at 350°C. (662°F.), yielding a vapor 8.8 times heavier than air with a characteristic odor of garlic and bitter almonds.

It is not dissolved by water and is hydrolyzed so slowly as to be negligible. Chemically very stable, it is readily soluble in the organic

fats and solvents, especially chloroform. Its vapor pressure is negligible and its volatility is even lower than its chlorine analogue, being only 0.0015 mg. per liter at 20°C. (68°F.).

The physical and chemical behavior and the physiological effect of diphenylcyanarsine are exactly like those of the chloro-compound except that the last is more intense and somewhat more enduring. The lowest irritant concentration of diphenylcyanarsine is 0.0001 mg. per liter, and its intolerable concentration (0.00025 mg. per liter) which is one-fourth that of diphenylchlorarsine. The toxicity of diphenylcyanarsine for 10 minutes' exposure is 1.00 mg. per liter as compared to 1.50 mg. per liter for the chlorine analogue. The former is, therefore, about 50 per cent more toxic than the latter, but this is not of great practical importance since these lethal concentrations are far above the limit of actual attainment in the field, except in very unusual circumstances, such as where a shell bursts in an inclosed space so that a supersaturated concentration is obtained. Such concentrations may also exist for a few seconds immediately adjacent to the point of burst of the shell, but on the whole are extremely rare, as is shown by the Allies' casualties from Blue Cross shell, which were surprisingly small in comparison with the vast quantities of these shell used, and the percentage of deaths was almost negligible.

On the other hand, owing to the ease with which diphenylcyanarsine penetrated gas-mask canisters in use in 1917 and the early part of 1918, it temporarily put out of action large numbers of troops during the initial period of a bombardment; where such bombardments were immediately followed by infantry assaults, considerable tactical advantage was thus derived. Also, the difficulty of retaining the mask after penetration by this agent undoubtedly increased the number of casualties from lung-injurant (Green Cross) agents which were simultaneously employed.

Owing to the fact that diphenylcyanarsine was effective in extremely small concentrations (1:10,000,000), it was the agent per excellence for general harassment of troops. Even a few shell, scattered over a wide area compelled all troops therein to mask and thus greatly hampered their combat efficiency and effectiveness. It was thus particularly effective against artillery and Blue Cross shell were largely employed in counterbattery fire.

Notwithstanding that the German Blue Cross shell did not disperse its chemical contents in a very efficient form, the Allies were so impressed with the possibilities of DA and CDA that they immediately started to work to devise the most effective means for their employment against the Germans.

The British were particularly active in pushing the development of a toxic candle which would by progressive burning distill off the chemical

as a true smoke, in which form it was found to be far more effective than when dispersed by explosion from artillery shells. Speaking of this development, General Foulkes says:

> When the DA was scattered by the high explosive it was liberated not in the form of a gas, but in fine particles; these were not sufficiently minute to penetrate the box respirator completely, and absolute protection was very soon obtained by adding an extension to the box which contained a cheesecloth filter.
>
> Colonel Watson, who was the head of the Central Laboratory at Hesdin, had suggested in September 1917 the study of particulate clouds; and one of my officers, Sisson, in a sp rit of investigation, put a pinch of DA which had been extracted from a German shell on the hot plate of a stove in his room at my headquarters. The result was so remarkable that everyone was driven out of the house immediately, and it was found that the latest pattern of German mask, even when fitted with the extension that had been supplied to give protection against Blue Cross shells, gave no protection whatever against the DA cloud produced in this way.
>
> This was the germ of a new and very valuable idea, and steps were taken immediately to investigate how DA could be best volatilized in the most highly effective and penetrant form by bringing it in contact with the heat evolved from the combination of a suitable mixture of chemicals; and a "thermo-generator" was soon designed, which consisted of a tin containing the DA and the heating mixture in separate compartments and which weighed two or three pounds.
>
> The plan of attack was similar to the one previously put forward for gas; but as the particulate cloud was effective in one-hundredth the concentration of the gas cloud, and the German protection against it was nonexistent, complete success was absolutely certain if only the secret could be kept.
>
> The proposed assembly of the infantry assaulting columns would be simpler than in the former proposal, because there was no longer any need to use a retired line for the discharge. In fact, it was not even desirable, because the discharge would now be a much shorter one, and the "M" device (as the thermo-generators came to be called) would have to be used on a grand scale—hundreds of thousands being set alight with a simple friction lighter, as in the case of the familiar smoke candles—so that the infantry themselves would be called upon to assist the Special Brigade in handling the tins. The latter were not dangerous under artillery bombardment, like gas cylinders, and in any case the hostile fire would be silenced in the course of a few minutes by the cloud and by our own intensive gas bombardment.
>
> The "M" device was never used in France; but if its secret had been kept there is not the slightest doubt that its effect on the enemy, both moral and physical, would have been overwhelming; and if it had been properly and fully exploited it would have had a more important bearing on the course of the war than any other measure that was put to a practical trial on the battlefield or that was even considered.

In diphenylcyanarsine, we have the extreme limit of effectiveness in low concentrations of all chemical agents used in the war. Thus, a concentration of 0.00025 mg. per liter is intolerable if inhaled for 1 minute. As a man at rest normally inhales 8 liters of air per minute, he would absorb only 0.0002 mg. of the substance in that time. This is, however, sufficient to incapacitate him for an hour. For an average man, weighing

154 lb. (70,000,000 mg.), this means that diphenylcyanarsine is effective in the ratio of 1:35,000,000 of body weight, which makes it the strongest

of all the known irritants.

Ethylcarbazol $((C_6H_4)_2NC_2H_5)$

The last of the simple respiratory irritants used in the World War was ethylcarbazol, introduced by the Germans at the battle of the Marne in July, 1918. This compound is a white flaky solid which melts at 68°C. (149°F.) and boils at 190°C. (374°F.), yielding a vapor seven times heavier than air. It is soluble in alcohol and ether, but is insoluble in water and is practically unaffected thereby.

Very little information is available concerning the use of this substance or the reason for its introduction since it was by no means as irritant as either diphenylchlorarsine or diphenylcyanarsine with which it was mixed in the Blue Cross shell. Hanslian says, "As a matter of fact, it was not irritant at all, but merely served as a solvent for the arsine." This explanation, however, throws little light upon the subject since ethylcarbazol was itself a solid and was loaded in mixture with solid diphenylchlorarsine as a solid charge in the Blue Cross shell. It is, therefore, not clear as to how it could be used as a solvent. Moreover, it did have a decided irritant effect alone, although much less than any of the other respiratory-irritant substances.

The appearance of ethylcarbazol on the scene in the World War remains as one of those peculiar phenomena which seem altogether lacking in justification. It was used only to a limited extent and did not achieve any notable results. It is mentioned here only to complete the record.

Diphenylaminechlorarsine $((C_6H_4)_2NHAsCl)$

American: "Adamsite"

When the Allies found that diphenylchlorarsine could be made very effective by distilling it into the air and projecting it as a particulate cloud, they decided to use it against the Germans in this manner, but they had had no previous experience in the mass production of this compound, or even of its principal intermediates. The German process was so complicated that it was soon realized that a simpler method of making it must be developed. In seeking to find such a method, the British and American chemists simultaneously discovered that a slightly different, though closely related, compound could be easily manufactured in large quantities, and that this substitute compound had very similar properties and seemed to be equally effective as a respiratory-irritant chemical agent. This new compound was diphenylaminechlorarsine which

212

differs from the German substance, diphenylchlorarsine, only by the addition of an amino (NH) group to the latter compound, thus

$$C_6H_5-As(Cl)-C_6H_5$$

(Diphenylchlorarsine)

$$C_6H_4\langle As(Cl),\ (H)(N) \rangle C_6H_4$$

(Diphenylaminechlorarsine)

While this chemical difference is very slight, it immensely simplified the problem of manufacture, since all that is required is to mix together and heat diphenylamine and arsenic trichloride and a smooth reaction proceeds in accordance with the following equation (see Chart XIV):

$$(C_6H_5)_2NH + AsCl_3 = (C_6H_4)_2NHAsCl + 2HCl$$

The resulting product is a dark green molten mass which can be purified by recrystallization from benzene and glacial acetic acid. The Americans named this compound "Adamsite," after its American discoverer, Major Roger Adams.

Not only is the process of manufacture simple but the two ingredients are readily obtainable in large quantities. Diphenylamine is a common intermediate widely used in the dye industry and is also required in large quantities in time of war as a stabilizer in the manufacture of smokeless powder, while arsenic trichloride is obtained by chlorinating white

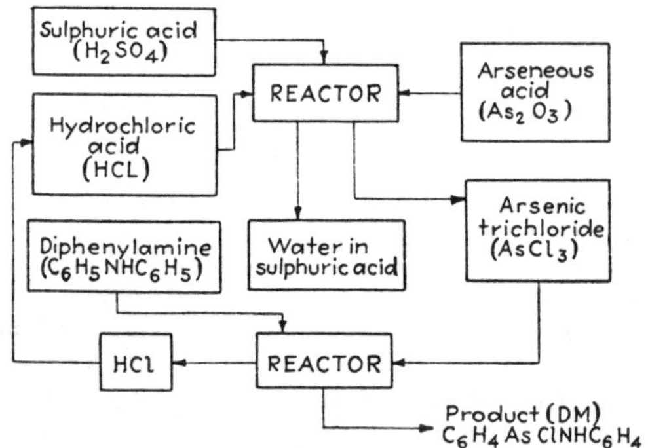

CHART XIV.—Manufacture of diphenylaminechlorarsine (flow sheet).

213

arsenic (AS_2O_3). Of all the arsenical chemical agents, diphenylaminechlorarsine is the most easily manufactured.

In addition to the research and development work of the British and Americans on diphenylaminechlorarsine during 1918, the Germans claim to have previously discovered, manufactured, and tested this compound. Thus, Dr. Mueller (21, page 108) says: "A method for its manufacture was patented by the Leverkusen Farbwerk as early as 1915 (German Patent 281,049)" and Dr. Hanslian says: "In Germany it was manufactured and tested even during the war by Wieland; however, it was not used in the field." Dr. Mueller says it was not used in the field because of the readiness with which it is decomposed when heated. In view, however, of the small difference in this regard between diphenylchlorarsine and diphenylaminechlorarsine, the substantially equal capability of the latter as a chemical agent, and its far greater ease of manufacture, it would seem that there was little justification for the German use of diphenylchlorarsine, which was so much more difficult to produce. Dr. Hanslian also says that the commercial method of manufacture of diphenylaminechlorarsine was greatly simplified and perfected by the Italian chemists Contardi and Fenaroli, and that certain Russian publications state that this compound was actually used by the Italians during the latter part of the war. This latter statement is, however, improbable as no Italian authorities make such a claim, nor is there any record of the tactical use of this compound by the Italians in the war.

When pure, diphenylaminechlorarsine is a yellow crystalline solid, of 1.65 specific gravity, which melts at 195°C. (387°F.) and boils (with decomposition) at 410°C. (770°F.) under normal pressure. It has practically no vapor pressure or vapor density, as it distills into the air in the form of minute solid particles. The impure commercial product used in chemical warfare is a dark brownish green crystalline mass which partially liquefies at 160°C. (320°F.), but the major portion does not melt until a temperature of 190°C. (374°F.) is reached. It is chemically a very stable compound, being unaffected by the humidity of the air or precipitation. It is insoluble in water and hydrolyzes very slowly and with great difficulty, yielding hydrochloric acid and a toxic oxide $[(C_6H_4)_2NHAs]_2O$. It is also very slightly soluble in the ordinary organic solvents and is not readily dissolved in any of the liquid chemical agents. The fumes of diphenylaminechlorarsine are much less inflammable than those from diphenylchlorarsine, so that there is much less risk of its inflaming when dispersed by heat. It acts on metals, corroding iron, steel, bronze, and brass. Upon dissemination in the air, it persists for about 10 minutes in both hot and cold weather, so that it is classed as a nonpersistent agent.

The physiological effects of diphenylaminechlorarsine are in general very similar to those of diphenylchlorarsine. Like the latter it strongly

214

irritates the eyes and mucous membranes of the nose and throat and causes violent sneezing and coughing. It then produces severe headaches, acute pains and tightness in the chest, and finally nausea and vomiting. The irritation of the eyes and the respiratory tract is at first weak, but within a minute or so it increases in severity so that it becomes unbearable. The acute effects usually last about 30 minutes after the victim has left the contaminated atmosphere. Qualitatively, the physiological effects of diphenylaminechlorarsine differ somewhat from those of diphenylchlorarsine, in that they appear more slowly and last longer; also coughing and a burning pain in the nose and throat are less intense. During the time of exposure, the effects of the latter are more apparent, but in higher concentrations the effects of the latter were more immediate and just as severe, but not as persistent as the former. The longest period of incapacitation from diphenylchlorarsine was about 1 hour, while that from diphenylaminechlorarsine was about 3 hours. The latter is then more efficient as a casualty producer since men gassed therewith are put out of action for three times as long a period.

To the average person, diphenylaminechlorarsine is odorless in ordinary field concentrations, and one is not aware of breathing this gas until sufficient has been absorbed to produce its typical physiological effects. It irritates the nose and throat in concentrations as low as 0.00038 mg. per liter (1:30,000,000), and causes irritation of the lower respiratory tract at a concentration of 0.0005 mg. per liter. A concentration of 0.65 mg. per liter is lethal on 30 minutes' exposure, while the lethal concentration for 10 minutes' exposure is 3.0 mg. per liter.

Like diphenylchlorarsine, diphenylaminechlorarsine is most effective when disseminated as a smoke, but when atomized, either by explosion or distillation, it readily penetrates the gas-mask canister unless fitted with the most efficient type of dust filter. Such filters have been developed by all modern armies but they always increase the breathing resistance of the canister and add to the difficulty of securing adequate protection.

As diphenylaminechlorarsine appears to be fully equal to diphenylchlorarsine and is much easier to make, it bids fair to remain as the standard respiratory-irritant compound, at least until it is replaced by a more effective one.

In addition to its value as a chemical-warfare agent, diphenylaminechlorarsine has proved to be very effective in suppressing riots and civil disturbances of a more serious character. For this purpose, it is usually mixed with tear gas (chloracetophenone) and loaded in hand grenades which function by progressive burning and distill off the irritant compound in its most effective form.

215

Phenyldichlorarsine ($C_6H_5AsCl_2$)

German: "Blue Cross No. 1"; French: "Sternite"

This compound is primarily a toxic lung injurant and is therefore treated in Chap. VII, page 165. In addition to its lung-injurant effect, however, it also exerts a considerable respiratory-irritant action, and for that reason, was used by the Germans in "Blue Cross 1" shell in mixture with, and as a solvent for, diphenylcyanarsine.

As phenyldichlorarsine was not used alone during the war, there is no war data available as to its effectiveness by itself. When mixed with diphenylchlorarsine or diphenylcyanarsine, in approximately equal proportions, as it was used in the war, the mixture appears to have a more irritating and toxic effect than either of the latter compounds when used alone. The 50–50 mixture produces toxic smokes similar in character to those produced by pure diphenylchlorarsine, but somewhat denser and slightly less penetrating as regards the gas mask.

Because of its high toxicity and not inconsiderable vesicant effect, in addition to its respiratory-irritant action, phenyldichlorarsine is to be ranked among the most valuable of the World War gases.

Ethyldichlorarsine ($C_2H_5AsCl_2$)

German: "Dick"

This compound is also primarily a toxic lung injurant and has been treated as such in Chap. VII. It is also a rather powerful respiratory irritant. A concentration as low as 0.0038 mg. per liter (1:1,900,000) produces a slight irritation of the throat; 0.0125 mg. per liter (1:570,000) strongly irritates the nose and throat and produces a burning sensation in the chest which persists for about an hour after exposure ceases.

Ethyldichlorarsine was introduced by the Germans in an attempt to produce a quick-acting nonpersistent vesicant and was first called "Yellow Cross 1." It was soon found, however, that it was not very effective as a vesicant, but proved to be highly toxic and its classification was changed to "Green Cross 3." It was thereafter used primarily as a lung-injurant agent.

Its combined toxic, irritant, and vesicant effects, together with its low persistency and quick action make it a valuable war gas for offensive use.

Ethyldibromarsine

This compound is the bromine analogue of ethyldichlorarsine and its properties are almost identical therewith. It was used in the war only as a mixture with ethyldichlorarsine in "Green Cross 3" shell and data

216

as to its effectiveness alone are lacking. From its chemical structure, it should be slightly more powerful than the chloro-compound, but as bromine compounds usually attack iron and steel, any such advantage would be more than offset by the disadvantage of its corrosive properties. The reason for its use in the war is not apparent.

COMPARATIVE EFFECTIVENESS OF RESPIRATORY IRRITANTS

The effectiveness of the respiratory irritants depends primarily upon their minimum effective concentrations, since such concentrations are generally sufficient to incapacitate men for the period during which the irritants are effective. Accordingly, the lower the minimum effective concentration, the greater the effectiveness of the respiratory-irritant agent. On this basis, the foregoing respiratory irritants are arranged below in descending order of their effectiveness.

Agent	Minimum effective concentration	
	Milligrams per liter	Parts per million
Diphenylcyanarsine	0.00020	1:50,000,000
Diphenylaminechlorarsine	0.00038	1:30,000,000
Diphenylchlorarsine	0.00043	1:25,000,000
Phenyldichlorarsine	0.00500	1:2,000,000
Ethyldichlorarsine	0.00716	1:1,000,000
Ethyldibromarsine	0.01080	1:1,000,000
Ethylcarbazol	0.01596	1:500,000

USE OF RESPIRATORY IRRITANTS IN THE WORLD WAR

Based upon the total amount used in battle, the respiratory irritants constitute the third largest group of chemical agents used in the war. The Germans loaded no less than 14,000,000 Blue Cross shells, of which only a very small part remained on hand at the time of the Armistice. It is estimated that a total of 6,500 tons of respiratory irritants were used in the war and produced 20,000 casualties, among which the deaths were negligible. On the basis of casualties, therefore, it required 650 lb. of respiratory irritants to produce one casualty, as compared to 230 lb. of lung injurants and 60 lb. of vesicants per casualty. However, the tactical value of the respiratory irritants was far greater than simply their casualty value, as they were certainly very effective in counter battery fire and for general harassment of troops. Also they undoubtedly helped to secure a far larger number of lung-injurant casualties by penetrating the mask and causing its removal in the presence of lung-injurant gas concentrations. All in all, the respiratory agents played a major

217

role in the last year of gas warfare; while they were not used in their most effective form technically, it cannot be said that they were not successful tactically.

FUTURE OF RESPIRATORY IRRITANTS

The future of the respiratory irritants is somewhat difficult to estimate. The experimental work done by the Allies toward the end of, and since, the World War showed conclusively that these compounds are tremendously effective when thermally distilled and disseminated as toxic smokes; while all modern masks contain special filters for protecting against these smokes, the protection is only relative and greatly adds to the breathing resistance of the mask. All things considered, it is believed that these compounds are destined to play an important part in gas warfare of the future.

For a summary of the principal properties of the respiratory irritants, see Table IV.

SUMMARY OF GASES

We have now completed a survey of the 38 compounds which constitute the entire group of World War toxic agents. For convenience of reference, a consolidated list of these compounds is given below, arranged in groups by physiological classification, in order of their chronological appearance (of the group) in the war, as treated in the foregoing chapters.

I. Lacrimators

Simple

1. Ethylbromacetate.
2. Xylyl bromide.
3. Benzyl bromide.
4. Brommethylethyl ketone.
5. Ethyliodoacetate.*
6. Benzyl iodide.
7. Brombenzyl cyanide.*
8. Chloracetophenone.*

Toxic

9. Chloracetone.
10. Bromacetone.*
11. Iodoacetone.
12. Acrolein.

II. Lung Injurants

Simple

1. Chlorine.*
2. Methylsulfuryl chloride.
3. Ethylsulfuryl chloride.
4. Monochlormethylchloroformate.

5. Dimethyl sulfate.
6. Perchlormethylmercaptan.
7. Phosgene.*
8. Trichlormethylchloroformate.*
9. Chlorpicrin.*
10. Phenylcarbylamine chloride.
11. Dichlormethyl ether.
12. Dibrommethyl ether.

Toxic

13. Phenyldichlorarsine.
14. Ethyldichlorarsine.*
15. Phenyldibromarsine.

III. Systemic Toxics

1. Hydrocyanic acid.
2. Cyanogen bromide.
3. Cyanogen chloride.

IV. Vesicants

1. Dichlorethyl sulfide.*
2. Chlorvinyldichlorarsine.
3. Methyldichlorarsine.
4. Dibromethyl sulfide.

V. Respiratory Irritants

1. Diphenylchlorarsine.*
2. Diphenylcyanarsine.*
3. Ethylcarbazol.
4. Diphenylaminechlorarsine.

The 38 compounds listed above were selected from over 3,000 substances which were investigated to determine their value in chemical warfare, but only a small number, marked with an asterisk (*), achieved any noteworthy results in the war. The few really successful compounds, however, produced such astonishing results as to change the whole character of modern warfare (see Chap. XXIV).

Even these successful agents were not used efficiently so as to really develop their full possibilities. Much work has been done in the principal countries since the war to develop more effective ways and means of using the successful World War agents, and great progress has been made in this field. Aside from perfecting the various means of projecting chemicals used in the war, great stress has been laid upon developing effective means of dispersing chemicals from airplanes. This new development bids fair to become one of the most formidable weapons of the future, the ultimate effect of which no man can safely predict.

In addition to increasing the effectiveness of the World War agents, all nations have continued research to find still more powerful compounds for chemical warfare. Necessarily, the results of this research are kept

profound secrets and nothing has been published concerning the progress made in this field except sensational articles in popular magazines and newspapers, which are not only grossly exaggerated, but are utterly unreliable. Hardly a month passes but the public is apprised under lurid headlines of some new supergas a few hundred pounds of which dropped from airplanes could destroy New York. These startling announcements are invariably the figments of the imaginations of sensation writers who really have no technical or professional knowledge of chemical warfare, and, when their statements are analyzed, they are found to be without the slightest foundation in fact.

While these press reports of supergases are not to be taken seriously, it should be borne in mind that industrial research is constantly producing chemical compounds of ever increasing physiological power. We have seen in our survey of the World War chemical agents how the effective strengths of these agents progressively increased as each new one was brought out. Thus, it required a concentration of 5.6 mg. per liter of chlorine to render a man a casualty on 10 minutes' exposure, while a concentration of only 0.0002 mg. per liter of diphenylcyanarsine would cause a casualty on a 1-minute exposure. It was also stated that the respiratory irritant agents are effective in the ratio of 1:35,000,000 of body weight. This was considered in the war as the extreme limit of effectiveness in low concentrations. Since the war, however, chemicals have been discovered which are effective in far smaller doses—now in the order of 1:1,000,000,000 of body weight. Thus, 1 oz. of irradiated ergosterol, the new cure for rickets, will produce the same effect on the human body as 6 tons of cod liver oil! When we remember that one tablespoonful is the normal dose of cod liver oil, we can readily appreciate how tremendously powerful is this new drug and what vast progress has been made in this field in the few years that have elapsed since the war. As General Hartley says:

> Scientists are making very rapid advances, and many of these will have a direct bearing on the next war. It is absolutely essential to make adequate provision to continue research on gas warfare problems, as otherwise all preparations for defence may prove valueless. . . . Such research can only be made effective by the closest sympathy and cooperation between soldiers and scientists, and unless their cooperation is much closer than it was before the late war, there will be little chance of success. It is for the scientists to explore the possibilities and to develop such as are thought likely to be of value, and for the soldiers to apply the results to their investigation of war problems.

CHAPTER XI

SMOKE AGENTS

CLASSIFICATION

Smoke is the second member of the tripartite chemical arm. From a chemical-warfare viewpoint, smoke is a concentration of exceedingly minute solid or liquid particles suspended in the air. Its purpose is to obscure the vision of the enemy or to screen friendly troops and terrain from enemy observation. Its mission is thus essentially defensive and in this respect is directly opposite to that of gas, for, while gas disables and kills men, smoke protects them by a sheltering mantle of obscurity.

Tactically, we distinguish two kinds of smoke, depending on how it is placed with respect to enemy or friendly troops. A smoke cloud laid close to an enemy for the purpose of blinding him, or at least greatly restricting observation and thus crippling his fighting power, is termed a *blanketing* cloud; a smoke cloud generated close to friendly troops to conceal and protect them from the sight and aimed fire of the enemy, is called a *screening* cloud.

Since the special group of *toxic* smokes are employed like gases for their physiological effects and not for their incidental obscuring powers, it is more logical to consider them as translucent gases and they are so treated in Chap. X. When the simple term "smoke" is used, it will be understood as referring only to harmless obscuring smoke.

Physically, we distinguish two general types of smoke, according to whether it consists of (1) solid particles or (2) liquid particles. The first type comprises the smokes of combustion, while the second comprises the fogs and mists produced by chemical reactions not involving combustion. Each type may be used either for blanketing or screening, so this physical classification has no tactical significance.

HISTORICAL

As with gas, the methodical planned use of smoke in battle was a development of the World War. History does record sporadic attempts to use smoke tactically in combat, as when, in 1700, King Charles XII of Sweden crossed the Dvina River in the face of the opposing Polish-Saxon army under the protection of a smoke screen generated by burning large quantities of damp straw. But the results of such early, isolated inci-
221
dents were always too uncertain to justify the adoption of smoke as a recognized agency of warfare.

As a matter of fact, for a century prior to the World War the dense clouds of smoke generated by the increasing quantities of black powder used in battle had been a growing nuisance. They obscured the field of vision, interfered with the aiming and firing of weapons, and hampered the movement and maneuver of troops. By the time of American Civil War, this had become such a formidable problem as to force the invention of smokeless powder in order to restore visibility to the field of battle.

Because smoke had so long been regarded as a tactical handicap to land warfare, development of methods for its artificial generation for military purposes prior to the World War had been constantly neglected. Actually, the first experiments in this direction were made under naval auspices, a fact testifying to the importance of concealment in naval tactics.

Two methods were employed to generate smoke screens at sea. One, used by the British and American navies, was the simple expedient of limiting the admission of air to fires under ships' boilers, so that, owing to incomplete combustion of the fuel, a dense black smoke issued from the funnels. This was done as early as August, 1913, in the course of United States Navy maneuvers off Long Island.

The second method was to produce a white smoke by the reaction of certain chemicals, such as sulfur trioxide and chlorsulfonic acid, in special generators placed on the aft deck of the ship. The German Navy made experiments with such chemical-smoke producers as early as 1906 to 1909.

According to Dr. Hanslian during the World War the German Navy used smoke screens with great success on several cruisers in 1915, particularly in the battle of Jutland in 1916, when smoke was generated from sulfur trioxide and chlorsulfonic acid on board ship and from floating containers. During the summer of 1916, the Austrian fleet also successfully covered its retreat from the French fleet in the Mediterranean by the skillful use of a smoke screen. The regularly planned tactical use of smoke on land commenced in the summer of 1915, closely coinciding with the introduction of gas warfare.

Without doubt, the gas-cloud method of attack directed attention to the possibilities of smoke for screening parts of the battlefield from enemy observation. The dense clouds produced in damp weather by the release of chlorine served to mask the advance of the German infantry which followed behind them, to demonstrate clearly the tactical advantage of concealment during the offensive.

The British were the first to use smoke clouds artificially generated from special apparatus so as to mask their gas attacks and lead the
222
Germans to believe a gas attack was being put over where actually no gas was used. In such operations the British were able to advance unmasked behind the harmless smoke while the Germans, fearing gas, were put to the disadvantage of wearing masks. Smoke was also used for other deceptive purposes such as to draw wasteful artillery fire on unoccupied sectors by generating a smoke screen to indicate that an attack was imminent. The Germans soon adopted these same tactics and in turn used them effectively.

The first special smoke device used on land during the war was the British smoke pot containing a mixture of pitch, tallow, black powder, and saltpeter, which was introduced in July, 1915. The first large-scale smoke operation occurred during the attack of the Canadians against Messines Ridge on Sept. 20, 1915, where several thousand smoke shell were fired from trench mortars.

During the latter part of 1915 and in 1916, the use of smoke extended rapidly throughout all the principal belligerent armies. Not only were special smoke generators employed by each, but smoke fillings were loaded into every form of projectile. By the end of 1916 smoke was a standard filling in hand and rifle grenades, trench-mortar bombs, artillery shell, and even aviation bombs, and smoke tactics contributed to the successes of both sides in many important battles.

By the fall of 1917, the tactical use of smoke on the Western Front had become so well established that General Pershing cabled the War Department on Nov. 3, 1917, asking that large quantities of phosphorus be quickly manufactured for filling smoke ammunition for the American Army.

Following are some outstanding examples of successful large-scale tactical use of smoke during the World War.

The capture of the German position on the edge of the Oppy Forest by the 15th British Infantry Brigade on June 23, 1917, under cover of a smoke screen erected with artillery and trench-mortar smoke shell, succeeded with few losses after previous assaults without smoke had failed.

The maneuvers of the 9th and 29th British Divisions south of Meteran on Aug. 25, 1918, and the advance of the 1st, 2d, and 3d Canadian Battalions, at Vis en Artois sector, were conducted with great success by the aid of smoke. In both cases, under the cover of a dense smoke screen, the German Front was penetrated and from 300 to 500 prisoners brought in.

In crossing rivers, constructing bridges, and establishing bridge heads, smoke was frequently employed with excellent results as in the following instances:

The Austrian crossing of the Piave from Vidor to San Giovanni on June 15, 1918, was, in the opinion of eyewitnesses, successfully made
223
chiefly because of a smoke screen so dense that it was impossible for the excellently located Italian machine-gun flanking units to see.

The success with which the Germans in 1918 screened with smoke their preparations for the transportation of troops over the Marne at Dormans Vincelles-Vernouil was most noteworthy.

Smoke was also successfully employed in a number of tank attacks by the Allies of which the following are outstanding examples:

In the battle at Malmaison, October, 1917, a smoke screen including in part natural mist, concealed the majority of the French tanks so that the German Artillery had little effect against them and their losses were correspondingly small.

The British tank attack at Cambrai on Nov. 20, 1917, was also favored by dense morning mist that was increased by intensive fire of smoke shell by the British Artillery. In this attack 350 British tanks moved forward in several waves and completely broke through the German defenses.

French army officers report that in the battle of Metz, June 9–12, 1918, the French counterattack against the right flank of the German advance, made with four divisions with 12 tank sections and two regiments of horse artillery, was able to surprise the Germans and force them to retreat because of the protection afforded the counterattack by smoke.

By the fall of 1918 the planned use of artillery smoke shell by the French had become normal. On Sept. 2, 1918, in the combats at Somey and Soissons, three battalions of light tanks advanced behind a rolling-smoke barrage; despite German heavy standing barrages and a well-organized tank defense, the German lines were broken and 1½ kilometers of ground gained. In the hard fighting of the French Fourth Army in 1918 in the Champagne, the loss in tanks from artillery fire was greatly reduced by the general use of artillery smoke shell.

Concerning the penetration of the German front by the British at Amiens, on Aug. 8, 1918, during which 330 tanks, most of them heavy, pushed through the German lines by surprise, General Fuller emphasizes that: "The only artificial element in this successful attack was the ordinary smoke barrage inserted into our artillery plan, which fire increased the haziness of the early morning hour and the confusion." In the battle of Cambrai-St. Quentin, Sept. 27 to Oct. 9, 1918, tanks of the Ninth Tank Battalion made repeatedly successful use of smoke screens produced from the exhausts of their own engines and thus prevented losses from the fire of German close-range guns.

During the German drives in the spring and summer of 1918, smoke shell were used in large quantities to blind observation posts and strong points of resistance. Also in the German retreats in the fall of 1918, smoke was used very generally to cover withdrawal from covering posi-

224

tions, notably after the retreat from the Marne in 1918 and from the hill to the east of Beaumont Hammel in the same year. On both of these latter occasions, by developing dense smoke screens, the Germans were able to escape with small losses.

Smoke was also widely employed by the British and by our own gas troops in conjunction with their gas attacks. In smoke operations the British Special (Gas) Brigade used over 40,000 4-in. Stokes smoke bombs, and in one such operation, just north of Armentières on Sept. 26, 1918, 15,000 smoke candles were lighted by a single company.

Although drop bombs filled with white phosphorus were used to some extent in the World War, the tactical employment of smoke by airplanes was not developed to any appreciable degree.

On the whole, the tactical use of smoke during the World War lagged behind the tactical use of gas. It is safe to say the possibilities of the planned use of smoke in battle were only beginning to be realized at the close of the war.

It is a fact that, while the Germans took and held the initiative in the use of gas throughout the World War, the Allies excelled the Germans in the use of smoke, both from a qualitative and quantitative standpoint. This is explained by the Germans as owing to the lack of phosphorus in Germany and its availability and employment in enormous quantities by the Allies.

Since phosphorus was lacking in Germany and Austria, these countries had to resort to sulfur trioxide and other smoke-producing acids which were inferior to phosphorus. Nevertheless, the Central Powers made extensive and generally effective use of smoke during the last two years of the war.

Since the war distinct progress in the development of smoke technique and tactics has been made, particularly in the United States, Great Britain, and Germany. Not only have the World War means of using smoke been greatly improved, but an entirely new method of laying smoke screens by spraying from airplanes has been developed in all important armies.

NATURE OF SMOKE

We have already pointed out that the military term "smoke" comprehends two basically different phenomena: (1) an aerial concentration of minute *solid* particles resulting from combustion, and (2) an aerial concentration of minute *liquid* particles resulting from chemical reactions not involving combustion. Neither of these phenomena can be scientifically classified into any of the three standard physical states of matter. On the contrary, both are "dispersed" forms of matter, known as *colloidal* suspensions or solutions.

225

The colloidal state of matter is characterized by an intimate admixture of at least two phases—the dispersed phase and the dispersion medium. by a *dispersion* of this kind is meant the regular distribution of one substance into another in such a way that the individual particles of the one substance are suspended separately from each other in the second substance—in this case, the air. In this sense smoke is to be regarded as a two-phase colloid whose dispersion medium (air) is in the gaseous state and whose dispersed phase is a *solid* or a *liquid*. So-called *colloidal* solutions of this kind have physical and chemical behavior entirely different from normal solutions (such as sugar in water), in that the size of the particles may vary within certain limits without causing the solution to lose its colloidal character.

The particles of a smoke or fog vary in size from those just large enough to be perceived by the unaided eye to those that approach the size of single molecules. In general, smoke particles are intermediate in size between dust particles (10^{-4} cm.) and gas particles (10^{-7} cm.) and average about 10^{-5} cm. in diameter. As a rule, the smaller the particles in a given quantity of smoke, the greater is their obscuring power; hence the aim is to generate a smoke consisting of the maximum number of particles of minimum size.

Since smoke is a suspension of minute solid or liquid particles, it is not a true gas and does not follow the law of gaseous diffusion. However, owing to the collisions of the molecules of air with the smoke particles, the latter exhibit Brownian movements as the result of which they gradually diffuse and spread. Because of their greater mass and inertia and the resistance of the air, the larger particles of smoke diffuse more slowly than the smaller ones. But, compared with the effects of wind and convection currents, diffusion plays an almost negligible part in the dispersion of smokes; even in very dense smokes, the weight of the smoke particles is only a small fraction of 1 per cent of the weight of the air it occupies, so that a smoke cloud is distinguished from the surrounding atmosphere only by the small amount of suspended foreign material.

If smoke is released in warm air, it will rise as the warm air expands, *i.e.*, becomes lighter than the surrounding air and rises. If released in cold air, where these upward convection currents are absent, the smoke will spread out in a horizontal layer and cling to the ground. The movement of the cloud is therefore merely the movement of the air, which accounts for the characteristic behavior of smoke clouds.

Since floating smoke particles are themselves heavier than air they gradually fall, although at a very slow rate that varies with the size of the particles. Thus, according to Grey and Patterson (31) a smoke particle having a diameter of 10^{-4} cm. (the most common size of smoke

226

particles) falls about 0.071 in. per minute, which is so slow as to be negligible for practical purposes.

In the same manner as particles in colloidal solution, smoke particles tend to unite and increase in size by cohesion and coalescence as they come in contact with each other by Brownian movements or air currents. This agglomeration takes place much more rapidly in a dense than in a thin smoke. When the smoke particles are completely dry, agglomeration is not observed; but when the particles are liquid, or of a deliquescent solid with condensed surface moisture, this is more pronounced. The increase in the number and size of the larger at the expense of the smaller particles increases the rate of settling and decreases the concentration of the cloud. Also, the smaller smoke particles vaporize more rapidly because their surfaces are greater in proportion to their weight. From the foregoing it follows that a smoke is most stable when its particles are of the minimum size and consist of a dry nondeliquescent solid material.

OBSCURING POWER

Smoke obscures visibility by obstructing the rays of light and diffracting them by reflection from the individual smoke particles. As the obstruction and diffraction of the light rays is dependent primarily upon the number of smoke particles in a given volume, a maximum number of the minimum-size particles produces the greatest obscuration.

The tactical value of a smoke is measured by its power to obscure objects behind it. The term for such measurement is T.O.P. (total obscuring power). The T.O.P. of any smoke is the product of (1) the volume produced per unit weight of material used and (2) the density of concentration. The *density* of a smoke is the reciprocal of the smoke layer (in feet) necessary to obscure the filament of a 40-watt Mazda lamp, and a cloud of unit density is one of which a 1-ft. vertical layer will just obscure the filament. If the volume of smoke per unit weight of inert smoke material is expressed in cubic feet per pound and the density in reciprocal feet, the unit of T.O.P. is square feet per pound. The T.O.P. of a smoke is therefore the area in square feet covered by the smoke from 1 lb. of smoke-producing material, spread out in a layer of such thickness and density that it will exactly obscure the filament of a standard 40-watt lamp.

Factors Affecting T.O.P.—The three factors that most affect the T.O.P. of a smoke are (1) rate of settling, (2) humidity, and (3) temperature.

By rate of settling is meant the velocity with which the smoke particles fall to the ground under the influence of gravity. This increases with the size and density of the smoke particle. For particles larger

227

than 10^{-4} cm. (the most common size), Stokes law gives for the rate of settling (in air of spheres of unit density) a velocity

$$V = 3 \times 10^{-3} \text{ cm. per second}$$

This law does not hold accurately for particles smaller than 10^{-4} cm., the steady velocity of fall here being greater than indicated by the law. But since convection currents are usually greater than the rate of settling

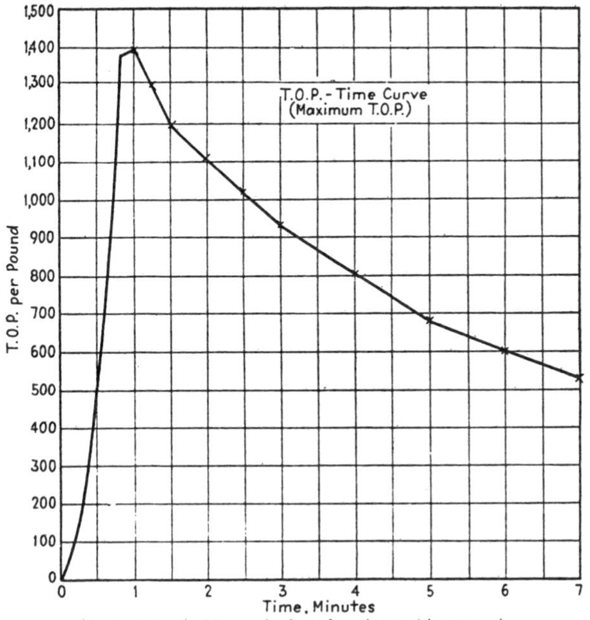

CHART XV.—B. M. standard smoke mixture (time curve).

of particles 10^{-4} cm. in diameter (11 cm. per hour), it is evident that such particles would never settle in ordinary atmosphere. Hence, except in very quiet air, smoke particles must grow to the order of 10^{-3} cm. before appreciable settling can occur. In quiet air, after some time, particles of order 10^{-4} cm. may settle out in appreciable quantities, but particles of order 10^{-5} cm. are probably precipitated only as a result of diffusion and convection (31).

Chart XV shows the relation between T.O.P. and elapsed *time* after initial formation of a standard smoke, due to settling out of the smoke

228

particles. Chart XVI shows the effect of *humidity* on the T.O.P. of a

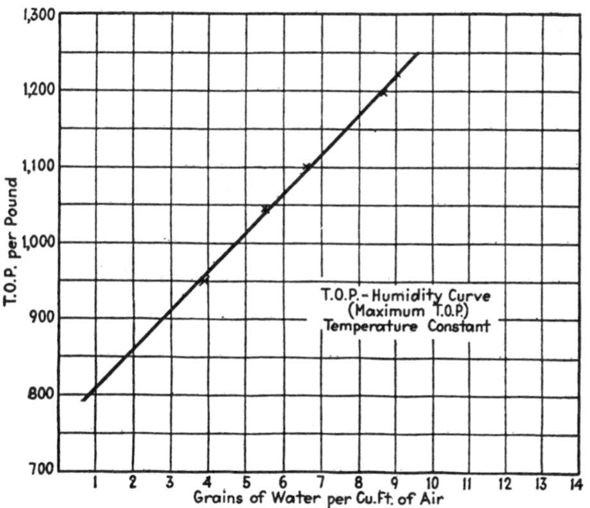

CHART XVI.—B. M. standard smoke mixture (humidity curve).

standard smoke, temperature being constant. Chart XVII shows the effect of *temperature* on the T.O.P. of a standard smoke mixture, humidity remaining constant.

From Chart XV it will be observed that T.O.P. at first sharply increases and then progressively decreases with elapsed time after generation of the smoke; Chart XVI shows that T.O.P. varies directly with humidity; Chart XVII shows that T.O.P. varies inversely with temperature.

These charts indicate typical relations between T.O.P. and the factors that principally affect it. While these relations apply in general to all smokes, there are some notable exceptions; the T.O.P. of phosphorus, *e.g.*, is unaffected by temperature, and the T.O.P. of ammonium chloride is unaffected by humidity. However, these are not important, for, while there are a few exceptions to the T.O.P.-temperature law shown in Chart XVII, ammonium chloride and carbon smokes (such as those generated by crude oil) are the only smokes that depart from the T.O.P.-humidity law, shown in Chart XVI.

Another useful measure for comparing the obscuring values of smokes is the so-called *standard smoke*, defined as one of such density that a

229

25-candle-power electric light is just invisible through a layer of smoke 100 ft. thick.

PRINCIPLES OF SMOKE PRODUCTION

A satisfactory smoke cloud requires, in the first place, density; a relatively thin layer of the smoke must completely obscure any object behind it. In the second place, the cloud must be inherently stable; it must not quickly dissipate or dilute, nor must it settle out. Third, the

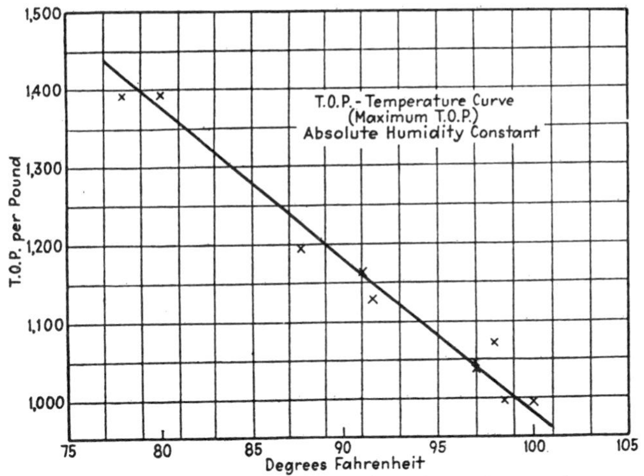

CHART XVII.—B. M. standard smoke mixture (temperature curve).

cloud must easily be produced without complicated apparatus or difficulties of manipulation. Finally, the materials required for producing the cloud must be readily available, easy of transportation, and not dangerous to handle.

Any smoke fulfilling these requirements must be composed of extremely small liquid or solid particles dispersed in the air. The individual particles must be large enough to disperse and diffuse light; but otherwise the smaller the particles, the greater the obscuring power for a given concentration of smoke in air and the more stable the smoke. The diffusing power of a given particle is probably not greatly influenced by its size, provided the particle is large enough to diffuse light at all. The problem of smoke formation, therefore, reduces itself to the problem of producing a suspension of extremely small particles of the smoke-forming substance in air. Successful smoke production depends upon appreciation and application of the following generalization.

230

Every particle of liquid, or solid, in contact with a gas is surrounded by a film of gas closely adhering to it and capable of removal or penetration only by the projection of another solid or liquid particle through it. This film serves as an effective insulator, separating the particle from the gas around it, and breaking down only through mechanical rupture. When such a particle travels through the gas, the film moves with it; when the gas moves past the particle, the film is distorted and made thin, but in no case completely removed. The protective action of this film upon the solid or liquid surface can never be lost sight of if the phenomena of cloud and smoke formation are to be appreciated.

Such particles of solid or liquid suspended in gas do not diffuse. This fact in connection with the insulating power of the gas film around them makes the removal of them from the gas extremely difficult. For example, gas containing a small amount of HCl can be washed free from the acid by bubbling through water, even though the rate of bubbling be very high. On the other hand, a gas containing a fume of NH_4Cl can be bubbled through water almost indefinitely without appreciable removal of the fume. The HCl being a gas, diffuses with extreme rapidity through the stationary film of air on the surface of the water in contact with the bubbles and in this way is effectively removed, and the solid particles incapable of diffusion pass through unabsorbed.

Such small suspended particles of either liquid or solid have also practically no tendency to coalesce. Even should two such particles tend to approach each other, they are held apart by the cushion or buffer effect of the air films around them. If, however, the particles be large, two particles approaching each other may have sufficient momentum to penetrate mechanically the surrounding gas films and in this way come together. Particles large enough to evidence this phenomenon to any considerable degree are too coarse to be described as smokes or fumes.

A smoke or fume, once formed, can undergo growth of the particles only through condensation of gaseous or vapor components in the air around them. Thus, a particle of NH_4Cl can grow only by the diffusion into it through the gas film surrounding it of gaseous NH_3 and HCl. A particle of water in a fog grows only by the infusion of atmospheric water vapor through the air film surrounding the drop. In other words, in order to build up a particle of smoke or fume, that particle must be formed by the condensation of gaseous components. It cannot be produced from liquid or solid reagents.

In illustration, a fume of NH_4Cl is formed only by the interaction of the vapors of its components; SO_3 cannot be absorbed by water because it reacts with the water vapor above the liquid surface to form a fog of sulfuric acid, the water vapor being continually replenished as fast as it is exhausted by evaporation of the water and diffusion of the water vapor

231

through the stationary film of air about the liquid; and HCl can be readily absorbed by aqueous ammonia, because of formation of a fog by interaction with the ammonia vapor from the solution. Only substances which volatilize before burning, such as soft coal, phosphorus, and the like, produce a cloud or smoke upon combustion.

To produce a smoke composed of particles of suitable minuteness, it is necessary that the components from which the smoke is formed be diluted with some inert gas before condensation. If this precaution is not observed, the particle of smoke initially formed will grow with extreme rapidity, owing to further condensation of its components, so that a large particle results. Only when the particle first formed finds the space around it depleted of its components, does it cease to grow. It is therefore self-evident that to produce a high-grade smoke, a diluted gas must be employed.

One of the most striking illustrations of this is the fact that phosphorus burned in a large excess of air, with good circulation, produces an extremely stable smoke; in insufficient air, with poor circulation, the smoke settles rapidly and has little obscuring power. Every smoke thus far studied shows very markedly the beneficial effect of dilution, even up to a dilution of several hundred times. Many reacting gases when diluted with 100 times their volume of air show from 20 to 50 times the T.O.P. obtained when the gases are diluted with but two or three volumes of air.

In general, dilution is beneficial up to a point where the reaction begins to be incomplete. This occurs much sooner when a large number of molecules must participate in the reaction than when the reaction is a simple one. For example, the first step of the reaction between chlorine and ammonia is $3Cl_2 + 2NH_3 = 6HCl + N_2$; the rate of this fifth-order reaction drops off as the fifth power of the concentration, and therefore begins to be complete before the full beneficial effects of dilution can be realized. On the other hand, HCl and NH_3 can be diluted to a very high degree without preventing complete reaction, and therefore the obscuring power per pound can be made three times as great as that for ammonia and chlorine, although the substances formed are exactly the same.

If the smoke consists of a nonvolatile solid, it makes practically no difference how the diluent air is distributed between the two reacting bases, any method of dilution being about equally effective in the production of a larger number of small particles. On the other hand, if there is the possibility of forming at any stage of the process liquid drops that grow in the presence of an excess of either component or if there is the possibility of forming two different compounds, the method of dilution becomes quite important and the best method must be determined by a study of the reaction in question.

232

In order that a smoke shall have reasonable stability, it must be nonvolatile, or nearly so. A smoke produced by the condensation of HCl and water vapor clears up rapidly in ordinary air, owing to complete evaporation of the mixture. The same is true of a smoke of ammonium carbonate and similar substances. Such smokes will also frequently block out the particles growing by the following mechanism; a small particle has a higher vapor pressure than a large one; such a small particle tends, therefore, to evaporate and to diffuse through the stationary air films surrounding it, condensing later upon some larger particle. This results in the disappearance of the smaller particles and growth of the larger ones. Thus, $SnCl_4$ reacts with water vapor to make a fog, consisting of a mixture of particles of stannic hydrate and a solution of HCl in water; this fog is poor because the stannic liquid particles rapidly and completely evaporate in unsaturated air. The use of ammonia in the production of this fog greatly improves it by introducing stable ammonium chloride particles.

Other things being equal, liquid particles are poorer than solid particles because they tend to condense into themselves any one of their components that may be present in excess, while a solid particle will only condense in a very small excess of one component before ceasing to grow. For example, a fume formed from HCl and water vapor will condense either water vapor or HCl almost indefinitely, whereas one of ammonium chloride will not grow in the presence of either component. Deliquescent solids are, of course, open to the same objection, since they continue to absorb moisture and grow to small drops of saturated solution.

SUBSTANCES USED AS SMOKE AGENTS

The substances that have been successfully used as smoke agents fall into five main groups, *viz.*, smokes that owe their obscuring power to: (I) particles of colloidal *carbon* suspended in air; (II) particles of phosphoric acid; (III) sulfuric acid; (IV) hydrochloric acid; and (V) zinc chloride.

Each of these groups appeared about in the order named and, except for phosphorus (the best of all smoke producers), each was an improvement upon its predecessor.

Group I

Crude Oil (CO)

The earliest modern method of producing artificial smoke was by the incomplete combustion of the crude-oil fuel under the boilers of naval vessels, especially destroyers. Crude-oil smoke was used by the Germans in the Battle of Jutland (1915) to cover a turning movement that enabled the German High Seas Fleet to escape from the pursuing British. It is now used by all navies to erect smoke screens at sea.

233

The oil used for this purpose is the mixture of hydrocarbons known by the trade name of *crude oil.* It is a liquid of 0.8 specific gravity which solidifies at −20°C. (−3°F.) and boils at 200°C. (392°F.). When incompletely burned it evolves a dense black smoke that derives its opacity from particles of colloidal carbon floating in the air. Oil smoke is slightly suffocating when dense, but has no other deleterious physiological effects. It is one of the few artificial smokes that are not affected by the humidity and is noncorrosive to material.

The smoke produced from crude oil may be generated in three ways:
1. The oil may be evaporated by heat and condensed again in the air to form small droplets. Such smokes are, however, very unstable owing to the vapor pressure of the oil, which causes it to assume the gaseous state with consequent disappearance of the colloidal carbon particles that constitute the smoke.
2. The oil may be only partially burned, the carbon thus separated in solid particles which at first float in the air and form a dense smoke. The solid particles soon coagulate into flakes that quickly settle out and drop to the ground. Such smoke is therefore quickly dissipated and has poor screening value.
3. The best method is a combination of the first two; *i.e.*, there is an imperfect combustion of the oil and at the same time an evaporation of the excess oil. In this case the liquid particles surround the solid particles of carbon and prevent their coagulation into flakes. Such a smoke is grayish black and is far more stable.

Notwithstanding the tendency to clog up the flues by depositing solid carbon therein, all modern navies use this method of producing smoke screens at sea. It requires no special apparatus, is cheap, and can readily generate large screens in a short time. Two ounces of crude oil are required to produce 1,000 cu. ft. of *standard smoke* and the cost is 8 cents; this is therefore the cheapest of all artificial smoke producers.

British Type S Mixture

The first material used in the World War for the generation of artificial smoke on land was the British Type S smoke mixture. This was used as a filling for the first smoke candles, called "Smoke Torch, Mark I, Type S," and consisted of the following ingredients:

	Per Cent by Weight
Potassium Nitrate	45
Sulfur	12
Pitch	30
Borax	9
Glue	4

234

Later in the war these ingredients were somewhat modified for the Smoke Candle, Mark II, Type S-I, to include:

	Per Cent, by Weight
Niter	40
Sulfur	14
Pitch (hard)	29
Borax	8
Coal dust	9

The ingredients were ground, mixed, screened, and, while still in a plastic condition, pressed into a 3-lb. tin container.

These candles burned vigorously for about 3 minutes and generated a large volume of yellowish brown smoke. The obscuring power of the smoke was due principally to the incomplete combustion of the solid carbon particles in the pitch. Its T.O.P. was quite low (460) and its screening properties were unreliable since the smoke had a tendency to rise rapidly, break up, and leave gaps in the screen. Yet the agent was cheap, easily produced from readily available materials, and had good keeping properties. These candles were therefore used in large quantities through the war by both the British and American armies.

Group II

White Phosphorus (WP)

One of the earliest and by far the most efficient material used in the war for generating artificial smoke was phosphorus. This element exists in two allotropic forms: white phosphorus and red phosphorus. White phosphorus, the normal and common form, was discovered in 1669 by the German chemist, Brand, who noted that it is spontaneously inflammable at ordinary temperatures and burns with a dense white smoke. While both white and red phosphorus were used in the war, white phosphorus was by far the most effective and the most widely employed and is the form now generally denoted by the word *phosphorus*.

Phosphorus is produced on a large scale in industry by heating phosphate rock (calcium phosphate) in an electric furnace. Such phosphates exist in enormous quantities in the United States and North Africa.

White phosphorus is formed by quickly cooling the vapors distilled from the phosphate rock. When pure it is a waxy solid, of 1.8 specific gravity, which melts at 44°C. (111°F.) and boils at 287°C. (549°F.). It is chemically very active and combines readily with oxygen in the air, even at room temperature. The greater the surface exposed to the air, the more rapid is the reaction. Upon oxidation the phosphorus becomes luminous and in a few minutes bursts into vigorous flames that can only be quenched by complete submersion in water. It must therefore be

235

stored and worked entirely under water. White phosphorus is insoluble in water but readily soluble in fats and in carbon bisulfide.

Red phosphorus is produced by heating white phosphorus to a temperature of from 250° to 300°C., out of contact with air, and then dissolving out the small traces of unchanged white phosphorus with suitable solvents. Red phosphorus is a reddish brown amorphous powder, of 2.3 specific gravity, which is chemically much less active than white phosphorus. In contact with air at ordinary temperatures, it remains unchanged for a long time; it does not appreciably dissolve in carbon bisulfide and the ordinary solvents for white phosphorus; it does not become luminous; and it can be heated to 260°C. before it ignites. Its vapors are not toxic as are the vapors of white phosphorus.

Both forms of phosphorus combine with oxygen in the air to form phosphorus pentoxide:

$$4P + 5O_2 = 2P_2O_5$$

The phosphorus pentoxide is then converted by the moisture in the air to phosphoric acid:

$$2P_2O_5 + 6H_2O = 4H_3PO_4$$

Thus 1 lb. of phosphorus combines with 1.33 lb. of oxygen and 0.9 lb. of water to form 3.23 lb. of phosphoric acid, which makes phosphorus the best smoke producer, pound for pound, of any known material. The red phosphorus does not equal white phosphorus for generating smoke and for that reason is seldom used alone, but it has been mixed with white phosphorus in the ratio of 1:2 in artillery and trench-mortar smoke shell.

While the vapors of white phosphorus are exceedingly toxic, these vapors are so quickly oxidized to phosphorus pentoxide and phosphoric acid as to be harmless to men and animals in ordinary field concentrations. There is some difference of opinion as to the physiological effect of phosphorus smoke because of the possibility of the continued presence of phosphorus vapors therein. Extensive field tests, however, have shown no injurious effects from phosphorus smoke under conditions which obtain in the field.

In addition to its smoke value, phosphorus is of tactical importance because of its burning effect upon both personnel and material. In contact with the body, phosphorus produces burns that are slow and difficult to heal; thus the firing of phosphorus against personnel has a psychological value that greatly increases its tactical effectiveness. Against material, however, the incendiary effect of phosphorus is limited, as it ignites only readily combustible materials, so that here it is inferior to thermite and other primarily incendiary materials.

236

The principal disadvantages of phosphorus are: (1) the difficulty of storage and handling; (2) the bright flame produced when burning; and (3) that it is a solid and cannot be sprayed without dissolving in highly inflammable and dangerous solvents. In spite of these drawbacks, phosphorus remains today one of the most efficient smoke-producing materials.

Group III

Sulfuric Trioxide (SO_3)

Sulfuric Anhydride

Next to phosphorus, sulfur trioxide was the best smoke producer used in the war, notwithstanding that it requires humid air to develop its full effect. It is prepared by passing a mixture of sulfur dioxide and oxygen over a catalyst (such as sponge platinum) at a temperature of from 400° to 450°C. It may also be obtained by the catalytic combustion of sulfurous acid in special contact ovens. When pure, sulfur trioxide is a mobile colorless liquid, of 1.92 specific gravity, which boils at 45°C. (113°F.) and freezes at 18°C. (60°F.) into a transparent solid of 2.75 specific gravity. It also polymerizes spontaneously into an asbestoid crystalline mass, $(SO_3)_2$, of 1.97 specific gravity, which melts at 40°C. (104°F.) into the liquid commercial product. On contact with the air it fumes vigorously and throws off dense white clouds composed of minute droplets of sulfurous and sulfuric acids.

Sulfur trioxide produces its smoke effect by the formation of fine droplets of sulfurous and sulfuric acids that remain suspended in the air for some time because of their minute size, and then are not volatilized because of the low vapor pressure of these acids. As the SO_3 fumes combine with moisture in the air, concentrated sulfuric acid is formed, which attracts more moisture and tends to become diluted, until finally an equilibrium is established between the moisture in the air and the sulfuric acid droplets, the latter being concentrated in proportion to the humidity of the air. Sulfuric acid is not so hygroscopic as the phosphoric acid formed by burning phosphorus, and the formation of its droplets stops sooner, so that sulfur trioxide smoke is less stable than phosphorus smoke.

Since sulfurous and sulfuric acid are corrosive, the SO_3 smoke has a somewhat irritant effect upon the respiratory organs and the skin. A concentration of even 0.010 mg. per liter causes a hacking cough which is much aggravated in higher concentrations. A concentration of 0.030 mg. per liter completely obscures objects 20 ft. distant. In humid weather sulfur trioxide has an obscuring value equal to 70 per cent of that of phosphorus.

During the war sulfur trioxide was used as a filling for German artillery and trench-mortar smoke shell. Since the war extensive experi-

237

ments have been made in Germany, England, and America in spraying sulfur trioxide and other liquid smoke-producing materials from airplane tanks for the production of smoke screens. Various portable devices have also been invented for evaporating and spraying SO^3 to form smoke concentrations on the ground.

Oleum ($SO_3 + H_2SO_4$)

Fuming Sulfuric Acid

Oleum is a solution of sulfur trioxide in concentrated sulfuric acid, the proportions of SO_3 varying from 20 to 40 per cent. It is a dense liquid that fumes vigorously on contact with air. During the war, for producing smoke screens on land and sea, the Germans used special smoke generators (*Nebelkalkraketen*), in which oleum was brought in contact with quicklime. In these generators the oleum was permitted to drip on a bed of quicklime, which in a few minutes became red hot from the heat of the reaction (68,600 calories per mol) and quickly evaporated the oleum which continued to drip on it. The smoke thus formed was vigorously emitted in a very finely atomized form, free from large drops.

Oleum was also used in the war by the Americans for generating smoke from airplanes and combat tanks by squirting a small stream of it into the hot exhaust manifolds of the engines. In this way, the engine exhaust heat was used to evaporate the oleum in lieu of the heat chemically generated by quicklime in the German smoke generators.

Experiments with oleum show that its smoke-producing power is due solely to its sulfur trioxide content, the sulfuric acid itself acting only as a solvent. Pure sulfur trioxide is superior as a filling for smoke shell, while oleum gives better results when progressively evaporated by heat.

Chlorsulfonic Acid ($HClSO_3$)

Chemically and as a smoke producer, chlorsulfonic acid is very similar to sulfur trioxide. It is obtained by acting on sulfur trioxide with gaseous hydrochloric acid:

$$SO_3 + HCl = HClSO_3$$

This is a colorless liquid, of 1.77 specific gravity, which boils at 158°C (316°F.) and fumes on contact with air, forming sulfuric and hydrochloric acids:

$$HClSO_3 + H_2O = H_2SO_4 + HCl$$

Chlorsulfonic acid was first used by the Germans, who adopted it as a smoke agent early in the war, using the oleum process of dripping on

238

quicklime. It produces a volatile and not very dense smoke and has now been superseded by other materials.

Sulfuryl Chloride (SO_2Cl_2)

A third smoke-producing substance closely related to sulfur trioxide is sulfuryl chloride. This compound is a colorless extremely pungent liquid, of 1.66 specific gravity, which boils at 70°C. (158°F.) and decomposes on contact with moisture in air to form sulfuric and hydrochloric acids. Its efficiency as a smoke producer is very much lower than the other substances in this group and for that reason was not used alone as a smoke agent. It was, however, extensively employed by the Allies in mixture with certain toxic gases, such as phosgene and chlorpicrin, as a "fumigant" to render the toxic-gas concentrations visible.

Sulfur Trioxide–Chlorsulfonic Acid Mixture ($SO_3 + SO_3HCl$)

American: "FS"

The several disadvantages of titanium tetrachloride led to search for a substitute liquid and finally resulted in the discovery that a mixture consisting of sulfur trioxide and chlorosulfonic acid produced a superior smoke agent.

This mixture, known by the symbol "FS," is a liquid of 1.91 specific gravity, which freezes at −30°C. (−22°F.), and has a T.O.P. of 2,550 as compared to 1,900 for titanium tetrachloride. FS costs only 7.5 cents per pound as compared to 30 cents per pound for FM; it deposits no solid residue on hydrolysis and therefore flows freely from nozzles without clogging the eduction ports. There is no marked difference in the rate of settling of the two smokes, so that they are about equal in persistency.

The only disadvantage of FS is its highly corrosive action on metals and airplane fabrics, although in this respect it appears to be no worse than FM. Because of its all-around superior qualities, FS has been adopted as the standard liquid-smoke agent of the United States Army and Navy.

Group IV

Tin Tetrachloride ($SnCl_4$)

British: "KJ"; French: "Opacite"

As phosphorus was very dangerous to work with and could not be used in liquid form for spraying without extreme hazard to using troops, and since the various SO_3 compounds oxidizing sulfuric acid were very corrosive, much effort was expended toward the end of the war in finding substitute smoke agents free from these disadvantages. This resulted

239

in the introduction of a series of metallic chlorides of which tin tetrachloride was the first.

This compound is obtained by the direct chlorination of metallic tin. It is a liquid of 2.28 specific gravity, which boils at 114°C. (237°F.). It fumes in the air and hydrolyzes into stannic hydroxide:

$$SnCl_4 + 4H_2O = Sn(OH)_4 + 4HCl$$

The smoke thus produced is only one-half as dense as sulfur trioxide smokes, but is less corrosive and far more penetrant to the gas-mask canisters used during the war. For this last reason tin tetrachloride was employed principally in mixtures with phosgene and chlorpicrin to increase the visibility and penetrability of the gas clouds generated therewith. It is very expensive and the scarcity of tin caused other compounds to be substituted toward the end of the war.

Silicon Tetrachloride ($SiCl_4$)

The next metallic chloride used as a smoke agent was silicon tetrachloride. This compound is prepared by heating silicon or silicon carbide with chlorine in an electric furnace. It is a colorless liquid, of 1.52 specific gravity, which boils at 60°C. (140°F.) and fumes strongly on contact with the moisture in the air by which it is hydrolyzed:

$$SiCl_4 + 4H_2O = Si(OH)_4 + 4HCl$$

At a concentration of 0.20 mg. per liter, no further hydrolysis takes place, but an equilibrium seems to be established in which the hydrochloric acid liberated prevents further decomposition. In fact, when the hydrochloric acid becomes too great the above reaction may even be reversed and the amount of smoke actually diminished. If, however, the excess hydrochloric acid is neutralized by reaction with ammonia, hydrolysis of the silicon tetrachloride proceeds smoothly

$$SiCl_4 + 4NH_3 + 4H_2O = Si(OH)_4 + 4NH_4Cl$$

and a dense smoke is obtained. Thus, while the value of silicon tetrachloride alone as a smoke producer is limited, its smoke-generating power with ammonia vapors is five times as great as silicon tetrachloride alone and exceeds even that of phosphorus. Moreover, the smoke thus generated is much less irritant to the respiratory organs.

So closely does this smoke resemble natural fog that, when it was employed by the British in their naval attack on Zeebrugge, the German defending forces thought the smoke coming in from the sea was a natural fog, and the British thus succeeded in approaching the harbor unseen. The so-called *smoke funnels* that the British used in this attack consisted of iron cylinders 2 ft. in diameter, into which gaseous ammonia and

240

silicon tetrachloride were injected, the latter by means of carbon dioxide. The results obtained were so satisfactory that small portable smoke knapsacks, embodying the same method of operation, were also constructed and frequently used with good results in the field.

The only disadvantage of the silicon tetrachloride-ammonia method of generating smoke is its complication, and for this reason other simpler methods of smoke production were developed for field use.

Owing to its comparatively high volatility, silicon tetrachloride has also been used to lay smoke screens by spraying from airplane tanks. The droplets are volatilized after falling a very short distance and good results are obtained. However, ammonia is also necessary in these devices, which constitutes an undersirable complication in the apparatus. Except for this drawback, the silicon tetrachloride-ammonia mixture is one of the most effective smoke producers so far devised.

Because of the shortage of tin toward the end of the war, silicon tetrachloride was substituted for tin tetrachloride in gas shells.

Titanium Tetrachloride ($TiCl_4$)

German: "F-Stoff"; American: "FM"

The complications involved in producing dense smoke by use of ammonia with silicon tetrachloride caused the introduction of titanium tetrachloride by the Allies, near the end of the war, as a substitute for tin and silicon tetrachlorides.

This compound is obtained from rutile TiO_2 which is found in natural beds in Norway and in Virginia. The rutile ore is first mixed with 30 per cent carbon and heated to 650°C. in an electric furnace. A fused mass is formed, consisting of titanium carbonitride ($Ti_5C_4N_4$) and titanium carbide (TiC), which is converted to $TiCl_4$ by heating with gaseous chlorine. The product is a colorless highly refractory liquid, of 1.7 specific gravity, which boils at 136°C. (277°F.) and solidifies into white crystals at −23°C. (−9°F.). It reacts vigorously with the moisture in the air, forming titanic acid hydrate and hydrochloric acid:

$$TiCl_4 + 4H_2O = Ti(OH)_4 + 4HCl$$

with the evolution of dense clouds of acrid white smoke. The titanic acid hydrate forms finely divided solid particles in the smoke while the hydrochloric acid is in the gaseous state.

Like silicon tetrachloride, complete decomposition of the titanium tetrachloride, according to the above equation, is inhibited by an excess of hydrochloric acid. Therefore, the best smoke is formed when the titanium tetrachloride is present in low concentrations and there is an excess of moisture in the air (five parts of water to one of the tetrachloride,

241

instead of the theoretical four parts). Owing to these peculiarities, when it is used in concentrations under 0.060 mg. per liter and when the humidity is high, titanium tetrachloride is superior in obscuring power to sulfur trioxide; but when the concentrations are high and the humidity low, it is inferior.

On account of its hydrochloric acid content, titanium tetrachloride smoke is acrid, but in ordinary field concentrations it is not sufficiently irritating to the respiratory system as to cause coughing or other unpleasant physiological effects. The smoke can be neutralized and rendered completely harmless by the simultaneous use of ammonia which fixes the hydrochloric acid and greatly increases the density of the smoke by the addition of ammonium chloride. While the addition of ammonia almost doubles the obscuring effect of the titanium tetrachloride, the total amount of material required is doubled, so that no advantage is gained from the standpoint of weight. Also the apparatus employing two liquids is much more complicated and, as titanium tetrachloride alone is an excellent smoke producer when used in the proper proportion to the moisture content of the air, the use of ammonia is not necessary.

Because of its high boiling point and not too great volatility, titanium tetrachloride is peculiarly adapted for use in laying smoke screens from airplanes since each individual droplet can move through a great distance before it is completely volatilized and hydrolyzed. For this reason it was adopted as the standard American liquid-smoke agent for several years following the war. Because of its relatively high cost (about twenty times as much as sulfur trioxide for equal smoke effect), the fact that in hydrolyzing it deposits a gummy solid residue that clogs up the emission orifices of the sprayer, and its corrosive action (in liquid form) on metals, titanium tetrachloride has been displaced by the much cheaper and more generally satisfactory smoke agent FS.

It requires 0.15 oz. of titanium tetrachloride to produce 1,000 cu. ft. of *standard smoke,* as against 0.06 oz. of phosphorus, so that, on a basis of equal weights, the former is about 40 per cent as efficient a smoke producer as the latter.

Titanium tetrachloride, although more expensive and not otherwise superior to FS, is nevertheless used as a filler in artillery and mortar-smoke shell.

Group V

Berger Mixture (Zn + CCl_4 + ZnO + Kieselguhr)

The next group of substances employed during the World War as smoke agents were compounds and mixtures containing zinc that generated the so-called *zinc smokes.* The first substance of this type to be

242

introduced was a mixture containing carbon tetrachloride and zinc dust, called "Berger Mixture" after the French chemist, Berger, who invented it. The original Berger Mixture as used by the French government during the war had the following composition:

	Per Cent, by Weight
Zinc (dust)	25
Carbon tetrachloride	50
Zinc oxide	20
Kieselguhr	5

The theory of this mixture is as follows: Finely divided metallic zinc reacts vigorously with organic chlorine compounds (*e.g.* carbon tetrachloride or hexachlorethane), forming zinc chloride:

$$2Zn + CCl_4 = 2ZnCl_2 + C$$

This reaction liberates a large quantity of heat, which instantly evaporates the zinc chloride and generates a dense cloud of smoke. As the reaction quickly raises the temperature to 1,200°C., it has to be moderated by the addition of a volatile substance, such as an excess of carbon tetrachloride, that absorbs heat during evaporation. In order to prevent the heavy zinc dust from settling to the bottom of the liquid carbon tetrachloride, an absorbent, kieselguhr, is added, forming a smooth paste which cannot again be separated into its constituents. The zinc oxide used in the original mixture was practically useless as its absorbent power is small.

In order to ignite and start the Berger Mixture to burning, an igniting composition consisting of iron dust and potassium permanganate was employed. This ignition composition was started with an ordinary match head. About 3 lb. of Berger Mixture were pressed into a tin container about the size of a large tomato can and covered with a layer of igniting mixture; in this way were obtained the smoke candles used in the World War.

Smoke candles made with Berger Mixture had many advantages over the liquid smoke producers. They were chemically inert and entirely harmless until ignited and could not be fired even if hit by projectiles. They could be stored for long periods without deterioration, occupied a relatively small storage space, and could be easily transported, handled, and operated. The smoke generated was quite harmless and produced no irritant effects until the concentration exceeded 0.100 mg. per liter, which was far in excess of ordinary field concentrations. The principal disadvantages of the Berger Mixture smoke candles were: (1) high reaction temperature and the dispersion of sparks that caused fires; (2) the mixture was somewhat erratic in burning and did not utilize all its ingredients to their full values; (3) the smoke generated was light gray with

243

considerable carbon in the residue. Berger Mixture was also not suitable for use in smoke grenades, artillery shell, or airplane bombs, as it is too slow in igniting and burning.

In order to improve the performance of the original Berger Mixture, a great deal of experimenting was done and a large number of formulas for this mixture are found in chemical-warfare literature. Regardless, however, of the variations in the mixture, the general principles of operation are the same; one part by weight of zinc dust to two parts by weight of carbon tetrachloride furnish the main reaction, to which is added enough absorbent material, such as kieselguhr, to form a doughlike paste which cannot be reduced to its original ingredients.

"B.M. Mixture" ($Zn + CCl_4 + NaClO_3 + NH_4Cl + MgCO_2$)

The American improvement on the original Berger Mixture was worked out in 1917 by the U.S. Bureau of Mines, and was therefore known as "B.M. Mixture." It had the following composition:

	Per Cent, by Weight
Zinc (dust)	35.4
Carbon tetrachloride	41.6
Sodium chlorate	9.3
Ammonium chloride	5.4
Magnesium carbonate	8.3

The changes in the original Berger Mixture, shown in the foregoing formula, were made for the following reasons: The original Berger Mixture produced a gray smoke and lacked vigor in reaction. The first step, then, was to add a substance to oxidize the carbon, thereby changing the color of the smoke from gray to white and at the same time accelerating the reaction. For economic reasons, sodium chlorate was chosen for this purpose. The addition of sodium chlorate greatly increased the quantity and quality of the smoke produced, but made the rate of burning too rapid, the heat of reaction too great, and the smoke too hot. The next step was therefore the substitution of ammonium chloride for the zinc oxide of the original Berger Mixture. By absorbing a great deal of heat in its volatilization, this cooled the smoke and considerably retarded its rate of burning. It also added materially to the density of the smoke, as the obscuring power of the chloride itself is high. The last step was the substitution of magnesium carbonate for the kieselguhr in the original mixture. Kieselguhr was not satisfactory as an absorbing agent. It lacked constancy of composition, contained variable amounts of moisture and organic matter, and swelled, caked, and arched badly upon burning, thereby causing irregularities in the rate of combustion of the mixture. Magnesium carbonate proved a better absorbent, gave a smoother burn-

244

ing mixture, and added to the density of the smoke by virtue of the magnesium mechanically expelled.

By reason of these changes, the T.O.P. of the smoke was increased from 1,250 to 1,400 and the smoke had far better hanging properties, was not as easily disturbed by air currents, and did not dissipate as rapidly.

In order to give a quick puff of smoke at the beginning of the reaction, when the standard B.M. Mixture was just starting to burn, a "fast" mixture was employed, having the following composition:

	Per Cent, by Weight
Zinc (dust)	30.2
Carbon tetrachloride	35.1
Sodium chlorate	24.9
Zinc oxide	9.8

This burns much more rapidly than the standard mixture, as ammonium chloride and magnesium carbonate are absent and the zinc oxide acts as the absorbent.

B.M. Mixture was employed in smoke candles, grenades, and floating boxes for naval use. These devices, in addition to the standard and fast B.M. smoke mixture, also contained two starting mixtures, as follows:

Starting Mixture 1 served to start the reaction and was of the following composition:

	Per Cent, by Weight
Powdered sulfur	20.7
Zinc (dust)	63.1
Zinc oxide	16.2

Starting Mixture 2 received the flash from the igniting match head, served to burn through the igniting cup, and ignited the Starting Mixture 1. It consisted of:

	Per Cent, by Weight
Powdered iron (reduced)	46.6
Potassium permanganate	53.4

As compared to the British smoke mixture, the B.M. smoke mixture had certain definite advantages. It burned more uniformly and freely, left a much smaller residue, and the smoke had better hanging properties and greater persistency. Moreover the T.O.P. of the B.M. smoke was 1,400 as compared to 460 for the British Type S smoke mixture. Its disadvantages were: (1) absorbents that constituted about 25 per cent of inert material; and (2) the necessity for an absolutely airtight container to prevent the evaporation of carbon tetrachloride. Nevertheless, the B.M. Mixture was the most efficient smoke producer of this type developed during the war.

245

HC Mixture ($Zn + C_2Cl_6 + ZnO$)

Since the war efforts have continued in America to produce a better zinc-smoke producer by improving the B.M. Mixture.

Solid hexachlorethane (C_2Cl_6) was substituted for and found to be much superior to carbon tetrachloride. It proved to be an equally good source of chlorine and, being itself a solid, eliminated the necessity for an inert filler such as magnesium carbonate.

As an absorbent in place of sodium chlorate and ammonia chloride, zinc oxide was substituted.

The new mixture, used in smoke candles HC, MI, contained the following constitutentents:

	Per Cent, by Weight
Zinc (dust)	28
Hexachlorethane	50
Zinc oxide	22

This mixture was ignited by a starting mixture composed of:

	Per Cent, by Weight
Antimony	76.4
Zinc (dust)	11.8
Potassium perchlorate	11.8

The original HC smoke mixture, as a result of continued development and improvement, has evolved to the following composition used in smoke candles HC, MII:

	Per cent	
	Fast mixture	Slow mixture

Zinc (dust)	36	36
Hexachlorethane	43	44
Ammonium perchlorate	15	10
Ammonium chloride	6	10

The filling of this smoke candle consists of about nine-tenths slow-burning mixture and one-tenth fast-burning mixture. The fast-burning mixture is placed as a layer over the slow-burning mixture and is ignited by a starting mixture consisting of:

	Per Cent, by Weight
Potassium nitrate	42
Antimony trisulfide	26
Ferrous sulfide	26
Dextrin	6

246

The chemical reaction in the HC Mixture is as follows:

$$3Zn + C_2Cl_6 = 3ZnCl_2 + 2C$$

The ignition and burning processes are similar to those of the B.M. Mixture, but the reaction is less violent and no delaying agents are necessary. The mixture is also more stable and more efficient per unit weight than the B.M. Mixture.

This HC Mixture, MII, is now the standard smoke producer for smoke candles and pots in the United States Army. It requires only 0.12 oz. to produce 1,000 cu. ft. of *standard smoke* and represents the most advanced development of the zinc-smoke type of smoke agents.

COMPARISON OF SMOKE AGENTS

On the basis of total obscuring power (T.O.P.), the smoke agents discussed above, as well as other substances that have been used since the War for producing smoke, are arranged below in the descending order of their T.O.P.'s.

White phosphorus	4,600
Titanium tetrachloride and ammonia	3,030
Sulfur trioxide	3,000
Sulfur trioxide and chlorsulfonic acid (FS)	2,550
Hydrochloric acid and ammonia	2,500
HC Mixture	2,100
Silicon tetrachloride and ammonia	1,960
Titanium tetrachloride (FM)	1,900
Oleum*	1,890
Tin tetrachloride (KJ)	1,860
Phosphorus trichloride and ammonia	1,800
Chlorsulfonic acid and ammonia	1,600
Silicon tetrachloride	1,500
Sulfur chloride and ammonia	1,425
Chlorsulfonic acid*	1,400
B.M. Mixture	1,400
Berger Mixture	1,250
Titanium tetrachloride and ethylene dichloride	1,235
Sulfuryl chloride	1,200
Chlorine and ammonia	750
Arsenic trichloride	460
Type S mixture	460
Crude oil	200

* Heating to 450°F. increases T.O.P.'s from 30 to 50 per cent.

In comparing the T.O.P.'s for different smokes, the rate of burning must be considered, since a slow-burning smoke may not reach its maximum density before its particles begin to settle out. Humidity and temperature also have an important influence on the T.O.P.'s of many chemical smokes. The values given above are for average conditions of

247

temperature and humidity and may vary greatly with variations of either or both.

FUTURE OF SMOKE AGENTS

During the World War obscuring smoke proved its tactical value on land and sea and won for itself an assured place as a military weapon. Since the war the development of air forces has still further enhanced the value of obscuring smoke, for not only are airplanes a means par excellence for putting down smoke screens on the field of battle, but their power of observation has greatly increased the need for obscuration. So greatly has aircraft increased the facility of observing enemy dispositions and maneuvers and of attacking troops in march and other concentrated formations, that it has become increasingly necessary to find some means of concealing and protecting ground troops from air observation and attack. Obscuring smoke is a most effective means for this purpose.

All nations are impressed with the importance of obscuring smoke and are busily engaged in developing the superior smoke agents and in devising technical means of employing them. The rapid strides made in this direction during and since the World War plainly indicate the possibilities of this field.

Detailed data concerning the most important smoke agents are presented in Table IV. The technical apparatus for producing smoke and the tactical principles involved in its use are treated in Chap. XIV.

248

CHAPTER XII

INCENDIARY AGENTS

CLASSIFICATION

Incendiaries, the third member of the chemical arm, are substances used to set fire to enemy material in the Theater of War. Unlike gas and smoke, which are directed against personnel and are used chiefly on the field of battle, incendiaries are directed primarily against material, and their employment is not limited to the battle front, but extends to targets anywhere in the Theater of War that can be reached by bombing airplanes. Incendiaries may also be used to a limited extent against personnel, as in the World War, when air-burst trench-mortar shell, filled with phosphorus and thermite, were fired against enemy machine gunners sheltered from rifle and machine-gun fire.

Tactically, we distinguish two types of incendiaries: (1) the intensive type, where the heat and flames are concentrated in a limited space, in order to set fire to heavy construction and targets generally difficult to ignite; (2) the scatter type, where the incendiary materials are scattered in a number of small burning masses over a relatively large area, in order to initiate fires at a number of points simultaneously in large targets of inflammable or easily ignited materials. Another convenient tactical classification of incendiaries is by the using arm, thus:

Using Arm	Munition
Infantry	Small-arms incendiary bullets Incendiary grenades and other hand devices
Chemical troops	Chemical-mortar incendiary projectiles Livens projector incendiary drums Flame projectors
Artillery	Incendiary shell
Air force	Incendiary aircraft bombs

Technically, we distinguish four classes of incendiaries, as follows:

1. Spontaneously inflammable materials.
   a. *Solids*, such as phosphorus and sodium.
   b. *Liquids*, such as phosphorus dissolved in carbon bisulfide and zinc ethyl.
2. Metallic oxides, such as thermite.
3. Oxidizing combustible mixtures, such as barium peroxide and magnesium powder, or barium nitrate, magnesium, and linseed oil.
4. Flammable materials, used as such, *e.g.*, resins, pitch, celluloid, "solid oil," and flammable liquids and oil.

249

HISTORICAL

Unlike gas and smoke, the systematic use of incendiaries in warfare is not modern, but extends back into ancient times. The early use of incendiaries in combat is easily understood when it is remembered that, from the earliest times, fire has been the most ruthless enemy of mankind, and its application to war is but further evidence of the universal dread of the Great Destroyer which has come down through the ages.

The idea of using incendiaries in battle dates back to early Biblical times when armies attacking and defending fortified cities threw upon each other burning oils and flaming fire balls consisting of resin and straw. The first flame projector was used at Delium in 424 B.C. It consisted of a hollow tree trunk to the lower end of which was attached a basin filled with glowing coals, sulfur, and pitch. A bellows blew the flame from the tree trunk in the form of a jet, setting fire to the enemy fortifications and aiding the besiegers in the capture of the city.

The next recorded use of incendiaries was by the Trojan king, Æneas, about 360 B.C. He made use of fire compositions consisting of pitch, sulfur, tow, resinous wood, and other highly inflammable substances which were easily ignited and hard to extinguish. The incendiary composition was poured burning into pots, which were fired from the walls of besieged cities upon the attacking troops below.

Somewhat later the Romans hurled from catapults crude iron laticework bombs, about 2 ft. in diameter, filled with highly inflammable materials. These were ignited and thrown as flaming projectiles upon the enemy fortifications. Later, incendiary arrows came into use as a means of setting fire to the wooden forts sheltering the enemy. These incendiary arrows were subsequently enlarged and shot from catapults. Behind the arrowhead they carried a perforated tube containing a mixture of tow, resin, sulfur, and petroleum, which was ignited just before being shot.

The greatest impetus to the use of incendiaries in war came with the introduction of "Greek Fire," which was said to have been invented by the Syrian, Callinicus, about the year 660 A.D., although there is evidence of the use of similar materials as early as the time of Constantine the Great, in the fourth century A.D. The exact formula for "Greek Fire" has never been definitely established. The process for making it was kept a secret for several centuries and no detailed information as to its composition seems to have survived. It is certainly known to have contained readily inflammable substances such as pitch, resin, and petroleum, as well as quicklime and sulfur. The quicklime, on contact with water, generated sufficient heat to ignite the petroleum, the burning of which ignited the other combustible materials. The light vapors from the petroleum caused explosions which still further spread the flames.

250

It was difficult to extinguish "Greek Fire" because water increased the reaction of the quicklime and spread the petroleum. The troops of the Byzantine Empire made such effective use of "Greek Fire" against the Saracens that it is frequently said to have saved the empire from Mohammedan domination for nearly a thousand years. At any event, "Greek Fire" was extensively employed in the wars of the Middle Ages, and its use survived until the introduction of gunpowder in the fifteenth century.

From the beginning of modern times down to the World War, incendiaries were not extensively employed, as the introduction of firearms caused armies to engage in battle at such distances that they could not be effectively reached by incendiaries. Moreover, the defensive use of armor and later of earthworks left little of combustible material on the field of battle. So formidable were the technical difficulties created by these new conditions that the successful use of incendiaries in war remained an unsolved problem until the advent of the World War, when the vast resources of modern science were utilized to effect a solution. So, while fire has been considered of military value from antiquity, means for scientifically using it in warfare were not developed until the World War.

The effectiveness of incendiaries in war is dependent upon the character of the materials employed and upon the devices used for carrying them to the target and setting them in action there. Because of the generally adverse conditions of modern warfare, the development of successful incendiary armament involves chemical and mechanical problems of great complexity, as will be appreciated from the consideration of the many rigid technical and tactical requirements which must be met. At the same time, the introduction of the military airplane has greatly increased the field of application of incendiaries, as it is now possible by such means to reach large and vulnerable incendiary targets at practically any point in the Theater of War. This was exemplified in the German air raids on Paris and London in 1915, in which incendiary bombs were frequently employed.

Although the French and Germans both had developed incendiary artillery shell before the World War, one French model dating back to 1878, such shell were not used to any extent in the early days of the war, probably because they were largely ineffective. The earliest incendiary munitions used in the war appear to be incendiary bullets and antiaircraft artillery shell directed against observation balloons.

The first incendiary attacks against ground troops were by means of flame projectors. These devices were invented by the Germans before the war (20, page 7) but do not appear to have been used until 1915.

251

General Foulkes says that the Germans used their *Flammenwerfer* (flame projectors) on the French front on June 25, 1915, but it is probable that their first use was several months earlier, for it is known that the Germans had an organized detachment of *Flammenwerfer* troops as early as January, 1915, and the French made a formal protest against the use of these devices under date of Apr. 29, 1915.

The initial use of incendiaries from aircraft occurred during the first German Zeppelin raid over London on May 31, 1915, during which one airship dropped 90 incendiary bombs.

By the end of 1915, improved types of incendiary artillery shell were in use by both sides. These were soon followed by the introduction of incendiary grenades, trench-mortar shell, and projector bombs. Throughout the war, all the principal belligerents engaged in the energetic development of incendiary armament and much progress was made in improving all types of incendiary munitions, particularly aviation drop bombs.

SUBSTANCES USED AS INCENDIARY AGENTS

GROUP I. SPONTANEOUSLY INFLAMMABLE MATERIALS

Solids

Phosphorus (P)

American and British: "W.P."

While white phosphorus is primarily a smoke producer, its property of igniting spontaneously and burning vigorously when exposed to the air made it one of the first materials proposed for incendiary munitions. Experience showed that against readily combustible materials and substances which can be ignited by a brief exposure to a small flame, phosphorus is undoubtedly effective, and it was therefore the principal incendiary agent used against balloons and aircraft and for setting fire to woods, grain fields, etc. However, against wooden structures and materials relatively difficult to ignite, phosphorus proved of little value, principally because of its low temperature of combustion and the excellent fireproof protection of the phosphoric oxides formed by burning phosphorus.

In addition to its incendiary effect on material, phosphorus proved very effective in use against personnel. When scattered from overhead bursts of grenades and trench-mortar bombs, the phosphorus rained down in flaming particles, which stuck to clothing and could not be brushed off or quenched. The larger particles quickly burned through clothing and produced painful burns that were slow and difficult to heal. These properties soon became known to troops and phosphorus was justly

252

dreaded and always caused a demoralizing effect far beyond the actual casualties produced.

During the war, phosphorus was extensively used in small-arms incendiary bullets and in hand and rifle grenades by all the principal belligerents; in artillery incendiary shell by the French and Germans; and in trench-mortar bombs by the British and Americans. In all munitions, except small-arms bullets, the phosphorus produced both obscuring smoke and incendiary effects and they were, therefore, variously classified as either smoke or incendiary projectiles. The physical and chemical properties of phosphorus are given in Chap. XI, page 234.

Sodium (Na)

Sodium is a light soft ductile metal of 0.97 specific gravity, which melts at 97.6°C. (208°F.) and boils at 750°C. (1382°F.). It is obtained by the electrolysis of molten sodium chloride (common salt). On contact with water, sodium decomposes it with vigorous evolution of hydrogen. The heat of reaction is sufficient to ignite the hydrogen and, hence, in the presence of moisture, sodium is spontaneously inflammable.

Sodium was used as a filling for the German 17.5-cm. incendiary shell. In that shell, which was the largest incendiary shell used during the war, the sodium was ignited by thermite. Sodium was also used in some of the spontaneously inflammable liquids of the World War to ignite the mixture on contact with water. Except for this latter use, sodium was not an effective incendiary material, as it required considerable moisture to ignite it, which generally prevented the ignition of other materials.

Liquids

As liquids generally give better and more uniform dispersion on explosion of the container, and also have a tendency to adhere and penetrate into combustible materials, with greater chance of igniting them, they are preferred to solids as incendiary agents. Also, since spontaneously inflammable substances require no igniting device and initiate fires in several places simultaneously, a *spontaneously inflammable liquid* was sought which would: (1) ignite after short exposure to the atmosphere; (2) have a positive and effective incendiary action; and (3) be safe to transport and handle.

As phosphorus was spontaneously inflammable and was also readily soluble in carbon disulfide, this mixture was among the first spontaneously inflammable liquids tried out. It failed, however, to meet requirements in a number of particulars. First, it was no more effective as an incendiary agent than the phosphorus it contained, and therefore, had the disadvantages mentioned for phosphorus. It was also dangerous to

253

transport and handle and was so volatile that it frequently burned out before heating the contacting material to the ignition point.

To correct the deficiencies of the phosphorus–carbon disulfide solution, mixtures were made by adding various combustible oils in such proportions that a homogenous mass was secured and no separation of any of the constituents occurred. It was then found that these mixtures lacked intensity of combustion, so various nitrated organic compounds were added to accelerate the reaction. Of these compounds, trinitrotoluene (TNT) was found to be the most satisfactory. As a final result of this research, a mixture containing phosphorus, carbon disulfide, crude benzene, fuel oil, gas-tar oil, and trinitrotoluene was developed. This was found to be satisfactory from the standpoints of simplicity of preparation, safety, and effectiveness; also, by varying the proportions of the ingredients, the ignition could be regulated to occur either almost instantly upon exposure to the air, or after a considerable delay.

The speed and spread of combustion of the mixture are secured by its readily volatile constituents, and the duration and intensity of the flame, by its heavier combustibles. With proper precautions, the preparation and handling of the mixture can be done without danger of accidental ignition. Also, it is not subject to detonation by shock, and its low coefficient of expansion (0.0174 per degree centigrade) and low vapor pressure (58 cm. at 50°C.) will not cause undue pressure in the container. The mixture may be used alone or with an absorbent, (*e.g.*, cotton waste) in any sort of device designed to carry liquid material, such as 8-in. Livens projectiles.

In the course of the research on spontaneously inflammable liquids, many substances, such as zinc ethyl, phosphine, silicine, chromyl chloride, fuming nitric acid, permanganates, and phosphorus, were fully investigated. In the end, it was found that phosphorus–carbon disulfide solution was the best material to initiate the fire, and the fuel and tar oils were the best materials to propagate and sustain the flames. While the problem of spontaneously inflammable liquids was considered reasonably solved during the World War, the solution was not effected in time for use on the field of battle, at least insofar as American munitions were concerned. There is, however, no reason to believe that the solution indicated above would not be satisfactory in war.

A satisfactory spontaneously inflammable liquid has a great field of application from aircraft, for not only should drop bombs filled with such a liquid prove very effective on targets, and even on cities of light wooden construction, but by regulating the ignition to occur after the lapse of sufficient time for the liquid to reach the target, such a liquid could also be sprayed at night from low-flying attack planes over relatively large areas with tremendous effectiveness.

254

Group II. Metallic Oxides

Thermite

For several years prior to the late war, a mixture of iron oxide and finely divided aluminum, known under the proprietary name of "Thermite," was used in industry for welding iron and steel. When ignited, this mixture reacts as follows:

$$8Al + 3Fe_3O_4 = 4Al_2O_3 + 9Fe$$

and produces an enormous heat (758,000 calories per gram molecule). This heat is sufficient to raise the temperature of the reaction to about 3,000°C., and the resulting molten slag prolongs the heating effect after the reaction ceases. However, when thermite is used alone, it has the disadvantage that its incendiary action is confined to a small area, and a very large percentage of its heat energy is wasted because of the fact that it is set free so rapidly. Against readily ignitable material which allows the conflagration to spread easily, thermite is very effective, but as such material is not often present in a target, the method of placing it with the thermite in the incendiary device was early adopted.

For igniting and starting the conflagration, thermite proved to be by far the most effective material used in the war; for a secondary incendiary material to continue the conflagration, thermite was found to be inferior to an inflammable liquid, either used as such or incorporated in a suitable absorbent carrier, and to specially prepared combustible materials, such as *solid oil*, which burned with a large flame and effectively set fire to a difficultly ignitable target. By using thermite as a primary igniting incendiary agent, the large amount of heat suddenly released is utilized and the secondary material begins its action with a tremendous burst of flame which is most effective. The proper secondary incendiary material is capable of not only burning with a large hot flame, but actually renders the target inflammable.

The thermite used in industry is generally composed of three parts by weight of aluminum powder to ten parts of magnetic iron oxide, but for military purposes a mixture consisting of 24 per cent aluminum and 76 per cent by weight of magnetic iron oxide was found to be most suitable. Ordinary granulation produced the best results, but special limits had to be placed on purity of materials, presence of moisture, and foreign substances.

As commercial thermite is simply a loose mixture of aluminum dust and coarse particles of iron oxide—materials of quite different densities—it could not be used in military devices that must withstand severe jarring, without some means of preventing segregation. To prevent segregation, the mixture may be either consolidated by pressure or bound

255

together in a hard mass by such binding substances as sodium silicate, sulfur, and celluloid.

Segregation may be successfully prevented by compressing ordinary thermite under a pressure of 12,000 lb. per square inch, which doubles its density and holds the compressed mass together even when subject to severe jarring. However, this increase in density causes the ignition to become more difficult, makes the propagation of the reaction uncertain and increases the time of burning. Moreover, since the compressed thermite does not materially increase the incendiary effect over the same volume of thermite bound together with sodium silicate, the cost of obtaining the same results with compressed thermite is greater. For these reasons we did not adopt it for general military use and the British employed it only in their special flame mixture which contains barium nitrate.

On the other hand, the use of sodium silicate as a binder was found to give several advantages. Besides preventing segregation, it caused the thermite blocks to react completely regardless of the point of ignition, and the material so bound is insensitive to shock and shot and may, therefore, be utilized in high velocity projectiles and bombs. The optimum amount of sodium silicate (of 40°Bé.) was found to be 15 per cent by weight of thermite. The liquid silicate is simply mixed with the thermite which is then molded and baked until thoroughly dry. Because of its advantages, sodium (or potassium) silicate was generally used as a thermite binder by most of the nations in the World War.

In binding thermite with sodium silicate, it is very essential that all the water be driven out, and, because of the difficulty of completely drying the silicate-bound thermite, a number of other binders were tried. Sulfur was highly recommended as a binder, since a unit of weight of mixture made up according to the equation

$$8Al + 3Fe_3O_4 + 9S = 4Al_2O_3 + 9FeS$$

theoretically generates the same amount of heat as an equal weight of thermite containing no sulfur so that the binder does not reduce the heat efficiency of the mixture. However, in actual tests of incendiary value the sulfur-bound thermite did not show up well, owing to the fact that it burned with explosive violence and spattered as small drops over a considerable area, thus lessening its incendiary effect. Also, the molten products from the silicate-bound thermite were more effective in penetrating metal and prolonging incendiary action upon inflammable materials. Notwithstanding these drawbacks, the French used sulfur-bound thermite, which they called "Daisite," in an incendiary drop bomb in which the explosive property of the thermite was utilized to scatter the other incendiary materials in the bomb.

Celluloid, dissolved in a suitable solvent,[256] proved to be fairly successful as a binder, particularly where it was desired to get a long flame and uniform burn of the thermite. It was also used as an envelope for the incendiary units of scatter-type drop bombs, chiefly by the Germans. Various organic materials, such as resin, paraffin, and hard pitch, were also investigated as binders, but did not give satisfactory results.

For the ignition of thermite used in devices where it is not desired to scatter the contents, the commercial igniter, consisting of finely divided aluminum and barium peroxide mixed with a certain amount of coarse aluminum and black iron oxide, was found to be most satisfactory. This igniter has no explosive reaction and can be ignited by a black powder flash, although better results are obtained by the use of a "booster" charge composed of reduced iron and potassium nitrate pressed on top of it.

For the ignition of thermite in devices where it is desired to scatter the contents, an entirely different type of igniter is required. For this purpose, an igniter should react with such rapidity and explosive violence as to simultaneously ignite and scatter the reaction products and, at the same time, should be as safe as the slow igniter. The best World War solution of the quick igniter was the British "Ophorite" which consisted of an intimate mixture of 9 parts of magnesium powder to 13 parts of potassium perchlorate. Ophorite was much easier to ignite than the commercial igniter and was extensively used by the British and ourselves as an igniting and bursting charge for incendiary projectiles and also as an explosive in certain types of gas shell. Ophorite was, however, not altogether safe to manufacture and the British had several very serious explosions and fires in their manufacturing and loading plants during the war.

Modified Thermite

Since the general military requirements of a thermite mixture are that it should function properly under all conditions of use and that the reaction should produce the desired effects, and since it matters little what the reaction products are, it is obvious that the composition of the mixture may be varied greatly. A number of mixtures, in which copper, nickel, manganese, and lead oxides were used in place of iron oxide, were tested but were found to be no better for military purposes than the ordinary thermite mixture, although the Germans used, in certain early incendiary bombs, a mixture containing manganese dioxide and magnesium.

Later in the war, alumino-thermite mixtures, in which oxidizing agents other than the oxides were incorporated, were investigated, and a special flaming thermite was developed by the British and used in their "baby incendiary" bombs. This mixture consisted of:[257] aluminum, powdered, 3 parts; barium nitrate, 6 parts; hammerscale (Fe_3O_4) 8 parts; and was compressed to half its original volume in the bombs.

Thermite mixtures containing oxidizing agents other than those necessary for the thermite reaction were also investigated but none were found to possess special merit for military purposes, and it was concluded after many tests that a simple mixture of magnetic iron oxide and aluminum was the most satisfactory for general military uses. Of all the incendiary materials adopted by the Allies, thermite was probably the most widely used. On the other hand, the Germans did not use thermite very extensively, although many German incendiary drop bombs and artillery shell contained thermite or an alumino-thermite mixture.

Group III. Oxidizing Combustible Mixtures

Incendiary mixtures which contain an *inorganic oxidizing agent,* such as potassium or barium nitrate, barium or lead oxide, or potassium perchlorate, together with such *combustible substances* as carbon, sulfur, magnesium, aluminum, or organic combustibles, are designated by the generic name of *oxidizing combustible mixtures.* Such mixtures have been used successfully in two widely different types of incendiary munitions, *viz.:* (1) small-arms incendiary bullets, and (2) drop bombs and other special devices.

For devices as different as bullets and drop bombs, it is evident that very different types of mixtures are required for most effective results. Thus, a mixture for use in bullets must meet very rigid requirements as to weight per unit volume, time of reaction, change of weight during reaction, and character of incendiary effect.

For bullets, the ballistic requirements are even more important than the incendiary requirements since the bullet must be capable of accurate flight in order to reach the desired target and have any effect at all. On the other hand, the type of mixture desired for drop bombs must react to give considerable heat and flame when the bomb bursts.

In both types of munitions, it is, of course, important that the mixtures do not segregate, and this is accomplished either by compression or by binding the mass with some substance, such as sulfur, shellac, resin, pitch, paraffin, gum, etc., and then heating or compressing.

The following typical mixtures have been used with success in small-arms incendiary ammunition:

	Parts, by Weight
Barium peroxide	17
Magnesium (powder)	2

The magnesium powder mixed with alcohol is pressed into the bullets under a pressure of 2,500 lb., and is ignited by the propellant.[258]

Red lead	9
Magnesium	1

or

Red lead	15
Aluminum	1

Compressed into the shell under a pressure of 15 tons per sq. in. and ignited by a primer consisting of

Potassium nitrate	65
Sulfur	13.5
Antimony (powder)	19
Shellac (powder)	2.5

Another typical mixture comprising a different type of oxidizing agent, is

Barium nitrate	64
Magnesium	28
Linseed oil	8

The linseed oil acts as a binder and deterrent.

For use in projectiles where the tracing effect is important, a considerable number of the so-called *pyrotechnic mixtures* have been used. These give upon ignition a large amount of smoke and a very brilliant light, but have little or no real incendiary effect. These mixtures should, therefore, not be registered as true incendiaries.

The use of oxidizing combustible mixtures in drop bombs and other relatively large incendiary devices was less successful than in small-arms ammunition. Such mixtures were used early in the war in incendiary artillery shell and in drop bombs, but in many cases were later discarded for the thermite-type mixtures. As a primary incendiary material whose chief function was to ignite other materials in drop bombs, the following mixture was used:

	Parts, by Weight
Potassium perchlorate	80
Paraffin	20

For use in a small unit drop bomb designed to set fire to very inflammable targets, we developed a successful mixture consisting of the following ingredients:

Barium chlorate	54
Resin	16
Aluminum	14
Asphaltum varnish	16

This mixture was ignited by a mixture comprising reduced iron and potassium permanganate bound with paraffin.

259

Another celebrated World War mixture of the oxidizing-combustible type was the so-called "Scheelite" consisting of one part hexamethylenetetramine and two parts of sodium peroxide. It was named for its inventor, a Dr. Scheele, who claimed he had destroyed the cargoes of 32 vessels by its use. Our experiments with this formula showed that when ignited by sulfuric acid it reacts very rapidly in the open and generates great heat and flames, but, if confined, it explodes. On the whole, it was found unsatisfactory for use in the larger incendiary devices, but a modified form has possibilities for use in certain small drop bombs.

Group IV. Flammable Materials (Used as such)

This group comprises those incendiary materials that are used as such without admixture of oxidizing agents and includes the following substances: petroleum oils, carbon disulfide, wood distillation products, resins, pitch, celluloid, and various sorts of flammable oils and liquids not spontaneously inflammable.

The two principal uses of this class of substances are: (1) as secondary incendiary materials to propagate and prolong the incendiary action of the primary material in the larger size drop bombs and projectiles; and (2) as liquids used in flame projectors.

In the development of the intensive-type incendiary drop bomb, intended to set fire to heavy wooden structures and other targets relatively difficult to ignite, it was early found that such devices should contain some quick-acting great-heat-producing material, such as thermite, and a larger amount of flammable material which, when ignited by the thermite, would burn with a large hot flame for a considerable time and actually render the target more inflammable.

For this purpose, various oxidizing combustible mixtures, resins and pitches, and heavy oils were tried and found unsatisfactory. Then flammable oils, absorbed in cotton or jute waste, were experimented with in the hope that the absorbents would prevent too rapid volatilization and burning of the oil, but were found to possess many disadvantages. Thus, if the mass were scattered by an explosion, the intensive incendiary action is lost; if it is allowed to burn without scattering, the absorbent material protects the target to a considerable extent. Mixtures of paraffin and light oils were also tested and found to have objectionable hydrostatic effects when used in drop bombs and projectiles.

Systematic research was then undertaken to find and develop a more nearly ideal incendiary material for drop bombs and projectiles that would meet the following requirements:

1. Burn for a considerable time with a very large hot flame.
2. Actually render very inflammable not only the combustible material upon which it rests, but the material around it for a considerable area.

260

3. Contain practically no material which is not extremely inflammable or which would not aid in the combustion.
4. Present no great problems of manufacture, cost, transportation, or use.

Solid Oil

As a result of an extensive investigation of materials which would meet the foregoing requirements, it was found that the oils possessed the most desirable incendiary properties and their only drawback was their liquid state. To correct this defect, experiments were made to solidify satisfactory oil mixtures by the use of colloidal substances, and after considerable investigation a process was developed whereby a permanent solidified oil mixture, meeting all requirements, could be prepared simply and cheaply. This solidified mixture—called *solid oil*—contained a small percentage of liquid, having a relatively low fire point and a large percentage of a liquid having a moderately high fire point. Such a mixture burns readily, owing to the liquid of low fire point, and the burning of this liquid generates the necessary heat to melt and ignite the material of higher fire point which spreads over a large area, penetrates contacting material, and actually renders it inflammable. Best results were obtained from distillate fuel oils with a range of fire points of from 170° to 225°C.

The raw materials entering into the manufacture of solid oil were readily obtainable and its preparation and filling into 50 drops bombs presented no difficulties.

Solid oil is also suitable for use in other large incendiary devices, such as Livens projector drums, artillery shell, and trench-mortar bombs.

Flame-projector Liquids

For use in flame projectors, the principal requirements of a liquid mixture are: (1) it must be readily and easily ignited; (2) it must not have too low a specific gravity; and (3) combustion should not occur to any material extent until the stream has reached its objective, since the desired object is to throw upon the target an *ignited liquid* and not merely a flame.

After an extended investigation of liquid mixtures for use in American flame projectors, it was found that the most satisfactory mixture consisted of a heavy viscous oil or tar and a more fluid and flammable liquid. For the heavy component, water-gas tar (sp. gr. 1.044 and flash point 122°C.) proved to be the most satisfactory. For the light component, benzene heads (sp. gr. 0.756 and flash point 26°C.) or crude benzene were best. The optimum proportions were found to be 70 per cent water-gas tar and 30 per cent benzene heads, resulting in a liquid of 1.02 specific gravity, which gave an excellent trajectory, good range, and fierce flame. Ignition was effected by means of a hydrogen pilot lamp at the

261

nozzle which has the advantage of being nonluminous when not in action and positive ignition when needed. Approximately 30 per cent of this mixture remains unburned at the end of the trajectory, and a jet shooting 0.5 gal. can be thrown approximately 100 ft.

Other nations in the World War used various combinations of the most readily available heavy and light liquids, mostly petroleum distillates and coal-tar fractions, having an average specific gravity of about 0.90 at 15°C. They also used many methods of ignition, such as cartridges of slow-burning oxidizing combustible mixtures attached to the nozzle and ignited by electricity or friction.

INCENDIARY WEAPONS

A description of the construction and use of the various devices in which incendiary agents were employed in the World War is given in subsequent chapters in connection with the material pertaining to the several combat arms.

FUTURE OF INCENDIARIES

Modern warfare has left little on the field of battle that is combustible; hence suitable targets and opportunities for the use of incendiaries in the Combat Zone are very limited and will become increasingly so as armies are mechanized. On the other hand, the military airplane has opened up a vastly larger field of application for incendiaries in the areas behind the battle front and in the hinterlands of the belligerents. To an ever-increasing degree the successful waging of modern war depends upon the industrial organization of a nation to meet the enormous demands for military material. It is, therefore, not at all unlikely that in wars of the future military operations will be carried far into the interior territory of each belligerent in an effort to cripple and destroy the industries upon which modern armies depend. In the attack upon industrial centers and upon military concentration areas in the rear of armies, incendiaries will play a large and useful role.

The vast amount of research and development work on incendiaries in the World War went far toward solving the many and formidable technical problems created by the adverse conditions of modern warfare, and it may be said that, insofar as concerns the technical efficiency of the agents themselves, incendiary armament had reached a generally satisfactory state of performance. On the other hand, the tactical results from use of incendiaries in the late war were disappointing. This was chiefly due to two factors. First, the conditions on the Western Front and, to a somewhat less extent, on the Russian Front, were naturally very unfavorable to the use of incendiaries. Not only was the weather and much of the terrain wet and adverse to application of incendiaries,

262

but also the greater part of the possible targets were of masonry and other combustibly inert construction that afforded little or no chance for the successful use of incendiary agents.

In addition to these adverse conditions, many of the most effective incendiary devices were not perfected in time to be used in the war, and hence there was no opportunity to determine their real military value in that great conflict.

Since the World War, there has been little published concerning the development of incendiary armament. There is little doubt, however, that the use of those types of incendiary munitions which proved effective in the last war will be resumed in future wars. In fact it is not unlikely that with more efficient incendiary materials and devices these munitions will assume increased importance.

295

CHAPTER XIV

CHEMICAL TECHNIQUE AND TACTICS OF INFANTRY

TECHNIQUE

In considering the chemical technique and tactics of the several arms, we shall follow the organization of the Theater of Operations for chemical warfare, as presented in Chap. III, Diagram I, and discuss the chemical technique and tactics of each arm in the order of its proximity to the battle front of an army.

In connection with the normal chemical-warfare zones of operation, shown in Diagram I of Chap. III, it should be borne in mind that these zones are not rigidly delimited, nor are they even mutually exclusive. They are merely the zones in which the chemical-warfare activities of each arm may be most effectively and efficiently carried on, under average conditions. It will also be noted that some of the zones overlap. This indicates that chemical operations may be carried on conjointly by one arm to cover a zone normally assigned another arm, as for example, when no chemical troops are available the artillery carries out chemical missions in the zone usually covered by chemical troops.

Since infantry normally constitutes the front-line elements of an army, it is the arm chiefly concerned with chemical operations along the *immediate* battle front, particularly where such operations are for its own protection. We shall, accordingly, begin our consideration of the chemical technique and tactics of the several arms with a discussion of the chemical technique and tactics of infantry.

Chemical Armament of Infantry

Chemicals are used by infantry in the following munitions:

1. Chemical grenades { Gas grenades. / Smoke grenades. / Incendiary grenades.
2. Smoke candles and pots.
3. Infantry-mortar smoke shells.
4. Smoke generators on tanks.
5. Miscellaneous smoke devices.

Chemical Grenades—Gas

The grenade is a form of ammunition which came into extensive use during the late war, largely as a result of the requirements of trench warfare. Within certain limitations, the grenade is a convenient type of

296

ammunition to enable infantry to augment their primary weapons with a small missile similar, in general, to a shell or bomb. Grenades are classified according to the method of their projection, as:

1. Hand grenades.
2. Rifle grenades.
3. Combination hand-and-rifle grenades.

A chemical grenade is a grenade that is filled with a chemical agent, *i.e.*, a gas, smoke, or incendiary, dispersed by an igniting or exploding device, and thrown by hand or fired from a rifle.

Chemical warfare first made its appearance in the World War through the use of gas grenades. According to Hanslian, these earliest chemical weapons were in the form of 26-mm. rifle grenades, containing 19 cc. of tear gas (bromacetone), while Haber states that apparently at the same time (August, 1914), gas *hand* grenades, with the same kind of filling, were also used. These grenades were stated to be for use in attacking enfilading works, casemates, and passages of permanent field fortifications into which they could be shot through the narrow slits of the embrasures. As these grenades held such a small amount of gas, they were effective only in closed places and, since the first few months' fighting in the World War was almost altogether open warfare, they were not effective and were soon discarded.

In the second year of the war, after gas had been used on a large scale in cloud attacks and from artillery and trench-mortar projectiles, gas grenades, filled with more powerful gases, again made their appearance and continued to be used on both sides intermittently throughout the remainder of the war. Even with more powerful gases, gas grenades were never effective in the open and were used chiefly for raids during the period of trench warfare.

The following are the principal gas grenades used during the war:

Nation	Type	Chemical filling
German	Ball, glass, hand	Bromine; later FS; later BA
	Ball, Red B, hand	Brommethylethyl ketone
	Ball, Red C, hand	Methylsulfuryl chloride and 5 per cent dimethyl sulfate
	Stick, Blue C, hand	DA and HE
French	26-mm., rifle	BA and chloracetone
	6-cm., egg-shaped, hand	BA and chloracetone
	Suffocating and lacrimatory Mle. 1916, hand	Acrolein
British	Hand	Ethyliodoacetate
	No. 28, hand, Mk-I	Stannic chloride
	No. 28, hand, Mk-II	Stannic chloride and PS
United States	Gas, hand, Mk-II	Stannic chloride

297

United States Gas Hand Grenade, M-II (Fig. 10).—This grenade, which is typical of all the World War gas grenades, consisted of a sheet-steel body, steel bushing, detonator thimble, detonator, and automatic firing mechanism (*bouchon*), as shown in Fig. 10.

In throwing the grenade, it was first held firmly in the right hand with the firing mechanism up, in such a manner as to secure the lever. The safety pin was then pulled with the index finger of the left hand. The grenade was then armed. After it was thrown, the lever, which was no longer held by the safety pin, was thrown off and the striker pin, impelled by a strong spring, rotated around its hinge pin and struck the primer, first perforating the tinfoil disk which was sealed over the top of the cap to waterproof the primer. The end of the fuse was tipped by a priming

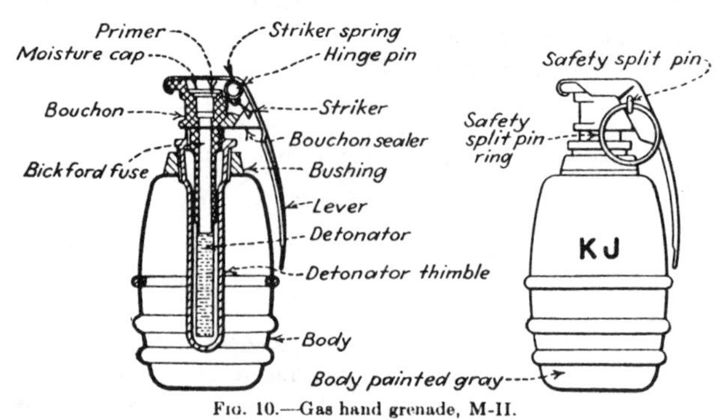

Fig. 10.—Gas hand grenade, M-II.

powder composition which ignited the primer and in turn the fuse. In 5 seconds the flame from the fuse exploded the detonator, which burst the grenade with sufficient force to scatter the chemical filling in fine droplets. The gas cloud produced was intensely irritating to the eyes and respiratory passages and caused lacrimation and violent coughing.

Postwar Development.—Since the late war several types of gas grenades have been developed in this country. The early postwar types utilized the grenade bodies manufactured during the war and were filled with CN, the American standard lacrimatory filling. These grenades were found to be unsatisfactory because of the small amount of chemical filling that could be loaded into the grenade body. To overcome this defect, the grenade body was redesigned to increase its capacity without making it too large or heavy to be thrown by hand. As a result of postwar development, two types of gas grenades have been developed and adopted as standard for the United States Army. These are known as:

298

1. Grenade, hand, tear (CN), M-7.
2. Grenade, hand, irritant (CN-DM), M-6.

United States Standard Tear-gas Grenade.—The standard *tear-gas* grenade (CN), M-7, consists of the container, igniting fuse, and filling (see Fig. 11). The container is a tin cylinder 2⅜ in. in diameter and 4½ in. high. Two thin disks are crimped and soldered to the wall forming the top and bottom of the container. The top has a ¾-in. hole punched in its center into which is inserted and soldered an adapter. The latter is internally threaded to take the igniting fuse. Small holes are punched

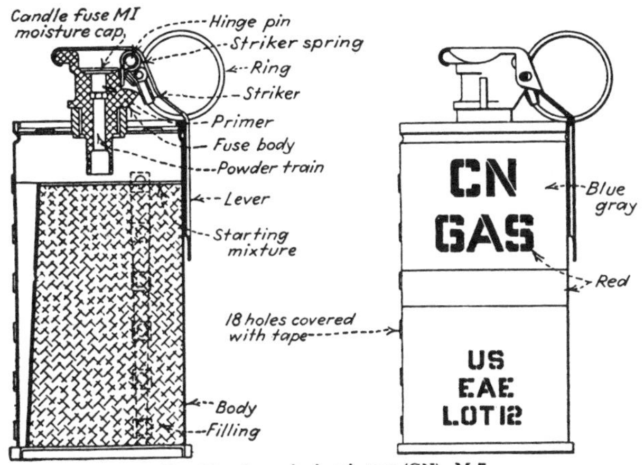

Fig. 11.—Grenade, hand, tear (CN), M-7.

in the top of the body around the adapter and, in the fast-burning type, in the wall of the container body. These are normally covered by small squares of adhesive tape.

The *fuse* consists of a fuse body which carries the firing mechanism and a 2-second fuse. The firing mechanism consists of a steel striker horizontally hinged on a steel hinge pin in a recess between the two wings of the fuse body and actuated by a steel-coil spring. A firing pin is attached to the striker. The striker is normally held away from the primer, against the tension of the spring, by a lever which forms a cover for the firing mechanism and extends downward over the top of the container. The lever hooks under a protruding lip of the fuse body and has two wings through which a split pin of annealed steel passes securing it to the body. This pin forms the safety device for the firing mechanism. The fuse assembly consists of a primer of fulminate of mercury and a

299

2-second-delay powder train in a lightly sealed lead container projecting downward from the fuse body.

The *filling* is a solid or solidified mixture. A starting mixture of potassium nitrate, antimony trisulfide ferrous sulfide, and dextrine is placed on top of the agent.

Operation. *Throwing by Hand.*—When the safety pin has been pulled, the lever, held in the palm of the hand, acts as a deterrent to prevent contact between the striker and the primer. As the grenade leaves the hand, the striker, actuated by its spring, throws the lever clear and strikes the primer. The primer flashes the fuse which in 2 seconds' time ignites the starting mixture. The starting mixture generates the heat required to start the chemical reaction of the agent. The pressure, resulting from the combustion, forces the adhesive tape from the small emission holes and the agent from the container.

To Fire from a Stationary Point of Release.—Place grenade on ground and hold the lever firmly in position while withdrawing the safety pin. When ready to fire, release lever and move rapidly upwind for a distance of 5 yd. The functioning is the same as indicated above.

The following are the principal characteristics of the standard tear-gas grenade:

Weight filled	1 lb. (approximately)
Shape	Cylindrical
Color	Blue-gray
Safety device	Safety pin
Igniter	Fuse, igniting M-I (a 2-second delay)
Filling	CN—10 oz. (mixture of chloracetophenone, oxide); a thin layer of starting mixture is placed on top of the filling
Identification	Red letters—CN Red word—Gas One red band
Characteristics of cloud	White to blue-gray to colorless vapor having a fruitlike pungent odor; an immediate lacrimatory effect on unprotected personnel; nontoxic except in extreme concentrations; practically no obscuring effect
Time of burning	25 to 40 seconds (comes to full volume within 5 seconds after firing); a small stream of vapor continues some 10 or 15 seconds longer.

United States Standard Irritant-gas Grenade.—The standard *irritant-gas* grenade (CN-DM), M-6, is identical with the standard tear-gas grenade (CN), M-7, except as to chemical filling. The irritant grenade contains a 50-50 mixture of CN and DM, instead of pure CN, as in the

300

tear-gas grenade. It therefore has both the lacrimatory effect of CN and the irritant (sternutatory) effect of DM. The following are the principal characteristics of the irritant grenade:

Weight filled	1 lb. (approximately)
Shape	Cylindrical
Color	Blue-gray
Safety device	Safety pin
Igniter	Fuse, igniting M-I (a 2-second delay)
Filling	CN-DM, approximately 10 oz. (a mixture of chloracetophenone and diphenylaminechlorarsine and smokeless powder and magnesium iodide); a thin layer of starter mixture is placed on top of the filling
Identification	Red letters—CN/DM Red word—Gas One red band
Characteristics of cloud	Blue-gray to yellow in color, with a pungent fruitlike odor; the smell of smokeless powder is also apparent; the vapor has an immediate lacrimatory and nauseating effect on unprotected personnel and may cause sneezing and vomiting
Time of burning	25 to 40 seconds (candle comes to full volume in about 5 seconds after ignition)

Chemical Grenades—Smoke

The principal smoke grenades used during the war were the following:

Nation	Type	Chemical filling
German	Ball (*Nebel*), hand	Chlorsulfonic acid
French	Incendiaire et Fumigène, Mle. 1916—Automatique, hand	Phosphorus (WP)
British	No. 27 Combination hand and rifle, M-I	Phosphorus (WP)
United States	Combination hand and rifle, M-I	Phosphorus (WP)
	Smoke, hand, M-II	Phosphorus (WP)

With the exception of the German, all the principal World War smoke grenades were filled with phosphorus. The American combination hand and rifle smoke grenade was identical with the British No. 27 smoke grenade, and these two were the only smoke grenades which could be projected with a rifle. The American hand smoke grenade was very similar to the combination hand-and-rifle smoke grenade, except that it had no base plate and rod.

301

United States Combination Hand-and-rifle Grenade, M-II (Fig. 12.) This grenade consisted chiefly of the following parts: the body (and rod), the gaine, and the firing mechanism.

The body of the grenade, cylindrical in form, was about 3¾ in. long and 2¼ in. in diameter. It was made of tinned plate and was capped on either end with dished tinned-plate stampings somewhat heavier than the metal forming the body. To the lower cap, forming the base, was soldered a steel base plate approximately ¼ in. thick. This steel plate was tapped to receive a rod 15 in. long and of the proper diameter to fit the bore of the service rifle. The rod was used only when the grenade was projected with a rifle. The rods were issued detached from the grenades in the ratio of 60 per cent of the grenades.

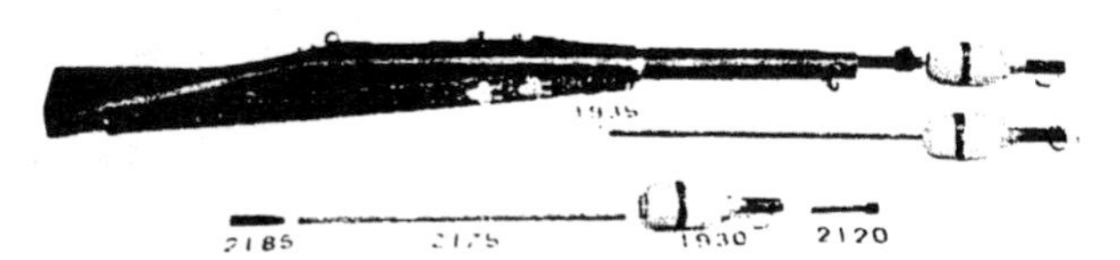

Fig. 12.—Grenade, combination hand and rifle, W.P., line, complete, showing assembly.

To the upper cap, forming the cover of the body, was soldered a striker chamber, externally threaded to hold the firing mechanism. The gaine was inserted through the striker-chamber cover and was soldered to the former.

The primer rested on top of, and was held in place by, the striker chamber. The primer was crimped to the fuse, on the other end of which was crimped the detonator, the fuse and detonator extending into the gaine. The striker was held by a shear wire. Over the entire firing mechanism was placed a metal cover to prevent accidental discharge, the cover being held in place by means of a retaining pin and ring. A small hole was provided in the cover cap for filling. This was sealed with a disc of tin. The filling charge was about 0.90 lb. of white phosphorus.

When used as a *hand grenade*, the cap over the firing mechanism was removed after withdrawing the retaining pin. The striker was then struck against any solid object, as the heel of the boot, the butt of the gun, a rock, etc., and the grenade was thrown immediately after striking. The shock sheared the small restraining wire and the striker point fired the primer and started the fuse burning.

When used as a *rifle grenade*, the stem was attached by screwing it into the base plate of the grenade as far as it would go. The protecting cap was then removed, exposing the striker. A blank cartridge furnished for this purpose was next loaded into the rifle, after which the grenade

302

rod was inserted into the muzzle of the rifle and pushed down as far as it would go. The butt of the gun was set against some solid object, such as the bottom of the trench, a sandbag, etc., and the elevation adjusted according to the range desired. Upon the discharge of the rifle, the set-back sheared the small restraining wire, permitting the striker pin to impinge upon the primer and thus ignited the fuse which in 5 seconds fired the detonator.

The maximum range was obtained with the rifle held at 45 degrees. Shorter ranges could be had by either raising or lowering this elevation. Under favorable conditions, ranges up to 230 yd. were obtained.

Postwar Development of Smoke Grenades.—The phosphorus combination hand-and-rifle grenade was a very successful munition and was by far the most effective and useful chemical grenade in the late war. Because it was so satisfactory in the war, nothing has been done since to develop a more effective smoke grenade, and the World War type of combination hand-and-rifle smoke grenade remains today the most effective device of its kind.

Chemical Grenades—Incendiary

In addition to the phosphorus grenades mentioned above which, although primarily smoke devices, had considerable incendiary effect, there was also used in the war a special incendiary grenade which was called by the French, "Grenade-Incendiaire A Main, Mle. 1916—Cylindrique," and by the Americans, "Thermite Hand Grenade, MK-I." These two grenades were identical, the American grenade being copied directly from the French as the most successful device of its kind.

United States Thermite Hand Grenade, M-I (Fig. 13).—This grenade consisted of the following parts:

1. A cylindrical shell of tin plate to which the top and bottom were attached by crimping and soldering. In the cover was a hole into which was soldered a metallic ring, tapped to receive the firing mechanism.
2. A percussion cap provided with a Bickford fuse.
3. A charge of thermite.
4. A mixture of special ignition material.

The grenade body was approximately 5⅞ in. long and 2½ in. in diameter. The total weight of the charged grenade was about 1.65 lb.

To use the grenade, it was grasped firmly in one hand, and the cover cap was removed with the other hand. The striker was then forced in sharply by striking it a keen blow against a hard body such as the heel, a rock, the butt of the gun, etc., and the grenade was then immediately thrown or placed against the object to be burned. The percussion of the primer ignited the Bickford fuse. Its combustion required 5 seconds, after which the quick match was lighted. This, in turn, ignited the

303

special igniting mixture. By reason of the delay and absence of explosion, the grenade could be placed by hand or thrown to a distance.

The thermite incendiary grenade was effective because of the intense heat of the molten material. It was placed by hand above the object to be burned and used principally for the destruction of noncombustible

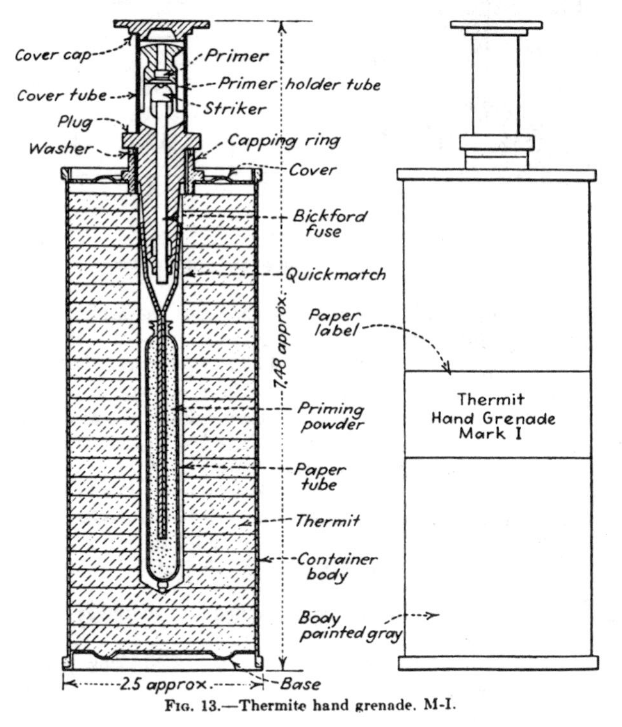

Fig. 13.—Thermite hand grenade, M-I.

material. It contained a thermite mixture which produced an exceedingly high temperature, the contents becoming a mass of white-hot molten metal.

Smoke Candles and Pots

Small portable nonmissile devices which produced smoke by progressive burning of a chemical filling were in the late war called *smoke candles*. If the device were of a larger size, not so readily portable, but producing a more enduring smoke cloud by longer burning, it was called a *smoke pot*.

304

These devices were among the first smoke producers used in the war. They proved very effective for supplementing the gas operations of chemical troops and were later more extensively employed in screening infantry operations.

Smoke candles were introduced by the British at the battle of Loos in September, 1915, being used by the British special gas companies in

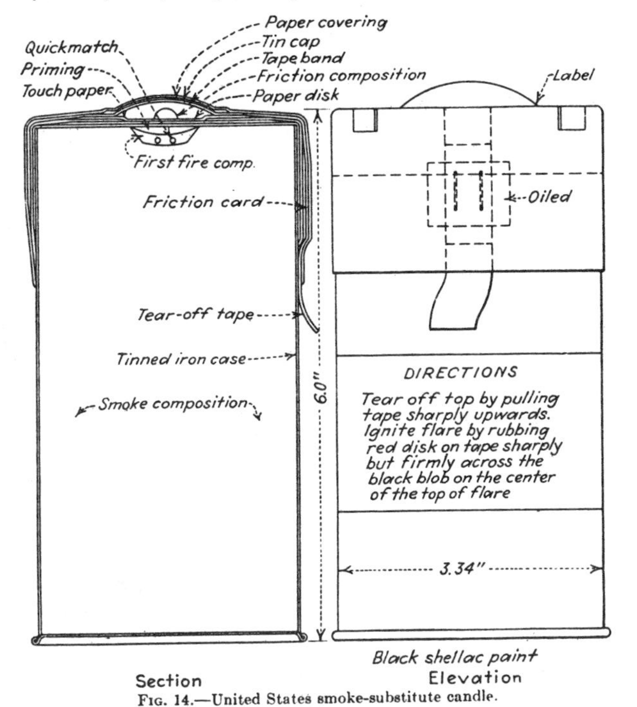

Fig. 14.—United States smoke-substitute candle.

conjunction with their gas operations at that time (12, page 56). These candles were known as "Smoke Candle, Mark I/L/Type S."

When the United States entered the war, it adopted a smoke candle, which was very similar to the British Type S Smoke Candle, and was known as "Candle, Smoke Substitute."

United States Candle, Smoke Substitute.—This candle consisted of a tin case, cylindrical in shape, 5⅞ in. high and 3⅜ in. in diameter, and filled with a solid smoke mixture, as shown in Fig. 14. To the top of the

305

case was fitted a case cover, containing a central circular hole 1 in. in diameter, through which the match head was inserted and from which the smoke escaped when the candle was fired. A cardboard disk containing the match head was placed on top of the case cover. The match head extended down through the hole in the case cover and acted as the igniter for the smoke mixture. A scratch block for igniting the match head was taped to the cardboard disk on one side of the match head and a small strip of wood, the same size as the scratch block, was placed on the other side of the match head in such a manner that they were easily

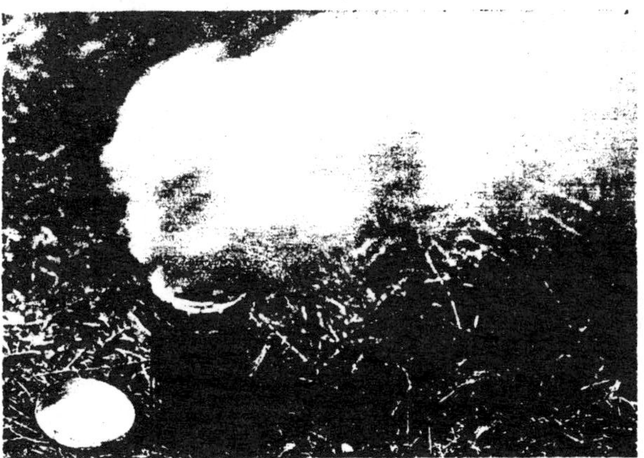
Fig. 15.—Candle, smoke substitute, in operation.

removable. The strip of wood, together with the scratch block, formed a protection for the match head. A metal cover was fitted over the top of the candle and sealed with adhesive tape.

The smoke mixture consisted of potassium nitrate, coal dust, sulfur, borax, and hard pitch, while the match head consisted of a mixture of potassium chlorate, antimony sulfide, and dextrine.

The candle completely assembled was 6½ in. high and 3⅜ in. in diameter, weighed 3½ lb., was painted black, and was not marked or stenciled in any way.

By drawing the scratch block quickly across the match head, the latter was ignited and flashed into the candle, igniting the smoke mixture. A delay of about 3 seconds occurred between the scratching of the match head and the evolution of smoke. The cardboard disk holding the match head burned off.

306

Smoke of a yellowish brown color was generated in considerable volume for a period of 4 minutes. A small cloud of vapor at the finish usually lasted for another half minute. Figure 15 shows the candle, smoke substitute, in operation.

These candles could be fired either singly with the scratch block or as a group with electric squibs. When fired individually, the adhesive tape from the cover of the candle was removed and the candle was placed in an upright position on the ground.

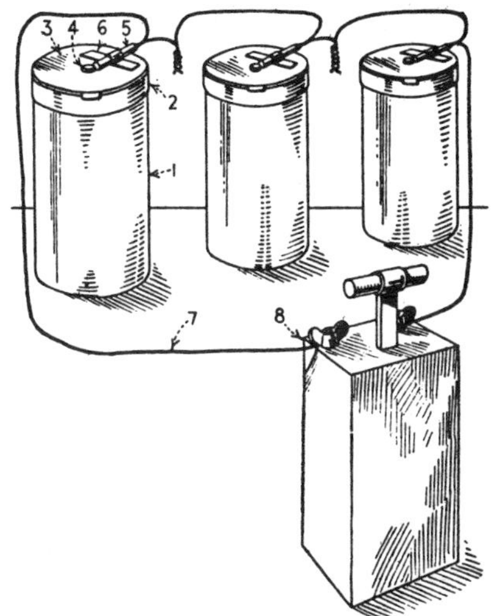

Fig. 16.—Illustration of electrical method of firing candles.

1. Candle. 2. Inner cover. 3. Cardboard disk. 4. Match head. 5. Squib. 6. Adhesive tape. 7. Lead wire. 8. Exploder.

After the tape was removed from the match head; the scratch block was drawn across the match head. When fired as a group, the adhesive tape from the cover of the candle and the cover were removed, also the scratch block and tape, exposing the match head. The plug from the base of an electric squib was removed and the squib with base (open end) was securely taped against the match head.

The candles were then connected in a series and attached to a blasting machine (see Fig. 16). The number of candles that may be fired electrically is limited only by the capacity of the exploder or blasting machine used.

The candle, smoke substitute, was painted black. Paint was applied by dipping the candle in asphaltum paint for the purpose of protecting

307

the container and preventing the access of moisture to the contents. No marking was placed on the candle, smoke substitute.

Postwar Development of Smoke Candles.—The postwar development of smoke candles has closely paralleled that of tear-gas candles. The first step was to substitute HC smoke mixture* for the British Type S smoke mixture. The next step was to standardize the size of the smoke candle so as to make it the same as the tear-gas candle and thus utilize the same container for both types. The result of this step in the develop-

* See Chap. XI, p. 245.

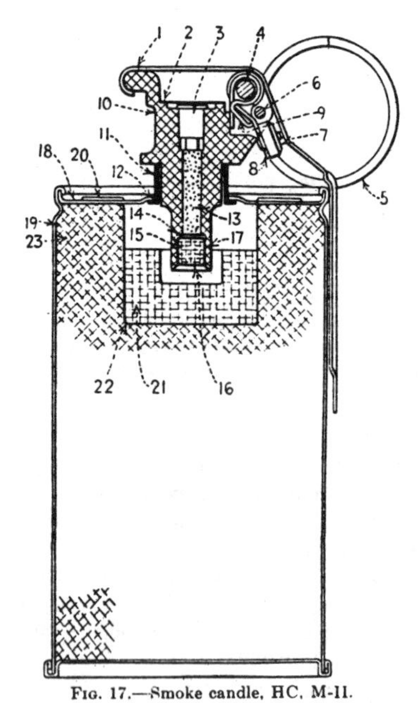

Fig. 17.—Smoke candle, HC, M-II.

1. Lever.
2. Disk.
3. New No. 4 primer.
4. Hinge pin.
5. Ring.
6. $\frac{1}{16}$-in. cotter pin.
7. Striker point.
8. Striker.
9. Spring.
10. Fuse body.
11. Adapter.
12. Solder.
13. Delay element.
14. 0.06-gram Army black powder.
15. 0.12-gram Army black powder.
16. Cup disk.
17. Cup.
18. Top.
19. Container body.
20. Zinc oxide adhesive tape.
21. Starter mixture.
22. Starter-mixture cup.
23. Smoke mixture.

308

ment was known as "Smoke Candle, HC, M-II," (later called "Smoke Grenade, HC, M8").

Smoke Candle, HC, M-II, consisted of a cylindrical tin container $2\frac{5}{16}$ in. in diameter and 4½ in. high, filled with a solid smoke mixture and a starting mixture and had a fuse mechanism for firing. With the fuse attached, the height of the candle is 5¾ in. For details see Fig. 17.

A zinc cup, circular in shape, 1⅛ in. in diameter, and ¾ in. deep, was placed in a depression left in the top of the smoke mixture. The top of the cup was flanged outward, the flange being $\frac{9}{16}$ in. wide. The flange of the starter cup covered the entire surface of the mixture.

The container top, in which there were four ¼ in. holes covered by squares of adhesive tape and to which a brass adapter was riveted, was fitted to the can on top of the zinc starter cup. Into the brass adapter was assembled a fuse, M-I.

The smoke mixture was composed of hexachlorethane, powdered zinc, ammonium perchlorate, and ammonium chloride, and the starting mixture consisted of potassium nitrate, antimony trisulfide, and dextrine.

The candle, with fuse attached, weighed approximately 1¾ lb.

When the safety pin of the fuse was pulled and the lever released, the striker fired the primer. This ignited the delay element which in turn ignited the starting mixture. The starting mixture burned through the zinc cup and started a chemical reaction of the smoke mixture, generating considerable heat with the formation of zinc chloride.

The zinc chloride escaped into the air as a dense white smoke, composed of finely divided solid particles, which readily absorbed moisture and became highly obscuring liquid particles.

The candle burned from 2½ to 3¼ minutes in full volume. A small stream of vapor lasted for possibly ¼ minute longer. Figure 18 shows Smoke Candle, HC, M-II, in operation.

To fire, the candle was grasped with lever held firmly against the candle body and the safety pin was withdrawn, keeping a firm grasp around the candle and lever. The candle was thrown with a full swing of the arm, like a grenade, or placed on the ground. As the candle was released from the hand, the lever dropped away, allowing the striker to fire the primer.

The candle could not be thrown into or placed within 5 ft. of dry grass or other readily inflammable material if a fire was to be avoided. After the candle was ignited, personnel remained at least 5 ft. away from the burning candle. While the candle was practically harmless, the smoke was evolved with great vigor, and there was a tendency to throw out hot particles of residue.

Smoke candle, HC, M-II, was painted gray. A yellow band 1½ in. wide was painted around the can, 2 in. from the top. Stenciled in yellow

309

in ½-in. letters was the symbol "HC," ½ in. from the top of the container, and the word "SMOKE" 1¼ in. from the top of the container. Below the yellow band, stenciled in yellow were the letters "U.S.," the manufacturer's identification mark, and the lot number.

HC Smoke Pot, M-I.—After several years' use of Smoke Candle, HC, M-II, it was found to be too small for the most economical generation of smoke, and a larger size device was developed. This device, known as "Smoke Pot, HC, M-I," uses HC smoke mixture as a filling and the scratch-block type of firing mechanism employed in the smoke-substitute candle. Smoke Pot, HC, M-I, is now the standard portable field screening smoke generator for the United States Army.

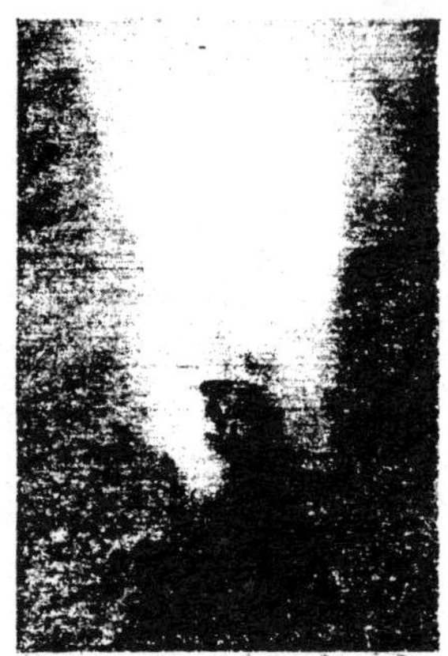

Fig. 18.—Smoke Candle, HC, M-II, in operation.

The present standard smoke pot (Smoke Pot, HC, M-I) is greatly superior to the World War types of smoke candles, both as regards quality and quantity of smoke generated. As indicated in Chap. XI (page 246), HC smoke mixture has a T.O.P. of 2,100, as compared to a T.O.P. of 460 for the World War Type S smoke mixture. Also the standard smoke pot contains 12.5 lb. of HC filling as against 3 lb. for the smoke-substitute candle. One standard pot, therefore, is equivalent to 20 smoke-substitute (Type S) smoke candles in obscuring capacity.

533

CHAPTER XIX

INDIVIDUAL PROTECTION

WORLD WAR DEVELOPMENT

To accomplish its mission in war, an army must protect itself; it must seek to keep itself intact and avoid an excessive drain in casualties upon its resources and fighting power. Hence there is both an individual and a collective demand for protection in war regardless of what means or weapons are employed. In consequence of this, the history of war might well be viewed as an age-long and continuing struggle between weapon development as a means of taking life, on the one hand, and protection as a measure for safeguarding life, on the other.

Broadly speaking, gas is used as a war weapon to contaminate the atmosphere about the enemy's position, rendering it dangerous to breathe. Certain chemical agents are so toxic that but a few breaths of them in high concentration will cause death by asphyxiation. Other gases attack the surface of the body and produce casualties by burns. It is therefore imperative that each individual be provided with a protective device to remove the noxious substances from the air before they are breathed or before they come in contact with the body. This is the problem of *individual protection.*

War gases are heavier than air. Hence they tend to hug the ground and flow more or less like water into ground depressions, such as ravines, hollows, and valleys, remaining effective in such places much longer than on high ground exposed to the wind. Gas seeps into trenches and dugouts and penetrates ordinary buildings just as does pure air. Woods contribute to their persistency. Hence it is that ordinary cover from gun fire is not only ineffective against gas but, to the extent that it causes "gas pockets," actually contributes to the effectiveness of chemical agents. The continuing action of gas after its release has also to be reckoned with for, unlike an H.E. shell, the effect of which is complete when the shell explodes and each of its fragments has come to rest, the action of a chemical shell merely begins upon its explosion.

These factors greatly complicate the problem of gas protection, for not only is it necessary to have special protective equipment, but there must be some means of giving warning in time for this equipment to be adjusted. Moreover, men cannot wear masks continuously. They can neither eat nor obtain much rest while wearing masks. Hence means

534

must be provided to enable soldiers to eat and sleep without masks and to enable staffs and special-duty men whose work requires freedom from the restrictions imposed by the gas mask to carry on their functions unmasked and yet protected from the all-pervading clutches of toxic gases. This is the problem of group or *collective protection.*

Finally, measures must always be taken to protect tactical units against chemical attack and to assist them in accomplishing their missions without excessive gas casualties. This is the problem of *tactical protection.*

From the foregoing it will be seen that defense against chemical attack presents three classes of problems: (1) individual, (2) collective, and (3) tactical protections. The first two of these involve protective measures of a generally passive nature, *i.e.*, principally the provision and use of individual protective equipment, discussed in this chapter, and installations for group protection, treated in Chap. XX. The third problem—tactical protection—concerns modes of action and troop leading, with the view to avoiding gas casualties in the conduct of military operations.

When the Germans launched the first chlorine cloud against the British and French in April, 1915, it caught them without any form of protection, and hence caused a tremendous number of casualties (15,000) and a high percentage of fatalities (33 per cent). So staggering was this blow that all the energies of the British and French Governments were concentrated during the next few weeks on improvising means of protection against gas, and the results achieved were nothing short of miraculous. Within the short space of two weeks, every British soldier at the front was issued a cotton pad soaked in a solution of sodium carbonate and thiosulfate, which could be tied over his face and which afforded protection against chlorine—the only gas then in use.

Concerning this early effort on the part of the British, General Foulkes says:

> Immediately after the first German gas attack . . . Lord Kitchener had sent two eminent scientists, Dr. Haldane and Professor Baker, to France to investigate the problem of protection on the spot; he had also appealed to the British public to supply pad respirators, such as were being improvised in the field, and in a very few days, thanks to the devoted efforts of British women and the organization of the Red Cross, every man in the B.E.F. had been supplied with some sort of protection against gas.

From the first big gas attack in April, 1915, to the end of the war, the resources of both sides, and particularly of the Allies, were strained almost to the limit to keep gas protection abreast of the rapid development in the offensive use of gas. It was truly a modern version (vastly accelerated) of the age-old race between armor and armor-piercing projectiles. During the three and a half years of the gas war the British Government alone issued 50,000,000 gas masks of seven different kinds to protect an

535

army of 2,000,000 men in France—an average of 25 masks per man. This was not waste; it was dire necessity, forced by the following sequence of events:

The Germans used:

1. *Chlorine*, on Apr. 21, 1915, against unprotected troops. By May 3, 1915, British troops were issued cotton cloth pads soaked in a solution of sodium carbonate, sodium thiosulfate, and water. These were supplemented with boxes of cotton waste from which each soldier took a handful to stuff in his mouth and nostrils before fastening the pad over his face. The pads required frequent soaking. This form of protection was never regarded as more than a temporary expedient.

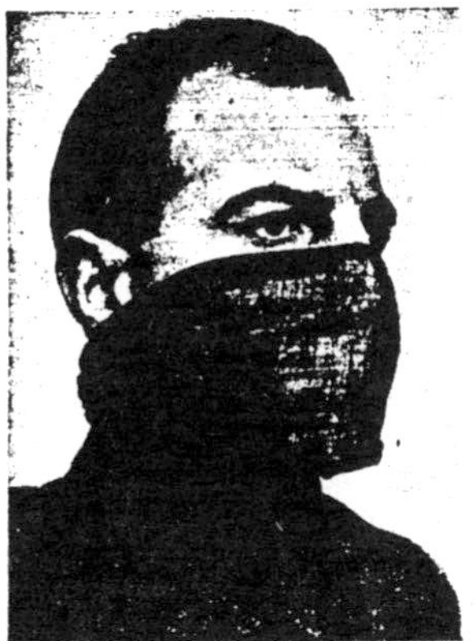

FIG. 108.—First British gas mask, Black Veil Respirator.

By May 10, 1915, British troops in the Ypres sector were provided with the *Black Veil Respirator* (see Fig. 108). This consisted of a fourfold piece of black veiling about 1 yd. long and 8 in. wide. The center portion was padded with cotton and saturated with sodium carbonate, glycerine, and water, the glycerine having been added to keep the pad moist. Tied about the face, this respirator, however, did not insure a gastight fit and was soon replaced with a new design.

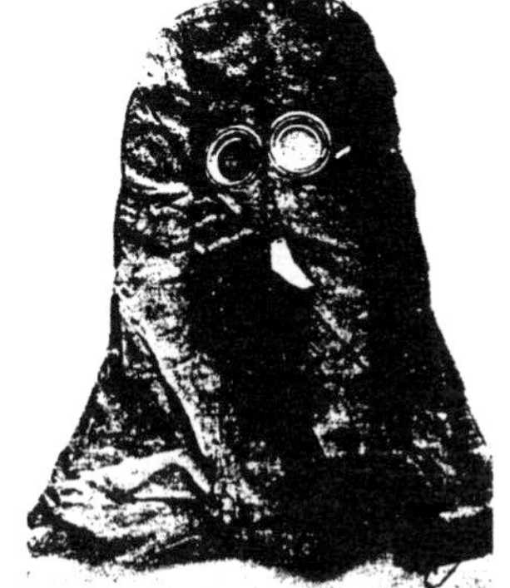

FIG. 109.—British Hypo, P., or P.H. Helmet, showing skirt effect.

2. *Tear gas* (T-Stoff), in shell beginning in January, 1915, but increasing to serious proportions in May and June. These tear gases caused very serious lacrimation (an unprotected man was helpless) when present in a concentration only one six-thousandth of the lethal concentration of chlorine. To meet this threat the British issued the *Hypo Helmet* (see Figs. 109 and 110). This helmet was made of flannel in the form of a sack which could be put over the head with the open ends tucked inside the blouse. The cloth was dipped in hypo (sodium thiosulfate), washing soda, and glycerine. A rectangular piece of

536

celluloid was inserted in the helmet for vision. This was easily cracked and the mask was otherwise defective in having no outlet valve to prevent the harmful accumulation of carbon dioxide inside the helmet. This mask was issued to all troops in the field by July 6, 1915.

3. *Phosgene*, on Dec. 11, 1915. Phosgene was ten times more poisonous than chlorine. By July, 1915, it was learned that phosgene would be employed by the Germans during the following December. The British Intelligence Service ascertained not only this important fact but also the exact area within which the attack would take place. With five months to prepare, the British developed the *P. Helmet.* This was similar in shape to the Hypo Helmet but was made of flannelette and was provided with two glass eyepieces. It also had an expiratory valve made of rubber, very similar to the outlet valve on present-day masks (see Figs. 109 and 110). The helmet was dipped in a solution of caustic soda, phenol, and glycerine. The first two of these substances react to form sodium phenolate which neutralized phosgene, hence the name *P.* or *Phenolate Helmet*. It was used by the British during the large phosgene attack near Pilckum on Dec. 19, 1915. It saved many lives though it was not fully satisfactory against high concentrations.

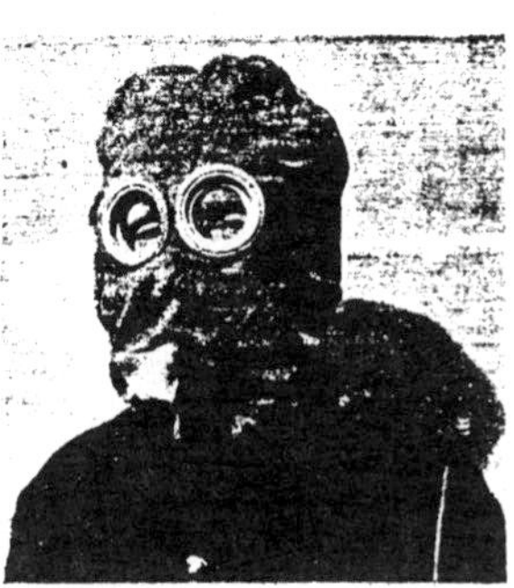

FIG. 110.—British Hypo, P., or P.H. Helmet in use, skirt buttoned under tunic.

Meanwhile the Russians had discovered that a substance known as urotropine or hexamethylenetetramine readily neutralized phosgene. With this information, the British now discarded the P. Helmet for the *P.H.* (phenate-hexamine) *Helmet*, similar except for the protective solution in which it was dipped (see Figs. 109 and 110). The new solution was urotropine, caustic soda, phenol, and glycerine. The P.H. Helmet gave much better protection than the P. Helmet, was effective for about 24 hours' continuous use, and would withstand a high concentration of phosgene.

By the latter part of 1915, the Germans had commenced the extensive employment of lacrimators either alone or in conjunction with lethal gas. The P.H. Helmet offered little protection against lacrimators. Accordingly in September, 1915, goggles made of rubber with mica eyepieces were issued for use in connection with the P.H. Helmet. This involved difficulties of adjustment which led to the development of the *P.H.G. Helmet*, having tight-fitting goggles attached to the mask. This helmet, however, was also difficult to adjust and was soon discarded. With the

537

subsequent invention and issuance of the box respirator, the P.H. Helmet was continued in service use for some little time as a substitute in case the respirator was lost or damaged.

4. *Increasing concentration of gas* early in 1916. The protection provided was inadequate. Having reached what they believed was the limit of protection with the helmet-type of mask, still not fully satisfactory, the British now turned to an entirely different principle, with the invention of the *Large Box* or *Tarbox Respirator*. This was the first British Army mask which included a canister of neutralizing chemicals. The canister contained granules of charcoal, soda lime, and potassium permanganate. It was connected by a rubber tube to the facepiece which covered only the chin, mouth, and nose. The facepiece was made of 24 thicknesses of muslin soaked in sodium zincate and urotropine. The facepiece included a nose clip to prevent breathing through the nose and a rubber mouthpiece for breathing with the mouth through the canister. Goggles were used for protection against lacrimators.

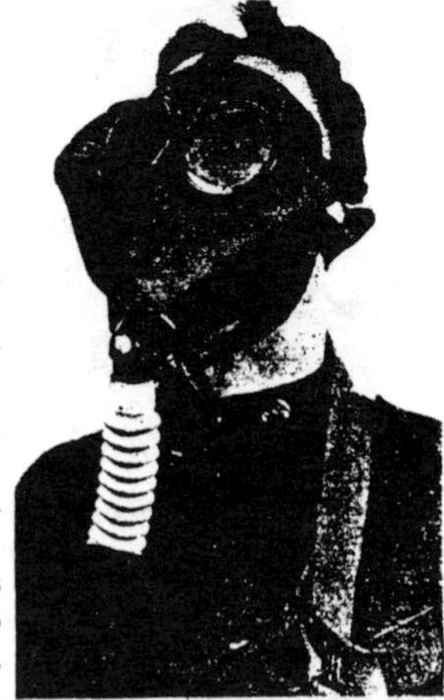
Fig. 111.—British Small Box Respirator.

5. *Chlorpicrin and similar* (*Green Cross*) *gases*, about Mar. 26, 1916. Chlorpicrin was about four times as poisonous as chlorine. It was also chemically very inert and was not efficiently absorbed by any respirator to this date.

The Large Box Respirator was cumbersome and deficient in protection against lacrimators. It, in turn, was supplanted by a mask of improved design called the *Small Box Respirator* (see Fig. 111). This was first issued to troops in April, 1916, and served the British, as well as many of the United States troops, to the end of the War. The Small Box Respirator consisted of a small canister containing layers of charcoal, soda lime, and potassium permanganate; a corrugated tube and a facepiece covered the entire face. The facepiece was made of rubber cloth and while a tight fit was depended upon for protection against lacrimators, the rubber mouthpiece and nose clip, to insure that only air from the canister was breathed, were retained.

6. *Mustard gas* (*Yellow Cross*), in July, 1917. Mustard gas is 36 times as poisonous as chlorine. The Small Box Respirator sufficiently protected the eyes and nose against mustard gas. The mustard gas

538

persisted for days in any locality where used and had very little odor and was not unpleasant at the time. The masks were very uncomfortable when worn for long periods. Also, the mustard gas affected all parts of the body, easily permeating the clothing. Hence tremendous casualties were caused by its use. Adequate protection never was devised. *Difficulties of manufacture fortunately limited the German supply.*

7. *Toxic smoke* (*Blue Cross*), in July 1917. Some of these toxic smokes produce intense and intolerable (an unprotected man could not fight) irritation of the nose and throat in concentrations only one twenty-thousandth of the lethal concentration of chlorine. All the masks previously mentioned permitted the penetration of smokes. The Germans discovered smokes terribly irritating to the nose and throat and commenced their use on a very large scale. The Germans manufactured 14,000,000 Blue Cross shell and expected extremely important results, hoping to force the removal of the mask and permit casualties to be readily produced by other gases.

The British had forseen this possibility and had provided a partial protection in the shape of an extension to the Small Box Respirator. Subsequently other changes were introduced. Really adequate protection never was devised. Fortunately the German shells were not effective. (Penetration of the mask is effective only when the particles are approximately of a certain size.)

The above facts illustrate grimly the strenuous race that took place between offensive and defensive gas warfare in the late war.

Mask Development

The evolution of the *British* wartime gas mask, as outlined above, is of special interest since it was the British type which was adopted by the American Army upon entry of the United States into the war.

The earliest *German* respirators consisted of pads of cloth soaked in a sodium thiosulfate—sodium carbonate solution. These were followed by masks of absorbent cloth made in the shape of a snout which fitted over the mouth and nose.

During the fall of 1915, the Germans turned to a canister-type respirator (see Fig. 112). The facepiece of this mask was made of leather treated with tar oil and tallow to render it gastight and watertight. The facepiece covered the entire face including the eyes. Eyepieces, consisting of an outer layer of glass and an inner layer of chemically treated celluloid which prevented dimming, were inserted. Screwed to a socket in the facepiece was a small cylindrical canister containing absorbent chemicals. The air was inhaled and expired directly through this canister. Originally the canister filling consisted of a layer of kieselguhr or granules of earth soaked in potassium carbonate covered with

539

powdered charcoal, a layer of charcoal granules, and a layer of pumice mixed with urotropine. In April, 1918, a layer of charcoal and zinc oxide was substituted for the layer of earth granules.

To protect against irritant smokes, a paper disk filter in a perforated metal container, which was fitted over the canister, was later issued.

This mask had the advantage of compactness, but as there was no outlet valve the wearer had to continually breathe a certain amount of his own expired air. Also the entire weight of the German mask and canister was carried by the head and produced fatigue of the neck muscles after a short period of wear.

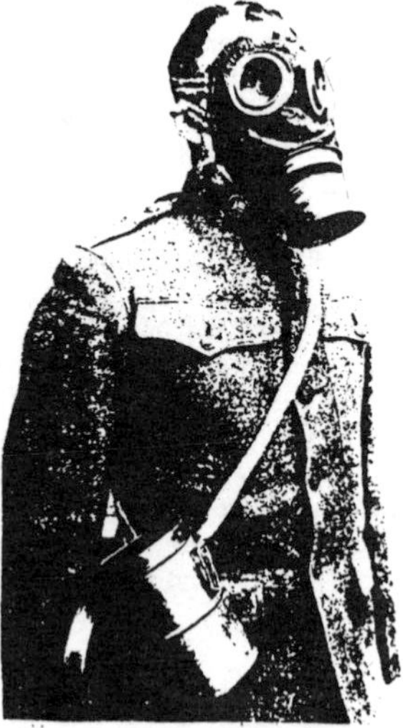
Fig. 112.—Early German gas mask.

The *French* developed three masks, the M2, the Tissot and the A.R.S. (*Appareil Respiratoire Spécial*).

The M2 Mask (see Fig. 113) was in the form of a snout covering the face. It was made of 32 layers of muslin impregnated with neutralizing chemicals. Celluloid eyepieces were provided for vision. There was no outlet valve. Air was inhaled and exhaled through the fabric.

The facepiece of the Tissot Mask (see Fig. 114) was made of pure rubber and was connected by a tube to a canister of absorbent chemicals carried on the back. The mask is noteworthy as being the first to provide for drawing the incoming air across the eyepieces to prevent them from dimming. It was used extensively by artillerymen and special observers in both the French and American armies. It was clumsy, however, and difficult to adjust and was hence unsuitable for front-line troops.

The French now turned to the German type of snout canister mask, developing the A.R.S. Mask, experimentation with which began in September, 1917. This mask was an improvement on the German in that it incorporated the Tissot principle of preventing dimming of the eyepieces by drawing the dry inspired air across them and it also included an outlet valve which the German type lacked. The French snout canister, however, gave somewhat less protection than the German. Moreover, the French did not furnish each soldier with an extra canister to carry with his mask as did the Germans.

540
The original *Italian* mask was somewhat similar to the French M2 type. This was soon discarded for the British Small Box Respirator which the Italians adopted for their troops during the war

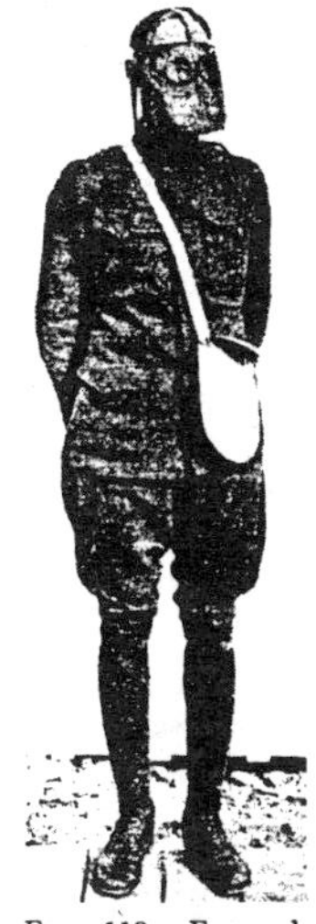

Fig. 113.—French M2 gas mask.

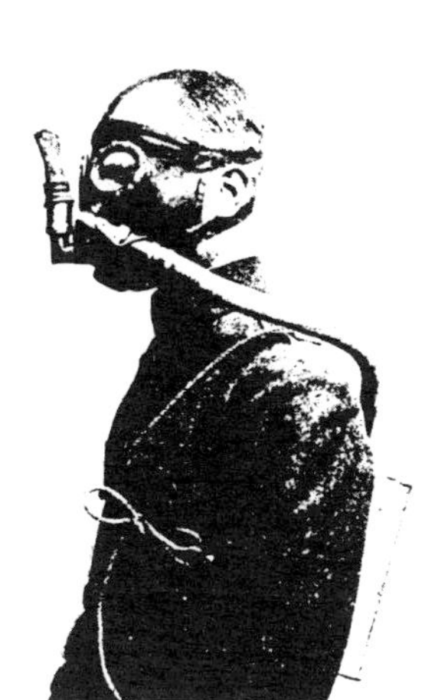

Fig. 114.—French Tissot gas mask.

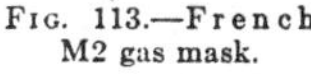

The *Russian* wartime gas mask (see Fig. 115) consisted of a headpiece which covered the head including the ears. It was connected directly to a canister box supported on the chest. The canister contained charcoal only. This mask had neither mouthpiece nor nose clip, but was still uncomfortable to wear.

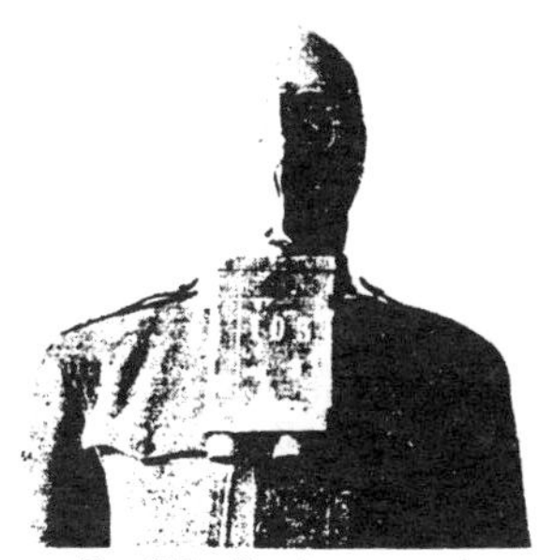

Fig. 115.—Russian gas mask.

Upon entry of the *United States* in the war, the War Department adopted the British Small Box Respirator (see Fig. 111), considering it the best of European masks which had been developed. However, in view of the then extensive use of mustard gas which necessitated the wearing of the mask for long periods of time, it was early realized by the American Gas Service that the uncomfortable mouthpiece and nose clip of the British type of mask should

541
be eliminated. Accordingly experimentation was immediately begun leading to development of a number of improved designs. None of these fully met requirements, and it was not until the close of the war that a satisfactory American mask of improved design was produced. All told a total of 5,692,499 masks were made in this country during the war. Of this number 4,210,586 were shipped to France.

The first American effort in gas-mask production was a lot of 25,000 masks of British type intended for use of the 1st Division. These were made without sufficient knowledge of British specifications and fabrication methods. They were shipped to France in 1917 but proved faulty and were never issued to troops.

Following receipt of more definite information, production of *masks* for *training* purposes, practically in exact duplication of the British type, was begun in this country in July, 1917. The facepiece of this type was made of rubberized cloth and included celluloid eyepieces. It had a rubber mouthpiece and nose clip similar to the British.

The Training Mask was followed in October, 1917, with the *C.E.* or *Corrected English Mask*. This included an improvement in the facepiece fabric, protecting against all gases, the previous type having been permeable to chlorpicrin. Other improvements were the addition of the flutter valve guard, use of coiled spring to hold the eyepieces in place, change in the angle tube giving lower breathing resistance, and the substitution of activated cocoanut charcoal in the canister, for the unactivated wood charcoal in the original British type. Before the Armistice, 1,864,000 of the C.E. Masks were turned out.

The *R.F.K. Mask* was a somewhat improved type designed by three men connected with the American Gas service, Richardson, Flory, and Kops. Noteworthy improvements of the C.E. mask were the use of spun-in aluminum eyepieces and a change in the shape and the facepiece binder frame to increase the comfort. From February, 1918, until the Armistice, 3,050,000 of these masks were produced.

To meet the demand for increased comfort and lower breathing resistance, there followed several types noteworthy as the forerunners of the present-day American Army mask. In all of these the mouthpiece and nose clip were dispensed with, and the Tissot principle of deflecting the incoming dry air across the eyepieces was incorporated. The A.T. (Akron Tissot) Mask, was designed by the Akron Rubber Company (see Fig. 116). The facepiece of this mask was made of molded rubber covered with stockinette. Inside the facepiece was a Y-shaped tube to deflect the incoming air across the eyepieces and a sponge-rubber chin rest was also provided. Production of this type started in June, 1917, a total of 197,000 being made before the Armistice.

542
Another improved type was designed by Kops and known as the *K.T.* or *Kops-Tissot Mask*. This mask contained a semiflexible facepiece binder frame and was provided with a butterfly shaped air deflector made of rubber. It had no angle tube, separate tubes for inlet and outlet of air being used. In place of the rubber chin rest of the A.T., it had an elastic chin rest strap. The self-centering adjustable head harness provided in the A.T. was incorporated in this mask. A total of 337,000 were made before the Armistice.

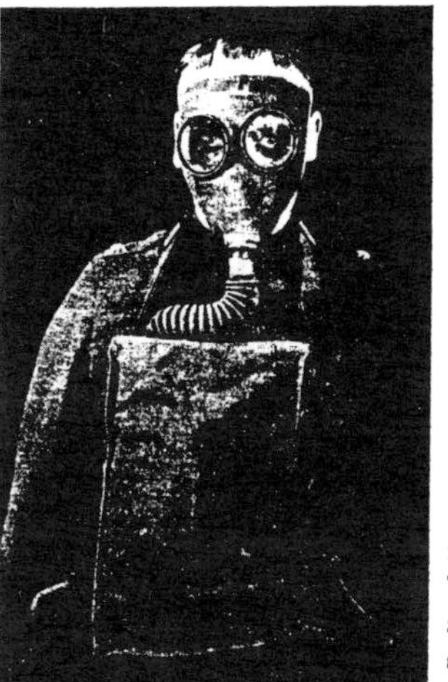

Fig. 116.—American A.T. (Akron-Tissot) gas mask.

The principal objection to the A.T. and K.T. Masks was that they were difficult to manufacture.

By October, 1919, production had begun on a further improved type known as the 1919 *Model* or *K.T.M. Mask*. About 2,000 of these were turned out before the Armistice, by which time preparations had been made for their manufacture at the rate of one million a month.

The facepiece of this mask was made of a special rubber compound. The outside surface was covered by a layer of thin cotton fabric called stockinette which was vulcanized to the rubber. The facepiece material with stockinette covering was manufactured in the form of sheets from which the facepieces were cut out by means of a special die. The die cutting was so shaped that when folded and two short edges were sewn together to form a chin seam, a properly fitting mask was obtained. This method of manufacture greatly facilitated mass production. Holes for the eyepieces were eliptical so that an uneven tension was produced around the cypieces causing the eyepieces to bulge forward as desired and insuring a proper fit about the temples. The mask had an angle tube similar to that of the A.T. and a deflector almost identical with that used in the K.T., but neither a chin rest nor a chin strap, the facepiece being so shaped that these were unnecessary. A head harness pad of canvas-covered felt and buckles for adjustment of the head harness straps were provided.

Canister Development (American)

The canisters of the early American type masks were filled with charcoal and soda lime in the proportion of 60 to 40 and were painted *black*.

543
They were about one-fourth larger than the British type, it having been feared that our charcoal was inferior and that hence a larger amount was

needed. It was later learned that American-made charcoal was in fact superior and the canister was accordingly reduced to the same size as the British.

The canisters of the C.E. Masks were of the reduced size and were painted *yellow*. By January, 1918, two cotton pads were inserted in the canister to protect against irritant smokes. These canisters were also painted yellow.

When the R.F.K. masks were being manufactured, it was found that the canister could be reduced still further in size and also that breathing resistance could be lowered. Canisters of this improved type were painted *green*.

Various sorts of irritant smoke filters were used during the World War, including paper, cellulose, and cotton. Felt was found to be the most efficient material, though it offered considerable resistance to breathing and was expensive. Accordingly, the next American improvement in canisters was the incorporation of a felt filter. This canister was painted *blue* and was used in the 1919 mask.

Carrier Development

For the early American types of gas masks, a square-shaped canvas satchel, carried slung over the shoulder, was provided. The sling or carrying strap for these carriers was so made that the satchel could be quickly transferred to the *alert position* across the chest, a cord being used to tie around the body and hold the satchel in place. This *two-position* carrier was not satisfactory in this respect and, moreover, when lying prone it was difficult to adjust the mask from the alert position of the carrier without undue exposure of the body. The side satchel was hence developed. Using a longer corrugated tube it was unnecessary, with the side satchel, to change its position before adjusting the mask.

POSTWAR DEVELOPMENT

The Gas Mask

Since the war, development work on gas masks has been mainly directed toward further improving the "1919 Model" Army service gas mask, brought out at the end of the war, and toward providing additional types of special masks needed for certain troops who have special duties to perform, such as communicating messages over telephones (the diaphragm mask), observing through optical instruments (optical mask), and piloting airplanes (aviation mask).

544

Our postwar mask-development work has been based upon certain practical requirements which control the design of the mask. These requirements may be summarized as follows:

1. The mask must protect against all chemical-warfare agents.
2. It must have a low breathing resistance.
3. It must be light in weight.
4. It must be comfortable.
5. It must be simple in design, easy to operate, and repair.
6. It must not interfere greatly with vision.
7. It must be rugged enough to withstand field conditions.
8. It must be reasonably easy to manufacture in quantity.
9. It must not deteriorate appreciably in storage for at least several years.
10. It must have a service life in the field for at least several months.

The ideal gas mask is one which affords complete protection against all known toxic gases. Theoretically such a mask is possible but it can not at the same time satisfy all of the practical requirements listed above. Thus, the requirements of maximum protection, low breathing resistance, and light weight, are essentially opposed, for protection varies directly with the amount of chemicals used and the capacity of the mechanical filter. But the more chemicals used and the larger the filter, the heavier the canister. Similarly, low breathing resistance requires a large superficial area for the filter which in turn increases the size and weight of the canister.

Again, if the canister is made small, the chemical filling must be reduced, which lowers protection, and the filter must be made smaller, which increases breathing resistance. Hence the military mask is a compromise, embodying an optimum balance among the ten requirements indicated above, particularly the first three.

In addition, the Army service gas mask is designed to protect only against substances suitable for war use as chemical agents. This should be thoroughly understood and the military mask should not be relied upon for any purposes other than those for which it is intended.

The Canister

The canister of the military gas mask is the means by which chemical agents present in the atmosphere are removed from air before it is breathed (see Fig. 117). It consists of three principal parts, *viz.*, a chemical container, usually made of sheet metal and provided with air inlet and outlet openings; a filter for the removal of solid and liquid particles by mechanical filtration; the chemical filling for the disposal of gases by physical adsorption, chemical neutralization, or by a combination of these processes.

As an integral part of the mask the canister itself must conform to the general requirements listed above. These requirements impose

545

decided limitations upon the number of materials or substances which may be used as components. The material used for the *mechanical filter* must be sufficiently dense to hold out the extremely minute solid or liquid particles of which the irritant gases and smokes are constituted. These particles, it may be said, are so small that they cannot be seen with an ordinary high-powered microscope while even with the ultramicroscope they are only visible as points of reflected light. On the other hand, the filter material must not be so dense as to impede unduly the flow of air through it. The chemical or chemicals used for the removal of gases must be highly porous in order to provide within small space a relatively enormous absorbent surface. They must not react with each other or corrode their metal container. Their effectiveness must not be appreciably lowered by exposure to air of high humidity.

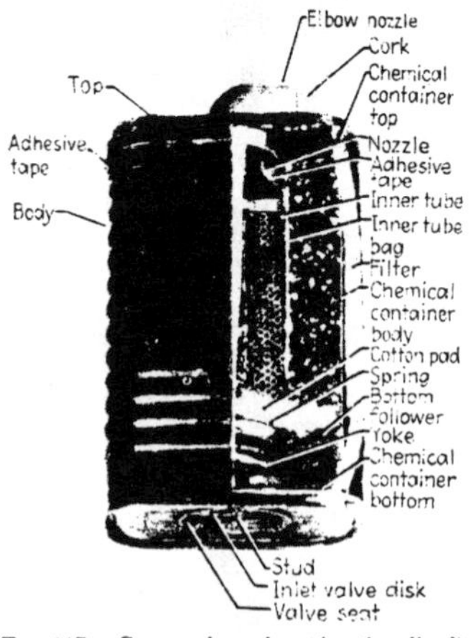

Fig. 117.—Gas-mask canister (sectionalized).

They must remove the gas very rapidly since any given portion of inspired air is in contact with the canister filling for but a fractional part of a second. They must have the capacity to dispose of large amounts of gas since the canister cannot be frequently replaced. They must be fairly cheap and available in great quantity. In turn, they, as well as the filter, must not cause high breathing resistance.

The only single substance which approximately fulfills all the requirements of a chemical filling for gas-mask canisters is activated charcoal in the form of small granules. Generally speaking the best charcoals for this purpose are made from very dense raw materials. The most satisfactory material found during the World War for canister charcoal was cocoanut shell. Various nut shells, fruit stones, and other substances, however, were also used. Since the war, improved methods of manufacture have made possible the use of more readily available materials. Charcoal is a highly porous substance consisting principally of carbon which is made by the carbonization of organic matter. As such, it is called *primary charcoal*. By subjecting primary charcoal to a certain process of heat and steam, called *activation*, the property of adsorption of gases, which primary charcoal possesses, is greatly increased.

When gas-laden air is passed through activated charcoal, the molecules of gas are attracted and held physically on the surface of the pores in the

546

charcoal granules, the purified air passing on through. This process of removal of the gas is called *adsorption*. It may roughly be compared to the action of a magnet in attracting and holding iron fillings on its surface. Activated charcoal which will adsorb half its own weight of toxic gas has been made on a large scale, while charcoals have been made in the laboratory which will adsorb more than their own weight of gas. The principal deficiency of charcoal as a canister filling is that it does not hold tenaciously certain highly volatile acid gases, notably phosgene, but gradually releases them to the passing air current. This deficiency is compensated for by the use of another substance mixed with the charcoal, *viz.*, soda lime.

Soda lime is a mixture consisting of hydrated lime, cement, kieselguhr, sodium hydroxide, and water in various proportions according to the formula used; there are several. Gases, which the charcoal does not hold firmly by adsorption and which are gradually given off by it, are caught by the soda lime, with which they enter into chemical combination. After continued exposure to certain gases, such as phosgene, a gradual transfer of the gas to the soda lime takes place, thus leaving the charcoal free to pick up more gas. It may therefore be said that the principal function of the soda lime is to act as a reservoir of large capacity for the permanent fixation of the more volatile acid and oxidizable gases, while the charcoal furnishes the required degree of activity for all gases as well as storage capacity for less volatile ones.

Another reason for the combination absorbent is that, while a rise in either temperature or humidity causes a decrease in the adsorptive capacity of charcoal, such conditions increase the reactivity of the soda lime.

The canister of the present military mask contains a mixture of soda lime and specially prepared charcoal as well as a highly efficient mechanical filter. It can thus be relied upon to give full protection against any gas likely to be encountered in the field. The function of the different components of the canister as regards the principal war gases is set forth below.

Gas	Neutralizing Agency
Brombenzyl cyanide	Charcoal
Chl rpicrin	Charcoal
Cyanogen chloride	Charcoal
Mustard gas	Charcoal
Chloracetophenone	Charcoal and filter
Chlorine	Charcoal–soda-lime mixture
Phosgene	Charcoal–soda-lime mixture
Diphosgene	Charcoal–soda-lime mixture
Hydrocyanic acid	Charcoal–soda-lime mixture
Lewisite	Charcoal–soda-lime mixture
Diphenylchlorarsine	Filter
Diphenylaminechlorarsine, etc	Filter

547

It should be impressed upon all concerned that the canister provided with the military gas mask is for protection against chemical warfare agents only. There are certain toxic gases unadapted for war use which may otherwise be encountered, especially in industry. The principal ones are carbon monoxide and ammonia. The Army canister does not protect against these gases and should never be relied upon for such purpose.

Carbon monoxide has neither odor nor color and a person subjected to a sufficient concentration of it loses consciousness without warning. Being lighter than air, high concentrations of this gas are generally limited to enclosed spaces. As it is one of the products of combustion of wood it is invariably present in burning buildings. Hence the military gas-mask canister should never be used in fire fighting. Carbon Monoxide is also present in automobile exhaust gas, in natural gas, artificial illuminating gas, blast-furnace gases, mine-explosion gases and in the gases resulting from the burning of smokeless powder in artillery.

Repair or rescue work about refrigeration plants and other places where there is leakage of ammonia gas should be undertaken with the military gas mask.

It should also be realized that the military gas mask does not supply or make air or oxygen and hence should never be used in an atmosphere deficient in oxygen. Tunnels and shafts of mines following an explosion, the holds of ships, and tanks and tank cars containing volatile liquids are places likely to be dangerous in this respect.

It should further be understood that *the Army service gas-mask canister is not designed to protect against concentrations of war gas greater than 1 per cent by volume.* It is most unlikely that concentrations as high as this will be encountered in the field. However, such concentrations may be found in the immediate vicinity of the explosion of the gas shell, for instance in a dugout when a shell bursts in the entrance to it. As additional precaution men, even though wearing masks, should move quickly from the immediate vicinity of the explosion holding their breath while so doing. Dangerously high concentrations may also be encountered through leakage in changing the valve on a cylinder containing a chemical agent liquefied by pressure, or in a tank containing a volatile solvent such as gasoline.

The Army Service Gas Mask

The gas mask now provided for the Army is known as the *Service Gas Mask* (see Fig. 118).

The principle upon which the gas mask functions is the purification of inspired air by removal of the gas or smoke. Perfect fit of the facepiece is depended upon to insure that only air which passes through the canister is drawn into the lungs. The mask consists of three main parts:

548

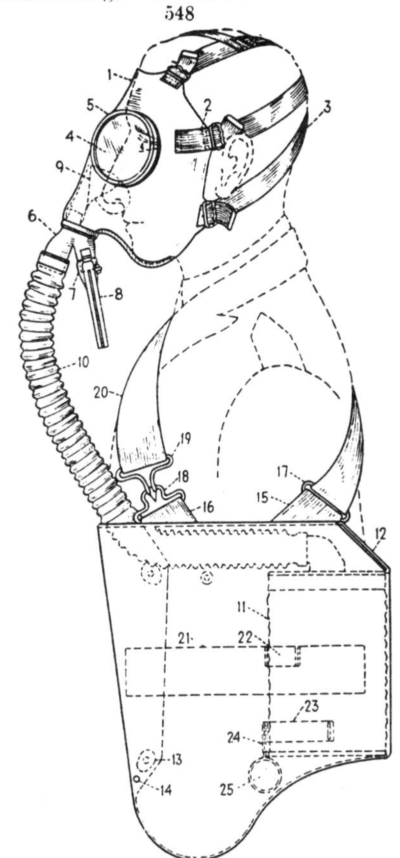

Fig. 118.—Army Service Gas Mask.

1. Rubber mask. 2. Harness attachment. 3. Head harness. 4. L. ns. 5. Eyepiece. 6. Angle tube. 7. Outlet valve. 8. Outlet valve guard. 9. Deflector. 10. Hose 11. Canister. 12. Carrier body. 13. Lift-the-dot fastener. 14. Rivet. 15. Chape 30°. 16. Chape 45°. 17. Strap loop. 18. Eye clasp. 19. Hook clasp. 20. Shoulder strap. 21. Body strap. 22. Upper can strap. 23. Lower can strap. 24. Antidim set strap. 25. Antidim set.

549

the facepiece, the canister, and the hose tube. The mask with the carrier weighs 5 lb.

The facepiece is made from molded-rubber blanks of approximately the correct size covered on the outside by a thin layer of cotton fabric called *stockinette* vulcanized to the rubber. The facepieces are cut out from the face blanks to exact size and shape by means of a die. These die cuttings are then folded, and two short edges are sewn together by a special zigzag stitch and taped with adhesive tape, thus forming a gastight seam at that portion of the mask which fits under the chin.

The eyepieces are made of two layers of glass separated by a thin layer of celluloid. Even if struck a sharp blow and badly cracked they will remain gastight and will not splinter. The lens are held in the facepiece by detachable screw-on typé retaining rims, so that they may easily be replaced.

When adjusted, the facepiece is held in place by an elastic head harness. The harness is made of strips of elastic tape held together in the center by a thin oblong piece of felt called the *head harness pad.* When the head harness is worn out a new harness can quickly be attached to the retaining buckles which are sewn to the facepiece itself.

Attached to the facepiece just above the chin seam is a metal casting called the *angle tube*. This tube has two passages, one connected with the hose tube for the passage of inhaled air, the other attached to the outlet valve is for the passage of exhaled air.

The outlet valve, protected by a metal guard, is made of rubber. It is a simple but effective device which allows the exhaled air to pass out of the facepiece but otherwise remains closed, preventing any air from being drawn into the mask through the outlet portion of the angle tube.

Inside the facepiece and connected to the air-inlet portion of the angle tube is a butterfly-shaped tube made of rubber. It is known as the *deflector*, its purpose being to deflect the incoming dry air across the eyepieces. This prevents the condensation of moisture from the breath on the glass surfaces. Without this device the eyepieces would soon become so fogged or dimmed that it would be impossible for a man wearing the mask to see.

To insure proper fit for any size or shape of face, facepieces until recently were furnished in a range of four sizes. A universal facepiece designed to fit any face has now been developed and is being supplied. This greatly simplifies the problem of fitting and also of supply.

The canister (see Fig. 117) is an oblong-shaped metal box, painted olive-drab color, and containing a combination gas and smoke filter. The filter consists of an oval-shaped perforated sheet-metal container filled with a mixture of 80 per cent activated charcoal and 20 per cent soda lime. The outer surface of the chemical container is covered with a material

550

which filters out irritant-smoke particles. Inspired air enters the canister through a one-way valve in the bottom called the *inlet valve*. From there it is drawn first through the smoke filter where solid and liquid particles, if present, are separated out. The air then passes to the interior of the chemical container where the toxic vapors are adsorbed by the charcoal or neutralized by the soda lime. The purified air passes out of the canister through a metal-elbow fitting at the top connected to the hose tube.

Fig. 119.—Army diaphragm gas mask.

The hose tube (see Fig. 118) is a corrugated tube of rubber covered with stockinette. It serves to conduct the purified air from the canister to the facepiece. The corrugations of the tube prevent it from collapsing or kinking and thus shutting off the flow of air.

The carrier (see Fig. 118) is a somewhat irregular-shaped satchel made of olive-drab canvas provided with adjustable shoulder and waist straps. It is carried at the left side, under the arm, the shoulder strap fitting over the right shoulder. The opening covered by a flap held in place by snap fasteners is at the front. The carrier not only serves for convenient carriage of the mask but protects it, especially the canister, from moisture and other harm. The mask is adjusted to the face from the carrier without change of the position of the carrier as was necessary with the wartime type.

Inside the carrier is a small cylindrical tin box containing a stick of soaplike substance, called *the antidim compound*, and a piece of cloth. When applied to the inner surfaces of the eyepieces and rubbed to a thin layer with a cloth this compound forms a transparent film over the glass surfaces which aids in preventing them from becoming fogged. The antidim container is held in place by a loop of fabric from which it can readily be detached when needed.

Special Masks

The Diaphragm Mask (Fig. 119) is especially designed to meet the requirements of personnel of the Army whose duties make ease in talking essential. The mask is identical with the service mask except for the facepiece which includes a diaphragm to facilitate the transmission of the sound of the voice. Instead of the angle tube as used in the Army service

551

facepiece, a metal part containing inlet and outlet air passages and also a seating for a diaphragm is employed. This metal piece, in addition, has two air-deflector tubes leading to the eyepieces which serve in lieu of the rubber deflector in the Army service mask. The voice transmission diaphragm consists of a thin disk of fabric treated with bakelite. It is held in place and protected by a perforated metal disk. For Army use, this type of mask is applicable for officers and for telephone operators.

The Diaphragm-optical Mask is designed for use by men whose duties require them to use optical instruments, such as range finders, telescopes, etc. For this purpose, the eye of the observer must be brought up into close and definite relationship to the observing optical instrument so the eyepieces of the mask are made small and are held in rigid though adjustable relation to each other and to the eyes of the wearer.

As observers requiring optical masks have also to transmit observed data by telephone, the optical mask is equipped with a special sound-transmitting diaphragm, similar to the Diaphragm Mask, and, since it embodies two special features, it is designated as the *Diaphragm-optical Mask*. The hose tube, canister, and carrier are the same as the Army service gas mask.

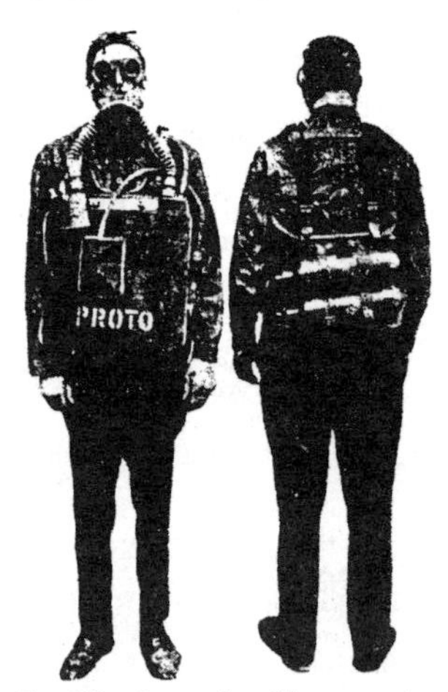

Fig. 120.—Oxygen-breathing apparatus (commercial type).

Oxygen-breathing Apparatus

Since air-purifying canisters on Army gas masks are effective only in atmospheres containing not over 1 per cent of toxic gases, they do not furnish adequate protection for certain personnel whose duties require them to enter or remain in closed places where higher toxic concentrations may accumulate. To protect such special personnel (only a very small fraction of combat troops), oxygen-breathing apparatus is required. Such apparatus is currently used in mine rescue work and in other hazardous occupations in industry where high toxic concentrations are encountered. For military use, the most suitable types of commercial oxygen-breathing apparatus are adapted to meet the special service requirements. The principal military characteristics are: (1) minimum weight; (2) maximum time of protection; (3) simplicity of operation; and (4) ruggedness of construction. Usually it is advantageous to combine

552

the service mask with an oxygen-breathing apparatus and provide a two-way valve so that either the service canister or oxygen may be used as the situation requires (see Fig. 120).

The Horse Mask

The horse mask (Fig. 121) is a device to protect the respiratory tract

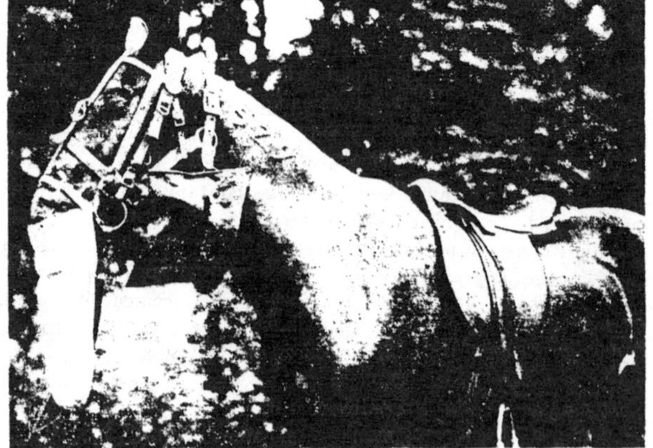

Fig. 121.—American horse mask in position (World War type).

of a horse or mule from lung injurants. It is a bag made of layers of cheese cloth treated with chemical which neutralize the gas when air is breathed through it.

As horses and mules never breathe through the mouth and as their eyes are not seriously affected by lacrimators, the mask covers the nostrils and upper jaw of the animal only.

The mask is provided with a canvas or leather pad which fits into the animal's mouth preventing him from biting through the mask; a drawstring to insure tight fit of the bag over the upper jaw; a simple head harness which fits over the head and ears and is retained in place by a throat latch. When not in use, the mask is carried in a waterproof burlap bag, which hangs under the lower jaw, attached to the halter.

To adjust the mask slip the mouthpiece pad well into the mouth, the open end of the bag covering the nostrils; adjust the head harness over the head; fasten the throat latch. The drawstring should be tightened so that the edge of the bag fits tightly over the upper jaw several inches above the nostrils.

553

Horse masks are primarily for protection of draft animals required for work through gas-contaminated areas. The mask greatly impedes the flow of air to the horse's lungs. As horses doing heavy work or running require a large volume of air, they should be given frequent rests while at work wearing masks and should not be required to run.

The Dog Mask

The dog mask is somewhat similar to the horse mask, except that it covers both jaws as well as the nostrils, since a dog breathes through both nose and mouth. As dogs are not used in the American Army, dog masks are not authorized.

The Pigeon Mask

Impregnated flannelette bags are provided for gas protection of pigeons used in war. The dimensions of the bag are 15 by 15 by 24 in. and it is designed to fit over the pigeon cage, the open end being drawn together tightly at the top by means of a drawstring. When for any reason pigeons cannot be protected they should be released at once.

Use of the Gas Mask

Gas masks are now made in but one (universal) size which has been specially designed to fit any type of face. The facepiece is made big enough to fit the largest face, on the principle of a flexible conical cap. It can be adjusted to fit smaller faces by entering the face further into the mask. The universal facepiece has been extensively tested and has been found to fit all sizes and types of faces to date. If subsequent experience should show that certain unusually variant types of faces, especially very small-sized faces, cannot be fitted with the universal facepiece, an additional small-size mask will also be supplied for such cases.

The World War type of mask with its uncomfortable nose clip and mouthpiece had a double line of protection. Proper fit of the facepiece was hence not vital as it is with the present mask. As the integrity of the present mask depends upon proper fitting, its importance cannot be too strongly emphasized.

There are two tests for *testing the fit* of a mask.

The *suction test* gives a good indication of the fit of the mask and should invariably be applied during the fitting procedure. It consists of three steps as follows:

1. Adjust the mask to the face.
2. Exhale fully.
3. Pinch the corrugated tube tightly and inhale.

The facepiece should now collapse tending to cling to the face and the wearer should be unable to breathe. If the vacuum thus formed inside

554

the facepiece breaks and air is felt to stream into the mask the fit is defective.

The only conclusive test of the fit of a gas mask is to test it in a gas atmosphere. This test is best carried out in a *gas chamber*.

The gas chamber is any room or other enclosed space in which a gas concentration may be set up and maintained by introducing a chemical agent readily detected at low concentrations (lacrimators are most frequently used). After fitting with masks and testing them by the

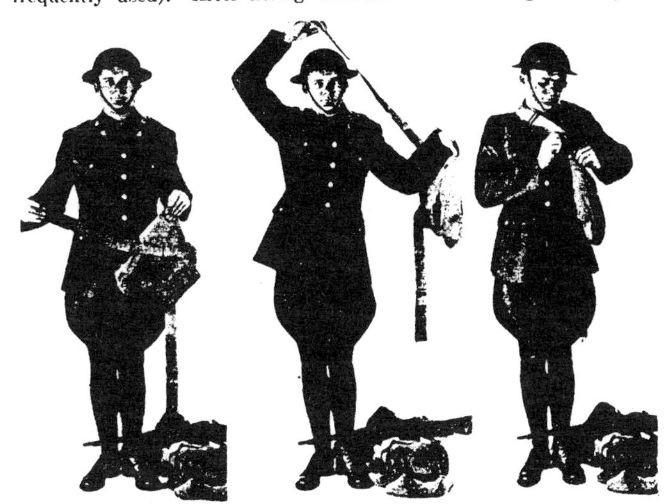

(1) (2) (3)
Fig. 122.—To sling the mask. (1) Position at the command "Sling." (2) Passing the shoulder sling behind the head and over the right shoulder at the command "Mask." (3) Fastening the hook and clasp together.

suction test described above, the masked men are marched into the gas chamber in small groups of from ten to twenty and remain in the gas concentration for a few minutes. If the facepiece does not fit correctly, or is adjusted improperly, warning is given in the gas chamber without any more serious effect than a momentary irritation.

Gas-mask Drill (17)

Preliminary drill is conducted "by the numbers" in order to develop proficiency in proper adjustment of the mask. Proficiency in this drill is then followed by practice without the numbers to insure as quick an adjustment as possible, and also to give practice in holding the breath. As a rule, careful adjustment is more essential than great speed.

555

Mask Drill. (1) *To Sling the Mask.*—1. Sling, 2. MASK. At the command "Sling," grasp with the left hand the metal hook, which is near the flap of the carrier, above the two snap fasteners, at the same time grasping with the right hand the metal clasp at the extremity of the shoulder sling. Hold the carrier waist high in front of the body with side containing snap fasteners next to the body (Fig. 122-1). At the command "Mask," extend the left arm sideways to full length. At the same time pass the shoulder sling behind the head and over the right shoulder with the right hand (Fig. 122-2); then bring the two hands together across the chest and fasten the hook and clasp together (Fig. 122-3). Adjust the carrier snugly under the left arm pit. Pass the waist strap around the waist and

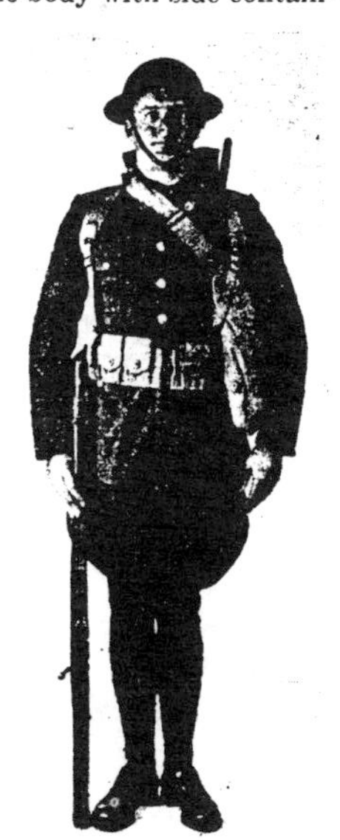

Fig. 123.—Mask in slung position. (The pack is put on after the mask is slung. The left front strap of pack is snapped to cartridge belt over the gas mask.)

fasten together in front (Fig. 123).

(2) *To Adjust the Mask.* *a. Dismounted.*—The headpiece adjusted with strap under the chin. 1. By the numbers, 2. GAS. Stop breathing. Place rifle (if unslung) between knees so that butt is off the ground; with left hand open flap of carrier; place fingers of left hand on chin above the chin strap; with the right hand knock off headpiece from behind (the headpiece being caught on the left arm by the chin strap) and continue the downward movement of the right hand until the latter is on a level with the opening of the carrier. Thrust the right hand into the carrier, grasping facepiece between the thumb and fingers just above the angle tube. Grasp the flap of the carrier with the left hand (Fig. 124-1).

TWO. Bring facepiece smartly out of carrier to height of chin, holding it firmly in both hands with the fingers of each extended and joined outside of the facepiece, the thumbs inside, midway between the two lower straps of the head harness. Thrust out the chin (Fig. 124-2).

THREE. Bring the facepiece toward the face, digging the chin into it. With the same motion guide straps of the harness over the head with the thumbs (Fig. 124-3).

FOUR. Feel around the edge to make sure the facepiece is well seated (Fig. 124-4). See that head harness is correctly adjusted.

FIVE. Close outlet valve by pinching between thumb and fingers of right hand to prevent passage of air through it and blow vigorously into

556

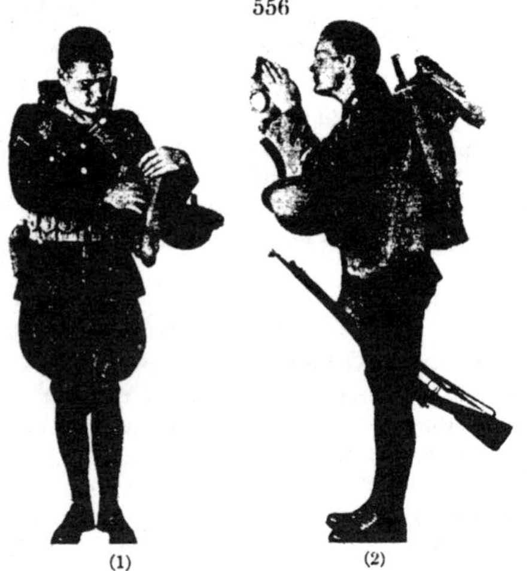

(1) (2)

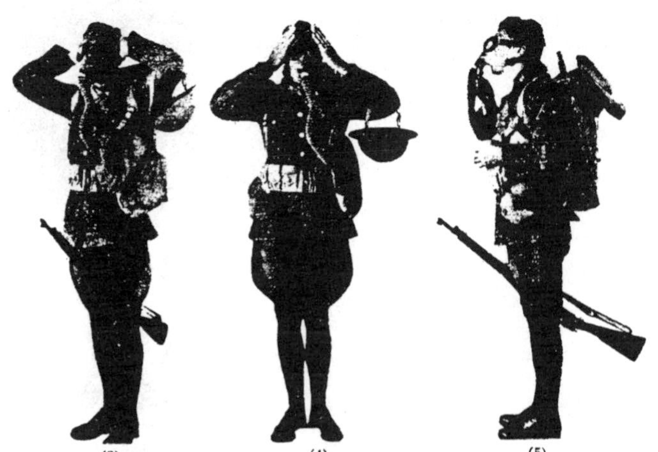

(3) (4) (5)

Fig. 124.—To adjust the facepiece by the numbers. (1) Position at the command GAS. (2) Position at the command TWO. (3) Position at the command THREE. (4) Position at the command FOUR. (5) Position at the command FIVE.

557

the mask, completely emptying the lungs, thus clearing the facepiece of gas (Fig. 124-5).

SIX. Replace headpiece, adjusting the chin strap to the back of the head. Pass the flap of the carrier around the hose and fasten on the outer snap fastener. Take the position of "Trail arms" (Fig. 125).

b. Mounted.—1. By the numbers, 2. GAS. Stop breathing. Drop the reins behind the pommel of the saddle. Continue as prescribed for the dismounted drill. Having fastened the flap of the carrier around the hose as prescribed, take the reins.

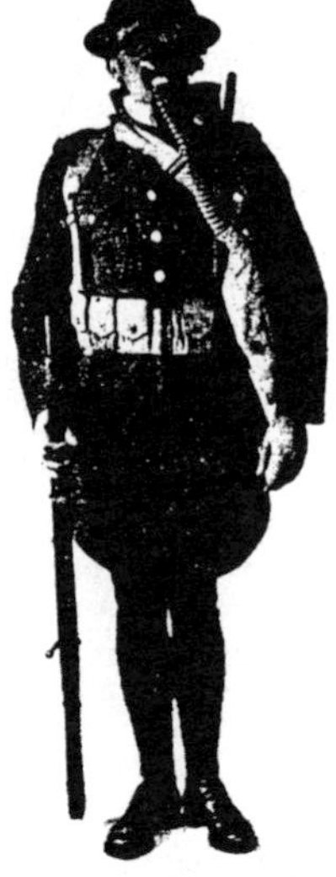

Fig. 125.—The mask adjusted to the face. (During the drill no equipment should touch the ground, which might be contaminated by a liquid agent.)

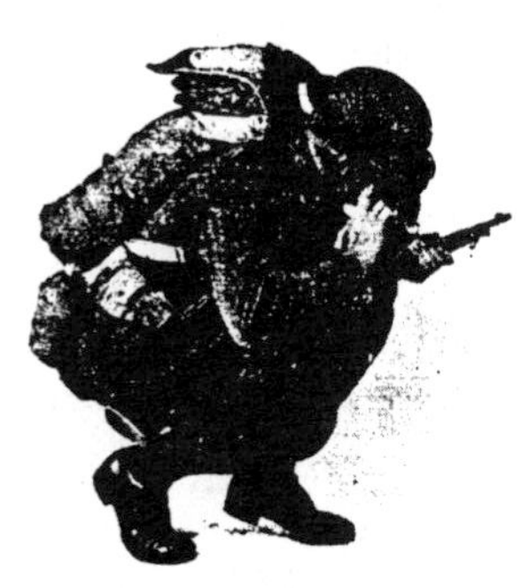

Fig. 126.—Position in testing for gas. (Knee or equipment should not touch the ground.)

(3) *To Test for Gas.*—Mask being adjusted, the command is: TEST FOR GAS. Dismount if mounted. Take a moderately full breath. Stoop down so as to bring the face close to the ground but do not kneel, care being taken that the rifle does not touch the ground. Insert two fingers of right hand under facepiece at right cheek. Pull the facepiece slightly away from right cheek and sniff gently (Fig. 126). If gas is smelled, readjust the facepiece and resume the erect position. Close outlet valve by pinching between thumb and fingers of right hand and blow out hard, thus clearing the facepiece of gas. Release hold on outlet valve.

(4) *To Remove the Mask.*—1. Remove, 2. MASK. At the command "Remove," drop the reins behind the pommel of the saddle if mounted; if

558

dismounted place rifle, if unslung, between knees so that the butt is off the ground; bend forward smartly and insert the left thumb under the pad of the head harness; grasp the headpiece with right hand (Fig. 127-1).

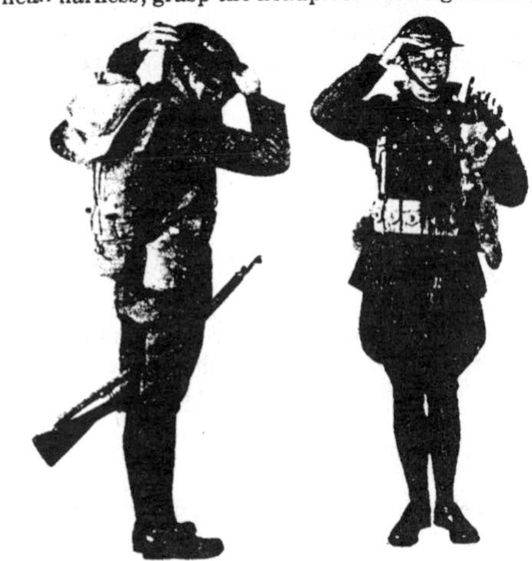

(1) (2)

Fig. 127.—To remove the mask. (1) Position at the command "Remove." (2) Position at the command "Mask."

At the command "Mask," lift the headpiece with right hand sufficiently to remove head harness, which is carried over the head with a forward circular motion of the left hand stretching the elastic fabric only enough to allow the head harness to pass over the head. The mask is retained by the thumb and forefinger of the left hand and held in front of the body. At the same time replace headpiece with right hand (Fig. 127-2).

(5) *To Replace the Mask.*—1. Replace, 2. MASK. At the command 'Replace," grasp the facepiece in right hand, palm up, and hold with edges of facepiece turned upward, the fingers under the left eyepiece and thumb under the right eyepiece. With the left hand, place head-harness pad inside the facepiece just above the eyepieces. With left hand, open flap of carrier (Fig. 128). At the command "Mask," feed and slide the corrugated tube into the bottom of the carrier with the left hand until the angle tube has passed the carrier entrance, then, with the right hand, turn the edges of the facepiece toward the back of the carrier and push the facepiece into the upper empty part of the carrier about the hose. With both hands, fasten the flap of the carrier on both snap fasteners,

559

the top of the flap on the inner or rear snap fastener. If mounted, take the reins. If dismounted, take position of "Train arms."

(6) *To Unsling the Mask.*—1. Unsling, 2. MASK. At the command "Mask," unfasten the body straps with both hands and then the shoulder strap with both hands. The mask is retained in the left hand by grasping the metal hook of the carrier just above the flap.

(7) *To Prepare for Mask Inspection.*—The mask being in the slung position, the command is: PREPARE FOR MASK INSPECTION.

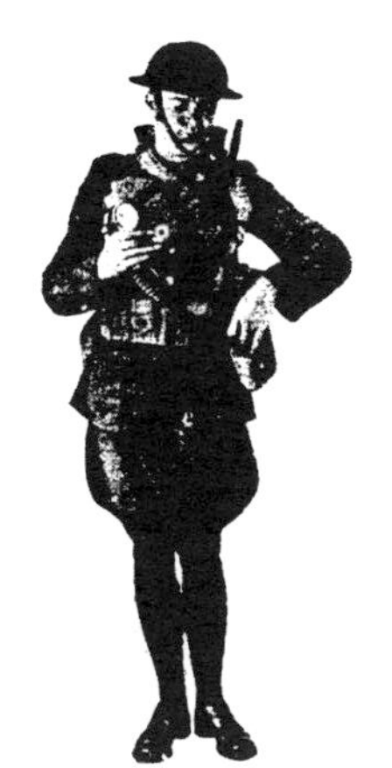

Fig. 128.—To replace the mask. Position at the command "Replace."

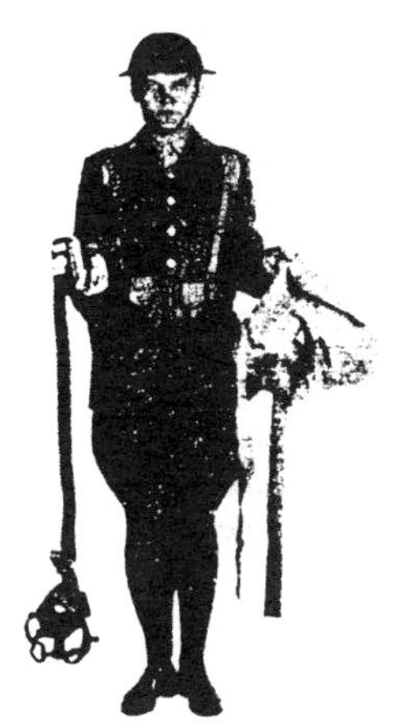

Fig. 129.—To prepare the mask for inspection. Position at the command "Prepare for mask inspection."

Place rifle (if unslung) between knees so that butt is off the ground. Unsling mask. Open flap of carrier and take out complete mask, including canister. Hold carrier in left hand and canister, with facepiece hanging downward, in right hand (Fig. 129).

(8) *Mask Inspection by the Numbers.*—Being prepared for mask inspection: 1. By the numbers, 2. Inspect, 3. MASK. Free right hand by holding canister in left arm pit, the hose and facepiece hanging over upper left arm (Fig. 130-1). Examine the sling and the exterior and interior of the carrier in turn to insure that there are no defective or missing parts; that all parts are securely fastened in place; that the body of the carrier contains an antidim tube and is free from holes, tears, and rips.

TWO. Fasten the hook and clasp of the shoulder sling together. Slip the left arm through the sling and allow the carrier to hang from over the left shoulder, at the same time removing the mask therefrom by

560

grasping the canister with the right hand (Fig. 130-2). Examine the canister for rust spots and weak places by pressing lightly with the fingers, beginning at the bottom and working toward the top; see that its contents do not rattle on shaking; see that rain shield is not loose and that the inlet valves are present.

THREE. Adjust the mask to the face. Then pinch together the walls of the hose just above the canister nozzle and inhale (Fig. 130-3).

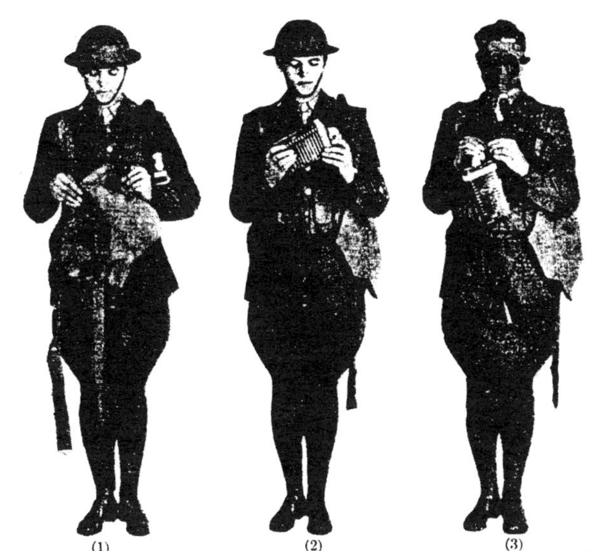

(1) (2) (3)

Fig. 130.—Mask inspection by the numbers. (1) Position at the command MASK. (2) Inspecting the canister at the command TWO. (3) Testing for leaks at the command THREE.

If air can be drawn in, a leak is present, and its approximate location may be determined as follows: Pinch the walls of the hose together at the angle tube. If a leak is no longer detected on inspiration, the leak is in the hose; otherwise it is elsewhere. This inspection is not conclusive as to the absence of a leak in the hose, and such a leak will be determined by the minute inspection indicated below. If the leak is found not to be in the hose, then pinch together the outlet valve at the angle tube and also the hose. If the leak is no longer detected on inspiration, the leak is in the outlet valve below where it was pinched; otherwise it must be above this point or in the facepiece. Having determined the approximate location of the leak, or its absence, next examine the hose for obvious

561

tears, punctures, or other defects. See that it is properly connected to the canister nozzle and to the angle tube and that the adhesive tape over the binding wires is present and in good condition.

FOUR. Examine the outlet valve for tears and pinholes by distending the rubber between the fingers (Fig. 130-4). Look especially for pinholes,

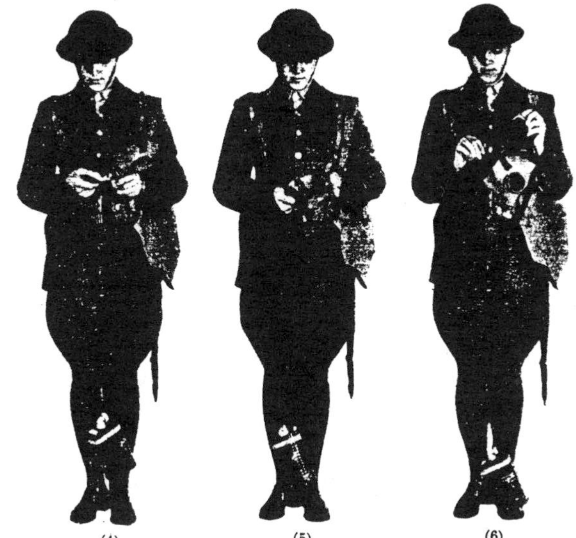

(4) (5) (6)

Fig. 130.—Mask inspection by the numbers (*Continued*). (4) Inspecting the outlet valve and guard at the command FOUR. (5) Inspecting the facepiece at the command FIVE. (6) Inspecting the head harness at the command SIX.

just below where the outlet valve is joined to angle tube, and for tears around valve opening. See that valve has no dirt or sand in it and that it is properly connected to the angle tube. See that the binding wire is properly taped. See that outlet-valve guard is not loose.

FIVE. Examine outside of facepiece for tears or other damage to stockinette. See that angle tube is properly connected to facepiece, with rubber band surrounding the binding. See that the fabric has not torn or pulled loose around the eyepiece frames. Examine the chin seam and see that it is in good condition and properly taped inside and outside. Examine the inside of the facepiece for pinholes (Fig. 130-5). See that the deflector is in good condition, properly connected to the angle tube, and properly cemented to the sides of the facepiece. Test the entire facepiece fabric for softness and pliability.

562

SIX. Examine the head harness (Fig. 130-6). Make sure that it is complete, that all its parts are properly attached, and that they are in a serviceable condition.

SEVEN. All men with defective masks step forward one pace. Others replace mask in the carrier, taking care to replace canister and facepiece in proper position (Fig. 131).

Care of the Mask

The importance of care of the mask, guarding it especially against moisture and rough handling, should be impressed upon troops. They should be made to understand the causes of deterioration of gas masks and realize that a defective mask affords no protection.

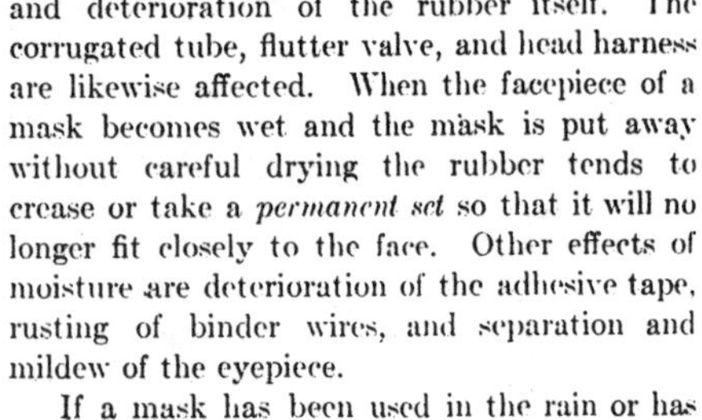

Fig. 131.—Replacing the canister in the carrier.

Excessive and prolonged *moisture* causes general deterioration of a gas mask finally rendering it useless altogether. Moisture in the canister materially reduces the adsorptive power of charcoal and is likely to result in caking with the opening up of large air passages through which the gas will freely flow owing to lack of sufficient contact with the absorbents.

Moisture causes rotting of the stockinette and deterioration of the rubber itself. The corrugated tube, flutter valve, and head harness are likewise affected. When the facepiece of a mask becomes wet and the mask is put away without careful drying the rubber tends to crease or take a *permanent set* so that it will no longer fit closely to the face. Other effects of moisture are deterioration of the adhesive tape, rusting of binder wires, and separation and mildew of the eyepiece.

If a mask has been used in the rain or has otherwise become wet, it should be slowly dried in a warm room. In no case should it be placed on a stove or near a fire as the rubber will be damaged.

Rubber parts of the mask gradually *deteriorate* with *age* though the use of antioxidents in the manufacture of rubber tends to prolong its life. If exposed to sunlight or heat the deterioration is greatly accelerated. Oil is also a cause of deterioration and oil from the hands and face are likely to accumulate on masks in service use.

Masks *in storage* should be kept in a cool dry place away from contact with sunlight, oils, corrosive liquids, or solvents. Packing in airtight

563

containers so as to leave a minimum amount of dead air space will retard oxidation. For long storage, masks should be kept in a neutral atmosphere. The method of storage of masks for war reserve is to pack each mask in a separate airtight metal container from which all air is removed and replaced by nitrogen.

When canisters are stored separately a cork should be placed in the nozzle of each canister and they should be placed in watertight boxes. Canisters so stored have shown no deterioration after eight years. It is probable that they can be preserved in this manner indefinitely.

Canisters of masks used *in training deteriorate slowly*, principally owing to absorption of carbon dioxide from the air. Tests, however, have shown that even after several years use many canisters are still in good condition. As a rule, in training use, other parts of the mask become unserviceable long before the canister begins to break down. The facepieces of masks which are frequently used, if properly cared for, last longer than those left in organization supply rooms. A training mask should give about five years' service.

It is probable that the average *life* of the gas mask *in field* service will be about six months. This is little more than a guess as it is impossible to say what concentrations masks may be exposed to in future war, and for how long a time. Frequent inspections should be made and new canisters obtained as required. The World War practice of attempting to have each soldier keep a record of exposures so as to determine the remaining service life of the canister is no longer considered practicable. Assuming new canisters are available there is no cause for apprehension in this respect since, when a canister begins to fail, gases penetrate it at first in most minute and harmless quantity. Their odor, however, can be detected thus giving warning that a new canister should be obtained.

From time to time, masks reported defective have been tested at Edgewood Arsenal with the result that in no case was a defective canister found among them. Failure of these masks to protect could be traced to one or several of the following causes: (1) poor fit of facepiece, (2) improper adjustment of facepiece, (3) leakage of valve or other facepiece defects. All such defects should have been detected in inspection.

The life of the facepiece of the mask will be prolonged if *talcum powder* is sprinkled frequently over the exposed rubber surfaces. The talcum tends to retard oxidation. Care should be exercised to prevent the powder from getting into the corrugated tube or the flutter valve.

There are two types of *repair kits*, the Mark II and Mark III. The Mark II kit is a small cardboard containing a tube of rubber cement and a roll of adhesive tape. It is designed for *company* use and is for minor repairs only. The Mark III kit contains materials, spare parts, and tools for all repairs which may be made outside the factory. The

564

kit is packed in a wooden box 23 by 10½ by 7¼ in. and weighs 32 lb. It is designed for issue to *regiments.*

A gas mask not used exclusively by one person should be *disinfected* immediately after use. The disinfection may be carried out as follows:

Material required: Two per cent solution of cresol or cresol liquor compound; several small rags.

To insure that no moisture will get into the canister during the disinfection, it should be elevated above the facepiece by placing the carrier containing the canister on a table or shelf with the facepiece hanging down. After disinfection, the facepiece should be left hanging until thoroughly dry before it is replaced in the carrier.

Saturate a rag with the disinfectant and sponge the entire inner surface of the facepiece, including the outer and inner side of the deflector. Apply disinfectant similarly to the outside of the flutter valve.

Pour about a teaspoonful of the disinfectant into the exit passage of the angle tube. Press the sides of the flutter valve with the thumb and finger so as to let the disinfectant run out. Do not shake off the excess.

Allow all disinfected parts to remain moist for about 15 minutes and then wipe out the inside of facepiece with a dry rag. The mask should dry thoroughly in the air before it is replaced in the carrier.

Rules for the care of the masks in the hands of troops may be briefly summarized as follows:

1. Keep mask dry.
2. If exposed to moisture dry mask carefully before replacing in carrier.
3. After using, sponge out inside of facepiece with cold water to remove saliva, dry thoroughly, and sprinkle with talcum powder.
4. Carry nothing in carrier but the mask and antidim compound.
5. Do not throw mask about.
6. When not in use see that mask is guarded against a blow or heavy weight.
7. Always replace mask properly in carrier to avoid kinking or creasing of corrugated tube or facepiece.
8. Inspect thoroughly at frequent regular intervals.
9. Repair damages to mask immediately.

INDIVIDUAL PROTECTION OTHER THAN MASKS

Protective Clothing

The gas mask protects only the respiratory organs, the eyes, and face. For protection of the body generally against the blistering action of vesicant agents which either in liquid or vapor form will readily penetrate ordinary cloth, special protective clothing is required.

Protective clothing is made of the so-called *linseed-oil cloth*, or cotton fabric treated with vegetable drying oils. The garment is a coverall with elastics at the ankles and wrists to insure tight fit at these places and a

565

zipper or other similar fastening in front. A hood is provided to be drawn over the head and fit tightly about the gas mask. Protective gloves and shoes complete the equipment (see Fig. 132).

Protective clothing is for protection against vesicants which may come in contact with the body. In the field it is suitable for decontamination work and for men detailed to clear passages through contaminated areas. It is also useful for men working in mustard-shell filling plants, etc. Once splashed with the liquid agent this clothing is very difficult to clean and generally must be discarded. Great care must be exercised in removing contaminated clothing to avoid touching the liquid agent. The wearer should be assisted by another man wearing both gas mask and protective gloves. Discarded contaminated clothing should be buried in a pit and covered with chloride of lime and earth.

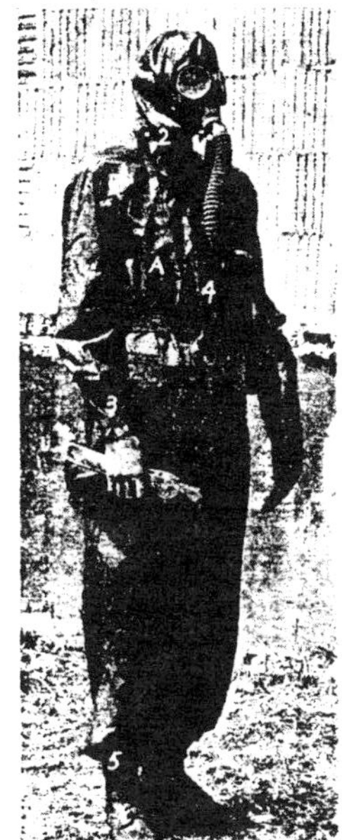

Fig. 132.—Protective suit, impermeable.

Protective clothing which is impervious to vesicant agents, such as mustard gas in either liquid or vapor form, is also impervious to air. It becomes very uncomfortable after short periods of wear since it interferes with the normal respiration of the body through the pores of the skin. It, therefore, can only be worn for a brief period at a time without injury to health. This period will vary from 15 to 30 minutes, depending upon the temperature and the amount of exercise.

Protective Salve

The idea of covering the body with some kind of salve or ointment which would protect it from vesicants was considered and tried during the World War. A salve called *sag paste* was developed and issued for this purpose. It was not a success as it absorbed mustard gas without decomposing it. Thus mustard soon penetrated the salve and came in contact with the body. At the present time, little prospect is entertained for protection against vesicants by the use of body salves or ointments.

Identification of Gases

Through Sense of Smell.—Development of ability to recognize the different chemical agents by their characteristic odors forms an important

566

part of training in individual protection. Characteristic odors of gases are covered in Chaps. V to X on chemical agents. They are also given in Table IV and hence need not be repeated here.

Through the odor, it is frequently possible to tell whether a gas is of the persistent or nonpersistent type, whether vesicant or nonvesicant. Quick perception of such facts is of paramount importance in the case of men detailed as gas sentries and on gas reconnaissance work. It is, however, important that each individual soldier be able to determine such facts himself. In war, many cases will arise in which an individual will have to rely upon his own knowledge. He should be able to distinguish *gas* from the odor of powder fumes; to know whether he should or should not wear a gas mask; to know whether the substance he smells is injurious or innocuous. Such knowledge is essential for the intelligent application of first-aid measures and for the elimination of fear and panic which arise from ignorance.

Chemical Detectors.—It is recognized that some men have a much more highly developed sense of smell than others and are hence able to detect gas in low concentrations that others fail to perceive at all. To eliminate the human equation in detection of the presence of gas, considerable effort has been made, both during the World War and since, to devise some sort of chemical detector. Such devices as have been produced, however, have not proved satisfactory. They have either been too complicated for use in the field by men with no technical training or else not sufficiently selective. The International Red Cross Society at Geneva has offered a reward of $25,000 to anyone who can produce a satisfactory war-gas detector, but so far no one has been able to claim the reward.

567

CHAPTER XX

COLLECTIVE PROTECTION

GENERAL CONSIDERATIONS

Measures of protection against chemical agents which apply generally to a group of persons, as distinguished from those measures which pertain solely to an individual, are classed under the heading of *Collective Protection*, (38) and comprise the following:

1. Provision and use of gasproof shelters where personnel may work, sleep, rest, and eat their meals in a gas-free atmosphere during gas attacks.
2. Removal of gas from enclosed spaces.
3. Decontamination of ground, buildings, clothing, and equipment.
4. Protection of weapons and ammunition.
5. Precautions with reference to food and water.
6. Provision of a protective organization to supply and issue protective equipment, to give warning of gas attacks, and to supervise training of personnel and the conduct of protective measures.

It will be noted that the measures listed above are generally of a passive nature. In addition to these there remain certain protective activities of a tactical nature which are involved in the handling of troops in combat operations. While these are sometimes included under Collective Protection, they pertain primarily to the combat elements rather than to the military force as a whole. Such measures are therefore considered separately in this text under the heading of Tactical Protection.

Collective Protection applies to all personnel in the Theater of Operations whether combatant or noncombatant. Group protective measures, however, should be regarded as merely supplemental to individual protection. The fundamental basis of all gas protection is still the individual mask and protective clothing.

In the combat zone, group protection by the use of gasproof shelters can be provided, at best, for a limited number at a time. Such shelters will afford means of carrying on certain activities during gas attacks which cannot be carried out by personnel wearing masks. They will affords places of temporary relief from gas where troops may be sent to eat their meals and rest. In rear areas, more extensive gas-protective arrangements will be possible; probably entire buildings, such as offices and storehouses, may be rendered gastight and habitable without necessity for the occupants to wear masks. The gas mask, however, must

568

always be close at hand for emergencies and for going to and from the sheltered enclosure.

GASPROOF SHELTERS

In war, especially in stabilized situations, large areas may be subjected to harassing or lethal concentrations of gas for long periods, possibly for several days at a time. Under such conditions, provision must be made for troops to eat, rest, and sleep without wearing gas masks. Places where work can be carried on without the encumbrance of the mask are also necessary, or at least most desirable, for headquarters, medical dressing stations, telephone and signal stations, observation posts, etc. In rear areas subject to shelling and bombing, offices and sleeping quarters for Lines of Communication personnel must likewise be made habitable under gas-attack conditions. The answer to these requirements is the gasproof shelter. Such a shelter is any enclosed space, dugout, part of a trench, a tent, building or room which is rendered gastight. It may be a simple nonventilated enclosure designed for only limited use or it may be an elaborate installation with a ventilating system enabling it to be occupied indefinitely.

Nonventilated shelters are for limited use only in the protection of personnel. Frequently they may be all that it is practicable to provide for front-line troops except in stabilized situations. Such shelters are merely enclosed spaces rendered as gastight as conditions and facilities permit.

The primary principle involved in the location or construction of a nonventilated shelter is the elimination of drafts. Insofar as practicable, such shelters should be protected from the wind, thus the lee side of a hill is preferable to the top or the windward side. Such shelters should always be provided with air-lock doorways, as described below.

In nonventilated shelters no fires can be allowed, since fires quickly consume the oxygen of the enclosed air and cause air from the outside to be drawn in through cracks and crevices and even through ordinary walls. Chimneys and all openings should be plugged up to render them as airtight as possible. The shelter should be located as high up as practicable, considering also other safety requirements. In the field, ravines, valleys, and wooded patches, where the concentration and persistency of gas are likely to be greatest, should be avoided. In buildings, the upper floors will be safer as regards gas concentration than the lower floor and cellar.

The *air-lock doorway* is an enclosed passageway with a door at each end, the passage being deep enough so that a man on entering or leaving cannot handle both doors at once. For medical dressing stations the passage must be sufficiently deep to accommodate two men carrying a stretcher. The doors hang on slanting frames and consist of weighted

569

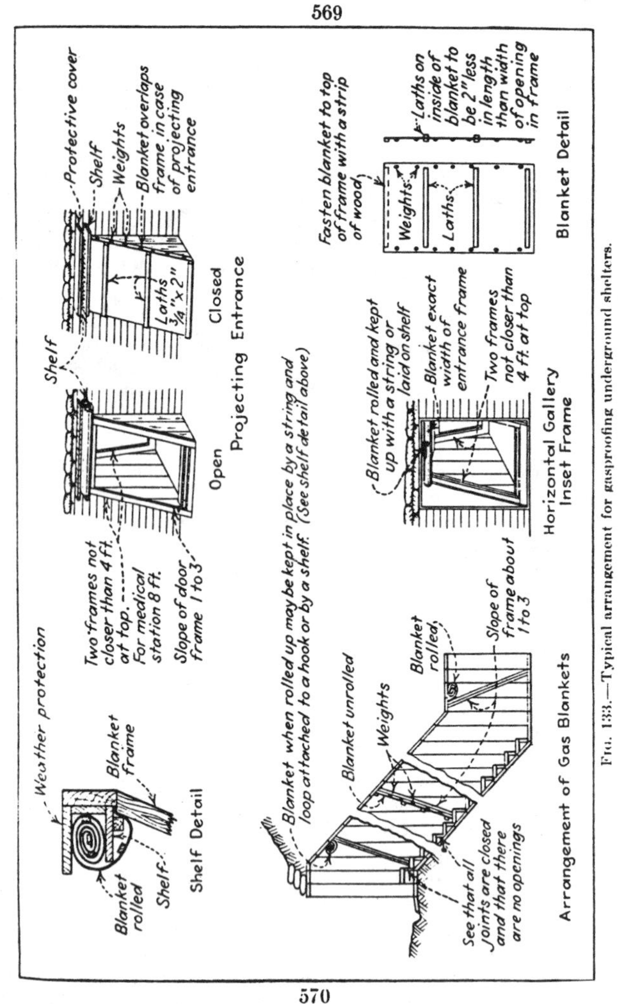

FIG. 133.—Typical arrangement for gasproofing underground shelters.

570

blankets which are raised up from the bottom to enter, the weights causing them to fall shut when released (see Fig. 133). The outside blanket is always lifted against the wind, as otherwise a gust of air will be blown into the passageway and raise the inner door admitting gas to the shelter. A box of chloride of lime (bleach) is kept in the passageway and is sprinkled over the floor of the passage. In case men entering the shelter have mustard gas on their shoes, they should shuffle their feet in the bleach. This will tend to neutralize the mustard and prevent a concentration of mustard vapor being built up in the enclosure. Otherwise a dangerous concentration may develop, and so gradually that its odor may not be detected by those inside. When practicable, shelters may be provided with anterooms where men can remove contaminated clothing and equipment before entering the inmost enclosure.

Nonventilated shelters are for limited use only in the protection of personnel. They may frequently be all that it is practicable to provide for front-line troops except in stabilized situations. Such shelters are merely enclosed spaces rendered as gastight as conditions and facilities permit. They should at least be provided with air-lock doors.

As there is no fresh air entering such a shelter, when occupied by personnel, the atmosphere inside will gradually become fouled owing to replacement of the oxygen by carbon dioxide given off in exhalation. Thus the length of time that such a shelter may be used depends upon the amount of air it contains, or its cubic capacity, and the number of persons occupying it. In making use of such spaces, it should be understood that the *minimum* amount of *air* required *for a man* is 1 *cu. ft. per minute*. Persons inside the chamber should remain quiet and not move about because muscular activity increases the consumption of oxygen, thus shortening the time which the place may be used with safety.

In the World War, many shelters of this type actually proved to be *gas traps*. This can be attributed to several causes. They were frequently dugouts leading from trenches into which gas tended to flow and remain in high concentration. Doorways were often poorly made and improperly used. Again, men were constantly entering and leaving these places each bringing in a certain amount of gas on his clothing or shoes so that gradually a dangerous concentration was built up inside. This was particularly true as regards mustard gas.

Nonventilated shelters are suitable for storage of food supplies, munitions, and equipment. They should be opened and ventilated as soon as the outside air is free of gas.

A *ventilated shelter* is one provided with apparatus for drawing in fresh air from the outside and filtering out the gas or irritant smoke in the same manner as a gas-mask canister. Such a filtration device is called a *collective protector*. For permanent installations, a collective protector

571

should consist of a large canister containing both chemical and mechanical filters, the air being drawn through the canister by a suction fan driven by an electric motor.

For use in the field, a collective protector should be portable on motor transportation and should be furnished in at least two sizes—one purifying sufficient air for small gasproof shelters in the forward part of the combat area, and one purifying sufficient air for larger shelters in the rear areas of the combat zone.

Coast-artillery plotting rooms, etc., can be rendered gasproof in this manner, though additional provisions are required in the way of blastproof doors and windows.

In all such shelters, the fact that the concentration of gas is invariably greater near the ground level should be remembered and, consequently, the air intake should be as high as it may be practicable to place it.

It is unnecessary to provide any special means of air outlet. It is necessary that a slightly higher air pressure be developed inside the shelter than outside. This will insure against seepage of gas through walls and crevices. As fresh air is drawn in through the filter and a positive pressure set up in the shelter, some air will be forced out through the walls and crevices so that there will be a gradual change of air in the enclosure.

Gas shelters in the forward part of the combat area will generally be bombproofed. In rear areas, when located near installations that are likely targets for air attack, bombproof shelters also probably will be required. Gas masks, of course, must be kept immediately at hand at all times.

647

CHAPTER XXIV

THE EFFECTIVENESS OF CHEMICAL WARFARE

Many factors enter into an evaluation of the relative effectiveness of war weapons. Chief among these are: (1) the belligerent's philosophy of battle; (2) the tactical objectives sought, *i.e.*, casualties, destruction of material, the occupation of important strategic positions, denial to the enemy of the use of vital land or water areas, etc.; (3) the military effort required to achieve the objectives sought; (4) the degree of preparation and training of the enemy's armed forces; and (5), last but not least, the morale and determination of the civil population. The strategical and tactical employment of chemicals in war and their effect upon the enemy's armed forces and civilian population has been discussed in preceding chapters. It is the purpose of this chapter to touch briefly on the other factors just mentioned, to discuss at some length the casualty value of chemicals in war, and to draw some comparisons between the results produced by the principal military agents used in the World War.

PHILOSOPHY OF BATTLE

Prior to the era of modern times, there do not seem to have been any generally recognized limits to the scope and character of warfare. On the contrary, in war, might made right, and those means which most expeditiously and utterly annihilated an enemy were preferred. Few if any checks or limitations appear to have been placed upon the powers of the commanders of armies in the field.

The first code of warfare which sought to define the limits within which armed conflict between civilized nations should be confined were the rules and instructions for the governance of the Union armies in the American Civil War (1861–1865). These were promulgated in the celebrated General Order 100 of the U.S. War Department in 1863, and eventually became the basis of what is now known as the Rules of Land Warfare. These "rules" are now accepted, at least in principle, by all civilized nations as the basis for the conduct of war.

There is, however, still a considerable divergence of viewpoint in the interpretation of many of the provisions in the Rules of Land Warfare. Perhaps the most fundamental of these differences is that concerning what might be termed the philosophy of battle. Here, there are two quite distinct schools of thought: One holds, in principle, that the ends

648

of war justify the means and that there is no limit to the degree of force which may be employed in order to attain victory. This philosophy of battle is typically illustrated in the German doctrine of war set forth in the German War Book of 1910, as follows:

> In the matter of making an end of the enemy's forces by violence it is an incontestable and self-evident rule that the right of killing and annihilating, hostile combatants is inherent in the war power, and its organs, and that all means which modern inventions afford, including the fullest, most dangerous, and the most massive means of destruction, may be utilized.

The other school of thought holds that no greater degree of force should be employed in war than is necessary to achieve victory in battle and that ruthless destruction of life and property is not warranted in the conduct of warfare. The United States Government has consistently held to this second viewpoint, and has always sought to wage war within the limitations thus imposed. As will be shown in this chapter, no weapons yet devised measure up to chemical agents in effectiveness in waging war in accordance with this philosophy of battle.

The object of war is to bring about the complete submission of the enemy as soon as possible by means of *regulated* violence. Manifestly, those means and instrumentalities which enable a nation at war to achieve this object with the minimum military effort and the least dislocation of its normal national life are, in general, the most effective. The choice of such means is not unlimited, however, since among modern civilized states the scope of armed conflict is measured by the recognized limits of military necessity. These limits are stated in the Rules of Land Warfare as follows:

> Military necessity admits of all direct destruction of life or limb of *armed* enemies, and of other persons whose destruction is incidentally *unavoidable* in the armed contests of war; it allows of the capturing of every armed enemy, and of every enemy of importance to the hostile government, or of peculiar danger to the captor; it allows of all destruction of property, and obstruction of ways and channels of traffic, travel, or communication, and of all withholding of sustenance or means of life from the enemy; of the appropriation of whatever the enemy's country affords that is necessary for the subsistence and safety of the army, and of such deception as does not involve the breaking of good faith, either positively pledged, regarding agreements entered into during the war, or supposed by the modern law of war to exist.

Despite the fact that airplanes, long-range artillery, and other modern inventions have vastly extended the scope and character of armed conflict, so that war is now no longer confined to the battle front, but extends far into the home territory of the enemy which supports the battle front by furnishing the means of war in both men and materials, nevertheless, the hostile army in the field is still the primary objective in military operations.

649

This being the case, it follows that the complete submission of an enemy will, in the future as in the past, be accomplished in the main by destroying the *combat strength* of his armed forces. How will this result be accomplished in future wars?

In ancient and medieval times, when wars were fought by professional armies small in comparison with the total population of a state, the most effective means of conquering an enemy was the more or less complete annihilation of his army. In modern times, however, wars are fought by enormous armies, raised by universal conscription, and composed of practically the entire able-bodied manhood of the nation. Also the vast quantities of munitions required in modern warfare tax the productive effort of the state as never before.

In the World War, not only were the armies of the various belligerents the largest ever raised, both in actual numbers and as percentages of the entire belligerent populations, but the effort to maintain these huge armies strained the economic life of each nation to the breaking point. Measures which increase this burden of maintenance will obviously contribute far more toward deciding the issues of future wars than the intrinsic loss of man power from battle deaths.

Based upon the mobilizations of the late war, military authorities variously estimate that modern war requires from three to six men behind the lines to keep one soldier at the front, and the difficulties of maintaining an army in the field are enormously increased by the task of caring for the sick and wounded.* Men put out of action by nonfatal battle wounds are (for the duration of their noneffective periods) military liabilities, instead of assets. The strategic value of battle deaths has thus greatly diminished, and modern military thought places chief emphasis upon *nonfatal* battle casualties. Those instrumentatilities which enable an army to inflict upon the enemy the greatest number of *nonfatal* battle casualties, in proportion to the military effort expended, are accordingly regarded as the most effective military agents.

* In the A.E.F. in France in 1918, the average annual strength of the Medical Department was 76,606, equal to *one-eighth* of our average total *combat* strength in France.

In order to ascertain the relative effectiveness of modern military agents, we cannot do better than examine and evaluate the casualties of the World War. We will accordingly devote the next few pages to a brief survey and comparison of the casualties sustained by both sides in the late war.

CASUALTIES

Before examining these casualty records, it might be well to define what is meant by the expression *casualty*. The popular idea of a war

650

casualty is a person who is either killed in action on the field of battle or who *died* from the effects of battle wounds. In a military sense, however, a casualty is any loss of personnel which reduces the effective fighting strength of a military unit. Military casualties are, therefore, those losses caused by death, wounds, sickness, capture, desertion, and discharge from the service. Casualties are usually divided into two general classes—battle casualties and nonbattle casualties. The former are those losses caused by enemy action in battle, while the latter include all other losses. Casualties may also be either permanent or temporary. Permanent casualties are those who are not returned to the army during the remainder of the war, while temporary casualties are those who are put out of action for temporary periods but are subsequently returned to the army during the war.

Very complete and accurate statistics have been compiled and published by the United States and British Governments concerning their World War casualties and many valuable military lessons have been learned as a result of the analytical study of these figures.

Unfortunately such excellent data have not been published by the other belligerents. Some have released partial statistics and have stated that they did not keep such detailed records of their casualties as to show cause of casualty and the result thereof, while others have published no figures at all and have made no explanation of their silence on the subject. The author has made every effort to secure the most accurate and reliable figures available, and has cited his principal authorities in each case. However, it must be borne in mind that statistics are always somewhat imperfect, especially where they have not been compiled from uniform viewpoints, as in this case.

Records of battle injuries from the very nature of the case cannot be complete. In most cases military casualty statistics are based upon hospital admissions and thus include only those men who were treated in the field hospitals. This necessarily leaves out of the record a very large number of men who were rendered *hors de combat* by battle injuries for which they received local treatment. While such men nominally remained with their units, they were militarily noneffective for considerable periods of time. This was particularly true of a large number of men who were sufficiently gassed to be put out of action, but who were not at the time thought to be so seriously injured as to require evacuation to the field hospitals.

Table IX shows the number of men mobilized by countries during the World War, together with the total casualties sustained by each. It also shows the number killed or dying from all causes, the wounded, those taken prisoner or missing, and the percentages of casualties in the total mobilizations of each country.

651

TABLE IX.—CASUALTIES IN THE WORLD WAR

	Total mobilized forces	Killed and died*	Wounded, excluding deaths	Prisoners and missing	Total casualties	Per cent
Allies:						
Russia	15.500.000	1.700.000	4.950.000	2.500.000	9.150.000	59.0
France	8.410.000	1.357.800	4,266.000	537,000	6.160.800	73.3
British Empire†	8.904.467	698.706	2.004.976	352.458	3.056.140	34.3
Italy	5.615.000	650.000	947.000	600.000	2.197.000	39.1
United States‡	4.137.828	116,902	219.296	4.500	340.698	8.2
Japan	800.000	300	907	3	1.210	0.2
Roumania	750.000	335,706	120.000	80,000	535.706	71.4
Serbia	707.343	45.000	133.148	152.958	331.106	46.9
Belgium	267.000	13.716	44.686	34,659	93.061	34.5
Greece	230.000	5,000	21.000	1,000	27.000	11.7
Portugal	100.000	7,222	13,751	12,318	33.291	33.3
Montenegro	50.000	3.000	10.000	7,000	20,000	40.0
Total	45,471,638	4,933,352	12.730.764	4.281,986	21,946,012	48.2
Central Powers:						
Germany	11.000.000	1,773,700	4.216.058	1.152.800	7,142,558	64.9
Austria-Hungary	7.800.000	1.200.000	3.620.000	2.200.000	7,020.000	90.0
Turkey	2.850.000	325,000	400.000	250.000	975.000	34.2
Bulgaria	1,200.000	87,500	152.390	27,029	266.919	22.2
Total	22,850,000	3.386,200	8,388,448	3.629,829	15,404.477	67.4
Grand total	68,321,638	8.319,552	21,119.212	7.911,725	37.350.489	54.7

* Killed and died includes deaths from *all* causes.

† British "Official Medical History of the War," H. M. Stationery Office, London, 1931.

‡ Figures for the United States include 80,727 United States Marines, but exclude United States Navy. Excluding United States Marines who served with the Army in France, the United States Army casualties were as follows: total mobilized forces, 4,057.101; killed and died, 114.095; wounded casualties, 210,398; excluding 13.691 who died of wounds; prisoners and missing, 4.423 (representing prisoners only, all missing cases cleared up; total casualties, 328.916; per cent, 8.1).

In order to arrive at the number of injuries inflicted by weapons ("battle injuries"), the "prisoners and missing" should be omitted, since obviously nothing definite is known as to their condition. In this connection, however, it should be pointed out the probabilities are that approximately the same percentages of "killed" and "wounded" would occur among the "prisoners and missing," as among the forces accounted for, so that, in arriving at the *total* "killed and wounded," it would be logical to extend the percentages of "killed and wounded" to apply also to the "prisoners and missing." On the other hand, in comparing casualties caused by various military agents, it is safer to exclude the "prisoners and missing," from the figures, in order to eliminate all conjecture, although it would not affect the relative percentages either way. Accord-

652

ingly the "prisoners and missing" are excluded in the following casualty statistics, unless otherwise stated.

Another important point to be noted in connection with Table IX is the fact that the figures in Column 3, showing "killed and died," include men who died from nonbattle injuries (including disease), as well as those who died from battle injuries. Exact figures are not available from all the countries shown in Table IX to permit these two classes of deaths to be separated. We have, however, the official figures for the United States and the British Empire and the approximate estimates for the other belligerents.

Table X shows (by country) the number of battle deaths and nonbattle deaths, the total wounded (including deaths), and the percentages of battle deaths to the total numbers wounded.

TABLE X.—BATTLE DEATHS IN WORLD WAR

Country	Battle deaths	Nonbattle deaths	Total wounded, including battle deaths	Per cent of "battle deaths" to "total wounded" (including "battle deaths")
Allies:				
Russia	1,416.700	283,300	6,366,700	22.2
France	1.131.500	226,300	5,397,500	21.0
British Empire	585.533	113.173	2,590,509*	22.6
Italy	541,500	108,500	1.488,500	36.4
United States	52.842	64.060	272,138	19.4
Japan	250	50	1,157	21.6
Roumania	279.756	55.950	399.756	70.0
Serbia	37,500	7.500	170.648	21.9
Belgium	11.430	2.286	56.116	20.4
Greece	4,000	1,000	25,000	16.0
Portugal	6,000	1.222	19,751	30.4
Montenegro	2.500	500	12.500	20.0
Total	4,069.511	863.841	16.800.275	24.2
Central Powers:				
Germany	1.478.000	295.700	5.694.058	25.9
Austria-Hungary	1.000.000	200.000	4.620.000	21.6
Turkey	270.000	55.000	670.000	40.3
Bulgaria	73.000	14.500	225.390	32.4
Total	2.821.000	565.000	11.209.448	25.2
Grand total	6.890.511	1.429.041	28.009.723	24.6

653

From Table X it is noted that the battle deaths were almost five-sixths of the total deaths, while less than one-fourth of the total wounded died.

While the figures in Tables IX and X show that the total casualties in the World War greatly exceeded, both in number and percentage of forces engaged, the casualties of all previous wars, and the ratio of *battle* injuries to *nonbattle* injuries was very much higher than ever before, the percentage of *deaths* due to battle injuries was much lower. The use of

TABLE XI.—GAS CASUALTIES IN THE WORLD WAR

Country	Battle casualties due to gas			Ratio of gas casualties to total wounded		Remarks
	Nonfatal injuries	Deaths	Totals	Including deaths	Excluding deaths	
				%	%	
Russia	419,340	56,000	475.340	7.5	8.5	1
France	182,000	8.000	190.000	3.5	4.3	1
British Empire	180.597	8.109	188.706	7.3	9.0	2
Italy	55.373	4.627	60.000	4.0	5.8	3
United States	71,345	1.462	72.807	26.8	32.5	4
Germany	191,000	9.000	200.000	3.5	4.5	5
Austria	97.000	3.000	100.000	2.2	2.7	6
Others	9,000	1.000	10.000	13.2	15.4	7
Total	1.205,655	91.198	1.296.853	4.6	5.7	

chemicals in the World War played a large part in reducing the percentage of deaths from battle injuries.

As gas was not used to any serious extent in the World War, except on the Western, Eastern, and Austro-Italian Fronts, only the countries which fought on those three fronts sustained any considerable number of gas casualties. It has been stated that Roumania and Bulgaria suffered a large number of gas casualties, but the author has been unable to verify this report or to ascertain any reliable figures concerning same. Accordingly, Table XI shows, for the countries engaged on the Western, Eastern, and Austro-Italian Fronts only, the number of *gas* casualties, the deaths resulting from battle gases, and the percentage of gas casualties to the total wounded, both including and excluding deaths.

[1] "A Comparative Study of World War Casualties," by Colonel (now Major General, Rtd.) H. L. Gilchrist, U.S. Government Printing Office, Washington, 1928. (46)

[2] The final volume of the British "Official Medical History of the War," published by His Majesty's Stationery Office, London, 1931, which deals with the statistical aspect of casualties, gives (Table 9, p. 111) the approximate total gas casualties admitted to Medical Units in France, 1915-1918, as 185,706 casualties (admissions) of which 5,899 were deaths. The figures for the year 1915, however,

654

include *British* troops only; the admissions and deaths among Dominion troops being unknown. Also since the casualties here reported are based upon hospital admissions, they do not include gas casualties who died on the battlefield. General Foulkes in his recent book, "Gas! The Story of the Special Brigade" (page 338), gives the total known British deaths from gas as 6,109, to which (he says) "must be added about 3,000 that were unrecorded, mostly dead, in April and May, 1915." These unrecorded casualties undoubtedly include the Dominion Troops (particularly Canadians) who were subjected to the first German gas-cloud attack at Ypres in April, 1915, and who were not included in the British official figures quoted above. The author has, accordingly, arrived at the total British gas casualties and deaths, given in Table XI above, by adding 3,000 casualties, including 2,000 deaths, to the British official casualty figures and to the total deaths stated by Foulkes.

[3] Gilchrist (46) gives the Italian gas casualties as 13,300, of which 4,627 (34.8 per cent) were deaths, but states that these figures are unreliable. From a study of the chemical attacks on the Italian Army and resulting gas casualties, it is believed that these figures are seriously in error. The author, after a careful estimate of the chemical-warfare situation on the Italian Front, is inclined to accept the stated deaths (4,627) as approximately correct, but believes the total number of Italian gas casualties were at least 60,000.

[4] "The Medical Department of the United States Army in the World War," Vol. XV, "Statistics," Part 2, Table 119, gives the complete casualty records of the United States Army during the World War. The figures, however, do not include the casualties of the United States Marines serving with the A.E.F. The figures, shown in Table III above, were arrived at by adding to the official Medical Department casualty records of the Army, the casualty figures for the Marine Corps, as follows: disabled by gas, 2,014; died of gas, 35; killed in action by gas, 6; total gassed, 2,055.

[5] Gilchrist (46) gives the German gas casualties as 78,663, of which only 2,280 died. Dr. Otto Muntsch, (48) quotes the same figures, but, in explanation of the relatively small number of German gas casualties, says:

"A great many of the gas casualties are to be found among those who were reported missing. In many cases, the casualty lists report as sick only the men who were treated in the field hospitals. The doubtless very great number of men who were only slightly affected by gas and who, although unfit for service, were able to remain with their units, receiving treatment in the ambulances, are thus left out of the statistics. Skin diseases caused by chemical substances are frequently classified in the statistics, not as gas injuries, but as skin affections."

It is also noted that Dr. Muntsch shows no gas casualties during the first year of the war (1915), although the British launched several very effective cloud-gas attacks against the Germans in the fall of 1915, and the French commenced the use of gas artillery shell against the Germans in September, 1915. Dr. Rudolph Hanslian (20) also quotes the same figures for the German gas casualties, thus: "The German casualties due to gas *are said* to have amounted to 78,663." He further states that 58,000 of these casualties occurred between Jan. 1 and Sept. 30, 1918! It has also been explained by other German writers that German battle casualties who were retained for treatment in regimental and corps areas (estimated at 30 per cent) were not included in the official casualty statistics. Even after making due allowances for all the various considerations mentioned above, the author is of the opinion that the published figures for the German gas casualties are far too low. Considering the great chemical activities of the British and French Armies and the known effectiveness of the British gas troops' attacks, it is impossible to believe that the German gas casualties could have been any less than either the British or French alone. After a careful estimate of the chemical-warfare situation on the Western Front, the author places the German gas casualties at 200,000, of which 9,000 were deaths.

[6] Considerable difficulty was encountered in obtaining reliable information concerning the Austrian gas casualties. A careful study was made of the Russian and Italian gas attacks against the Austrians and the conclusion was reached that the Austrian gas casualties approximated 100,000, including 3,000 deaths.

[7] In addition to the principal belligerents listed above, there were a number of troops of several smaller powers, such as Belgium and Portugal, which operated on the Western Front and sustained gas casualties. The gas casualties sustained by these troops are estimated collectively at 10,000, including 1,000 deaths.

From Tables IX, X, and XI, we extract the following significant figures. For the countries engaging in chemical warfare (*i.e.*, Russia, France, British Empire, Italy, United States, Belgium, Portugal, Germany and Austria-Hungary), the *total wounded* (including battle deaths) were 28,009,723, of which 1,296,853 (4.6 per cent) were due to gas, and 26,712,870 (95.4 per cent) were due to other military agents. Of the corresponding total of 21,119,212 *nonfatal* battle injuries, 1,205,655

655

(5.7 per cent) were due to gas, and 19,913,557 (94.3 per cent) were due to other military agents. For the same countries, the *total battle deaths* were 6,890,511, of which 91,198 (1.32 per cent) were due to gas, while 6,790,313 (98.68 per cent) were due to other military agents.

Thus, while gas caused 4.6 per cent of all battle injuries and 5.7 per cent of all *nonfatal* battle injuries, it caused only 1.32 per cent of all battle *deaths*. Gas was, therefore, over four times as effective in securing nonfatal battle injuries as in causing battle deaths. The military importance of *nonfatal* battle injuries, as distinguished from deaths, has already been pointed out, so that we may logically draw the conclusion that gas, as a military agent, responds in an outstanding degree to one of the most important requirements of modern warfare.

MILITARY EFFORT EXPENDED FOR GAS CASUALTIES

Having determined the battle casualties caused by gas, our next inquiry logically concerns the military effort expended in securing these casualties, as compared to the military effort expended in securing the sum total of battle casualties.

In connection with this inquiry, it should be borne in mind that the military effort here referred to is only that part of the total *combat* effort which was expended in securing *personnel* losses (*i.e.*, battle injuries and deaths), and does not concern *material* and other tactical losses inflicted on the enemy, although these latter are frequently of great importance in modern war.

Battle injuries and deaths are inflicted by the so-called *combat arms of armies*. As organized in the World War, the armies of the principal belligerents consisted of five combat arms in order of relative strength as follows: (1) infantry: (2) artillery; (3) combat engineers; (4) air corps; and (5) cavalry. These combat arms in all of the principal armies constituted about two-thirds of all troops in the Theater of Operations, and the relative strengths of these arms, in percentages of the total combat strengths, averaged approximately as follows:

	Per Cent
1. Infantry (including machine-gun and tank units)	50.0
2. Artillery (including heavy trench-mortar units)	25.0
3. Combat Engineers (including chemical units)	8.0
4. Air Corps (including observation-balloon units)	6.0
5. Cavalry (including mechanized units)	1.0
Miscellaneous (including headquarters and headquarters troops, M.P.'s, train headquarters, staffs, executive services, antiaircraft machine-gun units, and miscellaneous auxiliary combat units	10.0
Total *combat* strength	100.0

656

TABLE XII.—TOXIC GASES USED IN BATTLE DURING THE WORLD WAR*
(Tons)

Country	Arm	1914	1915	1916	1917	1918	Total used in battle
Germany	A	0.5	1.500	6.500	15.000	30.000	53.000.5
	C	0	1.650	1.200	1.250	500	4.600
France	A	0	350	3.000	7.000	15.650	26.000
	C	0	0	800	1.200	850	2.850
England	A	0	0	500	3.300	6.200	10.000
	C	0	170	1,205	2.065	2.260	5,700
United States	A	0	0	0	0	1.000	1,000
	C	0	0	0	0	100	100
Russia	A	0	200	1.500	2.000	0	3.700
	C	0	0	500	1.000	0	1.500
Austria	A	0	0	650	2.700	4.650	8.000
	C	0	0	230	320	250	800
Italy	A	0	0	350	2.500	3.500	6.350
	C	0	0	100	300	200	600
Total	A	0.5	2.050	12.500	32.500	61.000	108.050.5
Total	C	0	1.820	4.035	6,135	4.160	16,150
Grand total†		0.5	3.870	16.535	38.635	65.160	124.200.5

* In addition, smokes and incendiaries constituted about 20 per cent and 5 per cent, respectively, of the toxic-gas expenditures.

A indicates artillery, including trench mortars.

C indicates special chemical (engineer) troops.

† In the British and United States Armies the only trench mortars firing gas ammunition were the 4-in. Stokes mortars, especially designed for projecting chemicals. These mortars were manned by chemical troops. In all other armies a part of the ammunition fired by trench mortars was gas, and as trench mortar batteries were generally included under the artillery arm, the gas fired by trench mortars, (other than British and United States) is credited to the artillery.

As smoke agents and incendiaries were primarily employed for the protection of personnel and the destruction of enemy material, repectively, and caused only a negligible number of casualties, these two classes of chemical agents need not be further considered here.

Coming now to the war gases, we find two distinct classes—(1) the nonfatal lacrimators and irritants, which, while useful for many tactical purposes, caused no appreciable battle injuries, and (2), the lethal and

657

vesicant gases, which caused practically all the gas casualties. Again we eliminate the effects of noncasualty gases and consider only results produced by the casualty gases.

During the World War gases were employed offensively by *three* combat arms only, *viz.*, (1) artillery, (2) chemical troops (included above as engineers), and (3) infantry. As the infantry used gas only to a very limited extent in grenades, and these were nearly all of the lacrimatory and less irritant types, practically no gas casualties were caused by infantry action. This then left casualty gas warfare in the hands of the artillery and chemical troops.

Table XII shows the quantities of toxic gases used in battle by the artillery and chemical troops of the principal belligerents during the war.

From Table XII it will be noted that the artillery (including trench mortars) put over about 85 per cent, and the chemical troops about 15 per cent, of the gas used in the World War.

No artillery units were exclusively employed in chemical shoots, but all the light and medium artillery and part of the heavy artillery, on both sides, fired gas shell. The artillery effort devoted to gas warfare is accordingly measured by the ratio of gas shell fired to the total artillery ammunition expended during the war. The quantities of gas shell used were not uniform, even as percentages of the total shell fired, but varied considerably during the progress of the war. However, as indicated in Table XII, there was a rapidly expanding increase in the use of gas shell as the war progressed. In order, therefore, to arrive at any estimate as to the amounts and percentages of gas shell used, we should consider each year of the war separately and then strike an average for the whole war period.

No casualty-producing gas shell were used until near the end of the first year of the war (June, 1915), when the Germans brought out their K shell; the Allies did not commence firing such shell until January, 1916. From the beginning of 1916 to the end of the war, the percentage of gas shell used on both sides steadily increased, both in actual numbers and as percentages of the total artillery-ammunition fired (see Chart XIX, page 681).

The percentage of gas shell fired also varied greatly on the different fronts and even on various parts of the same front. By far the greatest part of all the gas shell used in the World War was fired on the Western Front. Next in gas artillery activity came the Eastern Front and the Austro-Italian Fronts in the order named. As far as can be ascertained, relatively few gas shells were used on other fronts in the late war. It is said that the Rumanians and Bulgarians sustained a considerable number of gas casualties, but neither the means employed nor the actual numbers involved could be verified.

658

Table XIII shows that 4.54 per cent of the artillery ammunition used in the war was gas. This means then that 4.54 per cent of the total artillery effort was devoted to gas warfare. As the strength of the artillery averaged about 25 per cent of the total combat strength of an army in the late war, we may say that artillery gas warfare constituted 4.54 per cent of 25 per cent, or 1.13 per cent of the total combat effort of each army engaged in gas warfare. To this figure for the artillery we must add the combat engineer (*chemical troops*) effort that was also devoted to gas warfare.

Table XIV shows the engineer troops that were organized and employed as special chemical troops during the war.

From Table XIV it is noted that the 23,765 engineers employed as gas (chemical) troops during the war constituted approximately 2.0 per cent of the total combat engineers, so we may say that 2.0 per cent of

Table XIII shows the estimated total artillery ammunition used during the war by the nations shown in Table XII.

TABLE XIII.—ESTIMATED TOTAL ARTILLERY AMMUNITION EXPENDED DURING THE WORLD WAR

Country	Gas shell		Other shell		Total	
	Number	Per cent	Number	Per cent	Number	Per cent*
Germany	33,000,000	6.37	485,000,000	93.63	518,000,000	35.6
France	16,000,000	4.57	334,000,000	95.43	350,000,000	24.05
England	4,000,000	2.2	178,000,000	97.8	182,000,000	12.51
United States	1,000,000	12.50	7,000,000	87.50	8,000,000	.55
Russia	3,000,000	4.17	69,000,000	95.83	72,000,000	4.95
Austria	5,000,000	2.86	170,000,000	97.14	175,000,000	12.03
Italy	4,000,000	2.67	146,000,000	97.33	150,000,000	10.31
Total	66,000,000	4.54	1,389,000,000	95.46	1,455,000,000	100.00

* Per cent of total shell fired by all the countries named.

the combat-engineer effort was devoted to chemical warfare, and that gas warfare by engineer (chemical) troops constituted 2 per cent of 8 per cent, or 0.16 per cent of the total combat effort of the armies. Adding the artillery effort (1.13 per cent) and engineer (0.16 per cent) together, we find that 1.29 per cent of the total combat effort of the armies was expended in gas-warfare operations from which were produced 4.6 per cent of the total battle injuries and 5.7 per cent of all the nonfatal battle injuries. We may, therefore, say that, on the basis of the ratio of casualties to military effort, *gas was from four to five times more effective* than the average of the military agents used in the war.

659

These are very remarkable results when we remember that gas warfare was not introduced until near the end of the first year of the war; it then went through a period of experimentation for the next two years and was not developed to a stage even remotely approaching its possibilities until almost the last year of the war when mustard gas was introduced in

TABLE XIV.—SPECIAL CHEMICAL TROOPS IN THE WORLD WAR

Country	Chemical units		Total chemical strength	Total combat engineer strength	Chemical per cent of combat engineers	Organization of chemical units
	Battalions	Companies				
Germany	9	36	7,000	320,000	2.0	4 Regiments of 2 battalions of 4 companies plus 1 additional battalion
England	5	21	7,365	106,000	6.9	1 Brigade of 5 battalions of 4 companies and 1 special company
France	6	18	3,600	175,000	2.0	6 Battalions of 3 companies each
United States	2	6*	1,700	85,000	2.0	1 Regiment of 2 battalions of 3 companies each
Russia	7	14	2,800	250,000	1.1	7 Battalions of 2 companies each
Austria	1	4	800	75,000	1.1	1 Battalion of 4 companies
Italy	1	3	500	150,000	0.3	1 Battalion of 3 companies
Total	31	102	23,765	1,161,000	2.0	

* Only two battalions of the 1st Gas Regiment arrived in France and took part in the operations on the Western Front in 1918. In March, 1918, the 1st Gas Regiment was increased to six battalions (of three companies each) with a total strength of 5,083 officers and men. Early in September, 1918, two additional six-battalion regiments were authorized, making a total of 15,000 chemical troops that would have been employed by the American Army in France in 1919, had the war continued.

July, 1917. Unlike H.E. shell which had been fully developed and were standard munitions for thirty years before the World War, gas shell had to be hastily improvised and developed under stress of war conditions. Many of the gases used in artillery shell proved unsuitable for such use or were not adapted to conditions met on the field of battle. Thus, out of a total of more than fifty chemical substances loaded into artillery shell. only four or five proved really effective under battle conditions.

660

Each time a new gas was tried out much effort was involved in preparing and firing the shell and in ascertaining their battle effectiveness. Often the efficiency of such shell was a matter of dispute and their real value could only be definitely ascertained after a large number of rounds had been fired. Perhaps the most noteworthy example of this kind was the French Vincennite shell, filled with a mixture of hydrocyanic acid and arsenic trichloride. This mixture had a very marked toxicity in the laboratory and great results were expected to be obtained in the field from its use. The French filled no less than 4,000,000 artillery shell with this filling, yet the consensus of opinion was that, owing to its extreme volatility and peculiar physiological reaction, it was not an effective gas under battle conditions, and hence only a very small percentage of casualties were actually obtained from a very large expenditure of this ammunition.

In addition to inefficient toxic gases, there were also a large number of shell containing gases of the lacrimatory and irritant types which were not intended to produce casualties, but to harass the enemy, causing him to mask or to penetrate the mask and cause its removal in the presence of toxic gas. Thus, Germany filled 14,000,000 shell with DA, a substance which, while highly irritant, was virtually not lethal and did not produce more than 20,000 casualties all told. When the various noncasualty-producing gas shells are substracted from the total, it discloses a very high casualty power for the remaining successful types such as the phosgene and mustard shells.

This is strikingly illustrated by the following comparison: Considering the seven countries which engaged in chemical warfare during the World War (listed in Table XIII), we find (from Table X) that the total casualties were 28,009,723, of which 1,296,853 were due to gas (Table XI). Of the 26,712,870 nongas casualties, it is estimated that approximately one-half were due to H.E. shell and shrapnel, or a total of 13,356,435. Since the total artillery ammunition (other than gas) expended by these countries during the war was 1,389,000,000 rounds (Table XIII), it follows that approximately *one casualty was produced by each* 100 *rounds of nongas artillery ammunition fired.*

On the other hand approximately 85 per cent of the 1,296,853 gas casualties (1,102,325) were due to artillery gas shell (see Table XI). These casualties were caused by the *toxic-gas* shell which were approximately 75 per cent of the total gas shell fired, so that we have 1,102,325 casualties produced by 49,500,000 toxic-gas shell, or an average of *one casualty for each* 45 *of such shell fired.* From this it follows that toxic gas shell were more than twice as effective as nongas (H.E.) shell in producing battle casualties.

661

RELATIVE CASUALTY VALUE OF GASES

In order to determine the relative casualty value of the principal battle gases, it is necessary to take into consideration the amounts of each that were used in battle during the World War. Table XV shows the amounts of battle gases of each class that were manufactured during the War.

Of the 150,000 tons of battle gases manufactured during the war, approximately 125,000 tons were used in battle and 25,000 tons were left on hand after the war in filled shell and in bulk storage, as indicated in Table XV.

Subtracting the stocks on hand at the end of the war from the totals manufactured during the war, we arrive at the tonnages of the various gases used in battle. Table XVI shows these tonnages and the corresponding number of casualties resulting from each.

From Table XVI, it is noted that all told about 125,000 tons of gas were used in the war and caused 1,296,853 casualties, or one casualty for each 192 lb. of gas. It must be remembered, however, that a large part of the early war gases were lacrimatory and irritant gases which caused no recorded casualties, so that the real casualty power of the later gases was considerably above this average.

Of all the casualty gases used in the war, mustard gas was by far the

TABLE XV.—BATTLE GASES MANUFACTURED DURING THE WORLD WAR (Tons)

Country	Gases				Totals
	Lacrimators	Lung injurants	Vesicants	Sternutators	
Germany	2,900	48,000	10,000	7,200	68,100
France	800	34,000	2,140	15	36,955
England	1,800	23,335	500	100	25,735
United States	5	5,500	710	0	6,215
Austria	245	5,000	0	0	5,245
Italy	100	4,000	0	0	4,100
Russia	150	3,500	0	0	3,650
Totals	6,000	123,335	13,350	7,315	150,000
Left on hand unused	0	22,835	1,350	815	25,000

most effective. It was not introduced until July 12, 1917, and hence was used by Germany only during the last sixteen months of the war. Owing to production difficulties, France was unable to fire mustard gas

662

shell until June, 1918, and Great Britain not until September, 1918—less than two months before the Armistice. Notwithstanding the short period of use, 1,200 tons of mustard gas (in artillery shell) caused 400,000 casualties, or one casualty for each 60 lb. of gas.

TABLE XVI.—BATTLE GASES USED IN WORLD WAR AND RESULTING CASUALTIES

Gases	Tons used in battle	Resulting casualties	Pounds of gas used per casualty
Lacrimators	6,000	0	0
Lung injurants	100,500	876,853	230
Vesicants	12,000	400,000	60
Sternutators	6,500	20,000	650
Totals	125,000	1,296,853	192 (average)

Altogether about 10,000,000 artillery shell were filled with mustard gas, and of these approximately 9,000,000 were fired in the late war. These 9,000,000 shell produced 400,000 casualties or one casualty for every 22.5 mustard shell fired. Thus, mustard gas shell proved to be twice as effective as the *average gas* shell and nearly five times as effective as shrapnel and high-explosive shell.

Contrast this record with high-explosive, rifle, and machine-gun casualty results. About 5,000,000,000 lb. of high explosives were used by all belligerents in the war, from which it is estimated 10,000,000 battle casualties resulted; thus each casualty required 500 lb. of high explosive. Again, a total of 50,000,000,000 rounds of rifle and machine-gun ammunition produced 10,000,000 casualties; thus each casualty required 5,000 rounds.

PRINCIPAL GAS ATTACKS IN WORLD WAR

Impressive as are the foregoing average results in the late war, many instances can be found where gas was used under favorable conditions and produced still more effective results. This was particularly true of the large-scale gas attacks put over by the chemical troops on both sides. These attacks comprised gas clouds released from cylinders or projected on the enemy by gas projectors.

Table XVII shows the principal gas attacks during the war, the approximate quantities of gas used, the means employed for putting over the gas, the casualties produced, and the average amount of gas casualty for each attack.

From the last column in Table XVII it will be noted that, in general, the early gas attacks were the most effective from the point of view of the

663

Amount of gas per casualty, lb.
22
94
60
60
215
63
58
169
58
205
223
275
150
330
215
60
87
63
67
33

664

TABLE XVII.—PRINCIPAL GAS ATTACKS IN WORLD WAR

Cloud-gas Operations

Date	Place	By	Against	Number of cylinders	Amount of gas, tons	Kind of gas	Casualties	
							Injuries	Deaths
1915	Western Front							
Apr 22	*Ypres (Bixchoote-Langemarck)*	*Germans*	*French*	5,730	168	Cl	15,000	(5,000)
24	Ypres (Bixchoote-Langemarck)	Germans	British					
25	Ypres (Bixchoote-Langemarck)	Germans	British					
May 1	Loos	Germans	British	15,000	330	Cl	7,000	(350)
6	Hill 160	Germans	British					
10	to							
24	South of Menin Road	Germans	British					
Sept. 25	Loos	British	Germans	2,400	70	Cl	2,400	(600)
Oct. 13	Hohenzollern Redoubt	British	Germans	1,225	36	Cl	1,200	(300)
19-20	*Rhiems at Fort Pompelle*	*Germans*	*French*	25,000	550	Cl	5,096	(815)
27	Marquises	Germans	French	2,000	44	Cl	1,400	(190)
Nov. 26	Forges-Bethincourt	Germans	French	500	11	Cl	387	(57)
Dec. 19	Flanders-Wieltje	Germans	British	4,000	88	Cl/CG	1,069	(120)
	Eastern Front							
May 2	*Bolimow*	*Germans*	*Russians*	12,000	264	Cl	9,100	(6,000)
1916	Western Front							
Feb. 21	Somme-(Fourges Bethincourt)	Germans	French	6,000	132	Cl/CG	1,289	(283)
Apr. 27	Flanders (Hulloch)	Germans	British	3,200	71	Cl/CG	1,260	(338)
29	Flanders (Hulloch)	Germans	British	3,200	71	Cl/CG		
30	Flanders (Wulverghem)	Germans	British	3,200	71	Cl/CG	512	(89)
May 19	Navarin-Somain			2,000	44	Cl/CG	584	(140)
21	Champagne-(Somme-Py)	Germans	French	4,500	100	Cl/CG	600	(155)
June 17	Flanders (Wulverghem)	Germans	British	2,750	60	Cl/CG	562	(95)
26	*Somme*	*British*	*Germans*	5,110	148	Cl/CG	5,000	(1,500)
Aug. 8	Flanders (Wieltje)	Germans	British	1,600	35	Cl/CG	804	(371)
Oct. 5	Flanders (Nieuport)	British	Germans	4,925	141	Cl/CG	4,500	(1,000)
8	Flanders	British	Germans	3,400	100	Cl/CG	3,000	(600)
	Italian Front							
June 29	Plateau of Doberdo	Austrians	Italians	3,000	100	Cl/CG	6,000	(5,000)

665

TABLE XVII.—PRINCIPAL GAS ATTACKS IN WORLD WAR.—(*Continued*)

Cloud-gas Operations

Date	Place	By	Against	Number of cylinders	Amount of gas, tons	Kind of gas	Casualties		Amount of gas per casualty, lb.
							Injuries	Deaths	
1916	Eastern Front								
Sept. 7	Barnowitschi	Germans	Russians	10,000	220	Cl/CG	6,000	(3,000)	73
Oct. 17	Witonize	Germans	Russians	10,000	220	Cl/CG	4,000	(1,200)	110
18	Kieselin	Germans	Russians	2,500	55	Cl/CG	1,500	(400)	73
24-25	Baronovichi	Russians	Germans	5,500	165	Cl/CG	1,100	(200)	300
December	*Riga-Minsk*	*Germans*	*Russians*	12,000	264	Cl/CG	7,791	(1,100)	68
1917									
Jan. 26	Aa on the Rigmitan Road	Russians	Germans	5,000	150	Cl/CG	1,500	(300)	200
	Western Front								
31	*Champagne (at the Prosnes)*	*Germans*	*French*	18,500	407	Cl/PS	2,062	(531)	395
Apr. 7	Remenauville	Germans	French	1,500	33	Cl/PS	458	(108)	144
23	Nieuport	Germans	French	1,000	22	Cl/PS	335	(52)	130
June 6	Nieuport	Germans	French	1,000	22	Cl/PS	375	(7)	60
July 1	Seichprey	Germans	French	2,000	44	Cl/CG	450	(136)	195
Sept. 26	Bethune Mines	Germans	French	400	9	Cl/PS	60	(12)	300
	Eastern Front								
Mar. 27	Kowel	Russians	Austrians	4,000	140	Cl/CG	800	(60)	350
Apr. 15	East of Kowel (Kichary)	Russians	Germans	5,000	150	Cl/CG	1,200	(700)	250
1918	Western Front								
May 13	La Bassee Canal-Scarpe	British	Germans	3,028	90	Cl/PS	1,500	(150)	120
24	La Bassee Canal-Scarpe	British	Germans	3,788	110	Cl/PS	2,000	(200)	110
June 10	La Bassee Canal-Scarpe	British	Germans	4,144	120	Cl/CG	3,000	(240)	80
July 13	La Bassee (Lens-Avion)	British	Germans	5,110	148	Cl/CG	4,200	(350)	70
			Total......	205,210	5,003	......	105,094	31,749	95 (average)

666

TABLE XVII.—PRINCIPAL GAS ATTACKS IN WORLD WAR.—(*Continued*)

Projector Operations

Date	Place	By	Against	Number of projectors	Amount of gas, tons	Kind of gas	Casualties		Amount of gas per casualty, lb.
							Injuries	Deaths	
1917	Western Front								
Apr. 4	*Arras*	*British*	*Germans*	3,827	48	CG	500	(100)	191
Dec. 5	Rechicourt	Germans	French	1,000	8	CG	100	(20)	160
11	Cambrai	Germans	British	1,000	8	CG	78	(21)	205
31	Givenchy	Germans	British	500	4	CG	34	(2)	235
	Italian Front								
Oct. 24	*Isonzo near Flitsch*	*Austrians*	*Italians*	1,000	8	CG	600	(500)	27
1918	Western Front								
Jan. 31	Lens	*Germans*	*British*	250	2	CG	19	(3)	200
Feb. 14	Bullecourt	Germans	British	500	4	CG	66	(4)	121
26	Ansauville (1st Division)	Germans	Americans	250	2	CG/PS	85	(8)	47
Mar. 6	Avion	Germans	British	500	4	CG	70	(13)	114
7	Gomielieu	Germans	British	500	4	CG	57	(13)	140
19	*St. Quentin*	*British*	*Germans*	5,649	85	CG	1,100	(250)	108
19	St. Elie	Germans	British	500	4	CG	75	(20)	107
21	*Lens*	*British*	*Germans*	3,728	57	CG	700	(150)	162
31	Hill 70	Germans	British	250	2	CG	17	(5)	235
Apr. 15	Pretre near Montauville	Germans	French	400	3	CG	26	(3)	230
17	Pretre near Montauville	Germans	French	750	6	CG	52	(24)	230
May 10	Apremont	Germans	French	1,000	8	CG	187	(20)	86
10	San Mihiel-Toul (26th Div)	Germans	Americans	500	4	CG	185	(23)	43
10	Bures, north of Parray	Germans	French	1,000	8	CG	120	(48)	133
26	N.E. of Bodonviller	Germans	French	1,000	8	CG	247	(40)	65
28	N.E. of Bodonviller	Germans	French	500	4	CG	70	(5)	114
June 23	Ypres	British	Germans	1,337	20	CG	500	(80)	80
July 12	Lens-Avion	British	Germans	1,462	22	CG	600	(85)	73
August	Dormans	Germans	British	1,000	8	CG	300	(50)	53
18	Meroillor near Baccarat	Americans	Germans	800	12	CG	250	(30)	100
			Total......	29,203	343	......	6,038	1,517	114 (average)

Casualties		Amount of gas per casualty, lb.
Injuries	Deaths	
1,600	(90)	343
1,100	(95)	340
600	(50)	500
750	(65)	500
2,490	(87)	100
1,250	(75)	400
14,726	(500)	340
13,158	(143)	380
1,200	(110)	225
1,000	(100)	350
900	(85)	267
2,330	(600)	300
{4,800	{(67)	275
2,423}	(20)}	
{11,860	{(66)	680
3,000}	(45)}	
542	(0)	258
8,242	(30)	485
8,470	(43)	492
693	(4)	430
4,980	(71)	600
3,918	(32)	750
443	(0)	54
600	(1)	50
518	(0)	770
2,600	(47)	770
3,400	(68)	500
759	(47)	470
1,060	(0)	10
1,892	(0)	5
1,000	(50)	400
24,363	(540)	328
10,600	(278)	300
137,267	3,409	94 (average)

TABLE XVII.—PRINCIPAL GAS ATTACKS IN WORLD WAR.—(*Continued*)
Artillery Operations

Date	Place	By	Against	Number of rounds	Amount of gas, tons	Kind of gas
1915	Eastern Front					
Jan. 31	Bolimow on Rawki	*Germans*	*Russians*	18,000	63	T-Stoff
1916	Western Front					
June 22	*Fleury*	Germans	French	110,000	225	GC
July 11	Verdun	Germans	French	75,000	137	GC
1917						
Mar. 25-Apr. 9	Arras offensive	British	Germans	60,000	150	PS
May 26-June 7	Messines offensive	British	Germans	75,000	162	PS
July 12	Ypres	Germans	British	50,000	125	HS
17-31	Ypres (third battle)	British	Germans	100,000	250	PS
14-Aug. 4	*Nieuport—Armentieres*	*Germans*	*British*	1,000,000	2,500	HS
Aug. 13-Sept. 24	*Meuse near Verdun*	*Germans*	*French*	1,000,000	2,500	HS
Oct. 15-22	Ailette Basin near Laffaux	Germans	French	90,000	135	CG
	Eastern Front					
Sept. 1	Duna River at Uxhull	Germans	Russians	116,400	175	CG/DA
Sept. 21	Jakbstadt	Germans	Russians	80,000	120	CG/DA
	Italian Front					
June 15	....	Austrians	Italians	170,000	350	CG
1918	Western Front					
	Somme offensive:					
Mar. 9-19	*Preparation bombardment* (Ypres-San Quentin)	*Germans*	*British & French*	500,000	1,000	HS/GC
Mar. 21-Apr. 6	*Attack bombardment* (Croiselles-La Fere)	*Germans*	*British & French*	2,000,000	4,000	HS/DA/CG
Mar. 21	Haute de la Faut (42nd Division)	Germans	Americans	3,000	7	HS
Apr. 9-27	*Lys offensive* (Lens-Armentiere)	*Germans*	*British-Portuguese*	1,000,000	2,000	HS/DA/CG
Apr. 20-25	(*Kemmel-Ypres*)	*Germans*	*British*	1,000,000	2,000	HS/DA/CG
May 3-4	Cantigny (1st Division)	Germans	Americans	10,000	15	HS
May 27-June 5	*Aisne offensive*	*Germans*	*French*	1,000,000	1,500	DA/CG
June 9-15	Noyon-Montdidier offensive	Germans	French	750,000	1,500	HS/DA/CG
18	Baccarat (42nd Division)	Germans	Americans	8,000	12	HS/CG/PS
July 14-15	Champagne-Marne (3rd Division)	Germans	Americans	7,500	15	HS/CG
14-17	Chateau Thierry (26th Division)	Germans	Americans	10,000	20	HS/CG
15-18	Champagne-Marne offensive	Germans	French	500,000	1,000	HS/DA/CG
31	Neuilly-Meuse	Germans	French	340,000	850	HS
Aug. 7-8	Siechprey (89th Division)	Germans	Americans	9,000	18	HS/DA
12-15	Vesle (77th Division)	Germans	Americans	2,000	5	HS
30-31	Fismes (28th Division)	Germans	Americans	2,000	5	HS/DA/CG
Sept. 12	San Mihiel	Americans	Germans	100,000	200	CG
Sept. 15-Nov. 11	*Autumn counteroffensive*	*Germans*	*British*	2,000,000	4,000	HS
Sept. 26-Nov. 11	*Meuse-Argonne*	*Americans*	*Germans*	800,000	1,600	CG/HS
			Total......	12,985,900	26,639	....

667

number of pounds of gas required per casualty. This, of course, was due to the absence of any effective protection from the first gases used in the war. As the means of protection increased in efficiency, the number of pounds of gas required to secure a casualty increased proportionately, although the results of successive gas attacks were by no means uniform; local conditions often entering largely into the relative effectiveness of each gas attack.

Another noteworthy point brought out in Table XVII is that on an average the large gas attacks were not as effective, per pound of gas used, as the smaller attacks. This was due primarily to the fact that, in general, in the small operations the targets were more definitely defined, and also the smaller the attack the better the execution could be controlled.

In considering the relative effectiveness of the various types of gases it must, of course, be borne in mind that the infliction of casualties is not the sole criterion. For example, lacrimators, being effective in much smaller concentrations than the other types, are far more efficient in forcing the enemy to mask than are any of the other gases. Indeed, so decided is the economy of the lacrimators for such use, it would be a tactical error to employ any of the other gases for this purpose. Since gas masks, no matter how much they may be improved, will always involve a material reduction in the physical vigor and fighting ability of troops, it is believed that lacrimators will always be used in war, although they cause no casualties.

Similarly, the sternutators (sneeze gases) cause relatively few casualties, but are so effective in extremely low concentrations in causing nausea and general physical discomfort that they fill a distinct tactical need for counterbattery work and in general harrassment of troops. Moreover, gases of this type are generally in the form of toxic smokes and have a marked mask-penetrative power. So penetrative are these gases that special mechanical filters are required to be added to gas-mask canisters in order to protect against them. Gas masks so equipped necessarily have a higher breathing resistance and thus tend still further to lower the physical vigor and combat ability of masked troops.

From what has just been said, it is apparent that while the infliction of casualties is the primary object of modern battle, it by no means follows that because a chemical agent does not possess a high casualty-producing power, it is of no tactical value in war. This point will be more fully appreciated when the tactical employment of chemical agents is taken into consideration.

AMERICAN GAS CASUALTIES

In the foregoing discussion we have considered the gas casualties of the late war from the general viewpoint of the total casualties of the

668

principal belligerents engaged in the war. While such a survey has the advantage of a broad point of view, it has the limitation that complete and accurate statistics concerning many aspects of the gas casualties of the principal belligerents are not available. We are, therefore, not able to draw definite conclusions as to the value of gas as compared with other military agents, or as to the relative values of the different gases. Fortunately, the excellent casualty records of the A.E.F. in France, compiled by our own medical department, are so accurate and complete that they afford ample material from which these omissions may be supplied and many valuable lessons may be learned from a careful analysis of these records.

While our battle experience was limited to the last nine months of the war, it embraced the period of greatest development in chemical attack, and hence most accurately reflects the real powers and limitations of this mode of warfare. The casualty records of the United States Army are for the year 1918 only, hence they indicate the results of chemical warfare after it had passed through its period of incubation and had reached a stage approximating its full effectiveness. We will, therefore, conclude our study of World War casualties by considering a few of the salient points indicated by our own casualties in the war.

A reference to Table XI will show that the United States had a far higher percentage of gas casualties than any other belligerent in the war. This has already been accounted for in the preceding paragraph and, if the casualty records of the other belligerents on the Western Front are considered for the year 1918 only, it will be found that the gas casualties of the other armies were about the same as our own. Thus the French sustained the following percentages of gas casualties during the great offensives of 1918,

	Per Cent
Mar. 1 to Apr. 6 (Somme offensive)........................	39.72
May 27 to June 5 (Aisne offensive)........................	11.17
June 9 to June 15 (Noyon-Montdidier offensive)..............	17.15
June 15 to July 31 (Aisne-Marne counteroffensive)............	30.14
Aug. 1 to Sept. 20 (Somme counteroffensive).................	23.39
Average..	24.3

These figures are very significant, as they clearly show the rapidly increasing casualty power of chemical agents as the war progressed. Thus, while the average gas casualties for the whole war period were only about 5 per cent of the total casualties, during the last year of the war, gas casualties had increased to approximately 25 per cent of the total casualties, including deaths, and an even greater percentage when deaths are excluded. This strikingly illustrates the point referred to above,

669

namely, that the experience of 1918 is far more indicative of the real and future power of chemicals than figures based upon the whole war period when chemical warfare was largely in the experimental stage.

The figures in Table XVIII show that gas ranked first among all the military agents in the production of nonfatal casualties, and second in production of total casualties. Table XVIII further shows that, with the single exception of *gunshot missiles* (a very generic and comprehensive class), *gas caused a far greater percentage of our casualties than any other military agent used in the war*, even including H.E. shells and shrapnel which were employed on a vastly larger scale.

This is a very impressive showing for any military agent, and is even more so for one which was hastily developed under stress of war and did not emerge from an experimental stage until the war was nearly half over.

It is noted that Table XVIII does not include those that died on the battlefields nor any casualties among the marines who served with the A.E.F. Supplying these omissions, we have the total battle casualties for the A.E.F. in Table XIX:

The official casualty reports of our medical department give the hospital admissions and deaths from battle injuries in the A.E.F. caused by the various military agents. These data have been extracted and consolidated in the following table:

TABLE XVIII.—BATTLE CASUALTIES AND DEATHS IN A.E.F. FROM VARIOUS MILITARY AGENTS*
(Based on Hospital Admissions)

Military agents	Battle casualties			Per cent of hospitalized casualties
	Nonfatal	Deaths	Totals	
Gunshot missiles	67,409	7,474	74,883	33.42
Gas	69,331	1,221	70,552	31.49
Shrapnel	31,802	1,985	33,787	15.08
Rifle ball	19,459	961	20,420	9.12
Shell	18,261	1,778	20,039	8.94
Hand grenade	824	56	880	0.40
Bayonet (cutting instruments)	369	5	374	0.16
Pistol ball	229	13	242	0.10
Airplane attacks	170	28	198	0.08
Saber	9	3	12	0.005
Miscellaneous, including agents not stated, crushing, falling objects indirect result	2,535	167	2,702	1.205
Totals	210,398	13,691	224,089	

* Excluding marines serving with the A.E.F.

670

TABLE XIX.—TOTAL BATTLE CASUALTIES IN A.E.F. FROM GAS AND NONGAS AGENTS

Military agent	U. S. Army casualties			U. S. marine casualties			Total casualties		
	Killed in action	Died in hospital	Wounded nonfatal	Killed in action	Died in hospital	Wounded nonfatal	Total deaths	Wounded nonfatal	Total casualties
Nongas	36,494	12,470	141,067	1,837	579	6,884	51,380	147,951	199,331
Gas	200	1,221	69,331	6	35	2,014	1,462	71,345	72,807
Totals	36,694	13,691	210,398	1,843	614	8,898	52,842	219,296	272,138

It will be seen from Table XIX that, while gas caused 26.75 per cent of all our casualties and 32.53 per cent of nonfatal casualties, only 2.00 per cent of the gas casualties died, whereas 25.78 per cent of the nongas casualties died. We may say from this that men wounded by gas had over twelve times the chance to escape with their lives than men wounded by other weapons.

This very low death rate from gas, as compared to other weapons, was also experienced by the other principal armies engaged in the gas war. Thus, British casualty records* show only 4.3 per cent deaths from gas as compared to 24.0 per cent deaths from nongas weapons; the French had 4.2 per cent deaths from gas as against 32.0 per cent deaths from nongas weapons; while the Germans had 4.5 per cent deaths from gas as against 36.5 per cent deaths from nongas weapons (see Plate I).

Not only were the deaths from gas comparatively low, but the percentage of those permanently put out of action by gas was equally low. This is indicated by the number of discharges for disability from battle injuries by various military agents, as shown in Table XX.

From Table XX it will be seen that gas caused only 11.3 per cent of the total discharges for disability, while it was responsible for 26.75 per cent of all casualties, and 32.55 per cent of all nonfatal casualties (see Table XIX). Dividing the number discharged for disability from each military agent, as indicated in Table XX, by the number of nonfatal casualties from each agent, as given in Table XVIII, we find the per cent of discharges among the casualties from the principal agents as follows:

25.4 per cent of those wounded by shell were discharged for disability.
21.9 per cent of those wounded by rifle balls were discharged for disability.
17.3 per cent of those wounded by shrapnel were discharged for disability.
10.8 per cent of those wounded by gunshot missiles were discharged for disability.
7.9 per cent of those wounded by gas were discharged for disability.

* France and Flanders only.

671

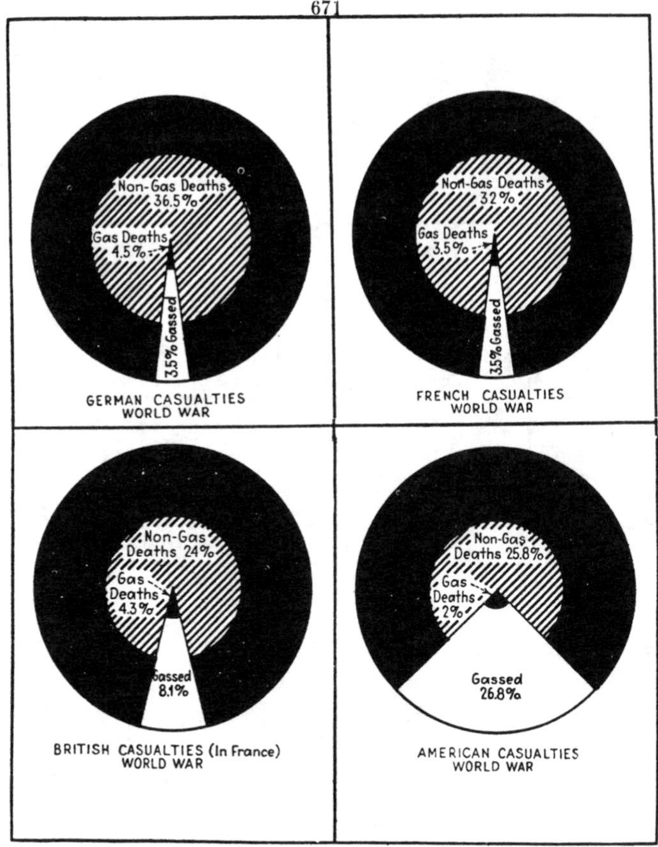

PLATE I.—Gas and nongas casualties in the World War.

672

TABLE XX.—DISCHARGES FOR DISABILITY AND DAYS LOST IN HOSPITAL IN A.E.F. FROM VARIOUS MILITARY AGENTS*

Military agent	Discharges for disability		Days lost in hospital	
	Number	Per cent	Number	Per cent
Gunshot missiles	7,280	29.0	6,157,451	35.2
Shrapnel	5,488	21.8	3,423,040	19.8
Shell	4,638	18.4	2,158,629	12.3
Rifle ball	4,264	16.9	2,373,692	13.5
Gas	2,857	11.3	2,947,308	16.8
Hand grenade	198	0.78	81,944	0.42
Airplane attacks	50	0.186	23,962	0.14
Pistol ball	26	0.1	23,153	0.13
Bayonet (cutting instruments)	14	0.056	16,151	0.1
Saber	2	0.008	1,577	0.01
Miscellaneous, including agents not stated, crushing, falling objects, indirect results, and others	370	1.47	284,937	1.6
Totals*	25,187	100.00	17,491,844	100.00

* Excluding marines serving with the A.E.F.

Stated in another way, we may say that as a casualty producer gas ranked first among all the weapons of war, but as regards eliminations through discharges for disability, it ranked *fifth* among the causative agents, being exceeded by gunshot missiles, shrapnel, shell, and pistol balls.

In view of the above, it might be inferred that, since such a small percentage of gas casualties were permanently put out of action, men gassed one day would return to their organizations the next day, and thus gas is too humane an agent to be a really effective war weapon. Such, however, is far from the fact, as is attested by the comparative number of days lost in hospital from the various military agents including gas. Referring again to Table XX, it will be noted that gas was responsible for

16.8 per cent of the total days lost in hospital, while it caused only 11.3 per cent permanent eliminations (discharges for disability) and 2.00 per cent deaths (Table XIX).

Stated in another way, we may say that gas ranked *third* among the causative agents as regards days lost in hospital, being exceeded only by gunshot missiles and shrapnel, while it ranked *fifth* as regards discharges for disability, and *fourth* as regards death (Table XVIII) (see Plate II).

What has just been said applies to all war gases as a group, but there is considerable variation among the several types of gases as regards the length of hospitalization from gas wounds. Thus the lethal or deadly

673

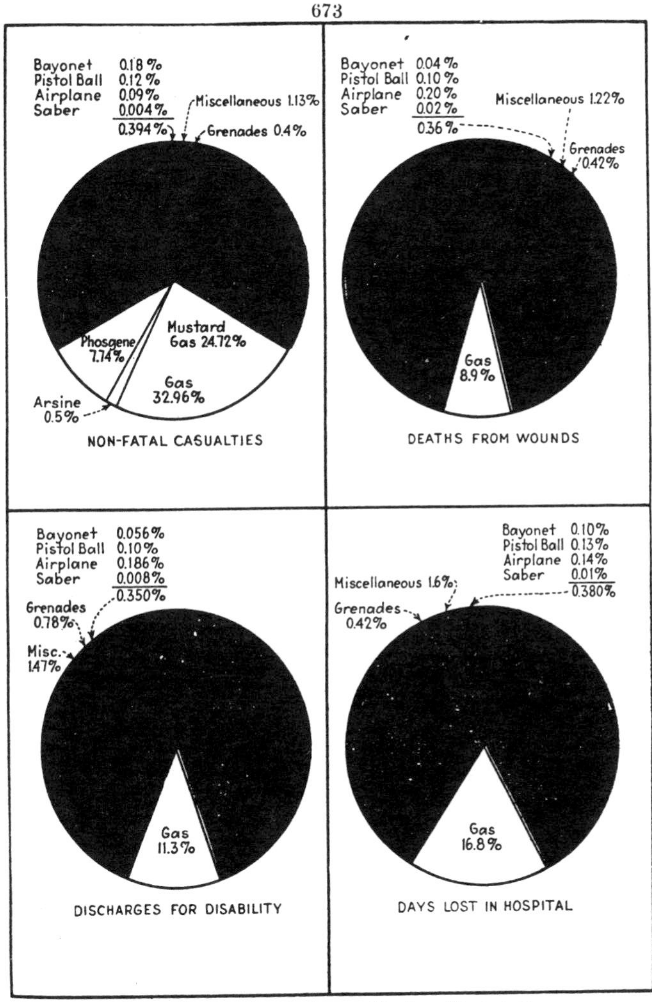

PLATE II.—American battle casualties by military agent.

674

gases, as a group, cause less loss of days in hospital than the vesicant-type gases, such as mustard gas. British statistics show that over 80 per cent of men fatally gassed with phosgene died on the first day in the hospital, whereas only 1 per cent of men fatally gassed with mustard died on the first day. On the other hand, among men nonfatally gassed with mustard, French statistics showed the percentages of those who recovered and returned to their units as follows:

	Per Cent
Within 30 days	0
Within 45 days	13
Within 60 days	35
Within 70 days	17
Total	65

The average American mustard-gas casualty lost 60 days in hospital.

From the viewpoint of modern warfare where the object of battle is not to destroy human life, but rather to put men out of action and thus not only decrease the enemy's combat power, but also increase his war burden by forcing him to maintain the maximum number of noneffectives, it is obvious that gas responds to an outstanding degree to every requirement of an effective military agent.

We will now conclude our consideration of casualties by a brief survey of the relative effectiveness of the principal World War gases. It has been variously estimated that between 50 and 100 chemical substances were used as chemical-warfare agents during the war. These may be conveniently grouped into the general classes:

Classes	Typical gas used by Allies	Typical gas used by Germans	Casualty effects
I. Lacrimators	Bromacetone	T-Stoff	None
II. Lung injurants	Phosgene	Green Cross	Fatal
III. Vesicants	Mustard	Yellow Cross	Seriously incapacitating
IV. Sternutators	None	Blue Cross	Slightly incapacitating

Reliable statistics showing the number of casualties inflicted by the various gases are not available. Aside from the British and American medical records, it does not appear that any effort was made in the World War to classify gas casualties in accordance with the kind of gas. There is, however, general agreement among the principal nations in the World War that mustard gas caused by far the majority of the gas casualties.

675

In the British Army 124,702 out of a total of 188,706 gas casualties (66 per cent) were due to mustard gas. In our own army the segregation is not quite so clear, as will be seen from Table XXI

TABLE XXI.—BATTLE INJURIES BY GASES IN A.E.F.
(Based on Hospital Admissions*)

Kind of gas	Class	Admissions Number	Admissions Per cent	Deaths Number	Deaths Per cent	Case fatality, per cent
Gas, kind not stated		33.587	47.6	546	44.7	1.63
Mustard gas	III	27.711	39.3	599	49.0	2.16
Phosgene gas	II	6.834	9.7	66	5.4	0.97
Chlorine gas	II	1.843	2.6	7	0.6	0.38
Arsine gas	IV	577	0.8	3	0.3	0.52
Total	..	70.552	100.0	1.221	100.0	1.73

* Excluding United States marines serving with A.E.F.

The information contained in Table XXI is not in a very satisfactory form and needs some revision in order to be properly evaluated. In the first place nearly one-half of the casualties reported are unclassified as to kind of gas. Then there is included a number of casualties charged to chlorine when, as a matter of fact, there is no known instance of where this gas was ever used against the American Army. Chlorine was only used in cloud-gas attacks and there were no such attacks against our troops in France, except possibly those serving with the British and French armies. Finally, the fatality rates in the last column of Table XXI make it appear that mustard gas was the most deadly of the war gases, when, as a matter of fact, it is quite generally known that phosgene was by long odds the most deadly gas and mustard was relatively low in fatalities.

The author accordingly believes the following revision of Table XXI would give a clearer picture of the actual facts. First, the chlorine casualties are merged with the phosgene, as the nearest allied type, and the one which most probably was actually used and caused the casualties charged to chlorine; then the unclassified cases are distributed in proportion to the relative casualties for the known gases, including the U.S. Marine casualties (Table XIX); finally, the 200 battle deaths from gas are added to the phosgene deaths since mustard has a delayed effect which would practically preclude battlefield deaths. Our gas casualties in the war then appear as follows:

676

TABLE XXII.—BATTLE CASUALTIES BY GASES IN A.E.F.
(Based on Author's Estimates*)

Kind of gas	Class	Nonfatal		Deaths		Case fatality, per cent
		Number	Per cent	Number	Per cent	
Mustard gas	III	53,500	75.0	1,114	76.2	2.04
Phosgene gas	II	16,700	23.4	342	23.4	2.50
Arsine gas	IV	1,145	1.6	6	0.4	.53
Totals	..	71,345	100.0	1,462	100.0	2.01

* Including United States marines serving with A.E.F.

A comparison of Tables XXI and XXII shows that, whereas in the former only 39.3 per cent of our gas casualties were charged to mustard gas, in the latter 75 per cent were so identified. This last percentage slightly exceeds the British experience (66 per cent mustard casualties) and is in very close agreement with the French experience with an estimated loss from mustard gas between 75 per cent and 80 per cent of their gas casualties. As high as these mustard-gas percentages were, they were (erroneously) thought by the Germans to be even higher. Thus, Hanslian (20, page 20) says: "We assume that the losses of the Allies through the Yellow Cross (mustard) shells were *eight* times as great as all the losses caused by the other gases."

THE AFTEREFFECTS OF CHEMICAL WARFARE

Up to this point we have considered the war effects of chemicals; but what of the aftereffects? Much time and effort have been expended in the years since the war in thoroughly investigating this subject, not only because it is important from a medical point of view, but also to settle the moot question as to whether gas really caused serious permanent disabilities, or predisposition toward such diseases as tuberculosis. A large amount of evidence has been gathered and carefully sifted and evaluated so that today these matters are no longer in doubt. Medical officers and scientists who have studied the data concerning this question are unanimous in their judgment that gas does not leave permanent disabilities or predisposing weakness to organic diseases.

To go very deeply into this matter here would extend beyond the scope of this chapter, but we cannot dismiss the subject without a few references to the leading authorities.

Unquestionably, in this country the foremost authority on the medical aspects of chemical warfare is Major General Harry L. Gilchrist, Rtd.,

677

late Chief of Chemical Warfare Service. General Gilchrist, then a Colonel of the Medical Department, was detailed in the fall of 1917 as Chief Medical Advisor of the Chemical Warfare Service A.E.F., and served as such throughout the war. In 1917 and 1918 Colonel Gilchrist spent much time inspecting troops and hospitals, not only of the A.E.F., but also of the French and British armies, and so gained a comprehensive, first-hand knowledge of the effects of battle gases during the progress of the War. After the War Colonel Gilchrist also devoted much time to an exhaustive study of the aftereffects of gas poisoning and has published several very illuminating papers on this subject. We cannot, therefore, do better than to quote a few extracts and conclusions from this eminent authority.

First, we shall consider blindness. It was frequently asserted during and just after the war that gas caused permanent blindness. General Gilchrist studied this matter very carefully and reported that, of the 812 cases of blindness in the A.E.F., 779 (96 per cent) were traceable to weapons other than gas, while gas caused only 33 cases (4 per cent). Since gas was responsible for about one-third of our nonfatal casualties, it is obvious that the percentage of cases of blindness from gas were far below the general percentage of gas casualties, and, therefore, blindness as a result of gassing was relatively infrequent.

Next, we shall consider tuberculosis. It was claimed that gas caused a marked predisposition toward tuberculosis, especially among those gassed by the lung-injurant gases. General Gilchrist, in collaboration with doctors from the U.S. Veterans' Bureau, examined the service records and clinical histories of nearly three thousand veterans with the following results:

Among the noteworthy effects of poison gas, as disclosed by the analysis of these cases, are the following: Preponderance of effects on the respiratory organs; the comparative rarity of persistent effects on the eyes and upper respiratory passages, and the greater proportion of deaths from the immediate or recent effects of mustard gas, while in its remote effects there is but little or no difference from those of chlorine or phosgene; and the death rate from pulmonary tuberculosis from it, over a period in excess of five years is less than the death rate as shown in the census report of 1920 for males of corresponding ages.

General Gilchrist then says, "The clinical experiences of many who have given this subject thorough study, as well as reports from laboratory experiments, now furnish evidence sufficient to serve the purpose of convincing anyone that pulmonary tuberculosis is not a common effect of gas poisoning and certainly not one of its later effects."

This opinion is confirmed by many able investigators in this field, as indicated by the references cited by General Gilchrist, while the

678

Surgeon General's Report for 1920 contains the following conclusive paragraph:

One hundred and seventy-three cases of tuberculosis occurred during 1918 among the 70,552 men who had been gassed in action. Of this number, 78 had been gassed by gas, kind not specified; 8 by chlorine; 65 by mustard; and 22 by phosgene. The number of cases of tuberculosis for each 1,000 men gassed was 2.45. Since the annual rate of occurrence for tuberculosis among enlisted men serving in France in 1918 was 3.50 and in 1919, 4.30 per 1,000, it would seem to be apparent that tuberculosis did not occur any more frequently among the soldiers who had been gassed than among those who had not been.

From this evidence, General Gilchrist concludes:

The above is a most remarkable showing. In brief, it shows that in the year 1918 there were one and one-half times as many cases of tuberculosis per 1,000 among all troops in France as there were among those gassed, and that in 1919 there were more than one and three-fourths times as many tuberculosis cases per 1,000 among all troops as there were among the gassed troops. This means that if gassing were not an actual deterrent to tuberculosis the small percentage of tubercular cases among the gassed can only be accounted for through the case of those patients in hospitals.

The total absence of direct sequential relation between gas poisoning and tuberculosis in the A.E.F. was also found to be true for the British Army in France. Quoting again from General Gilchrist:

The following analysis of information supplied by the ministry of pensions shows the general character of the more protracted disabilities seen after gas poisoning, it being impossible to distinguish in the records the precise type of gas by which each casualty was originally caused.

During the 12-month period, August 1919–1920, the resurvey boards made 26,156 examinations of cases of gas poisoning. Many of these men were examined more than once during that period, and the total number of individual cases examined is calculated to have been about 22,000. But of this number 3,136 were at once classed as "nil," since they showed no disability, leaving the total number of pensioners as about 19,000.

The known total of gas casualties in British Army is 180,983. But many of these were men who were gassed more than once, on each of which occasions a fresh casualty would be reported. It is impossible to determine the proportion of these, and the number of survivors from the early chlorine attacks is also unknown. As a reasonable approximation one may accept 150,000 as the total number of individuals surviving after gas poisoning, many of whom were, of course, very mild cases.

The number receiving disability pensions in 1920, two or more years after gassing, was approximately 19,000; that is, about 12 percent of the total gas casualties. Gas poisoning was responsible actually for 2 percent of all the disabilities after the war, 35 percent of all pensioners being classified as suffering from wounds and injuries and 65 percent as suffering from diseases.

The percentage degree of disablement from gas poisoning was generally low, as shown by actual assessments in a consecutive group of 2,416 examinations made by boards in a period of four weeks during September, 1920.

679

General Foulkes, Chief of British Gas Service in France, also gives some very impressive evidence on this subject. Two-thirds of the British gas casualties were from mustard gas; concerning these casualties General Foulkes says:

I have mentioned the low mortality amongst mustard-gas casualties; but it is not so widely known that of the 97½ percent which survive very few are rendered permanently unfit in the end. Towards the close of the war an examination of the medical records of 4575 of these cases which had been sufficiently severe to be sent to England for treatment (and were therefore rather more severe than the average) showed that 28.5 percent were transferred direct to Reserve battalions and 66 percent to convalescent depots—a total of 94.5 percent—within nine weeks of their arrival. Out of the total in this series of cases only 0.7 percent died; 9.4 percent were classified as permanently unfit; and less than 2 percent were reduced from Class A to a lower category. In fact, apart from about 2 percent which may be presumed to have died in France (to make up the average mortality of 2½ percent), only about 3 percent of the remainder were any the worse, say, after three months. I have reproduced this record because very mistaken ideas are held, even now, of the terrible effects of this gas. Even such a careful writer as Mr. H. G. Wells has stated recently (in his 'History of the next 100 years'): "It is doubtful if any of those affected by it" (mustard gas) "were ever completely cured. Its maximum effect was rapid torture and death; its minimum, prolonged misery and an abbreviated life."

HUMANITY OF CHEMICAL WARFARE

Much has been written both during and since the World War concerning the horrors of gas warfare and the cruel and inhuman consequences resulting from its uses. After a careful study of this matter and a close analysis of the casualties produced in the war, we now know the facts concerning the effects of gas and see that much of the alleged horrors of gas warfare were pure propoganda, deliberately disseminated during the World War for the purpose of influencing neutral world opinion, and had little sincerity or foundation in fact.

The measure of humaneness of any form of warfare is the comparison of (1) degree of suffering caused at the time of injury by the different weapons; the percentage of deaths to the total number of casualties produced by each weapon; and the permanent aftereffects resulting from the injuries inflicted by each particular method of warfare.

In general, gas causes less suffering than wounds from other weapons. It is unquestionably true that chlorine, the first gas used in the late war, did at first cause strangulation with considerable pain and a high mortality. But this was due mainly to the fact that the troops against whom these first gas attacks were launched were totally unprotected. Later when supplied with gas masks, chlorine became the most innocuous of the toxic gases and was the least feared by both sides.

The two other principal lethal gases used in the war, phosgene and chlorpicrin, when employed in high concentrations, caused instant col- 680 lapse with no suffering. With lower concentrations there is no pain. The pain caused by mustard gas is always delayed and depends upon the concentration, length of exposure, and parts affected. The very fact of the delay of several hours in the effects of mustard gas usually means that the soldiers are able to obtain medical treatment by the time the symptoms appear and much can be done to relieve the suffering. On the other hand, suffering from other wounds commences at once, and frequently wounded men have to endure hours of agony before medical aid can reach them and allay their sufferings.

Among those gassed the sufferings are less severe and of shorter duration than among those wounded by other war weapons. With the lung-injurant gases the casualties are fairly out of danger in 48 hours, while burns from mustard gas, although not painful after the first 24 hours, often hospitalize a man for several weeks. On an average, the period of hospitalization from gas was only about one-half that of those wounded by other weapons.

As to the ratio of deaths to total casualties, we have already shown that the mortality among those wounded by nongas weapons was over 12 times the mortality from gas, and further elaboration on this point seems unnecessary.

Finally, as to the relative aftereffects of gas as compared to other wounds, there can be no question. Gas not only produces practically no permanent injuries, so that if a man who is gassed survives the war, he comes out body whole, as God made him, and not the legless, armless, or deformed cripple produced by the mangling and rending effects of high explosives, gunshot wounds, and bayonet thrusts.

If any one has the slightest doubt on this point, he has only to take one glance at the horrible results of nonfatal gunshot wounds, as illustrated on Plate I of Colonel Vedder's book, "The Medical Aspects of Chemical Warfare".

History reveals that the death rate in war has constantly decreased as methods of warfare have progressed in efficiency as the result of scientific progress. Chemical warfare is the latest contribution to the science of war. The experience and statistics of the World War both indicate that it is not only one of the most efficient agencies for effecting casualties, but is the most humane method of warfare yet devised by man.

INCREASING USE OF GAS DURING WORLD WAR

One of the most convincing evidences of the effectiveness of chemical warfare was its rapidly increasing use as the World War progressed. This is strikingly illustrated in Chart XIX, which shows the amount of gas and gas shell used on both sides during each year of the war. 681

Owing to the large number of casualties which the Germans scored against the British and French with Yellow Cross (mustard) shell in the summer of 1917, and the great success attained against the Russians by their Colored Shoots, (mixed Green, Blue, and Yellow Cross shells) in the fall of 1917, the Germans based the artillery preparation for their great offensives in the spring of 1918 on the use of gas shell. Thus gas shell, which in 1915, 1916, and 1917 were used only in special operations for producing casualties and in the general harassment of troops, by the end of 1917 had become so effective that they were incorporated as an important part of the comprehensive tactical plans for the 1918 offensives.

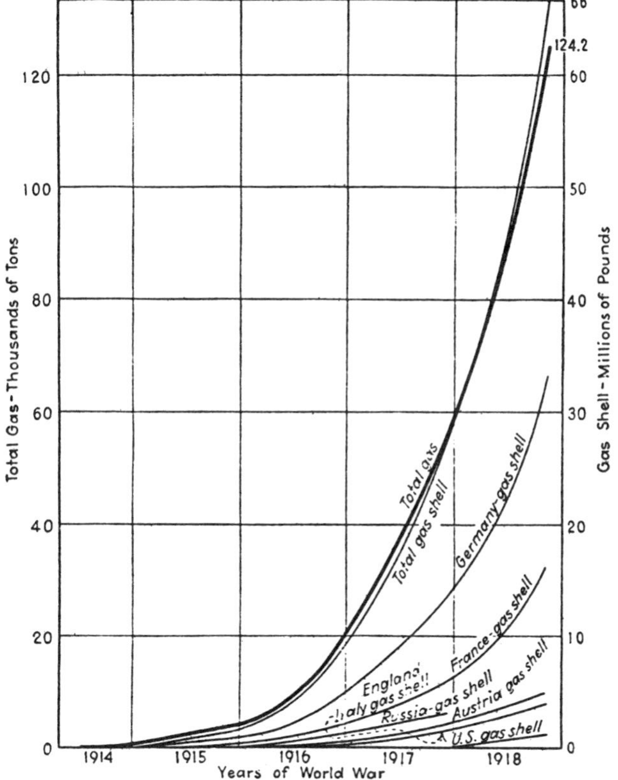

CHART XIX.—Gas and gas shell used in the World War.

682

In their first great offensive against the British in March, 1918, the Germans conducted a ten days' artillery bombardment in which they used over a half million gas shells (mostly Yellow Cross). In the ensuing attack which opened on Mar. 21, the Germans massed 1,705 batteries (about 7,500 guns) on a 44-mile front between Arras and La Fere and bombarded the British intensively for 5 hours. In this bombardment 25 to 30 per cent of the artillery shell were gas. General Ludendorff says of this attack: "Our artillery relied on gas for its effect."

The importance which the Germans attached to the use of gas shells in the artillery preparations for their great offensives in the spring of 1918 is further illustrated in a captured order of the German Seventh Army, dated May 8, 1918, which prescribed the proportions of gas shell to be used for the attack on the Aisne on May 27th, as follows:

a. Counterbattery and long-range bombardments:
Blue Cross, 70 per cent; Green Cross, 10 per cent; H.E., 20 per cent.
b. Against infantry:
Blue Cross, 30 per cent; Green Cross, 10 per cent; H.E., 60 per cent.
c. In the "box barrage:"
Blue Cross, 60 per cent; Green Cross, 10 per cent; H.E., 30 per cent.

No Yellow Cross shell were used immediately preceding an attack.

In commenting on the great German offensives of 1918, General Schwarte says: "During the big German attacks in 1918, gas was used against artillery and infantry in quantities which had never been seen before, and even in open warfare the troops were soon asking for gas."

Even after they were forced to take the defensive, the Germans continued to use a large percentage of gas shell, particularly, Yellow Cross. Thus General Hartley , referring to the German retreat in the fall of 1918 says:

Yellow Cross shell were used much further forward than previously. . . . The enemy attempted to create an impassable zone in front of our forward positions by means of mustard gas. . . . In Yellow Cross they had an extremely fine defensive weapon; which they did not use to the best advantage.

The enormous consumption of artillery gas shells by the Germans in 1918 gradually became such that they were no longer able to supply the demands, although, according to General Schwarte, at the time of the Armistice Germany was manufacturing monthly almost 1,000 tons of Yellow Cross (mustard) alone.

Commenting on this situation, Lefebure writes:

The normal establishment of a German divisional ammunition dump in July, 1918, contained about 50 per cent gas shell. The dumps captured later in the year contained from 30 per cent to 40 per cent. These figures are significant, for they show

683

how much importance the German Army attached to gas shell. When we think of the millions of shell and of the huge quantities of explosives turned out by our own factories to fill them, and when we realize that for a large number of gun calibers the Germans used as many shell filled with gas as with explosive, some idea of the importance of gas in the recent war and of its future possibilities can be obtained.

Confirming the shortage of German gas shell at the time of the Armistice, General Fries says: "Examination after the Armistice of German shell dumps captured during the advance revealed less than 1 per cent of mustard gas shell."

Throughout the war, with few exceptions, Germany maintained the initiative in chemical warfare, owing principally to her immensely superior chemical industry. Concerning this subject, Lefebure says:

As a general rule where the German lag between the approval of a substance and its use in the field covered weeks, our lag covered months. . . . The Germans used mustard gas in July, 1917. But the first fruits of allied production were not in the field for eleven months. British material was not used until a month or two before the Armistice.

And so the chemical warfare efforts of the Allies consisted largely of retaliatory measures in belated attempts to keep abreast of German initiative. For this reason the percentage of chemical shell in the German artillery-ammunition program was always ahead of that in the Allied programs.

At the time of the Armistice it is estimated that 50 per cent of the German, 35 per cent of the French, 25 per cent of the British, and 15 per cent of the American ammunition expenditures were chemical shell. The American chemical-shell program lagged considerably behind those of the other belligerents on the Western Front, principally because of production difficulties and the consequent lack of appreciation of the advantages of chemical shell in battle. However, shortly before the Armistice the American chemical-shell program was increased to 25 per cent of the artillery ammunition program to be effective Jan. 1, 1919. Gas-producing facilities in the United States were to be expanded so as to be able to provide 35 per cent chemical shell in 1919, had the war continued.

Regarding the British chemical-shell plans during the latter part of 1918, General Foulkes (12) writes:

. . . The opinion of our own General Staff of the value of gas was reflected in their last demand of the war, dated 9th August 1918, for gas shells and bombs for the 1919 campaign. 20 percent to 30 percent of all types of artillery shells were to have contained gas, the majority mustard gas, and pure lachrymators were eliminated entirely. Phosgene shells for the 18-pounder were demanded for the first time, the intention being to employ them in the moving barrage, not because any lethal effect was expected from them, but because it has been so often found advantageous to compel the enemy to meet our assaulting troops with their masks on.

684

Of the German chemical-shell program in 1918, Dr. Muntsch says: "In the year 1918, German Headquarters ordered 50% gas ammunition and 50% high explosive ammunition for the artillery."

All in all, it is clear from the plans of both sides that, had the war continued for another year, the campaign of 1919 would have been largely a chemical war. This phenomenal rise of chemicals from an unknown obscurity in 1915 to the position of a military agent of the first magnitude in 1918 is without parallel in the history of warfare.

697

CHAPTER XXVI

CONCLUSION

We have shown that chemical combat is a new mode of warfare which for the first time in recorded history departs from the physical blow as the fundamental principle of battle. Of all modern weapons, chemicals are destined to exert the most far-reaching effect in shaping the future character of warfare, for the action of chemicals over the areas in which they are employed is pervading as to space and is enduring in point of time, so that if aircraft may be said to have carried war into the third dimension, chemicals have extended it to the fourth dimension and no man can measure their ultimate possibilities.

Despite its crude and hastily improvised development, the remarkable effectiveness of chemical warfare was fully demonstrated in the World War, and clearly indicates that we are on the threshold of a new era in the evolution of war—an era of chemical rather than physical combat. Whereas in the late war, existing arms were employed to disseminate chemicals in addition to projectiles and explosives, in the future we may expect to see the requirements of chemical dissemination determine the character of the means employed in combat, and the resulting changes in armament will be more far-reaching than those brought about by the advent of gun powder.

We have also seen that chemical warfare is the most humane method of waging war heretofore employed, for by the use of chemicals not only may an enemy be overcome without annihilation or permanent injury, but the suffering caused by chemical action is, on the whole, far less than that resulting from the dismembering violence of explosives. Moreover, by chemical means alone may the blow be tempered and adjusted to the end in view, for with chemicals any effect can be produced from simple lacrimation to immediate death.

Also, unlike other means of combat, chemical warfare can be controlled and confined to the battlefield unless deliberately used elsewhere, for the laws governing the behavior of gases are as definite and well understood as the law of gravity.

While chemical combat immensely complicates modern war, it is susceptible to complete and adequate defense, and protection against it is essentially a matter of scientific skill. The chemical war of the future will, therefore, be primarily a contest between the scientific abilities of the

698

combatants, *i.e.*, a contest of brains and not brawn. This simple fact alone holds out the greatest hope for the future of civilization, for the destiny of man is safest in the hands of the most intelligent. One of the best safeguards of world peace today lies in an appreciation of the above facts and a consequent application of chemical resources to national defense.

Much confusion in the international situation has been engendered by plausible but misguided attempts to prohibit the use of chemicals in war. The history of such efforts clearly indicates both their impracticability and undesirability. Impracticable, because the gases generated by explosives are so closely akin to the gases used in chemical warfare that only hairline distinctions can be drawn between them. Such refined differentiation is impracticable of enforcement under the stress of war, even if good faith exists on both sides.

As was witnessed in the World War, sooner or later one side or the other will claim a violation of any treaty agreement against chemical warfare, because of a real or fancied encounter with toxic gases on the field of battle, such gases being impossible to exclude where high explosives are used.

Even if a convention against chemical warfare were possible of enforcement in war, on what real grounds is such an action desirable? Three objections to chemical warfare have been urged by those opposed to it: (1), that it is inhumane; (2) that it cannot be controlled and confined to armies in the field, but will run wild and decimate noncombatants and civilian populations generally; (3), that it is unsportsmanlike.

The casualty records of the late war and the united opinion of the medical profession and foremost toxicologists have shown conclusively that chemicals are not only more humane than other weapons, but that chemical combat is the one form of organized force that can be regulated to bring about the subjection of an opponent with a minimum of violence and injury. This is exemplified in the now widespread use of chemicals for quelling civil disturbances.

The experience of the World War and the results of extensive postwar experimentation have also shown the fallacy of the second objection—that chemical combat cannot be controlled and confined to the battlefield. Indeed, this evidence is so convincing, it may be safely said that the only danger to noncombatants and civilian populations from chemical warfare lies in the *deliberate* application of chemical weapons to such uses. In this respect there is no more to be feared from chemicals than from explosives and other weapons so misused.

The third charge that the use of chemicals is unsportsmanlike is hardly of sufficient weight to warrant serious consideration. It doubtless arose out of the situation early in the war, when gas was first used against

699

an unprotected enemy and was thus conceived to confer an unfair advantage upon the user. Such a situation cannot occur in the future for no government worthy of the name can fail to take steps in time of peace to protect itself against chemicals in war, unless it is lulled into a false sense of security by adherence to a treaty convention against chemical warfare and blindly fails in its duty to protect its people.

In the last analysis, war is not a sport, but a grim contest between states for national existence. War, therefore, cannot be conducted by any code of sportsmanship, but only by the law of military necessity, however much civilization may deplore the results. This being the case, the duty of any government is clear. It must take a practical and long-sighted view of the facts of war as they exist today; it must do everything in its power to insure that its armies and its people shall not be without the best possible protection against all modern weapons; and its armies shall be ready to employ the most effective means to bring to a speedy and successful conclusion any future war into which it may unfortunately be drawn.

What is chiefly needed today is a sane and rational outlook on the subject of chemical warfare, such as was voiced in one of the earliest suggestions concerning the use of toxic gas in war. In an article on "Greek Fire," which appeared in 1864, fifty years before the World War, a British writer says:

I feel it a duty to state openly and boldly, that if science were to be allowed her full swing, if society would really allow that "all is fair in war," war might be banished at once from the earth as a game which neither subject nor king dare play at. Globes that could distribute liquid fire could distribute also lethal agents, within the breath of which no man, however puissant, could stand and live. From the summit of Primrose Hill, a few hundred engineers, properly prepared, could render Regent's Park, in an incredibly short space of time, utterly uninhabitable; or could make an army of men, that should even fill that space, fall with their arms in their hands prostrate and helpless as the host of Sennacherib.

The question is, shall these things be? I do not see that humanity should revolt, for would it not be better to destroy a host in Regent's Park by making the men fall as in a mystical sleep, than to let down on them another host to break their bones, tear their limbs asunder and gouge out their entrails with three-cornered pikes; leaving a vast majority undead, and writhing for hours in torments of the damned? I conceive, for one, that science would be blessed in spreading her wings on the blast, and breathing into the face of a desperate horde of men prolonged sleep—for it need not necessarily be a death—which they could not grapple with, and which would yield them up with their implements of murder to an enemy that in the immensity of its power could afford to be merciful as Heaven.

The question is, shall these things be? I think they must be. By what compact can they be stopped? It were improbable that any congress of nations could agree on any code regulating means of destruction: but if it did, it were useless; for science becomes more powerful as she concentrates her forces in the hands of units, so that a nation could only act, by the absolute and individual assent of each of her repre-

700

sentatives. Assume, then, that France shall lay war to England, and by superior force of men should place immense hosts, well armed, on English soil. Is it probable that the units would rest in peace and allow sheer brute force to win its way to empire? Or put English troops on French soil, and reverse the question?

To conclude. War has, at this moment, reached, in its details, such an extravagance of horror and cruelty, that it cannot be made worse by an act, and can only be made more merciful by being rendered more terribly energetic. Who that had to die from a blow would not rather place his head under Nasmyth's hammer, than submit it to a drummer boy armed with a ferrule?

If the statesmen who control the destinies of nations could but achieve this enlightened viewpoint, the future of mankind would be far more secure.

701

APPENDIX

RELATION OF VOLATILITY TO VAPOR PRESSURE

The vapor pressures of many chemical compounds are given in chemical literature under the physical properties of the compounds. If the vapor pressure of a gas at any given temperature is known, the volatility of the substance may be obtained as follows:

Let M = the molecular weight of the gas, in grams.
T_1 = the temperature (absolute) at which the vapor pressure is known.
T = normal absolute temperature = 273°C.
P_1 = the vapor pressure at a temperature T, in mm. Hg.
P = normal atmospheric pressure = 760 mm. Hg.
V_1 = volatility of the gas at a temperature T, in grams per liter.

The gram molecule (*i.e.*, the molecular weight of the substance expressed in grams) of any gas occupies 22.4 liters at 0°C. and 760 mm. pressure.

Therefore

$$V = \frac{MTP_1}{22.4 \times 760T_1}$$

Thus, the molecular weight of phosgene is 99, its vapor pressure at 25°C. is 1,400 mm. Hg, and its volatility at 25°C. is

$$V = \frac{99 \times 273 \times 1{,}400}{22.4 \times 760 \times 298} = 7.488 \text{ grams}$$

or 7.488 mg. per liter (see Chart I, page 9).

Proceeding as above, the volatility curve for any gas may be constructed from its vapor pressure curve, as shown in Chart I.

RELATION OF VOLUMETRIC RATIOS TO WEIGHT RATIOS

The concentration of a toxic gas in the air is variously stated as: (1) grams of gas per cubic meter of air; (2) milligrams of gas per liter of air; (3) ounces of gas per 1,000 cu. ft. of air; and (4) parts of gas per million parts of air. In order to compare concentrations expressed in these different ways, it is necessary and convenient to know the conversion factors, which may be simply stated as follows:

Grams per cubic meter are numerically exactly the same as milligrams per liter, since a milligram is $\frac{1}{1000}$ gram and a liter is $\frac{1}{1000}$ cubic meter.

Since 1 oz. = 28.35 grams and 1 cu. ft. = 28.32 liters, 1 oz. per cubic foot = 1.001 grams per liter, and ounces per thousand cubic feet = 1.001 mg. per liter. Therefore, ounces per thousand cubic feet are numerically the same as milligrams per liter to the third decimal place.

Parts per million are converted to milligrams per liter as follows:
1 liter of air at 0°C. and 760 mm. weighs 1.293 grams.
1 cu. mm. of air at 0°C. and 760 mm. weighs 0.0001293 mg.

For air, or any gas of the same density, 1 part per million (1 p.p.m.) would be 1 cu. mm. per liter.

702

Hence under standard conditions 1 p.p.m. of any gas of the same density as air would weigh 0.001293 mg. per liter.

But the average molecular weight of air = 28.9; for any other gas the figure 0.001293 would vary in proportion to the molecular weight of the gas.

Therefore, if M = molecular weight of a gas, P = barometric pressure, and T = the absolute temperature, then

$$\text{Milligrams per liter} = \frac{M \times 0.001293 \times P \times 273}{28.9 \times 760 \times T} \text{ p.p.m.}$$

This may be reduced to the following:

$$\text{Milligrams per liter} = \frac{0.0000161MP}{T} \text{ p.p.m.}$$

or

$$\text{p.p.m.} = \frac{T}{0.0000161MP} \text{ mg. per liter.}$$

CHEMICALS IN WAR

A Treatise on Chemical Warfare

BY
AUGUSTIN M. PRENTISS, PH.D.
Brigadier General, Chemical Warfare Service
United States Army

INDEX

IMPROVISED MUNITIONS HANDBOOK

INDEX

TM 31-210

FOR OFFICIAL USE ONLY

IMPROVISED MUNITIONS HANDBOOK

TABLE OF CONTENTS

FRANKFORD ARSENAL

Philadelphia Pennsylvania

3

INTRODUCTION

1. Purpose and Scope

In Unconventional Warfare operations it may be impossible or unwise to use conventional military munitions as tools in the conduct of certain missions. It may be necessary instead to fabricate the required munitions from locally available or unassuming materials. The purpose of this Manual is to increase the potential of Special Forces and guerrilla troops by describing in detail the manufacture of munitions from seemingly innocuous locally available materials.

Manufactured, precision devices almost always will be more effective, more reliable, and easier to use than improvised ones, but shelf items will just not be available for certain operations for security or logistical reasons. Therefore the operator will have to rely on materials he can buy in a drug or paint store, find in a junk pile, or scrounge from military stocks. Also, many of the ingredients and materials used in fabricating homemade items are so commonplace or innocuous they can be carried without arousing suspicion. The completed item itself often is more easily concealed or camouflaged. In addition, the field expedient item can be tailored for the intended target, thereby providing an advantage over the standard item in flexibility and versatility.

The Manual contains simple explanations and illustrations to permit construction of the items by personnel not normally familiar with making and handling munitions. These items were conceived in-house or, obtained from other publications or personnel engaged in munitions or special warfare work. This Manual includes methods for fabricating explosives, detonators, propellants, shaped charges, small arms, mortars, incendiaries, delays, switches, and similar items from indigenous materials.

2. Safety and Reliability

Each item was evaluated both theoretically and experimentally to assure safety and reliability. A large number of items were discarded because of inherent hazards or unreliable performance. Safety warnings are prominently inserted in the procedures where they apply but it is emphasized that safety is a matter of attitude. It is a proven fact that men who are alert, who think out a situation, and who take correct precautions have fewer accidents than the careless and indifferent. It is important that work be planned and that instructions be followed to the letter; all work should be done in a neat and orderly manner. In the manufacture explosives, detonators, propellants and incendiaries, equipment must be kept clean and such energy concentrations as sparks,

4

friction, impact, hot objects, flame, chemical reactions, and excessive pressure should be avoided.

These items were found to be effective in most environments; however, samples should be made and tested remotely prior to actual use of assure proper performance. Chemical items should be used as soon as possible after preparation and kept free of moisture, dirt, and the above energy concentrations. Special care should be taken in any attempt at substitution or use of items for purposes other than that specified or intended.

5

Section I
No. 1
PLASTIC EXPLOSIVE FILLER

A plastic explosive filler can be made from potassium chlorate and petroleum jelly. This explosive can be detonated with commercial #8 or any military blasting cap.

MATERIAL REQUIRED	HOW USED
Potassium chlorate	Medicine Manufacture of matches
Petroleum jelly (Vaseline)	Medicine Lubricant
Piece of round stick	
Wide bowl or other container for mixing ingredients.	

PROCEDURE

1. Spread potassium chlorate crystals thinly on a hard surface. Roll the round stick over crystals to crush into a very fine powder until it looks like face powder or wheat flour.

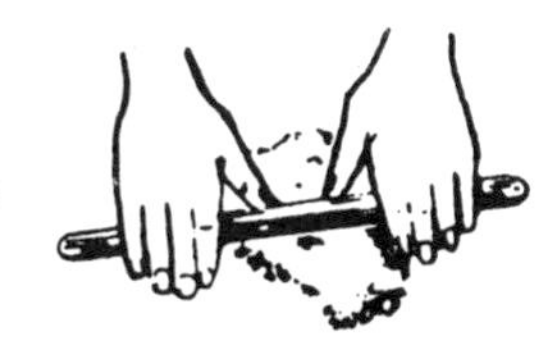

2. Place 9 parts powdered potassium chlorate and 1 part petroleum jelly in a wide bowl or similar container. Mix ingredients with hands (knead) until a uniform paste is obtained.

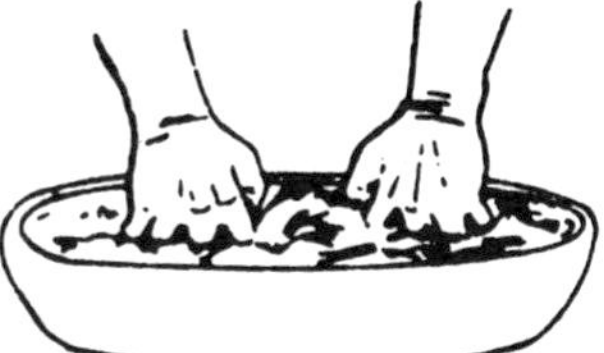

Store explosive in a waterproof container until ready to use.

Section I

6 No. 2

POTASSIUM NITRATE

Potassium nitrate (saltpeter) can be extracted from many natural sources and can be used to make nitric acid, black powder and many pyrotechnics. The yield ranges from .1 to 10% by weight, depending on the fertility of the soil.

MATERIALS	SOURCE
Nitrate bearing earth or other material, about 3-1/2 gallons (13-1/2 liters)	Soil containing old decayed vegetable or animal matter Old cellars and/or farm dirt floors Earth from old burial grounds Decayed stone or mortar building foundations
Fine wood ashes, about 1/2 cup (1/8 liter)	Totally burned whitish wood ash powder Totally burned paper (black)
Bucket or similar container, about 5 gallons (19 liters) in volume (Plastic, metal, or wood)	
2 pieces of finely woven cloth, each slightly larger than bottom of bucket	
Shallow pan or dish, at least as large as bottom of bucket	
Shallow heat resistant container (ceramic, metal, etc.)	
Water - 1-3/4 gallons (6-3/4 liters)	
Awl, knife, screwdriver, or other hole producing instrument	
Alcohol about 1 gallon (4 liters) (whiskey, rubbing alcohol, etc.)	
Heat source (fire, electric heater, etc.)	
Paper	
Tape	

NOTE: Only the ratios of the amounts of ingredients are important. Thus, for twice as much potassium nitrate, double quantities used.

7

PROCEDURE:

1. Punch holes in bottom of bucket. Spread one piece of cloth over holes inside of bucket.

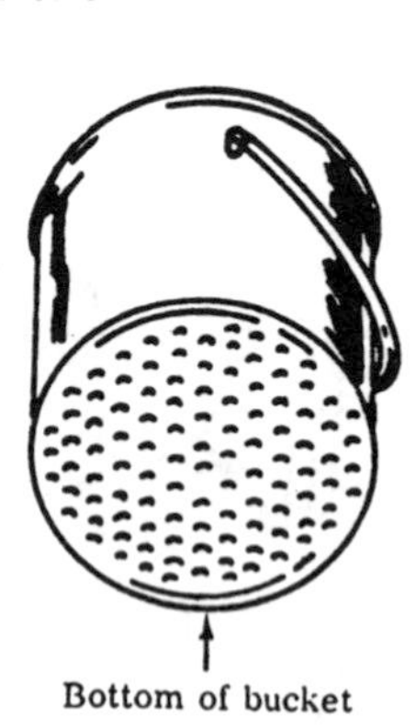

Bottom of bucket

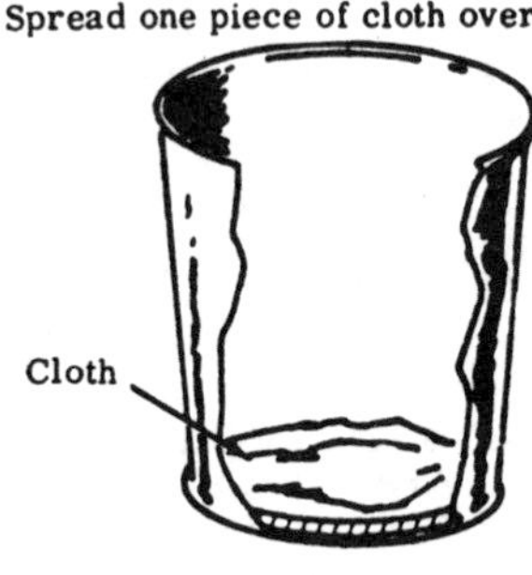

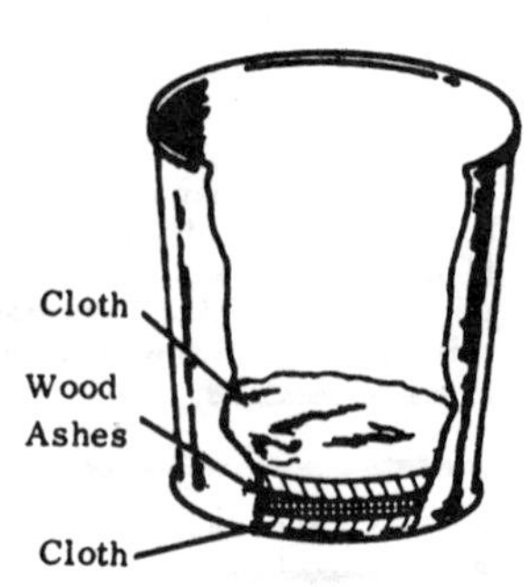

2. Place wood ashes on cloth and spread to make a layer about the thickness of the cloth. Place second piece of cloth on top of ashes.

3. Place dirt in bucket.

Earth
Cloth
Wood Ashes
Cloth

4. Place bucket over shallow container. Bucket may be supported on sticks if necessary.

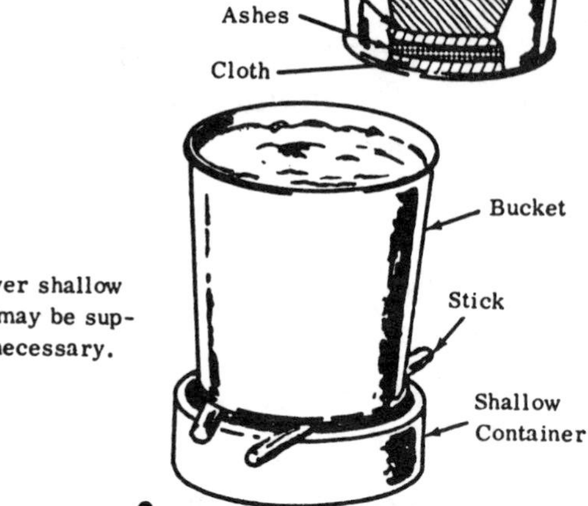

8

5. Boil water and pour it over earth in bucket a little at a time. Allow water to run through holes in bucket into shallow container. Be sure water goes through all of the earth. Allow drained liquid to cool and settle for 1 to 2 hours.

NOTE: Do not pour all of the water at once, since this may cause stoppage.

6. Carefully drain off liquid into heat resistant container. Discard any sludge remaining in bottom of the shallow container.

7. Boil mixture over hot fire for at least 2 hours. Small grains of salt will begin to appear in the solution. Scoop these out as they form, using any type of improvised strainer (paper, etc.).

Improvised Strainer
Heat Resistant Container
Heat Source

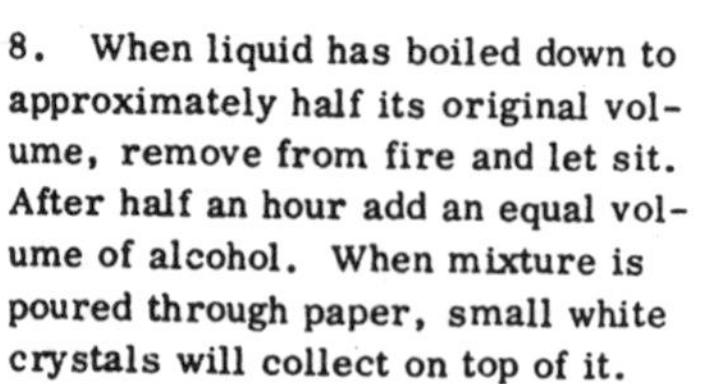

8. When liquid has boiled down to approximately half its original volume, remove from fire and let sit. After half an hour add an equal volume of alcohol. When mixture is poured through paper, small white crystals will collect on top of it.

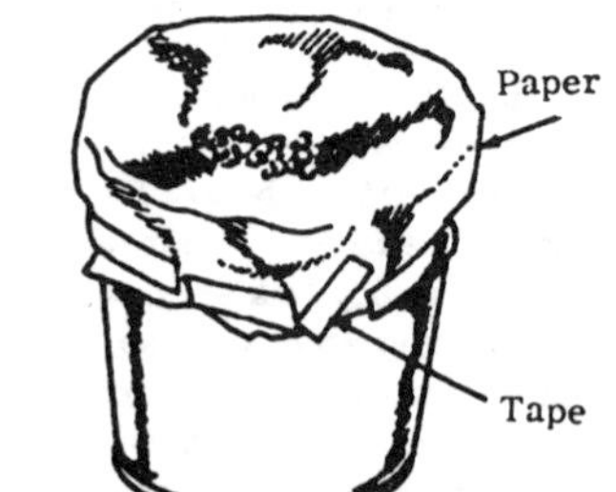

9. To purify the potassium nitrate, re-desolve the dry crystals in the smallest possible amount of boiled water. Remove any salt crystals that appear (Step 7); pour through an improvised filter made of several pieces of paper and evaporate or gently heat the concentrated solution to dryness.

10. Spread crystals on flat surface and allow to dry. The potassium nitrate crystals are now ready for use.

Section I
9 No. 4
NITRIC ACID

Nitric acid is used in the preparation of many explosives, incendiary mixtures, and acid delay timers. It may be prepared by distilling a mixture of potassium nitrate and concentrated sulfuric acid.

MATERIAL REQUIRED:	SOURCES:
Potassium nitrate (2 parts by volume)	Drug Store
	Improvised (Section I, No. 2)
Concentrated sulfuric acid (1 part by volume)	Motor vehicle batteries
	Industrial plants
2 bottles or ceramic jugs (narrow necks are preferable)	
Pot or frying pan	
Heat source (wood, coal, or charcoal)	
Tape (paper, electrical, masking, etc. but not cellophane)	
Paper or rags	

IMPORTANT: If sulfuric acid is obtained from a motor vehicle battery, concentrate it by boiling it until white fumes appear. DO NOT INHALE FUMES.

NOTE: The amount of nitric acid produced is the same as the amount of potassium nitrate. Thus, for 2 tablespoonsful of nitric acid, use 2 tablespoonsful of potassium nitrate and 1 tablespoonsful of concentrated sulfuric acid.

PROCEDURE:

1. Place dry potassium nitrate in bottle or jug. Add sulfuric acid. Do not fill bottle more than 1/4 full. Mix until paste is formed.

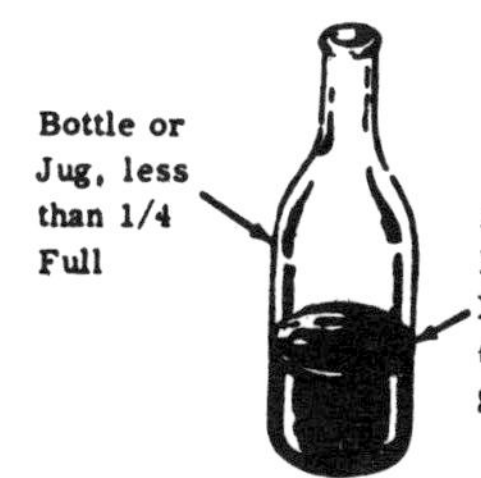

CAUTION: Sulfuric acid will burn skin and destroy clothing. If any is spilled, wash it away with a large quantity of water. Fumes are also dangerous and should not be inhaled.

10

2. Wrap paper or rags around necks of 2 bottles. Securely tape necks of bottles together. Be sure bottles are flush against each other and that there are no air spaces.

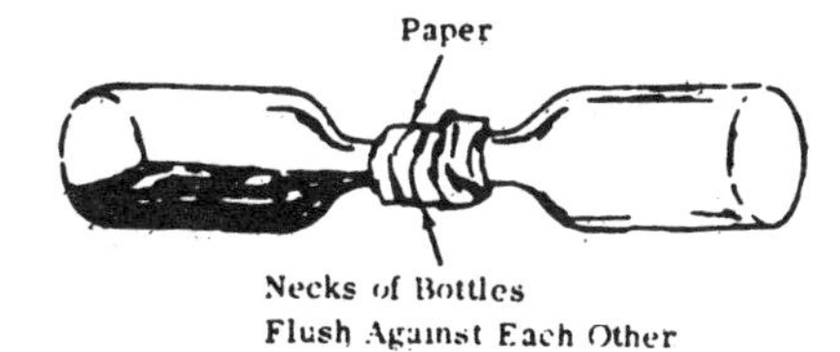

3. Support bottles on rocks or cans so that empty bottle is slightly lower than bottle containing paste so that nitric acid that is formed in receiving bottle will not run into other bottle.

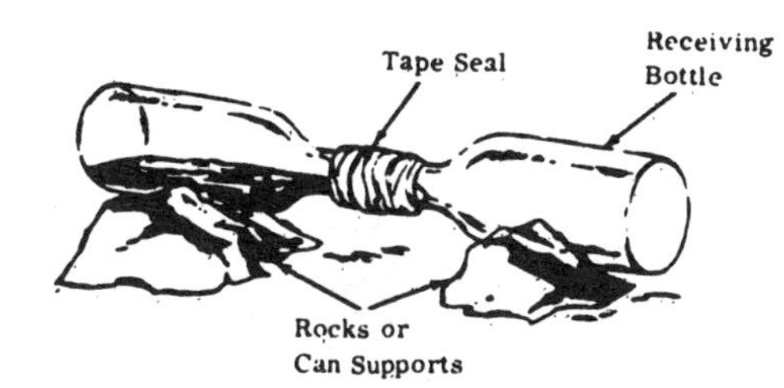

4. Build fire in pot or frying pan.

5. Gently heat bottle containing mixture by moving fire in and out. As red fumes begin to appear periodically pour cool water over empty receiving bottle. Nitric acid will begin to form in the receiving bottle.

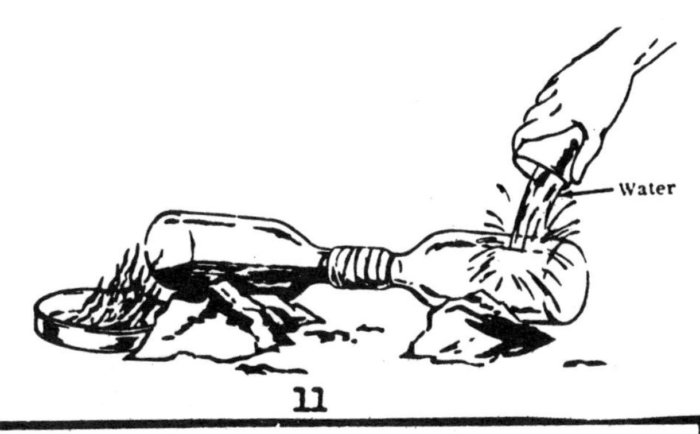

11

CAUTION: Do not overheat or wet bottle containing mixture or it may shatter. As an added precaution, place bottle to be heated in heat resistant container filled with sand or gravel. Heat this outer container to produce nitric acid.

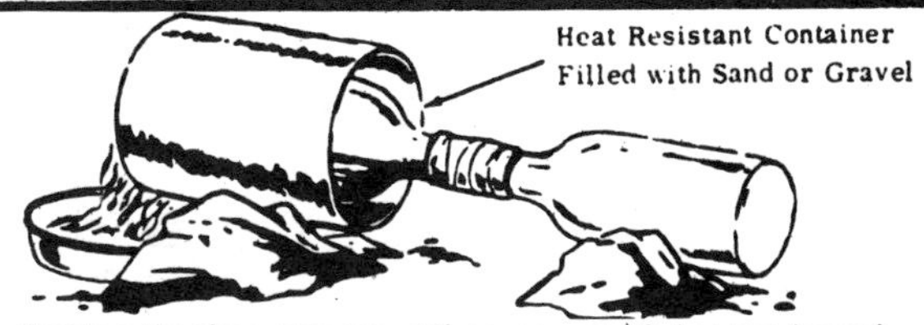

6. Continue the above process until no more red fumes are formed. If the nitric acid formed in the receiving bottle is not clear (cloudy) pour it into cleaned bottle and repeat Steps 2 - 6.

CAUTION: Nitric acid will burn skin and destroy clothing. If any is spilled, wash it away with a large quantity of water. Fumes are also dangerous and should not be inhaled.

Nitric acid should be kept away from all combustibles and should be kept in a sealed ceramic or glass container.

Section I
12 No. 5
INITIATOR FOR DUST EXPLOSIONS

An initiator which will initiate common material to produce dust explosions can be rapidly and easily constructed. This type of charge is ideal for the destruction of enclosed areas such as rooms or buildings.

MATERIAL REQUIRED:

A flat can, 3 in. (8 cm) diameter and 1-1/2 in. (3-3/4 cm) high. A 6-1/2 ounce Tuna can serves the purpose quite well.
Blasting cap
Explosive
Aluminum (may be wire, cut sheet, flattened can or powder
Large nail, 4 in. (10 cm) long
Wooden rod - 1/4 in. (6 mm) diameter
Flour, gasoline and powder or chipped aluminum

NOTE: Plastic explosives (Comp. C-4, etc.) produce better explosions than cast explosives (Comp. B, etc.).

PROCEDURE:

1. Using the nail, press a hole through the side of the Tuna can 3/8 to 1/2 inch (1 to 1-1/2 cm) from the bottom. Using a rotating and lever action, enlarge the hole until it will accommodate the blasting cap.

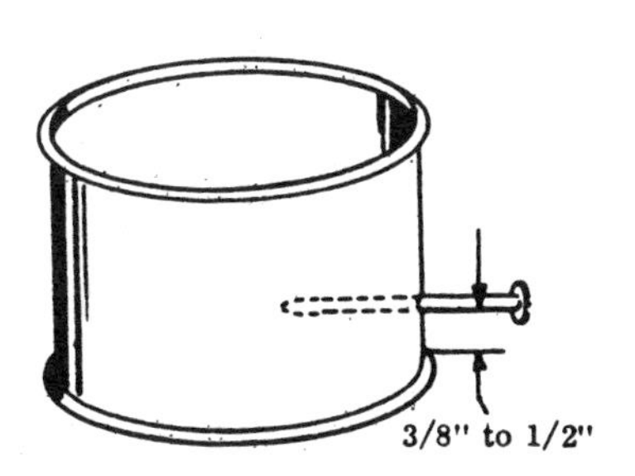

2. Place the wooden rod in the hole and position the end of the rod at the center of the can.

3. Press explosive into the can, being sure to surround the rod, until it is 3/4 inch (2 cm) from top of the can. Carefully remove the wooden rod.

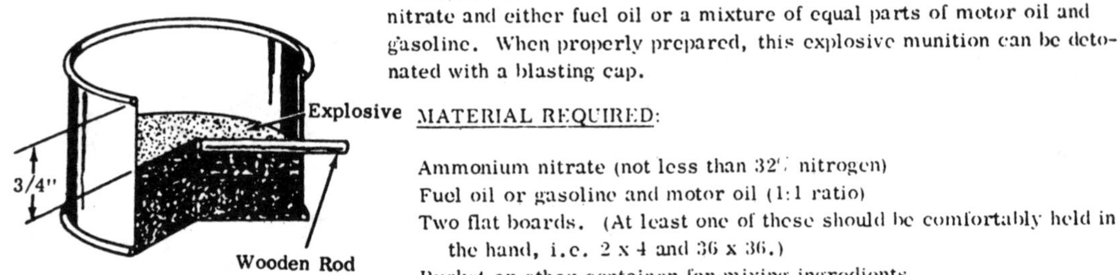

13

4. Place the aluminum metal on top of the explosive.

5. Just before use, insert the blasting cap into the cavity made by the rod. The initiator is now ready for use.

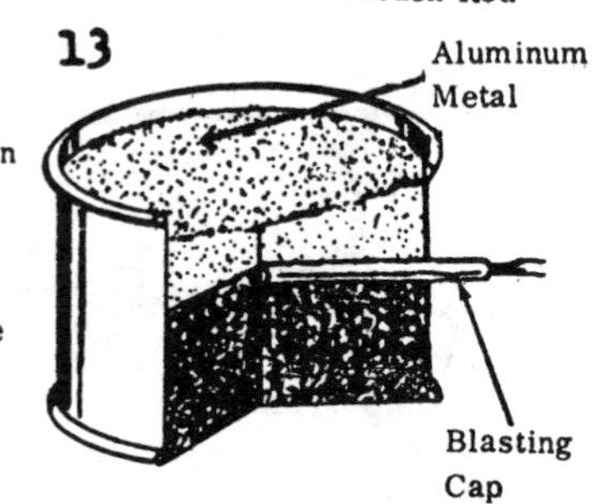

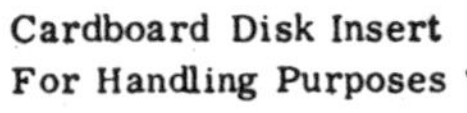

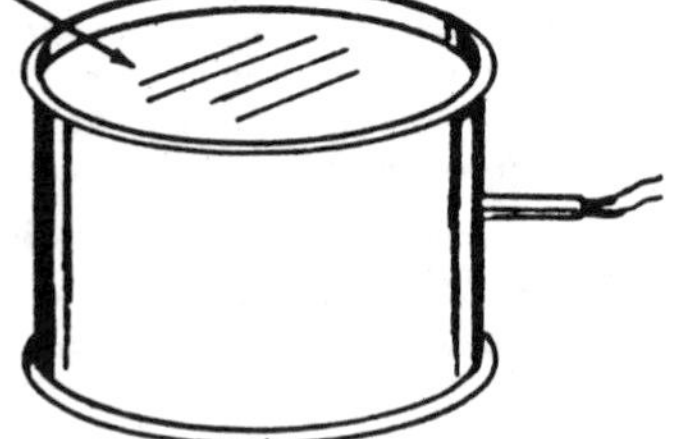

NOTE: If it is desired to carry the initiator some distance, cardboard may be pressed on top of the aluminum to insure against loss of material.

HOW TO USE:

This particular unit works quite well to initiate charges of five pounds of flour, 1/2 gallon (1-2/3 liters) of gasoline or two pounds of flake painters aluminum. The solid materials may merely be contained in sacks or cardboard cartons. The gasoline may be placed in plastic-coated paper milk cartons, plastic or glass bottles. The charges are placed directly on top of the initiator and the blasting cap is actuated electrically or by fuse depending on the type of cap employed. This will destroy a 2,000 cubic feet enclosure (building 10 x 20 x 10 feet).

NOTE: For larger enclosures, use proportionately larger initiators and charges.

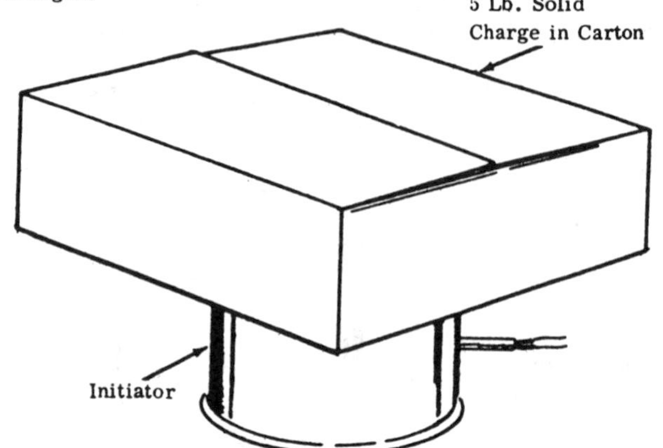

Section I

14 No. 6

FERTILIZER EXPLOSIVE

An explosive munition can be made from fertilizer grade ammonium nitrate and either fuel oil or a mixture of equal parts of motor oil and gasoline. When properly prepared, this explosive munition can be detonated with a blasting cap.

MATERIAL REQUIRED:

Ammonium nitrate (not less than 32% nitrogen)
Fuel oil or gasoline and motor oil (1:1 ratio)
Two flat boards. (At least one of these should be comfortably held in the hand, i.e. 2 x 4 and 36 x 36.)
Bucket or other container for mixing ingredients
Iron or steel pipe or bottle, tin can or heavy-walled cardboard tube
Blasting cap
Wooden rod - 1/4 in. diameter
Spoon or similar measuring container

PROCEDURE:

1. Spread a handful of the ammonium nitrate on the large flat board and rub vigorously with the other board until the large particles are crushed into a very fine powder that looks like flour (approx. 10 min).

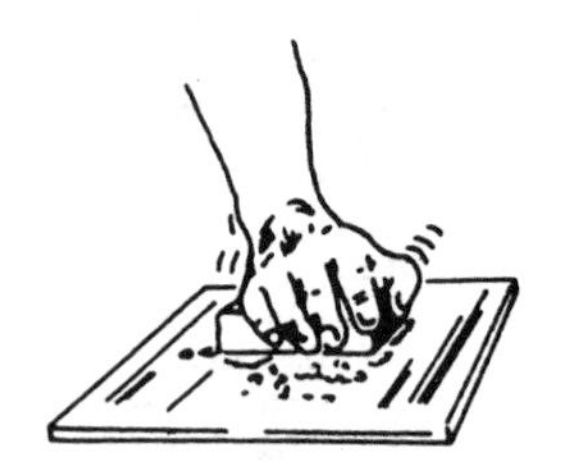

NOTE: Proceed with Step 2 as soon as possible since the powder may take moisture from the air and become spoiled.

2. Mix one measure (cup, tablespoon, etc.) of fuel oil with 16 measures of the finely ground ammonium nitrate in a dry bucket or other suitable container and stir with the wooden rod. If fuel oil is not available, use one half measure of gasoline and one half measure of motor oil. Store in a waterproof container until ready to use.

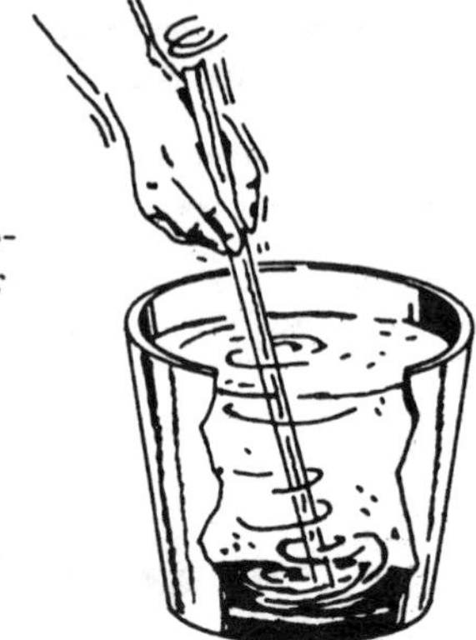

15

3. Spoon this mixture into an iron or steel pipe which has an end cap threaded on one end. If a pipe is not available, you may use a dry tin can, a glass jar or a heavy-walled cardboard tube.

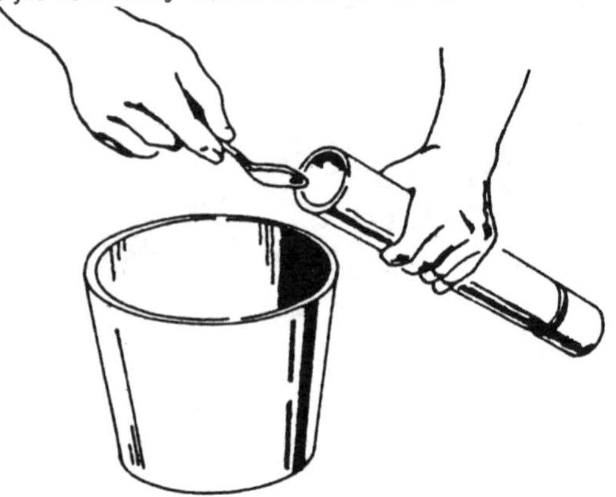

NOTE: Take care not to tamp or shake the mixture in the pipe. If mixture becomes tightly packed, one cap will not be sufficient to initiate the explosive.

Blasting Cap

4. Insert blasting cap just beneath the surface of the explosive mix.

Pipe

Mixture

NOTE: Confining the open end of the container will add to the effectiveness of the explosive.

16

Section I
No. 9
"RED OR WHITE POWDER" PROPELLANT

"Red or White Powder" Propellant may be prepared in a simple, safe manner. The formulation described below will result in approximately 2-1/2 pounds of powder. This is a small arms propellant and should only be used in weapons with 1/2 in. inside diameter or less, such as the Match Gun or the 7.62 Carbine, but not pistols.

MATERIAL REQUIRED:

Heat source (Kitchen stove or open fire)
2 gallon metal bucket
Measuring cup (8 ounces)
Wooden spoon or rubber spatula
Metal sheet or aluminum foil (at least 18 in. sq.)
Flat window screen (at least 1 ft. sq.)
Potassium nitrate (granulated) 2-1/3 cups
White sugar (granulated) 2 cups
Powdered ferric oxide (rust) 1/8 cup (if available)
Clear water, 3-1/2 cups

PROCEDURE:

1. Place the sugar, potassium nitrate, and water in the bucket. Heat with a low flame, stirring occasionally until the sugar and potassium nitrate dissolve.

2. If available, add the ferric oxide (rust) to the solution. Increase the flame under the mixture until it boils gently.

NOTE: The mixture will retain the rust coloration.

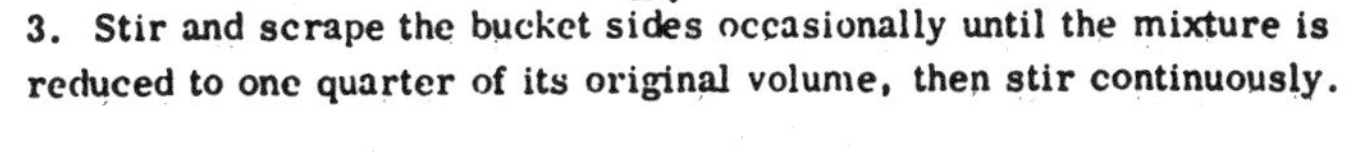

17

3. Stir and scrape the bucket sides occasionally until the mixture is reduced to one quarter of its original volume, then stir continuously.

4. As the water evaporates, the mixture will become thicker until it reaches the consistency of cooked breakfast cereal or homemade fudge. At this stage of thickness, remove the bucket from the heat source, and spread the mass on the metal sheet.

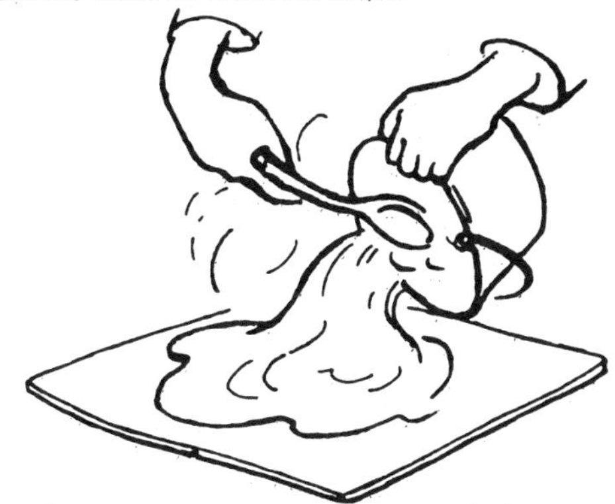

5. While the material cools, score it with the spoon or spatula in crisscrossed furrows about 1 inch apart.

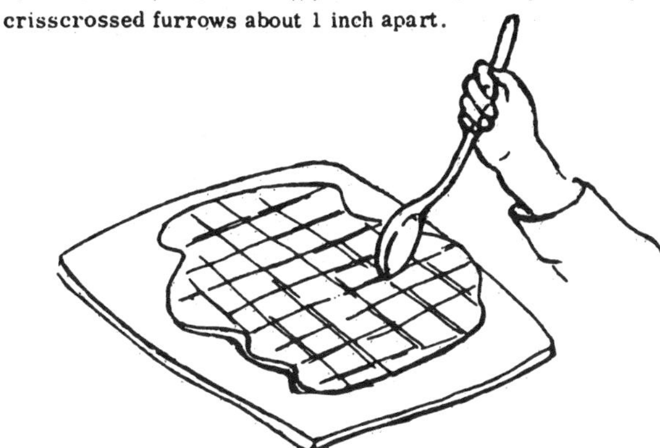

6. Allow the material to air dry, preferably in the sun. As it dries, rescore it occasionally (about every 20 minutes) to aid drying.

18

7. When the material has dried to a point where it is moist and soft but not sticky to the touch, place a small spoonful on the screen. Rub the material back and forth against the screen mesh with spoon or other flat object until the material is granulated into small worm-like particles.

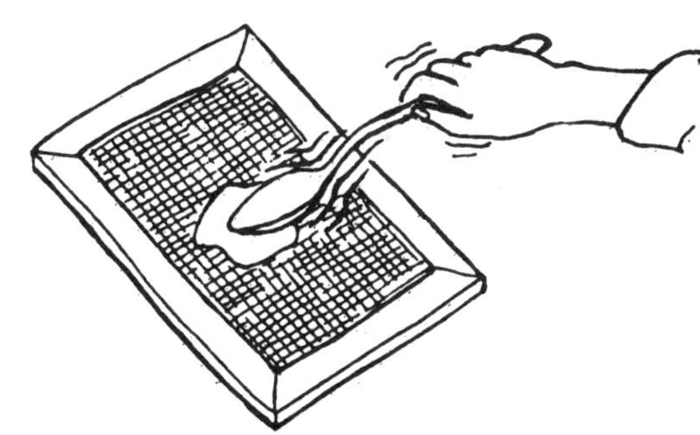

8. After granulation, return the material to the sun to dry completely.

19

Section II
No. 1
PIPE HAND GRENADE

Hand grenades can be made from a piece of iron pipe. The filler can be plastic or granular military explosive, improvised explosive, or propellant from shotgun or small arms ammunition.

MATERIAL REQUIRED

- Iron pipe, threaded ends, 1 1/2" to 3" diam., 3" to 8" long.
- Two (2) iron pipe caps.
- Explosive or propellant
- Nonelectric blasting cap. (Commercial or military)
- Fuse cord
- Hand drill
- Pliers

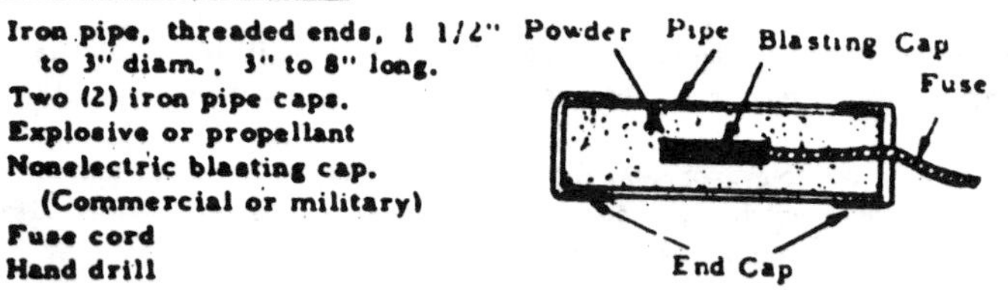

PROCEDURE

1. Place blasting cap on one end of fuse cord and crimp with pliers.

   NOTE: To find out how long the fuse cord should be, check the time it takes a known length to burn. If 12 inches burns in 30 seconds, a 6-inch cord will ignite the grenade in 15 seconds.

2. Screw pipe cap to one end of pipe. Place fuse cord with blasting cap into the opposite end so that the blasting cap is near the center of the pipe.

20

NOTE: If plastic explosive is to be used, fill pipe before inserting blasting cap. Push a round stick into the center of the explosive to make a hole and then insert the blasting cap.

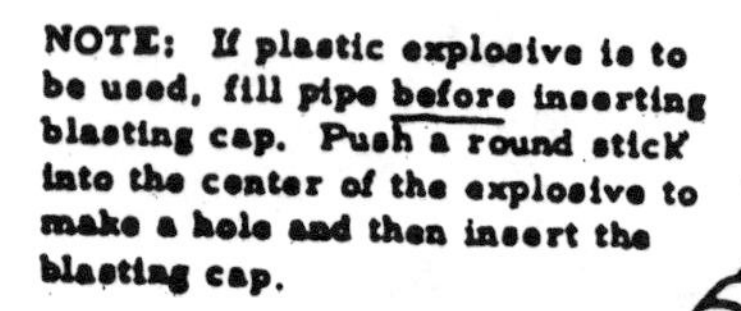

3. Pour explosive or propellant into pipe a little bit at a time. Tap the base of the pipe frequently to settle filler.

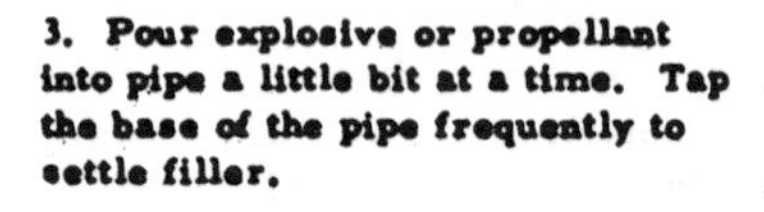

4. Drill a hole in the center of the unassembled pipe cap large enough for the fuse cord to pass through.

5. Wipe pipe threads to remove any filler material.

   Slide the drilled pipe cap over the fuse and screw handtight onto the pipe.

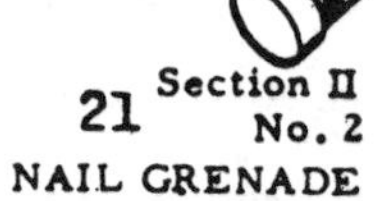

21 Section II No. 2

NAIL GRENADE

Effective fragmentation grenades can be made from a block of TNT or other blasting explosive and nails

MATERIAL REQUIRED:

- Block of TNT or other blasting explosive
- Nails
- Non-Electric Military blasting cap
- Fuse Cord
- Tape, string, wire or glue

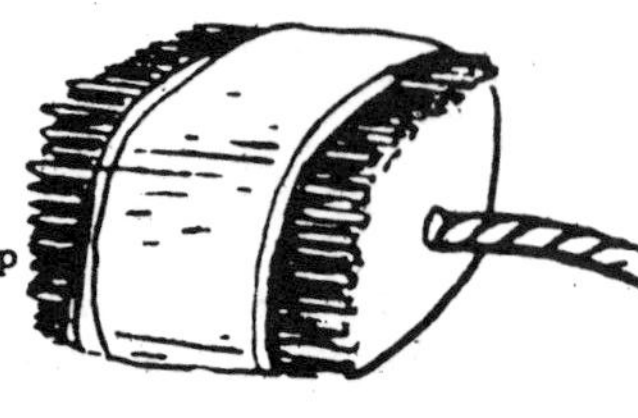

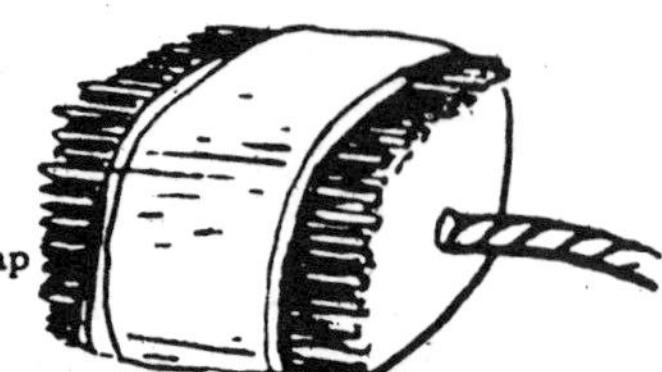

PROCEDURE:

1. If an explosive charge other than a standard TNT block is used, make a hole in the center of the charge for inserting the blasting cap. TNT can be drilled with relative safety. With plastic explosives, a hole can be made by pressing a round stick into the center of the charge. The hole should be deep enough that the blasting cap is totally within the explosive.

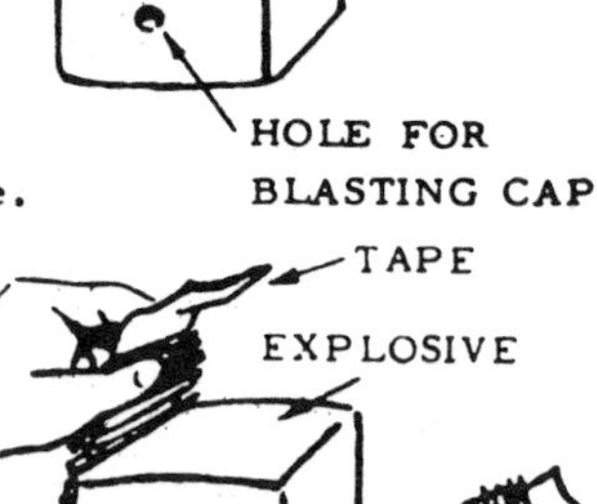

2. Tape, tie or glue one or two rows of closely packed nails to sides of explosive block. Nails should completely cover the four surfaces of the block.

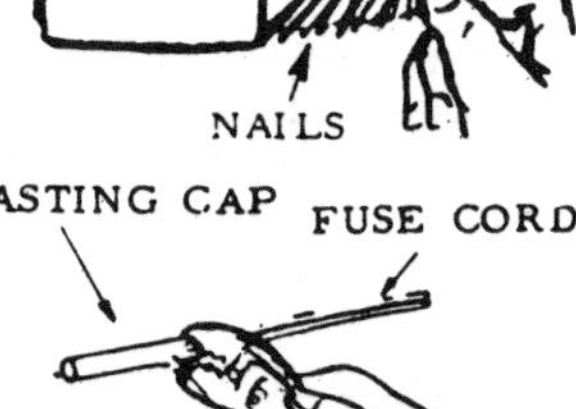

3. Place blasting cap on one end of the fuse cord and crimp with pliers.

NOTE: To find out how long the fuse cord should be, check the time it takes a known length to burn. If 12 inches (30 cm) burns for 30 seconds, a 10 second delay will require a 4 inch (10 cm) fuse.

22

4. Insert the blasting cap in the hole in the block of explosive. Tape or tie fuse cord securely in place so that it will not fall out when the grenade is thrown.

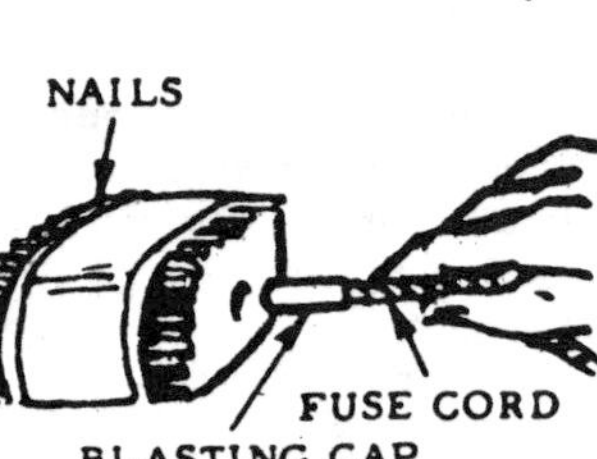

ALTERNATE USE:

An effective directional anti-personnel mine can be made by placing nails on only one side of the explosive block. For this case, an electric blasting cap can be used.

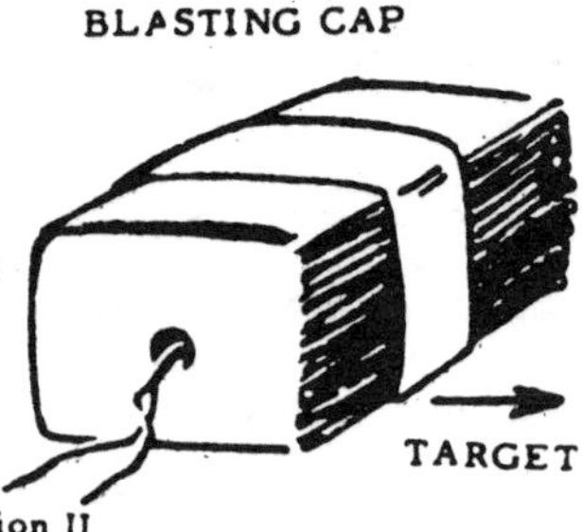

23 Section II No. 3

WINE BOTTLE CONE CHARGE

This cone charge will penetrate 3 to 4 inches of armor. Placed on an engine or engine compartment it will disable a tank or other vehicle.

MATERIAL REQUIRED:

- Glass wine bottle with false bottom (cone shaped)
- Plastic or castable explosive
- Blasting cap
- Gasoline or Kerosene (small amount)
- String
- Adhesive tape

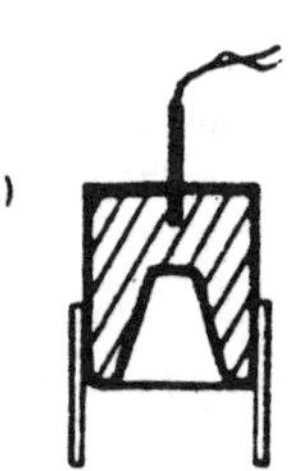

PROCEDURE:

1. Soak a piece of string in gasoline or kerosene. Double wrap this string around the wine bottle approximately 3 in. (7 1/2 cm) above the top of the cone.

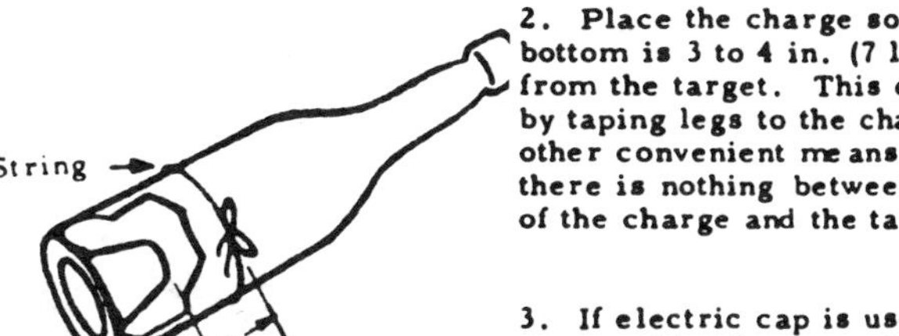

NOTE: A small amount of motor oil added to the gasoline or kerosene will improve results.

2. Ignite the string and allow to burn for 1 to 2 minutes. Then plunge the bottle into cold water to crack the bottle. The top half can now be easily removed and discarded.

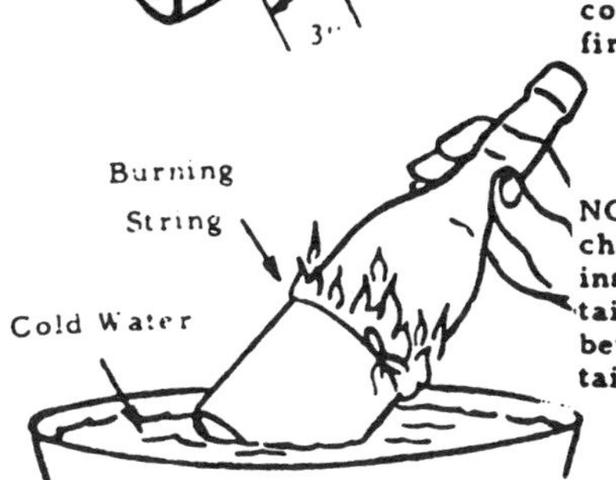

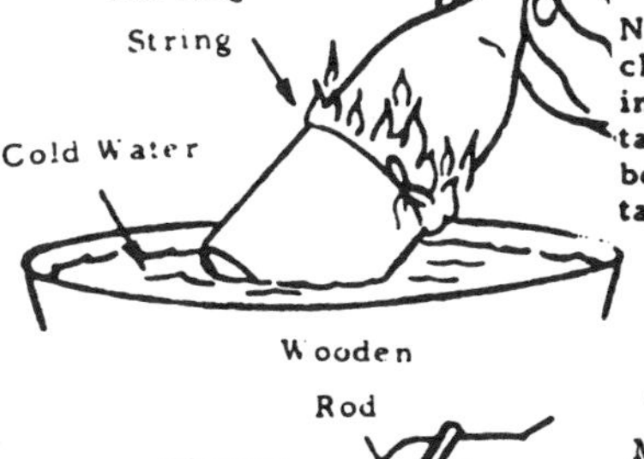

3. If plastic explosive is used:
(a) pack explosive into the bottle a little at a time compressing with a wooden rod. Fill the bottle to the top.

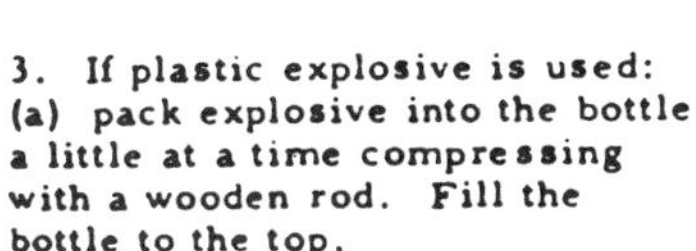

(b) press a 1/4 in. wooden dowel 1/2 in. (12mm) into the middle of the top of the explosive charge to form a hole for the blasting cap.

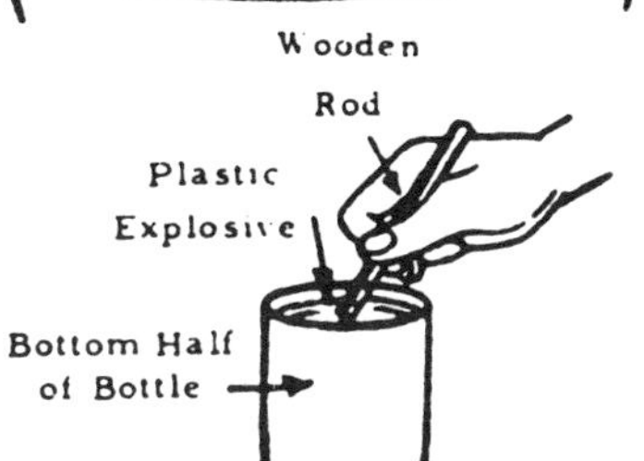

4. If TNT or other castable explosive is used:
(a) break explosive into small pieces using a wooden mallet or non-sparking metal tools. Place pieces in a tin can.

24

(b) Suspend this can in a larger container which is partly filled with water. A stiff wire or stick pushed through the smaller can will accomplish this.

Suspension Rod
Explosive
Inner Can
Outer Can
Water

CAUTION: The inner can must not rest on the bottom of the outer container.

(c) Heat the container on an electric hot plate or other heat source. Stir the explosive frequently with a wooden stick while it is melting.

CAUTION: Keep area well ventilated while melting explosive. Fumes may be poisonous.

(d) When all the explosive has melted, remove the inner container and stir the molten explosive until it begins to thicken. During this time the bottom half of the wine bottle should be placed in the container of hot water. This will pre-heat the bottle so that it will not crack when the explosive is poured.

(e) Remove the bottle from hot water and dry thoroughly. Pour molten explosive into the bottle and allow to cool. The crust which forms on top of the charge during cooling should be broken with a wooden stick and more explosive added. Do this as often as necessary until the bottle is filled to the top.

(f) When explosive has completely hardened, bore a hole for the blasting cap in the middle of the top of the charge about 1/2 in. (12mm) deep.

HOW TO USE:

1. Place blasting cap in the hole in the top of the charge. If non-electric cap is used be sure cap is crimped around fuze and fuze is long enough to provide safe delay.

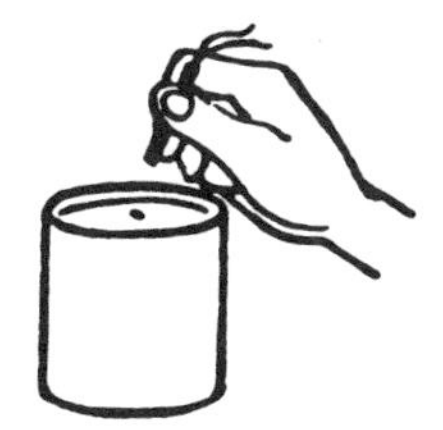

2. Place the charge so that the bottom is 3 to 4 in. (7 1/2 to 10 cm) from the target. This can be done by taping legs to the charge or any other convenient means as long as there is nothing between the base of the charge and the target.

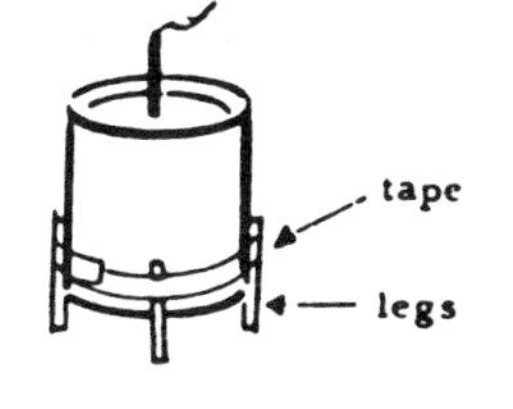

3. If electric cap is used, connect blasting cap wires to firing circuit.

NOTE: The effectiveness of this charge can be increased by placing it inside a can, box, or similar container and packing sand or dirt between the charge and the container.

Sand or Dirt
Container

Section II
25 No. 4
GRENADE-TIN CAN LAND MINE

This device can be used as a land mine that will explode when the trip wire is pulled.

MATERIAL REQUIRED:

Hand grenade having side safety lever
Sturdy container, open at one end, that is just large enough to fit over grenade and its safety lever (tin can of proper size is suitable).
Strong string or wire
NOTE: The container must be of such a size that, when the grenade is placed in it and the safety pin removed, its sides will prevent the safety lever from springing open. One end must be completely open.

PROCEDURE:

1. Fasten one piece of string to the closed end of container, making a strong connection. This can be done by punching 2 holes in the can, looping the string through them, and tying a knot.

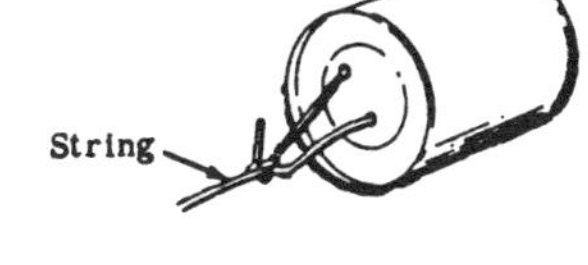

2. Tie free end of this string to bush, stake, fencepost, etc.

3. Fasten another length of string to the grenade such that it cannot interfere with the functioning of the ignition mechanism of the grenade.

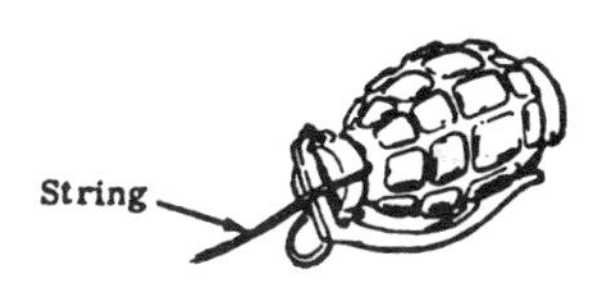

4. Insert grenade into container.

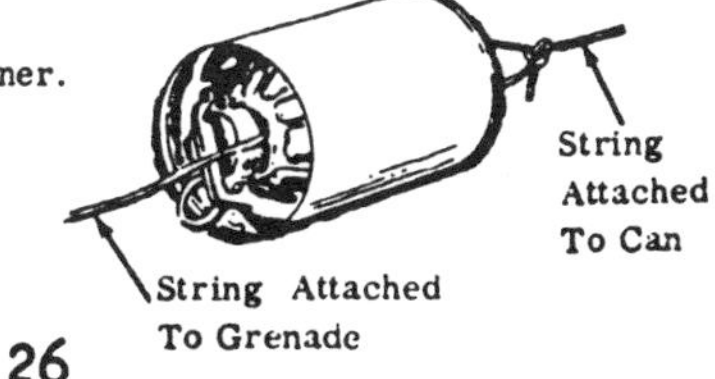

26

5. Lay free length of string across path and fasten to stake, bush, etc. The string should remain taut.

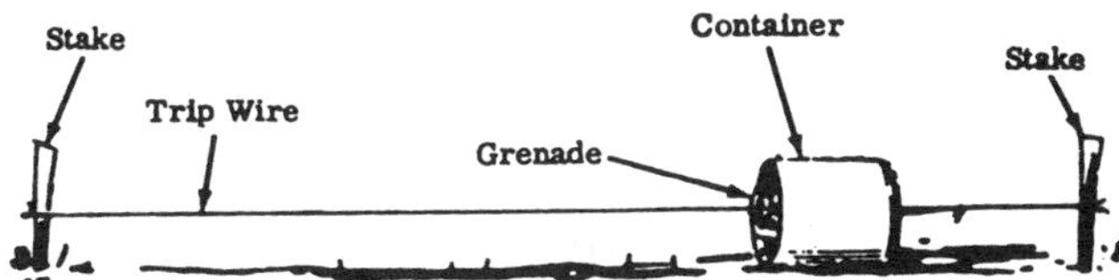

HOW TO USE:

1. Carefully withdraw safety pin by pulling on ring. Be sure safety lever is restrained during this operation. Grenade will function in normal manner when trip wire is pulled.

NOTE: In areas where concealment is possible, a greater effect may be obtained by suspending the grenade several feet above ground, as illustrated below.

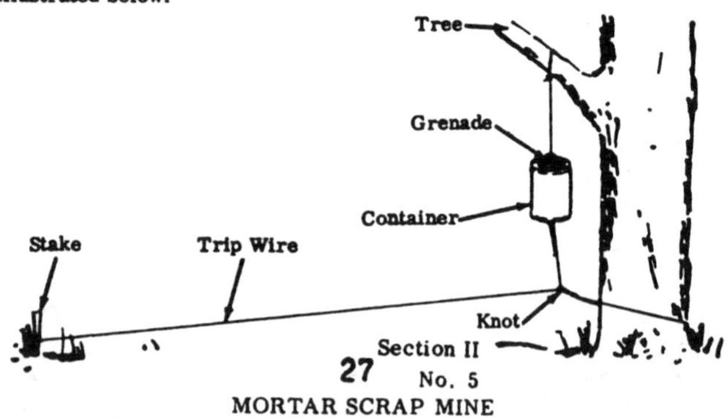

27

Section II
No. 5
MORTAR SCRAP MINE

A directional shrapnel launcher that can be placed in the path of advancing troops.

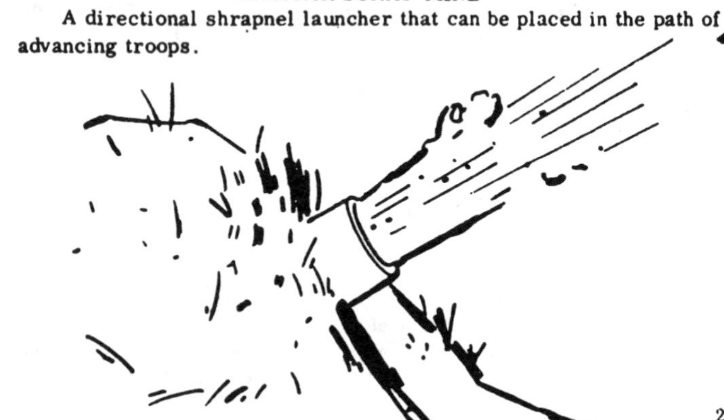

MATERIAL REQUIRED:

Iron pipe approximately 3 ft. (1 meter) long and 2 in. to 4 in. (5 to 10 cm) in diameter and threaded on at least one end. Salvaged artillery cartridge case may also be used.
Threaded cap to fit pipe.
Black powder or salvaged artillery propellant about 1/2 lb. (200 gms) total.
Electrical igniter (commercial SQUIB or improvised igniter, Section VI, No. 1). Safety or improvised fuse may also be used.
Small stones about 1 in. (2-1/2 cm) in diameter or small size scrap; about 1 lb. (400 gms) total.
Rags for wadding, each about 20 in. by 20 in. (50 cm x 50 cm)
Paper or bag
Battery and wire
Stick (non-metallic)

Note: Be sure pipe has no cracks or flaws.

28

PROCEDURE:

1. Screw threaded cap onto pipe.

2. Place propellant and igniter in paper or rag and tie package with string so contents will not fall out.

Igniter Leads

Propellant and igniter

3. Insert packaged propellant and igniter into pipe until package rests against threaded cap leaving firing leads extending from open end of pipe.

4. Roll rag till it is about 6 in. (15-1/2 cm) long and the same diameter as pipe. Insert rag wadding against packaged propellant igniter. With caution, pack tightly using stick.

5. Insert stones and/or scrap metal into pipe.

6. Insert second piece of rag wadding against stones and/or metal scrap. Pack tightly as before.

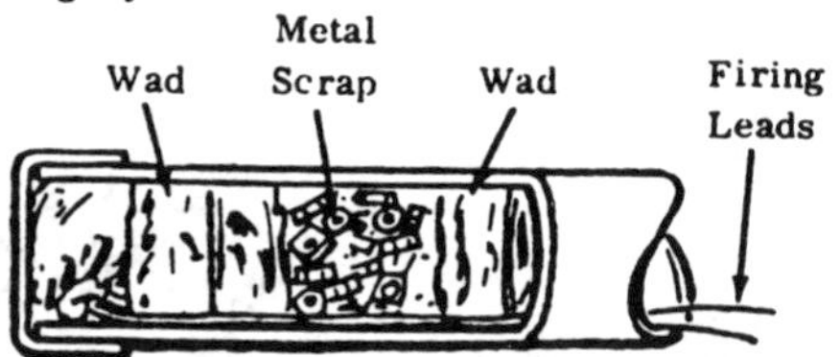

HOW TO USE:

1. Bury pipe in ground with open end facing the expected path of the enemy. The open end may be covered with cardboard and a thin layer of dirt or leaves as camouflage.

29

2. Connect firing leads to battery and switch. Mine can be remotely fired when needed or attached to trip device placed in path of advancing troops.

NOTE: A NON-ELECTRICAL ignition system can be substituted for the electrical ignition system as follows.

1. Follow above procedure, substituting safety fuse for igniter.

2. Light safety fuse when ready to fire.

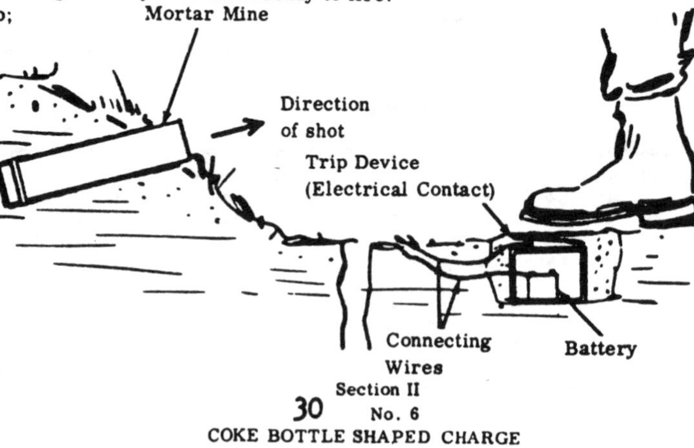

30

Section II
No. 6
COKE BOTTLE SHAPED CHARGE

This shaped charge will penetrate 3 in. (7-1/2 cm) of armor. (It will disable a vehicle if placed on the engine or engine compartment).

MATERIAL REQUIRED:

Glass Coke bottle, 6-1/2 oz. size
Plastic or castable explosive, about 1 lb. (454 gm)

Blasting cap
Metal cylinder, open at both ends, about 6 in. (15 cm) long and 2 in. (5 cm) inside diameter. Cylinder should be heavy walled for best results.
Plug to fit mouth of coke bottle (rags, metal, wood, paper, etc.)
Non-metal rod about 1/4 in. (6 mm) in diameter and 8 in. (20 cm) or more in length.
Tape or string
2 tin cans if castable explosive is used (See Section II, No. 3)

Coke Bottle

NOTE: Cylinder may be cardboard, plastic, etc. if castable explosive is used.

PROCEDURE:

Plug

1. Place plug in mouth of bottle.

Cylinder
Tape
Bottle

2. Place cylinder over top of bottle until bottom of cylinder rests on widest part of bottle. Tape cylinder to bottle. Container should be straight on top of bottle.

31

3. If plastic explosive is used:

a. Place explosive in cylinder a little at a time tamping with rod until cylinder is full.

b. Press the rod about 1/2 in. (1 cm) into the middle of the top of the explosive charge to form a hole for the blasting cap.

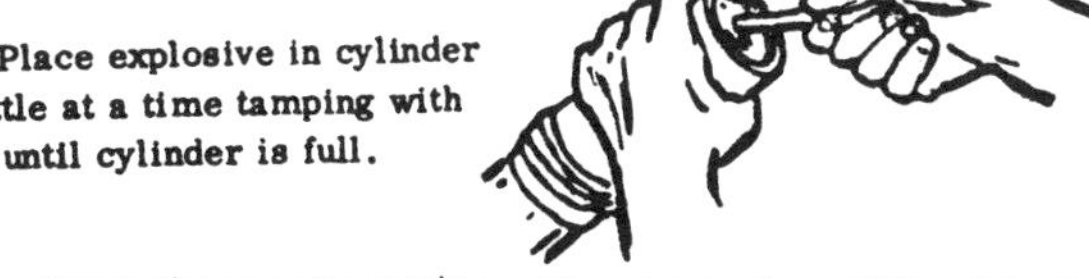

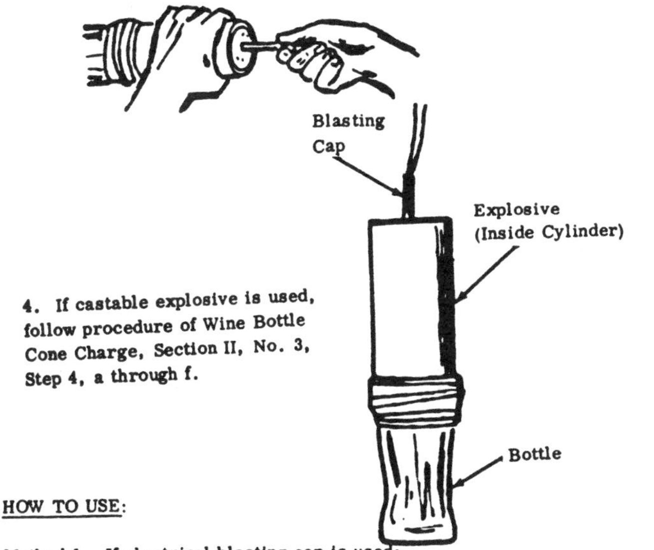

4. If castable explosive is used, follow procedure of Wine Bottle Cone Charge, Section II, No. 3, Step 4, a through f.

HOW TO USE:

Method 1. If electrical blasting cap is used:

1. Place blasting cap in hole in top of explosive.

> CAUTION: Do not insert blasting cap until charge is ready to be detonated.

32

2. Place bottom of Coke Bottle flush against the target. If target is not flat and horizontal, fasten bottle to target by any convenient means, such as by placing tape or string around target and top of bottle. Bottom of bottle acts as stand-off.

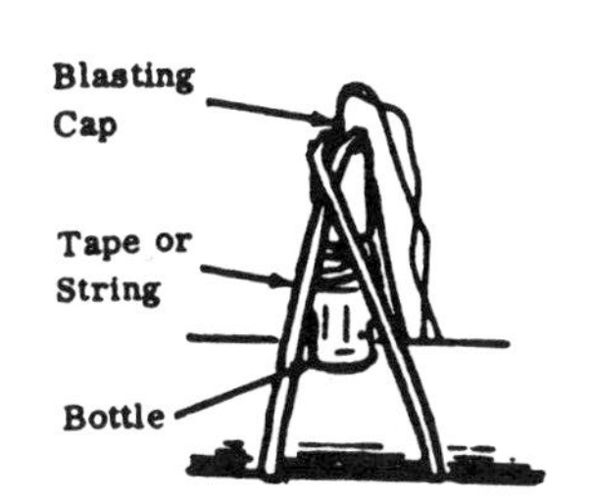

> CAUTION: Be sure that base of bottle is flush against target and that there is nothing between the target and the base of the bottle.

3. Connect leads from blasting cap to firing circuit.

Method II: If non-electrical blasting cap is used:

1. Crimp cap around fuse.

> CAUTION: Be sure fuse is long enough to provide a safe delay.

2. Follow steps 1, 2, and CAUTIONS of Method I.

3. Light fuse when ready to fire.

Section II
33 No. 7

CYLINDRICAL CAVITY SHAPED CHARGE

A shaped charge can be made from common pipe. It will penetrate 1-1/2 in. (3-1/2 cm) of steel, producing a hole 1-1/2 in. (3-1/2 cm) in diameter.

MATERIAL REQUIRED:

Iron or steel pipe, 2 to 2-1/2 in. (5 to 6-1/2 cm) in diameter and 3 to 4 in. (7-1/2 to 10 cm) long
Metal pipe, 1/2 to 3/4 in. (1-1/2 to 2 cm) in diameter and 1-1/2 in. (3-1/2 cm) long, open at both ends. (The wall of the pipe should be as thin as possible.)
Blasting cap
Non-metallic rod, 1/4 in. (6 mm) in diameter
Plastic or castable explosive
2 metal cans of different sizes } If castable explosive is used
Stick or wire }
Heat source }

PROCEDURE:

1. If plastic explosive is used:

a. Place larger pipe on flat surface. Hand pack and tamp explosive into pipe. Leave approximately 1/4 in. (6 mm) space at top.

Approximately 1/4 in. Empty Space
Large Pipe
Plastic Explosive
Flat Surface

b. Push rod into center of explosive. Enlarge hole in explosive to diameter and length of small pipe.

c. Insert small pipe into hole.

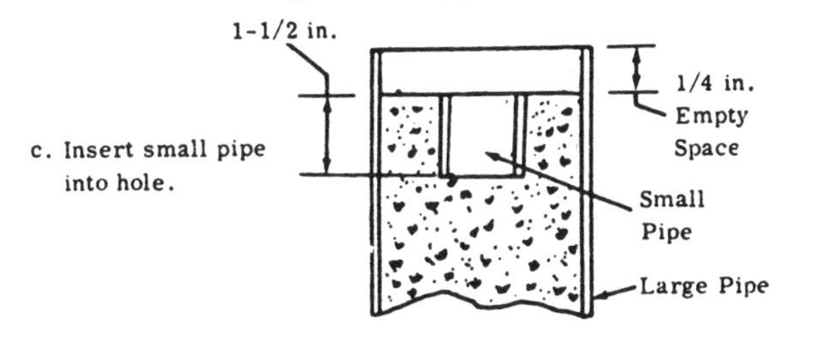

IMPORTANT: Be sure direct contact is made between explosive and small pipe. Tamp explosive around pipe by hand if necessary.

d. Make sure that there is 1/4 in. (6 mm) empty space above small pipe. Remove explosive if necessary.

e. Turn pipe upside down and push rod 1/2 in. (1-1/4 cm) into center of opposite end of explosive to form a hole for the blasting cap.

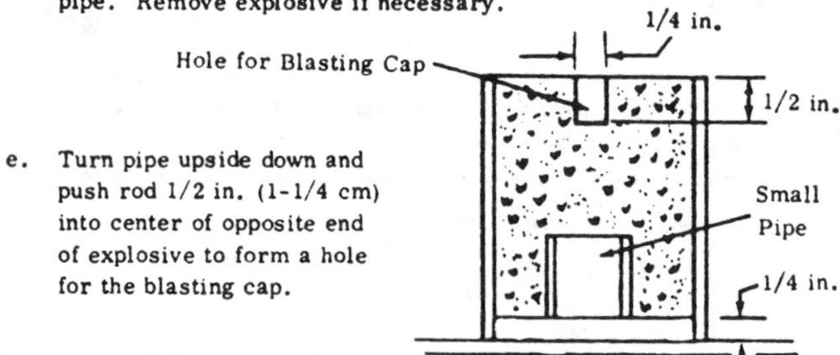

CAUTION: Do not insert blasting cap in hole until ready to fire shaped charge.

2. If TNT or other castable explosive is used:

a. Follow procedure, Section II, No. 3, Step 4, Parts a, b, c, including CAUTIONS.

b. When all the explosive has melted, remove the inner container and stir the molten explosive until it begins to thicken.

c. Place large pipe on flat surface. Pour explosive into pipe until it is 1-3/4 in. (4 cm) from the top.

d. Place small pipe in center of large pipe so that it rests on top of explosive. Holding small pipe in place, pour explosive around small pipe until explosive is 1/4 in. (6 mm) from top of large pipe.

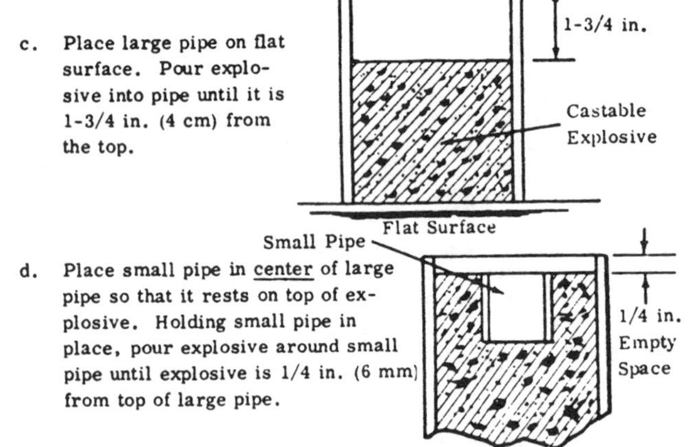

e. Allow explosive to cool. Break crust that forms on top of the charge during cooling with a wooden stick and add more explosive. Do this as often as necessary until explosive is 1/4 in. (6 mm) from top.

f. When explosive has completely hardened, turn pipe upside down and bore a hole for the blasting cap in the middle of the top of the charge about 1/2 in. (1-1/4 cm) deep.

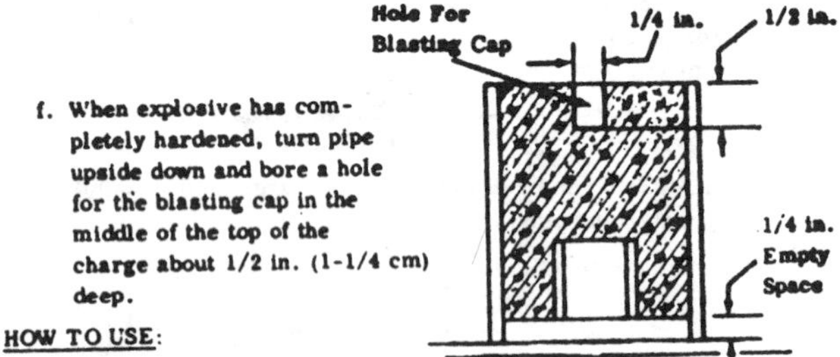

HOW TO USE:

Method I - If electrical blasting cap is used:

1. Place blasting cap in hole made for it.

CAUTION: Do not insert blasting cap until charge is ready to fire.

2. Place other end of pipe flush against the target. Fasten pipe to target by any convenient means, such as by placing tape or string around target and top of pipe, if target is not flat and horizontal

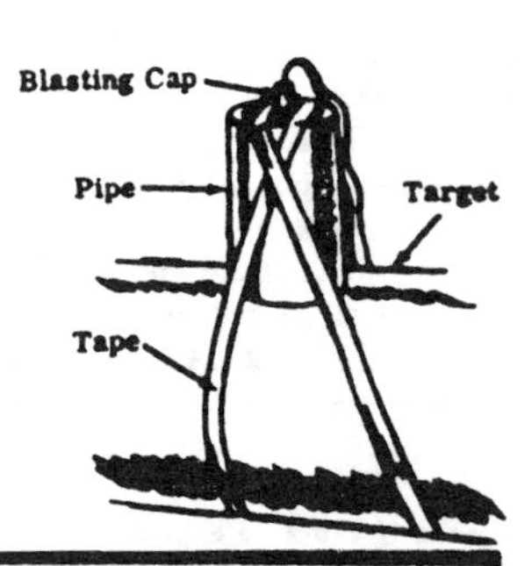

CAUTION: Be sure that base of pipe is flush against target and that there is nothing between the target and the base of the pipe.

3. Connect leads from blasting cap to firing circuit.

Method II - If non-electrical blasting cap is used:

1. Crimp cap around fuse.

CAUTION: Be sure fuse is long enough to provide a safe delay.

2. Follow Steps 1, 2, and CAUTION of Method I.

3. Light fuse when ready to fire.

Section III
No. 1
PIPE PISTOL FOR 9 MM AMMUNITION

A 9 mm pistol can be made from 1/4" steel gas or water pipe and fittings.

MATERIAL REQUIRED

- 1/4" nominal size steel pipe 4 to 6 inches long with threaded ends.
- 1/4" Solid pipe plug
- Two (2) steel pipe couplings
- Metal strap - roughly 1/8" x 1/4" x 5"
- Two (2) elastic bands
- Flat head nail - 6D or 8D (approx 1/16" diameter)
- Two (2) wood screws #8
- Wood 8" x 5" x 1"
- Drill
- 1/4" wood or metal rod, (approx 8" long)

PROCEDURE

1. Carefully inspect pipe and fittings.
   a. Make sure that there are NO cracks or other flaws in the pipe or fittings.
   b. Check inside diameter of pipe using a 9 mm cartridge as a gauge. The bullet should closely fit into the pipe without forcing but the cartridge case SHOULD NOT fit into pipe.
   c. Outside diameter of pipe MUST NOT BE less than 1 1/2 times bullet diameter (.536 inches; 1.37 cm)

2. Drill a 9/16" (1.43 cm) diameter hole 3/8" (approximately 1 cm) into one coupling to remove the thread.

Drilled section should fit tightly over smooth section of pipe.

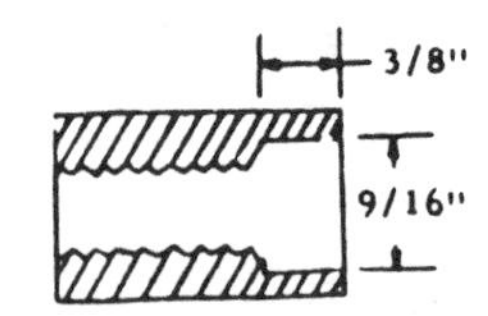

3. Drill a 25/64" (1 cm) diameter hole 3/4" (1.9 cm) into pipe. Use cartridge as a gauge; when a cartridge is inserted into the pipe, the base of the case should be even with the end of the pipe. Thread coupling tightly onto pipe, drilled end first.

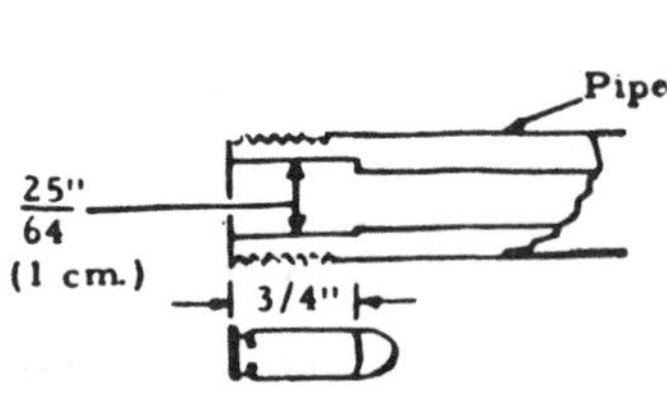

37

4. Drill a hole in the center of the pipe plug just large enough for the nail to fit through.

HOLE MUST BE CENTERED IN PLUG.

5. Push nail through plug until head of nail is flush with square end. Cut nail off at other end 1/16" (.158 cm) away from plug. Round off end of nail with file.

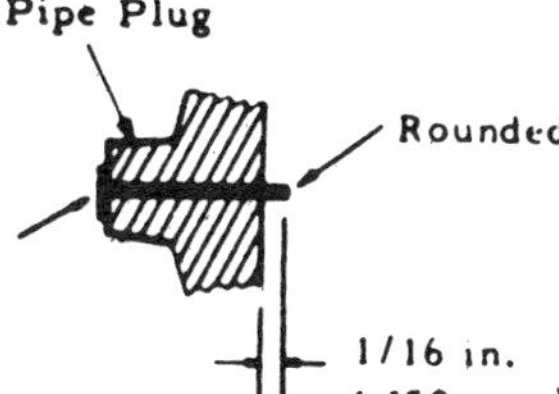

6. Bend metal strap to "U" shape and drill holes for wood screws. File two small notches at top.

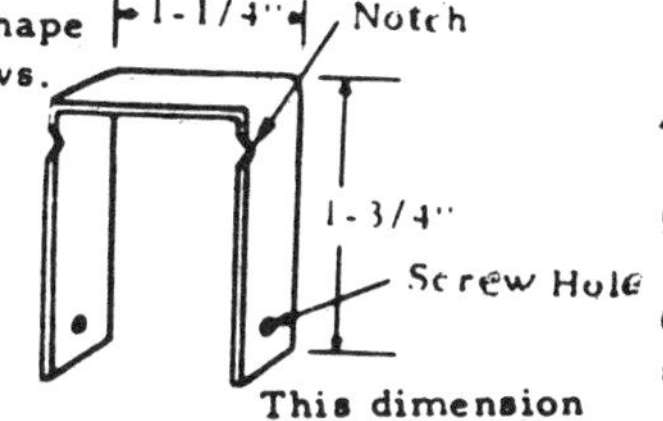

This dimension to be 2" greater than unassembled length of pipe.

7. Saw or otherwise shape 1" (2.54 cm) thick hard wood into stock.

English	Metric
1 in.	2.54 cm
1/2 in.	1.27 cm
9/16 in.	1.43 cm
2 in.	5.08 cm
6 in.	15.2 cm

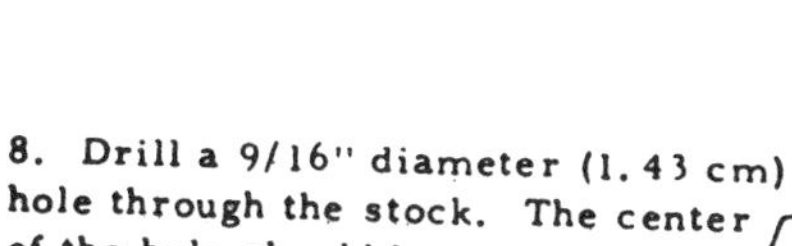

8. Drill a 9/16" diameter (1.43 cm) hole through the stock. The center of the hole should be approximately 1/2" (1.27 cm) from the top.

9. Slide the pipe through this hole and attach front coupling. Screw drilled plug into rear coupling.

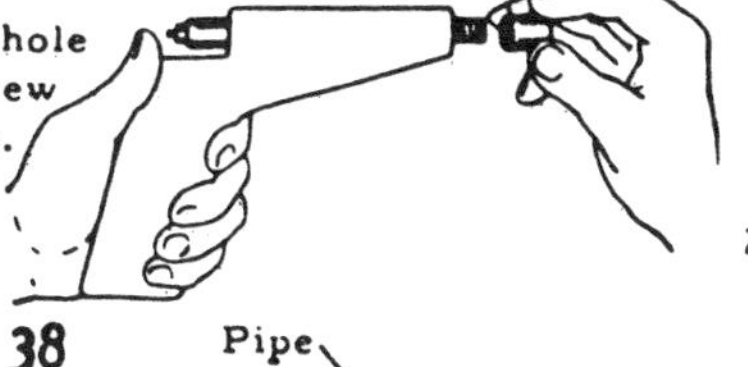

38

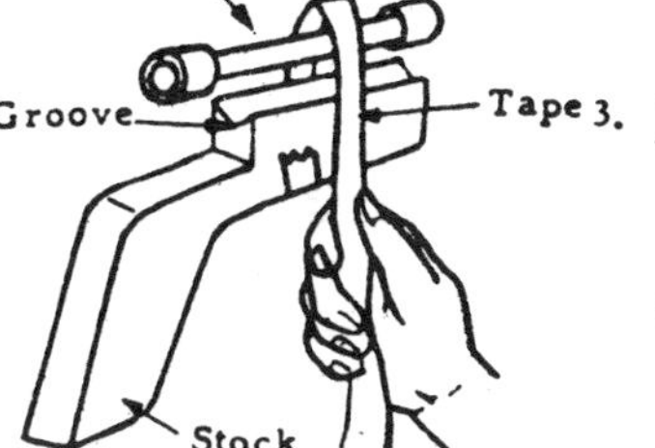

NOTE: If 9/16" drill is not available cut a "V" groove in the top of the stock and tape pipe securely in place.

10. Position metal strap on stock so that top will hit the head of the nail. Attach to stock with wood screw on each side.

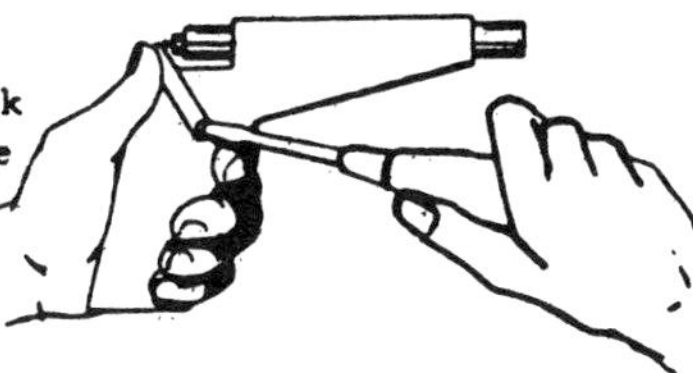

11. String elastic bands from front coupling to notch on each side of the strap.

SAFETY CHECK - TEST FIRE PISTOL BEFORE HAND FIRING

1. Locate a barrier such as a stone wall or large tree which you can stand behind in case the pistol ruptures when fired.

2. Mount pistol solidly to a table or other rigid support at least ten feet in front of the barrier.

3. Attach a cord to the firing strap on the pistol.

4. Holding the other end of the cord, go behind the barrier.

5. Pull the cord so that the firing strap is held back.

6. Release the cord to fire the pistol. (If pistol does not fire, shorten the elastic bands or increase their number.)

IMPORTANT: Fire at least five rounds from behind the barrier and then re-inspect the pistol before you attempt to hand fire it.

39

HOW TO OPERATE PISTOL

1. To Load

a. Remove plug from rear coupling.

b. Place cartridge into pipe.

c. Replace plug.

2. To Fire

a. Pull strap back and hold with thumb until ready.

b. Release strap.

3. To Remove Shell Case

a. Remove plug from rear coupling.

b. Insert 1/4" diameter steel or wooden rod into front of pistol and push shell case out.

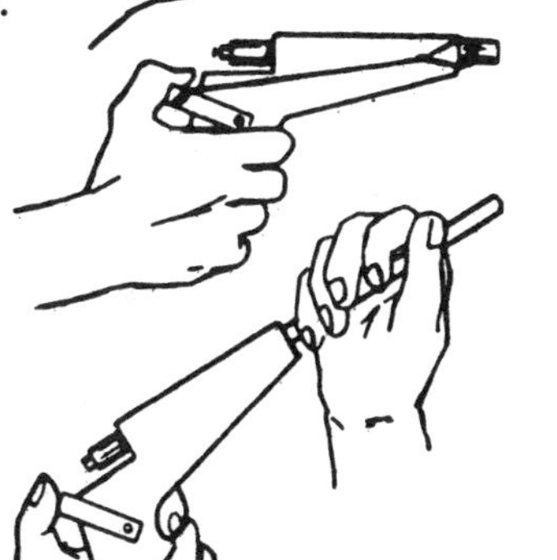

40
SHOTGUN (12 GAUGE)

A 12-gauge shotgun can be made from 3/4" water or gas pipe and fittings.

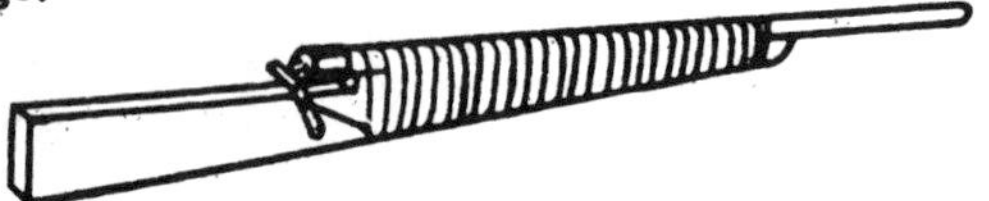

MATERIALS REQUIRED

Wood 2" x 4" x 32"
3/4" nominal size water or gas pipe 20" to 30" long threaded on one end.
3/4" steel coupling
Solid 3/4" pipe plug
Metal strap (1/4" x 1/16" x 4")
Twine, heavy (100 yards approximately)
3 wood screws and screwdriver
Flat head nail 6D or 8D
Hand drill
Saw or knife
File
Shellac or lacquer
Elastic Bands

PROCEDURE

1. Carefully inspect pipe and fittings.
   a. Make sure that there are no cracks or other flaws.
   b. Check inside diameter of pipe. A 12-gauge shot shell should fit into the pipe but the brass rim should not fit.
   c. Outside diameter of pipe must be at least 1 in. (2.54 cm).

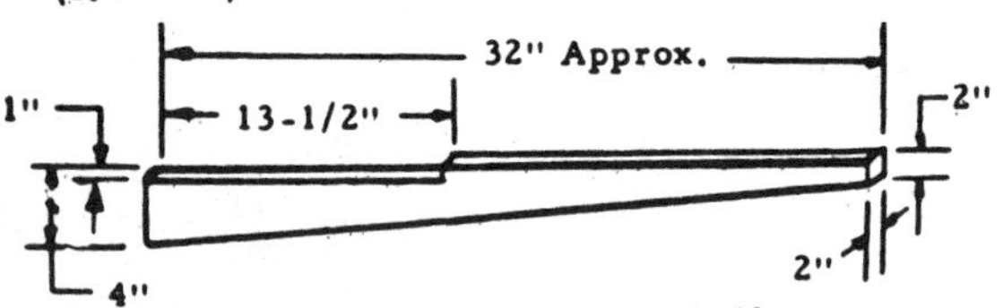

2. Cut stock from wood using a saw or knife.

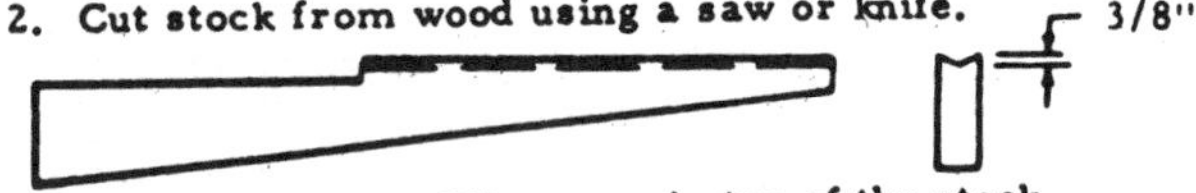

3. Cut a 3/8" deep "V" groove in top of the stock.

41

4. Turn coupling onto pipe until tight.

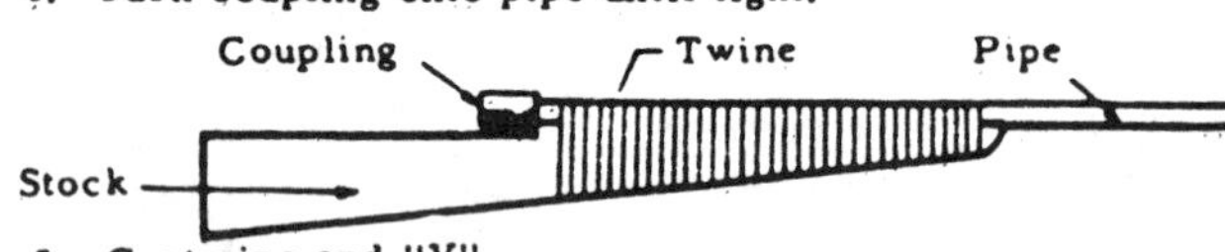

5. Coat pipe and "V" groove of stock with shellac or lacquer and, while still wet, place pipe in "V" groove and wrap pipe and stock together using two heavy layers of twine. Coat twine with shellac or lacquer after each layer.

6. Drill a hole through center of pipe plug large enough for nail to pass through.

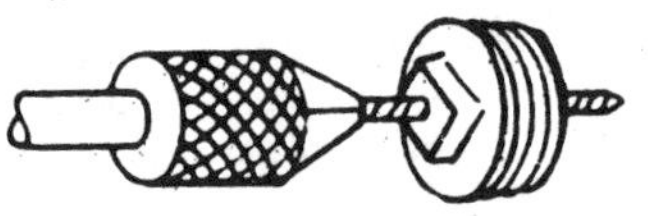

7. File threaded end of plug flat.

8. Push nail through plug and cut off flat 1/32" past the plug.

Pipe Plug
Flat
Nail
1/32 in.

9. Screw plug into coupling.

10. Bend 4" metal strap into "L" shape and drill hole for wood screw. Notch metal strap on the long side 1/2" from bend.

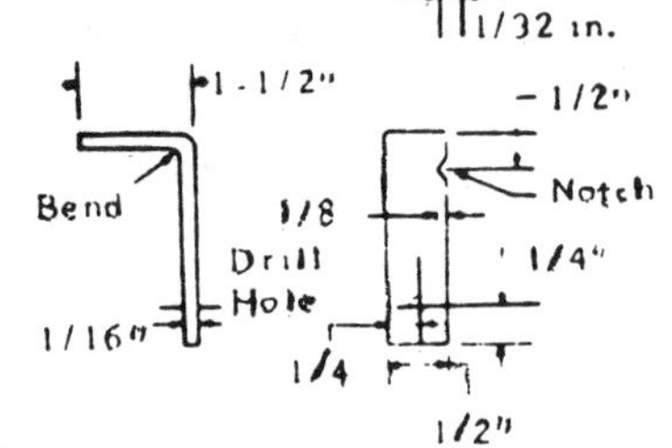

42

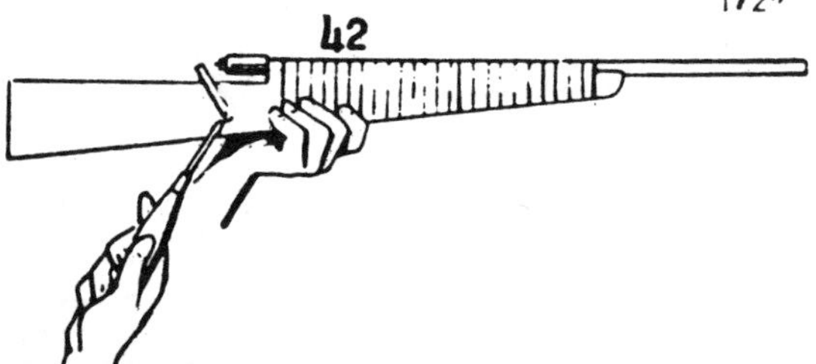

11. Position metal strap on stock so that top will hit the head of the nail. Attach to stock with wood screw.

Nail
Plug
Coupling
Elastic Bands
Firing Strap
Stock

12. Place screw in each side of stock about 4" in front of metal strap. Pass elastic bands through notch in metal strap and attach to screw on each side of the stock.

SAFETY CHECK - TEST FIRE SHOTGUN BEFORE HAND FIRING

1. Locate a barrier such as a stone wall or large tree which you can stand behind in case the weapon explodes when fired.

2. Mount shotgun solidly to a table or other rigid support at least ten feet in front of the barrier.

3. Attach a long cord to the firing strap on the shotgun.

4. Holding the other end of the cord, go behind the barrier.

5. Pull the cord so that the firing strap is held back.

6. Release the cord to fire the shotgun. (If shotgun does not fire, shorten the elastic bands or increase their number.)

IMPORTANT: Fire at least five rounds from behind the barrier and then re-inspect the shotgun before you attempt to shoulder fire it.

43

HOW TO OPERATE SHOTGUN

1. To Load

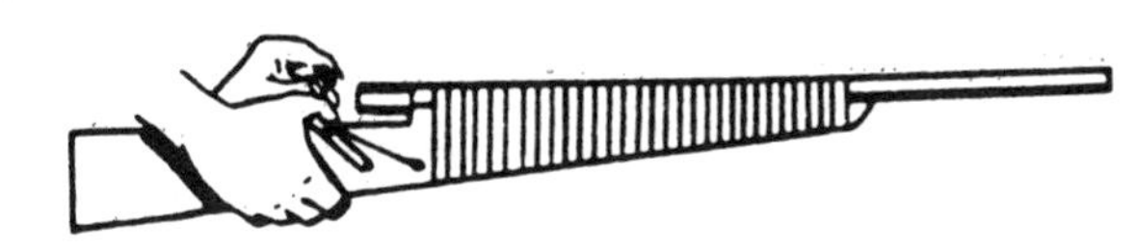

a. Take plug out of coupling.

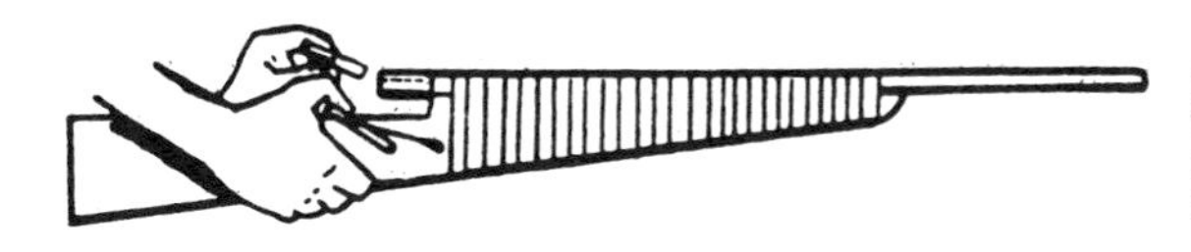

b. Put shotgun shell into pipe.

c. Screw plug hand-tight into coupling.

2. To Fire

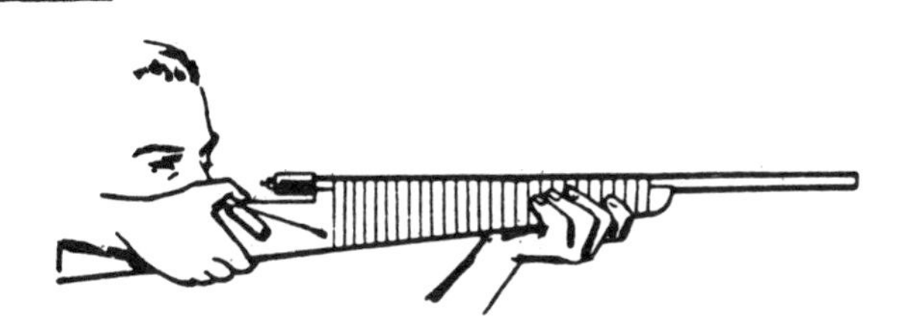

a. Pull strap back and hold with thumb.

b. Release strap.

3. To Unload Gun

a. Take plug out of coupling.

b. Shake out used cartridge.

44

Section III
No. 3
SHOTSHELL DISPERSION CONTROL

When desired, shotshell can be modified to reduce shot dispersion.

MATERIAL REQUIRED:

Shotshell
Screwdriver or knife
Any of the following filler materials:
- Crushed Rice
- Rice Flour
- Dry Bread Crumbs
- Fine Dry Sawdust

PROCEDURE:

STAR CRIMP

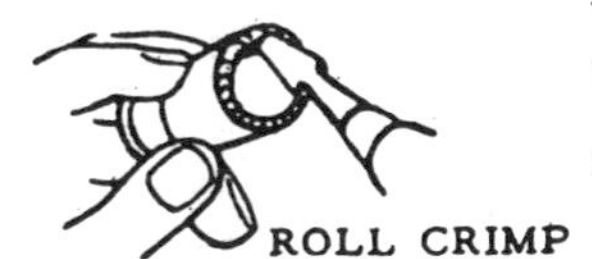

ROLL CRIMP

1. Carefully remove crimp from shotshell using a screwdriver or knife.

NOTE: If cartridge is of roll-crimp type, remove top wad.

2. Pour shot from shell.

3. Replace one layer of shot in the cartridge. Pour in filler material to fill the spaces between the shot.

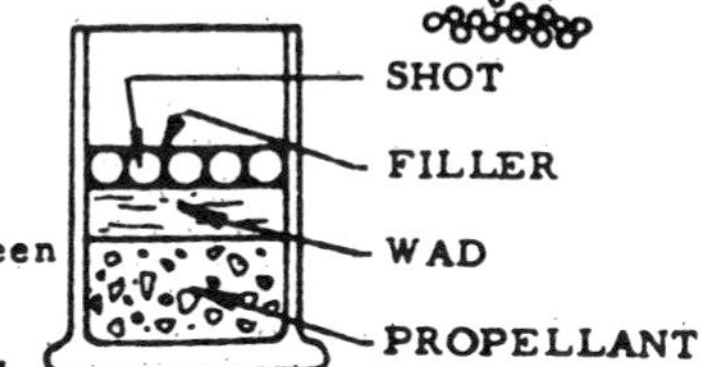

45

4. Repeat Step 3 until all shot has been replaced.

5. Replace top wad (if applicable) and re-fold crimp.

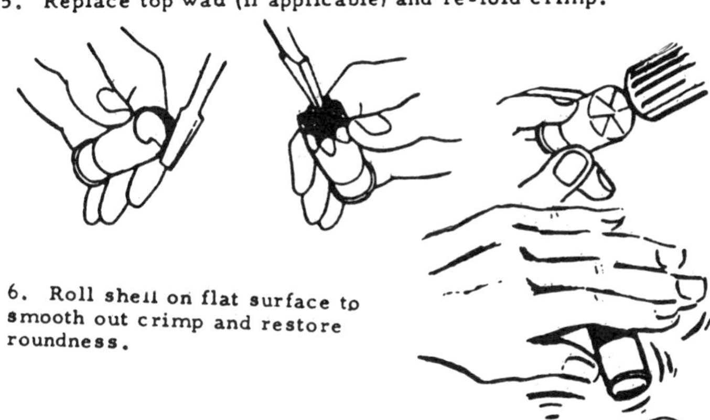

6. Roll shell on flat surface to smooth out crimp and restore roundness.

7. Seal end of case with wax.

CANDLE

HOW TO USE:

This round is loaded and fired in the same manner as standard shotshell. The shot spread will be about 2/3 that of a standard round.

46

Section III
No. 4
CARBINE (7.62 mm Standard Rifle Ammunition)

A rifle can be made from water or gas pipe and fittings. Standard cartridges are used for ammunition.

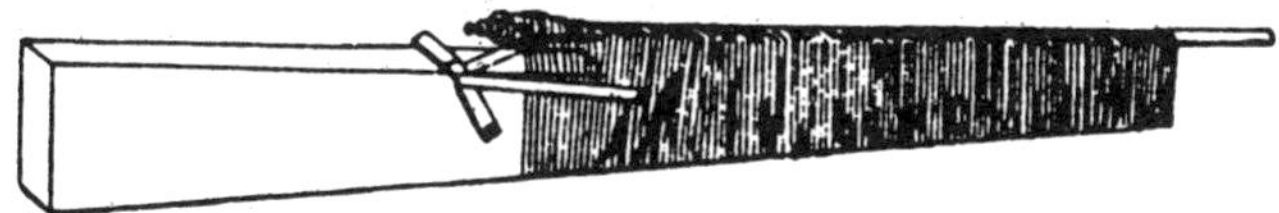

MATERIAL REQUIRED:

Wood approximately 2 in. x 4 in. x 30 in.
1/4 in. nominal size iron water or gas pipe 20 in. long threaded at one end.
Twine, heavy (100 yards approx.)
3 wood screws and screwdriver
Flat head nail about 1 in. long
Hand drill
Saw or knife

3/8 in. to 1/4 in. reducer
3/8 in. x 1-1/2 in. threaded pipe
3/8 in. pipe coupling
Metal strap approximately 1/2 in. x 1/16 in. x 4 in.
File
Pipe wrench
Shellac or lacquer
Elastic bands
Solid 3/8 in. pipe plug

PROCEDURE:

1. Inspect pipe and fittings carefully.

   a. Be sure that there are no cracks or flaws.

   b. Check inside diameter of pipe. A 7.62 mm projectile should fit into 3/8 in. pipe.

2. Cut stock from wood using saw or knife.

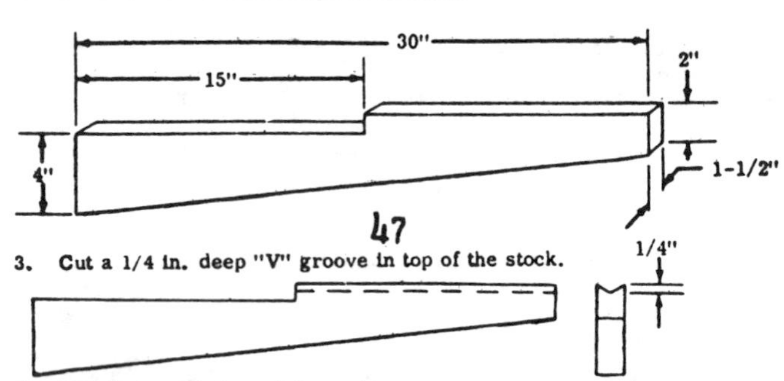

47

3. Cut a 1/4 in. deep "V" groove in top of the stock.

4. Fabricate rifle barrel from pipe.

   a. File or drill inside diameter of threaded end of 20 in. pipe for about 1/4 in. so neck of cartridge case will fit in.

   b. Screw reducer onto threaded pipe using pipe wrench.

   c. Screw short threaded pipe into reducer.

   d. Turn 3/8 pipe coupling onto threaded pipe using pipe wrench. All fittings should be as tight as possible. Do not split fittings.

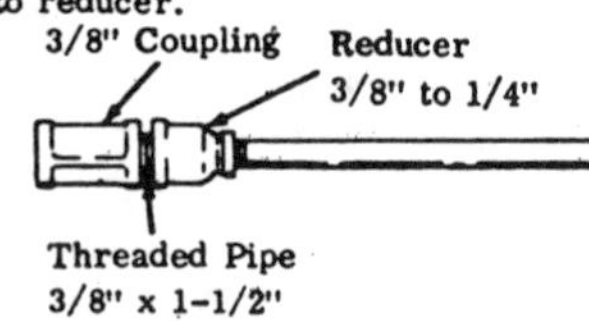

5. Coat pipe and "V" groove of stock with shellac or lacquer. While still wet, place pipe in "V" groove and wrap pipe and stock together using two layers of twine. Coat twine with shellac or lacquer after each layer.

6. Drill a hole through center of pipe plug large enough for nail to pass through.

7. File threaded end of plug flat.

48

8. Push nail through plug and cut off rounded 1/32 in. (2 mm) past the plug.

9. Screw plug into coupling.

10. Bend 4 in. metal strap into "L" shape and drill hole for wood screw. Notch metal strap on the long side 1/2 in. from bend.

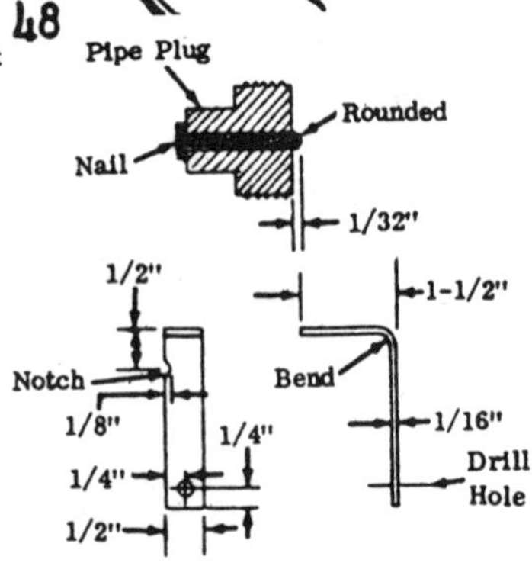

11. Position metal strap on stock so that top will hit the head of the nail. Attach to stock with wood screw.

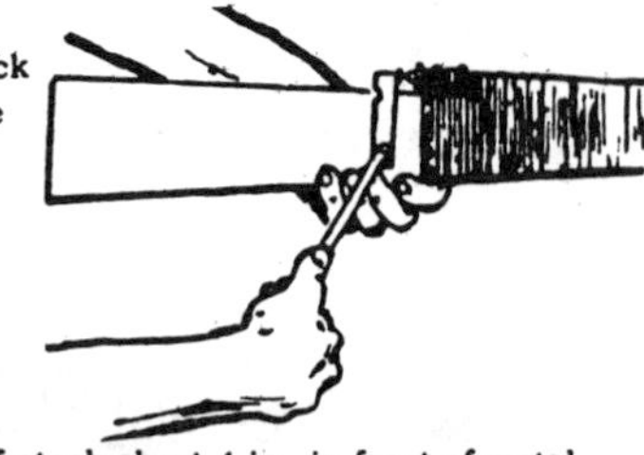

12. Place screw in each side of stock about 4 in. in front of metal strap. Pass elastic bands through notch in metal strap and attach to screw on each side of the stock.

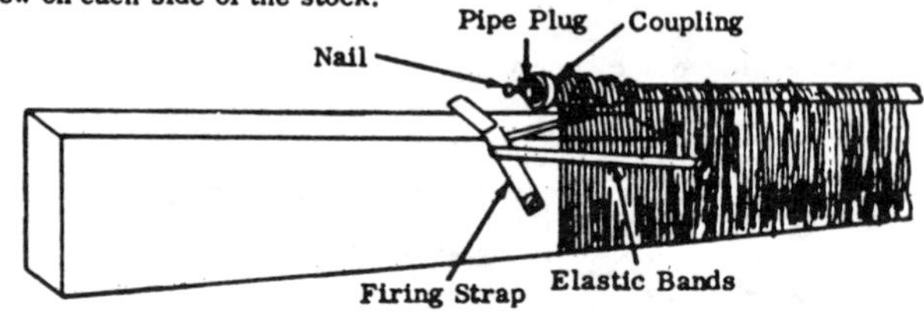

SAFETY CHECK - TEST FIRE RIFLE BEFORE HAND FIRING

1. Locate a barrier such as a stone wall or large tree which you can stand behind to test fire weapon.

2. Mount rifle solidly to a table or other rigid support at least ten feet in front of the barrier.

49

3. Attach a long cord to the firing strap on the rifle.

4. Holding the other end of the cord, go behind the barrier.

5. Pull the cord so that the firing strap is held back.

6. Release the cord to fire the rifle. (If the rifle does not fire, shorten the elastic bands or increase their number.)

> IMPORTANT: Fire at least five rounds from behind a barrier and then reinspect the rifle before you attempt to shoulder fire it.

HOW TO OPERATE RIFLE:

1. To Load

   a. Remove plug from coupling.

   b. Put cartridge into pipe.

   c. Screw plug hand-tight into coupling.

2. To Fire

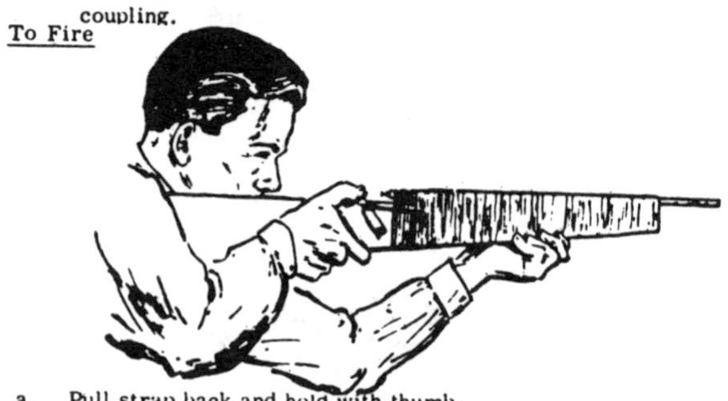

   a. Pull strap back and hold with thumb.

   b. Release strap.

3. To Unload Gun

   a. Take plug out of coupling.

   b. Drive out used case using stick or twig.

50 Section III
No. 5
REUSABLE PRIMER

A method of making a previously fired primer reusable.

MATERIAL REQUIRED:

Used cartridge case
2 long nails having approximately the same diameter as the inside of the primer pocket
"Strike-anywhere" matches - 2 or 3 are needed for each primer
Vise
Hammer
Knife or other sharp edged instrument

PROCEDURE:

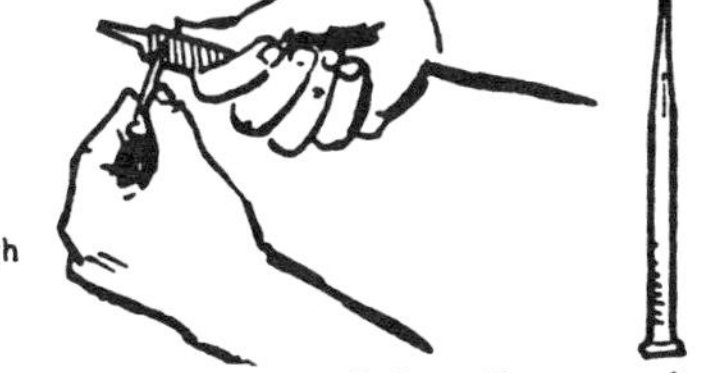

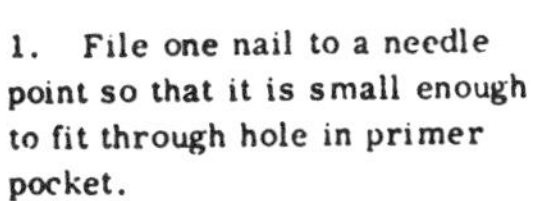
1. File one nail to a needle point so that it is small enough to fit through hole in primer pocket.

2. Place cartridge case and nail between jaws of vise. Force out fired primer with nail as shown:

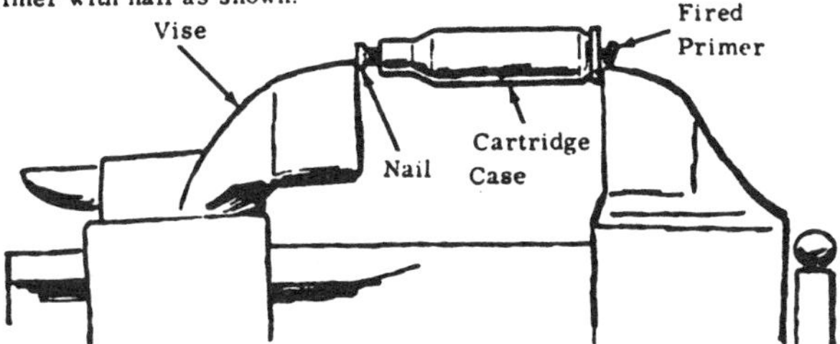

3. Remove anvil from primer cup.

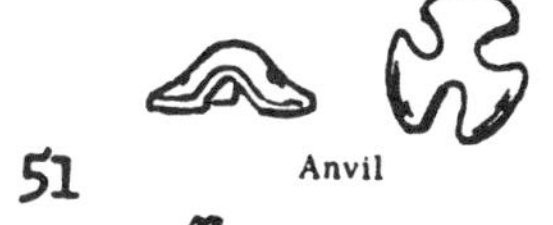

51

4. File down point of second nail until tip is flat.

5. Remove indentations from face of primer cup with hammer and flattened nail.

Nail
Primer Cup

6. Cut off tips of the heads of "strike-anywhere" matches using knife. Carefully crush the match tips on dry surface with wooden match stick until the mixture is the consistency of sugar.

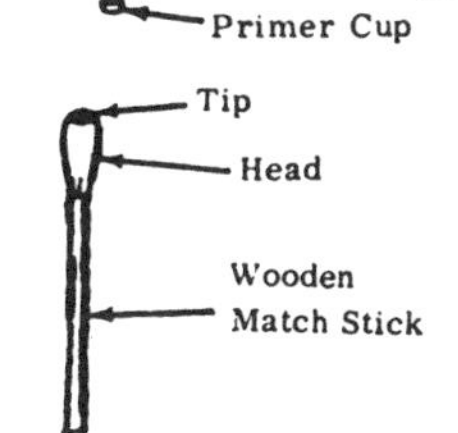

CAUTION: Do not crush more than 3 match tips at one time or the mixture may explode.

7. Pour mixture into primer cup. Compress mixture with wooden match stick until primer cup is fully packed.

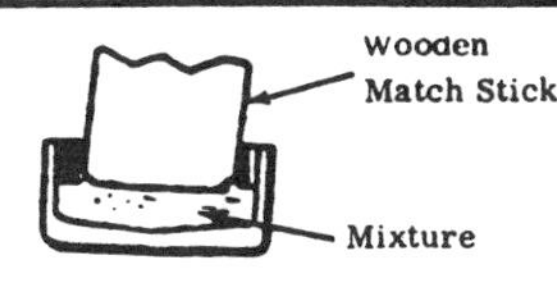

8. Place anvil in primer pocket with legs down.

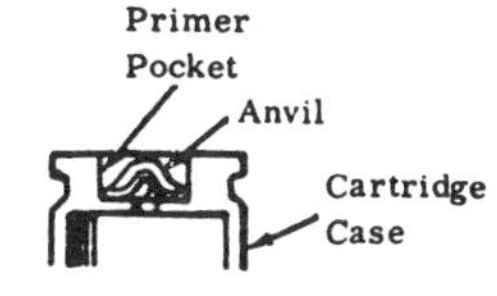

9. Place cup in pocket with mixture facing downward.

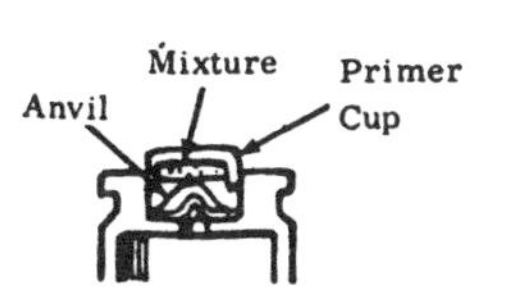

10. Place cartridge case and primer cup between vise jaws, and press slowly until primer is seated into bottom of pocket. The primer is now ready to use.

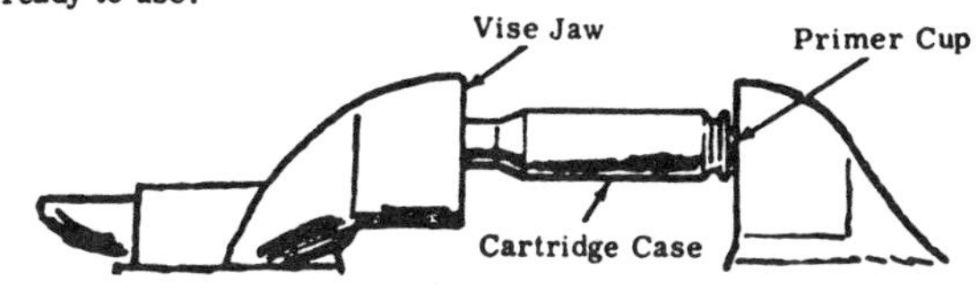

52 Section III
No. 6
PIPE PISTOL FOR .45 CALIBER AMMUNITION

A .45 caliber pistol can be made from 3/8 in. nominal diameter steel gas or water pipe and fittings. Lethal range is about 15 yards (13-1/2 meters).

MATERIAL REQUIRED:

Steel pipe, 3/8 in. (1 cm) nominal diameter and 6 in. (15 cm) long with threaded ends.
2 threaded couplings to fit pipe
Solid pipe plug to fit pipe coupling
Hard wood, 8-1/2 in. x 6-1/2 in. x 1 in. (21 cm x 16-1/2 cm x 2-1/2 cm)
Tape or string
Flat head nail, approximately 1/16 in. (1-1/2 mm) in diameter
2 wood screws, approximately 1/16 in. (1-1/2 mm) in diameter
Metal strap, 5 in. x 1/4 in. x 1/8 in. (12-1/2 cm x 6 mm x 1 mm)
Bolt, 4 in. (10 cm) long, with nut (optional).
Elastic bands
Drills, one 1/16 in. (1-1/2 mm) in diameter, and one having same diameter as bolt (optional).
Rod, 1/4 in. (6mm) in diameter and 8 in. (20 cm) long
Saw or knife

PROCEDURE:

1. Carefully inspect pipe and fittings.

a. Make sure that there are no cracks or other flaws in the pipe and fittings.

b. Check inside diameter of pipe using a .45 caliber cartridge as a gauge. The cartridge case should fit into the pipe snugly but without forcing.

c. Outside diameter of pipe MUST NOT BE less than 1-1/2 times the bullet diameter.

2. Follow procedure of Section III, No. 1, steps 4, 5, and 6.

53

3. Cut stock from wood using saw or knife.

Inches	Centimeters
1-1/2	4 cm
8-1/2	26-1/2
6	20
1-1/2	4
5	12-1/2

4. Cut a 3/8 in. (9-1/2 mm) deep groove in top of stock.

5. Screw couplings onto pipe. Screw plug into one coupling.

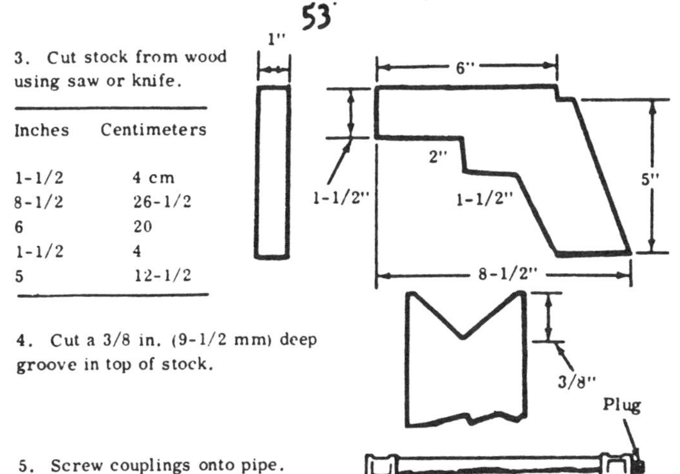

6. Securely attach pipe to stock using string or tape.

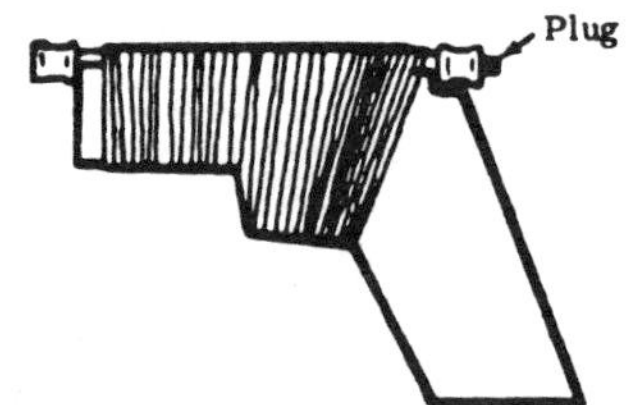

7. Follow procedures of Section III, No. 1, steps 10 and 11.

8. (Optional) Bend bolt for trigger. Drill hole in stock and place bolt in hole so strap will be anchored by bolt when pulled back. If bolt is not available, use strap as trigger by pulling back and releasing.

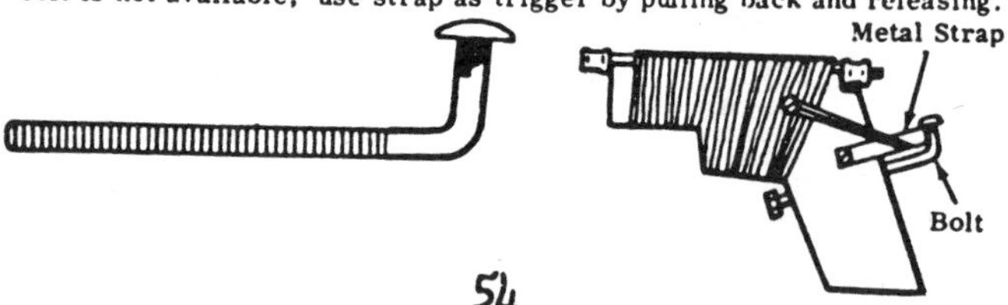

54

9. Follow SAFETY CHECK, Section III, No. 1

HOW TO USE:

1. To load:

a. Remove plug from rear coupling.

b. Wrap string or elastic band around extractor groove so case will seat into barrel securely.

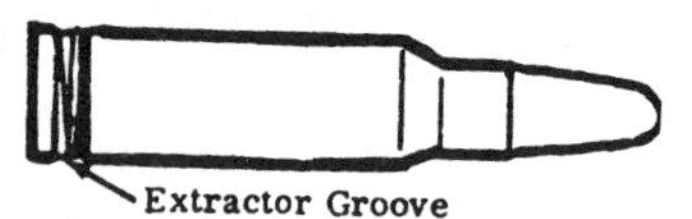

c. Place cartridge in pipe.

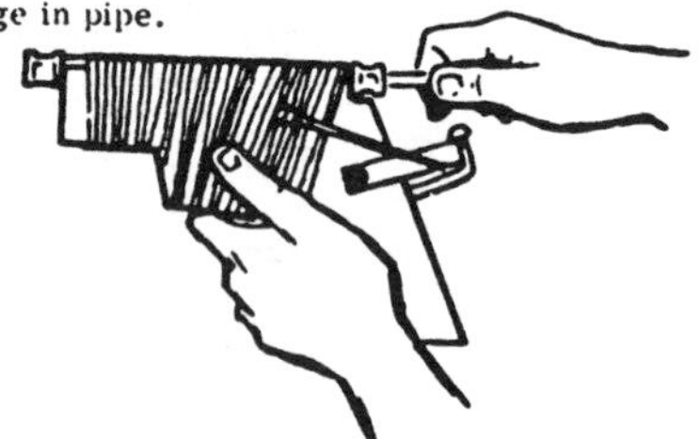

d. Replace plug.

2. To Fire:

a. Pull metal strap back and anchor in trigger.

b. Pull trigger when ready to fire.

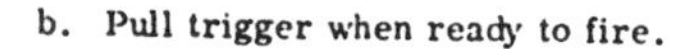

NOTE: If bolt is not used, pull strap back and release.

3. To remove cartridge case:

a. Remove plug from rear coupling.

b. Insert rod into front of pistol and push cartridge case out.

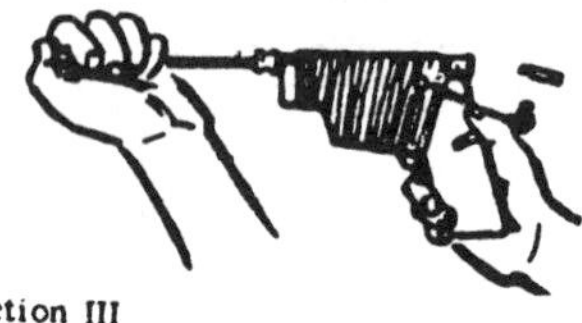

55 Section III
No. 7

MATCH GUN

An improvised weapon using safety match heads as the propellant and a metal object as the projectile. Lethal range is about 40 yards (36 meters).

MATERIAL REQUIRED:

Metal pipe 24 in. (61 cm) long and 3/8 in. (1 cm) in diameter (nominal size) or its equivalent, threaded on one end.
End cap to fit pipe
Safety matches - 3 books of 20 matches each.
Wood - 28 in. x 4 in. x 1 in. (70 cm x 10 cm x 2.5 cm)
Toy caps OR safety fuse OR "Strike-anywhere matches" (2)
Electrical tape or string
Metal strap, about 4 in. x 1/4 in. x 3/16 in. (10 cm x 6 mm x 4.5 mm)
2 rags, about 1 in x 12 in. and 1 in. x 3 in. (2-1/2 cm x 30 cm and 2-1/2 cm x 8 cm)
Wood screws
Elastic bands
Metal object (steel rod, bolt with head cut off, etc.), approximately 7/16 in. (11 mm) in diameter, and 7/16 in. (11 mm) long if iron or steel, 1-1/4 in. (31 mm) long if aluminum, 5/16 in. (8mm) long if lead.
Metal disk 1 in. (2-1/2 cm) in diameter and 1/16 in. (1-1/2 mm) thick
Bolt, 3/32 in. (2-1/2 mm) or smaller in diameter and nut to fit
Saw or knife

PROCEDURE:

1. Carefully inspect pipe and fittings. Be sure that there are no cracks or other flaws.

2. Drill small hole in center of end cap. If safety fuse is used, be sure it will pass through this hole.

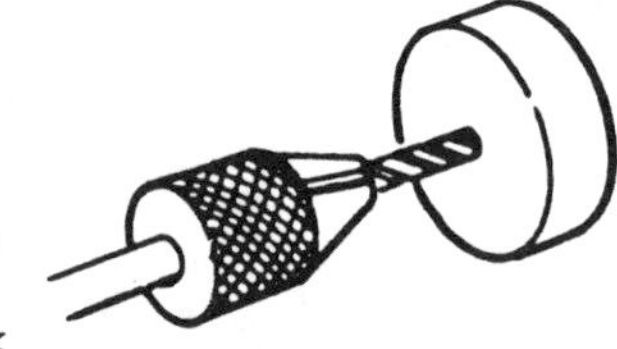

56

3. Cut stock from wood using saw or knife.

Metric	English
5 cm	2 in.
10 cm	4 in.
36 cm	14 in.
71 cm	28 in.

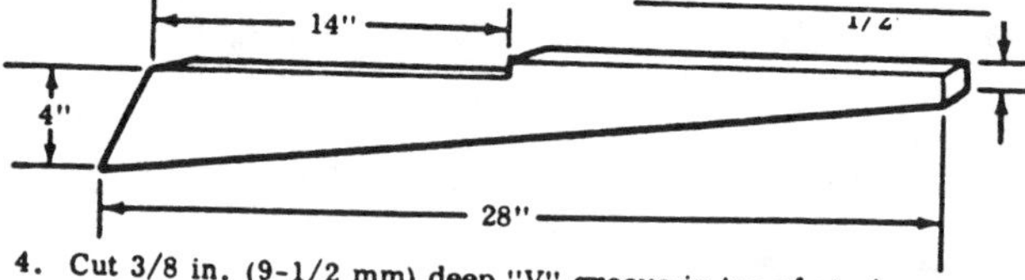

4. Cut 3/8 in. (9-1/2 mm) deep "V" groove in top of stock.

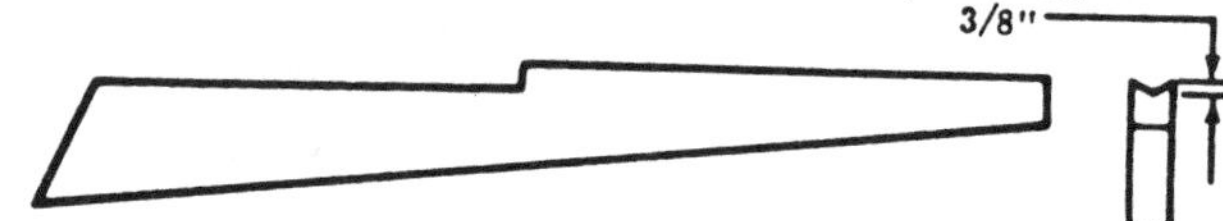

5. Screw end cap onto pipe until finger tight.

6. Attach pipe to stock with string or tape.

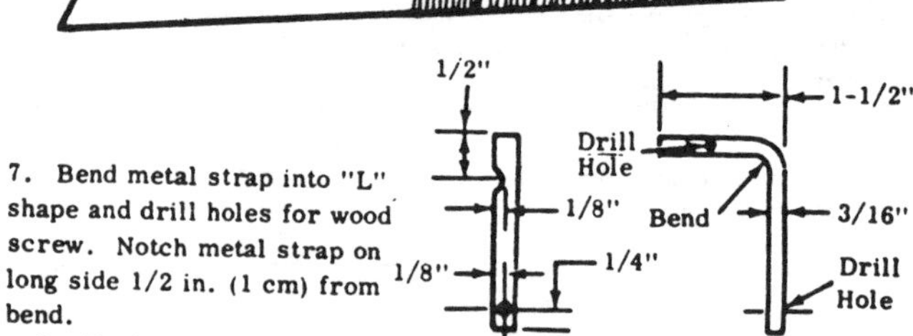

7. Bend metal strap into "L" shape and drill holes for wood screw. Notch metal strap on long side 1/2 in. (1 cm) from bend.

8. Position metal strap on stock so that the top will hit the center of hole drilled in end cap.

57

9. Attach metal disk to strap with nut and bolt. This will deflect blast from hole in end cap when gun is fired. Be sure that head of bolt is centered on hole in end cap.

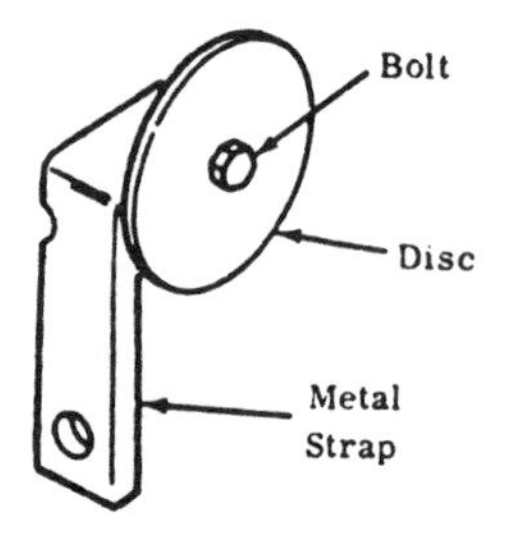

10. Attach strap to stock with wood screws.

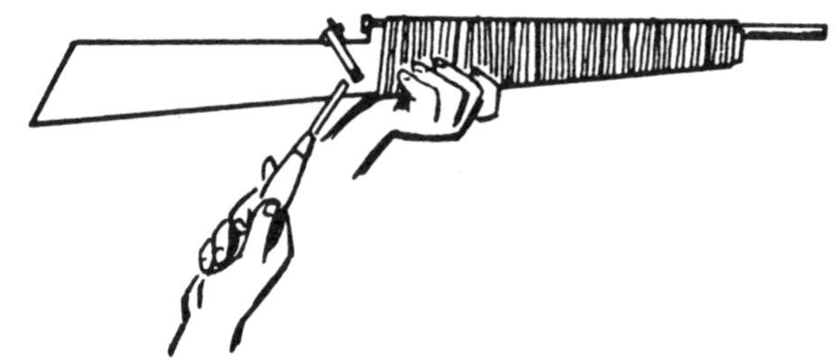

11. Place screw on each side of stock about 4 in. (10 cm) in front of metal strap. Pass elastic bands through notch in metal strap and attach to screw on each side of stock.

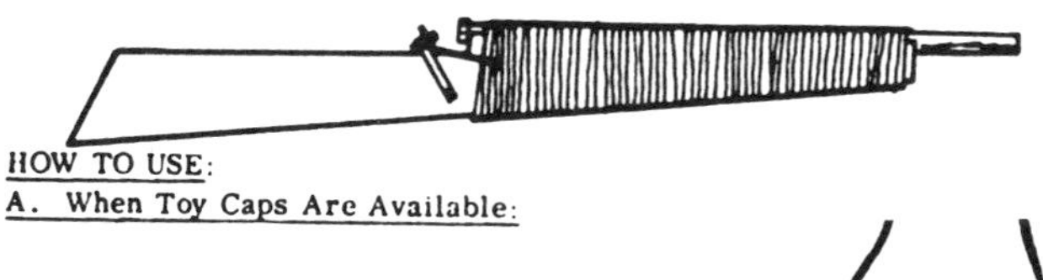

HOW TO USE:

A. When Toy Caps Are Available:

1. Cut off match heads from 3 books of matches with knife. Pour match heads into pipe.

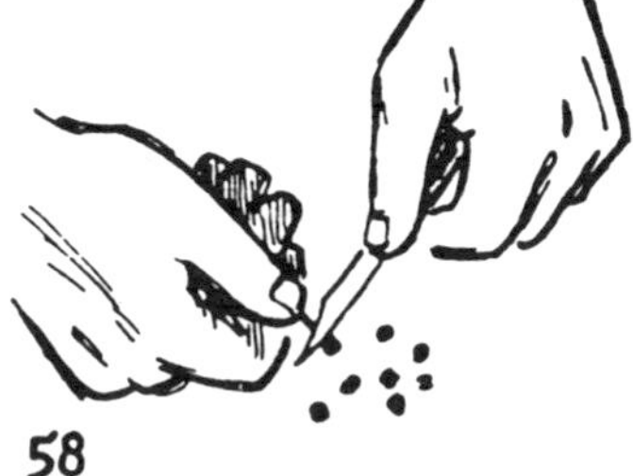

58

2. Fold one end of 1 in. x 12 in. rag 3 times so that it becomes a one inch square of 3 thicknesses. Place rag into pipe to cover match heads, folded end first. Tamp firmly WITH CAUTION.

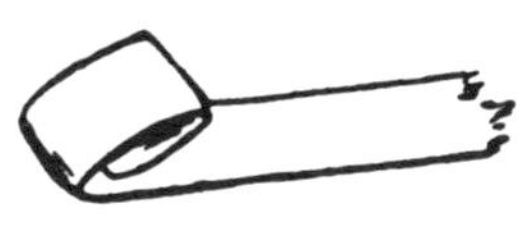

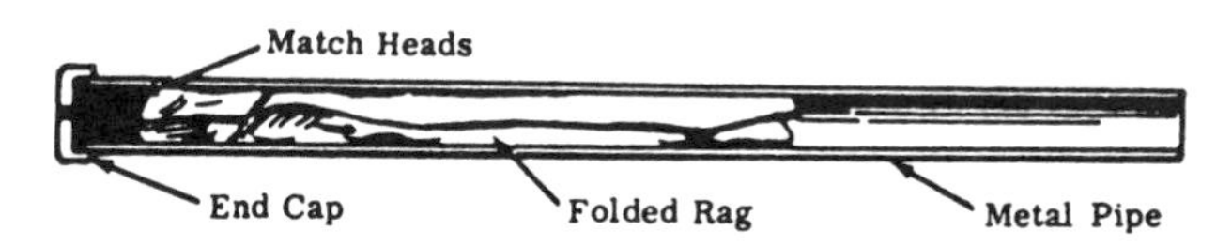

3. Place metal object into pipe. Place 1 in. x 3 in. rag into pipe to cover projectile. Tamp firmly WITH CAUTION.

4. Place 2 toy caps over small hole in end cap. Be sure metal strap will hit caps when it is released.

NOTE: It may be necessary to tape toy caps to end cap.

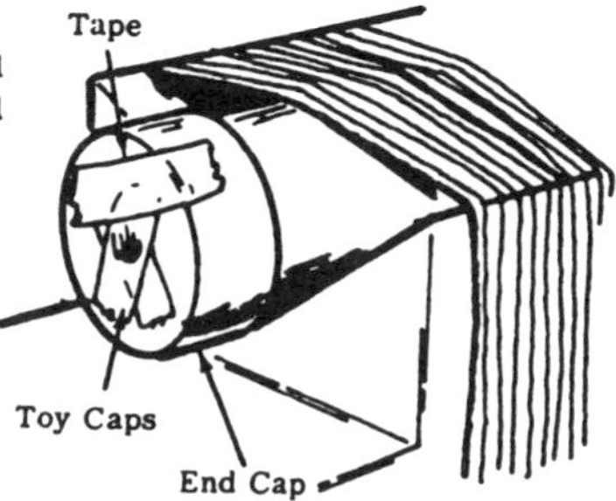

5. When ready to fire, pull metal strap back and release.

B. When "Strike-Anywhere" Matches Are Available:

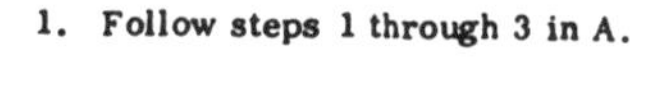

1. Follow steps 1 through 3 in A.

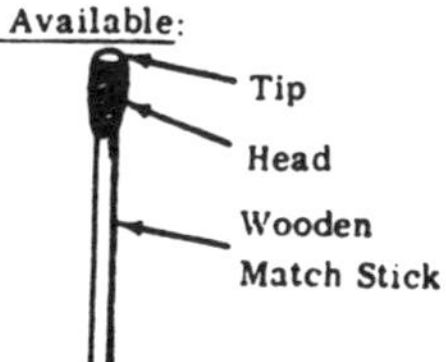

2. Carefully cut off tips of heads of 2 "strike-anywhere" matches with knife.

3. Place one tip in hole in end cap. Push in with wooden end of match stick.

59

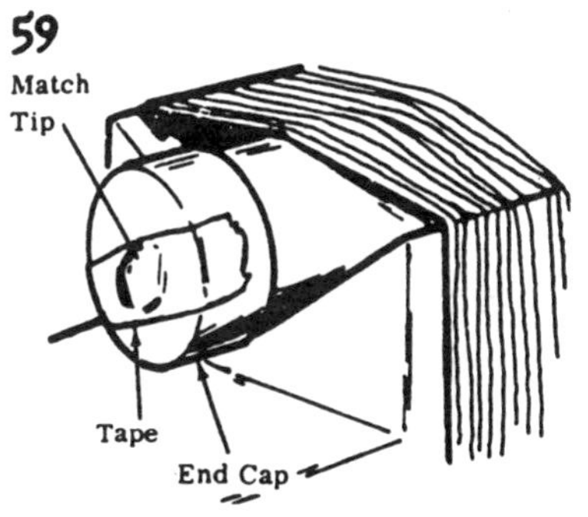

4. Place second match tip on a piece of tape. Place tape so match tip is directly over hole in end cap.

5. When ready to fire, pull metal strap back and release.

C. When Safety Fuse Is Available: (Recommended for Booby Traps)

1. Remove end cap from pipe. Knot one end of safety fuse. Thread safety fuse through hole in end cap so that knot is on inside of end cap.

2. Follow steps 1 through 3 in A.

3. Tie several matches to safety fuse near outside of end cap.
NOTE: Bare end of safety fuse should be inside match head cluster.

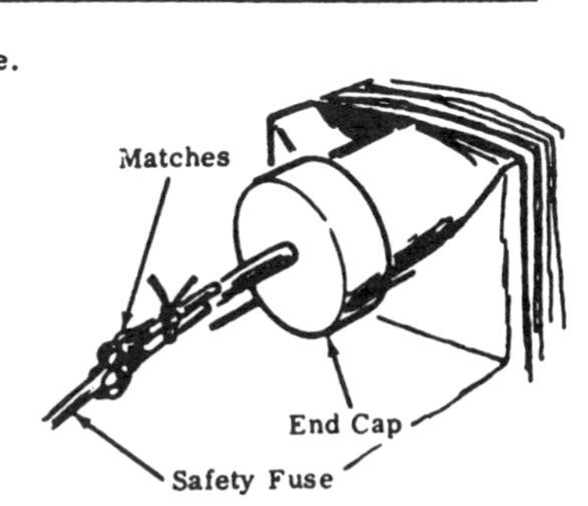

4. Wrap match covers around matches and tie. Striker should be in contact with match bands.

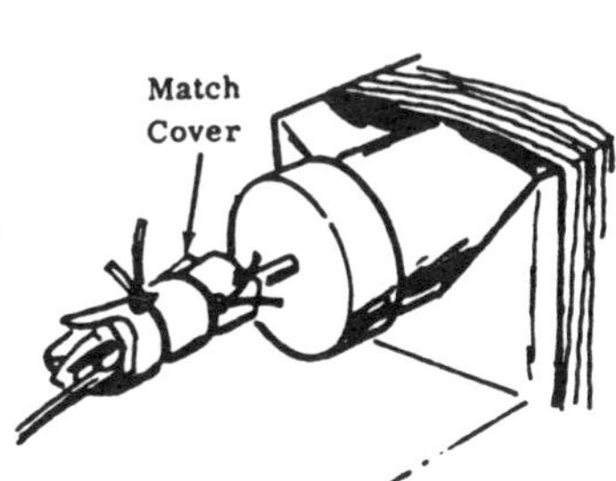

5. Replace end cap on pipe.

6. When ready to fire, pull match cover off with strong, firm, quick motion.

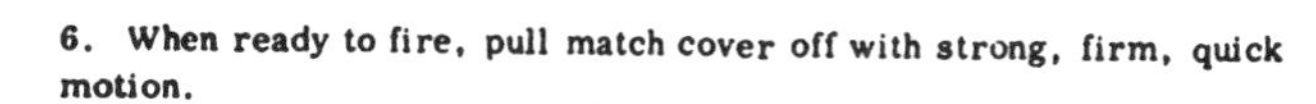

60

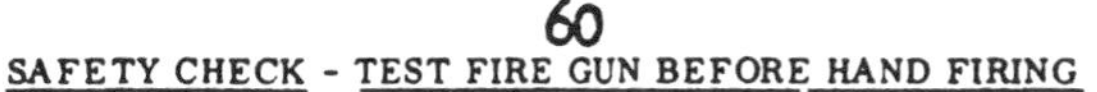

SAFETY CHECK - TEST FIRE GUN BEFORE HAND FIRING

1. Locate a barrier such as a stone wall or large tree which you can stand behind in case the weapon explodes when fired.

2. Mount gun solidly to a table or other rigid support at least ten feet in front of the barrier.

3. Attach a long cord to the firing strap on the gun.

4. Holding the other end of the cord, go behind the barrier.

5. Pull the cord so that the firing strap is held back.

6. Release the cord to fire the gun. (If gun does not fire, shorten the elastic bands or increase their number.)

IMPORTANT: Fire at least five rounds from behind the barrier and then re-inspect the gun before you attempt to shoulder fire it.

Section III
61 No. 8
RIFLE CARTRIDGE

NOTE: See Section III, No. 5 for reusable primer.

A method of making a previously fired rifle cartridge reusable.

MATERIAL REQUIRED:

Empty rifle cartridge, be sure that it still fits inside gun.
Threaded bolt that fits into neck of cartridge at least 1-1/4 in. (3 cm) long.
Safety or "strike-anywhere" matches (about 58 matches are needed for 7.62 mm cartridge)
Rag wad (about 3/4 in. (1-1/2 cm) square for 7.62 mm cartridge)
Knife
Saw

NOTE: Number of matches and size of rag wad depend on particular cartridge used.

PROCEDURE:

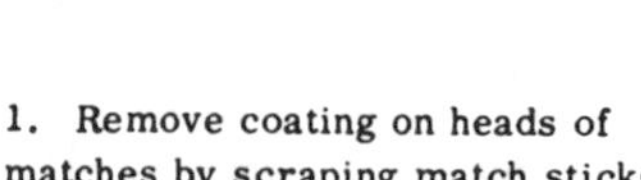

1. Remove coating on heads of matches by scraping match sticks with sharp edge.

CAUTION: If wooden "strike-anywhere" matches are used, cut off tips first. Discard tips or use for Reusable Primer, Section III, No. 5.

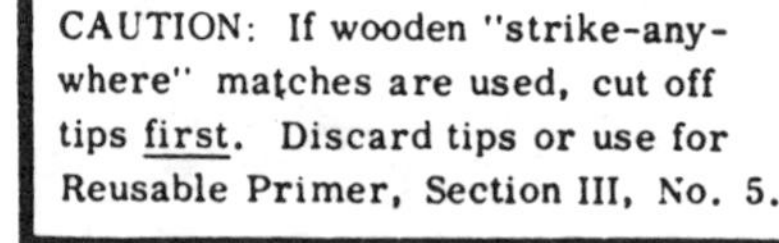

62

2. Fill previously primed cartridge case with match head coatings up to its neck. Pack evenly and tightly with match stick.

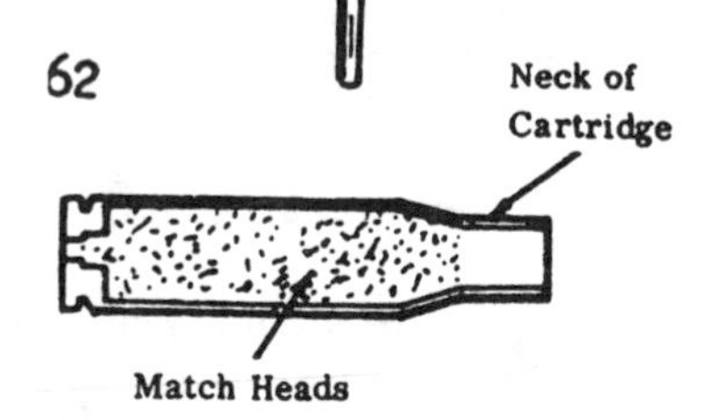

CAUTION: Remove head of match stick before packing. In all packing operations, stand off to the side and pack gently. Do not hammer.

3. Place rag wad in neck of case. Pack with match stick from which head was removed.

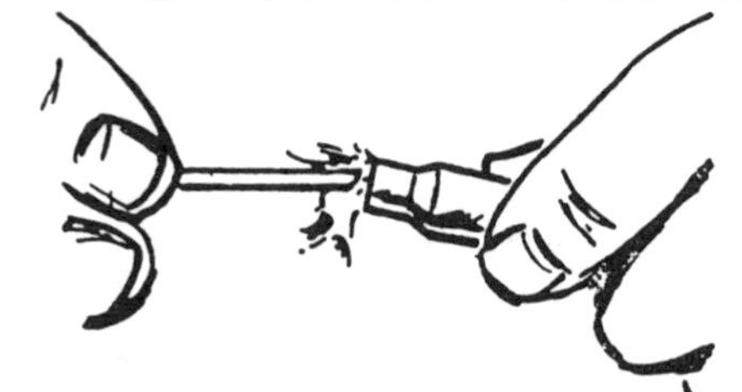

4. Saw off head end of bolt so remainder is approximately the length of the standard bullet.

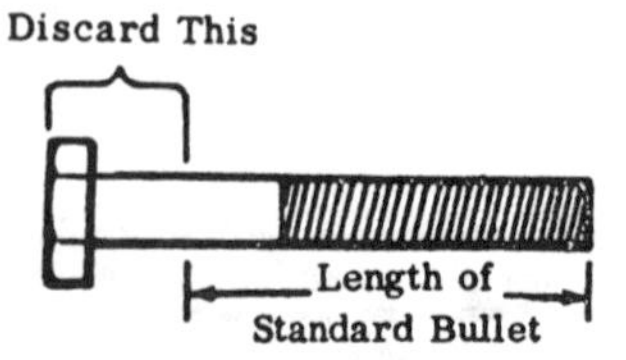

5. Place bolt in cartridge case so that it sticks out about the same length as the original bullet.

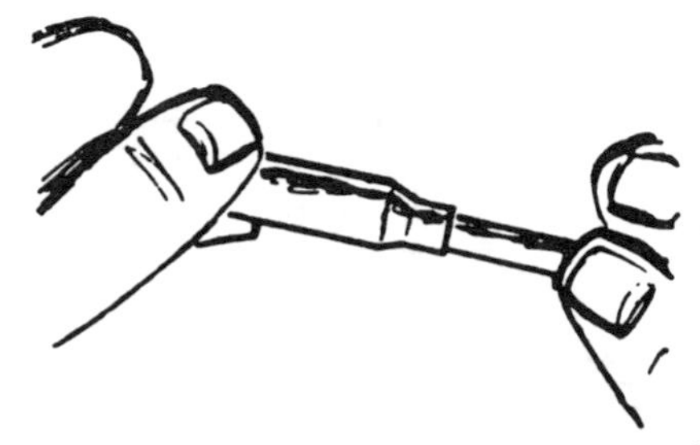

NOTE: If bolt does not fit snugly, force paper or match sticks between bolt and case, or wrap tape around bolt before inserting in case.

Section IV
63 No. 1
RECOILLESS LAUNCHER

A dual directional scrap fragment launcher which can be placed to cover the path of advancing troops.

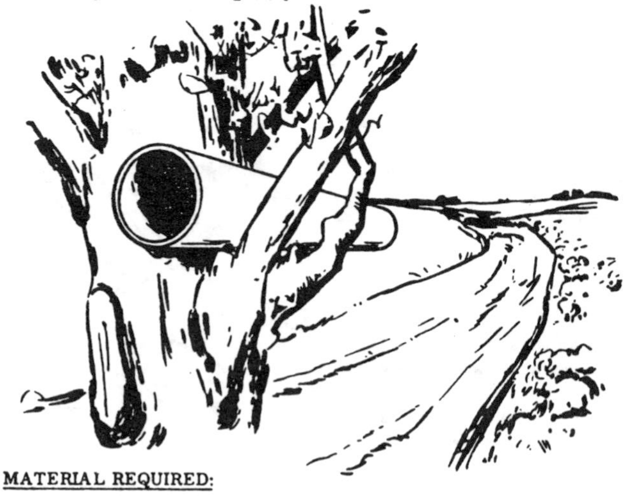

MATERIAL REQUIRED:

Iron water pipe approximately 4 ft. (1 meter) long and 2 to 4 in. (5 to 10 cm) in diameter
Black powder (commercial) or salvaged artillery propellant about 1/2 lb. (200 gms)
Safety or improvised fuse (Section VI, No. 7) or improvised electrical igniter (Section VI, No. 2)
Stones and/or metal scrap chunks approximately 1/2 in. (1 cm) in diameter - about 1 lb. (400 gms) total
4 rags for wadding, each about 20 in. by 20 in. (50 cm by 50 cm)
Wire
Paper or rag

NOTE: Be sure that the water pipe has no cracks or flaws.

64

PROCEDURE:

1. Place propellant and igniter in paper or rag and tie with string so contents cannot fall out.

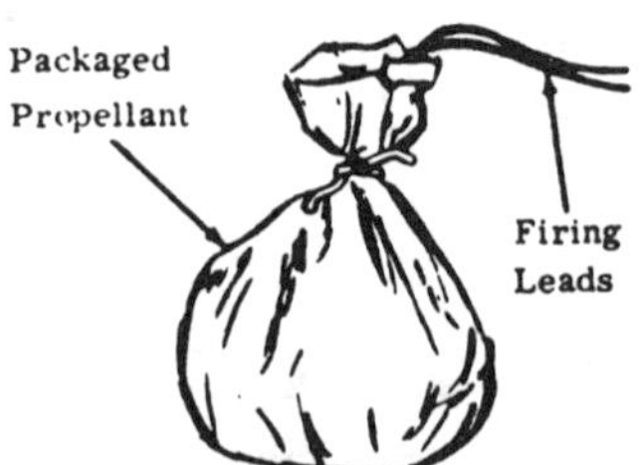

2. Insert packaged propellant and igniter in center of pipe. Pull firing leads out one end of pipe.

3. Stuff a rag wad into each end of pipe and lightly tamp using a flat end stick.

4. Insert stones and/or scrap metal into each end of pipe. Be sure the same weight of material is used in each side.

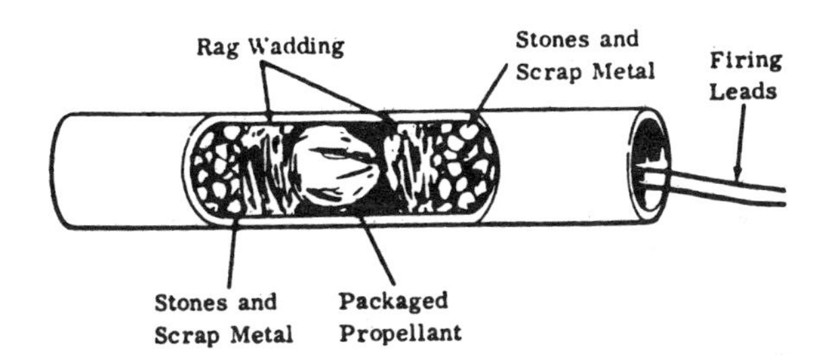

5. Insert a rag wad into each end of the pipe and pack tightly as before.

HOW TO USE:

1. Place scrap mine in a tree or pointed in the path of the enemy. Attach igniter lead to the firing circuit. The recoilless launcher is now ready to fire.

2. If safety or improvised fuse is used instead of the detonator, place the fuse into the packaged propellant through a hole drilled in the center of the pipe. Light free end of fuse when ready to fire. Allow for normal delay time.

CAUTION: Scrap will be ejected from both ends of the launcher.

65

Section IV

No. 2

SHOTGUN GRENADE LAUNCHER

This device can be used to launch a hand grenade to a distance of 160 yards (150 meters) or more, using a standard 12 gauge shotgun.

MATERIAL REQUIRED:

Grenade (Improvised pipe hand grenade, Section II, No. 1, may be used)
12 gauge shotgun
12 gauge shotgun cartridges
Two washers, (brass, steel, iron, etc.), having outside diameter of 5/8 in. (1-1/2 cm)
Rubber disk 3/4 in. (2 cm) in diameter and 1/4 in. (6 mm) thick (leather, neoprene, etc. can be used)
A 30 in. (75 cm) long piece of hard wood (maple, oak, etc.) approximately 5/8 in. (1-1/2 cm) in diameter. Be sure that wood will slide into barrel easily.
Tin can (grenade and its safety lever must fit into can)
Two wooden blocks about 2 in. (5 cm) square and 1-1/2 in. (4 cm) thick
One wood screw about 1 in. (2-1/2 cm) long
Two nails about 2 in. (5 cm) long
12 gauge wads, tissue paper, or cotton
Adhesive tape, string, or wire
Drill

PROCEDURE:

1. Punch hole in center of rubber disk large enough for screw to pass through.

2. Make push-rod as shown.

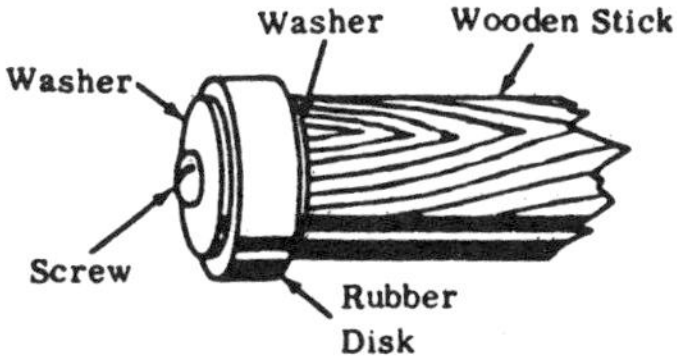

NOTE: Gun barrel is slightly less than 3/4 inch in diameter. If rubber disk does not fit in barrel, file or trim it very slightly. It should fit tightly.

3. Drill a hole through the center of one wooden block of such size that the push-rod will fit tightly Whittle a depression around the hole on one side approximately 1/8 in. (3 mm) and large enough for the grenade to rest in.

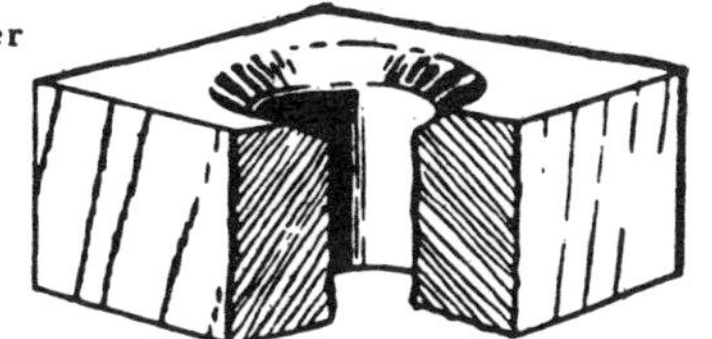

66

4. Place the base of the grenade in the depression in the wooden block. Securely fasten grenade to block by wrapping tape (or wire) around entire grenade and block.

NOTE: Be sure that the tape (or wire) does not cover hole in block or interfere with the operation of the grenade safety lever.

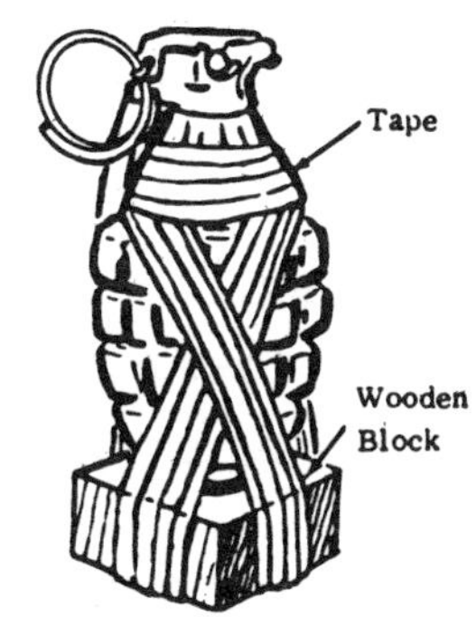

5. Drill hole through the center of the second wooden block, so that it will just slide over the outside of the gun barrel.

6. Drill a hole in the center of the bottom of the tin can the same size as the hole in the block.

7. Attach can to block as shown.

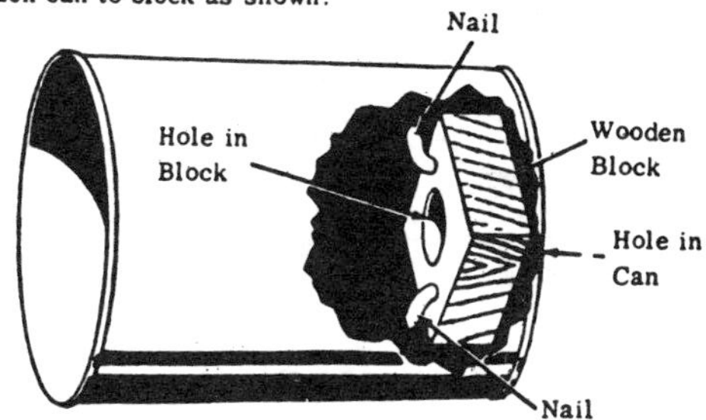

8. Slide the can and block onto the barrel until muzzle passes can open end. Wrap a small piece of tape around the barrel an inch or two from the end. Tightly wrapped string may be used instead of tape. Force the can and wooden block forward against the tape so that they are securely held in place. Wrap tape around the barrel behind the can

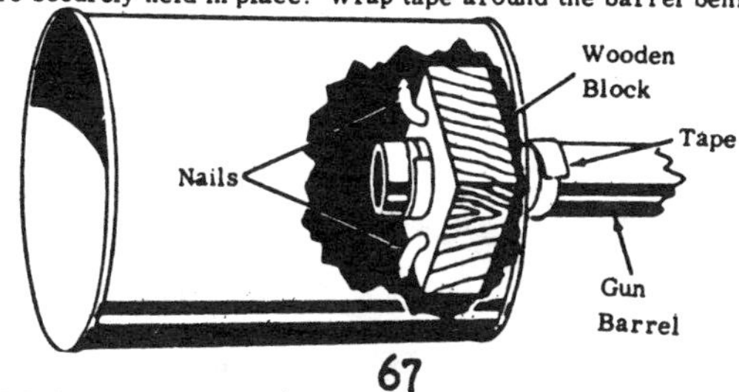

67

CAUTION: Be sure that the can is securely fastened to the gun barrel. If the can should become loose and slip down the barrel after the launcher is assembled, the grenade will explode after the regular delay time.

9. Remove crimp from a 12 gauge shotgun cartridge with pen knife. Open cartridge. Pour shot from shell. Remove wads and plastic liner if present.

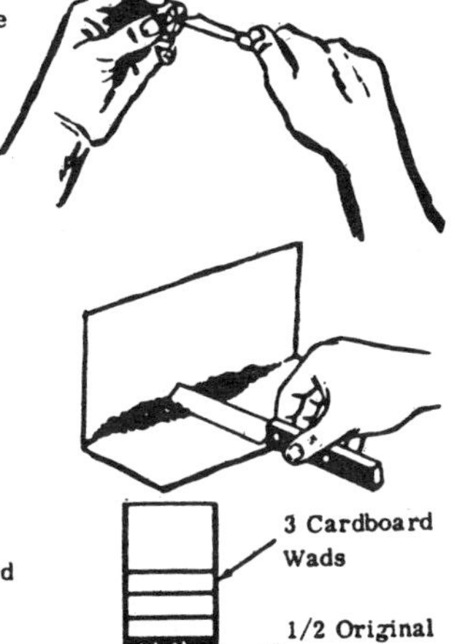

10. Empty the propellant onto a piece of paper. Using a knife, divide the propellant in half. Replace half of the propellant into the cartridge case.

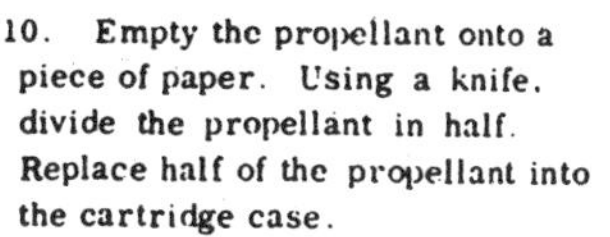

11. Replace the 12 gauge cardboard wads into cartridge case.

NOTE: If wads are not available, stuff tissue paper or cotton into the cartridge case. Pack tightly.

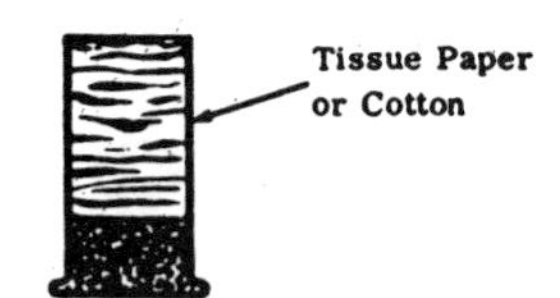

HOW TO USE:

Method I - When ordinary grenade is used:

1. Load cartridge in gun.

2. Push end of push-rod without the rubber disk into hole in wooden block fastened to grenade.

68

3. Slowly push rod into barrel until it rests against the cartridge case and grenade is in can. If the grenade is not in the can, remove rod and cut to proper size. Push rod back into barrel.

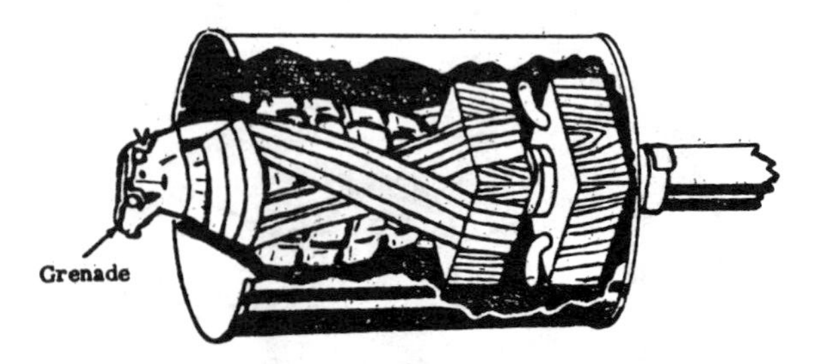

4. With can holding safety lever of grenade in place, carefully remove safety pin.

CAUTION: Be sure that the sides of the can restrain the grenade safety lever. If the safety lever should be released for any reason, grenade will explode after regular grenade delay time.

5. To fire grenade launcher, rest gun in ground at angle determined by range desired. A 45 degree angle should give about 150 meters (160 yds.)

Method II - When improvised pipe grenade is used:

An improvised pipe grenade (Section II, No. 1) may be launched in a similar manner. No tin can is needed.

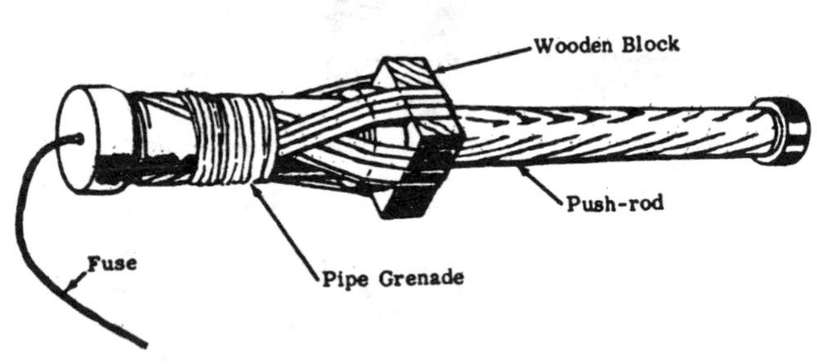

1. Fasten the grenade to the block as shown above with the fuse hole at the end opposite the block.

2. Push end of push-rod into hole in wooden block fastened to grenade.

3. Push rod into barrel until it rests against cartridge case.

69

4. Load cartridge in gun.

5. Follow step 5 of Method I.

6. Using a fuse with at least a 10 second delay, light the fuse before firing.

7. Fire when the fuse burns to 1/2 its original length.

70

Section IV

No. 3

GRENADE LAUNCHER (57 MM CARDBOARD CONTAINER)

An improvised method of launching a standard grenade 150 yds. (135 meters) or an improvised grenade 90 yds. (81 meters) using a discarded cardboard ammunition container.

MATERIAL REQUIRED:

Heavy cardboard container with inside diameter of 2-1/2 to 3 in. (5-1/2 to 8 cm) and at least 12 in. (30 cm) long (ammunition container is suitable)
Black powder - 8 grams (124 grains) or less
Safety or improvised fuse (Section VI, No. 7)
Grenade (Improvised hand grenade, Section II, No. 1 may be used)
Rag, approximately 30 in. x 24 in. (75 cm x 60 cm)
Paper

CAUTION: 8 grams of black powder yield the maximum ranges. Do not use more than this amount. See Improvised Scale, Section VII, No. 8, for measuring.

PROCEDURE: METHOD I - If Standard Grenade is Used.

1. Discard top of container. Make small hole in bottom.

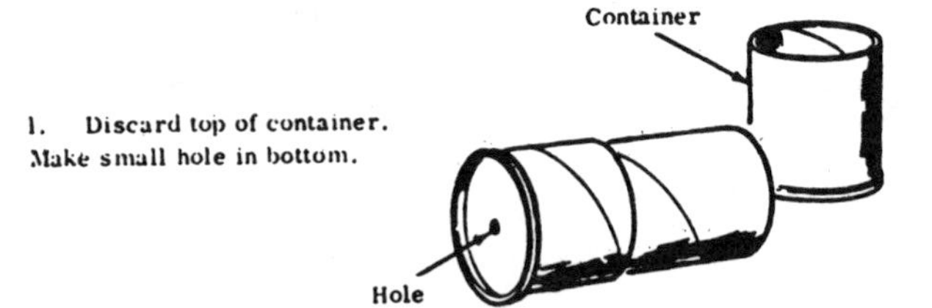

2. Place black powder in paper. Tie end with string so contents cannot fall out. Place package in container.

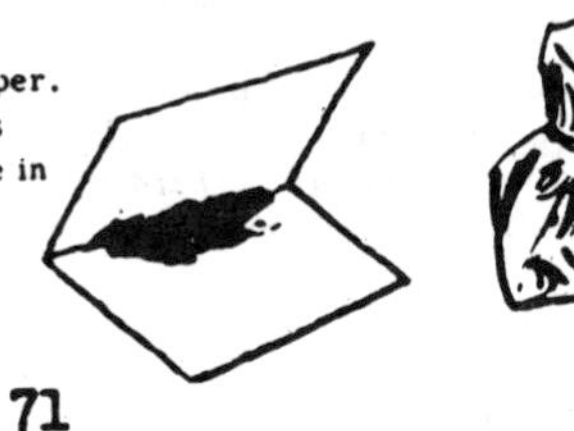

71

3. Insert rag wadding into container. Pack tightly with CAUTION.

4. Measure off a length of fuse that will give the desired delay. Thread this through hole in bottom of container so that it penetrates into the black powder package.

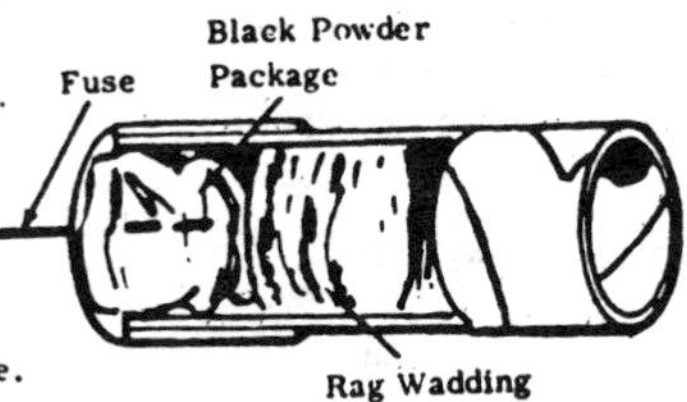

NOTE: If improvised fuse is used, be sure fuse fits loosely through hole in bottom of container.

5. Hold grenade safety lever and carefully withdraw safety pin from grenade. Insert grenade into container, lever end first.

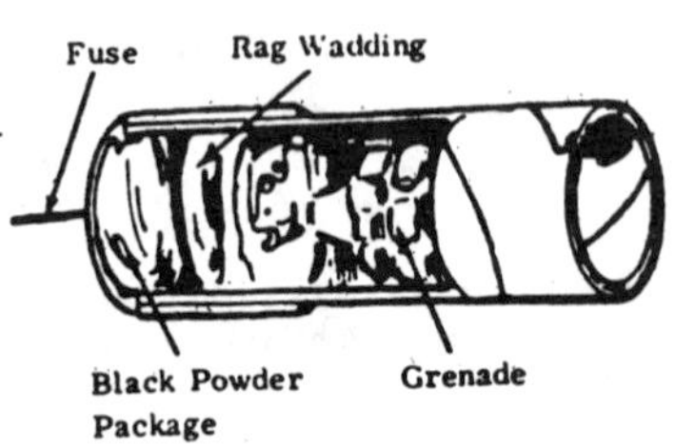

CAUTION: If grenade safety lever should be released for any reason, grenade will explode after normal delay time.

6. Bury container about 6 in. (15 cm) in the ground at 30° angle, bringing fuse up alongside container. Pack ground tightly around container.

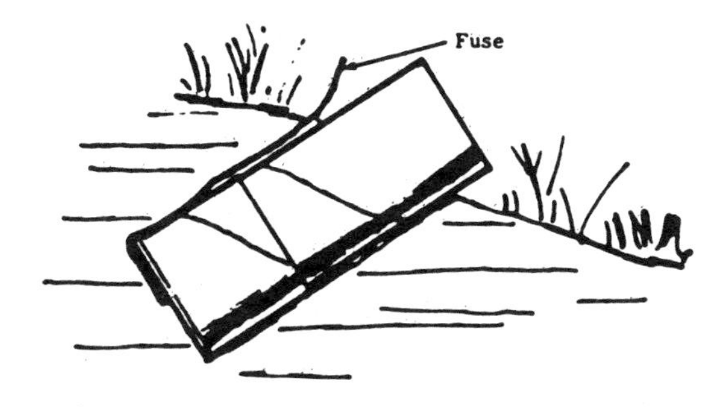

CAUTION: The tightly packed dirt helps to hold the tube together during the firing. Do not fire unless at least the bottom half of the container is buried in solidly packed dirt.

METHOD II - If Improvised Pipe Hand Grenade is Used.

1. Follow step 1 of above procedure.

72

2. Measure off a piece of fuse at least as long as the cardboard container. Tape one end of this to the fuse from the blasting cap in the improvised grenade. Be sure ends of fuse are in contact with each other.

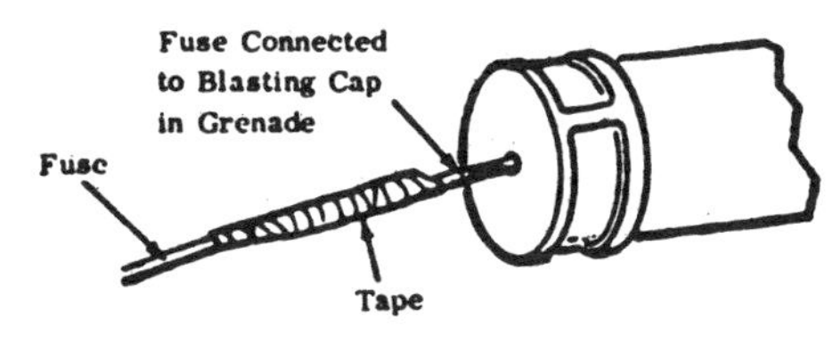

3. Place free end of fuse and black powder on piece of paper. Tie ends with string so contents will not fall out.

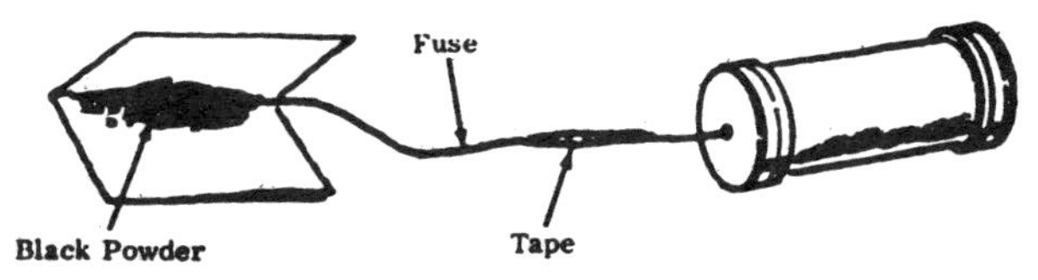

4. Place package in tube. Insert rag wadding. Pack so it fits snugly. Place pipe hand grenade into tube. Be sure it fits snugly.

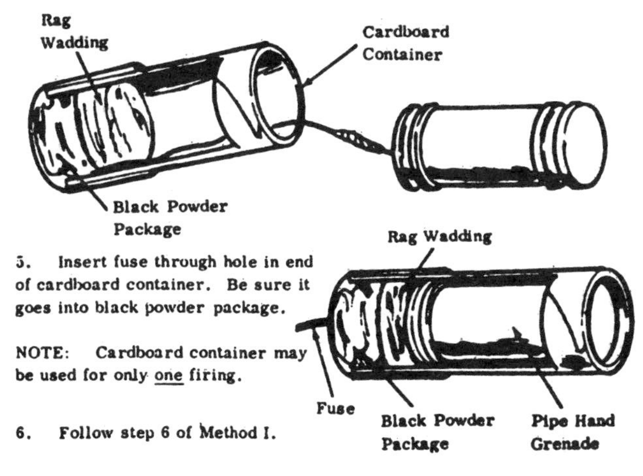

5. Insert fuse through hole in end of cardboard container. Be sure it goes into black powder package.

NOTE: Cardboard container may be used for only one firing.

6. Follow step 6 of Method I.

HOW TO USE:

Light fuse when ready to fire.

73 Section IV
No. 4
FIRE BOTTLE LAUNCHER

A device using 2 items (shotgun and chemical fire bottle) that can be used to start or place a fire 80 yards (72 meters) from launcher.

MATERIAL REQUIRED:

Standard 12 gauge or improvised shotgun (Section III, No. 2)
Improvised fire bottle (Section V, No. 1)
Tin can, about 4 in. (10 cm) in diameter and 5-1/2 in. (14 cm) high
Wood, about 3 in. x 3 in. x 2 in. (7-1/2 cm x 7-1/2 cm x 5 cm)
Nail, at least 3 in. (7-1/2 cm) long
Nuts and bolts or nails, at least 2-1/2 in. (6-1/2 cm) long
Rag
Paper
Drill

If Standard Shotgun is Used:

Hard wood stick, about the same length as shotgun barrel and about 5/8 in. (1-1/2 cm) in diameter. Stick need not be round.
2 washers (brass, steel, iron, etc.) having outside diameter of 5/8 in. (1-1/2 cm)
One wood screw about 1 in. (2-1/2 cm) long
Rubber disk, 3/4 in. (2 cm) in diameter and 1/4 in. (6 mm) thick, leather, cardboard, etc. can be used.
12 gauge shotgun ammunition

If Improvised Shotgun is Used:

Fuse, safety or improvised fast burning (Section VI, No. 7)
Hard wood stick, about the same length as shotgun barrel and 3/4 in. (2 cm) in diameter
Black powder - 9 grams (135 grains). See Section VII, No. 8.

74

PROCEDURE:

METHOD I - If Improvised Shotgun is Used:

1. Drill hole in center of wood block approximately 1 in. (2-1/2 cm) deep. Hole should have approximately the same diameter as the wooden stick.

2. Drill 2 small holes on opposite sides of the wooden block. Hole should be large enough for bolts to pass through.

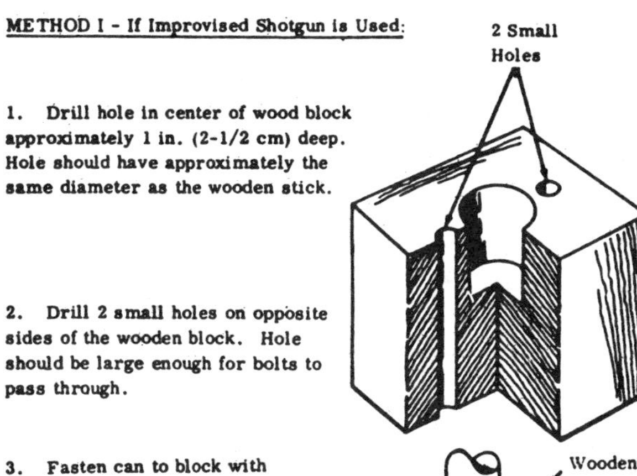

3. Fasten can to block with nuts and bolts.

NOTE: Can may also be securely fastened to block by hammering several nails through can and block. Do not drill holes, and be careful not to split wood.

4. Place wooden stick into hole in wooden block. Drill small hole (same diameter as that of 3 in. nail) through wooden block and through wooden stick. Insert nail in hole.

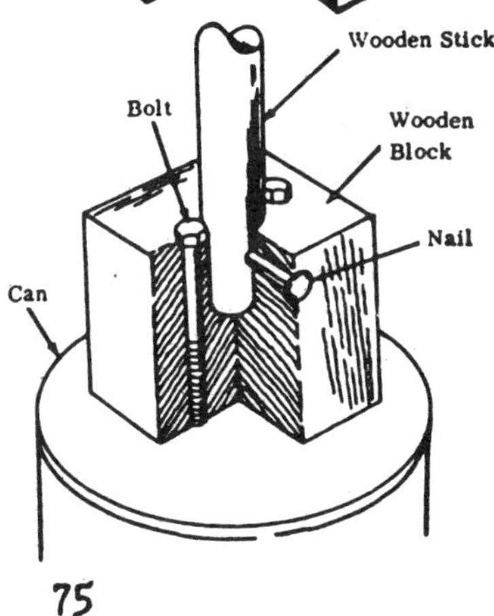

75

5. Crumple paper and place in bottom of can. Place another piece of paper around fire bottle and insert in can. Use enough paper so that bottle will fit snugly.

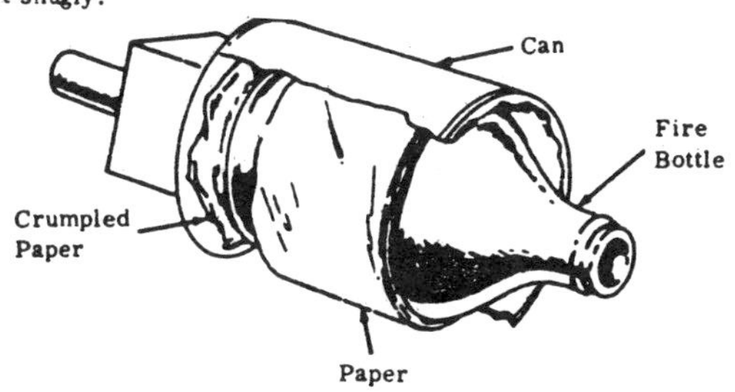

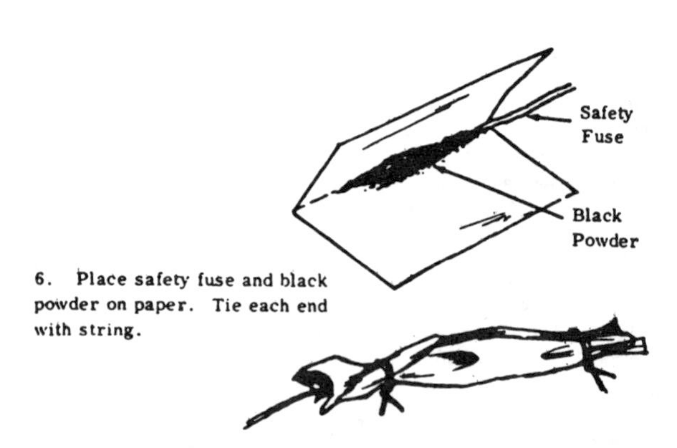

6. Place safety fuse and black powder on paper. Tie each end with string.

7. Thread fuse through hole in plug. Place powder package in rear of shotgun. Screw plug finger tight into coupling.

NOTE: Hole in plug may have to be enlarged for fuse.

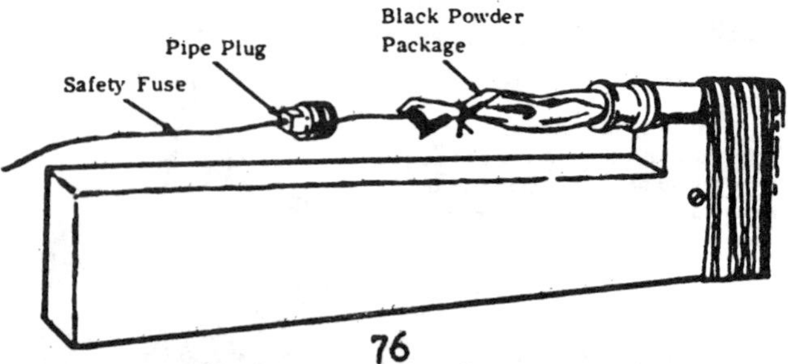

8. Insert rag into front of shotgun. Pack rag against powder package with stick. USE CAUTION.

METHOD II - If Standard Shotgun is Used:

1. Follow Steps 1 and 2, Shotgun Grenade Launcher, Section IV, No. 2.

2. Follow procedure of Method I, Steps 1 - 5.

3. Follow Steps 9, 10, 11, Shotgun Grenade Launcher, Section IV, No. 2, using 1/3 of total propellant instead of 1/2.

4. Load cartridge in gun.

HOW TO USE:

1. Insert stick and holder containing chemical fire bottle.

CAUTION: Do not tilt muzzle downward.

2. Hold gun against ground at 45° angle and light fuse.

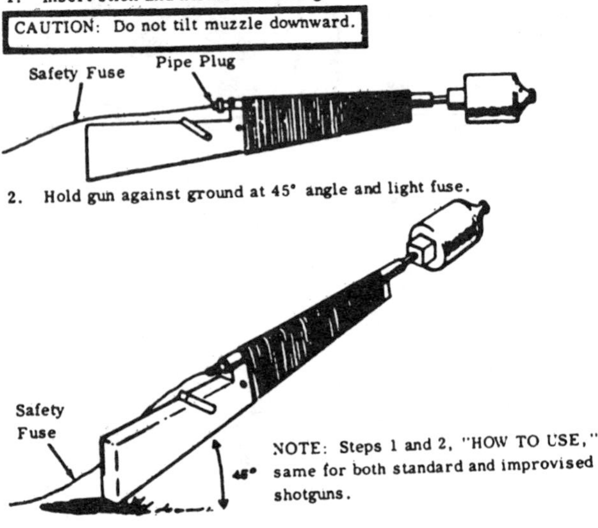

NOTE: Steps 1 and 2, "HOW TO USE," same for both standard and improvised shotguns.

CAUTION: Severe burns may result if bottle shatters when fired. If possible, obtain a bottle identical to that being used as the fire bottle. Fill about 2/3 full of water and fire as above. If bottle shatters when fired instead of being launched intact, use a different type of bottle.

Section IV
77 No. 5
GRENADE LAUNCHERS

A variety of grenade launchers can be fabricated from metal pipes and fittings. Ranges up to 600 meters (660 yards) can be obtained depending on length of tube, charge, number of grenades, and angle of firing.

MATERIAL REQUIRED:

Metal pipe, threaded on one end and approximately 2-1/2 in. (6-1/4 cm) in diameter and 14 in. to 4 ft. (35 cm to 119 cm) long depending on range desired and number of grenades used.
End cap to fit pipe
Black powder, 15 to 50 gm, approximately 1-1/4 to 4-1/4 tablespoons (Section I, No. 3)
Safety fuse, fast burning improvised fuse (Section VI, No. 7) or improvised electric bulb initiator (Section VI, No. 1 Automobile light bulb is needed)
Grenade(s) - 1 to 6
Rag(s) - about 30 in. x 30 in. (75 cm x 75 cm) and 20 in. x 20 in. (55 cm x 55 cm)
Drill
String

NOTE: Examine pipe carefully to be sure there are no cracks or other flaws.

PROCEDURE:

METHOD I - If Fuse is Used:

1. Drill small hole through center of end cap.

2. Make small knot near one end of fuse. Place black powder and knotted end of fuse in paper and tie with string.

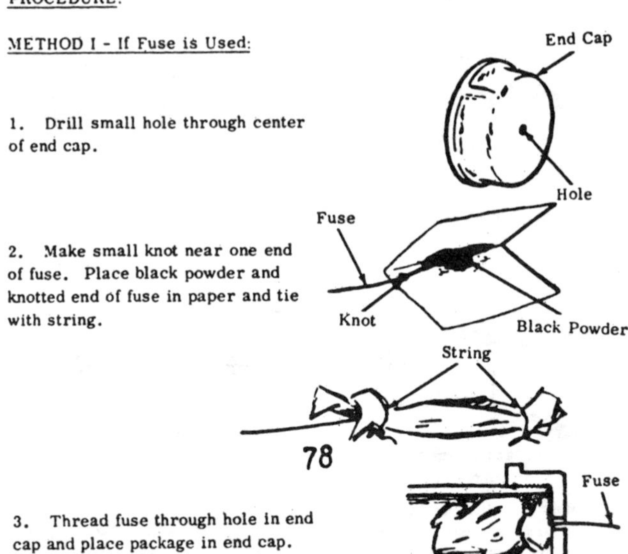

3. Thread fuse through hole in end cap and place package in end cap. Screw end cap onto pipe, being careful that black powder package is not caught between the threads.

4. Roll rag wad so that it is about 6 in. (15 cm) long and has approximately the same diameter as the pipe. Push rolled rag into open-end of pipe until it rests against black powder package.

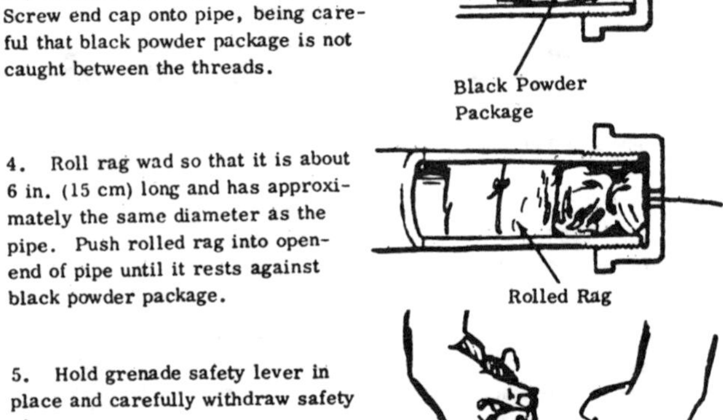

5. Hold grenade safety lever in place and carefully withdraw safety pin.

CAUTION: If grenade safety lever is released for any reason, grenade will explode after regular time. (4 - 5 sec.)

6. Holding safety lever in place, carefully push grenade into pipe, lever end first, until it rests against rag wad.

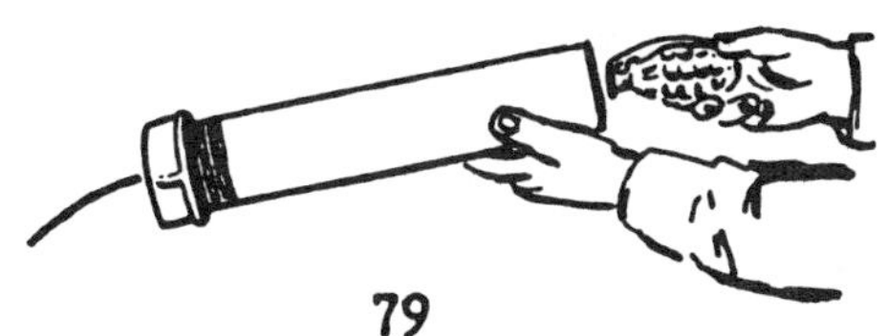

79

7. The following table lists various types of grenade launchers and their performance characteristics.

DESIRED RANGE	NO. OF GRENADES LAUNCHED	BLACK POWDER CHARGE	PIPE LENGTH	FIRING ANGLE
250 m	1	15 gm	14"	30°
500 m	1	50 gm	48"	10°
600 m (a)	1	50 gm	48"	30°
200 m	6 (b)	25 gm	48"	30°

(a) For this range, an additional delay is required. See Section VI, No. 11 and 12.

(b) For multiple grenade launcher, load as shown.

NOTE: Since performance of different black powder varies, fire several test rounds to determine the exact amount of powder necessary to achieve the desired range.

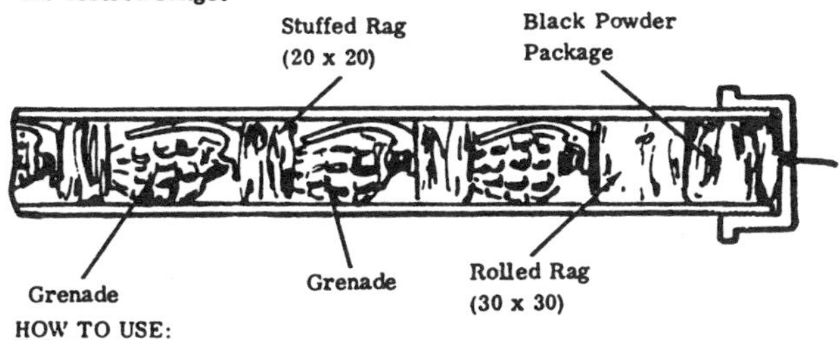

HOW TO USE:

1. Bury at least 1/2 of the launcher pipe in the ground at desired angle. Open end should face the expected path of the enemy. Muzzle may be covered with cardboard and a thin layer of dirt and/or leaves as camouflage. Be sure cardboard prevents dirt from entering pipe.

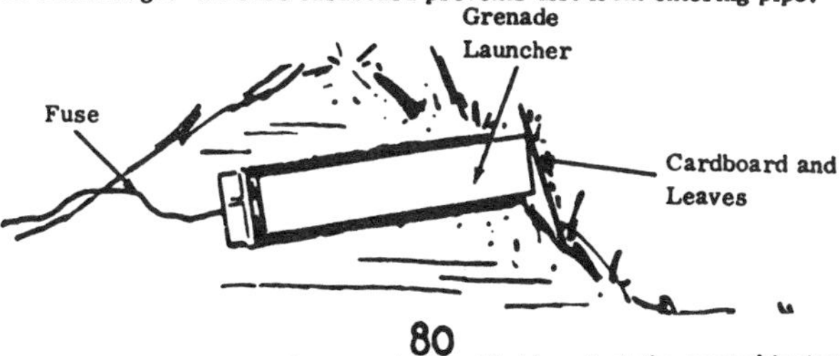

80

NOTE: The 14 in. launcher may be hand held against the ground instead of being buried.

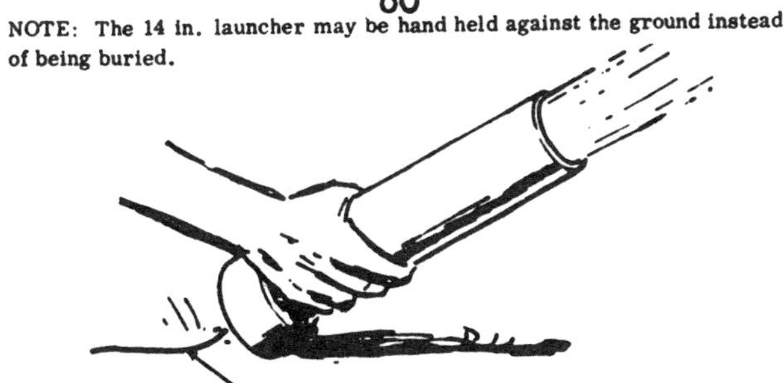

2. Light fuse when ready to fire.

METHOD II - If Electrical Igniter is Used:

NOTE: Be sure that bulb is in good operating condition.

1. Prepare electric bulb initiator as described in Section VI, No. 1.

2. Place electric initiator and black powder charge in paper. Tie ends of paper with string.

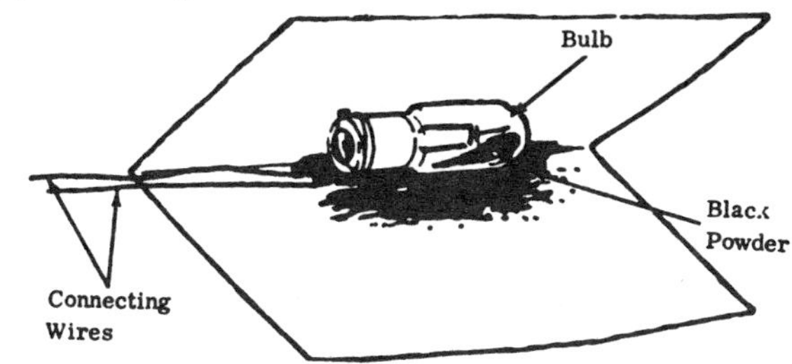

3. Follow above Procedure, Steps 3 to end.

HOW TO USE:

1. Follow above How to Use, Step 1.

2. Connect leads to firing circuit. Close circuit when ready to fire.

81

Section IV
No. 6
60 MM MORTAR PROJECTILE LAUNCHER

A device to launch 60 mm mortar rounds using a metal pipe 2-1/2 in. (6 cm) in diameter and 4 ft. (120 cm) long as the launching tube.

MATERIAL REQUIRED:

Mortar, projectile (60 mm) and charge increments
Metal pipe 2-1/2 in. (6 cm) in diameter and 4 ft. (120 cm) long, threaded on one end
Threaded end cap to fit pipe
Bolt, 1/8 in. (3 mm) in diameter and at least 1 in. (2-1/2 cm) long
Two (2) nuts to fit bolt
File
Drill

PROCEDURE:

1. Drill hole 1/8 in. (3 mm) in diameter through center of end cap.

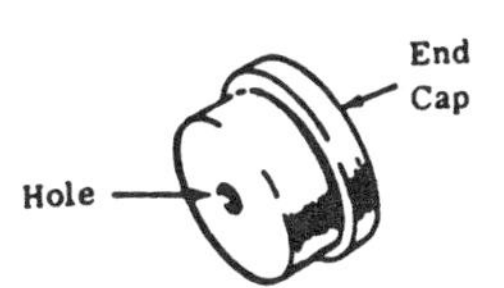

2. Round off end of bolt with file.

3. Place bolt through hole in end cap. Secure in place with nuts as illustrated.

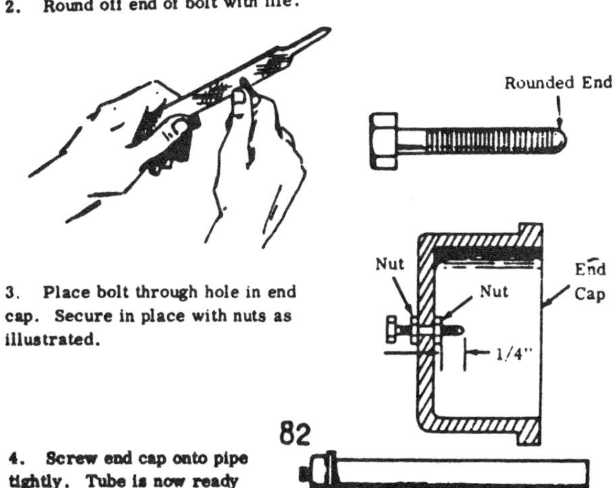

82

4. Screw end cap onto pipe tightly. Tube is now ready for use.

HOW TO USE:

1. Bury launching tube in ground at desired angle so that bottom of tube is at least 2 ft. (60 cm) underground. Adjust the number of increments in rear finned end of mortar projectile. See following table for launching angle and number of increments used.

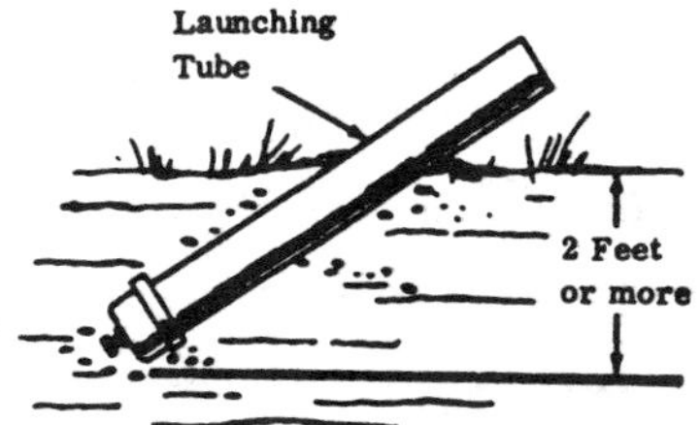

2. When ready to fire, withdraw safety wire from mortar projectile. Drop projectile into launching tube, FINNED END FIRST.

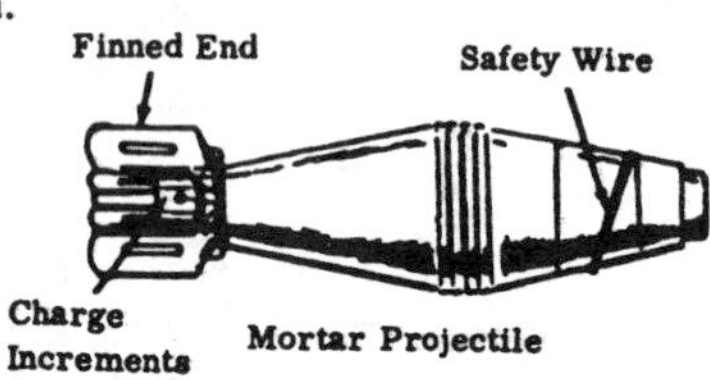

> CAUTION: Be sure bore riding pin is in place in fuse when mortar projectile is dropped into tube. A live mortar round could explode in the tube if the fit is loose enough to permit the bore riding pin to come out partway.

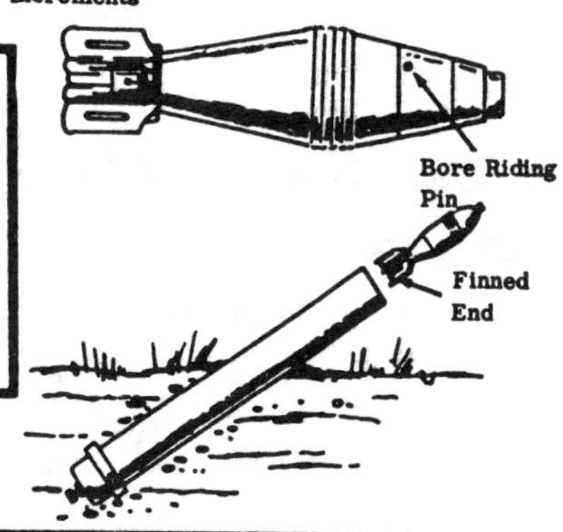

> CAUTION: The round will fire as soon as the projectile is dropped into tube. Keep all parts of body behind the open end of the tube.

83

DESIRED RANGE (YARDS)	MAXIMUM HEIGHT MORTAR WILL REACH (YARDS)	REQUIRED ANGLE OF ELEVATION OF TUBE (MEASURED FROM HORIZONTAL DEGREES)	CHARGE - NUMBER OF INCREMENTS
150	25	40	0
300	50	40	1
700	150	40	2
1000	225	40	3
1500	300	40	4
125	75	60	0
300	125	60	1
550	250	60	2
1000	375	60	3
1440	600	60	4
75	100	80	0
150	200	80	1
300	350	80	2
400	600	80	3
550	750	80	4

Section V
84 No. 1
CHEMICAL FIRE BOTTLE

This incendiary bottle is self-igniting on target impact.

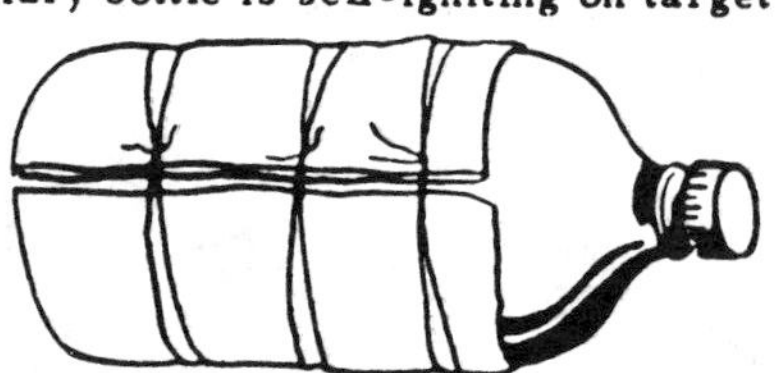

MATERIALS REQUIRED	How Used	Common Source
Sulphuric Acid	Storage Batteries	Motor Vehicles
Gasoline	Motor Fuel	Gas Station or Motor Vehicles
Potassium Chlorate	Medicine	Drug Store
Sugar	Sweetening Foods	Food Store

Glass bottle with stopper (roughly 1 quart size).
Small Bottle or jar with lid.
Rag or absorbent paper (paper towels, newspaper).
String or rubber bands.

PROCEDURE

1. Sulphuric Acid Must be Concentrated. If battery acid or other dilute acid is used, concentrate it by boiling until dense white fumes are given off. Container used should be of enamelware or oven glass.

> CAUTION
>
> Sulphuric acid will burn skin and destroy clothing. If any is spilled, wash it away with a large quantity of water. Fumes are also dangerous and should not be inhaled.

2. Remove the acid from heat and allow to cool to room temperature.

85

3. Pour gasoline into the large (1 quart) bottle until it is approximately 2/3 full.

4. Add concentrated sulphuric acid to gasoline slowly until the bottle is filled to within 1" to 2" from top. Place the stopper on the bottle.

5. Wash the outside of the bottle thoroughly with clear water.

> CAUTION
>
> If this is not done, the fire bottle may be dangerous to handle during use.

6. Wrap a clean cloth or several sheets of absorbent paper around the outside of the bottle. Tie with string or fasten with rubber bands.

Gasoline & Sulphuric Acid
Cap
Absorbent Paper
String

7. Dissolve 1/2 cup (100 gm) of potassium chlorate and 1/2 cup (100 gm) of sugar in one cup (250 cc) of boiling water.

8. Allow the solution to cool, pour into the small bottle and cap tightly. The cooled solution should be approx. 2/3 crystals and 1/3 liquid. If there is more liquid than this, pour off excess before using.

> CAUTION
>
> Store this bottle separately from the other bottle.

HOW TO USE

1. Shake the small bottle to mix contents and pour onto the cloth or paper around the large bottle.

Bottle can be used wet or after solution has dried. However, when dry, the sugar - Potassium chlorate mixture is very sensitive to spark or flame and should be handled accordingly.

2. Throw or launch the bottle. When the bottle breaks against a hard surface (target) the fuel will ignite.

Section V
86 No. 2
IGNITER FROM BOOK MATCHES

This is a hot igniter made from paper book matches for use with molotov cocktail and other incendiaries.

Material Required

Paper book matches.
Adhesive or friction tape.

Procedure

1. Remove the staple(s) from match book and separate matches from cover.

2. Fold and tape one row of matches.

3. Shape the cover into a tube with striking surface on the inside and tape. Make sure the folded cover will fit tightly around the taped match heads. Leave cover open at opposite end for insertion of the matches.

4. Push the taped matches into the tube until the bottom ends are exposed about 3/4 in. (2 cm).

87

5. Flatten and fold the open end of the tube so that it laps over about 1 in. (2-1/2 cm); tape in place.

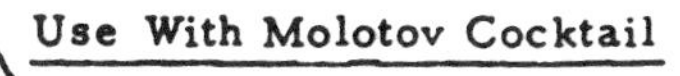

Use With Molotov Cocktail

Tape the "match end tab" of the igniter to the neck of the molotov cocktail.

OIL SOAKED RAG

Grasp the "cover end tab" and pull sharply or quickly to ignite.

General Use

The book match igniter can be used by itself to ignite flammable liquids, fuse cords and similar items requiring hot ignition.

CAUTION

Store matches and completed igniters in moistureproof containers such as rubber or plastic bags until ready for use. Damp or wet paper book matches will not ignite.

Section V
88 No. 3
MECHANICALLY INITIATED FIRE BOTTLE

The mechanically initiated Fire Bottle is an incendiary device which ignites when thrown against a hard surface.

MATERIALS REQUIRED

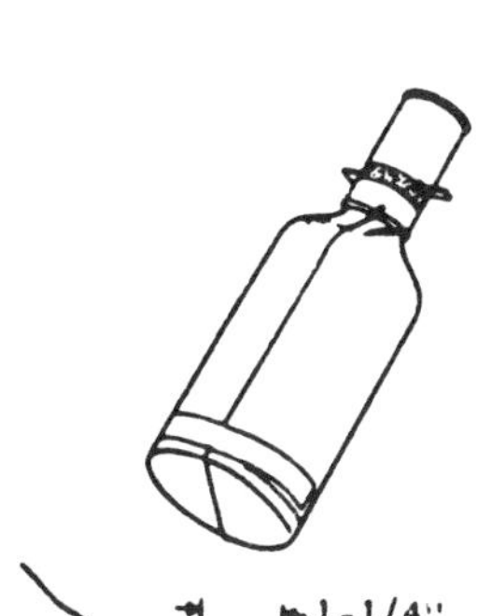

Glass jar or short neck bottle with a leakproof lid or stopper.
"Tin" can or similar container just large enough to fit over the lid of the jar.
Coil spring (compression) approximately 1/2 the diameter of the can and 1 1/2 times as long.
Gasoline
Four (4) "blue tip" matches
Flat stick or piece of metal (roughly 1/2" x 1/16" x 4")
Wire or heavy twine
Adhesive tape

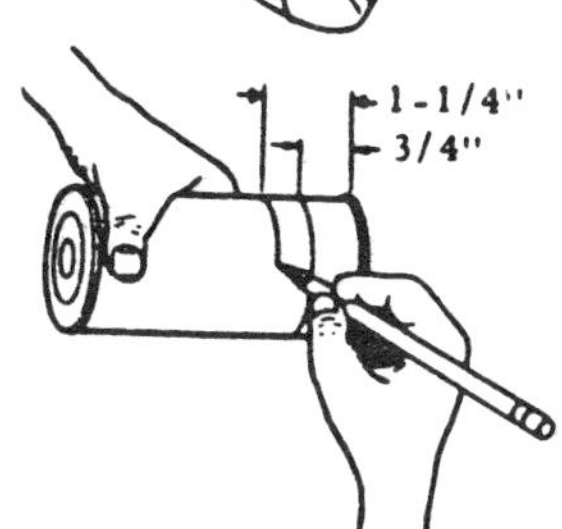

PROCEDURE

1. Draw or scratch two lines around the can - one 3/4" (19 mm) and the other 1 1/4" (30 mm) from the open end.

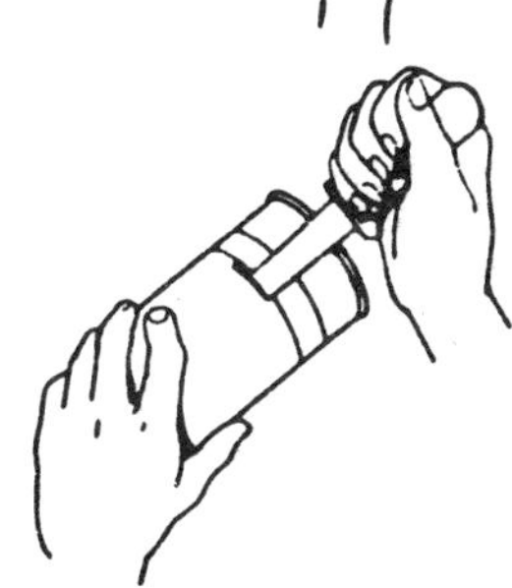

2. Cut 2 slots on opposite sides of the tin can at the line farthest from the open end. Make slots large enough for the flat stick or piece of metal to pass through.

89

3. Punch 2 small holes just below the rim of the open end of the can.

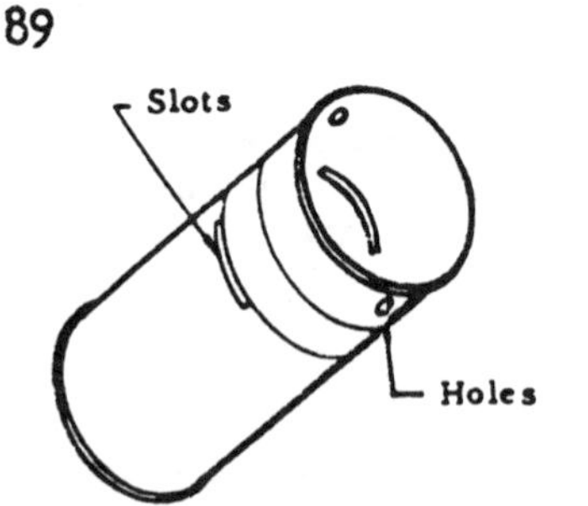

4. Tape blue tip matches together in pairs. The distance between the match heads should equal the inside diameter of the can. Two pairs are sufficient.

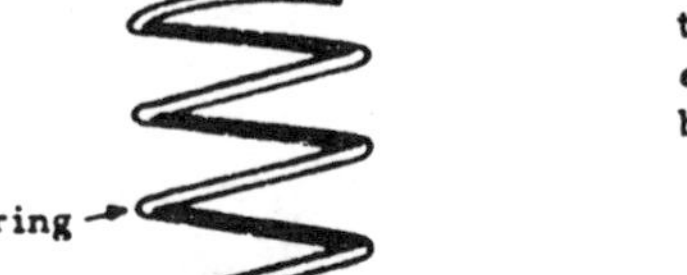

5. Attach paired matches to second and third coils of the spring, using thin wire.

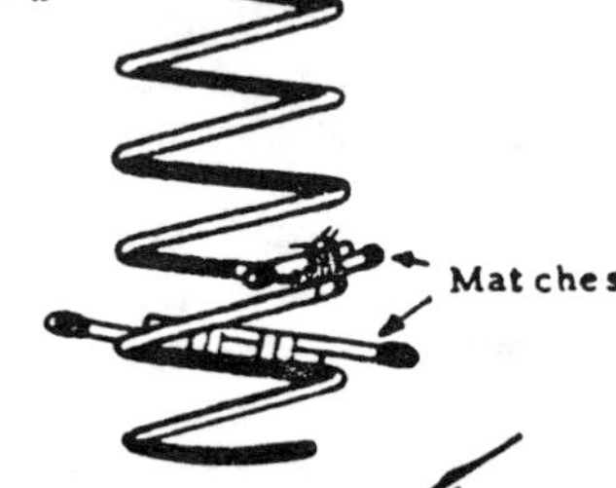

6. Insert the end of the spring opposite the matches into the tin can.

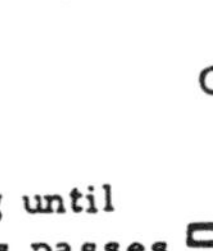

90

7. Compress the spring until the end with the matches passes the slot in the can. Pass the flat stick or piece of metal through slots in can to hold spring in place. This acts as a safety device.

8. Punch many closely spaced small holes between the lines marked on the can to form a striking surface for the matches. Be careful not to seriously deform can.

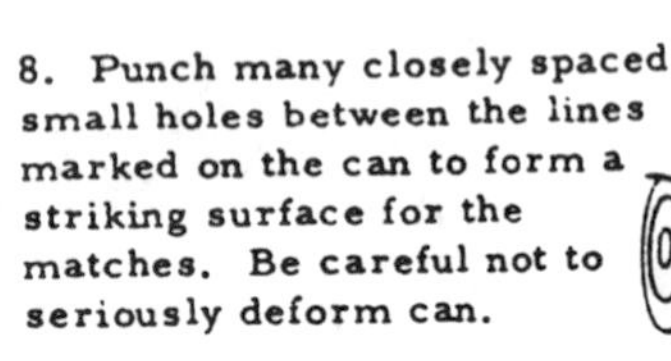

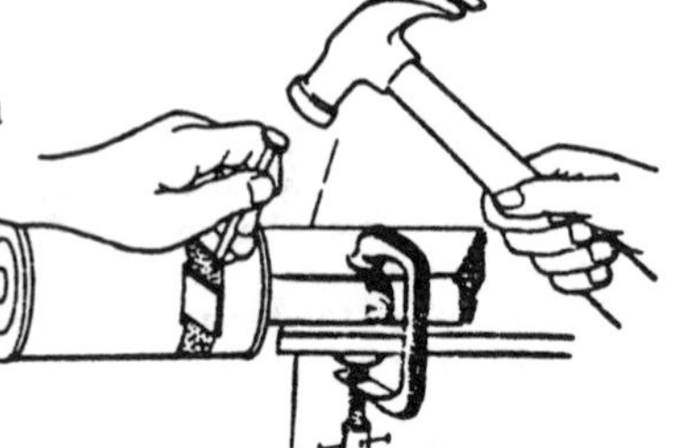

9. Fill the jar with gasoline and cap tightly.

10. Turn can over and place over the jar so that the safety stick rests on the lid of the jar.

91

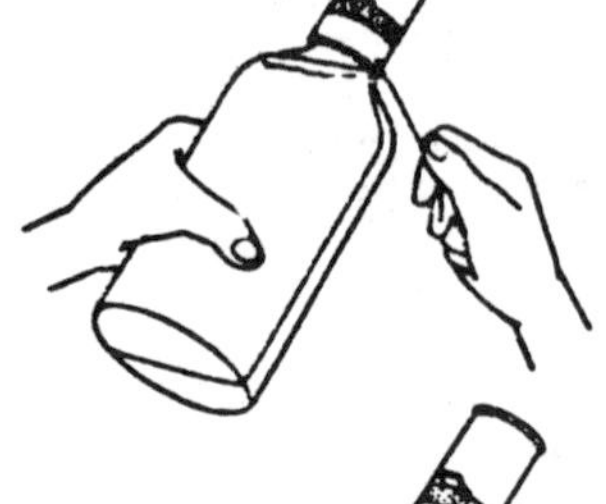

11. Pass wire or twine around the bottom of the jar. Thread ends through holes in can and bind tightly to jar.

12. Tape wire or cord to jar near the bottom.

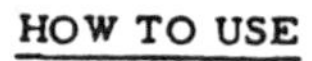

HOW TO USE

1. Carefully withdraw flat safety stick.

2. Throw jar at hard surface.

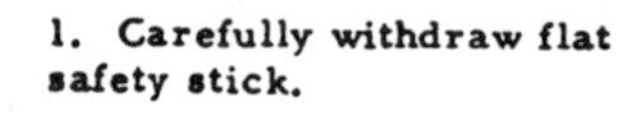

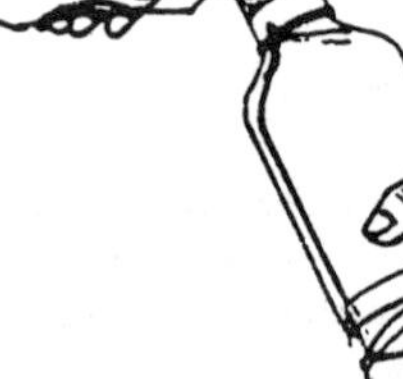

CAUTION:

DO NOT REMOVE SAFETY STICK UNTIL READY TO THROW FIRE BOTTLE.

The safety stick, when in place, prevents ignition of the fire bottle if it should accidentally be broken.

92 Section V
No. 4

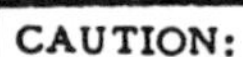

GELLED FLAME FUELS

Gelled or paste type fuels are often preferable to raw gasoline for use in incendiary devices such as fire bottles. This type fuel adheres more readily to the target and produces greater heat concentration.

Several methods are shown for gelling gasoline using commonly available materials. The methods are divided into the following categories based on the major ingredient:

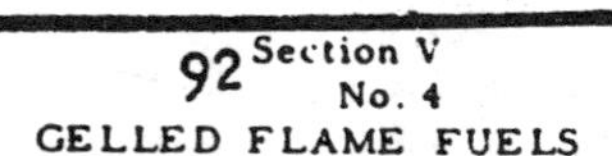

4.1 Lye Systems

4.2 Lye-Alcohol Systems

4.3 Soap-Alcohol Systems

4.4 Egg White Systems

4.5 Latex Systems

4.6 Wax Systems

4.7 Animal Blood Systems

93 Section V
No. 4.1
GELLED FLAME FUELS
LYE SYSTEMS

Lye (also known as caustic soda or Sodium Hydroxide) can be used in combination with powdered rosin or castor oil to gel gasoline for use as a flame fuel which will adhere to target surfaces.

NOTE: This fuel is not suitable for use in the chemical (Sulphuric Acid) type of fire bottle (Section V, No.1). The acid will react with the lye and break down the gel.

MATERIALS REQUIRED:

Parts by Volume	Ingredient	How Used	Common Source
60	Gasoline	Motor fuel	Gas station or motor vehicle
2 (flake) or 1 (powder)	Lye	Drain cleaner, making of soap	Food store Drug store
15	Rosin	Manufacturing Paint & Varnish	Naval stores Industry
	or		
	Castor Oil	Medicine	Food and Drug Stores

PROCEDURE:

CAUTION: Make sure that there are no open flames when mixing the flame fuel. NO SMOKING! in the area

1. Pour gasoline into jar, bottle or other container. (DO NOT USE AN ALUMINUM CONTAINER.)
2. If rosin is in cake form, crush into small pieces.
3. Add rosin or castor oil to the gasoline and stir for about five (5) minutes to mix thoroughly.
4. In a second container (NOT ALUMINUM) add lye to an equal volume of water slowly with stirring.

CAUTION: Lye solution can burn skin and destroy clothing. If any is spilled, wash away immediately with large quantities of water.

5. Add lye solution to the gasoline mix and stir until mixture thickens (about one minute).

NOTE: The sample will eventually thicken to a very firm paste. This can be thinned, if desired, by stirring in additional gasoline.

94 Section V
No. 4.2
GELLED FLAME FUELS

LYE-ALCOHOL SYSTEMS

Lye (also known as caustic soda or Sodium Hydroxide) can be used in combination with alcohol and any of several fats to gel gasoline for use as a flame fuel.

NOTE: This fuel is not suitable for use in the chemical (Sulphuric Acid) type of fire bottle (Section V, No. 1). The acid will react with the lye and break down the gel.

MATERIALS REQUIRED:

Parts by Volume	Ingredient	How Used	Common Source
60	Gasoline	Motor fuel	Gas station or motor vehicles
2 (flake) or 1 (powder)	Lye	Drain cleaner Making of soap	Food store Drug store
3	Ethyl Alcohol	Whiskey Medicine	Liquor store Drug store

NOTE: Methyl (wood) alcohol or isopropyl (rubbing) alcohol can be substituted for ethyl alcohol, but their use produces softer gels.

Parts by Volume	Ingredient	How Used	Common Source
14	Tallow	Food Making of soap	Fat rendered by cooking the meat or suet of animals.

NOTE: The following can be substituted for the tallow:

(a) Wool grease (Lanolin) (very good) -- Fat extracted from sheep wool.
(b) Castor oil (good).
(c) Any vegetable oil (corn, cottonseed, peanut, linseed, etc.)
(d) Any fish oil
(e) Butter or oleomargarine

It is necessary when using substitutes (c) to (e) to double the given amount of fat and of lye for satisfactory bodying.

PROCEDURE:

CAUTION: Make sure that there are no open flames in the area when mixing flame fuels. NO SMOKING!

1. Pour gasoline into bottle, jar or other container. (DO NOT USE AN ALUMINUM CONTAINER).

2. Add Tallow (or substitute) to the gasoline and stir for about 1/2 minute to dissolve fat.

95

3. Add alcohol to the gasoline mixture.

4. In a separate container (NOT ALUMINUM) slowly add lye to an equal amount of water. Mixture should be stirred constantly while adding lye.

CAUTION: Lye solution can burn skin and destroy clothing. If any is spilled, wash away immediately with large quantities of water.

5. Add lye solution to the gasoline mixture and stir occasionally until thickened (about 1/2 hour).

NOTE: The mixture will eventually (1 to 2 days) thicken to a very firm paste. This can be thinned, if desired, by stirring in additional gasoline.

96 Section V
No. 4.3
GELLED FLAME FUELS

SOAP-ALCOHOL SYSTEM

Common household soap can be used in combination with alcohol to gel gasoline for use as a flame fuel which will adhere to target surfaces.

MATERIAL REQUIRED:

Parts by Volume	Ingredient	How Used	Common Source
36	Gasoline	Motor fuel	Gas station, Motor vehicles
1	Ethyl Alcohol	Whiskey Medicine	Liquor store Drug store

NOTE: Methyl (wood) or isopropyl (rubbing) alcohols can be substituted for the whiskey.

Parts by Volume	Ingredient	How Used	Common Source
20 (powdered) or 28 (flake)	Laundry soap	Washing clothes	Stores

NOTE: Unless the word "soap" actually appears somewhere on the container or wrapper, a washing compound is probably a detergent. These Can Not Be Used.

PROCEDURE:

CAUTION: Make sure that there are no open flames in the area when mixing flame fuels. NO SMOKING!

1. If bar soap is used, carve into thin flakes using a knife.

2. Pour alcohol and gasoline into a jar, bottle or other container and mix thoroughly.

3. Add soap powder or flakes to gasoline-alcohol mix and stir occasionally until thickened (about 15 minutes).

97

Section V
No. 4.4

GELLED FLAME FUELS

EGG SYSTEMS

The white of any bird egg can be used to gel gasoline for use as a flame fuel which will adhere to target surfaces.

MATERIALS REQUIRED:

Parts by Volume	Ingredient	How Used	Common Source
85	Gasoline	Motor fuel Stove fuel Solvent	Gas station Motor vehicles
14	Egg Whites	Food Industrial processes	Food store Farms
Any One Of The Following:			
1	Table Salt	Food Industrial processes	Sea water Natural brine Food store
3	Ground Coffee	Food	Coffee plant Food store
3	Dried Tea Leaves	Food	Tea plant Food store
3	Cocoa	Food	Cacao tree Food store
2	Sugar	Sweetening foods Industrial processes	Sugar cane Food store
1	Saltpeter (Niter) (Potassium Nitrate)	Pyrotechnics Explosives Matches Medicine	Natural Deposits Drug store
1	Epsom salts	Medicine Mineral water Industrial processes	Natural deposits Kieserite Drug store Food store
2	Washing soda (Sal soda)	Washing cleaner Medicine Photography	Food store Drug store Photo supply store
1 1/2	Baking Soda	Baking Manufacture of: Beverages, Mineral waters and Medicines	Food store Drug store
1 1/2	Aspirin	Medicine	Drug store Food store

98

PROCEDURE:

CAUTION: Make sure that there are no open flames in the area when mixing flame fuels. NO SMOKING!

1. Separate egg white from yolk. This can be done by breaking the egg into a dish and carefully removing the yolk with a spoon.

NOTE: DO NOT GET THE YELLOW EGG YOLK MIXED INTO THE EGG WHITE. If egg yolk gets into the egg white, discard the egg.

2. Pour egg white into a jar, bottle, or other container and add gasoline.

3. Add the salt (or other additive) to the mixture and stir occasionally until gel forms (about 5 to 10 minutes).

NOTE: A thicker gelled flame fuel can be obtained by putting the capped jar in hot (65°C) water for about 1/2 hour and then letting them cool to room temperature. (DO NOT HEAT THE GELLED FUEL CONTAINING COFFEE).

99

Section V
No. 4.5

GELLED FLAME FUELS

LATEX SYSTEMS

Any milky white plant fluid is a potential source of latex which can be used to gel gasoline

MATERIALS REQUIRED:

Ingredient	How Used	Common Source
Gasoline	Motor fuel Solvent	Gas station Motor vehicle
Latex, commerical or natural	Paints Adhesives	Natural from tree or plant Rubber cement
One of the Following Acids:		
Acetic Acid (Vinegar)	Salad dressing Developing film	Food stores Fermented apple cider Photographic supply
Sulfuric Acid (Oil of Vitriol)	Storage batteries Material processing	Motor vehicles Industrial plants
Hydrochloric Acid (Muriatic Acid)	Petroleum wells Pickling and metal cleaning Industrial processes	Hardware store Industrial plants

NOTE: If acids are not available, use acid salt (alum, sulfates and chlorides other than sodium or potassium). The formic acid from crushed red ants can also be used.

PROCEDURE:

CAUTION: Make sure that there are no open flames in the area when mixing flame fuels. NO SMOKING!

1. With Commercial Rubber Latex:

a. Place 7 parts by volume of latex and 92 parts by volume of gasoline in bottle. Cap bottle and shake to mix well.

b. Add 1 part by volume vinegar (or other acid) and shake until gel forms.

CAUTION: Concentrated acids will burn skin and destroy clothing. If any is spilled, wash away immediately with large quantities of water.

100

2. With Natural Latex:

a. Natural latex should form lumps as it comes from the plant. If lumps do not form, add a small amount of acid to the latex.

b. Strain off the latex lumps and allow to dry in air.

c. Place 20 parts by volume of latex in bottle and add 80 parts by volume of gasoline. Cover bottle and allow to stand until a swollen gel mass is obtained (2 to 3 days).

101

Section V
No. 4.6

GELLED FLAME FUELS

WAX SYSTEMS

Any of several common waxes can be used to gel gasoline for use as a flame fuel which will adhere to target su-faces.

MATERIALS REQUIRED:

Parts by Volume	Ingredient	How Used	Common Source
80	Gasoline	Motor fuel Solvent	Gas station Motor vehicles
Any one of the following:			
20	Ozocerite Mineral wax Fossil wax Ceresin wax	Leather polish Sealing wax Candles Crayons Waxed paper Textile sizing	Natural deposits General stores Department store
	Beeswax	Furniture and floor waxes Artificial fruit and flowers Lithographing Wax paper Textile finish Candles	Honeycomb of bee General store Department store
	Bayberry wax Myrtle wax	Candles Soaps Leather polish Medicine	Natural form Myrica berries General store Department store Drug store

PROCEDURE:

1. Obtaining wax from Natural Sources: Plants and berries are potential sources of natural waxes. Place the plants and/or berries in boiling water. The natural waxes will melt.

Let the water cool. The natural waxes will form a solid layer on the water surface. Skim off the solid wax and let it dry. With natural waxes which have suspended matter when melted, screen the wax through a cloth.

2. Melt the wax and pour into jar or bottle which has been placed in a hot water bath.

3. Add gasoline to the bottle.

4. When wax has completely dissolved in the gasoline, allow the water bath to cool slowly to room temperature.

NOTE: If a gel does not form, add additional wax (up to 40% by volume) and repeat the above steps. If no gel forms with 40% wax, make a Lye solution by dissolving a small amount of Lye (Sodium Hydroxide) in an equal amount of water. Add this solution (1/2% by volume) to the gasoline wax mix and shake bottle until a gel forms.

102 Section V No. 4.7

GELLED FLAME FUELS

ANIMAL BLOOD SYSTEMS

Animal blood can be used to gel gasoline for use as a flame fuel which will adhere to target surfaces.

MATERIAL REQUIRED:

Parts by Volume	Ingredient	How Used	Common Source
68	Gasoline	Motor fuel Solvent	Gas station Motor vehicles
30	Animal blood Serum	Food Medicine	Slaughter House Natural habitat
Any one of the following:			
2	Salt	Food Industrial processes	Sea Water Natural brine Food store
	Ground Coffee	Food Caffeine source Beverage	Coffee plant Food store
	Dried Tea Leaves	Food Beverage	Tea plant Food store
	Sugar	Sweetening foods Industrial processes	Sugar cane Food store
	Lime	Mortar Plaster Medicine Ceramics Steel making Industrial processes	From calcium carbonate Hardware store Drug store Garden supply store
	Baking soda	Baking Beverages Medicine Industrial processes	Food store Drug store
	Epsom salts	Medicine Mineral water Industrial processes	Drug store Natural deposits Food store

103

PROCEDURE:

1. Preparation of animal blood serum:

a. Slit animal's throat by jugular vein. Hang up-side down to drain.

b. Place coagulated (lumpy) blood in a cloth or on a screen and catch the red fluid (serum) which drains through.

c. Store in cool place if possible.

CAUTION: Do not get aged animal blood or the serum into an open cut. This can cause infections.

2. Pour blood serum into jar, bottle, or other container and add gasoline.

3. Add the salt (or other additive) to the mixture and stir until a gel forms.

104 Section V No. 5

ACID DELAY INCENDIARY

This device will ignite automatically after a given time delay.

MATERIAL REQUIRED:

Small jar with cap
Cardboard
Adhesive tape
Potassium Chlorate
Sugar
Sulphuric Acid (Battery Acid)
Rubber sheeting (automotive inner tube)

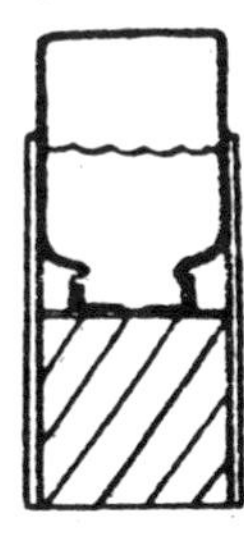

PROCEDURE:

1. Sulphuric acid must be concentrated. If battery acid or other dilute acid is used, concentrate it by boiling. Container used should be of enamelware or oven glass. When dense white fumes begin to appear, immediately remove the acid from heat and allow to cool to room temperature.

CAUTION: Sulphuric acid will burn skin and destroy clothing. If any is spilled, wash it away with a large quantity of water. Fumes are also dangerous and should not be inhaled.

2. Dissolve one part by volume of Potassium Chlorate and one part by volume of sugar in two parts by volume of boiling water.

3. Allow the solution to cool. When crystals settle, pour off and discard the liquid.

4. Form a tube from cardboard just large enough to fit around the outside of the jar and 2 to 3 times the height of the jar. Tape one end of the tube closed.

JAR

CARDBOARD

5. Pour wet Potassium Chlorate-sugar crystals into the tube until it is about 2/3 full. Stand the tube aside to dry.

POTASSIUM CHLORATE-SUGAR

CARBOARD TUBE

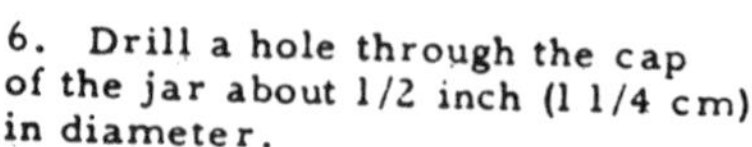

6. Drill a hole through the cap of the jar about 1/2 inch (1 1/4 cm) in diameter.

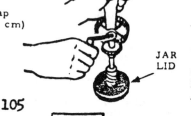

105

7. Cut a disc from rubber sheet so that it just fits snugly inside the lid of the jar.

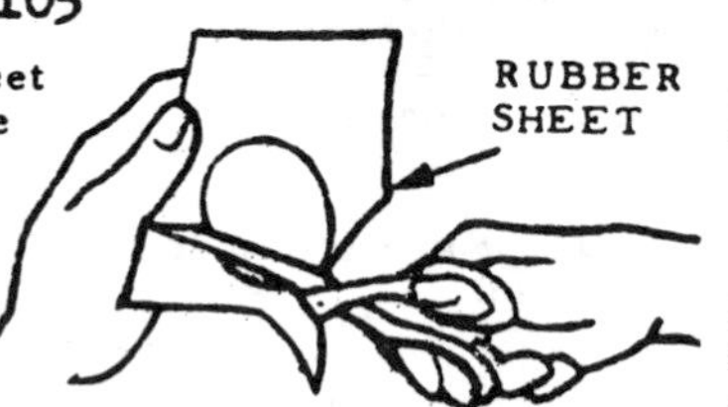

8. Partly fill jar with water, cover with rubber disc and cap tightly with the drilled lid. Invert bottle and allow to stand for a few minutes to make sure that there are no leaks. THIS IS EXTREMELY IMPORTANT.

9. Pour water from jar and fill about 1/3 full with concentrated sulphuric acid. Replace the rubber disc and cap tightly.

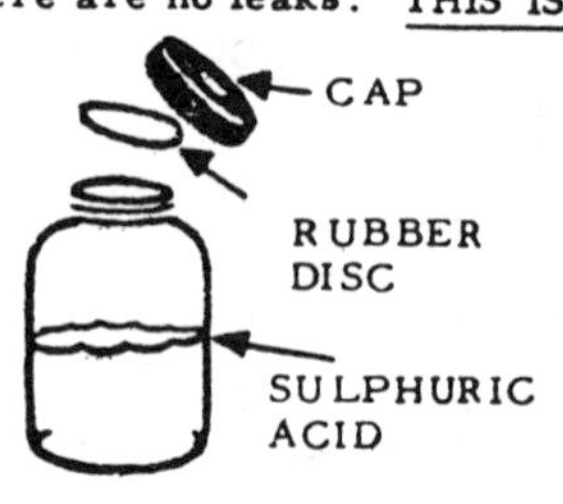

IMPORTANT: Wash outside of jar thoroughly with clear water. If this is not done, the jar may be dangerous to handle during use.

HOW TO USE:

1. Place the tube containing the Sugar Chlorate crystals on an incendiary or flammable material taped end down.

2. Turn the jar of sulphuric acid cap end down and slide it into the open end of the tube.

JAR WITH SULPHURIC ACID

TUBE OF SUGAR CHLORATE

INCENDIARY OR FLAMMABLE MATERIAL

After a time delay, the acid will eat through the rubber disc and ignite the sugar chlorate mix. The delay time depends upon the thickness and type of rubber used for the disc. Before using this device, tests should be conducte[illegible] determine the delay time that can be expected.

NOTE: A piece of standard automobile inner tube (about 1/32" thick) will provide a delay time of approximately 45 minutes.

Section VI
106 No. 1

ELECTRIC BULB INITIATOR

Mortars, mines and similar weapons often make use of electric initiators. An electric initiator can be made using a flashlight or automobile electric light bulb.

MATERIAL REQUIRED

Electric light bulb and mating socket
Cardboard or heavy paper
Black Powder
Adhesive tape

Bulb Base

Filament

Black Powder

Cardboard Tube

Cap or Tape

PROCEDURE

Method I

1. Break the glass of the electric light bulb. Take care not to damage the filament. The initiator will NOT work if the filament is broken. Remove all glass above the base of the bulb.

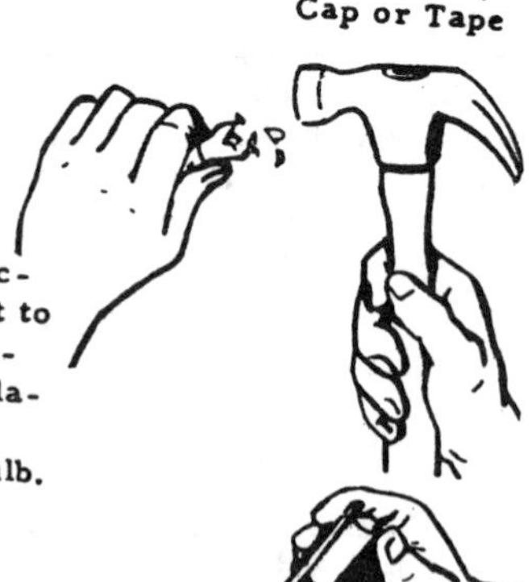

2. Form a tube 3 to 4 inches long from cardboard or heavy paper to fit around the base of the bulb. Join the tube with adhesive tape.

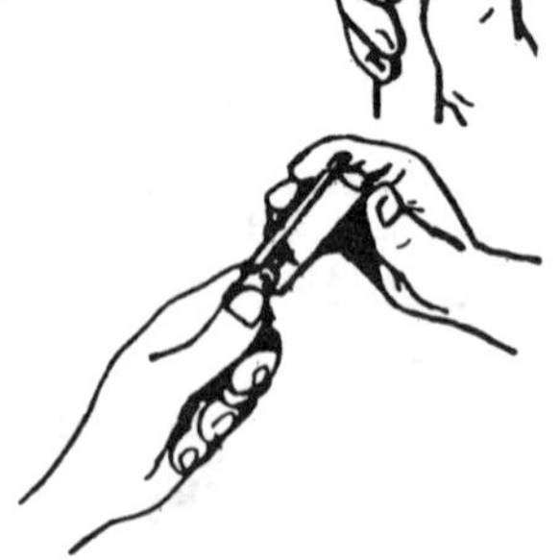

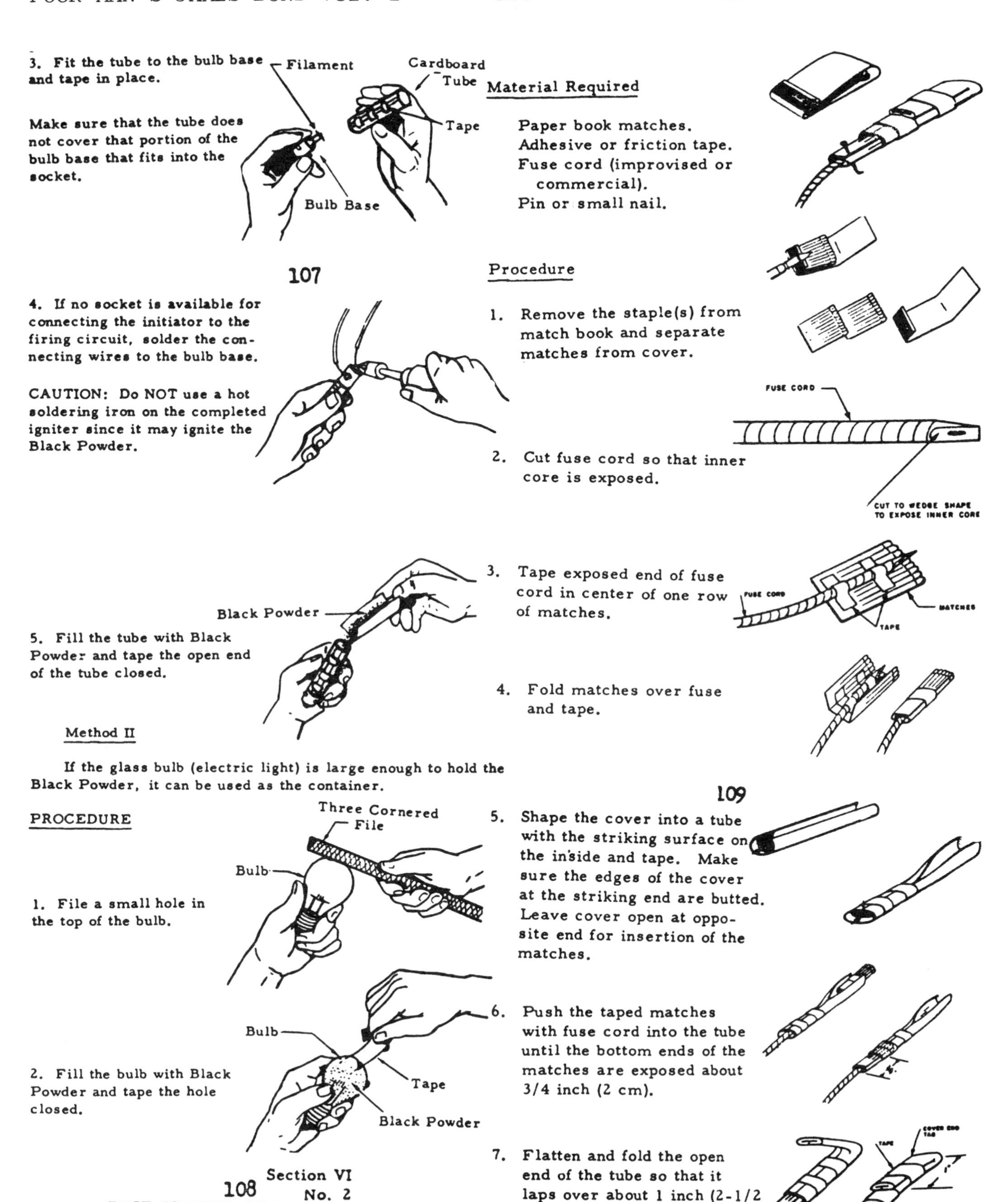

3. Fit the tube to the bulb base and tape in place.

Make sure that the tube does not cover that portion of the bulb base that fits into the socket.

4. If no socket is available for connecting the initiator to the firing circuit, solder the connecting wires to the bulb base.

CAUTION: Do NOT use a hot soldering iron on the completed igniter since it may ignite the Black Powder.

5. Fill the tube with Black Powder and tape the open end of the tube closed.

Method II

If the glass bulb (electric light) is large enough to hold the Black Powder, it can be used as the container.

PROCEDURE

1. File a small hole in the top of the bulb.

2. Fill the bulb with Black Powder and tape the hole closed.

Section VI
No. 2
FUSE IGNITER FROM BOOK MATCHES

A simple, reliable fuse igniter can be made from paper book matches.

Material Required

Paper book matches.
Adhesive or friction tape.
Fuse cord (improvised or commercial).
Pin or small nail.

Procedure

1. Remove the staple(s) from match book and separate matches from cover.
2. Cut fuse cord so that inner core is exposed.
3. Tape exposed end of fuse cord in center of one row of matches.
4. Fold matches over fuse and tape.
5. Shape the cover into a tube with the striking surface on the inside and tape. Make sure the edges of the cover at the striking end are butted. Leave cover open at opposite end for insertion of the matches.
6. Push the taped matches with fuse cord into the tube until the bottom ends of the matches are exposed about 3/4 inch (2 cm).
7. Flatten and fold the open end of the tube so that it laps over about 1 inch (2-1/2 cm); tape in place.

8. Push pin or small nail through matches and fuse cord. Bend end of pin or nail.

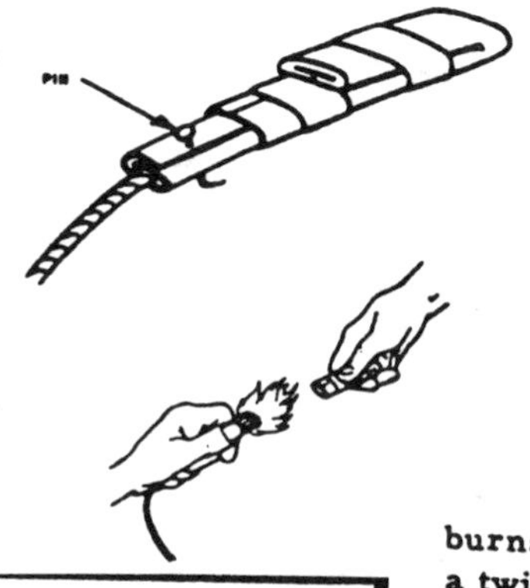

Method of Use

To light the fuse cord, the igniter is held by both hands and pulled sharply or quickly.

> **CAUTION**
>
> Store matches and completed fuse igniters in moistureproof containers such as plastic or rubber type bags until ready for use. Damp or wet paper book matches will not ignite. Fuse lengths should not exceed 12 in. (30 cm) for easy storage. These can be spliced to main fuses when needed.

Section VI
110 No. 3
DELAY IGNITER FROM CIGARETTE

A simple and economical time delay can be made with a common cigarette.

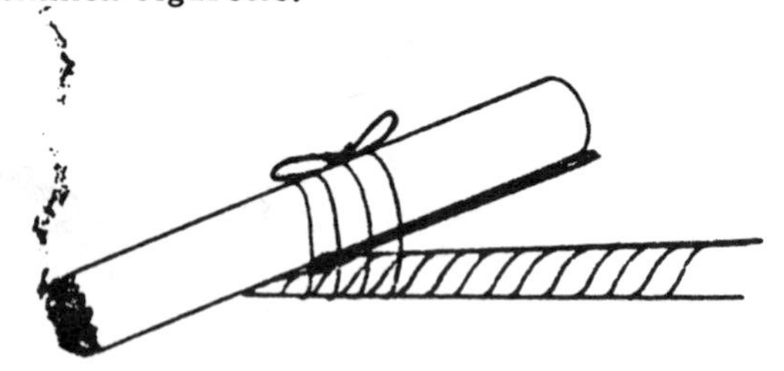

Materials Required

Cigarette.
Paper match.
String (shoelace or similar cord).
Fuse cord (improvised or commercial).

Procedure

CUT SO INNER CORE IS EXPOSED

1. Cut end of fuse cord to expose inner core.

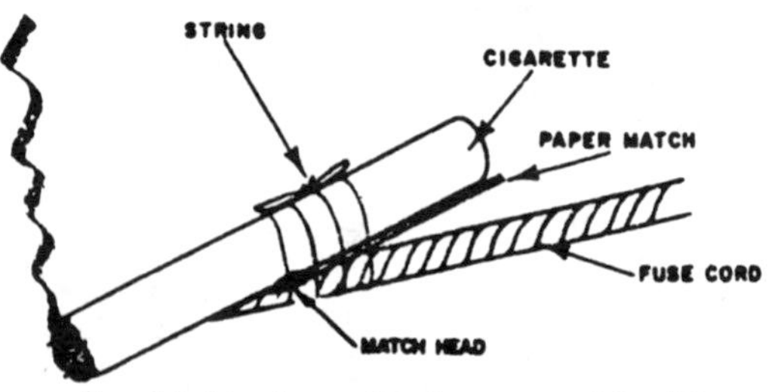

2. Light cigarette in normal fashion. Place a paper match so that the head is over exposed end of fuse cord and tie both to the side of the burning cigarette with string.

111

TWIG
STRING
TO INCENDIARY OR OTHER DEVICE
PUSH TWIG INTO GROUND

3. Position the burning cigarette with fuse so that it burns freely. A suggested method is to hang the delay on a twig.

NOTE

Common dry cigarettes burn about 1 inch every 7 or 8 minutes in still air. If the fuse cord is placed 1 inch from the burning end of a cigarette a time delay of 7 or 8 minutes will result.

Delay time will vary depending upon type of cigarette, wind, moisture, and other atmospheric conditions.

To obtain accurate delay time, a test run should be made under "use" conditions.

Section VI
112 No. 4
WATCH DELAY TIMER

A time delay device for use with electrical firing circuits can be made by using a watch with a plastic crystal.

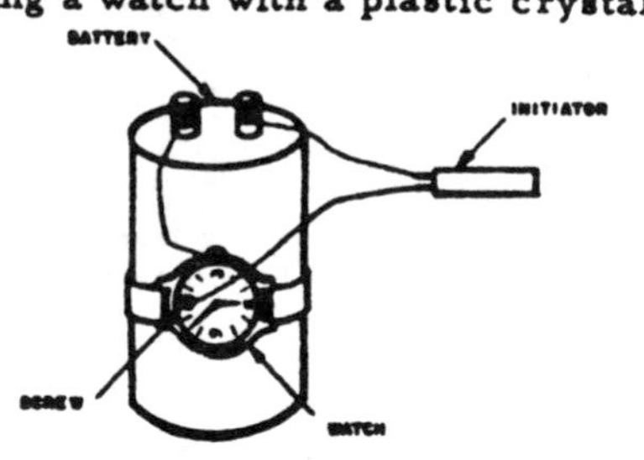

Material and Equipment Required

Watch with plastic crystal.
Small clean metal screw.
Battery.
Connecting wires.
Drill or nail.

Procedure

1. If watch has a sweep or large second hand, remove it. If delay time of more than one hour is required, also remove the minute hand. If hands are painted, carefully scrape paint from contact edge with knife.

2. Drill a hole through the crystal of the watch or pierce the crystal with a heated nail. The hole must be small enough that the screw can be tightly threaded into it.

113

3. Place the screw in the hole and turn down as far as possible without making contact with the face of the watch. If screw has a pointed tip, it may be necessary to grind the tip flat.

If no screw is available, pass a bent stiff wire through the hole and tape to the crystal.

IMPORTANT:	Check to make sure hand of watch cannot pass screw or wire without contacting it.

How to Use

1. Set the watch so that a hand will reach the screw or wire at the time you want the firing circuit completed.

2. Wind the watch.

3. Attach a wire from the case of the watch to one terminal of the battery.

4. Attach one wire from an electric initiator (blasting cap, squib, or alarm device) to the screw or wire on the face of the watch.

5. After thorough inspection is made to assure that the screw or the wire connected to it is not touching the face or case of the watch, attach the other wire from the initiator to the second terminal of the battery.

> CAUTION
>
> Follow step 5 carefully to prevent premature initiation.

Section VI
114 No. 5
NO-FLASH FUSE IGNITER

A simple no-flash fuse igniter can be made from common pipe fittings.

MATERIAL REQUIRED:

1/4 in. (6mm) Pipe Cap
Solid 1/4 in. (6mm) Pipe Plug
Flat head nail about 1/16 in. (1 1/2 mm) in diameter
Hand Drill
Common "Strike Anywhere" Matches
Adhesive Tape

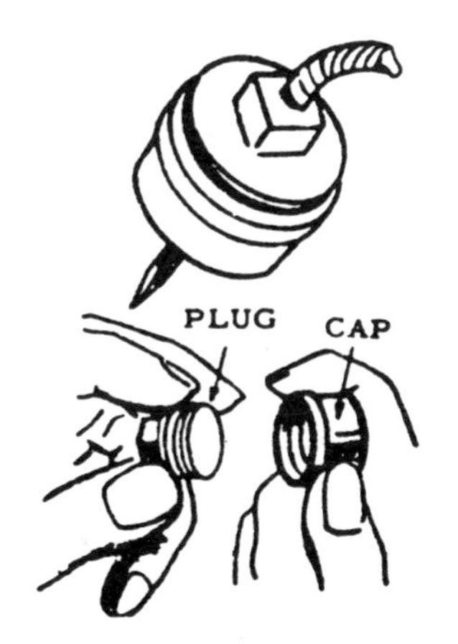

PROCEDURE:

1. Screw the pipe plug tightly into the pipe cap.

2. Drill hole completely through the center of the plug and cap large enough that the nail fits loosely.

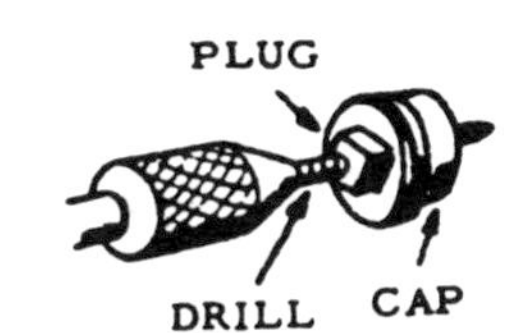

3. Enlarge the hole in the plug except for the last 1/8 in. (3 mm) so that the fuse cord will just fit.

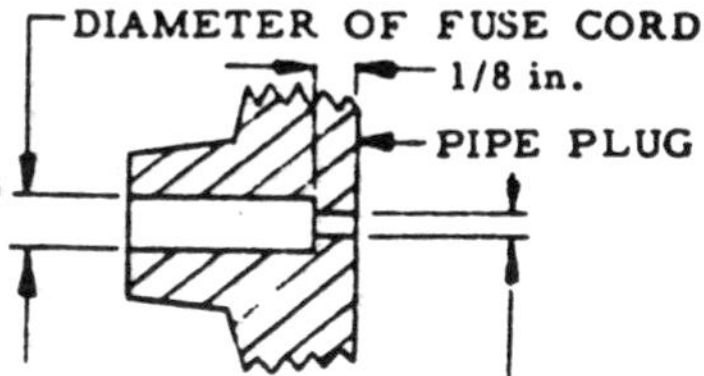

4. Remove the plug from the cap and push the flat head nail through the hole in the cap from the inside.

NAIL
PIPE CAP

115

5. Cut the striking tips from approximately 10 strike-anywhere matches. Place match tips inside pipe cap and screw plug in finger tight.

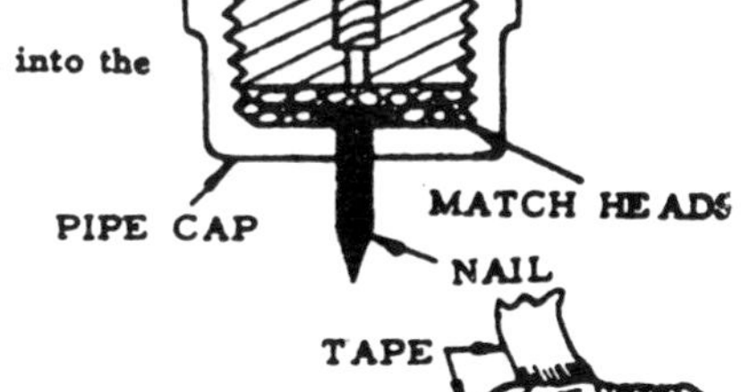

HOW TO USE:

1. Slide the fuse cord into the hole in the pipe plug.

2. Tape igniter to fuse cord.

TAPE

3. Tap point of nail on a hard surface to ignite the fuse.

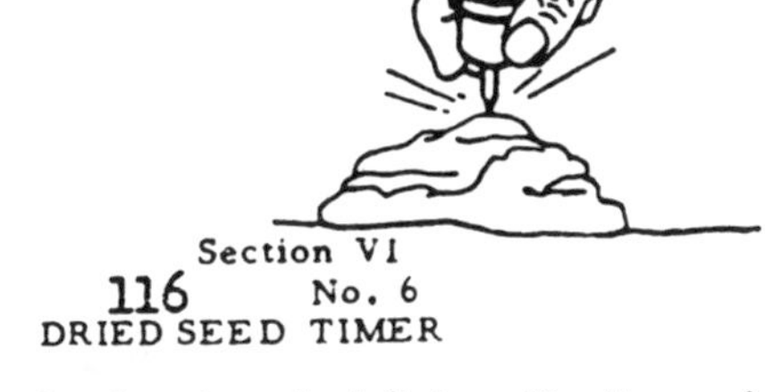

Section VI
116 No. 6
DRIED SEED TIMER

A time delay device for electrical firing circuits can be made using the principle of expansion of dried seeds.

MATERIEL REQUIRED:

Dried peas, beans or other dehydrated seeds

Wide mouth glass jar with non-metal cap
Two screws or bolts
Thin metal plate
Hand drill
Screwdriver

PROCEDURE:

1. Determine the rate of rise of the dried seeds selected. This is necessary to determine delay time of the timer.

   a. Place a sample of the dried seeds in the jar and cover with water.

   b. Measure the time it takes for the seeds to rise a given height. Most dried seeds increase 50% in one to two hours.

2. Cut a disc from thin metal plate. Disc should fit loosely inside the jar.

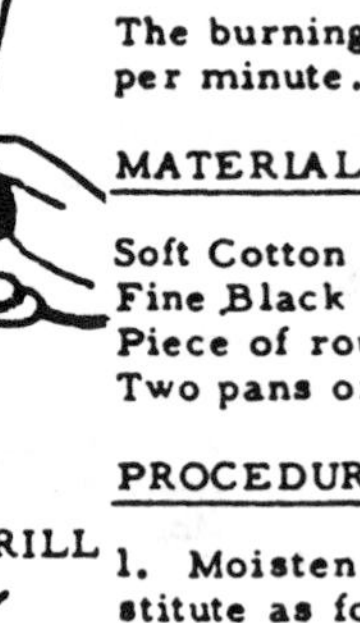

NOTE: If metal is painted, rusty or otherwise coated, it must be scraped or sanded to obtain a clean metal surface.

3. Drill two holes in the cap of the jar about 2 inches apart. Diameter of holes should be such that screws or bolts will thread tightly into them. If the jar has a metal cap or no cap, a piece of wood or plastic (NOT METAL) can be used as a cover.

DRILL

CAP

117

4. Turn the two screws or bolts through the holes in the cap. Bolts should extend about one in. (2 1/2 cm) into the jar.

IMPORTANT: Both bolts must extend the same distance below the container cover.

JAR CAP

BOLT

5. Pour dried seeds into the container. The level will depend upon the previously measured rise time and the desired delay.

METAL DISC

6. Place the metal disc in the jar on top of the seeds.

JAR

DRIED SEEDS

HOW TO USE:

1. Add just enough water to completely cover the seeds and place the cap on the jar.

2. Attach connecting wires from the firing circuit to the two screws on the cap.

CONNECTING WIRES

METAL DISC

DRIED SEEDS

Expansion of the seeds will raise the metal disc until it contacts the screws and closes the circuit.

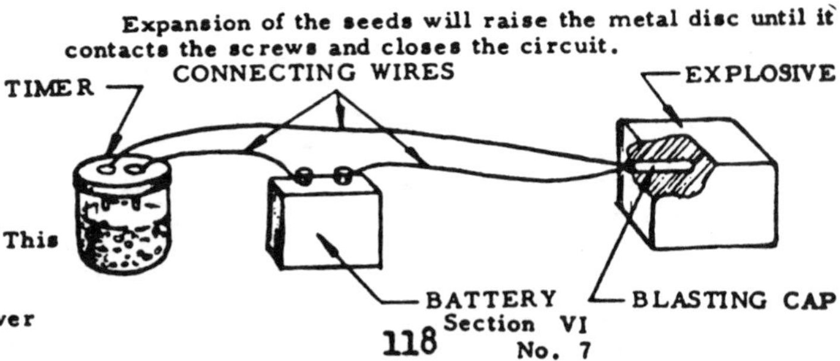

118 Section VI No. 7

FUSE CORDS

These fuse cords are used for igniting propellants and incendiaries or, with a non-electric blasting cap, to detonate explosives.

FAST BURNING FUSE

The burning rate of this fuse is approximately 40 in. (100 cm) per minute.

MATERIAL REQUIRED:

Soft Cotton String
Fine Black Powder --or-- { Potassium Nitrate (Saltpeter) 25 parts; Charcoal 3 parts; Sulphur 2 parts }
Piece of round stick
Two pans or dishes

PROCEDURE:

1. Moisten fine Black Powder to form a paste or prepare a substitute as follows:

   a. Dissolve Potassium Nitrate in an equal amount of water.

   b. Pulverize charcoal by spreading thinly on a hard surface and rolling the round stick over it to crush to a fine powder.

   c. Pulverize sulphur in the same manner.

   d. Dry mix sulphur and charcoal.

   e. Add Potassium Nitrate solution to the dry mix to obtain a thoroughly wet paste.

STRING NAIL

BOARD

2. Twist or braid three strands of cotton string together.

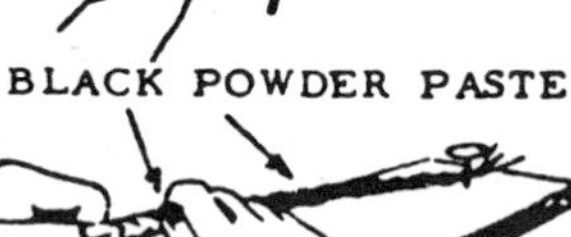

3. Rub paste mixture into twisted string with fingers and allow to dry.

119

4. Check actual burning rate of fuse by measuring the time it takes for a known length to burn. This is used to determine the length needed for a desired delay time. If 5 in. (12 1/2 cm) burns for 6 seconds, 50 in. (125 cm) of fuse cord will be needed to obtain a one minute (60 second) delay time.

SLOW BURNING FUSE

The burning rate of this fuse is approximately 2 in. (5 cm) per minute.

MATERIAL REQUIRED:

Cotton String or 3 Shoelaces
Potassium Nitrate or Potassium Chlorate
Granulated Sugar

PROCEDURE:

1. Wash cotton-string or shoelaces in hot soapy water; rinse in fresh water.

2. Dissolve 1 part Potassium Nitrate or Potassium Chlorate and 1 part granulated sugar in 2 parts hot water.

3. Soak string or shoelaces in solution.

4. Twist or braid three strands of string together and allow to dry.

5. Check actual burning rate of the fuse by measuring the time it takes for a known length to burn. This is used to determine the length needed for the desired delay time. If 2 in. (5 cm) burns for 1 minute, 10 in. (25 cm) will be needed to obtain a 5 minute delay.

NOTE: The last few inches of this cord (the end inserted in the material to be ignited) should be coated with the fast burning Black Powder paste if possible. This must be done when the fuse is used to ignite a blasting cap.

> REMEMBER: The burning rate of either of these fuses can vary greatly. Do Not Use for ignition until you have checked their burning rate.

Section VI
120 No. 8
CLOTHESPIN TIME DELAY SWITCH

A 3 to 5 minute time delay switch can be made from the clothespin switch (Section VII, No. 1) and a cigarette. The system can be used for initiation of explosive charges, mines, and booby traps.

MATERIAL REQUIRED:

Spring type clothespin
Solid or stranded copper wire about 1/16 in. (2 mm) in diameter (field or bell wire is suitable)
Fine string, about 6 inches in length
Cigarette
Knife

PROCEDURE:

1. Strip about 4 inches (10 cm) of insulation from the ends of 2 copper wires. Scrape copper wires with pocket knife until metal is shiny.

2. Wind one scraped wire tightly on one jaw of the clothespin, and the other wire on the other jaw so that the wires will be in contact with each other when the jaws are closed.

3. Measuring from tip of cigarette, measure a length of cigarette that will correspond to the desired delay time. Make a hole in cigarette at this point, using wire or pin.

Burning Length
Pin or Wire
121

NOTE: Delay time may be adjusted by varying the burning length of the cigarette. Burning rate in still air is approximately 7 minutes per inch (2.5 cm). Since this rate varies with environment and brand of cigarette, it should be tested in each case if accurate delay time is desired.

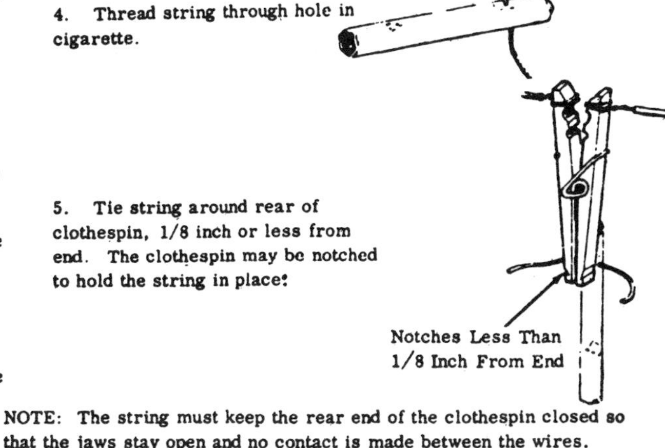

4. Thread string through hole in cigarette.

5. Tie string around rear of clothespin, 1/8 inch or less from end. The clothespin may be notched to hold the string in place.

NOTE: The string must keep the rear end of the clothespin closed so that the jaws stay open and no contact is made between the wires.

HOW TO USE:

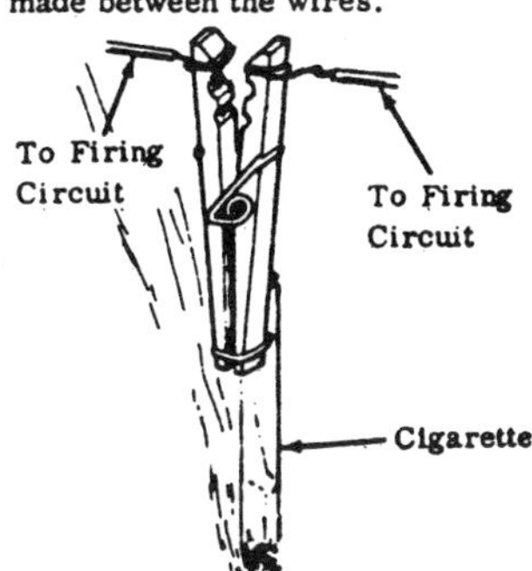

Suspend the entire system vertically with the cigarette tip down. Light tip of cigarette. Switch will close and initiation will occur when the cigarette burns up to and through the string.

NOTE: Wires to the firing circuit must not be pulled taut when the switch is mounted. This could prevent the jaws from closing.

SECTION VI
122 No. 9
TIME DELAY GRENADE

This delay mechanism makes it possible to use an ordinary grenade as a time bomb.

MATERIAL REQUIRED:

Grenade
Fuse Cord

IMPORTANT: Fuse cord must be the type that burns completely. Fast burning improvised fuse cord (Section VI, No. 7) is suitable. Safety fuse is not satisfactory, since its outer covering does not burn.

PROCEDURE:

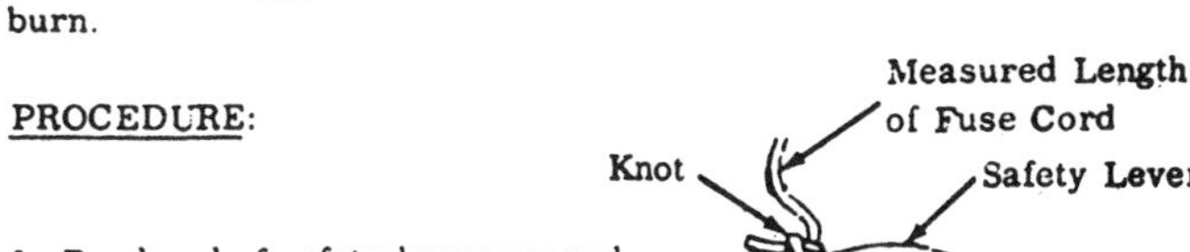

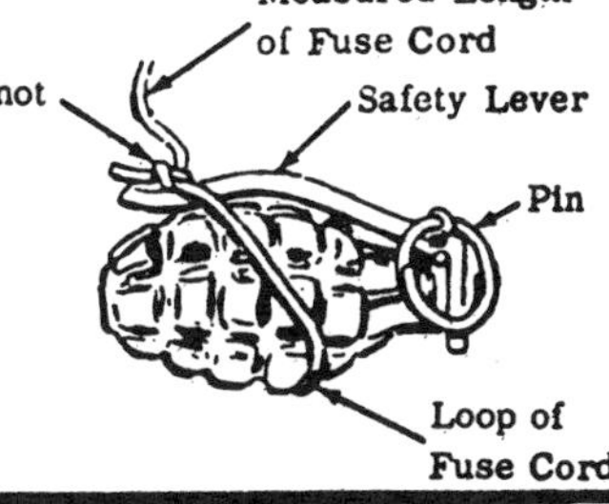

1. Bend end of safety lever upward to form a hook. Make a single loop of fuse cord around the center of the grenade body and safety lever. Tie a knot of the non-slip variety at the safety lever.

> NOTE: The loop must be tight enough to hold the safety lever in position when the pin is removed.

2. Measuring from the knot along the free length of the fuse cord, measure off a length of fuse cord that will give the desired delay time. Cut off the excess fuse cord.

HOW TO USE:

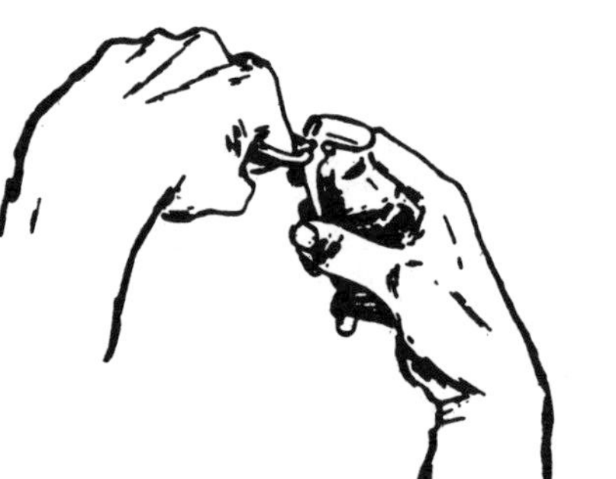

1. Place hand around grenade and safety lever so safety lever is held in place. Carefully remove pin.

2. Emplace grenade in desired location while holding grenade and safety lever.

3. Very carefully remove hand from grenade and safety lever, making sure that the fuse cord holds the safety lever in place.

123

> **CAUTION: If loop and knot of fuse cord do not hold for any reason and the safety lever is released, the grenade will explode after the regular delay time.**

4. Light free end of fuse cord.

Section VI

124 No. 10

CAN-LIQUID TIME DELAY

A time delay device for electrical firing circuits can be made using a can and liquid.

MATERIAL REQUIRED:

Can
Liquid (water, gasoline, etc.)
Small block of wood or any material that will float on the liquid used
Knife
2 pieces of solid wire, each piece 1 foot (30 cm) or longer

PROCEDURE:

1. Make 2 small holes at opposite sides of the can very close to the top.

2. Remove insulation from a long piece of wire for a distance a little greater than the diameter of the can.

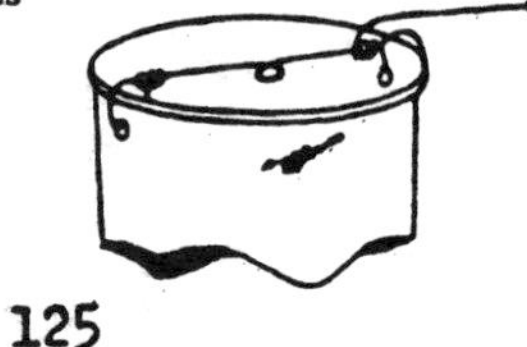

3. Secure the wire in place across the top of the can by threading it through the holes and twisting in place, leaving some slack. Make loop in center or wire. Be sure a long piece of wire extends from one end of the can.

125

4. Wrap a piece of insulated wire around the block of wood. Scrape insulation from a small section of this wire and bend as shown so that wire contacts loop before wood touches bottom of container. Thread this wire through the loop of bare wire.

5. Make a very small hole (pinhole) in the side of the container. Fill container with a quantity of liquid corresponding to the desired delay time. Since the rate at which liquid leaves the can depends upon weather conditions, liquid used, size of hole, amount of liquid in the container, etc., determine the delay time for each individual case. Delays from a few minutes to many hours are possible. Vary time by adjusting liquid level, type of liquid (water, oil) and hole size.

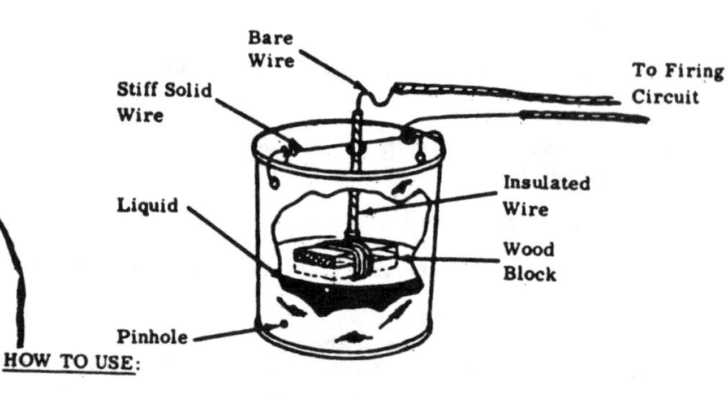

HOW TO USE:

1. Fill can with liquid to the same level as during experimental run (step 5 above). Be sure that wooden block floats on liquid and that wire is free to move down as liquid leaves container.

2. Connect wires to firing circuit.

NOTE: A long term delay can be obtained by placing a volatile liquid (gasoline, ether, etc.) in the can instead of water and relying on evaporation to lower the level. Be sure that the wood will float on the liquid used. DO NOT MAKE PINHOLE IN SIDE OF CAN!

Section VI

126 No. 11

SHORT TERM TIME DELAY FOR GRENADE

A simple modification can produce delays of approximately 12 seconds for grenades when fired from Grenade Launchers (Section IV, No. 5).

MATERIAL REQUIRED:

Grenade
Nail
Knife } may not be needed
Pliers }
Safety fuse

NOTE: Any safety or improvised fuse may be used. However, since different time delays will result, determine the burning rate of the fuse first.

PROCEDURE:

1. Unscrew fuse mechanism from body of grenade and remove. Pliers may have to be used.

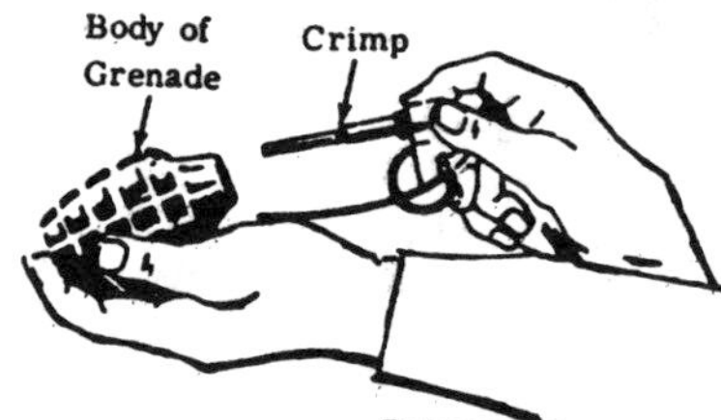

2. Carefully cut with knife or break off detonator at crimp and save for later use.

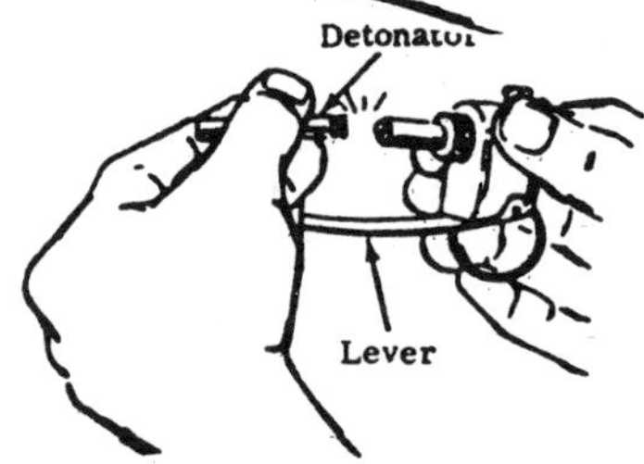

> CAUTION: If detonator is cut or broken below the crimp, detonation may occur and severe injuries could result.

3. Remove safety pin pull ring and lever, letting striker hit the primer. Place fuse mechanism aside until delay fuse powder mix in mechanism is completely burned.

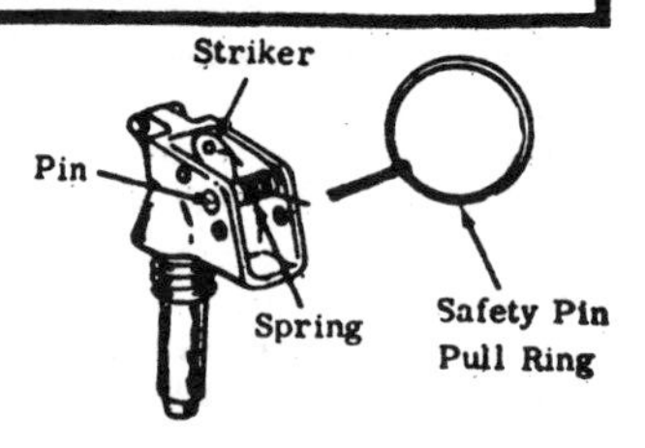

127

4. Remove pin, spring, and striker.

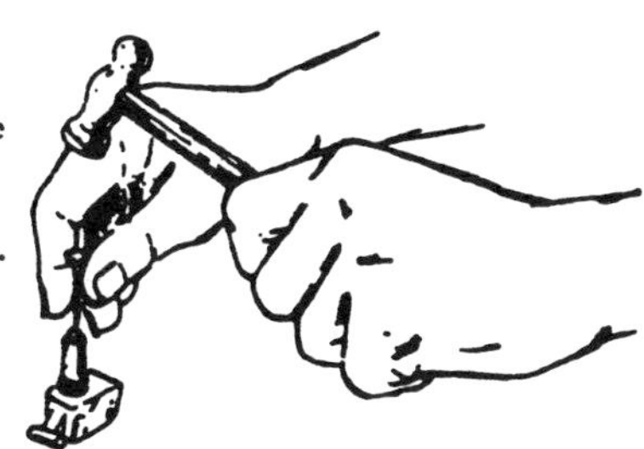

5. Remove primer from fuse mechanism by pushing nail through bottom end of primer hole and tapping with hammer.

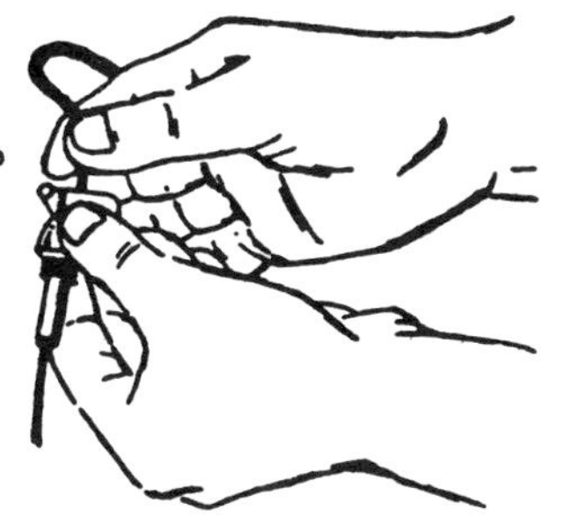

6. Insert safety fuse through top of primer hole. Enlarge hole if necessary. The fuse should go completely through the hole.

7. Insert fuse into detonator and tape it securely to modified fuse mechanism.

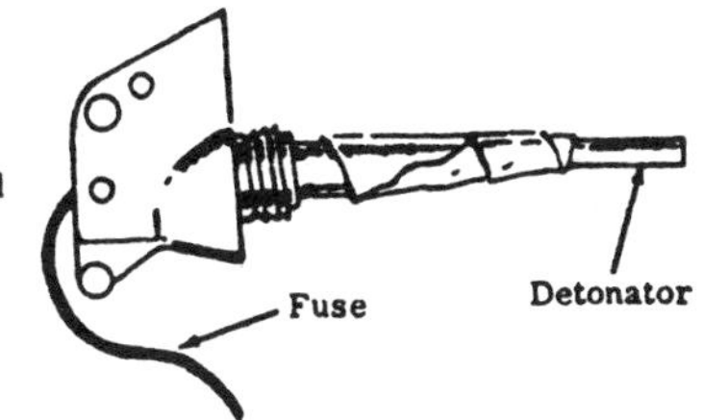

NOTE: Be sure that fuse rests firmly against detonator at all times.

8. Screw modified fuse mechanism back into grenade. Grenade is now ready for use.

128

NOTE: If time delay is used for Improvised Grenade Launchers (Section IV, No. 5) -

1. Wrap tape around safety fuse.
2. Securely tape fuse to grenade.
3. Load grenade in launcher. Grenade will explode in approximately 12 seconds after safety fuse burns up to bottom of grenade.

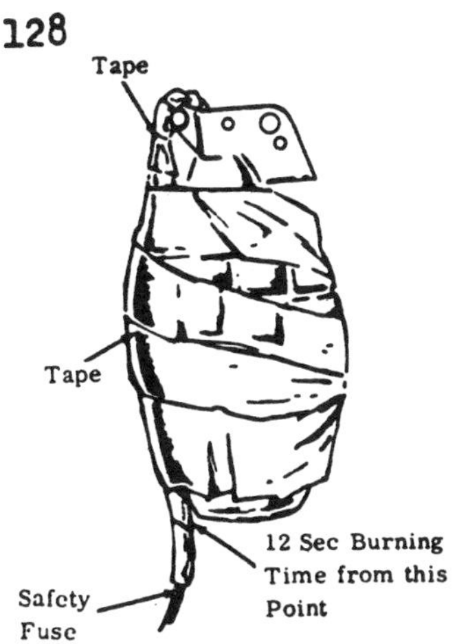

129 Section VI
No. 12

LONG TERM TIME DELAY FOR GRENADE

A simple modification can produce delays of approximately 20 seconds for grenades when fired from Grenade Launchers (Section IV, No. 5).

MATERIAL REQUIRED:

Grenade
Nail
"Strike-anywhere" matches, 6 to 8
Pliers (may not be needed)
Knife or sharp cutting edge
Piece of wood
Safety fuse

NOTE: Any safety or improvised fuse may be used. However, since different time delays will result, determine the burning rate of the fuse first.

PROCEDURE:

1. Unscrew fuse mechanism from body of grenade and remove. Pliers may have to be used.

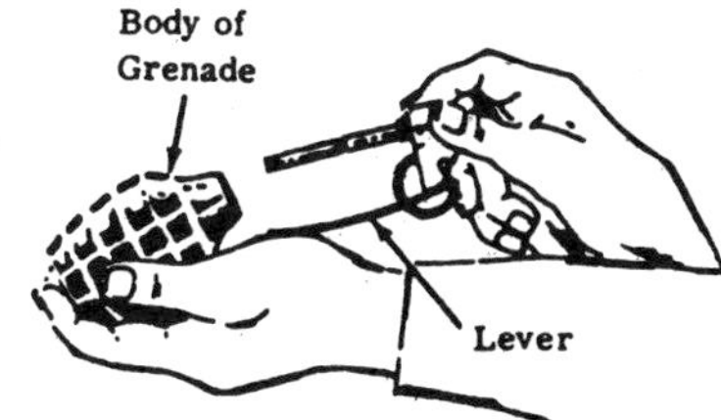

2. Insert nail completely through safety hole (hole over primer).

3. Carefully remove safety pin pull ring and lever, and allow striker to hit nail.

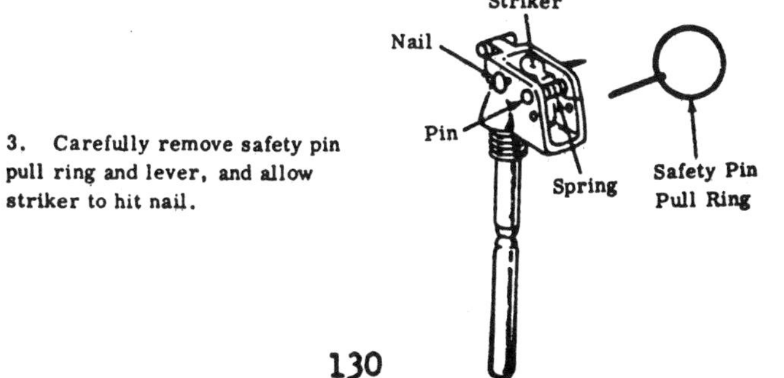

130

CAUTION: If for any reason, striker should hit primer instead of nail, detonator will explode after (4-5 sec.) delay time.

4. Push pin out and remove spring and striker. Remove nail.

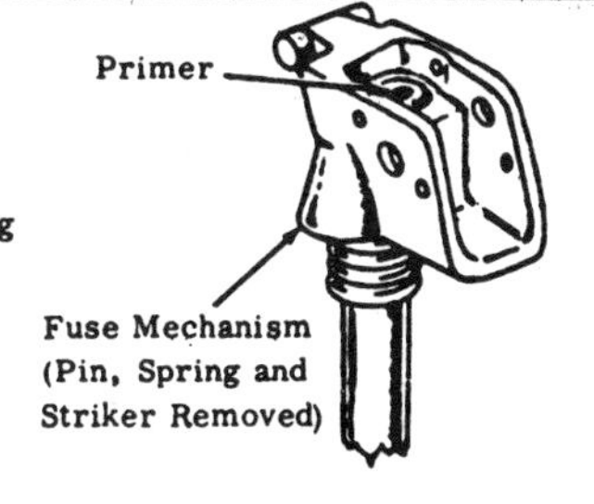

5. Carefully remove top section of fuse mechanism from bottom section by unscrewing. Pliers may have to be used.

CAUTION: Use extreme care - sudden shock may set off detonator.

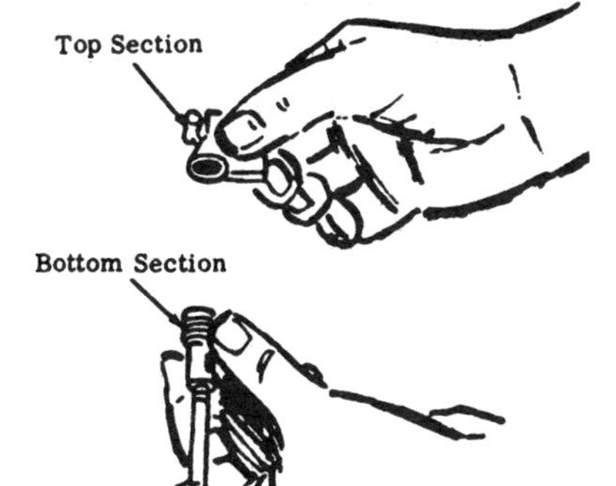

6. Fire primer by hitting nail placed against top of it. Remove fired primer (same as procedure 5 of Section VI, No. 11).

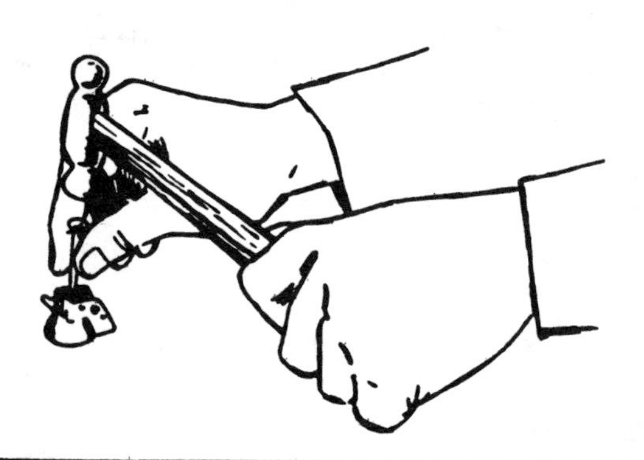

CAUTION: Do not hold assembly in your hand during above operation, as serious burns may result.

131

7. Scrape delay fuse powder with a sharpened stick. Loosen about 1/4 in. (6 mm) of powder in cavity.

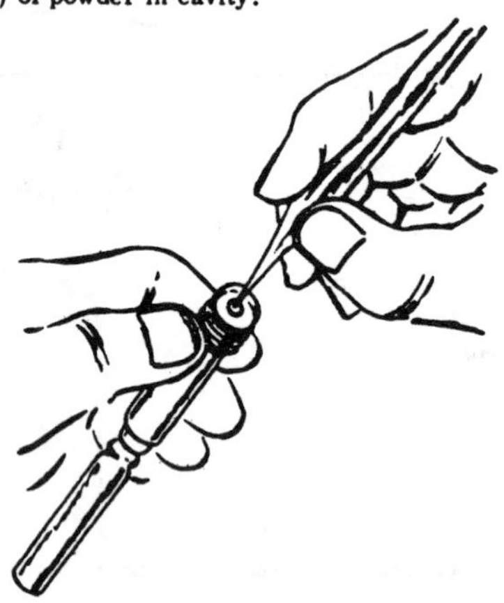

8. Cut off tips (not whole head) of 6 "strike-anywhere" matches with sharp cutting edge. Drop them into delay fuse hole.

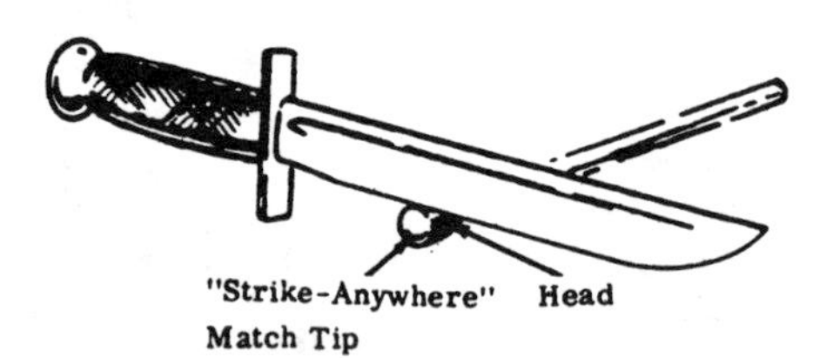

9. Place safety fuse in delay fuse hole so that it is flush against the match tips.

IMPORTANT: Be sure fuse remains flush against the match tips at all times.

10. Thread fuse through primer hole. Enlarge hole if necessary. Screw modified fuse mechanism back together. Screw combination back into grenade. Grenade modification is now ready for use. Light fuse when ready to use.

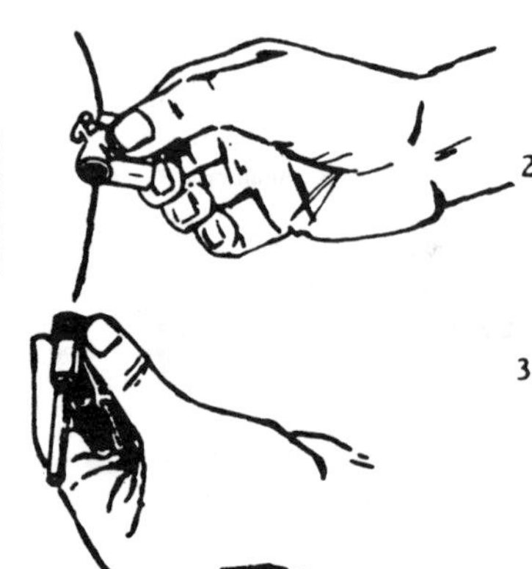

132

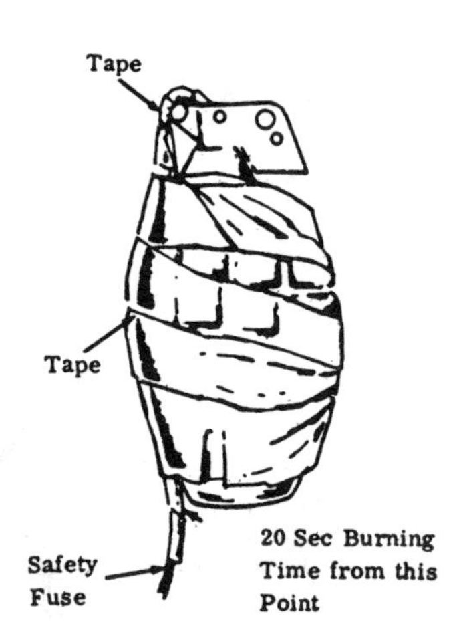

NOTE: If time delay is used for Improvised Grenade Launchers (Section IV, No. 5) -

1. Wrap tape around safety fuse.
2. Securely tape fuse to grenade
3. Load grenade in launcher. Grenade will explode in approximately 20 seconds after safety fuse burns up to bottom of grenade.

Section VII

133 No. 1

CLOTHESPIN SWITCH

A spring type clothespin is used to make a circuit closing switch to actuate explosive charges, mines, booby traps and alarm systems.

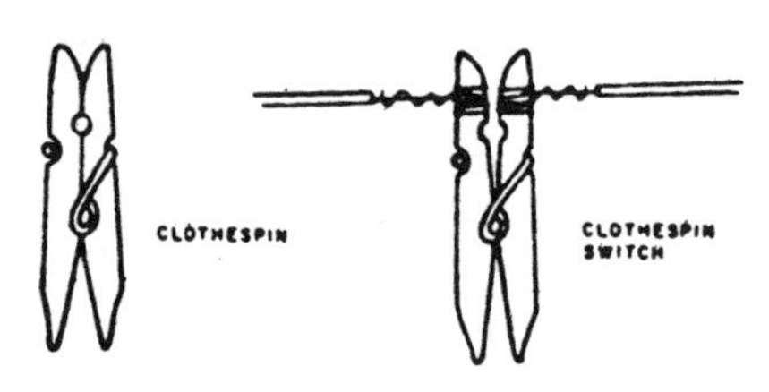

Material Required

Spring type clothespin.
Solid copper wire -- 1/16 in. (2 mm) in diameter.
Strong string on wire.
Flat piece of wood (roughly 1/8 x 1" x 2").
Knife.

Procedure

1. Strip four in. (10 cm) of insulation from the ends of 2 solid copper wires. Scrape copper wires with pocket knife until metal is shiny.

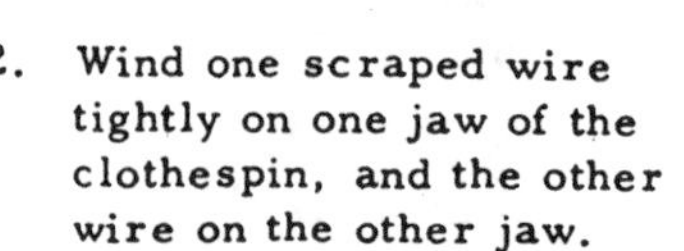

2. Wind one scraped wire tightly on one jaw of the clothespin, and the other wire on the other jaw.

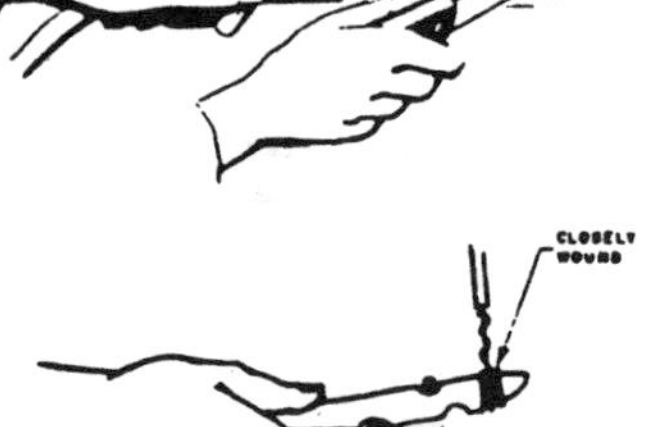

3. Make a hole in one end of the flat piece of wood using a knife, heated nail or drill Tie strong string or wire through the hole.

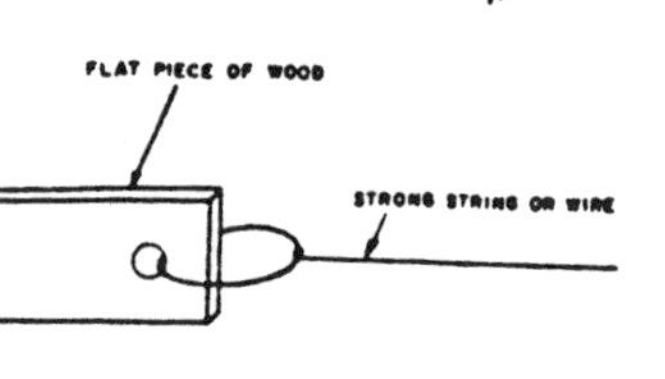

134

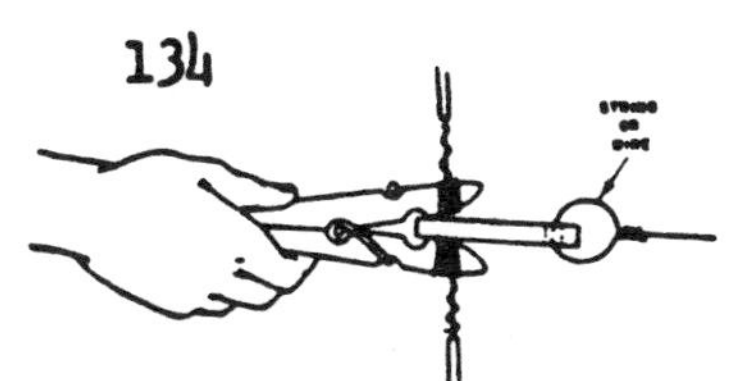

5. Place flat piece of wood between jaws of the clothespin switch.

Basic Firing Circuit

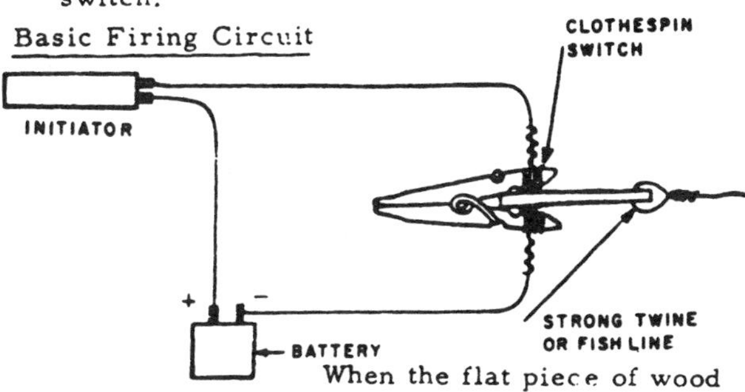

When the flat piece of wood is removed by pulling the string, the jaws of the clothespin will close completing the circuit.

CAUTION

Do not attach the battery until the switch and trip wire have been emplaced and examined. Be sure the flat piece of wood is separating the jaws of the switch.

A Method of Use

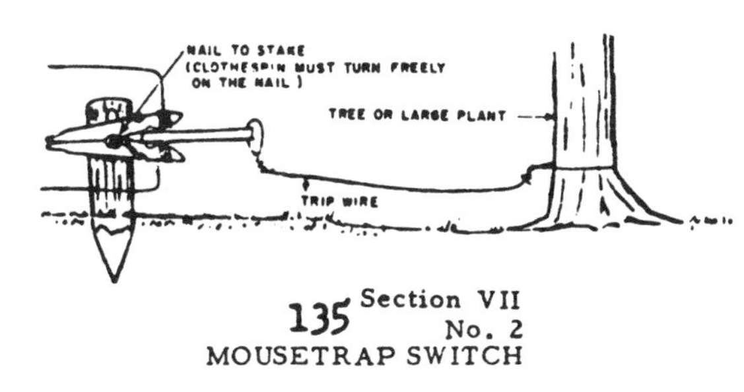

135 Section VII No. 2

MOUSETRAP SWITCH

A common mousetrap can be used to make a circuit closing switch for electrically initiated explosives, mines and booby traps.

MATERIEL REQUIRED:

Mousetrap
Hacksaw or File
Connecting wires

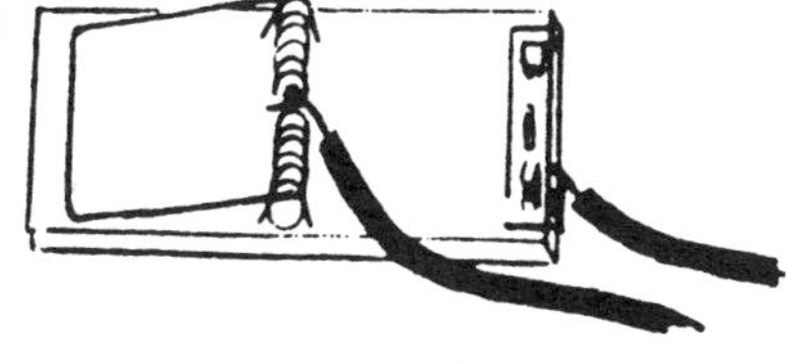

TRIP LEVER

STAPLE

PROCEDURE:

1. Remove the trip lever from the mousetrap using a hacksaw or file. Also remove the staple and holding wire.

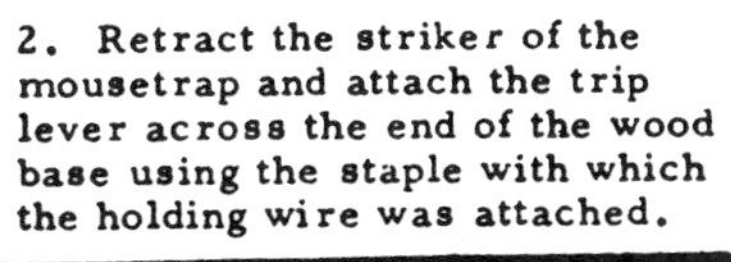

2. Retract the striker of the mousetrap and attach the trip lever across the end of the wood base using the staple with which the holding wire was attached.

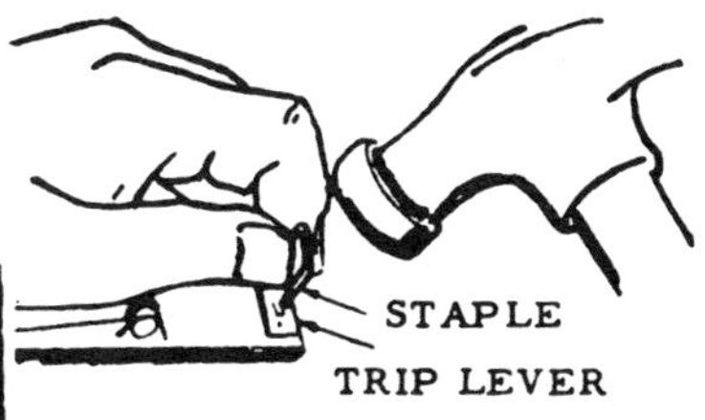

NOTE: If the trip lever is not made of metal, a piece of metal of approximately the same size should be used.

3. Strip one in. (2 1/2 cm) of insulation from the ends of 2 connecting wires.

4. Wrap one wire tightly around the spring loaded striker of the mousetrap.

136

5. Wrap the second wire around some part of the trip lever or piece of metal.

NOTE: If a soldering iron is available, solder both of the wires in place.

CONNECTING WIRES

HOW TO USE:

This switch can be used in a number of ways -- one typical method is presented here.

The switch is placed inside a box which also contains the explosive and batteries. The spring loaded striker is held back by the lid of the box and when the box is opened the circuit is closed.

Shelf Explosive Blasting Cap
Mousetrap Switch
Box
Battery

137 Section VII No. 3

FLEXIBLE PLATE SWITCH

This pressure sensitive switch is used for initiating emplaced mines and explosives.

MATERIAL REQUIRED:

Two flexible metal sheets
 one approximately 10 in. (25 cm) square
 one approximately 10 in. x 8 in. (20 cm)
Piece of wood 10 in. square by 1 in. thick
Four soft wood blocks 1 in. x 1 in. x 1/4 in.
Eight flat head nails, 1 in. long
Connecting wires
Adhesive tape

PROCEDURE:

1. Nail 10 in. x 8 in. metal sheet to 10 in. square piece of wood so that 1 in. of wood shows on each side of metal. Leave one of the nails sticking up about 1/4 in.

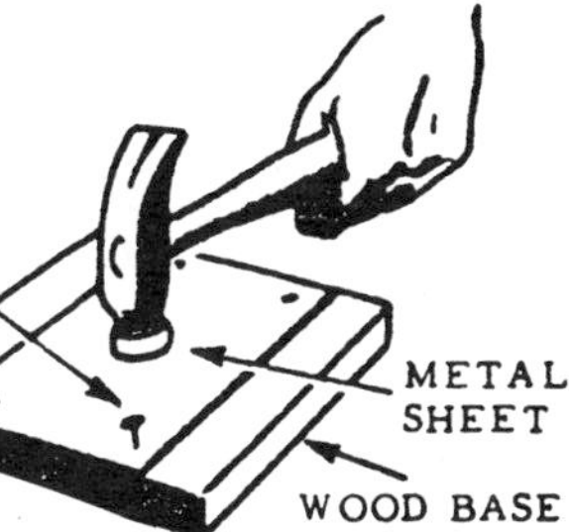

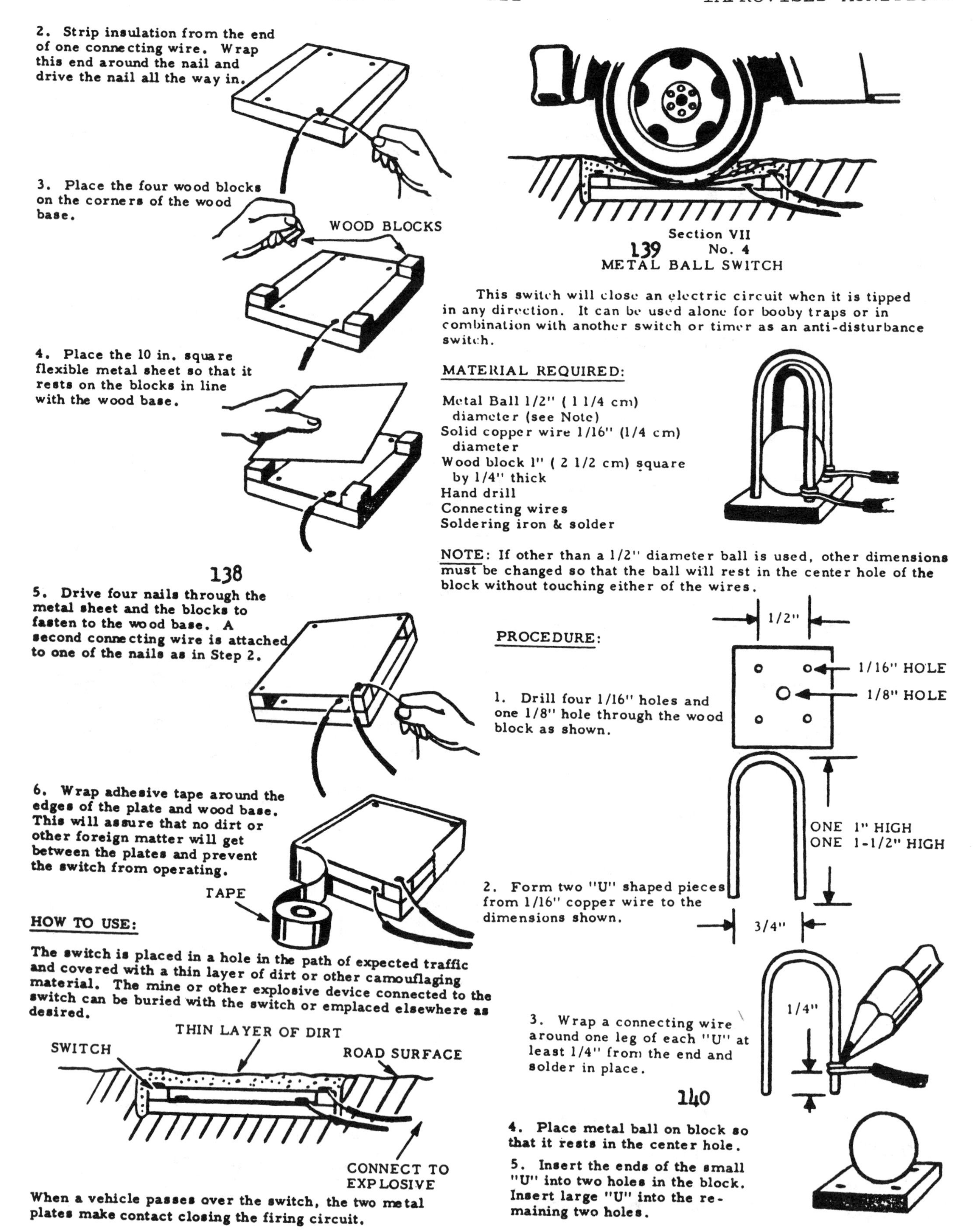

2. Strip insulation from the end of one connecting wire. Wrap this end around the nail and drive the nail all the way in.

3. Place the four wood blocks on the corners of the wood base.

4. Place the 10 in. square flexible metal sheet so that it rests on the blocks in line with the wood base.

138

5. Drive four nails through the metal sheet and the blocks to fasten to the wood base. A second connecting wire is attached to one of the nails as in Step 2.

6. Wrap adhesive tape around the edges of the plate and wood base. This will assure that no dirt or other foreign matter will get between the plates and prevent the switch from operating.

HOW TO USE:

The switch is placed in a hole in the path of expected traffic and covered with a thin layer of dirt or other camouflaging material. The mine or other explosive device connected to the switch can be buried with the switch or emplaced elsewhere as desired.

When a vehicle passes over the switch, the two metal plates make contact closing the firing circuit.

Section VII
139 No. 4
METAL BALL SWITCH

This switch will close an electric circuit when it is tipped in any direction. It can be used alone for booby traps or in combination with another switch or timer as an anti-disturbance switch.

MATERIAL REQUIRED:

Metal Ball 1/2" (1 1/4 cm) diameter (see Note)
Solid copper wire 1/16" (1/4 cm) diameter
Wood block 1" (2 1/2 cm) square by 1/4" thick
Hand drill
Connecting wires
Soldering iron & solder

NOTE: If other than a 1/2" diameter ball is used, other dimensions must be changed so that the ball will rest in the center hole of the block without touching either of the wires.

PROCEDURE:

1. Drill four 1/16" holes and one 1/8" hole through the wood block as shown.

2. Form two "U" shaped pieces from 1/16" copper wire to the dimensions shown.

3. Wrap a connecting wire around one leg of each "U" at least 1/4" from the end and solder in place.

140

4. Place metal ball on block so that it rests in the center hole.

5. Insert the ends of the small "U" into two holes in the block. Insert large "U" into the remaining two holes.

CAUTION: Make sure that the metal ball does not touch either "U" shaped wire when the switch is standing on its base. If the ball does touch, bend wires outward slightly.

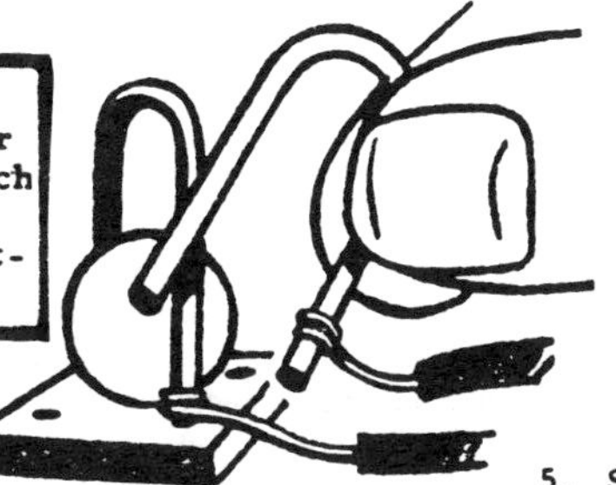

HOW TO USE:

Mount switch vertically and connect in electrical firing circuit as with any other switch. When tipped in any direction it will close the circuit.

CAUTION: Switch must be mounted vertically and not disturbed while completing connections.

141 Section VII
No. 5
ALTIMETER SWITCH

This switch is designed for use with explosives placed on aircraft. It will close an electrical firing circuit when an altitude of approximately 5000 ft (1-1/2 KM) is reached.

MATERIAL REQUIRED:

Jar or tin can
Thin sheet of flexible plastic or waxed paper
Thin metal sheet (cut from tin can)
Adhesive Tape
Connecting Wires

PROCEDURE:

1. Place sheet of plastic or waxed paper over the top of the can or jar and tape tightly to sides of container.

NOTE: Plastic sheet should not be stretched tight. A small depression should be left in the top.

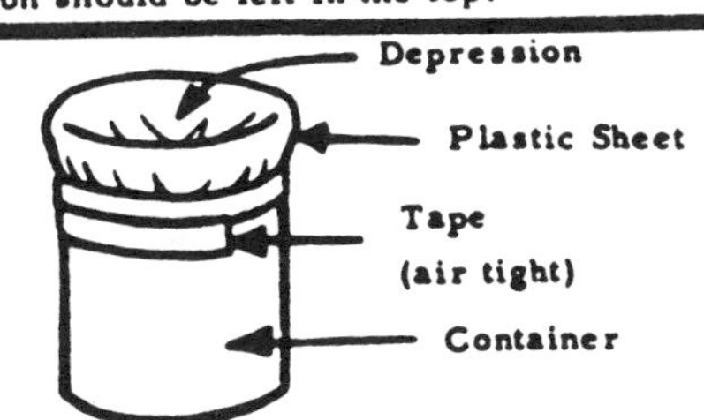

2. Cut two contact strips from thin metal and bend to the shapes shown.

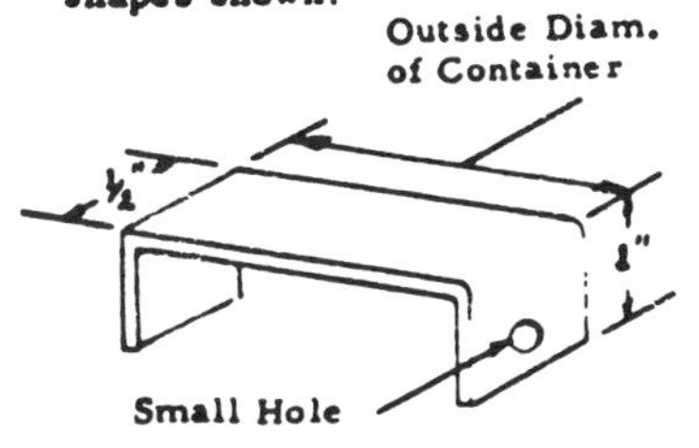

3. Strip insulation from the ends of two connecting wires. Attach one wire to each contact strip.

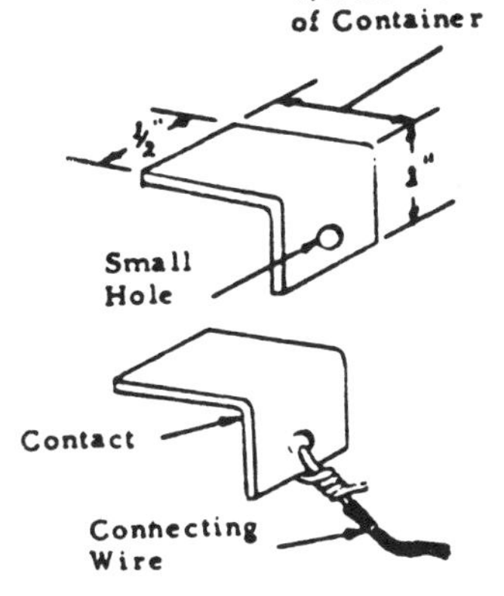

NOTE: If a soldering iron is available solder wires in place.

142

4. Place contact strips over container so that the larger contact is above the smaller with a very small clearance between the two.

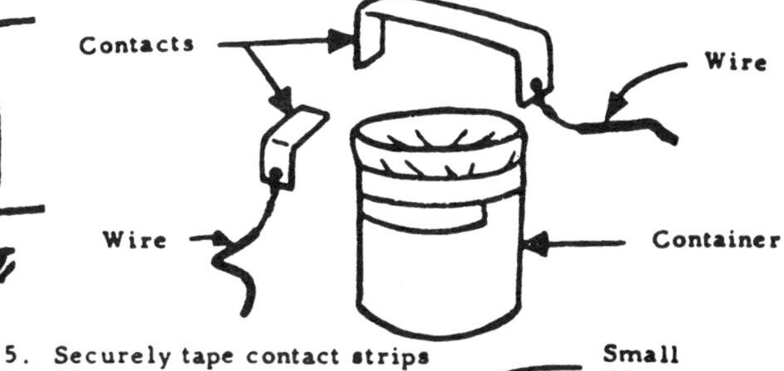

5. Securely tape contact strips to sides of container.

Small Clearance
Contacts Taped To Container

HOW TO USE:

1. Connect the altimeter switch in an explosive circuit the same as any switch.

2. Place the explosive package on airplane. As the plane rises the air inside the container will expand. This forces the plastic sheet against the contacts closing the firing circuit.

NOTE: The switch will not function in a pressurized cabin. It must be placed in some part of the plane which will not be pressurized.

143 Section VII
No. 6
PULL-LOOP SWITCH

This switch will initiate explosive charges, mines, and booby traps when the trip wire is pulled.

MATERIAL REQUIRED:

2 lengths of insulated wire
Knife
Strong string or cord
Fine thread that will break easily

PROCEDURE:

1. Remove about 2 inches of insulation from one end of each length of wire. Scrape bare wire with knife until metal is shiny.

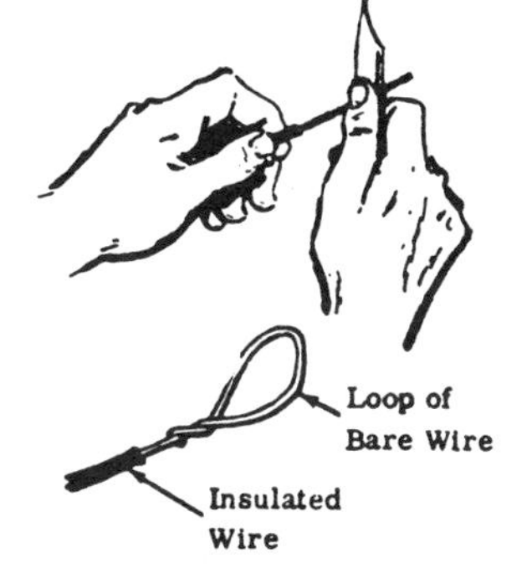

2. Make a loop out of each piece of bare wire.

3. Thread each wire through the loop of the other wire so the wires can slide along each other.

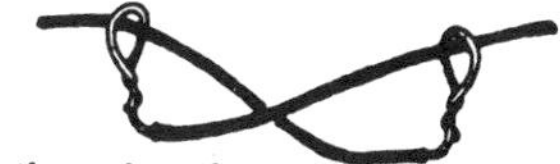

NOTE: The loops should contact each other when the two wires are pulled taut.

144

HOW TO USE:

1. Separate loops by about 2 inches. Tie piece of fine thread around wires near each loop Thread should be taut enough to support loops and wire, yet fine enough that it will break under a very slight pull.

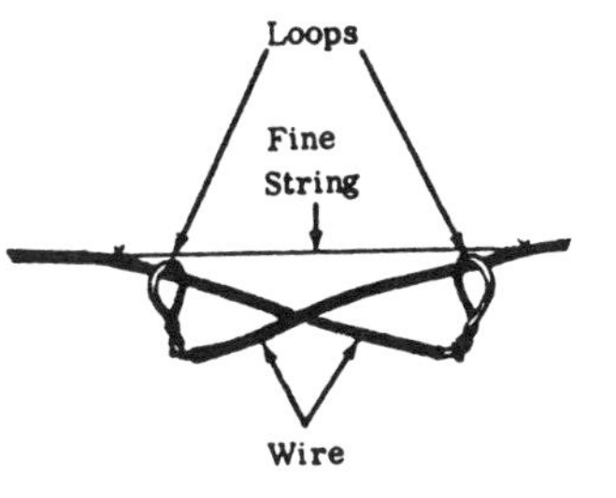

2. Fasten one wire to tree or stake and connect end to firing circuit.

3. Tie a piece of cord or string around the other piece of wire a few inches from the loop. Tie free end of cord around tree, bush, or stake. Connect the free end of the wire to the firing circuit. Initiation will occur when the tripcord is pulled.

CAUTION: Be sure that the loops do not contact each other when the wires are connected to the firing circuit.

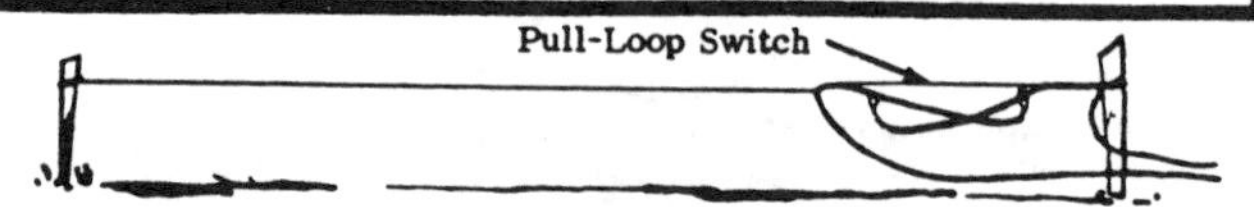

OTHER USES: The switch minus the fine thread may be used to activate a booby trap by such means as attaching it between the lid and a rigid portion of a box, between a door and a door jamb, and in similar manners.

145 Section VII No. 7

KNIFE SWITCH

This device will close the firing circuit charges, mines, and booby traps when the trip wire is pulled or cut.

MATERIAL REQUIRED:

Knife or hack saw blade
6 nails
Strong string or light rope
Sturdy wooden board
Wire

PROCEDURE:

1. Place knife on board. Drive 2 nails into board on each side of knife handle so knife is held in place.

2. Drive one nail into board so that it touches blade of knife near the point.

3. Attach rope to knife. Place rope across path. Apply tension to rope, pulling knife blade away from nail slightly. Tie rope to tree, bush, or stake.

4. Drive another nail into board near the tip of the knife blade as shown below. Connect the two nails with a piece of conducting wire. Nail should be positioned so that it will contact the second nail when blade is pulled about 1 inch (2-1/2 cm) to the side.

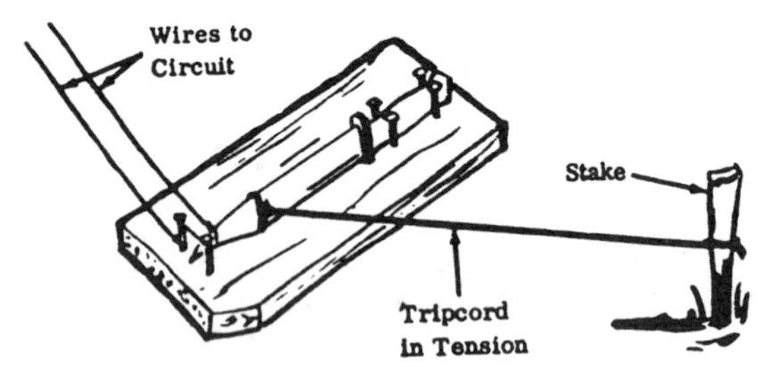

NOTE: Check position of nails to knife blade. The nails should be placed so that the knife blade will contact either one when the rope is pulled or released.

HOW TO USE:

Attach one wire from firing circuit to one of the nails and the other to the knife blade. The circuit will be completed when the tripcord is pulled or released.

146 Section VII No. 8

IMPROVISED SCALE

This scale provides a means of weighing propellant and other items when conventional scales or balances are not available.

MATERIAL REQUIRED:

Pages from Improvised Munitions Handbook
Straight sticks about 1 foot (30 cm) long and 1/4 in. (5 mm) in diameter
Thread or fine string

PROCEDURE:

1. Make a notch about 1/2 in. (1 cm) from each end of stick. Be sure that the two notches are the same distance from the end of the stick.

2. Find the exact center of the stick by folding in half a piece of thread the same length as the stick and placing it alongside the stick as a ruler. Make a small notch at the center of the stick.

3. Tie a piece of thread around the notch. Suspend stick from branch, another stick wedged between rocks, or by any other means. Be sure stick is balanced and free to move.

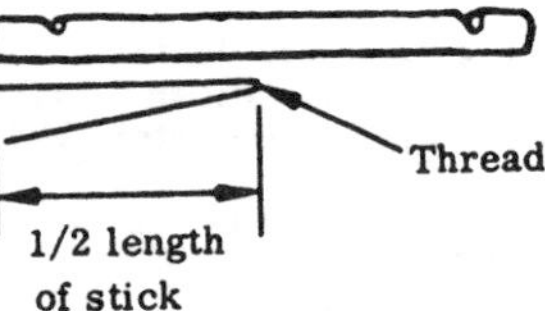

NOTE: If stick is not balanced, shave or scrape a little off the heavy end until it does balance. Be sure the lengths of the arms are the same.

4. Make a container out of one piece of paper. This can be done by rolling the paper into a cylinder and folding up the bottom a few times.

5. Punch 2 holes at opposite sides of paper container. Suspend container from one side of stick.

147

6. Count out the number of handbook pages equal in weight to that of the quantity of material to be weighed. Each sheet of paper weighs about 1.3 grams (20 grains or .04 ounce). Suspend these sheets, plus one, to balance container on the other side of the scale.

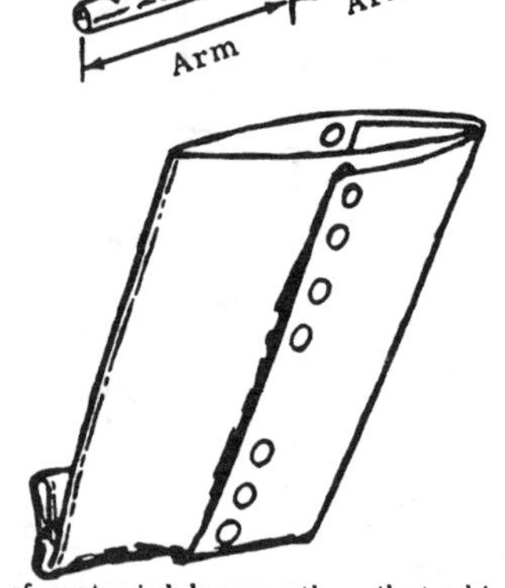

7. Slowly add the material to be weighed to the container. When the stick is balanced, the desired amount of material is in the container.

8. If it is desired to weigh a quantity of material larger than that which would fit in the above container, make a container out of a larger paper or paper bag, and suspend from one side of the stick. Suspend handbook pages from the other side until the stick is balanced. Now place a number of sheets of handbook pages equal in weight to that of the desired amount of material to be weighed on one side, and fill the container with the material until the stick is balanced.

9. A similar method may be used to measure parts or percentage by weight. The weight units are unimportant. Suspend equal weight containers from each side of the stick. Bags, tin cans, etc. can be used. Place one material in one of the containers. Fill the other container with the other material until they balance. Empty and refill the number of times necessary to get the required parts by weight (e.g., 5 to 1 parts by weight would require 5 fillings of one can for one filling of the other).

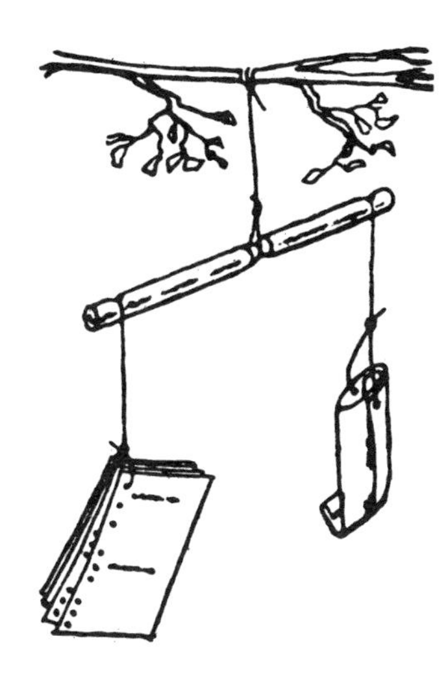

149

CAUTION: If safety lever should be released for any reason, grenade will explode after regular delay time (4-5 sec.).

NOTE: If diameter of safety fuse is too large to fit in hole (Step 4), follow procedure and How to Use of Time Delay Grenade, Section VI, No. 9, instead of Steps 3 and 4 above.

HOW TO USE:

1. Light fuse.

2. Whirl grenade overhead, holding knot at end of rope, until grenade picks up speed (3 or 4 turns).

3. Release when sighted on target.

CAUTION: Be sure to release grenade within 10 seconds after fuse is lit.

NOTE: It is helpful to practice first with a dummy grenade or a rock to improve accuracy. With practice, accurate launching up to 100 meters (300 feet) can be obtained.

148 Section VII
No. 9

ROPE GRENADE LAUNCHING TECHNIQUE

A method of increasing the distance a grenade may be thrown. Safety fuse is used to increase the delay time.

MATERIAL REQUIRED:

Hand grenade (Improvised pipe hand grenade, Section II, No. 1 may be used)
Safety fuse or fast burning Improvised Fuse, (Section VI, No. 7)
Light rope, cord, or string

PROCEDURE:

1: Tie a 4 to 6 foot (1 meter) length of cord to the grenade. Be sure that the rope will not prevent the grenade handle from coming off.

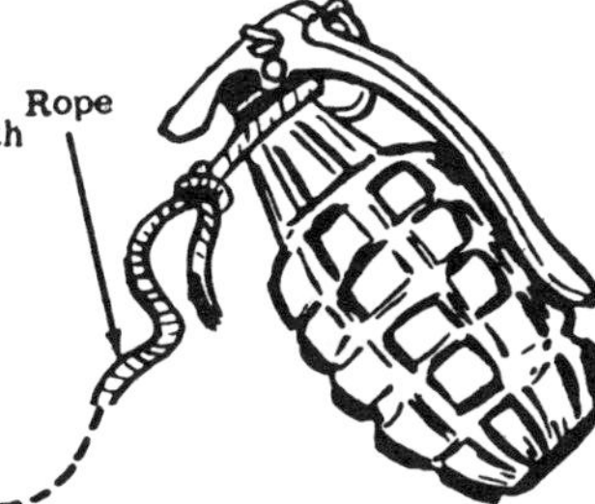

Note: If improvised grenade is used, tie cord around grenade near the end cap. Tape in place if necessary.

2. Tie a large knot in the other end of the cord for use as a handle.

3. Carefully remove safety pin from grenade, holding safety lever in place. Enlarge safety pin hole with point of knife, awl, or drill so that safety fuse will pass through hole.

4. Insert safety fuse in hole. Be sure that safety fuse is long enough to provide a 10 second or more time delay. Slowly release safety lever to make sure fuse holds safety lever in place.

Safety Fuse
Rope

150 Section VII
No. 10

BICYCLE GENERATOR POWER SOURCE

A 6 volt, 3 watt bicycle generator will set off one or two blasting caps (connected in series) or an igniter.

MATERIAL REQUIRED:

Bicycle generator (6 volts, 3 watt)
Copper wire
Knife

PROCEDURE:

1. Strip about 4 in. (10 cm) of coating from both ends of 2 copper wires. Scrape ends with knife until metal is shiny.

2. Connect the end of one wire to the generator terminal.

3. Attach the end of the second wire to generator case. This wire may be wrapped around a convenient projection, taped, or simply held against the case with the hand.

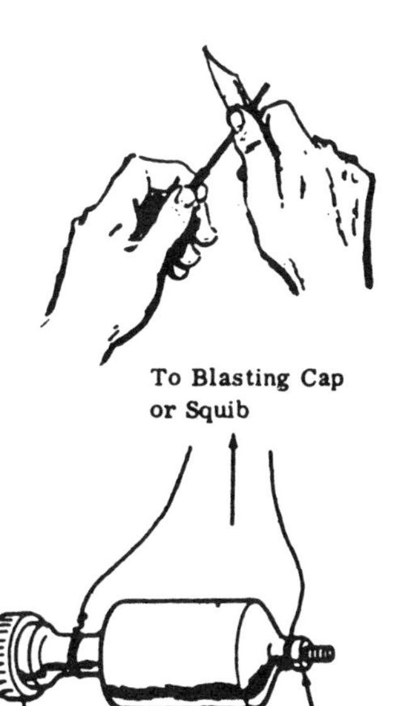

151

HOW TO USE:

1. Connect free ends of wires to blasting cap or squib leads.

> CAUTION: If drive wheel is rotated, explosive may be set off.

2. Run the drive wheel firmly and rapidly across the palm of the hand to activate generator.

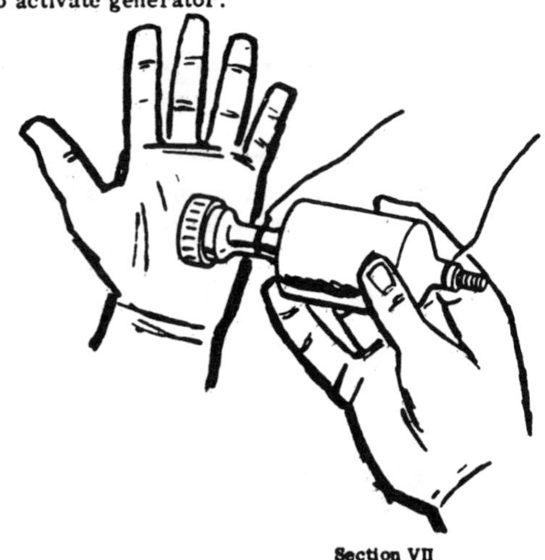

Section VII
152 No. 11
AUTOMOBILE GENERATOR POWER SOURCE

An automobile generator can be used as a means of firing one blasting cap or igniter. (Improvised Igniter, Section V, No. 2, may be used.)

MATERIAL REQUIRED:

Automobile generator (6, 12, or 28 volts). (An alternator will not work.)
Copper Wire
Strong string or wire, about 5 ft. (150 cm) long and 1/16 in. (1-1/2 mm) in diameter
Knife
Small light bulb requiring same voltage as generator, (for example, bulb from same vehicle as generator).

PROCEDURE:

1. Strip about 1 in. (2-1/2 cm) of coating from both ends of 3 copper wires. Scrape ends with knife until metal is shiny.

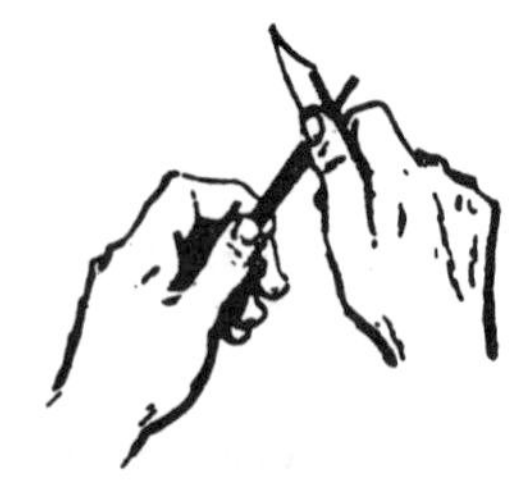

2. Connect the A and F terminals with one piece of wire.

3. Connect a wire to the A terminal. Connect another to the G terminal.

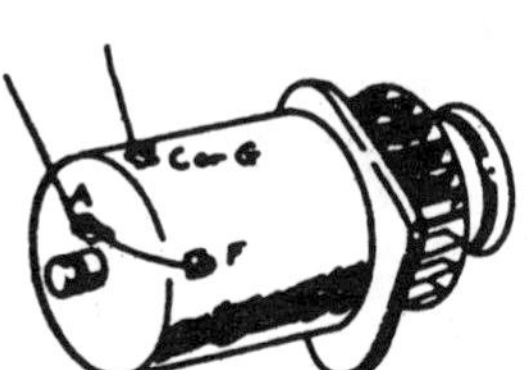

NOTE: The F and G or C terminals may not be labeled; in this case, connect wires as shown. The F terminal is usually smaller in size than the C or G terminal.

153

4. Wrap several turns of string or wire clockwise around the drive pulley.

HOW TO USE:

1. Connect the free ends of the wires to the light bulb.

2. Place one foot on the generator to secure it in place. Give the string or wire a very hard pull to light the bulb.

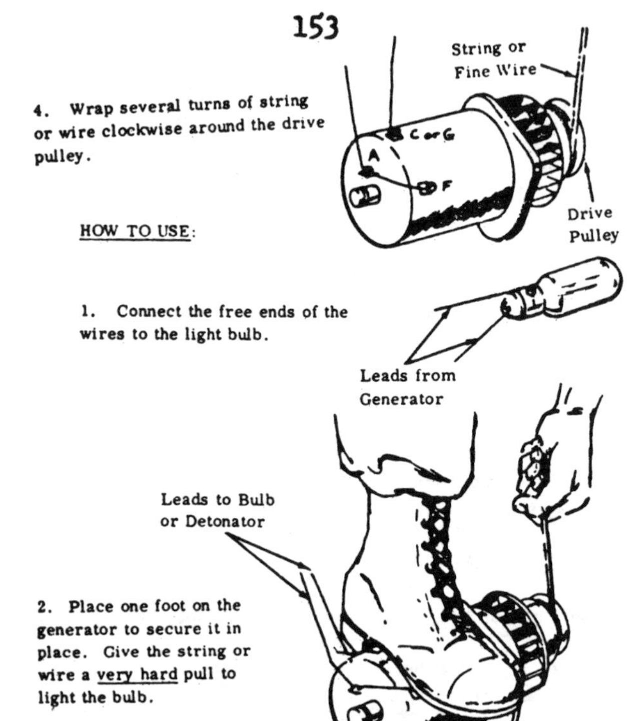

NOTE: If not successful at first, rewind string and try again several times. After repeating this operation and the bulb still does not light, follow Step 4, "How to Use."

3. If light bulb lights, follow Steps 1 and 2 of above, "How to Use," connecting free ends of wires to blasting cap or igniter instead of to light bulb.

4. If light bulb does not light after several pulls, switch leads connected to F and G terminals. Repeat above "How to Use," Steps 1 to 3.

Section VII
154 No. 12
IMPROVISED BATTERY (SHORT LASTING)

This battery is powerful but must be used within 15 minutes after fabrication. One cell of this battery will detonate one blasting cap or one igniter. Two cells, connected in series, will detonate two of these devices and so on. Larger cells have a longer life as well as greater power.

MATERIALS	COMMON SOURCE
Water	
Sodium hydroxide (lye, solid or concentrated solution)	Soap manufacturing Disinfectants Sewer cleaner
Copper or brass plate about 4 in. (10 cm) square and 1/16 in. (2 mm) thick	

Aluminum plate or sheet, same size as copper plate

Charcoal powder

Container for mixing

Knife

One of the following:

Potassium permanganate, solid	Disinfectants Deodorants
Calcium hypochlorite, solid	Disinfectants Water treating chemicals Chlorine bleaches
Manganese dioxide (pyrolucite)	Dead dry-cell batteries

NOTE: Be sure sodium hydroxide solution is at least a 45% solution by weight. If not, boil off some of the water. If solid sodium hydroxide is available, dissolve some sodium hydroxide in about twice as much water (by volume).

155

PROCEDURE:

1. Scrape coating off both ends of wires with knife until metal is shiny.

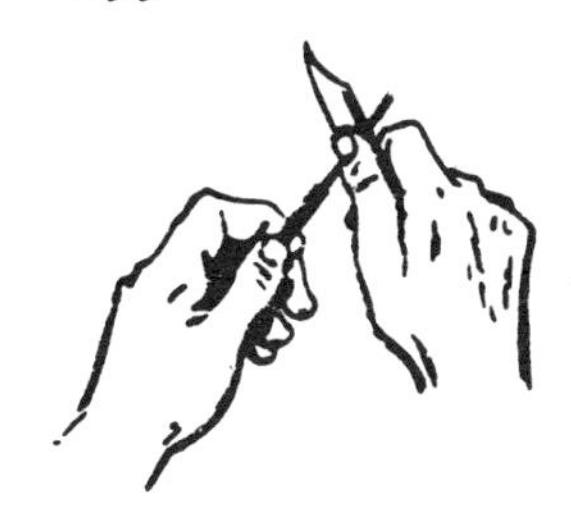

2. Mix thoroughly (do not grind) approximately equal volumes of powdered charcoal and one of the following: potassium permangenate, calcium hypochlorite, or manganese dioxide. Add water until a very thick paste is formed.

CAUTION: Avoid getting any of the ingredient on the skin or in the eyes.

3. Spread a layer of this mixture about 1/8 in. (2 mm) thick on the copper or brass plate. Be sure mixture is thick enough so that when mixture is sandwiched between two metal plates, the plates will not touch each other at any point.

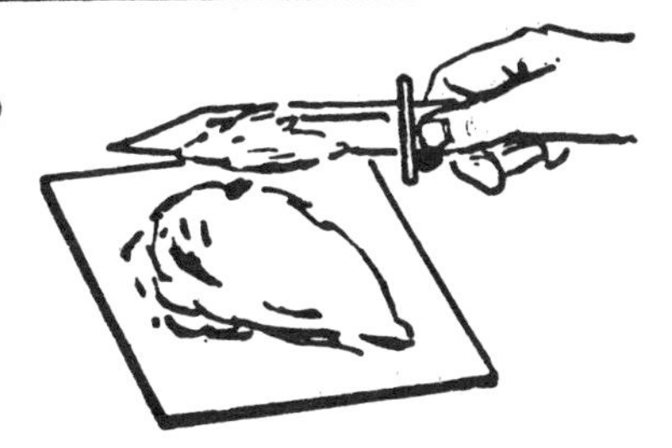

NOTE: If more power is required, prepare several plates as above.

HOW TO USE:

1. Just prior to use (no more than 15 minutes), carefully pour a small quantity of sodium hydroxide solution over the mixture on each plate used.

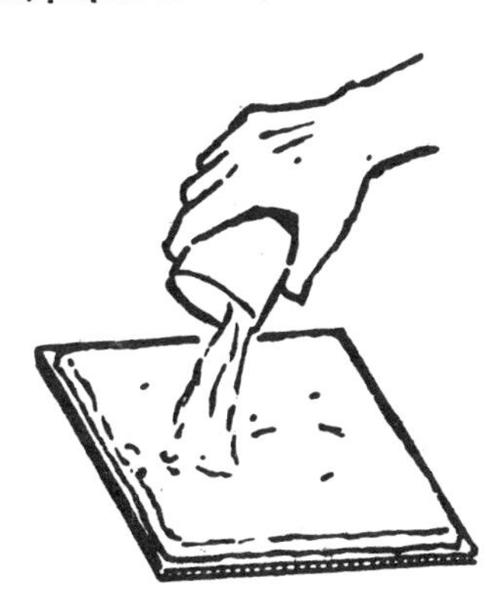

156

CAUTION: If solution gets on skin, wash off immediately with water.

2. Place an aluminum plate on top of the mixture on each copper plate. Press firmly. Remove any excess that oozes out between the plates.

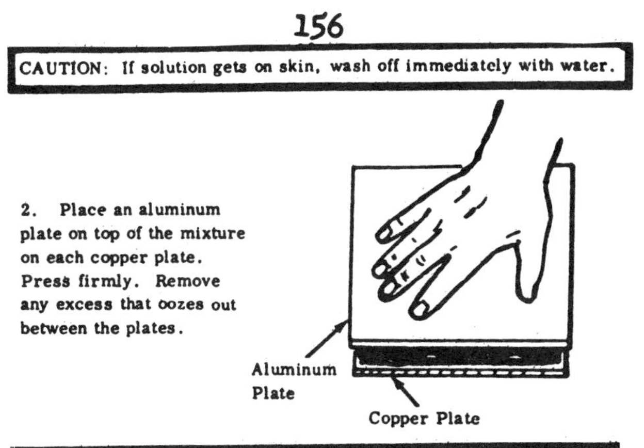

CAUTION: Be sure plates are not touching each other at any point.

3. If more than one cell is used, place the cells on top of each other so that unlike metal plates are touching.

Aluminum Plate

Copper Plate

Aluminum Plate

Copper Plate

4. When ready to fire, clean plates with knife where connections are to be made. Connect one wire to the outer aluminum plate. This may be done by holding the wires against the plates or by hooking them through holes punched through plates. If wires are hooked through plates, be sure they do not touch mixture between plates.

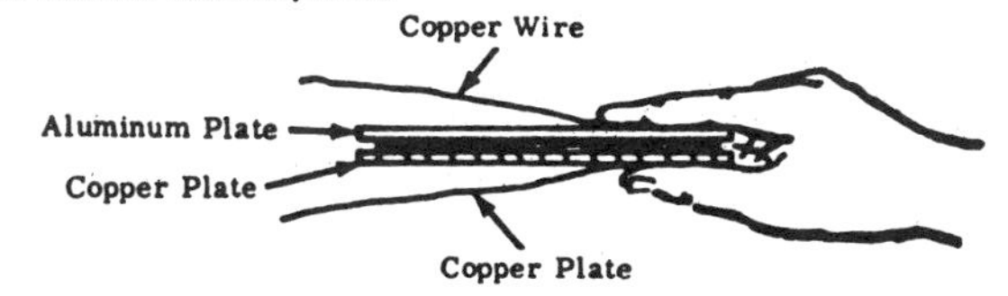

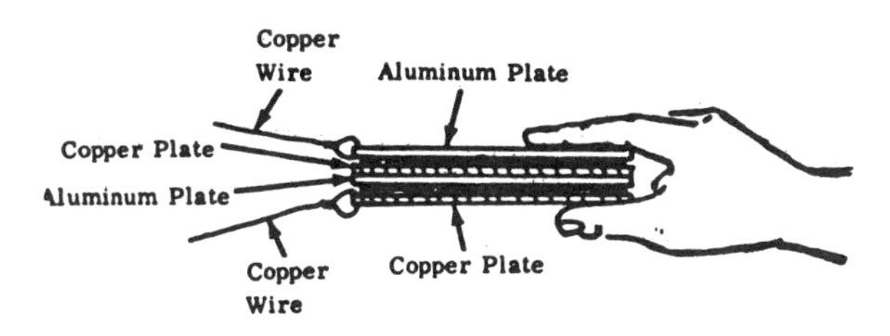

157 Section VII
No. 13

IMPROVISED BATTERY (2 HOUR DURATION)

This battery should be used within 2 hours and should be securely wrapped. Three cells will detonate one blasting cap or one igniter. Five cells, connected in series, will detonate two of these devices and so on. Larger cells have a longer life and will yield more power.

If depolarizing materials such as potassium permanganate or manganese dioxide cannot be obtained, ten cells without depolarizer, arranged as described below, (Step 4) will detonate one blasting cap.

MATERIALS	COMMON SOURCE
Water	
Ammonium chloride (sal ammoniac) (solid or concentrated solution)	Medicines Soldering fluxes Fertilizers Ice melting chemicals for roads

Charcoal powder

Copper or brass plate about 4 in. (10 cm) square and 1/16 in. (2 mm) thick

Aluminum plate same size as copper or brass plate

Wax and paper (or waxed paper) — Candles

Wire, string or tape

Container for mixing

Knife

One of the following:

Potassium permanganate, solid	Disinfectants Deodorants
Manganese dioxide	Dead dry batteries

NOTE: If ammonium chloride solution is not concentrated (at least 45% by weight) boil off some of the water.

158

PROCEDURE:

1. Mix thoroughly (do not grind) approximately equal volumes of powdered charcoal, ammonium chloride and one of the following: potassium permanganate or manganese dioxide. Add water until a very thick paste is formed. If ammonium chloride is in solution form, it may not be necessary to add water.

2. Spread a layer of this mixture, about 1/8 in. (3 mm) thick, on a clean copper or brass plate. The layer must be thick enough to prevent a second plate from touching the copper plate when it is pressed on top.

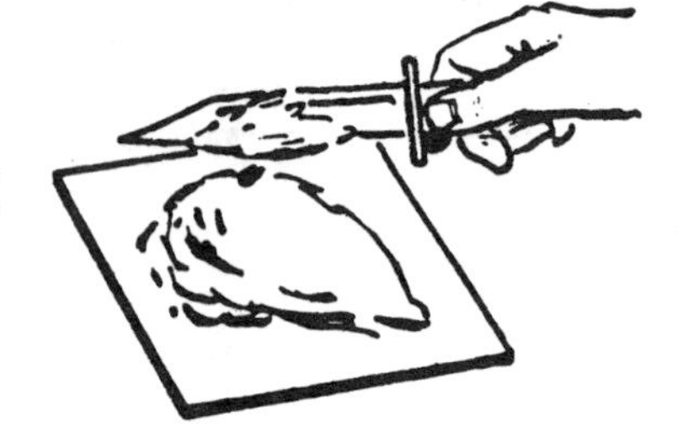

3. Press an aluminum plate very firmly upon the mixture on the copper plate. Remove completely any of the mixture that squeezes out between the plates. The plates must not touch.

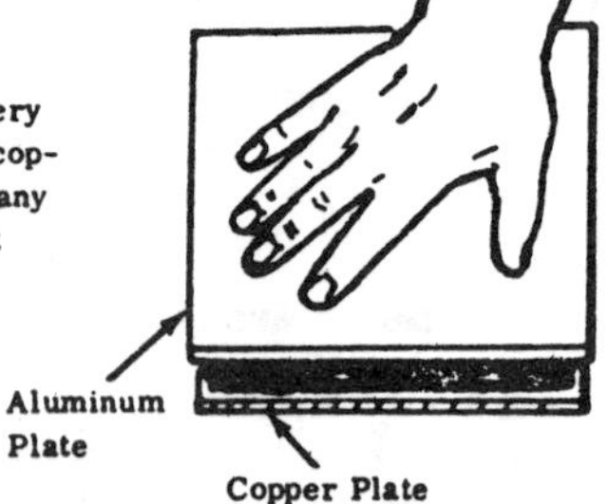

4. If more than one cell is desired:

   a. Place one cell on top of the other so that unlike metal plates are touching.

Aluminum Plate

Copper Plate

Aluminum Plate

Copper Plate

159

   b. Wrap the combined cells in heavy waxed paper. The waxed paper can be made by rubbing candle wax over one side of a piece of paper. Secure the paper around the battery with string, wire or tape. Expose the top and bottom metal plates at one corner.

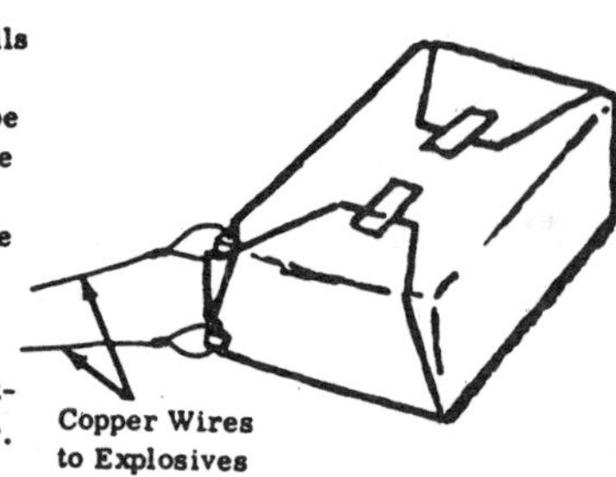

HOW TO USE:

1. Scrape a few inches off each end of two wires with knife till metal is shiny.

2. Clean plates with knife until metal is shiny where connections are to be made.

3. Connect one wire from the explosive to a copper or brass plate and the other wire to an aluminum plate. The connection can be made by holding the wire against the plate. A permanent connection can be made by hooking the wire through holes in the exposed corners of the plates. The battery is now ready for use.

NOTE: If battery begins to fail after a few firings, scrape the plates and wires where connections are made until metal is shiny.

160 Section VII No. 14

ARMOR MATERIALS

The following table shows the amount of indigenous materials needed to stop ball type projectiles of the 5.56 mm, .30 caliber, and .50 caliber ammunition fired from their respective weapons at a distance of 10 feet (3 m).

INDIGENOUS MATERIAL	THICKNESS OF MATERIALS: Inches			Centimeters		
	5.56 mm	.30 cal 7.62 mm	.50 cal 12.70 mm	5.56 mm	.30 cal 7.62 mm	.50 cal 12.70 mm
Mild steel (structural)	1/2	1/2	3/4	1 1/4	1 1/4	2
Mild aluminum (structural)	1	1	2	2 1/2	2 1/2	5
Pine wood (soft)	14	22	32	36	56	82
Broken stones (cobble gravel)	3	4	11	8	11	28
Dry sand	4	5	14	11	13	36
Wet sand or earth	6	13	21	16	33	54

NOTE: After many projectiles are fired into the armor, the armor will break down. More material must be added.

The Chemistry of Powder and Explosives

BY

TENNEY L. DAVIS, PH.D.

Emeritus Professor of Organic Chemistry
Massachusetts Institute of Technology
Director of Research and Development
National Fireworks, Inc.

COMPLETE IN ONE VOLUME

CONTENTS

1

CHAPTER I

PROPERTIES OF EXPLOSIVES

Definition

An explosive is a material, either a pure single substance or a mixture of substances, which is capable of producing an explosion by its own energy.

It seems unnecessary to define an explosion, for everyone knows what it is—a loud noise and the sudden going away of things from the place where they have been. Sometimes it may only be the air in the neighborhood of the material or the gas from the explosion which goes away. Our simple definition makes mention of the one single attribute which all explosives possess. It will be necessary to add other ideas to it if we wish to describe the explosive properties of any particular substance. For example, it is not proper to define an explosive as a substance, or a mixture of substances, which is capable of undergoing a sudden transformation with the production of heat *and* gas. The production of heat alone by the inherent energy of the substance which produces it will be enough to constitute the substance an explosive. Cuprous acetylide explodes by decomposing into copper and carbon and heat, no gas whatever, but the sudden heat causes a sudden expansion of the air in the neighborhood, and the result is an unequivocal explosion. All explosive substances produce heat; nearly all of them produce gas. The change is invariably accompanied by the liberation of energy. The products of the explosion represent a lower energy level than did the explosive before it had produced the explosion. Explosives commonly require some stimulus, like a blow or a spark, to provoke them to liberate their energy, that is, to undergo the change which produces the explosion, but the stimulus which "sets off" the explosive does not contribute to the energy of the explosion. The various stimuli to which explosives respond and the manners of their responses in producing explosions provide a convenient basis for the classification of these interesting materials.

2

Since we understand an explosive material to be one which is capable of producing an explosion by its own energy, we have opened the way to a consideration of diverse possibilities. An explosive perfectly capable of producing an explosion may liberate its energy without producing one. Black powder, for example, may burn in the open air. An explosion may occur without an explosive, that is, without any material which contains intrinsically the energy needful to produce the explosion. A steam boiler may explode because of the heat energy which has been put into the water which it contains. But the energy is not intrinsic to water, and water is not an explosive. Also, we have explosives which do not themselves explode. The explosions consist in the sudden ruptures of the containers which confine them, as happens in a Chinese firecracker. Fire, traveling along the fuse (note the spelling) reaches the black powder—mixture of potassium nitrate, sulfur, and charcoal—which is wrapped tightly within many layers of paper; the powder burns rapidly and produces gas. It burns very rapidly, for the heat resulting from the burning of the first portion cannot get away, but raises the temperature of the next portion of powder, and a rise of temperature of 10°C. more than doubles the velocity of a chemical reaction. The temperature mounts rapidly; gas is produced suddenly; an explosion ensues. The powder burns; the cracker explodes. And in still other cases we have materials which themselves explode. The molecules undergo such a sudden transformation with the liberation of heat, or of heat and gas, that the effect is an explosion.

Classification of Explosives

I. **Propellants** or *low explosives* are combustible materials, containing within themselves all oxygen needful for their combustion, which burn but do not explode, and function by producing gas which produces an explosion. Examples: black powder, smokeless powder. Explosives of this class differ widely among themselves in the rate at which they deliver their energy. There are slow powders and fast powders for different uses. The kick of a shotgun is quite different from the persistent push against the shoulder of a high-powered military rifle in which a slower-burning and more powerful powder is used.

II. **Primary explosives** or *initiators* explode or detonate when

they are heated or subjected to shock. They do not burn; sometimes they do not even contain the elements necessary for combustion. The materials themselves explode, and the explosion results whether they are confined or not. They differ considerably in their sensitivity to heat, in the amount of heat which they give off, and in their *brisance*, that is, in the shock which they produce when they explode. Not all of them are brisant enough to initiate the explosion of a high explosive. Examples: mercury fulminate, lead azide, the lead salts of picric acid and trinitroresorcinol, *m*-nitrophenyldiazonium perchlorate, tetracene, nitrogen sulfide, copper acetylide, fulminating gold, nitrosoguanidine, mixtures of potassium chlorate with red phosphorus or with various other substances, the tartarates and oxalates of mercury and silver.

III. **High explosives** *detonate* under the influence of the shock of the explosion of a suitable primary explosive. They do not function by burning; in fact, not all of them are combustible, but most of them can be ignited by a flame and in small amount generally burn tranquilly and can be extinguished easily. If heated to a high temperature by external heat or by their own combustion, they sometimes explode. They differ from primary explosives in not being exploded readily by heat or by shock, and generally in being more brisant and powerful. They exert a mechanical effect upon whatever is near them when they explode, whether they are confined or not. Examples: dynamite, trinitrotoluene, tetryl, picric acid, nitrocellulose, nitroglycerin, liquid oxygen mixed with wood pulp, fuming nitric acid mixed with nitrobenzene, compressed acetylene and cyanogen, ammonium nitrate and perchlorate, nitroguanidine.

It is evident that we cannot describe a substance by saying that it is "very explosive." We must specify whether it is sensitive to fire and to shock, whether it is really powerful or merely brisant, or both, whether it is fast or slow. Likewise, in the discussions in the present book, we must distinguish carefully between sensitivity, stability, and reactivity. A substance may be extremely reactive chemically but perfectly stable in the absence of anything with which it may react. A substance may be exploded readily by a slight shock, but it may be stable if left to itself. Another may require the shock of a powerful detonator

to make it explode but may be subject to spontaneous decomposition.

The three classes of explosive materials overlap somewhat, for the behavior of a number of them is determined by the nature of the stimuli to which they are subjected and by the manner in which they are used. Black powder has probably never been known, even in the hideous explosions which have sometimes occurred at black powder mills, to do anything but burn. Smokeless powder which is made from colloided nitrocellulose, especially if it exists in a state of fine subdivision, is a vigorous high explosive and may be detonated by means of a sufficiently powerful initiator. In the gun it is lighted by a flame and functions as a propellant. Nitroglycerin, trinitrotoluene, nitroguanidine, and other high explosives are used in admixture with nitrocellulose in smokeless powders. Fulminate of mercury if compressed very strongly becomes "dead pressed" and loses its power to detonate from flame, but retains its power to burn, and will detonate from the shock of the explosion of less highly compressed mercury fulminate. Lead azide, however, always explodes from shock, from fire, and from friction.

Some of the properties characteristic of explosives may be demonstrated safely by experiment.

A sample of commercial black powder of moderately fine granulation, say FFF, may be poured out in a narrow train, 6 inches or a foot long, on a sheet of asbestos paper or a wooden board. When one end of the train is ignited, the whole of it appears to burn at one time, for the flame travels along it faster than the eye can follow. Commercial black powder is an extremely intimate mixture; the rate of its burning is evidence of the effect of intimacy of contact upon the rate of a chemical reaction. The same materials, mixed together as intimately as it is possible to mix them in the laboratory, will burn much more slowly.

Six parts by weight of potassium nitrate, one of sulfur (roll brimstone), and one of soft wood (willow) charcoal are powdered separately and passed through a silk bolting-cloth. They are then mixed, ground together in a mortar, and again passed through the cloth; and this process is repeated. The resulting mixture, made into a train, burns fairly rapidly but by no means in a single flash. The experiment is most convincing if a train of commercial black powder leads into a train of this laboratory powder, and the black powder is ignited by means of a piece of *black match* leading from the end of the train and extending beyond the edge of the surface on which the powder is placed. The

black match may be ignited easily by a flame, whereas black powder on a flat surface is often surprisingly difficult to light.

Black match may be made conveniently by twisting three or four strands of fine soft cotton twine together, impregnating the resulting cord with a paste made by moistening *meal powder*[1] with water, wiping off the excess of the paste, and drying while the cord is stretched over a frame. A slower-burning black match may be made from the laboratory powder described above, and is satisfactory for experiments with explosives. The effect of temperature on the rate of a chemical reaction may be demonstrated strikingly by introducing a 12-inch length of black match into a 10-inch glass or paper tube (which need not fit it tightly); when the match is ignited, it burns in the open air at a moderate rate, but, as soon as the fire reaches the point where the tube prevents the escape of heat, the flame darts through the tube almost instantaneously, and the gases generally shoot the burning match out of the tube.

[1] Corning mill dust, the most finely divided and intimately incorporated black powder which it is possible to procure. Lacking this, black sporting powder may be ground up in small portions at a time in a porcelain mortar.

Cuprous acetylide, of which only a very small quantity may be prepared safely at one time, is procured by bubbling acetylene into an ammoniacal solution of cuprous chloride. It precipitates as a brick-red powder. The powder is collected on a small paper filter and washed with water. About 0.1 gram of the material, still moist, is transferred to a small iron crucible—the rest of the cuprous acetylide ought to be destroyed by dissolving in dilute nitric acid—and the crucible is placed on a triangle over a small flame. As soon as the material has dried out, it explodes, with a loud report, causing a dent in the bottom of the crucible.

A 4-inch filter paper is folded as if for filtration, about a gram of FFF black powder is introduced, a 3-inch piece of black match is inserted, and the paper is twisted in such manner as to hold the powder together in one place in contact with the end of the match. The black match is lighted and the package is dropped, conveniently, into an empty pail. The powder burns with a hissing sound, but there is no explosion for the powder was not really confined. The same experiment with about 1 gram of potassium picrate gives a loud explosion. All metallic picrates are primary explosives, those of the alkali metals being the least violent. Potassium picrate may be prepared by dissolving potassium carbonate in a convenient amount of water, warming almost to boiling, adding picric acid in small portions at a time as long as it dissolves with effervescence, cooling the solution, and collecting the crystals and drying them by exposure to the air. For safety's sake,

6

quantities of more than a few grams ought to be kept under water, in which the substance is only slightly soluble at ordinary temperatures.

About a gram of trinitrotoluene or of picric acid is heated in a porcelain crucible. The substance first melts and gives off combustible vapors which burn when a flame is applied but go out when the flame is removed. A small quantity of trinitrotoluene, say 0.1 gram, may actually be sublimed if heated cautiously in a test tube. If heated quickly and strongly, it decomposes or explodes mildly with a "zishing" sound and with the liberation of soot.

One gram of powdered picric acid and as much by volume of litharge (PbO) are mixed carefully on a piece of paper by turning the powders over upon themselves (not by stirring). The mixture is then poured in a small heap in the center of a clean iron sand-bath dish. This is set upon a tripod, a lighted burner is placed beneath it, and the operator retires to a distance. As soon as the picric acid melts and lead picrate forms, the material explodes with an astonishing report. The dish is badly dented or possibly punctured.

A Complete Round of Ammunition

The manner in which explosives of all three classes are brought into use will be made clearer by a consideration of the things which happen when a round of H.E. (high-explosive) ammunition is fired. The brass cartridge case, the steel shell with its copper driving band and the fuze screwed into its nose are represented diagrammatically in the accompanying sketch. Note the spelling of fuze: a *fuze* is a device for initiating the explosion of

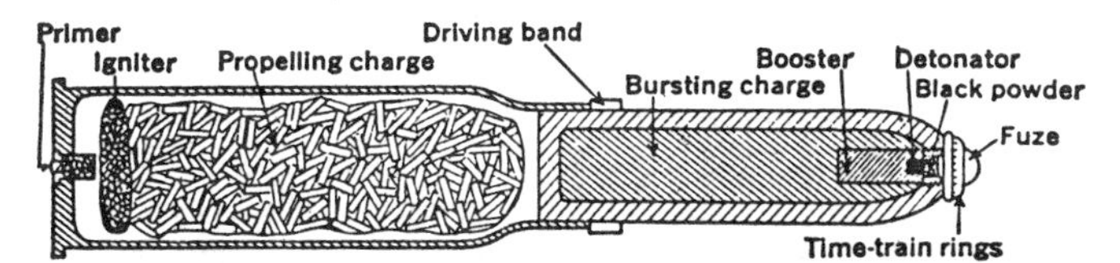

FIGURE 1. Diagram of an Assembled Round of High-Explosive Ammunition. The picture is diagrammatic, for the purpose of illustrating the functions of the various parts, and does not correspond exactly to any particular piece of ammunition.

high-explosive shells or of bombs, shrapnel, mines, grenades, etc.; a *fuse* is a device for communicating fire. In cases where the shell is expected to penetrate armor plate or other obstruction, and not to explode until after it has penetrated its target, the nose

7

of the shell is pointed and of solid steel, and the fuze is screwed into the base of the shell—a base-detonating fuze. The fuze which we wish here to discuss is a point combination fuze, *point* because it is at the nose of the shell, and *combination* because it is designed to explode the shell either after a definite interval of flight or immediately on impact with the target.

The impact of the *firing pin* or trigger upon the *primer cap* in the base of the cartridge case produces fire, a quick small spurt of flame which sets fire to the black powder which is also within the primer. This sets fire to the powder or, in the case of bagged charges, to the *igniter*—and this produces a large hot flame which sweeps out into the chamber of the gun or cartridge, sweeps around the large grains of smokeless powder, and sets fire to them all over their surface. In a typical case the primer cap contains a mixture of mercury fulminate with antimony sulfide and potassium chlorate. The fulminate explodes when the mixture is crushed; it produces fire, and the other ingredients of the composition maintain the fire for a short interval. The igniter bag in our diagram is a silk bag containing black powder which takes fire readily and burns rapidly. The igniter and the bag containing the smokeless powder are made from silk because silk either burns or goes out—and leaves no smoldering residue in the barrel of the gun after the shot has been fired. For different guns and among different nations the igniters are designed in a variety of ways, many of which are described in the books which deal with guns, gunnery, and ammunition. Sometimes the igniter powder is contained in an integral part of the cartridge case. For small arms no igniter is needed; the primer ignites the propellant. For large guns no cartridge case is used; the projectile and the propelling charge are loaded from the breech, the igniter bag being sewed or tied to the base end of the bag which contains the powder, and the *primer* being fitted in a hole in the breechblock by which the gun is closed.

The smokeless powder in our diagram is a dense, progressive-burning, colloided straight nitrocellulose powder, in cylindrical grains with one or with seven longitudinal perforations. The flame from the igniter lights the grains, both on the outer surfaces which commence to burn inward and in the perforations which commence to enlarge, burning outward. The burning at first is slow. As the pressure increases, the projectile starts to move.

8

The rifling in the barrel of the gun bites into the soft copper driving band, imparting a rotation to the projectile, and the rate of rotation increases as the projectile approaches the muzzle. As heat accumulates in the chamber of the gun, the powder burns faster and faster; gas and heat and pressure are produced for some time at an accelerated rate, and the projectile acquires acceleration continuously. It has its greatest velocity at the moment when it leaves the muzzle. The greatest pressure, however, occurs at a point far back from the muzzle where the gun is of correspondingly stronger construction than at its open end. The duration of the burning of the powder depends upon its *web thickness*, that is, upon the thickness between the single central perforation and the sides of the cylindrical grain, or, in the multiperforated powders, upon the thickness between the perforations. The powder, if properly designed, is burned completely at the moment when the projectile emerges from the muzzle.

The combination fuze contains two primer caps, and devices, more or less free to move within the fuze, by which these may be fired. When the shell starts to move, everything within it undergoes *setback*, and tends to lag because of its inertia. The fuze contains a piece of metal with a point or firing pin on its rearmost end, held in place by an almost complete ring set into its sides and in the sides of the cylindrical space through which it might otherwise move freely. This, with its primer cap, constitutes the *concussion* element. The setback causes it to pull through the ring; the pin strikes the cap; fire is produced and communicates with a train of slow-burning black powder of special composition (fuze powder) the length of which has been previously adjusted by turning the *time-train rings* in the head of the fuze. The powder train, in a typical case, may burn for any particular interval up to 21 seconds, at the end of which time the fire reaches a chamber or magazine which is filled with ordinary black powder. This burns rapidly and produces a large flame which strikes through to the detonator, containing mercury fulminate or lead azide, which explodes and causes the shell to detonate while it is in flight. The head of the fuze may also be adjusted in such manner that the fire produced by the concussion element will finally burn to a dead end, and the shell in that case

will explode only in consequence of the action of the *percussion* element when it hits the target.

When the shell strikes any object and loses velocity, everything within it still tends to move forward. The percussion element consists of a metal cylinder, free to move backward and forward through a short distance, and of a primer cap, opposite the forward end of the cylinder and set into the metal in such fashion that the end of the cylinder cannot quite touch it. If this end of the cylinder should carry a firing pin, then it would fire the cap, and this might happen if the shell were dropped accidentally—with unfortunate results. When the shell starts to move in the gun, the cylinder lags back in the short space which is allotted to it. The shell rotates during flight. Centrifugal force, acting upon a mechanism within the cylinder, causes a firing pin to rise up out of its forward end. The fuze becomes *armed*. When the shell meets an obstacle, the cylinder rushes forward, the pin strikes the cap, fire is produced and communicates directly to the black powder magazine and to the detonator—and the shell is exploded forthwith.

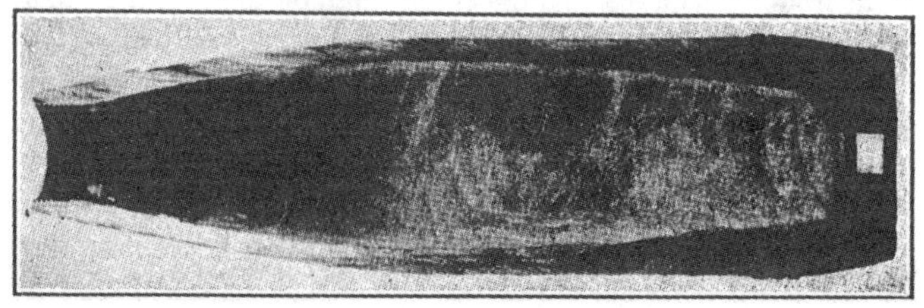

FIGURE 2. Cross Section of a 155-mm. High-Explosive Shell Loaded with TNT.

The high explosive in the shell must be so insensitive that it will tolerate the shock of setback without exploding. Trinitrotoluene (TNT) is generally considered to be satisfactory for all military purposes, except for armor-piercing shells. The explosive must be tightly packed within the shell. There must be no cavities, lest the setback cause the explosive to move violently across the gap and to explode prematurely while the shell is still within the barrel of the gun, or as is more likely, to pull away from the detonator and fail to be exploded by it.

Trinitrotoluene, which melts below the boiling point of water,

is generally loaded by pouring the liquid explosive into the shell. Since the liquid contracts when it freezes, and in order to prevent cavities, the shell standing upon its base is supplied at its open end with a paper funnel, like the neck of a bottle, and the liquid TNT is poured until the shell and the paper funnel are both full. After the whole has cooled, the funnel and any TNT which is in it are removed, and the space for the *booster* is bored out with a drill. Cast TNT is not exploded by the explosion of fulminate, which, however, does cause the explosion of granular and compressed TNT. The explosion of granular TNT will initiate the explosion of cast TNT, and the granular material may be used as a booster for that purpose. In practice, tetryl is generally preferred as a booster for military use. It is more easily detonated than TNT, more brisant, and a better initiator. Boosters are used even with high explosives which are detonated by fulminate, for they make it possible to get along with smaller quantities of this dangerous material.

Propagation of Explosion

When black powder burns, the first portion to receive the fire undergoes a chemical reaction which results in the production of hot gas. The gas, tending to expand in all directions from the place where it is produced, warms the next portion of black powder to the *kindling* temperature. This then takes fire and burns with the production of more hot gas which raises the temperature of the next adjacent material. If the black powder is confined, the pressure rises, and the heat, since it cannot escape, is communicated more rapidly through the mass. Further, the gas- and heat-producing chemical reaction, like any other chemical reaction, doubles its rate for every 10° (approximate) rise of temperature. In a confined space the combustion becomes extremely rapid, but it is still believed to be combustion in the sense that it is a phenomenon dependent upon the transmission of heat.

The explosion of a primary explosive or of a high explosive, on the other hand, is believed to be a phenomenon which is dependent upon the transmission of pressure or, perhaps more properly, upon the transmission of shock.[2] Fire, friction, or shock,

[2] The effects of static pressure and of the rate of production of the pressure have not yet been studied much, nor is there information concerning the pressures which occur within the mass of the explosive while it is exploding.

acting upon, say, fulminate, in the first instance cause it to undergo a rapid chemical transformation which produces hot gas, and the transformation is so rapid that the advancing front of the mass of hot gas amounts to a wave of pressure capable of initiating by its shock the explosion of the next portion of fulminate. This explodes to furnish additional shock which explodes the next adjacent portion of fulminate, and so on, the explosion advancing through the mass with incredible quickness. In a standard No. 6 blasting cap the explosion proceeds with a velocity of about 3500 meters per second.

If a sufficient quantity of fulminate is exploded in contact with trinitrotoluene, the shock induces the trinitrotoluene to explode, producing a shock adequate to initiate the explosion of a further portion. The explosive wave traverses the trinitrotoluene with a velocity which is actually greater than the velocity of the initiating wave in the fulminate. Because this sort of thing happens, the application of the principle of the booster is possible. If the quantity of fulminate is not sufficient, the trinitrotoluene either does not detonate at all or detonates incompletely and only part way into its mass. For every high explosive there is a minimum quantity of each primary explosive which is needed to secure its certain and complete denotation. The best initiator for one high explosive is not necessarily the best initiator for another. A high explosive is generally not its own best initiator unless it happens to be used under conditions in which it is exploding with its maximum *velocity of detonation.*

Detonating Fuse

Detonating fuse consists of a narrow tube filled with high explosive. When an explosion is initiated at one end by means of a detonator, the explosive wave travels along the fuse with a high velocity and causes the detonation of other high explosives which lie in its path. Detonating fuse is used for procuring the almost simultaneous explosion of a number of charges.

Detonating fuse is called *cordeau dêtonant* in the French language, and *cordeau* has become the common American designation for it. Cordeau has been made from lead tubes filled with trinitrotoluene, from aluminum or block tin tubes filled with picric acid, and from tubes of woven fabric filled with nitrocellulose or with pentaerythrite tetranitrate (PETN). In this country the Ensign-Bickford Company, at Simsbury, Connecticut, manufac-

12

tures *Cordeau-Bickford*, a lead tube filled with TNT, and *Primacord-Bickford*,[3] a tube of waterproof textile filled with finely powdered PETN. The cordeau is made by filling a large lead pipe (about 1 inch in diameter) with molten TNT, allowing to cool, and drawing down in the manner that wire is drawn. The finished tube is tightly packed with finely divided crystalline TNT. Cordeau-Bickford detonates with a velocity of about 5200 meters per second (17,056 feet or 3.23 miles), Primacord-Bickford with a velocity of about 6200 meters per second (20,350 feet or 3.85 miles). These are not the maximum velocities of detonation of the explosives in question. The velocities would be greater if the tubes were wider.

[3] These are not to be confused with *Bickford fuse* or *safety fuse* manufactured by the same company, which consists of a central thread surrounded by a core of black powder enclosed within a tube of woven threads, surrounded by various layers of textile, waterproof material, sheathing, etc. This is *miner's fuse*, and is everywhere known as Bickford fuse after the Englishman who invented the machine by which such fuse was first woven. The most common variety burns with a velocity of about 1 foot per minute. When the fire reaches its end, a spurt of flame about an inch long shoots out for igniting black powder or for firing a blasting cap.

Detonating fuse is fired by means of a blasting cap held snugly and firmly against its end by a *union* of thin copper tubing crimped into place. Similarly, two ends are spliced by holding them in contact within a *coupling*. The ends ought to touch each other, or at least to be separated by not more than a very small space, for the explosive wave of the detonating fuse cannot be depended upon to throw its initiating power across a gap of much more than ⅛ inch.

When several charges are to be fired, a single main line of detonating fuse is laid and branch lines to the several charges are connected to it. The method by which a branch is connected to a main line of cordeau is shown in Figures 3, 4, 5, 6, and 7. The main line is not cut or bent. The end of the branch is slit in two (with a special instrument designed for this purpose) and is opened to form a V in the point of which the main line is laid—and there it is held in place by the two halves of the slit branch cordeau, still filled with TNT, wound around it in opposite directions. The connection is made in this manner in order that the explosive wave, traveling along the main line, may strike the

13

branch line squarely against the length of the column of TNT, and so provoke its detonation. If the explosive wave were traveling from the branch against the main line (as laid), it would

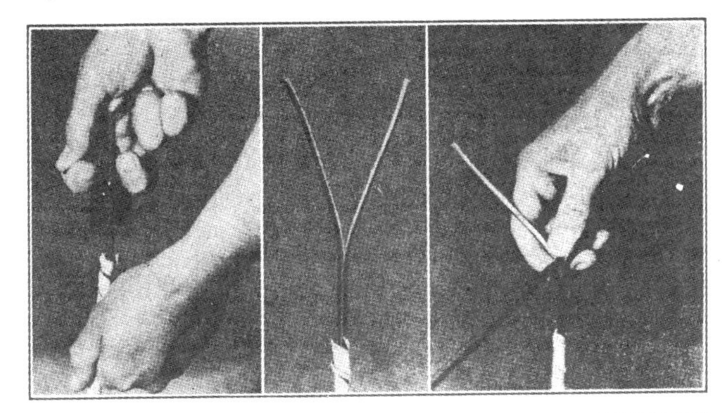

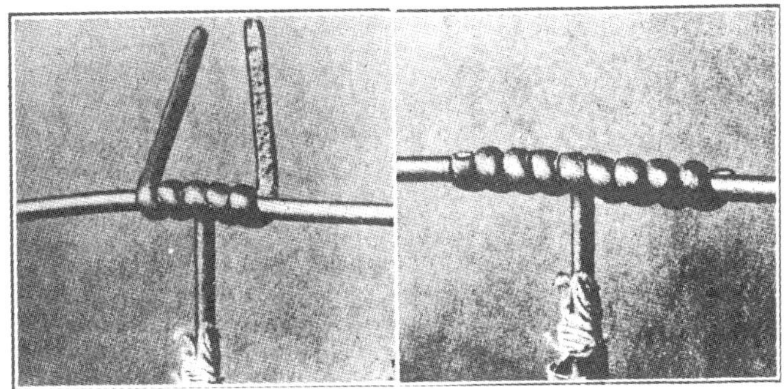

FIGURES 3, 4, 5, 6, and 7. Method of Connecting a Branch to a Main Line of Cordeau. (Courtesy Ensign-Bickford Company.) FIGURE 3. Slitting the Branch Line. FIGURE 4. The Slit End Open. FIGURE 5. The Main Line in Place. FIGURE 6. Winding the Splice. FIGURE 7. The Finished Junction.

strike across the column of TNT and would shatter it, but would be less likely to make it explode. For connecting a branch line of Primacord, it is satisfactory to make a half hitch of the end around the main line.

A circle of detonating fuse around a tree will rapidly strip off a belt of heavy bark, a device which is sometimes useful in the

14

control of insect pests. If the detonating fuse is looped successively around a few blocks of TNT or cartridges of dynamite, and if these are strung around a large tree, the tree may be felled very quickly in an emergency. In military operations it may be desirable to "deny a terrain to the enemy" without occupying it oneself, and the result may be accomplished by scattering mustard gas over the area. For this purpose, perhaps during the night, a long piece of Primacord may be laid through the area, looped here and there in circles upon which tin cans of mustard gas (actually a liquid) are placed. The whole may be fired, when desired, by a single detonator, and the gas adequately dispersed.

Velocity of Detonation

If the quantity of the primary explosive used to initiate the explosion of a high explosive is increased beyond the minimum necessary for that result, the velocity with which the resulting explosion propagates itself through the high explosive is correspondingly increased, until a certain optimum is reached, depending upon the physical state of the explosive, whether cast or powdered, whether compressed much or little, upon the width of the column and the strength of the material which confines it, and of course upon the particular explosive which is used. By proper adjustment of these conditions, by pressing the powdered explosive to the optimum density (which must be determined by experiment) in steel tubes of sufficiently large diameter, and by initiating the explosion with a large enough charge of dynamite or other booster (itself exploded by a blasting cap), it is possible to secure the maximum velocity of detonation. This ultimate maximum is of less interest to workers with explosives than the maximum found while experimenting with paper cartridges, and it is the latter maximum which is generally reported. The physical state and density of the explosive, and the temperature at which the determinations were made, must also be noted if the figures for the velocity of detonation are to be reproducible.

Velocities of detonation were first measured by Berthelot and Vieille, who worked first with gaseous explosives and later with liquids and solids. They used a Boulengé chronograph the precision of which was such that they were obliged to employ long

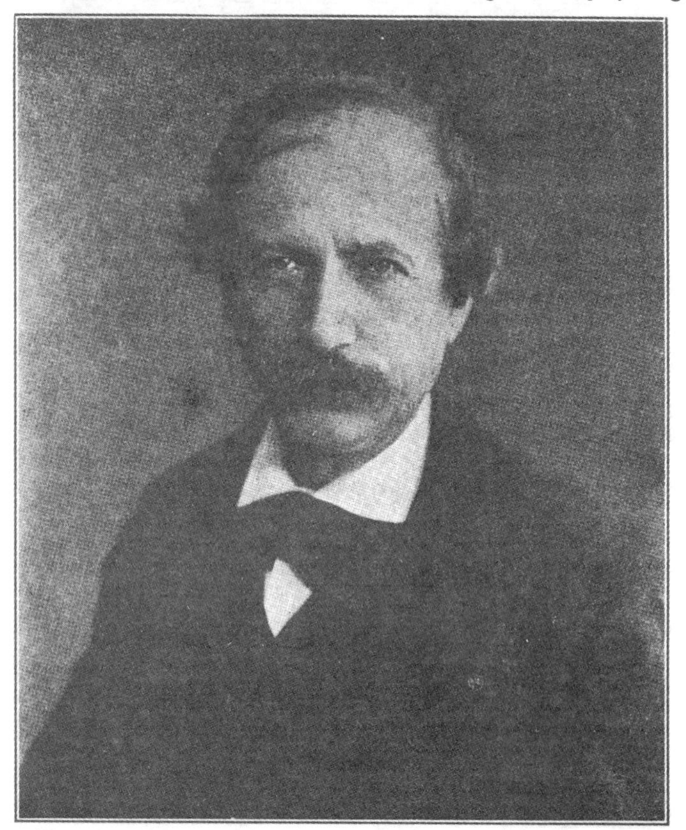

FIGURE 8. Pierre-Eugène Marcellin Berthelot (1827-1907) (Photo by P. Nadar, Paris). Founder of thermochemistry and the science of explosives. He synthesized acetylene and benzene from their elements, and alcohol from ethylene, studied the polyatomic alcohols and acids, the fixation of nitrogen, the chemistry of agriculture, and the history of Greek, Syriac, Arabic, and medieval chemistry. He was a Senator of France, Minister of Public Instruction, Minister of Foreign Affairs, and Secretary of the Academy of Sciences, and is buried in the Panthéon at Paris.

16

columns of the explosives. The Mettegang recorder now commonly used for these measurements is an instrument of greater precision and makes it possible to work with much shorter cartridges of the explosive materials. This apparatus consists essentially of a strong, well-turned and balanced, heavy cylinder of steel which is rotated by an electric motor at a high but exactly known velocity. The velocity of its smoked surface relative to a platinum point which almost touches it may be as much as 100 meters per second. The explosive to be tested is loaded in a cylindrical cartridge. At a known distance apart two thin copper wires are passed through the explosive at right angles to the axis of the cartridge. If the explosive has been cast, the wires are bound tightly to its surface. Each of the wires is part of a closed circuit through an inductance, so arranged that, when the circuit is broken, a spark passes between the platinum point and the steel drum of the chronograph. The spark makes a mark upon the smoked surface. When the explosive is now fired by means of a detonator at the end of the cartridge, first one and then the other of the two wires is broken by the explosion, and two marks are made on the rotating drum. The distance between these marks is measured with a micrometer microscope. The duration of time which corresponds to the movement of the surface of the rotating drum through this distance is calculated, and this is the time which was required for the detonation of the column of known length of explosive which lay between the two wires. From this, the velocity of detonation in meters per second is computed easily.

Since a chronograph is expensive and time-consuming to use, the much simpler method of Dautriche, which depends upon a comparison of the unknown with a standard previously measured by the chronograph, finds wide application. Commercial cordeau is remarkably uniform. An accurately measured length, say 2 meters, of cordeau of known velocity of detonation is taken, its midpoint is marked, and its ends are inserted into the cartridge of the explosive which is being tested, at a known distance apart, like the copper wires in the absolute method (Figure 9). The middle portion of the loop of cordeau is made straight and is laid upon a sheet of lead (6-8 mm. thick), the marked midpoint being

17

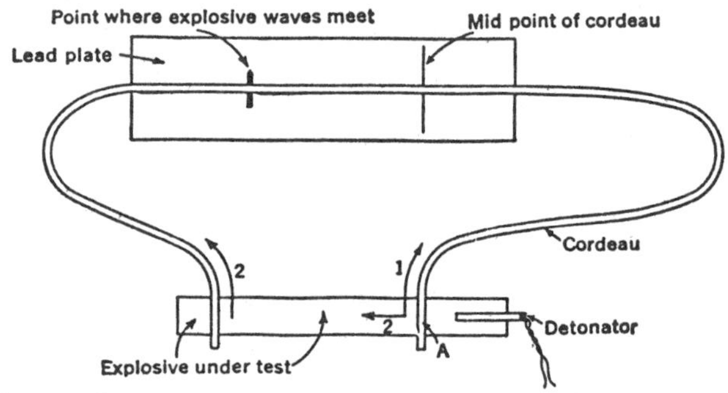

FIGURE 9. Dautriche Method of Measuring Velocity of Detonation. From the point *A* the explosion proceeds in two directions: (1) along the cordeau (of known velocity of detonation), and (2) through the cartridge

of explosive which is being tested and then along the cordeau. When the two waves in the cordeau meet, they make a mark in the lead plate upon which the cordeau is resting.

placed upon a line scratched in the lead plate at right angles to the direction of the cordeau. When the detonator in the end of the cartridge of explosive is fired, the explosive wave first encounters one end of the cordeau and initiates its explosion from this end, then proceeds through the cartridge, encounters the other end of the cordeau, and initiates its explosion from that end. The explosive waves from the two ends cf the cordeau meet one another and mark the point of their meeting by an extra-deep, sharp furrow in the lead plate, perhaps by a hole punched through it. The distance of this point is measured from the line where the midpoint of the cordeau was placed. Call this distance *d*. It is evident that, from the moment when the near end of the cordeau started to detonate, one explosive wave traveled in the cordeau for a distance equal to one-half the length of the cordeau plus the distance *d*, while the other explosive wave, during the same interval of time, traveled in the explosive under examination a distance equal to the distance between the inserted ends of cordeau, then in the cordeau a distance equal to one-half its length minus the distance *d*. The times required for the passage of the explosive waves in the cordeau are calculated from the known velocity of detonation of the cordeau used; thence the time required for the detonation of the column of explosive which

stood between the ends of the cordeau; thence the velocity of detonation in meters per second.

Velocities of detonation have recently been measured by high-speed photography of the explosions through a slit, and by other devices in which the elapsed times are measured by means of a cathode-ray oscillograph.

The Munroe Effect

The mark which explosive waves, traveling toward each other on the same piece of cordeau, make at the point where they meet is evidently due to the fact that they spread out sideways at the point of their encounter. Their combined forces produce an effect greater than either alone could give. The behavior of jets of water, shot against each other under high pressure, supplies a very good qualitative picture of the impact of explosive waves. If the waves meet at an angle, the resultant wave, stronger than either, goes off in a direction which could be predicted from a consideration of the parallelogram of forces. This is the explanation of the Munroe effect.

Charles Edward Munroe, while working at the Naval Torpedo Station at Newport, discovered in 1888 that if a block of guncotton with letters countersunk into its surface is detonated with its lettered surface against a steel plate, the letters are indented into the surface of the steel. Similarly, if the letters are raised above the surface of the guncotton, by the detonation they are reproduced in relief on the steel plate, embossed and raised above the neighboring surface. In short, the greatest effects are produced on the steel plate at the points where the explosive material stands away from it, at the points precisely where explosive waves from different directions meet and reinforce each other. Munroe found that by increasing the depth of the concavity in the explosive he was able to produce greater and greater effects on the plate, until finally, with a charge which was pierced completely through, he was able to puncture a hole through it. By introducing lace, ferns, coins, etc., between the flat surface of a

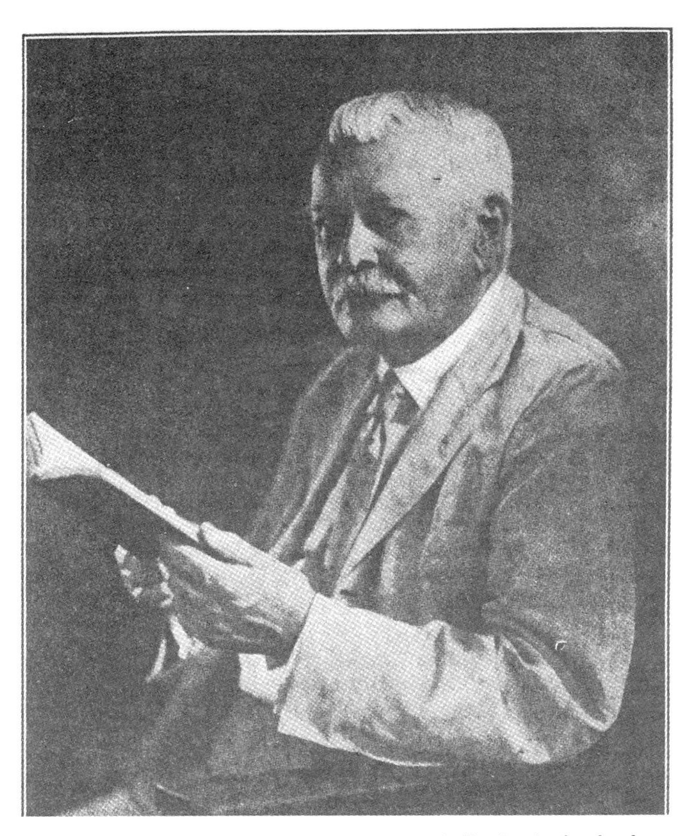

FIGURE 10. Charles Edward Munroe (1849-1938). Leader in the development of explosives in the United States. Invented *indurite*, a variety of smokeless powder, and discovered the Munroe effect. Professor of chemistry at the U. S. Naval Academy, Annapolis, Maryland, 1874-1886; chemist at the Naval Torpedo Station and Naval War College, Newport, Rhode Island, 1886-1892; professor of chemistry at George Washington University, 1892-1917; and chief explosives chemist of the U. S. Bureau of Mines in Washington, 1919-1933. Author and co-author of many very valuable publications of the Bureau of Mines.

block of explosive and pieces of armor plate, Munroe was able to secure embossed reproductions of these delicate materials. Several fine examples of the Munroe effect, prepared by Munroe himself, are preserved in a fire screen at the Cosmos Club in Washington.

The effect of hollowed charges appears to have been rediscovered, probably independently, by Egon Neumann, who claimed it as an original discovery, and its application in explosive technique was patented by the Westfälisch-Anhaltische Sprengstoff-

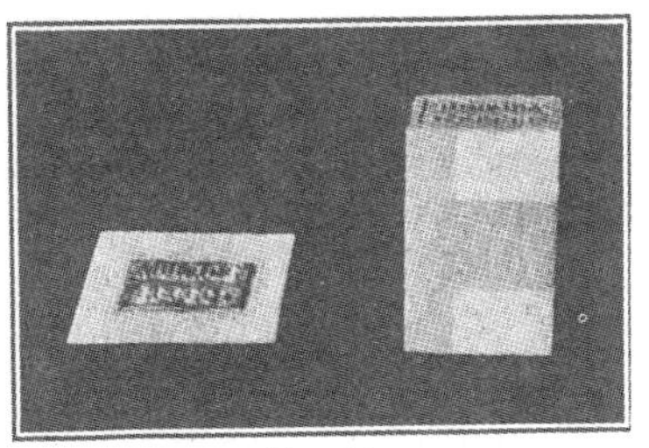

FIG. 11

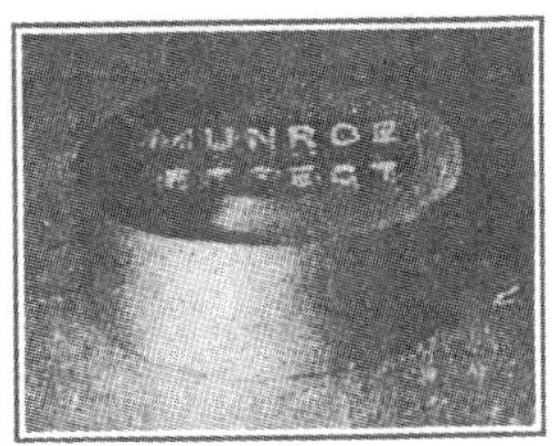

FIG. 12

FIGURES 11 and 12. Munroe Effect. (Courtesy Trojan Powder Company). FIGURE 11. Explosive Enclosed in Pasteboard Wrapper. Note that the letters incised into the surface of the explosive are in mirror writing, like words set in type, in order that the printing may be normal. A steel plate after a charge like that pictured was exploded against it, the incised surface being next to the plate. FIGURE 12. A section of steel shafting after

a charge like that represented in FIGURE 11 had been exploded upon it, the incised surface of the explosive being next to the steel.

A. G. in 1910. Neumann, working with blocks of TNT having conical indentations but not complete perforations, found that such blocks blew holes through wrought-iron plates, whereas solid blocks of greater actual weight only bent or dented them.

It has been recommended that torpedoes be loaded with charges hollowed in their forward ends. Advantage is taken of the Munroe effect in the routine blasting of oil wells, and, intentionally or not, by every explosives engineer who initiates an explosion by means of two or more electric blasting caps, fired simultaneously, at different positions within the same charge.

21

Sensitivity Tests

Among the important tests which are made on explosives are the determinations of their sensitivity to impact and to temperature, that is, of the distance through which a falling weight must drop upon them to cause them to explode or to inflame, and of the temperatures at which they inflame, explode, or "puff" spontaneously. At different places different machines and apparatus are used, and the numerical results differ in consequence from laboratory to laboratory.

For the falling weight or *impact* or *drop test* a 2-kilogram weight is generally used. In a typical apparatus the explosive undergoing the test is contained in a hole in a steel block, a steel plunger or piston is pressed down firmly upon it, and it is directly upon this plunger that the weight is dropped. A fresh sample is taken each time, and material which has not exploded from a single impact is discarded. A drop of 2 to 4 cm. will explode mercury fulminate, one of about 70 to 80 cm. will cause the inflammation of black powder, and one of 60 to 180 cm. will cause the explosion of TNT according to the physical state of the sample.

For determining the *temperature of ignition*, a weighed amount of the material is introduced into a copper capsule (a blasting cap shell) and this is thrust into a bath of Wood's metal previously heated to a known temperature. If no explosion occurs within 5 seconds (or other definite interval), the sample is removed, the temperature of the bath is raised 5° (usually), and a fresh sample in a fresh copper capsule is tried. Under these conditions (that is, within a 5-second interval), 4F black powder takes fire at 190° ± 5°, and 30-caliber straight nitrocellulose smokeless powder at 315° ± 5°. In another method of carrying out the test, the capsule containing the explosive is introduced into the metal bath at 100°, the temperature is raised at a steady and regulated rate, and the temperature at which the explosive decomposition occurs is noted. When the temperature is raised more rapidly, the inflammation occurs at a higher temperature, as indicated by the following table. The fact that explosives are more sensitive to shock and to friction when they are warm is doubtless due to the same ultimate causes.

22

TEMPERATURE OF IGNITION
Heated from 100°

	at 20° per minute	at 5° per minute
Trinitrotoluene	321°	304°
Picric acid	316°	309°
Tetryl	196°	187°
Hexanitrodiphenylamine	258°	250°
Hexanitrodiphenyl sulfide	319°	302°
Hexanitrodiphenyl sulfone	308°	297°

Substances like trinitrotoluene, picric acid, and tetryl, which are intrinsically stable at ordinary temperatures, decompose slowly if they are heated for considerable periods of time at temperatures below those at which they inflame. This, of course, is a matter of interest, but it is a property of all samples of the substance, does not vary greatly between them, and is not made the object of routine testing. Nitrocellulose and many nitric esters, however, appear to be intrinsically unstable, subject to a spontaneous decomposition which is generally slow but may be accelerated greatly by the presence of impurities in the sample. For this reason, nitrocellulose and smokeless powder are regularly subjected to *stability tests* for the purpose, not of establishing facts concerning the explosive in question, but rather for determining the quality of the particular sample.[10]

[10] The routine tests which are carried out on military explosives are described in U. S. War Department Technical Manual TM9-2900, "Military Explosives." The testing of explosives for sensitivity, explosive power, etc., is described in the *Bulletins* and *Technical Papers* of the U. S. Bureau of Mines. The student of explosives is advised to secure from the Superintendent of Documents, Washington, D. C., a list of the publications of the Bureau of Mines, and then to supply himself with as many as may be of interest, for they are sold at very moderate prices. The following are especially recommended. Several of these are now no longer procurable from the Superintendent of Documents, but they may be found in many libraries.

23

Tests of Explosive Power and Brisance

For estimating the total energy of an explosive, a test in the manometric bomb probably supplies the most satisfactory single indication. It should be remembered that total energy and actual effectiveness are different matters. The effectiveness of an explosive depends in large part upon the rate at which its energy is liberated.

The high pressures developed by explosions were first measured by means of the Rodman gauge, in which the pressure caused a hardened-steel knife edge to penetrate into a disc of soft copper. The depth of penetration was taken as a measure of the pressure to which the apparatus had been subjected. This gauge was improved by Nobel, who used a copper cylinder placed between a fixed and a movable steel piston. Such *crusher gauges* are at present used widely, both for measuring the maximum pressures produced by explosions within the confined space of the manometric bomb and for determining the pressures which exist in the barrels of guns during the proof firing of powder. The small copper cylinders are purchased in large and uniform lots, their deformations under static pressures are determined and plotted in a chart, and the assumption is made that the sudden pressures resulting from explosions produce the same deformations as static pressures of the same magnitudes. Piezoelectric gauges, in which the pressure on a tourmaline crystal or on discs of quartz produces an electromotive force, have been used in work with manometric bombs and for measuring the pressures which exist in the chambers of guns. Other gauges, which depend

24

upon the change of electrical resistance of a conducting wire, are beginning to find application.

The manometric bomb is strongly constructed of steel and has a capacity which is known accurately. In order that the pressure resulting from the explosion may have real significance, the *density of loading*, that is, the number of grams of explosive per cubic centimeter of volume, must also be reported. The pressures produced by the same explosive in the same bomb are in general not directly proportional to the density of loading. The temperatures in the different cases are certainly different, and the compositions of the hot gaseous mixtures depend upon the pressures which exist upon them and determine the conditions of the equilibria between their components. The water in the gases can be determined, their volume and pressure can be measured at ordinary temperature, and the temperature of the explosion can be calculated roughly if the assumptions are made that the gas laws hold and that the composition of the cold gases is the same as that of the hot. If the gases are analyzed, and our best knowledge relative to the equilibria which exist between the components is assumed to be valid for the whole temperature range, then the temperature produced by the explosion can be calculated with better approximation.

Other means of estimating and comparing the capacity of explosives for doing useful work are supplied by the tests with the *ballistic pendulum* and by the Trauzl and small lead block tests. The first of these is useful for comparing a new commercial explosive with one which is standard; the others give indications which are of interest in describing both commercial explosives and pure explosive substances.

In the *Trauzl lead block test* (often called simply the lead-block test) 10 grams of the explosive, wrapped in tinfoil and stemmed with sand, is exploded by means of an electric detonator in a cylindrical hole in the middle of a cylindrical block of lead, and the enlargement of the cavity, measured by pouring in water from a graduate and corrected for the enlargement which is ascribable to the detonator alone, is reported. For the standard test, the blocks are cast from chemically pure lead, 200 mm. in height and 200 mm. in diameter, with a central hole made by the mold, 125 mm. deep and 25 mm. in diameter.[25] The test is applicable only to explosives which detonate. Black powder and other explosives which burn produce but little effect, for the gases blow out the stemming and escape. The test is largely one of brisance, but for explosives of substantially equal brisance it gives some indication of their relative power. An explosive of great brisance but little power will create an almost spherical pocket at the bottom of the hole in the block, while one of less brisance and greater power will enlarge the hole throughout its

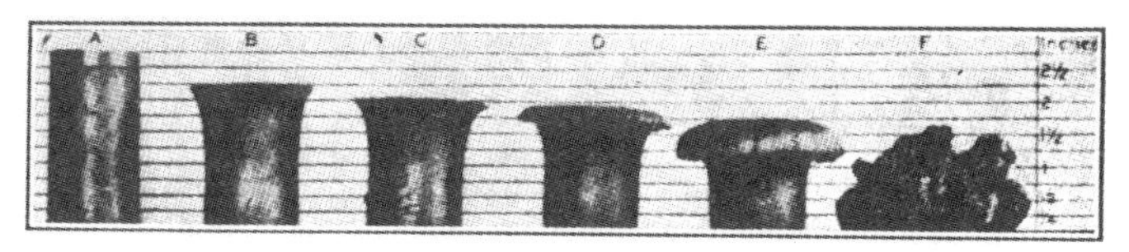

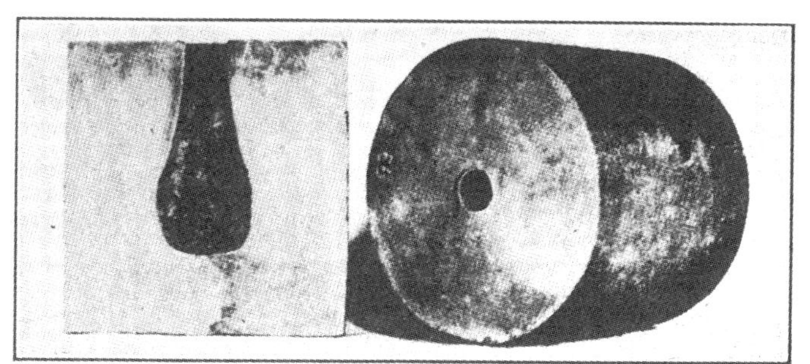

FIGURE 13. Lead Block Tests (above), and Trauzl Tests (below). (Courtesy U. S. Bureau of Mines.)

length and widen its throat at the top of the block. The form of the hole, then, as shown by sectioning the block, is not without significance. The Trauzl test does not give reliable indications with explosives which contain aluminum (such as *ammonal*) or with others which produce very high temperatures, for the hot gases erode the metal, and the results are high.

A small Trauzl block is used for testing commercial detonators.

Another test, known as the *small lead block test*, is entirely a test of brisance. As the test is conducted at the U. S. Bureau of Mines,[26] a lead cylinder 38 mm. in diameter and 64 mm. high is set upright upon a rigid steel support; a disc of annealed steel 38 mm. in diameter and 6.4 mm. thick is placed upon it; a strip of manila paper wide enough to extend beyond the top of the composite cylinder and to form a container at its upper end is wrapped and secured around it; 100 grams of explosive is placed

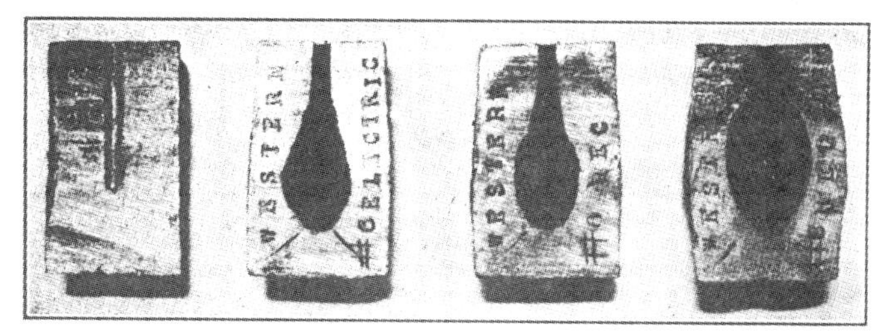

FIGURE 14. Small Trauzl Tests of Detonators. (Courtesy Western Cartridge Company.)

in this container and fired, without tamping, by means of an electric detonator. The result is reported as the compression of the lead block, that is, as the difference between its height before and its height after the explosion. The steel disc receives the force of the explosion and transmits it to the lead cylinder. Without it, the lead cylinder would be so much deformed that its height could not be measured.

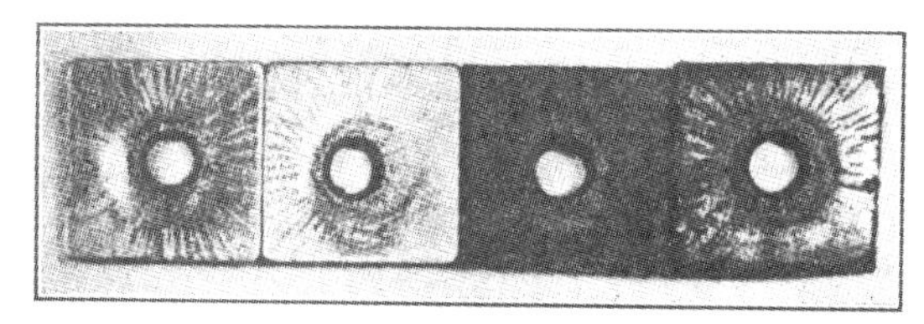

FIGURE 15. Aluminum Plate and Lead Plate Tests of Detonators. (Courtesy Atlas Powder Company.)

In the *lead plate test of detonators*, the detonator is fired while standing upright on a plate of pure lead. Plates 2 to 6 mm. thick are used, most commonly 3 mm. A good detonator makes a clean-cut hole through the lead. The metal of the detonator case is blown into small fragments which make fine and characteristic markings on the lead plate radiating away from the place where[27]

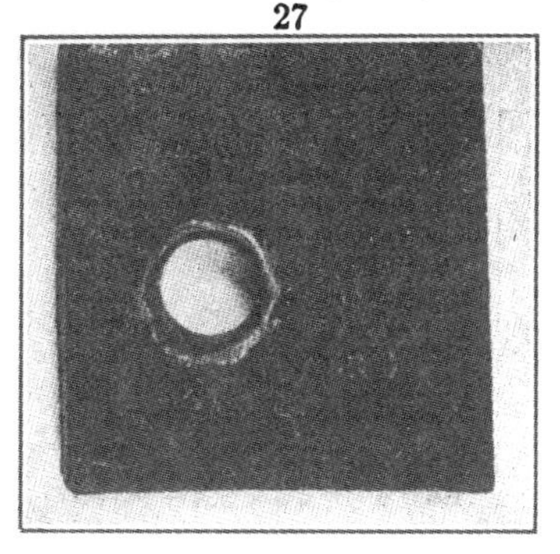

FIGURE 16. Effect of Detonator on Lead Plate 10 cm. Distant from Its End. The diameter of the hole is about 1½ times the diameter of the detonator which was fired. The lead has splashed up around the hole in much the same fashion as placid water splashes when a pebble is dropped into it. Note the numerous small splashes on the lead plate where it was struck by fragments of the detonator casing.

the detonator stood. With a good detonator, the surface of the lead plate ought to show no places where it has been torn roughly by large fragments of the case. Similar tests are often carried out with plates of aluminum.

28

CHAPTER II

BLACK POWDER

The discovery that a mixture of potassium nitrate, charcoal, and sulfur is capable of doing useful mechanical work is one of the most important chemical discoveries or inventions of all time. It is to be classed with the discovery or invention of pottery, which occurred before the remote beginning of history, and with that of the fixation of nitrogen by reason of which the ecology of the human race will be different in the future from what it has been throughout the time that is past. Three great discoveries signalized the break-up of the Middle Ages: the discovery of America, which made available new foods and drugs, new natural resources, and new land in which people might multiply, prosper, and develop new cultures; the discovery of printing, which made possible the rapid and cheap diffusion of knowledge; and the discovery of the controllable force of gunpowder, which made huge engineering achievements possible, gave access to coal and to minerals within the earth, and brought on directly the age of iron and steel and with it the era of machines and of rapid transportation and communication. It is difficult to judge which of these three inventions has made the greatest difference to mankind.

Black powder and similar mixtures were used in incendiary compositions, and in pyrotechnic devices for amusement and for war, long before there was any thought of applying their energy usefully for the production of mechanical work. The invention of guns—and it seems to be this invention which is meant when "the discovery of gunpowder" is mentioned—did not follow immediately upon the discovery of the composition of black powder. It is possible that other applications antedated it, that black powder was used in petards for blowing down gateways, drawbridges, etc., or in simple operations of blasting, before it was used for its ballistic effect.

29

Berthold Schwarz

The tradition that the composition of black powder was discovered and that guns were invented about 1250 (or 1350 or even later) by Berthold Schwarz, a monk of Freiburg i. Br., in Germany, is perpetuated by a monument at that place. Constantin Anklitzen assumed the name of Berthold when he joined the Franciscan order, and was known by his confreres as *der schwarzer Berthold* because of his interest in black magic. The records of the Franciscan chapter in Freiburg were destroyed or scattered before the Reformation, and there are no contemporaneous accounts of the alleged discovery. Concerning the absence of documents, Oesper says:

> If he is a purely legendary inventor the answer is obvious. However, history may have taken no interest in his doings because guns were said to be execrable inventions and their employment (except against the unbelievers) was decried as destructive of manly valor and unworthy of an honorable warrior. Berthold was reputed to have compounded powder with Satan's blessing, and the clergy preached that as a coworker of the Evil One he was a renegade to his profession and his name should be forgotten. There is a tradition that he was imprisoned by his fellow monks, and some say he made his diabolic invention while in prison. According to another legend, Berthold blew himself up while demonstrating the power of his discovery; another states that he was executed.

The lovers of fine points may argue over Berthold's existence, but it can be historically established that Freiburg in the fourteenth and fifteenth centuries was a flourishing center for the casting of cannon and the training of gunners.

Boerhaave on Black Powder

Although black powder has done immeasurable good through its civil uses, it has nevertheless been regarded as an evil discovery because of the easy and unsportsmanlike means which it provides for the destruction of life. Boerhaave, more than two centuries ago, wrote in the modern spirit on the importance of chemistry in war and condemned black powder in a manner

30

similar to that in which some of our latest devices of warfare have been decried in public print.

> It were indeed to be wish'd that our art had been less ingenious, in contriving means destructive to mankind; we mean those instruments of war, which were unknown to the ancients, and have made such havoc among the moderns. But as men have always been bent on seeking each other's destruction by continual wars; and as force, when brought against us, can only be repelled by force; the chief support of war, must, after money, be now sought in chemistry.
>
> *Roger Bacon*, as early as the twelfth century,[3] had found out gunpowder, wherewith he imitated thunder and lightning; but that age was so happy as not to apply so extraordinary a discovery to the destruction of mankind. But two ages afterwards, *Barthol. Schwartz*,[4] a *German* monk and chemist, happening by some accident to discover a prodigious power of expanding in some of this powder which he had made for medicinal uses, he apply'd it first in an iron barrel, and soon after to the military art, and taught it to the *Venetians*. The effect is, that the art of war has since that time turned entirely on this one chemical invention; so that the feeble boy may now kill the stoutest hero: Nor is there anything, how vast and solid soever, can withstand it. By a thorough acquaintance with the power of this powder, that intelligent *Dutch* General *Cohorn* quite alter'd the whole art of fighting; making such changes in the manner of fortification, that places formerly held impregnable, now want defenders. In effect, the power of gun-powder is still more to be fear'd. I tremble to mention the stupendous force of another

[3] Bacon lived in the thirteenth century; we quote the passage as it is printed.

[4] Shaw's footnote (*op. cit.*, p. 190) states:

> What evidently shews the ordinary account of its invention false, is, that *Schwartz* is held to have first taught it to the *Venetians* in the year 1380; and that they first used it in the war against the *Genoese*, in a place antiently called *Fossa Caudeana*, now *Chioggia*. For we find mention of fire arms much earlier: *Peter Messius*, in his *variae lectiones*, relates that *Alphonsus XI.* king of Castile used mortars against the *Moors*, in a siege in 1348; and *Don Pedro*, bishop of *Leon*, in his chronicle, mentions the same to have been used above four hundred years ago, by the people of *Tunis*, in a sea fight against the *Moorish* king of *Sevil*. *Du Cange* adds, that there is mention made of this powder in the registers of the chambers of accounts in *France*, as early as the year 1338.

31

> powder, prepar'd of sulfur, nitre, and burnt lees of wine;[5] to say nothing of the well-known power of *aurum fulminans*. Some person taking a quantity of fragrant oil, chemically procured from spices, and mixing it with a liquor procured from salt-petre, discover'd a thing far more powerful than gun-powder itself; and which spontaneously kindles and

[5] This is *fulminating powder*, made, according to Ure's "Dictionary of Chemistry," first American edition, Philadelphia, 1821:

by triturating in a warm mortar, three parts by weight of nitre, two of carbonate of potash, and one of flowers of sulfur. Its effects, when fused in a ladle, and then set on fire, are very great. The whole of the melted fluid explodes with an intolerable noise, and the ladle is commonly disfigured, as if it had received a strong blow downwards.

Samuel Guthrie, Jr. (cf. *Archeion*, 13, 11 ff. [1931]), manufactured and sold in this country large quantities of a similar material. In a letter to Benjamin Silliman dated September 12, 1831 (*Am. J. Sci. Arts*, 21, 288 ff. [1832]), he says:

I send you two small phials of nitrated sulphuret of potash, or yellow powder, as it is usually called in this country. . . . I have made some hundred pounds of it, which were eagerly bought up by hunters and sportsmen for *priming* fire arms, a purpose which it answered most admirably; and, but for the happy introduction of powder for priming, which is ignited by percussion, it would long since have gone into extensive use.

With this preparation I have had much to do, and I doubt whether, in the whole circle of experimental philosophy, many cases can be found involving dangers more appalling, or more difficult to be overcome, than melting fulminating powder and saving the product, and reducing the process to a business operation. I have had with it some eight or ten tremendous explosions, and in one of them I received, full in my face and eyes, the flame of a quarter of a pound of the composition, just as it had become thoroughly melted.

The common proportions of 3 parts of nitre, 2 parts of carbonate of potash and 1 part of sulphur, gave a powder three times quicker than common black powder; but, by *melting together* 2 parts of nitre and 1 of carbonate of potash, and when the mass was cold adding to 4½ parts of it, 1 part of sulphur—equal in the 100, to 54.54 dry nitre, 27.27 dry carbonate of potash and 18.19 sulphur—a greatly superior composition was produced, burning no less than eight and one half times quicker than the best common powder. The substances were intimately ground together, and then melted to a *waxy* consistence, upon an iron plate of one inch in thickness, heated over a muffled furnace, taking care to knead the mass assiduously, and remove the plate as often as the bottom of the mass became pretty slippery.

By the previously melting together of the nitre and carbonate of potash, a more intimate union of these substances was effected than could possibly be made by mechanical means, or by the slight melting which was admissible in the after process; and by the slight melting of the whole upon a *thick* iron plate, I was able to conduct the business with facility and safety.

The melted mass, after being cold, is as hard and porous as pumice stone, and is grained with difficulty; but there is a stage when it is cooling in which it is very crumbly, and it should then be powdered upon a board, with a small wooden cylinder, and put up hot, without sorting the grains or even sifting out the flour.

32

burns with great fierceness, without any application of fire.[6] I shall but just mention a fatal event which lately happen'd in *Germany*, from an experiment made with balsam of sulphur terebinthinated, and confined in a close chemical vessel, and thus exploded by fire; God grant that mortal men may not be so ingenious at their own cost, as to pervert a profitable science any longer to such horrible uses. For this reason I forbear to mention several other matters far more horrible and destructive, than any of those above rehearsed.

[6] Shaw's footnote (*op. cit.*, p. 191): "A drachm of compound spirit of nitre being poured on half a drachm of oil of carraway seeds *in vacuo*; the mixture immediately made a flash like gun-powder, and burst the exhausted receiver, which was a glass six inches wide, and eight inches deep."

Greek Fire

Fire and the sword have been associated with each other from earliest times. The invention of Greek fire appears to have consisted of the addition of saltpeter to the combustible mixtures already in use, and Greek fire is thus seen as the direct ancestor both of black gunpowder and of pyrotechnic compositions.

The Byzantine historian, Theophanes the Confessor, narrates that "Constantine [Constantine IV, surnamed Pogonatus, the Bearded], being apprised of the designs of the unbelievers against Constantinople, commanded large boats equipped with cauldrons of fire (tubs or vats of fire) and fast-sailing galleys equipped with siphons." The narrative refers to events which occurred in the year 670, or possibly 672. It says for the next year: "At this time Kallinikos, an architect (engineer) from Heliopolis of Syria, came to the Byzantines and having prepared a sea fire (or marine fire) set fire to the boats of the Arabs, and burned these with their men aboard, and in this manner the Byzantines were victorious and found (discovered) the marine fire." The Moslem fleet was destroyed at Cyzicus by the use of this fire which for several centuries afterwards continued to bring victory to the Byzantines in their naval battles with the Moslems and Russians.

Leo's *Tactica*, written about A.D. 900 for the generals of the empire, tells something of the manner in which the Greek fire was to be used in combat.

33

And of the last two oarsmen in the bow, let the one be the *siphonator*, and the other to cast the anchor into the sea. . . . In any case, let him have in the bow the *siphon* covered with copper, as usual, by means of which he shall shoot the *prepared fire* upon the enemy. And above such siphon (let there be) a false bottom of planks also surrounded by boards, in which the warriors shall stand to meet the oncoming foes. . . . On occasion [let there be] formations immediately to the front [without maneuvers] so, whenever there is need, to fall upon the enemy at the bow and set fire to the ships by means of the *fire of the siphons*. . . . Many very suitable contrivances were invented by the ancients and moderns, with regard to both the enemy's ships and the warriors on them—such as at that time the *prepared fire* which is ejected (thrown) by means of *siphons* with a roar and a lurid (burning) smoke and filling them [the ships] with smoke. . . . They shall use also the other method of small *siphons* thrown (i.e., directed) by hand from behind iron shields and held [by the soldiers], which are called *hand siphons* and have been recently manufactured by our state. For these can also throw (shoot) the *prepared fire* into the faces of the enemy.

Leo also described the use of *strepta*, by which a liquid fire was ejected, but he seemed to have been vague upon the details of construction of the pieces and upon the force which propelled the flame, and, like the majority of the Byzantine writers, he failed to mention the secret ingredient, the saltpeter, upon which the functioning of the fires undoubtedly depended, for their flames could be directed downward as well as upward.

The Byzantines kept their secret well and for a long time, but the Moslems finally learned about it and used the fire against the Christians at the time of the Fifth Crusade. In the Sixth Crusade the army of Saint Louis in Egypt was assailed with incendiaries thrown from ballistae, with fire from tubes, and with grenades of glass and metal, thrown by hand, which scattered fire on bursting. Brock thinks that the fire from tubes operated in the manner of Roman candles. The charge, presumed to be a nonhomogeneous mixture of combustible materials with saltpeter, "will, in certain proportions, if charged into a strong tube, give intermittent bursts, projecting blazing masses of the mixture to a

34

considerable distance. The writer has seen this effect produced in a steel mortar of 5½ inches diameter, the masses of composition being thrown a distance of upwards of a hundred yards, a considerable range in the days of close warfare." There is no reason to believe that the fire tubes were guns.

Marcus Graecus

In the celebrated book of Marcus Graecus, *Liber ignium ad comburendos hostes,* Greek fire and other incendiaries are described fully, as is also black powder and its use in rockets and crackers. This work was quoted by the Arabian physician, Mesue, in the ninth century, and was probably written during the eighth.

> Greek fire is made as follows: take sulfur, tartar, sarcocolla, pitch, melted saltpeter, petroleum oil, and oil of gum, boil all these together, impregnate tow with the mixture, and the material is ready to be set on fire. This fire cannot be extinguished by urine, or by vinegar, or by sand. . . .
>
> Flying fire (rockets) may be obtained in the following manner: take one part of colophony, the same of sulfur, and two parts of saltpeter. Dissolve the pulverized mixture in linseed oil, or better in oil of lamium. Finally, the mixture is placed in a reed or in a piece of wood which has been hollowed out. When it is set on fire, it will fly in whatever direction one wishes, there to set everything on fire.

Another mixture corresponds more closely to the composition of black powder. The author even specifies grapevine or willow charcoal which, with the charcoal of black alder, are still the preferred charcoals for making fuze powders and other grades where slow burning is desired.

> Take one pound of pure sulfur, two pounds of grapevine or willow charcoal, and six pounds of saltpeter. Grind these three substances in a marble mortar in such manner as to reduce them to a most subtle powder. After that, the powder in desired quantity is put into an envelope for flying (a rocket) or for making thunder (a cracker). Note that the envelope for flying ought to be thin and long and well-filled with the above-described powder tightly packed, while the envelope for making thunder ought to be short and thick,
>
> 35
>
> only half filled with powder, and tightly tied up at both ends with an iron wire. Note that a small hole ought to be made in each envelope for the introduction of the match. The match ought to be thin at both ends, thick in the middle, and filled with the above-described powder. The envelope intended to fly in the air has as many thicknesses (ply) as one pleases; that for making thunder, however, has a great many.

Toward the end of the *Liber ignium* the author gives a slightly different formula for the black powder to be used in rockets.

> The composition of flying fire is threefold. The first composition may be made from saltpeter, sulfur, and linseed oil. These ground up together and packed into a reed, and lighted, will make it ascend in the air. Another flying fire may be made from saltpeter, sulfur, and grapevine or willow charcoal. These materials, mixed and introduced into a papyrus tube, and ignited, will make it fly rapidly. And note that one ought to take three times as much charcoal as sulfur and three times as much saltpeter as charcoal.

Roger Bacon

Roger Bacon appears to have been the first scholar in northern Europe who was acquainted with the use of saltpeter in incendiary and explosive mixtures. Yet the passage in which he makes specific mention of this important ingredient indicates that toy firecrackers were already in use by the children of his day. In the "Opus Majus," Sixth Part, On Experimental Science, he writes:

> For malta, which is a kind of bitumen and is plentiful in this world, when cast upon an armed man burns him up. The Romans suffered severe loss of life from this in their conquests, as Pliny states in the second book of the Natural History, and as the histories attest. Similarly yellow petroleum, that is, oil springing from the rock, burns up whatever it meets if it is properly prepared. For a consuming fire is produced by this which can be extinguished with difficulty; for water cannot put it out. Certain inventions disturb the hearing to such a degree that, if they are set off suddenly at night with sufficient skill, neither city nor army can endure them. No clap of thunder could compare with such noises. Certain of these strike such terror to the sight that the coruscations of the clouds disturb it incomparably less. . . . We have an example of this in that toy of children which is made in many parts of the world, namely an instrument as
>
> 36

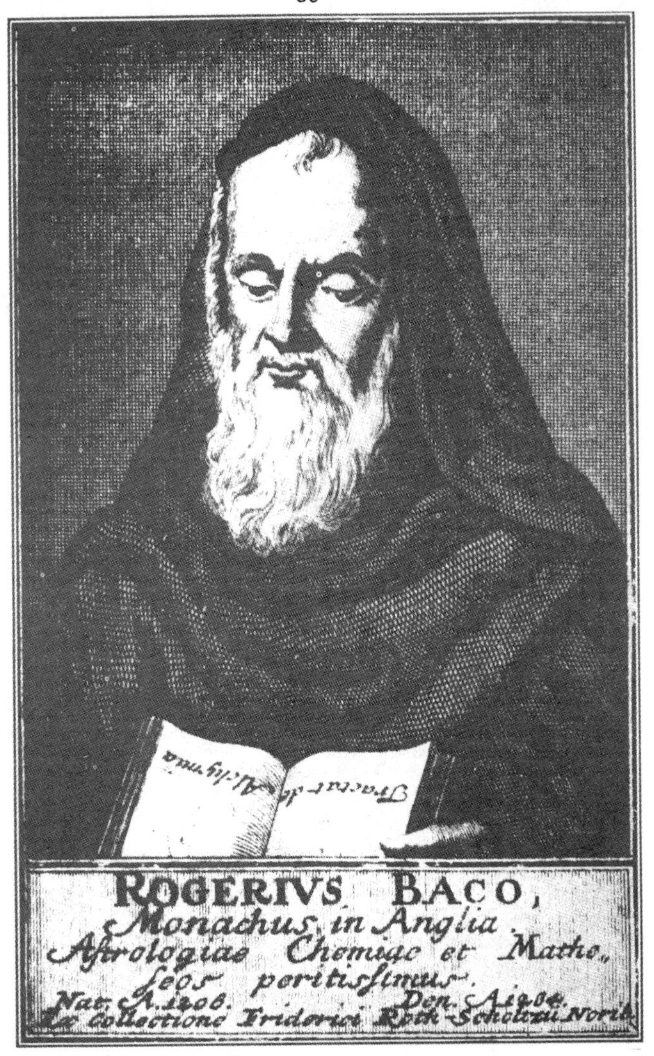
ROGERIVS BACO,
Monachus in Anglia
Astrologiae Chemiae et Matheseos peritissimus.

FIGURE 17. Roger Bacon (c. 1214-1292). Probably the first man in Latin Europe to publish a description of black powder. He was acquainted with rockets and firecrackers, but not with guns.

37

> large as the human thumb. From the force of the salt called saltpeter so horrible a sound is produced at the bursting of so small a thing, namely a small piece of parchment, that we perceive it exceeds the roar of sharp thunder, and the flash exceeds the greatest brilliancy of the lightning accompanying the thunder.

A description in cypher of the composition of black powder in the treatise "De nullitate magiae" which is ascribed to Roger Bacon has attracted considerable attention. Whether Bacon wrote the treatise or not, it is certain at any rate that the treatise dates from about his time and certain, too, that much of the material which it contains is to be found in the "Opus Majus." The author describes many of the wonders of nature, mechanical, optical, medicinal, etc., among them incendiary compositions and firecrackers.

We can prepare from saltpeter and other materials an artificial fire which will burn at whatever distance we please. The same may be made from red petroleum and other things, and from amber, and naphtha, and white petroleum, and from similar materials. . . . Greek fire and many other combustibles are closely akin to these mixtures. . . . For the sound of thunder may be artificially produced in the air with greater resulting horror than if it had been produced by natural causes. A moderate amount of proper material, of the size of the thumb, will make a horrible sound and violent coruscation.

Toward the end of the treatise the author announces his intention of writing obscurely upon a secret of the greatest importance, and then proceeds to a seemingly incoherent discussion of something which he calls "the philosopher's egg." Yet a thoughtful reading between the lines shows that the author is describing the purification of "the stone of Tagus" (saltpeter), and that this material is somehow to be used in conjunction with "certain parts of burned shrubs or of willow" (charcoal) and with the "vapor of pearl" (which is evidently sulfur in the language of the medieval

38

chemists). The often-discussed passage which contains the black powder anagram is as follows:

Sed tamen salis petrae LVRV VO PO VIR CAN VTRIET sulphuris, et sic facies tonitruum et coruscationem: sic facies artificium.

A few lines above the anagram, the author sets down the composition of black powder in another manner. "Take then of the bones of Adam (charcoal) and of the Calx (sulfur), the same weight of each; and there are six of the Petral Stone (saltpeter) and five of the Stone of Union." The Stone of Union is either sulfur or charcoal, probably sulfur, but it doesn't matter for the context has made it evident that only three components enter into the composition. Of these, six parts of saltpeter are to be taken, five each of the other two. The little problem in algebra supplies a means of checking the solution of the anagram, and it is evident that the passage ought to be read as follows:

Sed tamen salis petrae R. VI. PART. V. NOV. CORVLI. ET V. sulphuris, et sic facies tonitruum et coruscationem: sic facies artificium.

But, however, of saltpeter take six parts, five of young willow (charcoal), and five of sulfur, and so you will make thunder and lightning, and so you will turn the trick.

The 6:5:5 formula is not a very good one for the composition of black powder for use in guns, but it probably gave a mixture which produced astonishing results in rockets and firecrackers, and it is not unlike the formulas of mixtures which are used in certain pyrotechnic pieces at the present time.

Although Roger Bacon was not acquainted with guns or with the use of black powder for accomplishing mechanical work, yet he seems to have recognized the possibilities in the mixture, for the treatise "On the Nullity of Magic" comes to an end with the statement: "Whoever will rewrite this will have a key which opens and no man shuts, and when he will shut, no man opens."[13]

[13] Compare *Revelations*, 3: 7 and 8. "And to the angel of the church in Philadelphia write: These things saith he that is holy, he that is true, he that hath the key of David, he that openeth, and no man shutteth; and shutteth, and no man openeth; I know thy works: behold, I have set before thee an open door, and no man can shut it."

39

Development of Black Powder

Guns apparently first came into use shortly after the death of Roger Bacon. A manuscript in the Asiatic Museum at Leningrad, probably compiled about 1320 by Shems ed Din Mohammed, shows tubes for shooting arrows and balls by means of powder. In the library of Christ Church, Oxford, there is a manuscript entitled "De officiis regum," written by Walter de Millemete in 1325, in which a drawing pictures a man applying a light to the touch-hole of a bottle-shaped gun for firing a dart. On February 11, 1326, the Republic of Venice ordered iron bullets and metal cannon for the defense of its castles and villages, and in 1338 cannon and powder were provided for the protection of the ports of Harfleur and l'Heure against Edward III. Cannon were used in 1342 by the Moors in the defense of Algeciras against Alphonso XI of Castile, and in 1346 by the English at the battle of Crécy.

When guns began to be used, experiments were carried out for determining the precise composition of the mixture which would produce the best effect. One notable study, made at Bruxelles about 1560, led to the selection of a mixture containing saltpeter 75 per cent, charcoal 15.62 per cent, and sulfur 9.38 per cent. A few of the formulas for black powder which have been used at various times are calculated to a percentage basis and tabulated below:

	Saltpeter	Charcoal	Sulfur
8th century, Marcus Graecus	66.66	22.22	11.11
8th century, Marcus Graecus	69.22	23.07	7.69
c. 1252, Roger Bacon	37.50	31.25	31.25
1350, Arderne (laboratory recipe)	66.6	22.2	11.1
1560, Whitehorne	50.0	33.3	16.6
1560, Bruxelles studies	75.0	15.62	9.38
1635, British Government contract	75.0	12.5	12.5
1781, Bishop Watson	75.0	15.0	10.0

It is a remarkable fact, and one which indicates that the improvements in black powder have been largely in the methods of manufacture, that the last three of these formulas correspond very closely to the composition of all potassium nitrate black powder for military and sporting purposes which is used today. Any considerable deviation from the 6:1:1 or 6:1.2:0.8 formulas

40

produces a powder which burns more slowly or produces less vigorous effects, and different formulas are used for the com-

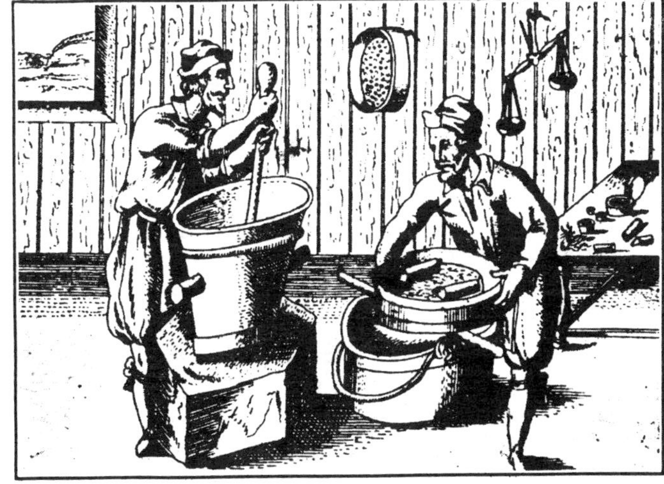

Figure 18. Gunpowder Manufacture, Lorrain, 1630. After the materials had been intimately ground together in the mortar, the mixture was moistened with water, or with a solution of camphor in brandy, or with other material, and formed into grains by rubbing through a sieve.

pounding of powders for blasting and for other special purposes. In this country blasting powder is generally made from sodium nitrate.

John Bate early in the seventeenth century understood the individual functions of the three components of black powder when he wrote: "The Saltpeter is the Soule, the Sulphur the Life, and the Coales the Body of it." The saltpeter supplies the oxygen for the combustion of the charcoal, but the sulfur is the life, for this inflammable element catches the first fire, communicates it throughout the mass, makes the powder quick, and gives it vivacity.

Hard, compressed grains of black powder are not porous—the sulfur appears to have colloidal properties and to fill completely

41

the spaces between the small particles of the other components—and the grains are poor conductors of heat. When they are lighted, they burn progressively from the surface. The area of the surface of an ordinary grain decreases as the burning advances, the grain becomes smaller and smaller, the rate of production of gas decreases, and the duration of the whole burning depends upon the dimension of the original grain. Large powder grains which required more time for their burning were used in the larger guns. Napoleon's army used roughly cubical grains 8 mm. thick in its smaller field guns, and cubical or lozenge-shaped grains twice as thick in some of its larger guns. Grains in the form of hexagonal prisms were used later, and the further improvement was introduced of a central hole through the grain in a direction parallel to the sides of the prism. When these single-perforated hexagonal prisms were lighted, the area of the outer surfaces decreased as the burning advanced, but the area of the inner surfaces of the holes actually increased, and a higher rate of production of gas was maintained. Such powder, used in rifled guns, gave higher velocities and greater range than had ever before been possible. Two further important improvements were made: one, the use of multiple perforations in the prismatic grain by means of which the burning surface was made actually to increase as the burning progressed, with a resultant acceleration in the rate of production of the gases; and the other, the use of the slower-burning *cocoa powder* which permitted improvements in gun design. These, however, are purely of historical interest, for smokeless powder has now entirely superseded black powder for use in guns.

If a propellent powder starts to burn slowly, the initial rise of pressure in the gun is less and the construction of the breech end of the gun need not be so strong and so heavy. If the powder later produces gas at an accelerated rate, as it will do if its burning surface is increasing, then the projectile, already moving in the barrel, is able to take up the energy of the powder gases more advantageously and a greater velocity is imparted to it. The desired result is now secured by the use of progressive-burning colloided smokeless powder. Cocoa powder was the most successful form of black powder for use in rifled guns of long range.

Cocoa powder or brown powder was made in single-perforated

42

hexagonal or octagonal prisms which resembled pieces of milk chocolate. A partially burned brown charcoal made from rye straw was used. This had colloidal properties and flowed under pressure, cementing the grains together, and made it possible to manufacture powders which were slow burning because they contained little sulfur or sometimes even none. The compositions of several typical cocoa powders are tabulated below:

	Saltpeter	Brown Charcoal	Sulfur
England	79	18	3
England	77.4	17.6	5
Germany	78	19	3
Germany	80	20	0
France	78	19	3

Cocoa powder was more sensitive to friction than ordinary black powder. Samples were reported to have inflamed from shaking in a canvas bag. Cocoa powder was used in the Spanish-American war, 1898. When its use was discontinued, existing stocks were destroyed, and single grains of the powder are now generally to be seen only in museums.

Burning of Black Powder

Black powder burns to produce a white smoke. This, of course, consists of extremely small particles of solid matter held temporarily in suspension by the hot gases from the combustion. Since the weight of these solids is equal to more than half of the weight of the original powder, the superiority of smokeless powder, which produces practically no smoke and practically 100 per cent of its weight of hot gas, is immediately apparent. The products of the burning of black powder have been studied by a number of investigators, particularly by Noble and Abel, who showed that the burning does not correspond to any simple chemical reaction between stoichiometrical proportions of the ingredients. Their experiments with RLG powder having the percentage composition indicated below showed that this powder burned to produce (average results) 42.98 per cent of its weight of gases, 55.91 per cent solids, and 1.11 per cent water.

43

Potassium nitrate			74.430
Potassium sulfate			0.133
Sulfur			10.093
Charcoal	Carbon	12.398	14.286
	Hydrogen	0.401	
	Oxygen	1.272	
	Ash	0.215	
Moisture			1.058

Their mean results from the analysis of the gaseous products (percentage by volume) and of the solid products (percentage by weight) are shown in the following tables.

Gas	%	Solid	%
Carbon dioxide	49.29	Potassium carbonate	61.03
Carbon monoxide	12.47	Potassium sulfate	15.10
Nitrogen	32.91	Potassium sulfide	14.45
Hydrogen sulfide	2.65	Potassium thiocyanate	0.22
Methane	0.43	Potassium nitrate	0.27
Hydrogen	2.19	Ammonium carbonate	0.08
		Sulfur	8.74
		Carbon	0.08

One gram of the powder in the state in which it was normally used, that is, while containing 1.058 per cent of moisture, produced 718.1 calories and 271.3 cc. of permanent gas measured at 0° and 760 mm. One gram of the completely desiccated powder gave 725.7 calories and 274.2 cc. These results indicate by calculation that the explosion of the powder produces a temperature of about 3880°.

Uses of Black Powder

Where smoke is no objection, black powder is probably the best substance that we have for communicating fire and for producing a quick hot flame, and it is for these purposes that it is now principally used in the military art. Indeed, the fact that its flame is filled with finely divided solid material makes it more efficient as an igniter for smokeless powder than smokeless powder itself. Standard black powder (made approximately in accordance with the 6:1:1 or the 6:1.2:0.8 formula) is used in *pétards*, as a base charge or expelling charge for shrapnel shells, in saluting and blank fire charges, as the bursting charge of practice shells and bombs, as a propelling charge in certain pyrotechnic pieces, and, either with or without the admixture of other substances which modify the rate of burning, in the time-train

44

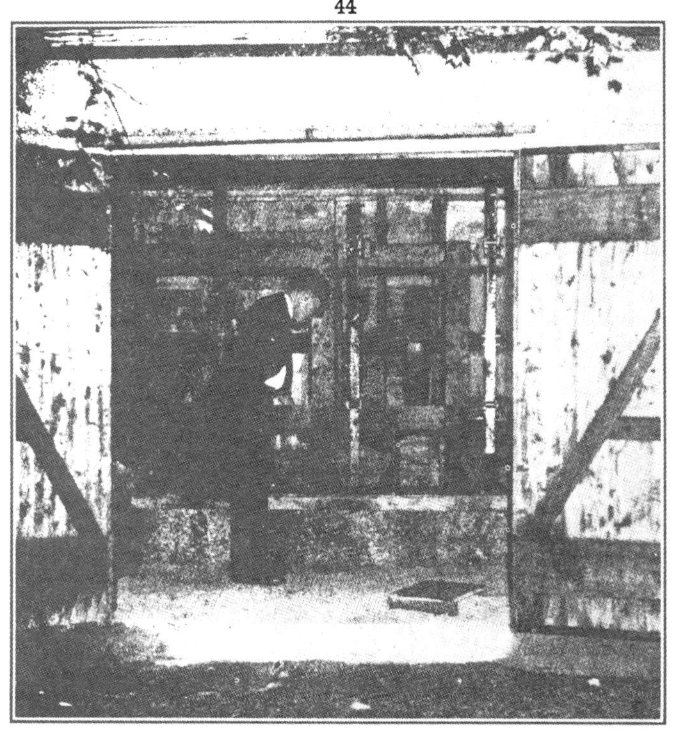

FIGURE 19. Stamp Mill for Making Black Powder. (Courtesy National Fireworks Company and the *Boston Globe*.) This mill, which makes powder for use in the manufacture of fireworks, consists of a single block of granite in which three deep cup-shaped cavities have been cut. The stamps which operate in these cups are supplied at their lower ends with cylindrical blocks of wood, sections cut from the trunk of a hornbeam tree. These are replaced when worn out. The powder from the mill is called "meal powder" and is used as such in the manufacture of fireworks. Also it is moistened slightly with water and rubbed through sieves to form granular gunpowder for use in making rockets, Roman candles, aerial bombshells, and other artifices.

45

rings and in other parts of fuzes. Modified black powders, in which the proportion of the ingredients does not approximate to the standard formulas just mentioned, have been used for blasting, especially in Europe, and have been adapted to special uses in pyrotechny. Sodium nitrate powder, *ammonpulver*, and other more remote modifications are discussed later in this chapter or in the chapter on pyrotechnics.

Manufacture

During the eighteenth century, stamp mills (Figure 19) for incorporating the ingredients of black powder largely superseded the more primitive mortars operated by hand. The meal powder, or *pulverin* as the French call it, was made into gunpowder by moistening slightly and then pressing through sieves.[17] The powder grains were not uniform with one another either in their composition or their density, and could not be expected to give very uniform ballistic results. The use of a heavy wheel mill for grinding and pressing the materials together, and the subsequent pressing of the material into a hard cake which is broken up into grains, represent a great advance in the art and produce hard grains which are physically and ballistically uniform.[18] The operations in the manufacture of black powder as it is carried out at present are briefly as follows:

1. *Mixing* of the powdered materials is accomplished by hand or mechanical blending while they are dampened with enough water to prevent the formation of dust, or the powdered sulfur and charcoal are stirred into a saturated solution of the requisite amount of potassium nitrate at a temperature of about 130°, the hot mass is spread out on the floor to cool, and the lumps are broken up.

2. *Incorporating or Milling.* The usual wheel mill has wheels which weigh 8 or 10 tons each. It takes a charge of 300 pounds of

[17] The French still make *pulverin*, for the preparation of black match and for use in pyrotechnics, by rolling the materials with balls, some of lead and some of lignum vitae, in a barrel of hardwood. They also sometimes use this method for mixing the ingredients before they are incorporated more thoroughly in the wheel mill.

[18] The black powder wheel mill is also used for reducing (under water) deteriorated smokeless powder to a fine meal in order that it may be reworked or used in the compounding of commercial explosives, and for the intimate incorporation of such explosives as the French *schneiderite*.

46

the mixture. The wheels rotate for about 3 hours at a rate of about 10 turns per minute. Edge runners turn back under the tread of the wheels material which would otherwise work away from the center of the mill. Considerable heat is produced during the milling, and more water is added from time to time to replace that which is lost by evaporation in order that the material may always be moist. The "wheel cake" and "clinker" which result from the milling are broken up into small pieces for the pressing.

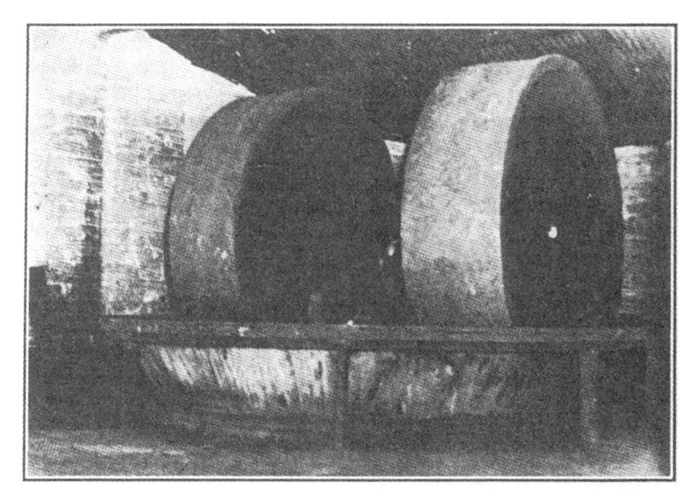

FIGURE 20. Modern Wheel Mill for Making Black Powder. (Courtesy Atlas Powder Company.) The large wheels weigh 10 tons each.

3. *Pressing* is done in a horizontal hydraulic press. Layers of powder are built up by hand between plates of aluminum, and the whole series of plates is pressed in one operation. The apparatus is so designed that fragments of powder are free to fall out at the edges of the plates, and only as much of the material remains between them as will conveniently fill the space. An effective pressure of about 1200 pounds per square inch is applied, and the resulting press cakes are about ¾ inch thick and 2 feet square.

4. *Corning or granulating* is the most dangerous of the operations in the manufacture of black powder. The corning mill is usually situated at a distance from the other buildings, is barri-
47
caded, and is never approached while the machinery, controlled from a distance, is in operation. The press cake is cracked or granulated between crusher rolls. Screens, shaken mechanically, separate the dust and the coarse pieces from the grains which are of the right size for use. The coarse pieces pass between other crusher rolls and over other screens, four sets of crusher rolls being used. Corning mill dust is used in fuse powder and by the makers of fireworks, who find it superior for certain purposes to other kinds of meal powder.

5. *Finishing.* The granulated powder from the corning mill is rounded or polished and made "bright" by tumbling in a revolving wooden cylinder or barrel. Sometimes it is dried at the same time by forcing a stream of warm air through the barrel. Or the polished powder is dried in wooden trays in a dry-house at 40°. If a glazed powder is desired, the glaze is usually applied before the final drying. To the polished powder, still warm from the tumbling, a small amount of graphite is added, and the tumbling is continued for a short time. Black powder of commerce usually contains about 1 or 1.5 per cent moisture. If it contains less than this, it has a tendency to take up moisture from the air; if it contains much more, its efficiency is affected.

6. *Grading.* The powder is finally rescreened and separated into the different grain sizes, C (coarse), CC, CCC, F (fine), FF or 2F, 3F, 4F, etc. The word *grade* applied to black powder, refers to the grain size, not to the quality.

Analysis[19]

A powdered sample for analysis may be prepared safely by grinding granulated black powder, in small portions at a time, in a porcelain mortar. The powder may be passed through a 60-mesh sieve and transferred quickly to a weighing bottle without taking up an appreciable amount of moisture.

[19] A test which from ancient times has been applied to black powder is carried out by pouring a small sample onto a cold flat surface and setting fire to it. A good powder ought to burn in a flash and leave no "pearls" or residue of globules of fused salt. A solid residue indicates either that the ingredients have not been well incorporated, or that the powder at some time in its history has been wet (resulting in larger particles of saltpeter than would be present in good powder, the same result as poor incorporation), or that the powder at the time of the test contains an undue amount of moisture.

48
Moisture is determined by drying in a desiccator over sulfuric acid for 3 days, or by drying to constant weight at 60° or 70°, at which temperature 2 hours is usually long enough.

For determining *potassium nitrate*, the weighed sample in a Gooch crucible is washed with hot water until the washings no longer give any test for nitrate,[20] and the crucible with its contents is dried to constant weight at 70°. The loss of weight is equal to potassium nitrate *plus* moisture. In this determination, as in the determination of moisture, care must be taken not to dry the sample too long, for there is danger that some of the sulfur may be lost by volatilization.

Sulfur is determined as the further loss of weight on extraction with carbon disulfide in a Wiley extractor or other suitable apparatus. After the extraction, the crucible ought to be allowed to dry in the air away from flames until all the inflammable carbon disulfide has escaped. It is then dried in the oven to constancy of weight, and the residue is taken as *charcoal*. *Ash* is determined by igniting the residue in the crucible until all carbon has burned away. A high result for ash may indicate that the water extraction during the determination of potassium nitrate was not complete. The analytical results may be calculated on a moisture-free basis for a closer approximation to the formula by which the manufacturer prepared the powder.

Blasting Powder

The 6:1:1 and 6:1.2:08 formulas correspond to the quickest and most vigorous of the black-powder compositions. A slower and cheaper powder is desirable for blasting, and both these desiderata are secured by a reduction in the amount of potassium nitrate. For many years the French government has manufactured and sold three kinds of blasting or mining powder, as follows:

	Saltpeter	Charcoal	Sulfur
Forte........	72	15	13
Lente........	40	30	30
Ordinaire.....	62	18	20

In the United States a large part of all black powder for blast-

[20] A few drops, added to a few cubic centimeters of a solution of 1 gram of diphenylamine in 100 cc. of concentrated sulfuric acid, give a blue color if a trace of nitrate is present.

49
ing is made from sodium nitrate. This salt is hygroscopic, but a heavy graphite glaze produces a powder from it which is satisfactory under a variety of climatic conditions. Analyses of samples of granulated American blasting powder have shown that the compositions vary widely, sodium nitrate from 67.3 to 77.1 per cent, charcoal from 9.4 to 14.3 per cent, and sulfur from 22.9 to 8.6 per cent. Perhaps sodium nitrate 73, charcoal 11, and sulfur 16 may be taken as average values.

Pellet powders, made from sodium nitrate, are finding extensive use. These consist of cylindrical "pellets," 2 inches long, wrapped in paraffined paper cartridges, 1¼, 1⅜, 1½, 1¾, and 2 inches in diameter, which resemble cartridges of dynamite. The cartridges contain 2, 3, or 4 pellets which are perforated in the direction of their axis with a ⅜-inch hole for the insertion of a squib or fuse for firing.

Ammonpulver

Propellent powder made from ammonium nitrate is about as powerful as smokeless powder and has long had a limited use for military purposes, particularly in Germany and Austria. The Austrian army used Ammonpulver, among others, during the first World War, and it is possible that the powder is now, or may be at any time, in use.

Gäns of Hamburg in 1885 patented a powder which contained no sulfur and was made from 40 to 45 per cent potassium nitrate, 35 to 38 per cent ammonium nitrate, and 14 to 22 per cent charcoal. This soon came into use under the name of *Amidpulver,* and was later improved by decreasing the proportion of potassium nitrate. A typical improved Amidpulver, made from potassium nitrate 14 per cent, ammonium nitrate 37 per cent, and charcoal 49 per cent, gives a flashless discharge when fired in a gun and only a moderate amount of smoke. Ammonpulver which contains no potassium nitrate—in a typical example ammonium nitrate 85 per cent and charcoal 15 per cent, or a similar mixture containing in addition a small amount of aromatic nitro compound—is flashless and gives at most only a thin bluish-gray smoke which disappears rapidly. Rusch has published data

50

which show that the temperature of the gases from the burning of ammonpulver (ammonium nitrate 80 to 90 per cent, charcoal 20 to 10 per cent) is below 900°, and that the ballistic effect is approximately equal to that of ballistite containing one-third of its weight of nitroglycerin.

Ammonpulver has the advantages of being cheap, powerful, flashless, and smokeless. It is insensitive to shock and to friction, and is more difficult to ignite than black powder. In use it requires a strong igniter charge. It burns rapidly, and in gunnery is used in the form of single-perforated cylindrical grains usually of a diameter nearly equal to that of the space within the cartridge. It has the disadvantages that it is extremely hygroscopic and that it will not tolerate wide changes of temperature without injury. The charges must be enclosed in cartridges which are effectively sealed against the ingress of moisture from the air. Ammonium nitrate has a transition point at 32.1°. If Ammonpulver is warmed above this temperature, the ammonium nitrate which it contains undergoes a change of crystalline state; this results in the crumbling of the large powder grains and consequent high pressures and, perhaps, bursting of the gun if the charge is fired. At the present time Ammonpulver appears to be the only modification of black powder which has interesting possibilities as a military propellant.

Other Related Propellent Explosives

Guanidine nitrate powders have not been exploited, but the present availability of guanidine derivatives from the cyanamide industry suggests possibilities. The salt is stable and non-hygroscopic, and is a flashless explosive—cooler indeed than ammonium nitrate. Escales cites a German patent to Gäns for a blasting powder made from potassium nitrate 40 to 60 per cent, guanidine nitrate 48 to 24 per cent, and charcoal 12 to 16 per cent.

Two other powders, now no longer used, are mentioned here as historically interesting examples of propellants made up in accordance with the same principle as black powder, namely, the principle of mixing an oxidizing salt with a combustible material.

Raschig's white blasting powder was made by dissolving 65 parts of sodium nitrate and 35 parts of sodium cresol sulfonate

51

together in water, running the solution in a thin stream onto a rotating and heated steel drum whereby the water was evaporated, and scraping the finished powder off from the other side of the drum. It was cheap, and easy and safe to make, but was hygroscopic. For use in mining, it was sold in waterproof paper cartridges.

Poudre Brugère was made by grinding together 54 parts of ammonium picrate and 46 parts of potassium nitrate in a black powder wheel mill, and pressing and granulating, etc., as in the manufacture of black powder. The hard grains were stable and non-hygroscopic. The powder was used at one time in military weapons. It was more powerful than black powder and gave less smoke.

52

CHAPTER III

PYROTECHNICS

The early history of pyrotechnics and the early history of black powder are the same narrative. Incendiary compositions containing saltpeter, and generally sulfur, mixed with combustible materials were used both for amusement and for purposes of war. They developed on the one hand into black powder, first used in crackers for making a noise and later in guns for throwing a projectile, and on the other into pyrotechnic devices. The available evidence indicates that fireworks probably developed first in the Far East, possibly in India earlier than in China, and that they were based upon various compositions of potassium nitrate, sulfur, and charcoal, with the addition of iron filings, coarse charcoal, and realgar (As_2S_2) to produce different visual effects. The nature of the composition and the state of subdivision of its ingredients determine the rate of burning and the appearance of the flame. In Chinese fire, coarse particles of hard-wood charcoal produce soft and lasting sparks; filings of cast iron produce bright and scintillating ones. The original Bengal lights were probably made more brilliant by the addition of realgar.

The manufacture of pyrotechnics from the Renaissance onward has been conducted, and still is practiced in certain places, as a household art or familiar craft. The artificer[1] needs patience and skill and ingenuity for his work. For large-scale factory production, the pyrotechnist has few problems in chemical engineering but many in the control of craftsmanship. His work, like that of the wood-carver or bookbinder, requires manual dexterity but transcends artistry and becomes art by the free play of the imagination for the production of beauty. He knows the kinds of effects, audible and visible, which he can get from his materials. He knows this as the graphic artist knows the appearance of his

[1] In the French language the word *artificier* means fireworks maker, and *artifice* means a pyrotechnic device.

53

colors. His problem is twofold: the esthetic one of combining these effects in a manner to produce a result which is pleasing, and the wholly practical one of contriving devices—and the means for the construction of devices—which shall produce these results. Like the graphic artist, he had but few colors at first, and he created designs with those which he had—lights, fountains, showers, Roman candles, rockets, etc. As new colors were discovered, he applied them to the production of better examples of the same or slightly modified designs. At the same time he introduced factory methods, devised improvements in the construction of his devices, better tools, faster and more powerful machinery, and learned to conduct his operations with greater safety and with vastly greater output, but the essential improvements in his products since the beginning of the seventeenth century have been largely because of the availability of new chemical materials.

Development of Pyrotechnic Mixtures

The use of antimony sulfide, Sb_2S_3, designated in the early writings simply as antimony, along with the saltpeter, sulfur, and charcoal, which were the standard ingredients of all pyrotechnic compositions, appears to have been introduced in the early part of the seventeenth century. John Bate's "Book of Fireworks," 1635, containing information derived from "the noted Professors, as Mr. Malthus, Mr. Norton, and the French Authour, Des Récreations Mathématiques," mentions no mixtures which contain antimony. Typical of his mixtures are the following.

> *Compositions for Starres.* Take saltpeter one pound, brimstone half a pound, gunpowder foure ounces, this must be bound up in paper or little ragges, and afterwards primed.
>
> *Another receipt for Starres.* Take of saltpeter one pound, gunpowder and brimston of each halfe a pound; these must be mixed together, and of them make a paste, with a sufficient quantity of oil of peter (petroleum), or else of faire water; of this paste you shal make little balles, and roll

them in drie gunpowder dust; then dry them, and keepe them for your occasions.

The iron scale which John Bate used in certain of his rocket

54

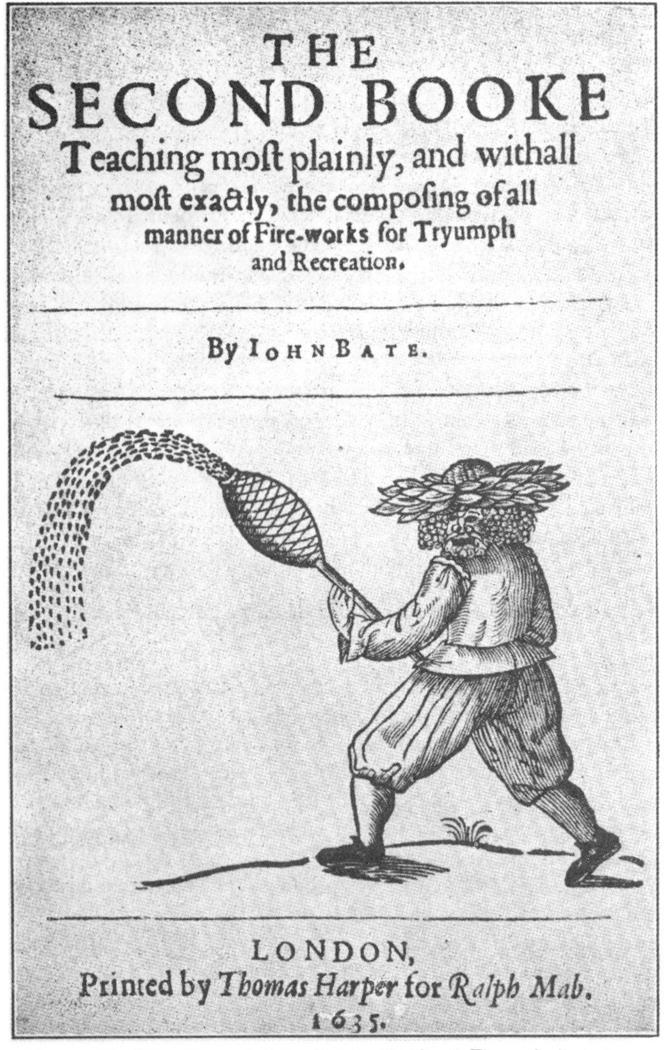

THE
SECOND BOOKE
Teaching most plainly, and withall
most exactly, the composing of all
manner of Fire-works for Tryumph
and Recreation.

By IOHN BATE.

LONDON,
Printed by Thomas Harper for Ralph Mab.
1635.

FIGURE 21. Title Page of John Bate's "Book of Fireworks." A "green man," such as might walk at the head of a procession, is shown scattering sparks from a fire club. The construction of this device is described as follows: "To make . . . you must fill diverse canes open at both ends (and of a foot long, or more, or lesse, as you think fit) with a slow composition, and binde them upon a staffe of four or five foot long; prime them so that one being ended, another may begin: you may prime them with a stouple or match (prepared as before). Make an osier basket about it with a hole in the very top to fire it by, and it is done."

55

compositions probably produced no brilliant sparks but only glowing globules of molten slag which gave the rocket a more luminous tail. Hanzelet Lorrain in 1630 showed a more advanced knowledge of the art and gave every evidence of being acquainted with it by his own experience. He described several mixtures containing antimony sulfide and compositions, for balls of brilliant fire to be thrown from the hand, which contain orpiment (As_2S_3) and verdigris.

Stars of the only two compositions which are well approved. Take of powder (gunpowder) four ounces, of saltpeter two ounces, of sulfur two ounces, of camphor half an ounce, of steel filings two *treseaux*, of white amber half an ounce, of antimony (sulfide) half an ounce, of (corrosive) sublimate half an ounce. For double the efficacy it is necessary to temper all these powders with gum *agragante* dissolved in brandy over hot cinders. When you see that the gum is well swollen and fully ready to mix with the said brandy, it is necessary forthwith to mix them in a mortar with the powder, the quicker the better, and then to cut up the resulting paste into pieces. These stars are very beautiful and very flowery. Note that it is necessary to put them to dry in a pastry or baking oven after the bread has been taken off of the hearth.

Second star composition. Take of saltpeter in fine and dry flour ten ounces, of charcoal, of sulfur, of powder (gunpowder), of antimony (sulfide), and of camphor each two *treseaux*. Temper the whole with oil of turpentine, and make it into a powdery (mealy) paste which you will put into little cartridges; and you will load them in the same manner as rockets [that is, by pounding in the charge]. When you wish to use them, it is necessary to remove the paper wrapper and to cut them into pieces setting a little black match (*mèche d'estoupin*) in the middle (of each piece) through a little hole which you will pierce there.

How fire-balls are made so white that one can scarcely look at them without being dazzled. Take a pound of sulfur, three pounds of saltpeter, half a pound of gum arabic, four ounces of orpiment: grind all together, and mix well by hand,

56

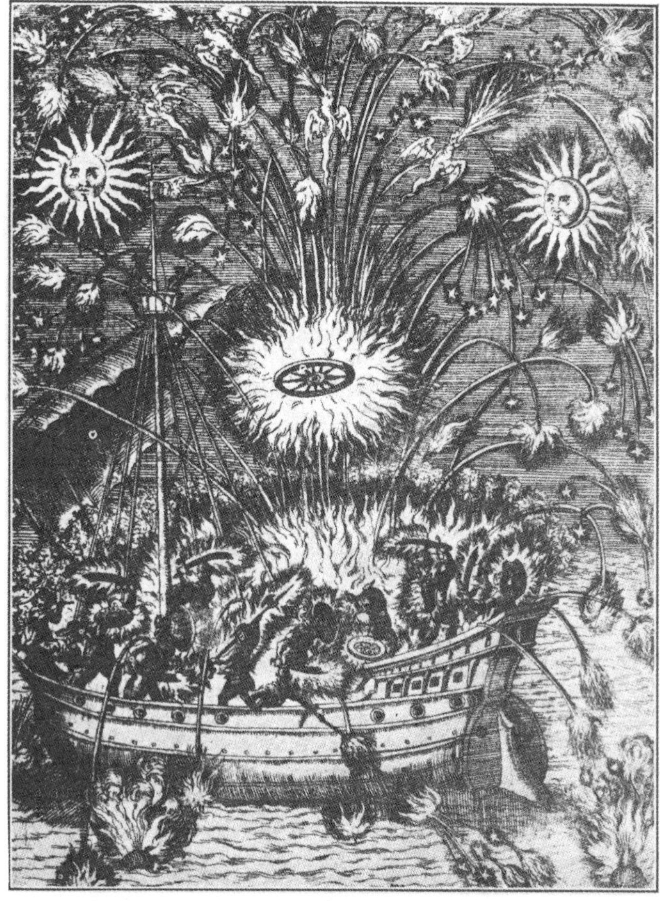

FIGURE 22. Seventeenth-Century Fireworks Display, Lorrain, 1630. Flaming swords, shields and pikes, wheel of fire, rockets, stars, candles, serpents, water fireworks. The sun and the moon which are pictured are presumably aerial bombs, and the dragons are probably dragon rockets running on ropes but may possibly be imaginative representations of serpents of fire. The picture is convincing evidence that many of the varieties of fireworks which are now used (in improved form) for display purposes were already in use three centuries ago.

57

and moisten with brandy and make into a stiff paste into which you will mix half a pound of ground glass, or of crystal in small grains, not in powder, which you will pass through a screen or sieve. Then, mixing well with the said paste, you will form balls of it, of whatever size you please and as round as you can make them, and then you will let them dry. If you wish to have green fire, it is necessary merely to add a little verdigris to the composition. This is a very beautiful fire and thoroughly tested, and it needs no other primer to fire it than the end of a lighted match, for, as soon as the fire touches it, it inflames forthwith. It is beautiful in saluting a prince or nobleman to have such agreeable hand fire balls before setting off any other fireworks.

Audot, whose little book we take to be representative of the state of the art at the beginning of the nineteenth century, had a slightly larger arsenal of materials.

Iron and steel filings. "They give white and red sparks. It is necessary to choose those which are long and not rolled up, and to separate them from any dirt. They are passed through two sieves, in order to have two sizes, fine filings and coarse filings. Those of steel are in all respects to be preferred. It is easy to procure them from the artisans who work in iron and steel."

Ground and filed cast iron. "Cast iron is used in the fires which are designated by the name of *Chinese fire*. Two kinds, fine and coarse. The cast iron is ground in a cast iron mortar with a cast iron or steel pestle, and then sifted."

Red copper filings. "This gives greenish sparks."

Zinc filings "produce a beautiful blue color; it is a substance very difficult to file."

Antimony (sulfide) "gives a blue flame. It is ground up and passed through a screen of very fine silk."

Yellow amber. "Its color, when it burns, is yellow. It is used only for the fire of lances. It is very common in the drug trade. It ought to be ground and passed through a sieve."

Lampblack. "It gives a very red color to fire, and it gives rose in certain compositions."

Yellow sand or gold powder. "It is used in suns where it produces golden yellow rays. It is a reddish yellow sand mixed with

58

little brilliant scales. The paperers sell it under the name of gold powder. It is very common in Paris."

Some of Audot's compositions are as follows:

Common fire: meal powder 16 parts, coarse and fine charcoal 5 parts.

Chinese fire: meal powder 16 parts, cast iron 6 parts.

Brilliant fire: meal powder 16 parts, steel filings 4 parts.

Blue fire for cascades: meal powder 16 parts, saltpeter 8, sulfur 12, and zinc filings 12 parts.

Fixed star: saltpeter 16 parts, sulfur 4, meal powder 4, and antimony (sulfide) 2 parts.

Silver rain for a turning sun or fire wheel: meal powder 16 parts, saltpeter 1, sulfur 1, steel filings 5 parts.

Green fire for the same: meal powder 16 parts, copper filings 3 parts.

Chinese fire for the same: meal powder 16 parts, saltpeter 8, fine charcoal 3, sulfur 3, fine and coarse cast iron 10 parts.

Composition for lances. Yellow: saltpeter 16 parts, meal powder 16, sulfur 4, amber 4, and colophony 3 parts. *Rose:* saltpeter 16 parts, lampblack 1, meal powder 3. *White:* saltpeter 16 parts, sulfur 8, meal powder 4. *Blue:* saltpeter 16 parts, antimony (sulfide) 8, very fine zinc filings 4. *Green:* saltpeter 16 parts, sulfur 6, verdigris 16, and antimony (sulfide) 6 parts.

Bengal flame: saltpeter 16 parts, sulfur 4, and antimony (sulfide) 2 parts. This mixture was to be lighted by quickmatch and burned in small earthenware pots for general illumination.

The Ruggieri, father and son, contributed greatly to the development of fireworks by introducing new, and often very elaborate, pieces for public display and by introducing new materials into the compositions. They appear to have been among the first who attempted to modify the colors of flames by the addition of salts. The compositions which we have cited from Audot are similar to some of those which the elder Ruggieri undoubtedly used at an earlier time, and the younger Ruggieri, earlier than Audot's book, was using materials which Audot does not mention, in particular, copper sulfate and ammonium chloride for the green fire of the palm-tree set piece. The use of ammonium chloride was a definite advance, for the chloride helps to volatilize the copper and to produce a brighter color. But ammonium

59

chloride is somewhat hygroscopic and tends to cake, and it is now no longer used; indeed, the chloride is unnecessary in compositions which contain chlorate or perchlorate. In the Ruggieri "we have two pyrotechnists who can be considered to represent the best skill of France and Italy; in fact, it was Ruggieri whose arrival in France from Italy in or about 1735 marked the great advance in pyrotechny in the former country." The elder Ruggieri conducted a fireworks display at Versailles in 1739. In 1743 he exhibited for the first time, at the Théâtre de la Comédie Italienne and before the King, the passage of fire from a moving to a fixed piece. "This ingenious contrivance at first astonished the scientists of the day, who said when it was explained to them that nothing could be more simple and that any one could have done it at once." In 1749 he visited England to conduct, with Sarti, a fireworks display in Green Park in celebration of the peace of Aix-la-Chapelle. The younger Ruggieri conducted many public pyrotechnic exhibitions in France during the years 1800-1820, and wrote a treatise on fireworks which was published both in French and in German.

Potassium chlorate had been discovered, or at least prepared in a state of purity, by Berthollet in 1786. It had been tried unsuccessfully and with disastrous results in gunpowder. Forty years elapsed before it began to be used in pyrotechnic mixtures, where, with appropriate salts to color the flame, it yields the brilliant and many-colored lights which are now familiar to us. At present it is being superseded for certain purposes by the safer perchlorate.

James Cutbush, acting professor of chemistry and mineralogy at West Point, in his posthumous "System of Pyrotechny," 1825, tells of the detonation of various chlorate mixtures and of their use for the artificial production of fire. "Besides the use of nitre in pyrotechnical compositions, as it forms an essential part of all

60

of them, there is another salt . . . that affords a variety of amusing experiments. This salt is the hyperoxymuriate or chlorate of potassa. Although it has neither been used for fire-works on an extensive scale, nor does it enter into any of the compositions usually made for exhibition, yet its effect is not the less amusing." At a later place Cutbush says: "M. Ruggieri is of opinion, that chlorate, or hyperoxymuriate of potassa may be employed with advantage in the composition of rockets, but we have not heard that it has been used. It is more powerful in its effects, and probably for this reason he recommended it. This salt, mixed with other substances, will produce the *green fire* of the palm-tree, in imitation of the Russian fire."

Ruggieri's Russian fire, as his son later described it, consisted of crystallized copper acetate 4 parts, copper sulfate 2 parts, and ammonium chloride 1 part, all finely pulverized and mixed with alcohol, and placed upon cotton wick attached to spikes upon the thin metal pieces which were the leaves of the palm tree. The resulting display would not be impressive according to modern standards.

Cutbush also knew how to color the flame, for he says:

> We are of opinion, that many of the nitrates might be advantageously employed in the manufacture of fire works. Some, as nitrate of strontian, communicate a red color to flame, as the flame of alcohol. Nitrate of lime also might be used. . . . Muriate of strontian, mixed with alcohol, or spirit of wine, will give a carmine-red flame. For this experiment, one part of the muriate is added to three or four parts of alcohol. Muriate of lime produces, with alcohol, an orange-coloured flame. Nitrate of copper produces an emerald-green flame. Common salt and nitre, with alcohol, give a yellow flame.

According to Brock, the use of chlorate in pyrotechnic mixtures, initiating the modern epoch in the art, first occurred about 1830. Lieut. Hippert of the Belgian artillery published at Bruxelles in 1836 a French translation, "Pyrotechnie raisonnée," of a work by Prussian artillery Captain Moritz Meyer in which one chapter is devoted to colored fires, and listed several com-

61

positions which contain potassium chlorate. Meyer states, incidentally, that the English at that time used colored rockets for signaling at sea and were able to produce ten distinguishable shades. His descriptions of his compositions give one reason to suspect that he had had little experience with them himself. The first, a mixture of potassium chlorate and sugar, burns, he says, with a red light; but the color is actually a bluish white.

> A powder which burns with a green flame is obtained by the addition of nitrate of baryta to chlorate of potash, nitrate of potash, acetate of copper. A white flame is made by the addition of sulfide of antimony, sulfide of arsenic, camphor. Red by the mixture of lampblack, coal, bone ash, mineral oxide of iron, nitrate of strontia, pumice stone, mica, oxide of cobalt. Blue with ivory, bismuth, alum, zinc, copper sulfate purified of its sea water [*sic*]. Yellow by amber, carbonate of soda, sulfate of soda, cinnabar. It is necessary in order to make the colors come out well to animate the combustion by adding chlorate of potash.

Although Meyer's formulas are somewhat incoherent, they represent a definite advance. Equally significant with the use of chlorate is his use of the nitrates of strontium and barium.

The second German edition of Ruggieri's book (we have not seen the first) contains a *Nachtrag* or supplement which lists nine compositions, of which four contain *Kali oxym.* or potassium chlorate. These are: (1) for red fire, strontium nitrate 24 parts, sulfur 3, fine charcoal 1, and potassium chlorate 5; (2) for green fire, barium carbonate 20 parts, sulfur 5, and potassium chlorate 8 parts; (3) for green stars, barium carbonate 20 parts, sulfur 5, and potassium chlorate 9 parts; and (4) for red lances, strontium carbonate 24 parts, sulfur 4, charcoal 1, and potassium chlorate 4 parts. Ruggieri says:

> The most important factor in the preparation of these compositions is the fine grinding and careful mixing of the several materials. Only when this is done is a beautiful flame to be expected. And it is further to be noted that the potassium chlorate, which occurs in certain of the compositions, is to be wetted with spirit for the grinding in order to avoid an explosion.

62

The chlorate compositions recommended by Ruggieri would undoubtedly give good colors, but are not altogether safe and would probably explode if pounded into their cases. They could be loaded with safety in an hydraulic press, and would probably not explode if tamped carefully by hand.

F. M. Chertier, whose book "Nouvelles recherches sur les feux d'artifice" was published at Paris in 1854, devotes most of his attention to the subject of color, so successfully that, although new materials have come into use since his time, Brock says that "there can be no doubt that Chertier stands alone in the literature of pyrotechny and as a pioneer in the modern development of the art." Tessier, in his "Chimie pyrotechnique ou traité pratique des feux colores," first edition, Paris, 1859, second edition 1883, discusses the effect of individual chemicals upon the colors of flames and gives excellent formulas for chlorate and for non-chlorate compositions which correspond closely to present practice. He used sulfur in many but not in all of his chlorate mixtures. Pyrotechnists in France, with whom the present writer talked during the first World War, considered Tessier's book at that time to be the best existing work on the subject of colored fires—and this in spite of the fact that its author knew nothing of the use of magnesium and aluminum. The spectroscopic study of the colors produced by pure chemicals, and of the colors of pyrotechnic devices which are best suited for particular effects, is the latest of current developments.

Chlorate mixtures which contain sulfur give brighter flames than those which lack it, and such mixtures are still used occasionally in spite of their dangerous properties. The present tendency, however, is toward chlorate mixtures which contain no sulfur, or toward potassium nitrate mixtures (for stars, etc.) which contain sulfur but no chlorate, or toward nitrates, such as those of strontium and barium, which supply both color for the flame and oxygen for the combustion and are used with magnesium or aluminum to impart brilliancy. Magnesium was first used for pyrotechnic purposes about 1865 and aluminum about 1894, both of them for the production of dazzling white light. These metals were used in the compositions of colored airplane

63

flares during the first World War, but their use in the colored fires of general pyrotechny is largely a later development.

Tessier introduced the use of cryolite ($AlNa_3F_6$) for the yellow coloring of stars, lances, and Bengal lights. In his second edition he includes a chapter on the small pyrotechnic pieces which are known as Japanese fireworks, giving formulas for them, and another on the picrates, which he studied extensively. The picrates of sodium, potassium, and ammonium crystallize in the anhydrous condition. Those of barium, strontium, calcium, magnesium, zinc, iron, and copper are hygroscopic and contain considerable water of crystallization which makes them unfit for use in pyrotechnic compositions. Lead picrate, with 1 H_2O, detonates from fire and from shock, and its use in caps and primers was patented in France in 1872. Potassium and sodium picrate deflagrate from flame, retaining that property when mixed with other substances. Ammonium picrate detonates from fire and from shock when in contact with potassium chlorate or lead nitrate, but in the absence of these substances it has the special advantage for colored fires that the mixtures give but little smoke and this without offensive odor. Tessier recommends ammonium picrate compositions for producing colored lights in the theater and in other places where smoke might be objectionable. "Indoor fireworks" have been displaced in the theater by electric lighting devices, but are still used for certain purposes. Tessier's formulas, which are excellent, are described later in the section on picrate compositions.

Colored Lights

Colored light compositions are used in the form of a loose powder, or are tamped into paper tubes in torches for political parades, for highway warnings, and for railway and marine signals, in Bengal lights, in airplane flares, and in lances for set pieces, or are prepared in the form of compact pellets as stars for Roman candles, rockets, and aerial bombs, or as stars to be shot from a special pistol for signaling.

Colored fire compositions intended for burning in conical heaps or in trains are sometimes sold in paper bags but more commonly in boxes, usually cylindrical, of pasteboard, turned wood, or tinned iron. The mixtures are frequently burned in the boxes in which they are sold.[64] Compositions which contain no chlorate (or perchlorate) are the oldest, and are still used where the most brilliant colors are not necessary.

	White					Red	Pink		Yellow
Potassium nitrate	5	3	32	8	14	..	12	14	..
Sulfur	2	1	15	2	4	5	5	4	3
Strontium nitrate	..	..	..	..	..	18	48	36	..
Barium nitrate	..	..	..	..	..	..	..	..	36
Sodium oxalate	..	..	..	..	..	..	..	..	6
Antimony metal	..	1	12	..	..	..	..	..	..
Antimony sulfide	1	1	..	..	..	..	..	..	..
Realgar	..	..	..	1	5	..	..	..	..
Minium	..	..	10	..	..	..	..	..	..
Lampblack	..	..	..	..	..	1	..	..	..
Charcoal	..	..	..	..	..	..	4	1	..
Red gum	..	..	..	..	..	..	..	4	5
Dextrin	..	..	1	..	..	..	..	1	..

The chlorate compositions listed below, which contain no sulfur, burn rapidly with brilliant colors and have been recommended for indoor and theatrical uses.

	White	Red	Yellow	Green
Potassium chlorate	12	1	6	2
Potassium nitrate	4	..	6	..
Strontium nitrate	..	4	..	..
Barium nitrate	..	..	..	1
Barium carbonate	1	..	..	..
Sodium oxalate	..	..	5	..
Cane sugar	4	..	..	1
Stearine	1	..	..	..
Shellac	..	1	3	..

The following are brilliant, somewhat slower burning, and suitable for outdoor use and general illumination. The smokes from the compositions which contain calomel and Paris green are poisonous. In mixing Paris green, care must be exercised not to inhale the dust.[65]

	Red			Green		Blue		
Potassium chlorate	10	4	8	4	4	6	8	16
Strontium nitrate	40	10	16	..	..	..	..	..
Barium nitrate	..	..	..	8	8	4	..	14
Paris green	..	..	..	..	..	4	..	12
Shellac	..	..	3	..	3	..	..	1
Stearine	..	..	..	..	..	1	..	2
Red gum	6	3	..	2	..	..	..	..
Calomel	..	..	..	..	..	..	6	2
Sal ammoniac	..	..	..	1	..	1	..	..
Copper ammonium chloride	..	..	..	..	..	..	2	..
Fine sawdust	6	..	..	..	..	..	..	..
Rosin	..	1	..	..	..	..	..	..
Lampblack	1	1	..	..	..	..	..	..
Milk sugar	..	..	..	..	..	..	3	..

Railway Fusees (Truck Signal Lights)

Motor trucks are required by law to be equipped with red signal lights for use as a warning in case an accident causes them to be stopped on the road at night without the use of their electric lights. Similar lights are used for signaling on the railways. The obvious requirement is that the signal should burn conspicuously and for a long time. A. F. Clark recommends a mixture of:

	Parts
Strontium nitrate (100 mesh)	132
Potassium perchlorate (200 mesh)	15
Prepared maple sawdust (20 mesh)	20
Wood flour (200 mesh)	1
Sulfur (200 mesh)	25

The prepared maple sawdust is made by cooking with miner's wax, 10 pounds of sawdust to 1 ounce of wax, in a steam-jacketed kettle. The mixture is tamped dry into a paper tube, 7/8 inch in external diameter, 1/32 inch wall, and burns at the rate of about 1 inch per minute. The fusee is supplied at its base with a pointed piece of wood or iron for setting it up in the ground, and it burns best when set at an angle of about 45°. In order to insure certain ignition, the top of the charge is covered with a primer or *starting fire*, loaded while moistened with alcohol,[66] which consists of potassium chlorate 16 parts, barium chlorate 8, red gum (gum yacca) 4, and powdered charcoal 1. This is covered with a piece of paper on which is painted a *scratch mixture* similar to that which composes the head of a safety match. The top of the fusee is supplied with a cylindrical paper cap, the end of which is coated with a material similar to that with which the striking surface on the sides of a box of safety matches is coated. To light the fusee, the cap is removed and inverted, and its end or bottom is scratched against the mixture on the top of the fusee.

Weingart recommends the first four of the following compositions for railway fusees; Faber reports the fifth. Weingart's mixtures are to be moistened with kerosene before they are tamped into the tubes.

Potassium chlorate	..	..	..	..	12
Potassium perchlorate	..	..	..	5	..
Strontium nitrate	48	36	16	36	72
Saltpeter	12	14	4	..	..
Sulfur	5	4	5	5	10
Fine charcoal	4	1	1	..	..
Red gum	10	4	..	..	4
Dextrin	..	1	..	..	..
Sawdust	..	..	..	2	..
Sawdust and grease	..	..	..	..	4
Calcium carbonate	..	..	..	..	1

Scratch Mixture

Typical scratch mixtures are the pair: (*A*) potassium chlorate 6, antimony sulfide 2, glue 1; and (*B*) powdered pyrolusite (MnO_2) 8, red phosphorus 10, glue 3, recommended by Weingart; and the pair: (*A*) potassium chlorate 86, antimony sulfide 52, dextrin 35; and (*B*) red phosphorus 9, fine sand 5, dextrin 4, used with gum arabic as a binder, and recommended by A. F. Clark.

Marine Signals

Other interesting signal lights, reported by Faber,[67] are as follows.

	Marine Flare Torch	Pilot's Blue Light
Barium nitrate	16	..
Potassium nitrate	8	..
Potassium chlorate	..	46
Strontium carbonate	1	..
Copper oxychloride	..	32
Sulfur	2	28
Red gum	2	..
Shellac	..	48
Calomel	..	3

Parade Torches

Parade torches are made in various colors; they are of better quality than railway fusees, burn with a deeper color and a brighter light, and are generally made with more expensive compositions. Below are a few typical examples. Parade torches are

	Red			Green		Purple	Amber	Blue
Strontium nitrate	16	5	9	..	..	7	36	..
Barium nitrate	..	..	..	40	30	..	..	..
Potassium chlorate	8	1	..	11	..	..	..	..
Potassium perchlorate	..	..	2	..	6	9	10	5
Sodium oxalate	..	..	..	..	..	..	8	..
Cupric oxide	..	..	..	..	..	6	..	..
Paris green	..	..	..	..	..	..	..	2
Sal ammoniac	..	..	..	1	..	..	..	..
Calomel	..	..	..	..	..	3	..	1
Sulfur	..	..	2	..	3	5	3	..
K.D. gum	..	..	..	6	2	..	..	..
Shellac	3	..	..	..	..	..	5	..
Red gum	..	1	1	..	..	..	..	..
Dextrin	..	..	..	..	..	..	..	1

equipped with wooden handles at the lower ends, and are sealed at their upper ends with a piece of cloth or paper, pasted on, through which a hole has been punched into the composition to a depth of about 1 inch—and through this a piece of *black match*[21] has been inserted and fixed in[68] place by a blob of paste of meal powder with gum-arabic water.

[21] The match, prepared by dipping a few strands of cotton twine, twisted together, into a paste of meal powder and allowing to dry while stretched on a frame, is called *black match* by the pyrotechnists. When this is enclosed in a paper tube, it burns almost instantaneously and is then known as *quickmatch*. Such *quickmatch* is used for communicating fire in set pieces, Catherine wheels, etc.

Aluminum and Magnesium Flares

When barium and strontium nitrates are used in colored lights, these substances serve the twofold purpose of coloring the flame and of supplying oxygen for its maintenance. The materials which combine with the oxygen to yield the flame, in the compositions which have been described, have been sulfur and carbonaceous matter. If, now, part or all of these materials is substituted by magnesium or aluminum powder or flakes, the resulting composition is one which burns with an intensely bright light. A mixture of potassium perchlorate 7 parts, mixed aluminum powder and flakes 5 parts, and powdered sulfur 2 parts burns with a brilliant light having a lilac cast. A balanced mixture of barium and strontium nitrates, that is, of green and red, gives a light which is practically white. Such lights are used in parade torches and signals, but are so bright as to be trying to the eyes. They find important use in aviation for signaling and for illuminating landing fields and military objectives.

Magnesium is attacked fairly rapidly by moisture, and pyrotechnic mixtures containing this metal do not keep well unless the particles of magnesium are first coated with a protecting layer of linseed oil or similar material. Aluminum does not have the same defect and is more widely used. An excellent magnesium light, suitable for illumination, is described in a patent recently granted to George J. Schladt. It consists of a mixture of 36 to 40 per cent barium nitrate, 6 to 8 per cent strontium nitrate, 50 to 54 per cent flake magnesium coated with linseed oil, and 1 to 4 per cent of a mixture of linseed and castor oils.

The airplane wing-tip flares which were used for signaling during the first World War are good examples of aluminum compositions. They were loaded in cylindrical paper cases 4¼ inches in length and 1⅝ inches in internal diameter. The white light composition consisted of 77 parts of barium nitrate, 13 of flake aluminum, and 5 of sulfur intimately mixed and secured by a binder of shellac, and burned in the cases mentioned, for 1 minute with an illumination of[69] 22,000 candlepower. The red light was made from 24 parts of strontium nitrate, 6 of flake aluminum, and 6 of sulfur with a shellac binder and burned for 1 minute with an illumination of 12,000 to 15,000 candlepower. The compositions were loaded into the cases by means of a pneumatic press, and filled them to within 5/16 inch of the top. The charge was then covered with a ⅛-inch layer of starting fire or *first fire composition*, made from saltpeter 6 parts, sulfur 4, and charcoal 1, dampened with a solution of shellac in alcohol, and this, when the device was used, was fired by an electric squib.

Lances

Lances are paper tubes, generally thin and of light construction, say, ¼ to ⅜ inch in diameter and 2 to 3½ inches long, filled with colored fire composition, loaded by tamping, not by ramming, and are used in set pieces, attached to wooden frameworks, to outline the figure of a temple or palace, to represent a flag, to spell words, etc. When set up, they are connected by quickmatch (black match in a paper tube) and are thus lighted as nearly simultaneously as may be. They are often charged in such manner as to burn with a succession of color, in which event the order of loading the various colors becomes important. Green should not be next to white, for there is not sufficient contrast. And green should not burn after red, for the color of the barium flame appears to one who has been watching the flame of strontium to be a light and uninteresting blue. The order of loading (the reverse of the order of burning) is generally white, blue (or yellow or violet, green, red, white. In the tables on page 70 a number of lance compositions are listed, illustrative of the various types and corresponding to considerable differences in cost of manufacture.

Picrate Compositions

Ammonium picrate is used in the so-called indoor fireworks which burn with but little smoke and without the production of objectionable odor. On page 71 some of the compositions recommended by Tessier for Bengal lights are tabulated.

70

WHITE	Potassium nitrate	33	5	9	8	11
	Antimony sulfide	5	..	2	..	1
	Antimony metal	..	1	..	..	3
	Realgar	..	..	..	1	..
	Sulfur	11	2	1	2	3
	Meal powder	2	1	..	..	..
RED	Potassium chlorate			10	6	36
	Strontium nitrate			..	..	54
	Strontium carbonate			3	2	..
	Sulfur			..	..	13
	Lampblack			..	..	2
	Shellac			2	..	12
	Paraffin			..	1	..
YELLOW	Potassium perchlorate		..	..	..	24
	Potassium chlorate		8	4	4	..
	Barium nitrate		1	..	22	..
	Sodium oxalate		..	2	..	8
	Sodium bicarbonate		2	..	..	..
	Cryolite		..	..	2	..
	Sulfur		4	..	5	..
	Lampblack		..	..	1	..
	Shellac		..	1	..	3
GREEN	Potassium chlorate		..	..	7	..
	Barium nitrate		12	4	7	..
	Barium chlorate		9	5	..	6
	Lampblack		1	..	..	..
	Shellac		10	1	2	1
BLUE	Potassium perchlorate			16	..	..
	Potassium chlorate			..	32	5
	Copper oxychloride			..	..	2
	Paris green			6	10	..
	Calomel			1	6	..
	Shellac			1	..	1
	Stearine			..	3	..
LILAC	Potassium chlorate					26
	Strontium sulfate					10
	Basic copper sulfate					6
	Lead nitrate					5
	Sulfur					4
	Shellac					1
	Stearine					1
VIOLET	Potassium chlorate					25
	Strontium sulfate					20
	Basic copper sulfate					1
	Sulfur					20

71

To be burned without compression, in the open, in trains or in heaps:

	Red		Green		Aurora	Yellow	White
Ammonium picrate	5	10	8	5	10	20	5
Strontium nitrate	25	40	..	..	31	12	..
Barium nitrate	..	..	32	25	..	58	30
Cryolite	..	..	..	..	3	7	..
Antimony metal	..	..	..	..	..	..	5
Lampblack	1	2	1	..	2	4	1
Paraffin	1	1	1	1	1	2	1

To be compressed in paper cartridges, 25-30 mm. internal diameter, to be burned in a horizontal position in order that the residue may not interfere with the burning:

	Red		Green			Aurora	Yellow		White	
Ammonium picrate	1	20	5	5	11	20	20	24	6	5
Strontium nitrate	1	60	..	..	..	60	10	3	..	..
Barium nitrate	..	..	6	28	36	..	60	20	4	30
Cryolite	..	..	..	..	..	7	7	4	..	..
Calcium fluoride	..	7	..	..	..	..	..	..	..	..
Antimony metal	..	..	..	..	..	..	..	..	..	4
Antimony sulfide	..	..	..	..	..	..	..	..	3	1
Lampblack	..	4	..	1	1	4	4	..	..	1
Paraffin	..	2	..	1	1	2	2	..	..	1

Picric acid added in small quantities to colors deepens them and increases their brilliancy without making them burn much faster. Stars containing picric acid ought not to be used in aerial shells, for they are likely to detonate either from the shock of setback or later from being ignited in a confined space. Mixtures which contain picric acid along with potassium chlorate or salts of heavy metals are liable to detonate from shock.

Weingart lists two "smokeless tableau" fires which contain picric acid, as follows:

72

	Red	Green
Strontium nitrate	8	..
Barium nitrate	..	4
Picric acid	5	2
Charcoal	2	1
Shellac	1	..

The picric acid is to be dissolved in boiling water, the strontium or barium nitrate added, the mixture stirred until cold, and the solid matter collected and dried. The same author gives picric acid compositions for stars, "not suitable for shells," as follows:

	Red		Green
Strontium nitrate	8	..	..
Strontium carbonate	..	3	..
Barium chlorate	..	..	12
Potassium chlorate	4	10	8
Picric acid	1.5	1.5	2
Calomel	..	..	6

Shellac	1.5	0.75	2
Fine charcoal	1	1	..
Lampblack	..	..	1.5
Dextrin	0.5	0.75	0.5

Picrate Whistles

An intimate mixture of finely powdered dry potassium picrate and potassium nitrate, in the proportion about 60/40, rammed tightly into paper, or better, bamboo tubes from ¼ to ¾ inch in diameter, burns with a loud whistling sound. The mixture is dangerous, exploding from shock, and cannot be used safely in aerial shells. Whistling rockets are made by attaching a tube of the mixture to the outside of the case in such manner that it burns, and whistles, during the flight—or by loading a small tube, say ¼ inch in diameter and 2½ inches long, into the head of the rocket to produce a whistle when the rocket bursts. The mixture

73

is used in whistling firecrackers, "musical salutes," "whistling whizzers," "whistling tornados," etc. The effect of a whistle as an accompaniment to a change in the appearance of a burning wheel is amusing. Whistles are perhaps most effective when six or eight of them, varying in size from the small to the large, are fired in series, the smallest caliber and the highest pitch being first.

Non-Picrate Whistles

Non-picrate whistles, made from a mixture of 1 part powdered gallic acid and 3 parts potassium chlorate, are considered to be safer than those which contain picrate. The mixture is charged into a ½-inch case, 5/16 inch in internal diameter. The case is loaded on a 1-inch spindle, and the finished whistle has a 1-inch length of empty tube which is necessary for the production of the sound. Whistles of this sort, with charges of a chlorate or perchlorate explosive at their ends, are used in "chasers," "whizzers," etc., which scoot along the ground while whistling and finally explode with a loud report.

Rockets

The principle of the rocket and the details of its design were worked out at an early date. Improvements have been in the methods of manufacture and in the development of more brilliant and more spectacular devices to load in the rocket head for display purposes. When rockets are made by hand, the present practice is still very much like that which is indicated by Figure 23. The paper casing is mounted on a spindle shaped to form the long conical cavity on the surface of which the propelling charge will start to burn. The composition is rammed into the space surrounding the spindle by means of perforated ram rods or *drifts* pounded by a mallet. The base of the rocket is no longer choked by crimping, but is choked by a perforated plug of clay. The clay, dried from water and moistened lightly with crankcase oil, is pounded or pressed into place, and forms a hard and stable mass. The tubular paper cases of rockets, *gerbs,*[27] etc., are now often made by machinery, and the compositions are loaded into them automatically or semi-automatically and pressed by hydraulic presses.

[27] Pronounced *jurbs.*

74

John Bate and Hanzelet Lorrain understood that the heavier rockets require compositions which burn more slowly.

It is necessary to have compositions according to the greatness or the littleness of the rockets, for that which is proper for the little ones is too violent for the large—because the fire, being lighted in a large tube, lights a composition of great amplitude, and burns a great quantity of material,

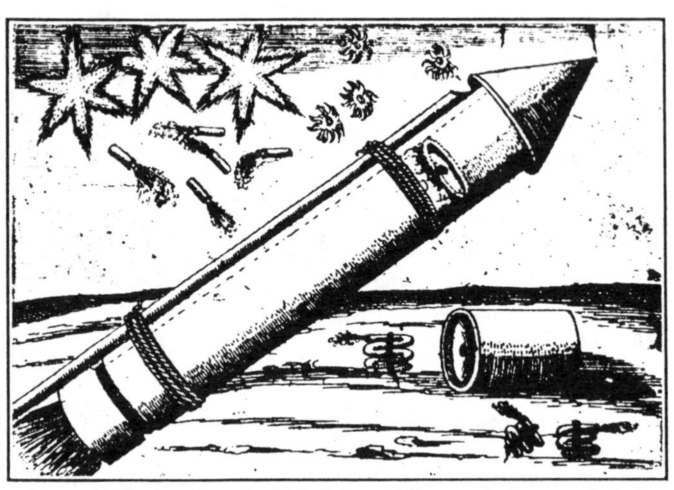

FIGURE 23. Rocket, Lorrain, 1630. Substantially as rockets are made today. After the propelling charge has burned completely and the rocket has reached the height of its flight, the fire reaches the charge in the head which bursts and throws out large and small stars, serpents and grasshoppers, or English firecrackers. The container, which is loaded into the head of the rocket, is shown separately with several grasshoppers in the lower right-hand corner of the picture.

and no geometric proportionality applies. Rockets intended to contain an ounce or an ounce and a half should have the following for their compositions.

Take of fine powder (gunpowder) passed through a screen or very fine sieve four ounces, of soft charcoal one ounce, and mix them well together.[28]

[28] The charcoal makes the powder burn more slowly, and produces a trail of sparks when the rocket is fired.

Otherwise. Of powder sieved and screened as above one pound, of saltpeter one ounce and a half, of soft charcoal

75

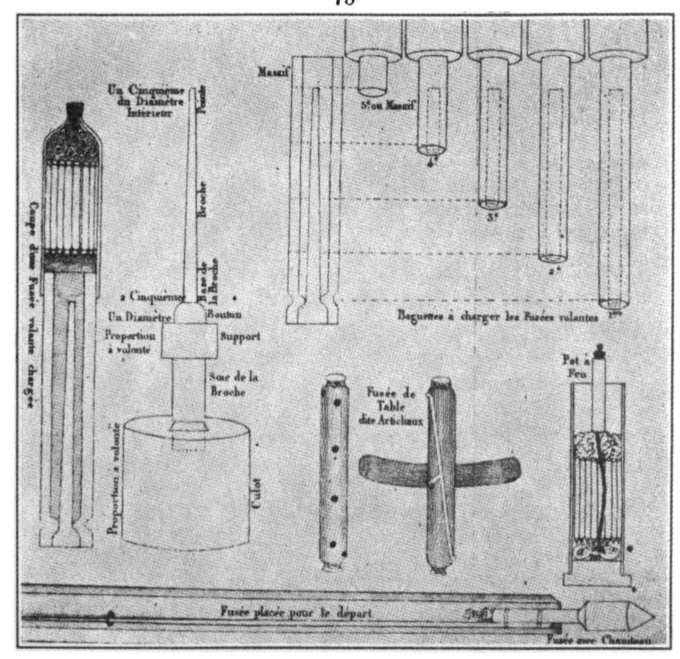

FIGURE 24. Details of Construction of Rocket and of Other Pieces, Audot, 1818. The rocket case, already crimped or constricted, is placed upon the

spindle (*broche*); the first portion of the propelling charge is introduced and pounded firmly into place by means of a mallet and the longest of the *drifts* pictured in the upper right-hand corner; another portion of the charge is introduced, a shorter drift is used for tamping it, and so on until the case is charged as shown at the extreme left. A tourbillion (table rocket or artichoke) and a mine charged with serpents of fire are also shown.

one ounce and a half. It does not matter what charcoal it is; that of light wood is best, particularly of wood of the vine.

For rockets weighing two ounces. Take of the above-said powder four ounces and a half, of saltpeter one ounce.

Otherwise for the same weight. Take powder two ounces, of soft charcoal half an ounce.

Composition for rockets weighing from 4 to 8 ounces. Take powder as above seventeen ounces, of saltpeter four ounces, of soft charcoal four ounces.

76

Otherwise and very good. Of saltpeter ten ounces, of sulfur one ounce, of powder three ounces and a half, of charcoal three ounces and a half.

To make them go up more suddenly. Take of powder ten ounces, of saltpeter three ounces and a half, of sulfur one ounce, of charcoal three ounces and a half.

For rockets weighing one pound. Take of powder one pound, of soft charcoal two ounces, and of sulfur one ounce.

Otherwise. Of saltpeter one pound four ounces, of sulfur two ounces, of soft charcoal five ounces and a half.

For rockets weighing three pounds. Of saltpeter 30 ounces, of charcoal 11 ounces, of sulfur 7 ounces and a half.

For rockets weighing four, five, six, and seven pounds. Of soft charcoal ten pounds, of sulfur four pounds and a half, of saltpeter thirty one pounds.

Present practice is illustrated by the specifications tabulated below for 1-ounce, 3-ounce, and 6-pound rockets as now manufactured by an American fireworks company. The diameter of

		Ounce	Ounce	Pound
Size		1	3	6
Composition of charge	Saltpeter	36	35	30
	Sulfur	6	5	5
	No. 3 charcoal	..	5	12
	No. 5 charcoal	12	..	..
	Charcoal dust	7	17	12
		Inch	Inch	Inch
Length of case		3	4 1/4	13
Outside diameter		1/2	11/16	2 3/8
Inside diameter		5/16	7/16	1 1/2
Overall length of spindle		2 3/4	4	12 3/4
Length of taper		2 1/2	3 23/32	12
Choke diameter		5/32	1/4	3/4

the base of the spindle is, of course, the same as the inside diameter of the case. That of the hemispherical tip of the spindle is half the diameter of the choke, that is, half the diameter of the hole in the clay plug at the base of the rocket. The clay rings and plugs, formed into position by high pressure, actually make grooves in the inner walls of the cases, and these grooves hold them in place against the pressures which arise when the rockets are used. The propelling charge is loaded in several successive small portions by successive pressings with hydraulic presses

77

which handle a gross of the 1-ounce or 3-ounce rockets at a time but only three of the 6-pound size. The presses exert a total pressure of 9 tons on the three spindles when the 6-pound rockets are being loaded.

Rockets of the smaller sizes, for use as toys, are closed at the top with plugs of solid clay and are supplied with conical paper caps. They produce the spectacle only of a trail of sparks streak-

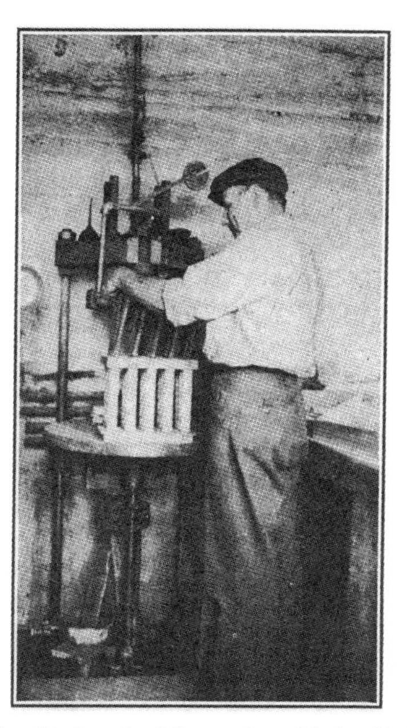

FIGURE 25. Loading Rockets by Means of an Hydraulic Press.

ing skyward. Rockets are generally equipped with sticks to give them balance and direct their flight and are then fired from a trough or frame, but other rockets have recently come on the market which are equipped with vanes and are fired from a level surface while standing in a vertical position.

Large exhibition rockets are equipped with heads which contain stars of various kinds (see below), parachutes, crackers (see grasshoppers), serpents (compare Figure 23), and so on. In these,

78

the clay plug which stands at the top of the rocket case is perforated, and directly below it there is a *heading* of composition which burns more slowly than the propelling charge. In a typical example this is made from a mixture of saltpeter 24 parts, sulfur 6, fine charcoal 4, willow charcoal dust 1½, and dextrin 2; it is loaded while slightly moist, pressed, and allowed to dry before the head of the rocket is loaded. When the rocket reaches the top of its flight, the heading burns through, and its fire, by means of several strands of black match which have been inserted in the perforation in the clay plug, passes into the head. The head is filled with a mixture, say, of gunpowder, Roman candle composition (see below), and stars. When the fire reaches this mixture, the head blows open with a shower of sparks, and the stars, which have become ignited, fall through the air, producing their own specialized effects.

In another example, the head may contain a charge of gunpowder and a silk or paper parachute carrying a flare or a festoon of lights or colored *twinklers*, the arrangement being such that the powder blows the wooden head from the rocket, ejects the parachute, and sets fire to the display material which it carries. In order that the fire may not touch the parachute, the materials which are to receive the fire (by match from the bursting charge) are packed softly in cotton wool and the remaining space is rammed with bran.

The very beautiful liquid fire effect is produced by equipment which is fully assembled only at the moment when it is to be used. The perforation in the clay plug at the top of the rocket is filled with gunpowder, and this is covered with a layer of waterproof cloth well sealed, separating it from the space in the empty head. When the piece is to be fired, the pyrotechnist, having at hand a can containing sticks of yellow phosphorus preserved under water, removes the wooden head from the rocket, empties the water from the can of phosphorus, and dumps the phosphorus, still wet, into the head case, replaces the wooden head, and fires. The explosion of the gunpowder at the top of the rocket's flight tears through the layer of waterproof cloth, ignites the phosphorus, blows off the wooden head, and throws out the liquid fire. A similar effect, with a yellow light, is obtained with metallic sodium.

79

Roman Candles

Roman candles are repeating guns which shoot projectiles of colored fire and send out showers of glowing sparks between the shots. To the pyrotechnists of the seventeenth century they were known as "star pumps" or "pumps with stars."

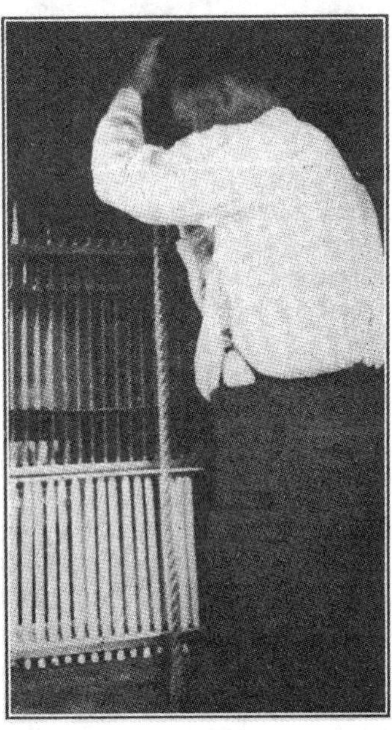

FIGURE 26. Ramming Roman Candles. (Courtesy National Fireworks Company.)

For the manufacture of Roman candles, gunpowder and stars and a modified black powder mixture which is known as Roman candle composition, or *candle comp*, are necessary. The candle comp is made from:

	PARTS	
Saltpeter	34	(200 mesh)
Sulfur	7	(200 mesh)
No. 4 Charcoal (hardwood)	15	(about 24 mesh)
No. 3 Charcoal (hardwood)	3	(about 16 mesh)
No. 2 Charcoal (hardwood)	3	(about 12 mesh)
Dextrin	1	

80

The materials are mixed thoroughly, then moistened slightly and rubbed for intimate mixture through a 10-mesh sieve, dried quickly in shallow trays, and sifted through a 10-mesh sieve. Candle comp burns more slowly than black powder and gives luminous sparks. The case is a long, narrow, strong tube of paper plugged at the bottom with clay. Next to the clay is a small quantity of gunpowder (4F); on top of this is a star; and on top of this a layer of candle comp. The star is of such size that it does not fit the tube tightly. It rests upon the gunpowder, and

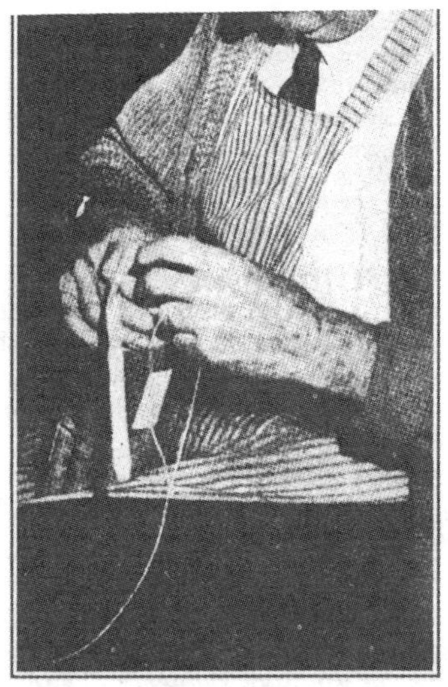

FIGURE 27. Matching a Battery of 10 Ball Roman Candles.

81

the space between the star and the wall of the tube is partly filled with candle comp. When the three materials have been introduced, they are rammed tightly into place. Then gunpowder, a star, and candle comp again are loaded into the tube and rammed down, and so on until the tube is charged. Damp candle comp, with a piece of black match leading to it and into it, is loaded at the top, pressed tightly into place, and allowed to dry. When a Roman candle is lighted, the candle comp begins to burn and to throw out a fountain of sparks. The fire soon reaches the star, ignites it, and flashes along the side of the star to light the gunpowder which blows the burning star, like a projectile, out of the tube.

Stars

Stars are pellets of combustible material. Those which contain neither aluminum nor magnesium nor Paris green have nothing in their appearance to suggest even remotely the magic which is in them. They are, however, the principal cause of the beauty of aerial pyrotechnic displays.

The components of star composition are mixed intimately and dampened uniformly with some solution which contains a binder, perhaps with gum-arabic water, perhaps with water alone if the composition contains dextrin, perhaps with alcohol if it contains shellac. Several different methods are used for forming the stars.

To make *cut stars,* the damp mixture is spread out in a shallow pan, pressed down evenly, cut into cubes, say 1/4 to 3/4 inch on the side, allowed to dry, and broken apart. Because of their corners, cut stars take fire very readily and are well suited for use in rockets and small aerial bombshells. Cylindrical stars are preferred for Roman candles.

For the preparation of a small number of stars, a *star pump* is a convenient instrument. This consists of a brass tube with a plunger which slides within it. The plunger has a handle and, on its side, a peg which works within a slot in the side of the tube—in such manner that it may be fixed in position to leave at the open end of the tube a space equal to the size of the star which it is desired to make. This space is then tightly packed with the damp mixture; the plunger is turned so that the peg may move through the longitudinal slot, and the handle is pushed to eject the star.

82

For large-scale production, a *star plate* or *star mold* assembly is best. This consists of three flat rectangular plates of hard wood or metal, preferably aluminum. One has a perfectly smooth surface. The second, which rests upon this, has many circular holes of the size of the stars which are desired. The damp mixture is dumped upon this plate, rubbed, pressed, and packed into the holes, and the surface of the plate is then wiped clean. The third

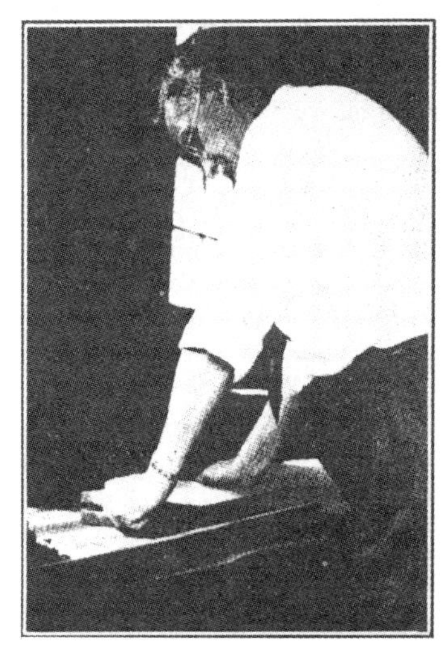

FIGURE 28. A Star Plate or Star Board in Use. (Courtesy National Fireworks Company.)

plate is supplied with pegs, corresponding in number and position to the holes of the second plate, the pegs being slightly narrower than the holes and slightly longer than their depth. The second plate is now placed above a tray into which the stars may fall, and the stars are pushed out by putting the pegged plate upon it. In certain conditions it may be possible to dispense with the pegged plate and to push out the stars by means of a roller of soft crêpe rubber.

Box stars are less likely to crumble from shock, and are accordingly used in large aerial bombshells. They are also used for festoons and for other aerial tableaux effects. Short pieces of 83 4-ply manila paper tubing, say ¾ inch long and ½ inch in diameter, are taken; pieces of black match long enough to protrude from both ends of the tubes are inserted and held in this position by the fingers while the tubes are pressed full of the damp composition. Box stars require a longer drying than those which are not covered.

White stars, except some of those which contain aluminum, are generally made with potassium nitrate as the oxidizing agent. Various white star compositions are tabulated below. The last three are for white *electric stars*. The last formula, containing perchlorate, was communicated by Allen F. Clark.

Potassium nitrate	70	28	180	20	42	14	28	..
Potassium perchlorate	..	..	..	..	..	..	..	30
Barium nitrate	..	..	..	..	..	..	..	5
Aluminum	..	..	..	..	..	3	5	22
Antimony sulfide	20	..	10	..	..	3	7	..
Antimony metal	..	5	40	..	..	..	..	..
Zinc dust	..	..	..	..	6	..	..	..
Realgar	..	..	..	6	6	..	..	..
Meal powder	..	..	..	..	12	6	3	..
Sulfur	20	8	50	6	23	..	8	..
Charcoal dust	..	..	3	..	..	..	..	..
Dextrin	3	1	6	1	..	1	1	..
Shellac	..	..	..	..	..	..	..	3

Stars which contain aluminum are known as electric stars because of the dazzling brilliancy of their light, which resembles that of an electric arc. Stars which contain chlorate and sulfur or antimony sulfide or arsenic sulfide or picric acid are dangerous to mix, likely to explode if subjected to too sudden shock, and unsafe for use in shells. They are used in rockets and Roman candles. Perchlorate compositions, and chlorate compositions without sulfur, sulfides, and picric acid, will tolerate considerable shock and are used in aerial bombshells.

The following star compositions which contain both chlorate and sulfur are among those recommended by Tessier. Mixtures which contain chlorate and sulfur have a tendency to "sour" with the production of sulfuric acid after they have been wetted, 84 and to deteriorate, but the difficulty may be remedied by the addition of an anti-acid, and some of these compositions do in-

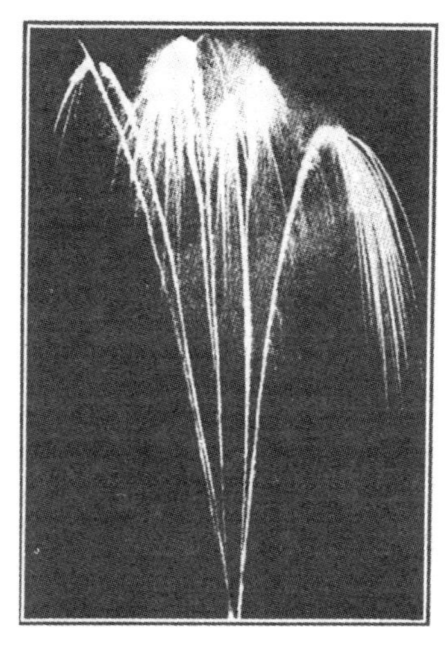

FIGURE 29. Aluminum Stars from a Single Rocket.

deed contain carbonates or basic salts which act in that capacity. Tessier recommends that the mixtures be made up while dampened with small quantities of 35 per cent alcohol.

	Red	Lilac	Lilac Mauve	Violet	Blue	Green
Potassium chlorate	167	17	17	56	24	48
Strontium carbonate	54	9	9	..	..	..
Strontium sulfate	..	..	..	16	..	..
Barium nitrate	..	..	..	..	..	80
Copper oxychloride	..	2	4	..	..	..
Basic copper sulfate	..	..	..	8	12	..
Lead chloride	..	1	1	3	2	10
Charcoal dust (poplar)	..	..	..	3	..	..
Sulfur	35	7	7	20	8	26
Dextrin	7	1	1	3	1	3
Shellac	16	..	..	..	..	2
Lampblack	..	..	..	..	..	2

85

Weingart reports compositions for cut, pumped, or candle stars which contain chlorate but no sulfur or sulfides, as follows:

	Red		Blue	Green	Yellow	
Potassium chlorate	12	48	48	12	32	16

Strontium nitrate	12	..	..	..	..	..
Strontium carbonate	..	8	..	..	..	..
Barium nitrate	..	..	16	12	12	..
Paris green	..	..	18	..	..	..
Calomel	..	..	..	1	..	..
Sodium oxalate	..	..	..	..	2	7
Fine charcoal	4	8	..	4	8	1
Dextrin	1	3	3	1	3	1
Shellac	2	6	10	2	6	3

For the following perchlorate star formulas the author is indebted to Allen F. Clark.

	Rose	Amber	Green		Violet	
Potassium perchlorate	12	10	..	44	12	41
Potassium nitrate	6	..	..	..	..	..
Barium perchlorate	..	..	32	90	..	..
Calcium carbonate	..	..	..	..	..	12
Strontium oxalate	1	..	..	..	9	3
Copper oxalate	..	..	..	..	5	..
Sodium oxalate	..	4	..	..	..	..
Calomel	..	..	..	..	..	3
Sulfur	..	..	..	..	..	14
Lampblack	1	..	..	..	..	..
Dextrin	1	..	..	6	..	..
Shellac	..	2	3	15	3	..

Illustrative of electric star compositions are the following; those which contain potassium chlorate are reported by Faber, the others, containing perchlorate, were communicated by Allen F. Clark. The last-named authority has also supplied two for-
86

	Red		Gold	Green			Blue	
Potassium perchlorate	..	12	..	..	..	6	..	14
Potassium chlorate	24	..	6	8	..	..	32	..
Barium perchlorate	..	..	..	..	12	12	..	..
Barium chlorate	..	..	4	16	..	..	..	..
Barium nitrate	..	..	..	16	..	..	..	..
Strontium chlorate	..	3	..	..	..	..	..	..
Strontium carbonate	4	..	..	..	..	..	..	..
Aluminum	8	3	4	12	5	8	8	6
Sodium oxalate	..	..	2	..	..	..	..	..
Calcium carbonate	..	..	..	..	..	..	..	1
Magnesium carbonate	..	..	1	..	..	..	..	..
Paris green	..	..	..	..	..	..	16	10
Calomel	..	..	..	..	..	..	..	2
Fine charcoal	1	..	..	3	..	..	..	..
Dextrin	2	1	..	2	..	1	2	1
Red gum	..	..	..	4	..	..	..	..
Shellac	2	1	2	..	1	2	1	2

	Amber	Green
Potassium perchlorate	4	..
Barium perchlorate	..	12
Magnesium	1	2
Sodium oxalate	2	..
Lycopodium powder	..	1
Shellac	1	2

mulas for magnesium stars. The compositions are mixed while dampened with alcohol which insures that the particles of magnesium are covered with a protective layer of shellac.

Lampblack stars burn with a rather dull soft light. Discharged in large number from a rocket or aerial shell, they produce the beautiful willow-tree effect. They are made, according to Allen F. Clark, by incorporating 3 pounds of lampblack, 4 pounds of meal powder, and ½ pound of finely powdered antimony sulfide with 2 ounces of shellac dissolved in alcohol.

Stars compounded out of what is essentially a modified black
87
powder mixture, given a yellowish or whitish color by the addition of appropriate materials, and used in rockets and shells in the same manner as lampblack stars, produce *gold* and *silver showers*, or, if the stars are larger and fewer in number, *gold* and *silver streamers*. The following formulas are typical.

	Gold	Silver
Potassium nitrate	16	10
Charcoal	1	2
Sulfur	4	3
Realgar	..	3
Sodium oxalate	8	..
Red gum	1	1

Twinklers are stars which, when they fall through the air, burn brightly and dully by turns. A shower of twinklers produces an extraordinary effect. Weingart in a recent letter has kindly sent the following formula for yellow twinklers:

Meal powder	24
Sodium oxalate	4
Antimony sulfide	3
Powdered aluminum	3
Dextrin	1

The materials are mixed intimately while dampened with water, and the mixture is pumped into stars about ¾ inch in diameter and ⅞ inch long. The stars are dried promptly. They function only when falling through the air. If lighted on the ground they merely smolder, but when fired from rockets or shells are most effective.

Spreader stars contain nearly two-thirds of their weight of powdered zinc. The remaining one-third consists of material necessary to maintain an active combustion. When they are ignited, these stars burn brightly and throw off masses of burning zinc (greenish white flame) often to a distance of several feet. Weingart gives the two following formulas for spreader stars, the first for "electric spreader stars," the second for "granite stars," so called because of their appearance.
88

Zinc dust	72	80
Potassium nitrate	..	28
Potassium chlorate	15	..
Potassium dichromate	12	..
Granulated charcoal	12	..
Fine charcoal	..	14
Sulfur	..	5
Dextrin	2	2

The first of these formulas is the more difficult to mix and the more expensive. All its components except the charcoal are first mixed and dampened; the granulated charcoal, which must be free from dust, is then mixed in, and the stars are formed with

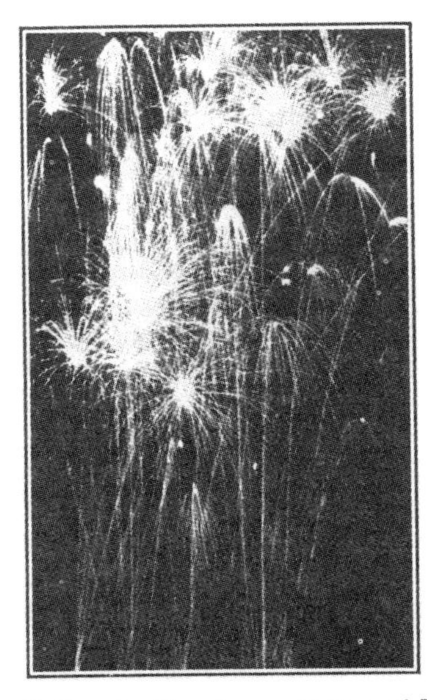

FIGURE 30. Spreader Stars from a Battery of Rockets.

a pump. They throw off two kinds of fire when they burn, masses of brightly burning zinc and particles of glowing charcoal. Weingart recommends that the second formula be made into cut stars ⅜ inch on the side. Spreader stars because of the zinc which they contain are much heavier than other stars. Rockets and aerial bombs cannot carry as many of them.

Gerbs

Gerbs produce jets of ornamental and brilliant fire and are used in set pieces. They are rammed or pressed like rockets, on a short nipple instead of a long spindle, and have only a slight depression within the choke, not a long central cavity. They are choked to about one-third the diameter of the tube. The simplest gerbs contain only a modified black powder mixture, say meal powder 4 parts, saltpeter 2, sulfur 1, and charcoal dust 1 or mixed charcoal 2; and are used occasionally for contrast in elaborate set pieces. Similar composition is used for the starting fire of steel gerbs which are more difficult to ignite. If antimony sulfide is used in place of charcoal, as in the mixtures:

Meal powder	2	3
Saltpeter	8	8
Sulfur	3	4
Antimony sulfide	1	2

the gerbs yield compact whitish flames and are used in star and floral designs. Gold gerbs appropriately arranged produce the sunburst effect. Colored gerbs are made by adding small cut stars. In loading the tube, a scoopful of composition is introduced

	Steel		Colored Steel	Gold	Colored Gold
Meal powder	6	4	8	40	40
Potassium nitrate	2	..	7	..	..
Sulfur	1	..	..	..	..
Fine charcoal	1	1	2	..	..
Steel filings	1	2	5	..	..
Stars	..	..	5	..	5
Sodium oxalate	..	..	..	6	6
Antimony sulfide	..	..	..	8	9
Aluminum	..	..	..	4	..
Dextrin	..	..	..	..	4

and rammed down, then a few stars, then more composition which is rammed down, and so on. Care must be exercised that no stars containing chlorate are used with compositions which contain sulfur, for an explosion might occur when the charge is rammed. The following compositions are typical. The steel filings

90

must be protected from rusting by previous treatment with paraffin or linseed oil.

Prismatic fountains, floral bouquets, etc., are essentially colored gerbs. Flower pots are supplied with wooden handles and generally contain a modified black powder composition with lampblack and sometimes with a small amount of granulated black powder. In the charging of fountains and gerbs, a small charge of gunpowder is often introduced first, next to the clay plug which closes the bottom of the tube and before the first scoopful of composition which is rammed or pressed. This makes them finish with a report or *bounce.*

Fountains

Fountains are designed to stand upon the ground, either upon a flat base or upon a pointed wooden stick. They are choked slightly more than gerbs, and have heavier, stronger cases to withstand the greater pressures which eject the fire to greater distances.

The "Giant Steel Fountain" of Allen F. Clark is charged with a mixture of saltpeter 5 parts (200 mesh), cast-iron turnings 1 part (8 to 40 mesh), and red gum 1 part (180 to 200 mesh). For loading, the mixture is dampened with 50 per cent alcohol. The case is a strong paper tube, 20 inches long, 4 inches in external diameter, with walls 1 inch thick, made from Bird's hardware paper. It is rolled on a machine lathe, the paper being passed first through a heavy solution of dextrin and the excess of the gum scraped off. The bottom of the case is closed with a 3-inch plug of clay. The composition will stand tremendous pressures without exploding, and it is loaded very solidly in order that it may stay in place when the piece is burned. The charge is rammed in with a wooden rammer actuated by short blows, as heavy as the case will stand, from a 15-pound sledge. The top is closed with a 3-inch clay plug. A ⅞-inch hole is then bored with an auger in the center of the top, and the hole is continued into the charge to a total depth of 10 inches. The composition is difficult to light, but the ignition is accomplished by a bundle of six strands of black match inserted to the full depth of the cavity and tied into place. This artifice produces a column of scintillating fire, 100 feet or more in height, of the general shape of a red cedar tree. It develops considerable sound, and ends sud-

91

denly with a terrifying roar at the moment of its maximum splendor. If loaded at the hydraulic press with a tapered spindle (as is necessary), it finishes its burning with a fountain which grows smaller and smaller and finally fades out entirely.

Wheels

Driving tubes or *drivers,* attached to the periphery of a wheel or to the sides of a square or hexagon of wood which is pivoted at its center, by shooting out jets of fire, cause the device to rotate and to produce various ornamental effects according to the compositions with which they are loaded. When the fire reaches the bottom of one driver, it is carried by quickmatch to the top of the next. Drivers are loaded in the same manner as gerbs, the compositions being varied slightly according to the size as is done with rockets. A gross of the 1-ounce and 2-ounce sizes in

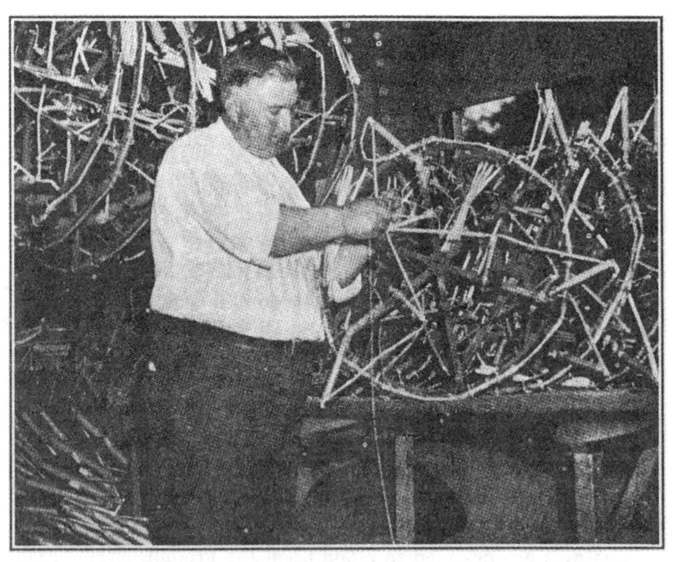

FIGURE 31. Matching Display Wheels.

present American practice is loaded at one time by the hydraulic press. Typical wheel turning compositions (Allen F. Clark) for use in 1-ounce and 2-ounce drivers are reported below, the first for a *charcoal spark effect*, the second for an *iron and steel effect*. The speed of the mixtures may be increased by increasing the proportion of gunpowder.

92

Saltpeter (210 mesh)	10	46
Sulfur (200 mesh)	2	19
Meal powder	6	..
Charcoal dust	..	16
Charcoal (80 mesh)	1	..
6F gunpowder	6	..
7F gunpowder	..	24
Cast-iron turnings (16 mesh)	..	30
Dextrin	..	8

Wheels, gerbs, and colored fires are the parts out of which such display pieces as the "Corona Cluster," "Sparkling Caprice," "Flying Dutchman," "Morning Glory," "Cuban Dragon," "Blazing Sun," and innumerable others are constructed.

Saxons

Saxons are strong paper tubes, plugged with clay at their middles and at both ends, and filled between the plugs with composition similar to that used in drivers. A lateral hole is bored through the middle of the tube and through the central clay plug, and it is around a nail, passed through this hole and driven into a convenient support, that the artifice rotates. Other holes, at right angles to this one, are bored from opposite sides near the ends of the tube, just under the end plugs, through one wall of the tube and into the composition but not through it. A piece of black match in one of these holes ignites the composition. The hot gases, sparks, etc., rushing from the hole cause the device to turn upon its pivot. When the fire reaches the bottom of the charge, it lights a piece of quickmatch, previously connected through a hole at that point and glued to the outside of the case, which carries the fire to the other half of the saxon.

Saxons are generally matched as described, the two halves burning consecutively and rotating it in the same direction. Sometimes they burn simultaneously, and sometimes one half turns it in one direction and the other afterwards "causes the rapid spinning to reverse amid a mad burst of sparks." This effect "is very pleasing and is considered one of the best to be obtained for so small an expenditure."

93

Pinwheels

To make pinwheels, manila or kraft paper tubes or *pipes*, about 12 inches long and 3/16 inch in diameter, are needed. One end is closed by twisting or folding over. The tubes are filled with composition, the other ends are closed in the same way, and the tubes are wrapped in a moist towel and set aside until they are thoroughly flabby. In this condition they are passed between rollers and flattened to the desired extent. Each tube is then wound in an even spiral around the edge of a cardboard disc which has a hole in its center for the pin, and the whole is placed in a frame which prevents it from uncoiling. Four drops of glue, at the four quarters of the circle, are then brushed on, across the pipes and onto the center disc, and the device is allowed to dry.

Weingart recommends for pinwheels the compositions which are indicated below. The first of these produces both steel and charcoal effects, the second steel with much less of the charcoal, the third aluminum and charcoal, and the fourth a circle merely of lilac-colored fire.

Meal powder	..	10	8	2
Gunpowder (fine)	8	5	8	..
Aluminum	..	..	3	..
Saltpeter	14	4	16	1
Steel filings	6	6	..	..
Sulfur	4	1	3	1
Charcoal	3	1	8	..

Tessier thought highly of pinwheels (*pastilles*). They were, he says,

> formerly among the artifices which were called *table fireworks*, the use of which has wholly fallen away since the immense apartments have disappeared which alone provided places where these little pyrotechnic pieces might be burned without too much inconvenience.
>
> The manner of use of these pastilles calls only for small calibers; also their small dimensions make it possible to turn them out at a low price, and the fireworks makers have always continued to make them the object of current manufacture. But what they have neglected, they still neglect: and that is, to seek to bring them to perfection. Those that

94

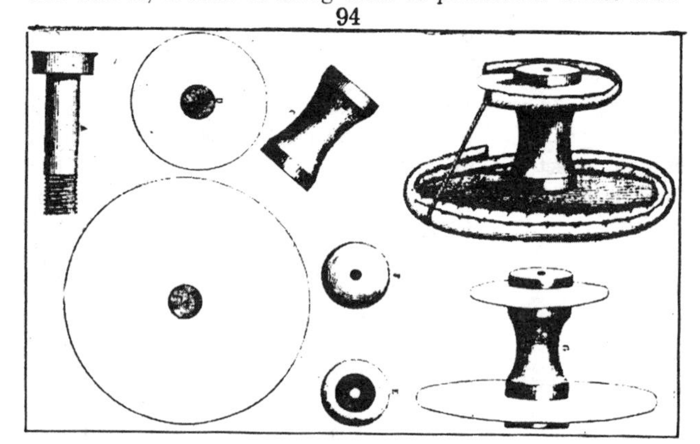

FIGURE 32. Pinwheels, Tessier, 1883. Wheels which show an inner circle of colored fire. Plate 1 (below) pictures pinwheels which are intended to be sold as completely consumable. The instrument represented at the bottom of the plate is the ramrod for tamping the charges in the pipes. Plate 2 (above) represents pinwheels which are intended to be exhibited by the pyrotechnist himself: the wooden parts are to be recovered and used again.

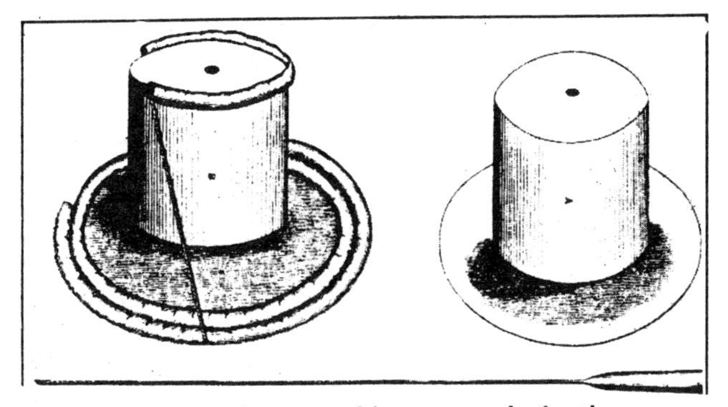

they confine themselves to making serve only for the amusement of children.

However, pastilles may become charming pieces of fireworks, fit to refresh all eyes. They can be made to produce truly marvellous effects, considering the conditions imposed by their size, effects all the more remarkable in as much as, by the very reason of these same conditions, they have no

95

need of a vast theater in which to be fired. The least little garden suffices for them. They burn under the very eye of the spectator, who loses nothing of their splendor, whereas, in general, large pieces of fireworks can be enjoyed only at a distance from the place of firing. Finally, they have over these last the advantage of their low price and the advantage that they can be transported without embarrassment and set in place at the moment of being fired.

Tessier describes ordinary pastilles, diamond pastilles, and pastilles with colored fires. The shorter and more central tubes (Figure 32), wound part way around discs 40 mm. in diameter, hold the colored fire compositions. The longer tubes, forming the larger circles around discs 72 mm. in diameter, are the turning tubes. The latter, it will be seen, are so arranged that they burn for a time before the fire reaches the colored compositions. "The charging of the tubes is commenced, up to a height of about 17 cms., with the four compositions, Nos. 142, 126, 128, and 129, in the order named. The rest of the tube is charged entirely with composition No. 149, or with No. 152, both of which produce scintillating aureoles." The charges are tamped tightly in the tubes by means of a long, thin ramrod and mallet. The compositions in question, designated by Tessier's own numbers, are indicated below.

	142	126	128	129	149	152
Meal powder	16	16	16	32	..	..
Potassium nitrate	1	1	1	4	..	..
Oak charcoal	1	..	..	..	..	..
Litharge	..	2	..	..	..	..
Powdered mica	..	..	2	..	..	..
Antimony sulfide	..	..	..	5	..	..
Plumbic powder No. 1	..	..	..	..	17	17
Cast-iron filings	..	..	..	..	3	..
Steel wool	..	..	..	..	..	3

No. 142 is a composition for ordinary pastilles. Tessier says that it produces "numerous sparks forming a feeble aureole. As this composition is not lively, and as it is not able to make the

96

pastilles turn conveniently, care is taken not to load more of it than a length of 15 mm. in the tube."

Nos. 126, 128, and 129 are also for ordinary pastilles. No. 126 "has not much force; it is incapable alone of making a pastille turn with the necessary rapidity. Hence care is taken in charging it to introduce only a small quantity into the tube." It burns with a white flame "forming a crown, more or less lacy-edged, from which rays and sparks are thrown out."

The two compositions, Nos. 142 and 126, evidently burn while the pastille is turning from the initial twirl given it by the hand. When the fire reaches the next composition, No. 128, the pastille accelerates by its own power. This gives "reddish rays, very straight and very numerous," and No. 129 gives "a white flame around the disc, and numerous and persistent sparks which fall down forming a sort of cascade on each side of the pastille."

Neither No. 128 nor 129 is bright enough to make much of a show if the colored fire is also burning. When they burn to an end, the fire is communicated to the colored composition; at the same time the bright diamond composition, either No. 149 or 152, commences to burn. No. 149 produces "a splendid aureole of silver-white flowers. These flowers are less developed than those produced by steel wool and make a different effect from the latter." No. 152 produces a "splendid effect—no inflamed disc, no reddish sparks—numerous jasmine flowers of all dimensions forming a vast aureole of a striking white."

Plumbic powder No. 1 is made from lead nitrate 12 parts, potassium nitrate 2 parts, and black alder charcoal 3 parts. The materials are powdered and mixed, and then rolled in a wooden ball-mill with balls of hard lead (Pb 5, Sb 1) or brass or bronze.

Tessier gives credit to the earlier French pyrotechnist, Chertier, for the introduction into pyrotechny of lead nitrate (which had been used before his time only for the preparation of slow-

97

match or fire wick), for the invention of plumbic powder by which a silver shower (*pluie d'argent*) is produced, and for originating the idea of the diamond pastille with colored fires which Chertier called the *dahlia pastille* but for the making of which he did not give precise directions.

Mines

Mines are paper mortars—commonly strong paper tubes each standing vertically on a wooden base into which it is countersunk and glued—arranged to throw into the air a display of stars, serpents, etc. They are often equipped with fountains, Roman candles, etc., which make a display on the ground before the final explosion occurs.

A *serpent mine* (*pot à feu*) is represented in Figure 24. This starts with a steel fountain. When the fire has reached the bottom of the fountain, it is carried by quickmatch to a charge of gunpowder in the paper bag, *a*. Immediately above the paper bag are the serpents. These are small paper tubes, rammed with a mixture of meal powder, gunpowder, saltpeter, sulfur, and mixed charcoal, crimped or plugged with clay at one end, supplied with match (as in the diagram) or merely left open-ended at the other. The lower, matched or open, ends of the serpents take fire from the burning of the gunpowder, which also blows them into the air where they dart and squirm about like little tailless rockets leaving a trail of sparks. In Audot's diagram, directly below the fountain and above the closed ends of the serpents, is a mass of wadding. This tends to offer a slight resistance to the force of the gunpowder, with the result that the serpents receive the fire more surely and are shot farther into the air before they begin to go their several ways.

Saucissons are constructed in the same way as serpents, but are larger, and have, next to the closed end, a small charge of gunpowder which makes them end with a bang. They are used in mines and in rockets.

Mines which discharge serpents, stars, English crackers, etc., are often made by loading these materials into the same paper bags which contain the blowing charges of granulated gunpowder. About two level teaspoonfuls of blowing powder is used per ounce of stars.[98] For making the bags, a board is taken which has had holes bored into it slightly smaller than the internal diameter of the mine case and of a depth suited to the caliber of the mine. A disc of tissue paper is placed over a hole and then punched down into it by a wooden punch or rod with slightly rounded edges which fits rather loosely in the hole. This makes a paper cup into which one end of the fuse is inserted, and around it the stars and blowing charge. The edges of the paper cup are then gathered together and tied with string or wire.

Mines are often made up with a single Roman candle, lacking the plug of clay at the bottom, mounted in the center of the mine case. The fuse leading from the charge in the paper bag is thrust into the bottom of the Roman candle. A mine with a large and short case, carrying a charge of tailed stars, serpents, and English crackers, and having one Roman candle in its center and four others, matched to burn simultaneously, attached to the outside of the case, is known as a *devil among the tailors.*

Comets and Meteors

These are virtually mines which shoot a single large star. A pumped star 1½ inches in diameter is fired, for example, from a tube or mortar 10 inches long and 1¾ inches in internal diameter. A piece of quickmatch (wrapped black match) about 6 inches longer than the mortar is taken; an inch of black match is made bare at one end, bent at right angles, and laid against the base of the star; and the star, with the quickmatch lying along its side, is then enclosed in the middle of a paper cylinder by wrapping a strip, say 4 inches wide, of pasted tissue paper around it. A half teaspoonful of granulated black powder is put into the cup thus formed on the (bottom) side of the star where the black match has been exposed, and the edges of the paper cylinder are brought together over it and tied. The other (upper) end of the paper cylinder is similarly tied around the quickmatch. In using this piece, and in using all others which are lighted by quickmatch, care must be taken that a few inches of the quickmatch have been opened and the black match exposed, before the fire is set to it; otherwise it will be impossible to get away quickly enough. This, of course, is already done in pieces which are offered for public sale.

Comets burn with a charcoal or lampblack effect, meteors with[99] an electric one. The two comet star compositions given below are due to Weingart; that of the green meteor to Allen F. Clark.

	Comets		Green Meteor
Potassium nitrate	6	..	..
Barium perchlorate	..	..	4
Barium nitrate	..	..	2
Meal powder	6	3	..
Sulfur	1	..	..
Fine charcoal	3	1	..
Antimony sulfide	3	1	..
Lampblack	..	2	..
Aluminum	..	..	1
Dextrin	..	..	1

Some manufacturers apply the name of meteors to artifices which are essentially large Roman candles, mounted on wooden bases and shooting four, six, eight, and ten stars 1½ inches in diameter. They are loaded in the same way as Roman candles except that a special device is used to insure the certain ignition of the stars. Two pieces of black match at right angles to each other are placed under the bottom of the star; the four ends are turned up along the sides of the star and are cut off even with the top of it. The match being held in this position, the star is inserted into the top of the case and pushed down with a rammer onto the propelling charge of gunpowder which has already been introduced. Then coarse candle comp is put in, then gunpowder, then another star in the same manner, and so on. The black match at the side of the star keeps a space open between the star and the walls of the tube, which space is only partly or loosely filled with candle comp. The black match acts as a quickmatch, insuring the early ignition of the propelling charge as well as the sure ignition of the star. Electric stars, spreader stars, and *splitters* are used in meteors. Splitter stars are made from the same composition as snowball sparklers (see below); the composition for stars, however, is moistened with much less water than for sparklers. They split into bright fragments while shooting upward and burst at the top to produce a palm-tree effect.[100]

Bombshells

Bombshells are shot from mortars by means of a charge of black powder and burst high in the air with the production of reports, flashes, showers, and other spectacular effects. The smaller ones are shot from paper mortars; the larger, most commonly from mortars of iron. In the past they have often been made in a spherical shape, wood or paper or metal hemispheres pasted heavily over with paper, but now in this country they are made almost exclusively in the form of cylinders. For the same caliber, cylindrical bombshells will hold more stars or other display material than spherical ones, and it is much easier to contrive them in a manner to procure multiple bursts. The materials of construction are paper, paste, and string. The shells are supplied with *Roman fuses* timed to cause them to burst at the top of their flight. The success and safety of bombshells depend upon carefully constructed fuses.

Roman fuses are made by pounding the fuse powder as firmly as is possible into hard, strong, tightly rolled paper tubes. These are commonly made from Bird's hardware paper, pasted all over before it is rolled, and are dried carefully and thoroughly before they are loaded with ramrod and mallet. "When a number of these cases are rolled," says Weingart, "they must be dried in the shade until they are as hard as wood and rattle when struck together." He recommends the first of the following-listed compositions, the Vergnauds the others:

Potassium nitrate	2	4	2
Sulfur	1	2	1
Meal powder	4	6	3
Antimony sulfide	..	1	..

The length of the column of composition determines the duration of the burning. The composition in the fuse must be as hard and as firmly packed as possible; otherwise it will blow through into the shell when in use and will cause a premature explosion. Some manufacturers load the tubes and cut them afterwards with a fine-tooth hack saw. Others prefer to cut them to the desired lengths with a sharp knife while they are prevented from collapsing by a brass rod through them, and afterwards to load the short pieces separately.[101] Different size tubes are often used for the fuses of different size shells; those for a 4-inch shell (that is, for a shell to be shot from a 4-inch mortar) are commonly made from tubes 5/16 inch in internal diameter and ⅝

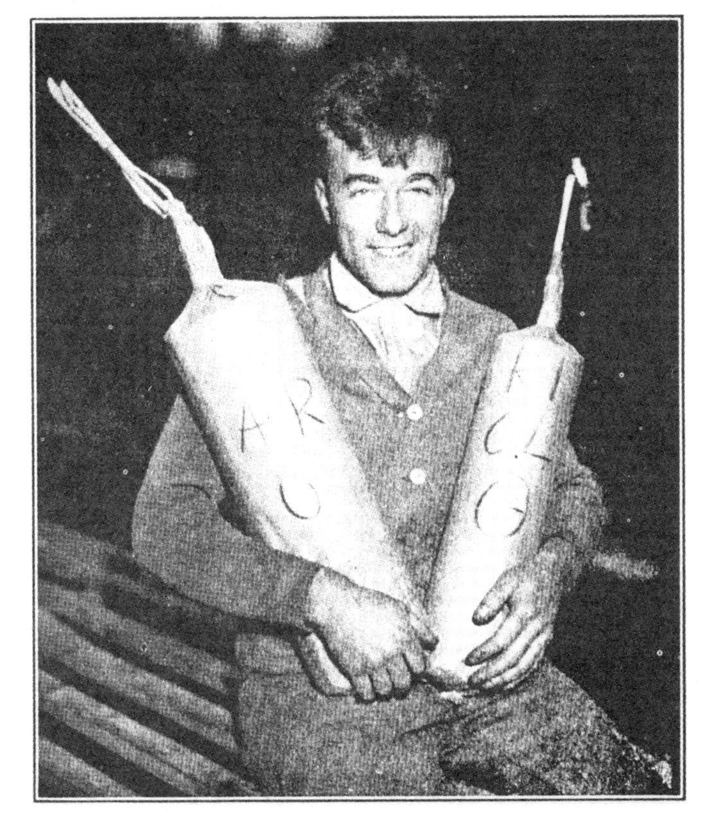

FIGURE 33. Bombshells for 4- and 6-inch Mortars. (Courtesy National Fireworks Company and the *Boston Globe*.)

inch in external diameter. Fuses are generally attached to the front end of the bombshell. The forward-pointing end of the tube, which is outside the shell and receives the fire, is filled flush with the composition. The other backward-pointing end, inside the shell, is empty of composition for ¾ inch of its length; a bundle of stiff 2-inch pieces of black match[102] is inserted into this space and is held in position by a rolled wrapper of paper, glued to the fuse case and tied with a string near the ends of the match, in order that it may not be dislodged by the shock of setback. The match serves to bring the fire more satisfactorily to the bursting charge within the shell.

The preparation of the bombshell is hand work which requires much skill and deserves a fairly full description. We describe the construction of a 4-inch shell to produce a single burst of stars. A strip of bogus or news board paper is cut to the desired length and is rolled tightly on a form without paste. When it is nearly all rolled, a strip of medium-weight kraft paper, 4 inches wider than the other strip, is rolled in and is rolled around the tube several times and is pasted to hold it in position. Three circular discs of pasteboard of the same diameter as the bogus tube (3½ inches) are taken, and a ⅝-inch hole is punched in the center of two of them. The fuse is inserted through the hole in one of them and glued heavily on the inside. When this is thoroughly dry, the disc is glued to one end of the bogus tube, the matched end of the fuse being outside; the outer wrapper of kraft paper is folded over carefully onto the disc, glued, and rubbed down smoothly; and the second perforated disc is placed on top of it.

The shell case is now turned over, there being a hole in the bench to receive the fuse, and it is filled with as many stars (½-inch diameter, ½ inch long) as it will contain. A mixture of 2F gunpowder and candle comp is then added, shaken in, and settled among the stars until the case is absolutely full. A disc of pasteboard is placed over the stars and powder, pressed down against the end of the bogus body and glued, and the outer kraft paper wrapper is folded and glued over the end.

At this point the shell is allowed to dry thoroughly before it is wound with strong jute twine. It is first wound lengthwise; the twine is wrapped as tightly as possible and as firmly against the fuse as may be; each time that it passes the fuse the plane of the winding is advanced by about 10° until 36 turns have been laid on, and then 36 turns are wound around the sides of the cylinder at right angles to the first winding. The shell is now ready to be "pasted in." For this purpose, 50-pound kraft paper is cut into strips of the desired dimensions, the length of the strips being across the grain of the paper. A strip of this paper is folded, rubbed, and twisted[103] in paste until it is thoroughly impregnated. It is then laid out on the bench and the shell is rolled up in it. The cylinder is now stood upright, the fuse end at the top, and the portion of the wet pasted kraft paper wrapper which extends above the body of the shell is torn into strips about ¾ inch wide; these, one by one, are rubbed down carefully and smoothly, one overlapping the other, upon the end of the shell case. They extend up the fuse tube for about ½ inch and are pressed down firmly against it. The shell is now turned over, the fused end resting against a tapered hole in the bench, and a corresponding operation is performed upon the other end. The body of the shell is now about ¼ inch thick on the sides of the cylinder, about ⅜ inch thick at the top end, and about ½ inch at the base end. It is dried outdoors in the sun and breeze, or in a well-ventilated dry-house at 100°F., and, when thoroughly dry, is ready to be supplied with the propelling or *blowing charge*.

A piece of *piped match* (black match in a paper tube) is laid along the side of the bombshell; both are rolled up without paste in 4 thicknesses of 30-pound kraft paper wide enough to extend about 4 inches beyond the ends of the cylinder, and the outer wrapper is tied lightly in place by two strings encircling the cylinder near the ends of the shell case. The cylinder is turned bottom end up. About 3 inches of the paper pipe of the quickmatch is removed to expose the black match, a second piece of black match is inserted into the end of the paper pipe, and the pipe is tied with string to hold the match in place. The propelling charge of 2F gunpowder is next introduced; the two inner layers of the outer kraft paper wrapper are folded down upon it and pressed firmly, then the two outer layers are pleated to the center of the cylinder, tied, and trimmed close to the string. The cylinder is then turned to bring the fuse end uppermost. The end of the fuse is scraped clean if it has been touched with paste. Two pieces of black match are crossed over the end of the fuse, bent down along the sides of the fuse tube, and tied in this position with string. The piped match which leads to the blowing charge is now laid down upon the end of the cylinder, up to the bottom of the fuse tube, then bent up along the side of the fuse tube, then bent across its end and down the other side, and then bent

104

back upon itself, and tied in this position. Before it is tied, a small hole is made in the match pipe at the point where it passes the end of the Roman fuse, and a piece of flat black match is inserted. The two inner layers of the kraft paper wrapper are now pleated around the base of the fuse and tied close to the shell. The two outer layers are pleated and tied above the top of the fuse, a 3-foot length of piped match extending from the upper end of the package. A few inches of black match is now bared at the end and an extra piece of black match is inserted and tied in place by a string about 1 inch back from the end of the pipe. The black match, for safety's sake, is then covered with a piece of lance tube, closed at the end, which is to be removed after the shell has been placed in the mortar and is ready for firing.

Maroons

Bombs which explode with a loud report, whether they are intended for use on the ground or in the air, are known as maroons. They are called *marrons* in French, a name which also means large chestnuts in that language—and chestnuts sometimes explode while being roasted.

Maroons are used for military purposes to disconcert the enemy by imitating the sounds of gunfire and shell bursts, and have at times been part of the standard equipment of various armies. A cubical pasteboard box filled with gunpowder is wound in three directions with heavy twine, the successive turns being laid close to one another; an end of miner's fuse is inserted through a hole made by an awl, and the container, already very strong, is made still stronger by dipping it into liquid glue and allowing to dry.

For sharper reports, more closely resembling those of a high-explosive shell, fulminating compositions containing chlorate are used. With these, the necessity for a strong container is not so great; the winding may be done with lighter twine, and the successive turns of twine need not make the closest possible contact. Faber reports two compositions, as follows:

Potassium chlorate	4	1
Sulfur	1	..
Soft wood charcoal	1	..
Antimony sulfide	..	1

105

"It is to be noted," he says, "that, while the first formula affords a composition of great strength, the second is still more violent. It is also of such susceptibility that extraordinary care is required in the handling of it, or a premature explosion may result."

Chlorate compositions are not safe for use in maroons. Black powder is not noisy enough. Allen F. Clark has communicated the following perchlorate formulas for reports for maroons. For

Potassium perchlorate	12	6	32
Sulfur	8	2	..
Antimony sulfide	..	3	..
Sawdust	1	..	..
Rosin	..	..	3
Fine charcoal	..	..	3

a *flash report* he uses a mixture of 3 parts of potassium permanganate and 2 of aluminum.

Toy Caps

Toy caps are commonly made from red phosphorus and potassium chlorate, a combination which is the most sensitive, dangerous, and unpredictable of the many with which the pyrotechnist has to deal. Their preparation ought under no conditions to be attempted by an amateur. Powdered potassium chlorate 20 parts is made into a slurry with gum water. It is absolutely essential that the chlorate should be wetted thoroughly before the red phosphorus is mixed with it. Red phosphorus, 8 parts, is mixed with powdered sulfur 1 part and precipitated calcium carbonate 1 part, and the mixture is made into a slurry separately with gum water, and this is stirred into the other until thoroughly mixed. The porridgelike mass is then spotted on paper, and a piece of pasted tissue paper is placed over the spotted surface in a manner to avoid the enclosure of any air bubbles between the two. This is important, for, unless the tissue paper covers the spots snugly, the composition is likely to crumble, to fall out, and to create new dangers. (A strip of caps, for example, may explode between the fingers of a boy who is tearing it.) The moist sheets of caps are piled up between moist blankets in a press, or with a board and weights on top of the pile, and are pressed for an hour or so. They are then cut into strips

106

of caps which are dried, packaged, and sold for use in toy repeating pistols. Or they are cut in squares, one cap each, which are not dried but are used while still moist for making Japanese torpedoes (see below). The calcium carbonate in this mixture is an anti-acid, which prevents it from deteriorating under the influence of moisture during the rather long time which elapses, especially in the manufacture of torpedoes, before it becomes fully dry.

Mixtures of potassium chlorate and red phosphorus explode from shock *and from fire*. They do not burn in an orderly fashion as do black powder and most other pyrotechnic mixtures. No scrap or waste ought ever to be allowed to accumulate in the building where caps are made; it ought to be removed hourly, whether moist or not, and taken to a distance and thrown upon a fire which is burning actively.

Silver Torpedoes

These contain silver fulminate, a substance which is as sensitive as the red phosphorus and chlorate mixture mentioned above, but which, however, is somewhat more predictable. They are made by the use of a *torpedo board*, that is, a board, say ⅞ inch thick, through which ¾-inch holes have been bored. A 2-inch square of tissue paper is placed over each hole and punched into the hole to form a paper cup. A second board of the same thickness, the *gravel board*, has ½-inch holes, bored not quite through it, in number and position corresponding to the holes in the torpedo board. Fine gravel, free from dust, is poured upon it; the holes are filled, and the excess removed. The torpedo board, filled with paper cups, is inverted and set down upon the gravel board, the holes matching one another. Then the two boards, held firmly together, are turned over and set down upon the bench. The gravel falls down into the paper cups, and the gravel board is removed A small amount of silver fulminate is now put, on top of the gravel, into each of the paper cups. This is a dangerous operation, for the act of picking up some of the fulminate with a scoop may cause the whole of it to explode. The explosion will be accompanied by a loud noise, by a flash of light, and by a tremendous local disturbance damaging to whatever is in the immediate neighborhood of the ful-

107

minate but without effect upon objects which are even a few

inches away.

In one plant which the present writer has visited, the fulminate destined to be loaded into the torpedoes rests in a small heap in the center of a piece of thin rubber (dentist's dam) stretched over a ring of metal which is attached to a piece of metal weighing about a pound. This is held in the worker's left hand, and a scoop made from a quill, held in the right hand, is used to take up the fulminate which goes into each torpedo. If the fulminate explodes, it destroys the piece of stretched rubber—nothing else. And the rubber, moreover, cushions it so that it is less likely to explode anyway. The pound of metal is something which the worker can hold much more steadily than the light-weight ring with its rubber and fulminate, and it has inertia enough so that it is not jarred from his hand if an explosion occurs. After the fulminate has been introduced into the paper cups, the edges of each cup are gathered together with one hand and twisted with the thumb and forefinger of the other hand which have been moistened with paste. This operation requires care, for the torpedo is likely to explode in the fingers if it is twisted too tightly.

Torpedoes, whether silver, Japanese, or globe, ought to be packed in sawdust for storage and shipment, and they ought not to be stored in the same magazine or shipped in the same package with other fireworks. If a number of them are standing together, the explosion of one of them for any reason is practically certain to explode the others. Unpacked torpedoes ought not to be allowed to accumulate in the building in which they are made.

Japanese Torpedoes

The so-called Japanese torpedoes appear to be an American invention. They contain a paper cap placed between two masses of gravel, and in general require to be thrown somewhat harder than silver torpedoes to make them explode. The same torpedo board is used as in the manufacture of silver torpedoes, but a gravel board which holds only about half as much gravel. After the gravel has been put in the paper cups, a paper cap, still moist, is placed on top of it; more gravel, substantially equal in amount to that already in the cup, is added to each, and the tops are twisted.

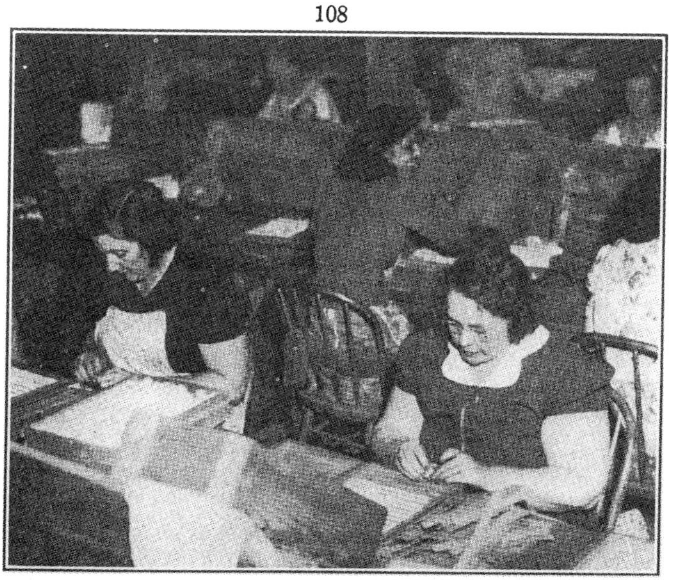

FIGURE 34. Manufacture of Globe Torpedoes. Introducing gravel and closing the paper capsules.

Globe Torpedoes

Small cups of manila paper, about 3/4 inch in diameter and 7/8 inch deep, are punched out by machine. They are such that two of them may be fitted together to form a box. The requisite amount of powdered potassium chlorate is first introduced into the cups; then, on top of it and without mixing, the requisite amount, already mixed, of the other components of the flash fulminating mixture is added. These other components are antimony sulfide, lampblack, and aluminum. Without disturbing the white and black powders in the bottoms of the cups, workers then fill the cups with clean coarse gravel and put other cups down upon them to form closed 3/4 by 3/4 inch cylindrical boxes. The little packages are put into a heated barrel, rotating at an angle with the horizontal, and are tumbled together with a solution of water-glass. The solution softens the paper (but later

hardens it), and the packages assume a spherical shape. Small discs of colored paper (punchings) are added a few at a time until the globes are completely covered with them and have lost all tendency to stick together. They are then emptied out of the

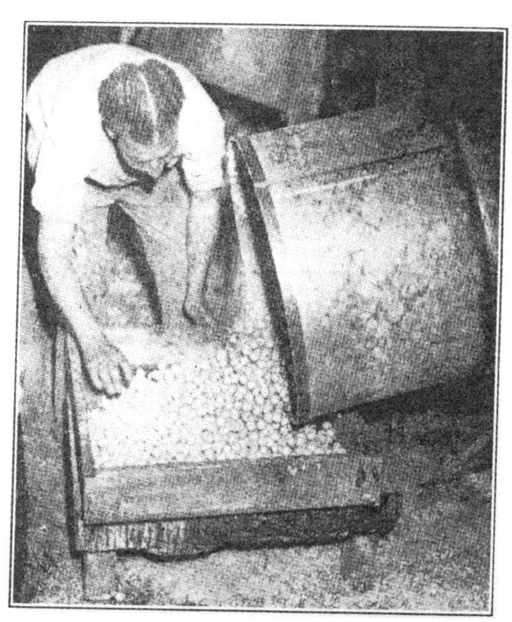

FIGURE 35. Manufacture of Globe Torpedoes. Removing the moist spheres from the tumbling barrel. (Courtesy National Fireworks Company and the *Boston Globe.*)

tumbler, dried in steam-heated ovens, and packed in wood shavings for storage and shipment.

Railway Torpedoes

A railway torpedo consists of a flat tin box, of about an ounce capacity, filled with a fulminating composition and having a strip of lead, soldered to it, which may be bent in order to hold it in place upon the railroad track. It explodes when the first wheel of the locomotive strikes it, and produces a signal which is audible to the engineer above the noise of the train. Railway tor-

pedoes were formerly filled with compositions containing chlorate and red phosphorus, similar to those which are used in toy caps; but these mixtures are dangerous and much more sensitive than

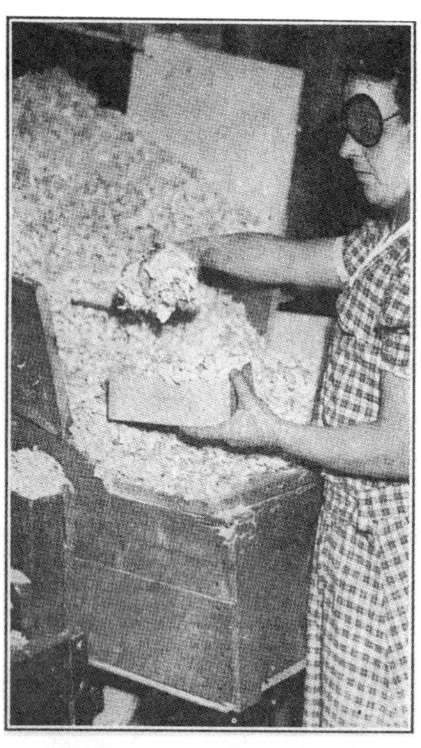

FIGURE 36. Packing Globe Torpedoes in Wood Shavings. (Courtesy National Fireworks Company and the *Boston Globe*.)

is necessary. At present, safer perchlorate mixtures without phosphorus are used. The following compositions (Allen F. Clark) can be mixed dry and yield railway torpedoes which will not explode from ordinary shock or an accidental fall.

Potassium perchlorate	6	12
Antimony sulfide	5	9
Sulfur	1	3

English Crackers or Grasshoppers [111]

These devices are old; they were described by John Bate and by Hanzelet Lorrain. English crackers are represented in the lower right-corner of Figure 23, reproduced from Lorrain's book of 1630. They are used in bombshells and, as Lorrain used them, in rockets, where they jump about in the air producing a series of flashes and explosions. Children shoot them on the ground like firecrackers where their movements suggest the behavior of grasshoppers.

English crackers are commonly loaded with granulated gunpowder, tamped into paper pipes like those from which pinwheels are made. The loaded pipes are softened by moisture in the same way, passed between rollers to make them flatter, folded in frames, and, for the best results, tied each time they are folded and then tied over the whole bundle. They are generally supplied with black match for lighting. They produce as many explosions as there are ligatures.

Chinese Firecrackers

Firecrackers have long been used in China for a variety of ceremonial purposes. The houseboat dweller greets the morning by setting off a bunch of firecrackers, for safety's sake in an iron kettle with a cover over it, to keep all devils away from him during the day. For their own use the Chinese insist upon firecrackers made entirely of red paper, which leave nothing but red fragments, for red is a color particularly offensive to the devils. Firecrackers for export, however, are commonly made from tubes of cheap, coarse, brown paper enclosed in colored wrappers. Thirty years ago a considerable variety of Chinese firecrackers was imported into this country. There were "Mandarin crackers," made entirely from red paper and tied at the ends with silk thread; cheaper crackers plugged at the ends with clay (and these never exploded as satisfactorily); "lady crackers," less than an inch long, tied, and no thicker than a match stem; and "cannon crackers," tied with string, 6, 8, and 12 inches long, made of brown paper with brilliant red wrappers. All these were loaded with explosive mixtures of the general nature of black powder, were equipped with fuses of tissue paper twisted around black powder, and were sold, as Chinese firecrackers are now sold, in bunches with their fuses braided together. The composition [112] 4 parts potassium nitrate, 1 of charcoal, and 1 of sulfur has been reported in Chinese firecrackers; more recently mixtures containing both potassium nitrate and a small amount of potassium chlorate have been used; and at present, when the importation of firecrackers over 1¾ inches in length is practically[51] prohibited, flash powders containing aluminum and potassium

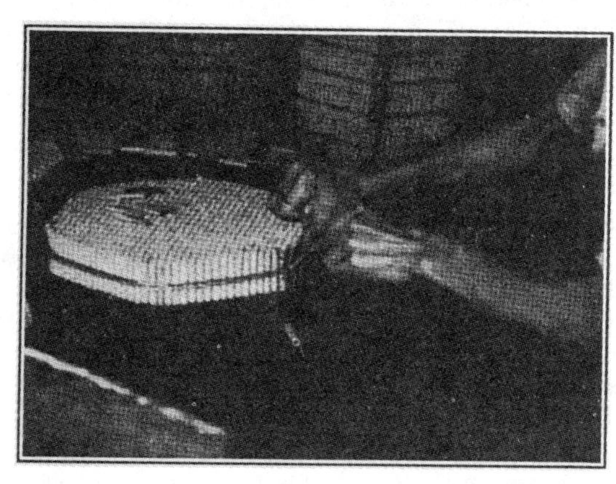

FIGURE 37. Chinese Firecrackers. Tying the Tubes into Bundles.

chlorate are commonly used, for they give a sharper explosion than black powder.

[51] Firecrackers not exceeding 1¾ inches in length and 5/16 inch in diameter carry a duty of 8 cents per pound. For longer crackers the duty is 25 cents per pound, which practically prohibits their importation.

The Chinese firecracker industry formerly centered in Canton but, since the Japanese occupation, has moved elsewhere, largely to French Indo-China and Macao in Portuguese territory. Its processes require great skill and manual dexterity, and have long been a secret and a mystery to Europeans. So far as we know, they had not been described in English print until Weingart's book published an account of the manufacture of clay-plugged crackers based upon information received from the manager of a fireworks company at Hong Kong. His account is illustrated with three pen sketches, two of them of workmen carrying out manual operations [113] and a third which shows some of the tools and instruments. The brief account which follows is based upon conversations with Wallace Clark of Chicago and upon still and moving pictures which he took at a large factory in French Indo-China in January, 1939.

The tubes for the firecrackers are rolled and cut to length in outlying villages, and are brought to the factory for loading.

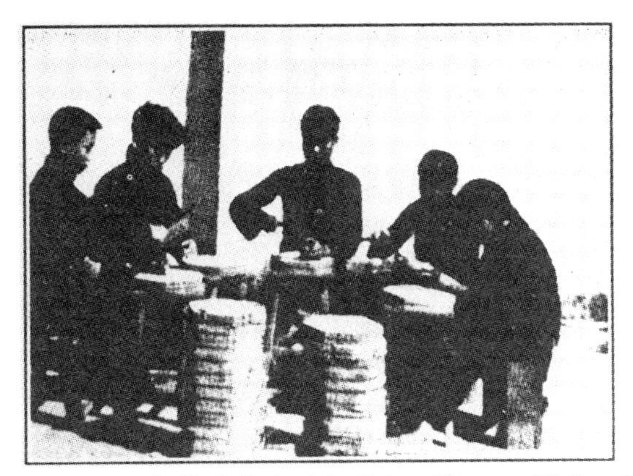

FIGURE 38. Crimping the Back Ends of the Tubes. (Courtesy Wallace Clark.)

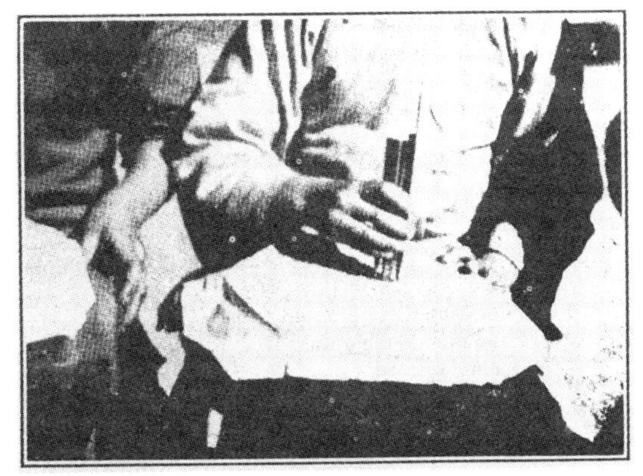

FIGURE 39. Punching Holes for Loading. (Courtesy Wallace Clark.)

114

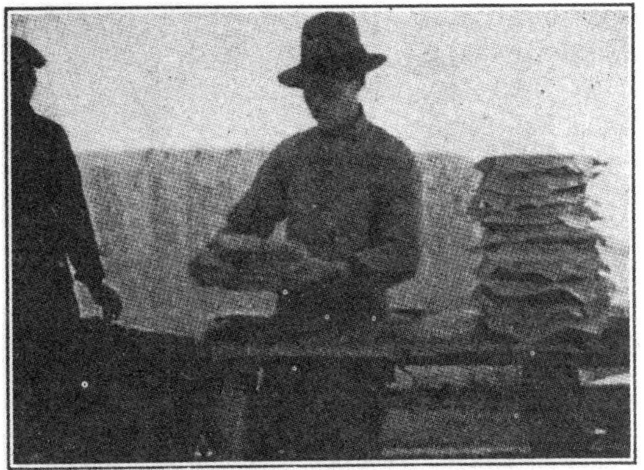

FIGURE 40. Loading. Filling the Tubes with Powder.

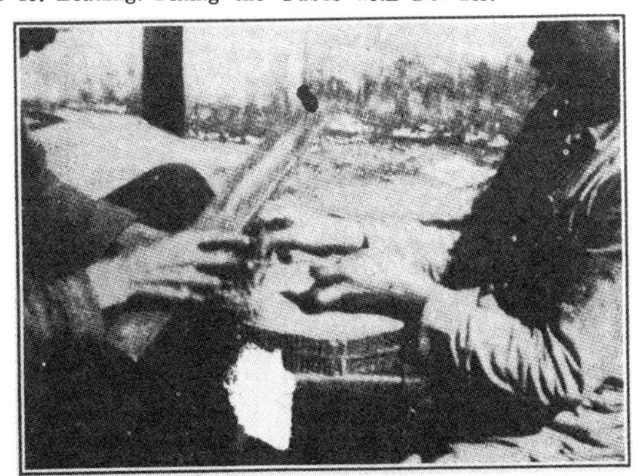

FIGURE 41. Fusing and Crimping. (Courtesy Wallace Clark.)

They are tied in hexagonal bundles, Figure 37, each containing 1006 tubes. Since the twine tied tightly around the bundle crushes the 6 tubes at the corners of the hexagon, and since these are discarded, each bundle contains tubes for 1000 finished crackers.

The back ends of the crackers are then crimped; Figure 38. A bamboo stick is placed against the end of the tube and is

115

struck a sharp blow; this forces some of the paper down into the tube and closes it effectively. The operation, like all the other

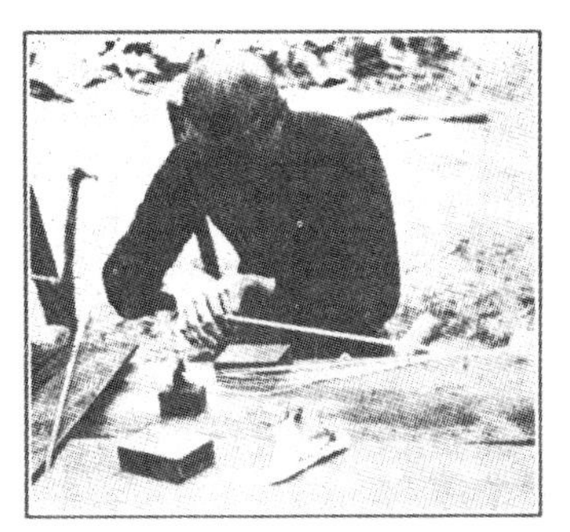

FIGURE 42. Making the Fuse. (Courtesy Wallace Clark.)

operations in the manufacture of the crackers, is carried out very rapidly.

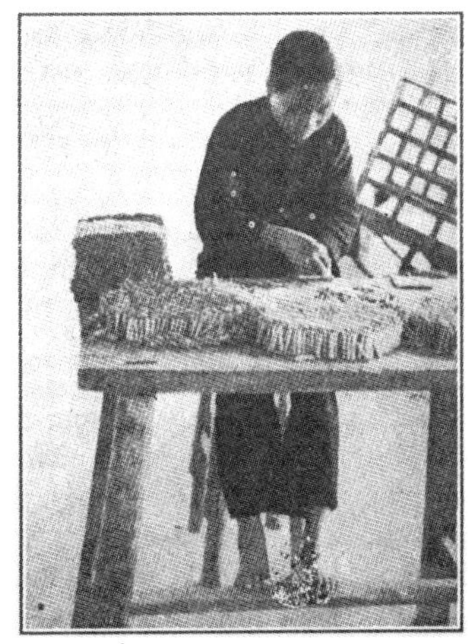

FIGURE 43. Making the Crackers into Bunches by Braiding Fuses Together. (Courtesy Wallace Clark.)

A sheet of paper is then pasted over the other side of the hexagonal bundle of tubes, closing the ends which are later to

116

carry the fuses. When this is dry, holes corresponding to the tubes are punched in the paper. The operation is carried out by young girls who punch the holes four at a time by means of four bamboo sticks held in one hand while they hold the bundle of tubes steady with the other; Figure 39. The edges of the paper are then bent slightly upward, giving it the form of a shallow saucer with 1000 holes in its bottom. The powder for charging the crackers is then introduced into this saucer, and the whole is

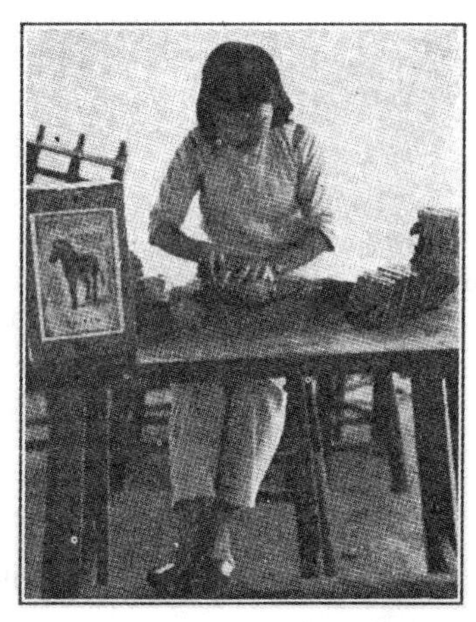

FIGURE 44. Wrapping the Bunches. (Courtesy Wallace Clark.)

shaken gently until all the tubes are full; Figure 40. Then, by a deft movement of the worker's hands and wrists, the excess powder in the saucer, and a portion of the powder in each of the tubes, is emptied out quickly, each of the tubes being left partly full of powder with enough empty space at the top for the fuse and the crimp. This operation, of all those in the manufacture, is considered to be the one which requires the greatest skill. Day after day the average consumption of powder per 1000 or per 100,000 crackers is remarkably constant.

The paper is then torn off from the hexagonal bundle, and the fuses, cut to length, are put in place by one workman while another with a pointed bamboo stick rapidly crimps the paper around them; Figure 41. The fuse is made from narrow strips of tissue paper about 2 feet long. While one end of the strip is clamped to the bench and the other is held in the hand, the strip

117

is shaped by a motion of the worker's other hand into the form of a trough which is then filled with a narrow train of powder, and, by another motion of the hand, the fingers being moistened, is twisted into the finished fuse; Figure 42. This is set aside to dry and is cut into lengths for use in the crackers. The fuses of the finished crackers are braided or pleated together, Figure 43, making the crackers into bunches, and the bunches are wrapped and labeled, Figure 44.

Flash Cracker Composition

Chinese firecrackers and American machine-made salutes are loaded with compositions which contain powdered aluminum and potassium chlorate or perchlorate. They produce a bright flash and an extremely sharp report when they explode. The compositions listed below are typical. The first four in the table have been used in Chinese firecrackers. For the last four the author is indebted to Allen F. Clark.

Potassium perchlorate	..	..	..	..	6	1	7	..
Potassium chlorate	2	3	..	7	..	..	..	..
Potassium nitrate	..	..	5	..	..	..	..	..
Barium nitrate	..	..	..	..	3	1	..	4
Aluminum (fine powder)	1	4	2	1	5	1	5	2
Sulfur	1	3	3	2	..	1	..	1
Antimony sulfide	..	..	..	1	..	..	..	..

The compositions which contain barium nitrate produce a green flash, the others a white one. All of them burn with great rapidity in the open. It is debatable whether the phenomenon of the burning is not really an explosion, or would be one if the material were not allowed to scatter while being burned. With the exception of the third and the last, they are all fulminating explosives when confined. All the mixtures which contain sulfur along with chlorate or perchlorate can be exploded on an iron anvil by a moderately strong blow with an iron hammer.

Sparklers

Snowball sparklers (Allen F. Clark) are made from:

Potassium nitrate	64
Barium nitrate	30
Sulfur	16
Charcoal dust	16
Antimony sulfide	16
Fine aluminum powder	9
Dextrin	16

118

The ingredients are all powdered to pass a 200-210 mesh sieve. The dry materials are mixed thoroughly and sifted, then moistened little by little with water with thorough mixing until the mixture attains the consistency of heavy molasses. Iron wires (20 gauge) of convenient length are dipped in the mixture and are hung up to dry for 24 hours. These are dipped a second time for size, and allowed to dry for another 24 hours. The sparklers burn with a bright white light and throw out "soft sparks" from the charcoal and occasionally scintillating sparks from the burning of the iron wire.

Other mixtures which produce similar effects are as follows:

Potassium nitrate	64	..
Potassium perchlorate	3	16
Barium nitrate	..	6
Sulfur	18	4
Lampblack	5	..
Red gum	4	4
Fine aluminum powder	6	6
Coarse aluminum powder	..	4

The first of these burns with a lilac-colored flame as contrasted with the flame of the second which appears white. These compositions are applied by adding the intimately mixed dry ingredients to a liquid known as "black wax," procured by melting together 3 pounds of rosin and 1 gallon of liquid roofing-paper tar. The iron wires are dipped two or three times in the resulting slurry, and allowed to dry between dips.

The use of iron and steel filings in the compositions produces a more brilliant display of scintillating sparks. The following formulas are typical. Water is used for applying the compositions. The iron and steel filings which are used in these com-

Barium nitrate	48	48	..
Potassium perchlorate	..	..	6
Fine aluminum powder	7	7	1
Fine iron filings	24	18	..
Fine steel filings	..	9	12
Manganese dioxide	2	1	..
Dextrin	12	12	2
Glucose	..	1	..

positions are coated, before the mixing, with paraffin or linseed oil to protect them from rusting.

119

Wire Dips and Colored Fire Sticks

These devices are made in the same way as sparklers, by dipping wires or twisted narrow strips of iron or thin sticks of wood, and generally burn with a tranquil flame except for the sparks that come from the burning of the iron wire or strip. Several typical compositions are listed. Alcohol is used for applying the compositions which contain shellac; water, for applying the others which contain dextrin.

	Red			Green	White
Potassium chlorate	..	2	3	..	..
Potassium perchlorate	..	..	..	..	10
Strontium nitrate	5	6	16	..	..
Barium chlorate	..	..	..	16	..
Fine aluminum powder	..	..	..	..	7
Coarse aluminum powder	..	6	..	24	..
Shellac	1	1	..	3	..
Red gum	..	..	4	..	..
Dextrin	..	..	3	..	3

Pharaoh's Serpents

Wöhler in 1821 first reported the remarkable property of mercurous thiocyanate that it swells up when it is heated, "winding out from itself at the same time worm-like processes, to many times its former bulk, of a very light material of the color of graphite, with the evolution of carbon disulfide, nitrogen, and mercury." Mercuric thiocyanate, which gives better snakes than the mercurous compound, came early into use for this purpose in pyrotechnic toys. When a heap or pellet of either of these compounds is set on fire, it burns with an inconspicuous blue flame, producing sulfur dioxide and mercury vapor. The resulting pale brown or pale gray snake, if broken, is found to be much darker in the interior, and evidently consists of paracyanogen and mercuric sulfide, the mercury having been burned and vaporized from the outer layer.

Mercuric thiocyanate is prepared by adding a solution of[120] potassium, sodium, or ammonium thiocyanate to a solution of mercuric nitrate, a ferric chloride or ferric alum indicator being used to indicate by a red color when enough of the former solution has been added. This is necessary since mercuric thiocyanate is soluble in an excess of either of the reagents by the interaction of which it is produced. The precipitate is collected, washed, dried, powdered, moistened with gum-arabic water in which a little potassium nitrate is dissolved, and made into small pellets by means of a device like a star board or by a pelleting machine. The small pellets are known as *Pharaoh's serpent's eggs.*

Snakes-in-the-grass, volcano snakes, etc., depend upon the use of ammonium dichromate. If this material in the form of a powder is made into a conical heap, and a flame applied to the top of it, a visible but not violent "combustion" proceeds through the mass, which "boils up" to form a large volume of green material resembling tea leaves.

$$(NH_4)_2Cr_2O_7 \longrightarrow N_2 + 4H_2O + Cr_2O_3$$

In practice, more flame is desired than ammonium dichromate alone will give. Weingart recommends a mixture of 2 parts of ammonium dichromate with 1 of potassium nitrate and 1 of dextrin. Tinfoil cones are made from circles of tinfoil shaped on a former, and are introduced by means of the former into conical cavities in a block of wood; they are then about half filled with the powdered mixture, a Pharaoh's serpent's egg is pressed in, and the edges of the tinfoil are turned down upon it to form the base of the cone.

While the fumes from burning mercuric thiocyanate are offensive because of their sulfur dioxide, the small amount of mercury vapor which they contain probably presents no serious danger. The possibility, however, that children may swallow the pellets, with fatal consequences, is a real hazard. For this reason, the sale of mercury snakes has been forbidden by law in many states, and black non-mercury snakes, which are essentially non-poisonous, have come into general use.

Black Non-Mercury Snakes

These are used in the form of *barrel snakes, hat snakes* (black[121] pellets affixed to black discs of pasteboard to form what look like miniature broad-brimmed black hats), *colored fire snakes,* etc. The best which we have seen are prepared from naphthol pitch by a process described by Weingart. The naphthol pitch is a by-product in the manufacture of β-naphthol. The method of "nitration by kneading" is so unusual that it appears worth while to describe the process in detail.

Preparation of Black Non-Mercury Snakes. Thirty grams of powdered naphthol pitch is mixed intimately with 6 grams of linseed oil, and the material is chilled in a 200-cc. Pyrex beaker surrounded by cracked ice. Twenty-one cubic centimeters of fuming nitric acid (*d.* 1.50) is added in small portions, one drop at a time at first, and the material is stirred over, kneaded, and kept thoroughly mixed at all times by means of a porcelain spatula. The addition of each drop of acid, especially at the beginning of the process, causes an abundance of red fumes, considerable heating, and some spattering. It is recommended that goggles and rubber gloves be worn, and that the operation be carried out in an efficient hood. The heat of the reaction causes the material to assume a plastic condition, and the rate of addition of the acid ought to be so regulated that this condition is maintained. After all the acid has been added, the dark brown, doughlike mass becomes friable on cooling. It is broken up under water with the spatula, washed thoroughly, and allowed to dry in the air. The product is ground up in a porcelain mortar with 10.5 grams of picric acid, made into a moist meal with gum-arabic water, pelleted, and dried. A pellet ½ inch long and ⅜ inch in diameter gives a snake about 4 feet long, smooth-skinned and glossy, with a luster like that of coke, elastic, and of spongy texture within.

The oxidized linseed oil produced during the nitration appears to play an important part in the formation of the snakes. If naphthol pitch alone is nitrated, ground up with picric acid, and made into pellets after moistening with linseed oil, the pellets when fresh do not yield snakes, but do give snakes after they have been kept for several months, during which time the linseed oil oxidizes and hardens. Weingart states in a letter that he has obtained satisfactory results by using, instead of naphthol pitch, the material procured by melting together 60 parts of Syrian asphalt and 40 of roofing pitch. Worked up in the regular way this "yielded fairly good snakes which were improved by rubbing[122] the finished product up with a little stearine before forming into pellets." The present writer has found that the substitution of β-naphthol for naphthol pitch yields fairly good snakes which, however, are not so long and not so shiny, and are blacker and covered with wartlike protuberances.

Smokes

Smoke shells and rockets are used to produce *smoke clouds* for military signaling and, in daylight fireworks, for ornamental effects. The shell case or rocket head is filled with a fine powder of the desired color, which powdered material need not necessarily be one which will tolerate heat, and this is dispersed in the form of a colored cloud by the explosion of a small bag of gunpowder placed as near to its center as may be. Artificial vermilion (red), ultramarine (blue), Paris green, chrome yellow, chalk, and ivory black are among the materials which have been used, but almost any material which has a bright color when powdered and which does not cake together may be employed.

Colored smokes strictly so called are produced by the burning, in *smoke pots* or smoke cases, of pyrotechnic compositions which contain colored substances capable of being sublimed without an undue amount of decomposition. The substances are volatilized by the heat of the burning compositions to form colored vapors which quickly condense to form clouds of finely divided colored dust. Colored smokes are used for military signaling, and recently have found use in colored moving pictures. Red smokes, for example, were used in the "Wizard of Oz." Colored smoke compositions are commonly rammed lightly, not packed firmly, in cases, say 1 inch in internal diameter and 4 inches long, both ends of which are closed with plugs of clay or wood. Holes, 1/4 inch in diameter, are bored through the case at intervals on a spiral line around it; the topmost hole penetrates well into the composition and is filled with starting fire material into which a piece of black match, held in place by meal powder paste, is inserted. According to Faber, the following-listed compositions were used in American airplane smoke-signal grenades during the first World War.
123

	Red	Yellow	Green	Blue
Potassium chlorate	1	33	33	7
Lactose	1	24	26	5
Paranitraniline red	3	..	..	..
Auramine	..	34	15	..
Chrysoidine	..	9	..	..
Indigo	..	..	26	8

The following (Allen F. Clark) are illustrative of the perchlorate colored smoke compositions which have come into use more recently.

	Red	Green	Blue
Potassium perchlorate	5	6	5
Antimony sulfide	4	5	4
Rhodamine red	10	..	..
Malachite green	..	10	..
Methylene blue	..	..	10
Gum arabic	1	1	1

Many other dyestuffs may be used. Paranitraniline Yellow gives a canary yellow smoke, and Flaming Red B gives a crimson-colored smoke by comparison with which the smoke from Paranitraniline Red appears to be scarlet. None of the colored smoke compositions are adapted to indoor use. All the smokes are unpleasant and unwholesome.

White smoke is produced by burning a mixture of potassium chlorate 3 parts, lactose 1, and finely powdered ammonium chloride 1. The smoke, which consists of finely divided ammonium chloride, is not poisonous, and has found some use in connection with the study of problems in ventilation.

For use in trench warfare, for the purpose of obscuring the situation from the sight of the enemy, a very satisfactory dense *white* or *gray smoke* is procured by burning a mixture of zinc dust and hexachloroethane. The mixture requires a strong starting fire. The smoke consists largely of finely divided zinc chloride. For a grayer smoke naphthalene or anthracene is added to the mixture. Torches for *black smoke* have also been used, charged with a mixture of potassium nitrate and sulfur with rosin or pitch and generally with such additional ingredients as sand, powdered chalk, or glue to modify the rate of their burning. 124

When shells are loaded with certain high explosives which produce no smoke (such as amatol), *smoke boxes* are generally inserted in the charges in order that the artilleryman, by seeing the smoke, may be able to judge the position and success of his fire. These are cylindrical pasteboard boxes containing a mixture of arsenious oxide and red phosphorus, usually with a small amount of stearine or paraffin.
125

CHAPTER IV

AROMATIC NITRO COMPOUNDS

Aromatic nitro compounds are generally stable but are frequently reactive, especially if they contain groups other than nitro groups in the *meta* position with respect to one another. As a class they constitute the most important of the military high explosives. They are also used as components of smokeless powder, in compound detonators, and in primer compositions. Liquid nitro compounds, and the mixtures which are produced as by-products from the manufacture of pure nitro compounds for military purposes, are used in non-freezing dynamite and other commercial explosives. The polynitro compounds are solvents for nitrocellulose.

The nitro compounds are poisonous. Nitrobenzene, known also as "oil of mirbane," is absorbed through the skin and by breathing its vapors, and has been reported to cause death by the careless wearing of clothing upon which it had been spilled. The less volatile polynitro compounds, like trinitrotoluene, are absorbed through the skin when handled, and may cause injury by the inhalation of their dust or of their vapors when they are melted. Minor TNT sickness may manifest itself by cyanosis, dermatitis, nose bleeding, constipation, and giddiness; the severer form, by toxic jaundice and aplastic anemia. One of the nitro groups is reduced in the body, and dinitrohydroxylaminotoluene may be detected in the urine. Trinitrobenzene is more poisonous than trinitrotoluene, which, in turn, is more poisonous than trinitroxylene, alkyl groups in this series having the same effect as in the phenols, cresol, xylenol, etc., where they reduce the toxicity of the substances but increase their antiseptic strength.
126

In the manufacture of explosives the nitro groups are always introduced by the direct action of nitric acid on the aromatic substances. The simple reaction involves the production of water and is promoted by the presence of sulfuric acid which thus functions as a dehydrating agent. We shall later see cases in which sulfuric acid is used as a means of hindering the introduction of nitro groups. In consequence of the reaction, the nitrogen

$$C_6H_5\text{—}H + HO\text{—}NO_2 \longrightarrow C_6H_5\text{—}NO_2 + H_2O$$

atom of the nitro group becomes attached to the carbon atom of the aromatic nucleus. Nitro groups attached to the nucleus, unless *ortho* and *para* to other nitro groups, are not affected by sulfuric acid as are nitro groups attached to oxygen (in nitric esters) and to nitrogen (in nitroamines), or, ordinarily, by hydrolytic agents as are nitro groups attached to oxygen. Nitric acid is a nitrating agent both at low and at elevated temperatures; its vigor in this respect depends upon the concentration. But it is an oxidizing agent even in fairly dilute solution, and becomes more vigorous if the temperature is raised. Further, it decomposes when heated to produce nitrous acid, which is also a powerful oxidizing agent and may reduce the yield of the desired product. Nitrous acid present in the nitrating acid may also result in the formation of nitrophenols from aromatic amines. Aromatic nitro compounds, such as TNT and picric acid, on refluxing for some hours with nitric acid (*d.* 1.42) and then distilling the mixture, yield appreciable quantities of tetranitromethane, formed by the rupture of the ring and the nitration of the individual carbon atoms. The nitro group "strengthens" the ring against attack by acid oxidizing agents, but makes it more accessible to attack by alkaline ones. The polynitro compounds are destroyed rapidly by warm alkaline permanganate yielding oxalic acid. They combine with aniline, naphthylamine, etc., to form brightly colored molecular compounds. All aromatic nitro compounds give colors, yellow, orange, red, even purple, with alkaline reagents.

The position which the nitro group takes on entering the aromatic nucleus and the ease with which the substitution is accomplished depend upon the group or groups already present

127

on the nucleus. We are accustomed to speak of the orienting or directing effect of the groups already present and of their influence in promoting or inhibiting further substitution. The two simple rules which summarize these effects have important implications and wide applications in the chemistry of aromatic substances.

Effect of Groups on Further Substitution

1. Orienting Effect. *The Modified Rule of Crum Brown and Gibson.* If the atom attached to the aromatic nucleus is attached to some other atom by an unsaturated linkage (i.e., by any bond which we commonly write as double or triple), then the next entering group takes the *meta* position; otherwise it takes the *ortho* and *para* positions.

The rule relieves us of the necessity for remembering which groups orient *meta* and which *ortho-para*; we may write them down on demand, thus: the $—NO_2$, —NO, —CO—, —COOH, —CHO, $—SO_2—OH$, —CN groups orient *meta*; and the $—NH_2$, —NHR, $—NR_2$, —OH, —OR, $—CH_3$, $—CH_2—CH_3$, —Cl, —Br groups orient *ortho-para*. It is necessary, however, to take note of three or four exceptions, only one of which is important in the chemistry of explosives, namely, that the azo group, —N=N—, orients *ortho-para*; the trichloromethyl group, $—CCl_3$, *meta*; that such conjugate systems as occur in cinnamic acid, —CH=CH—CO—, orient *ortho-para*; and further that a large excess of strong sulfuric acid reverses to a greater or less extent the normal orienting effects of the methoxy and ethoxy groups, of the amino group wholly and of the monosubstituted and disubstituted amino groups in part.

In all discussions of the application of the rule we make reference to the principal products of the reaction; substitution occurs for the most part in accordance with the rule, or with the exceptions, and small amounts of other materials are usually formed as by-products. In the mononitration of toluene, for example, about 96 per cent of the product is a mixture of *o-* and *p*-nitrotoluene, and about 4 per cent is the *m*-compound. Under the influence of *ortho-para* orienting groups, substitution occurs in the two positions without much preference for either one, but it appears to be the case that, when nitro groups are introduced, low temperatures favor the formation of *p*-compounds. The effect

128

of temperature on sulfonations appears to be exactly the opposite.

2. Ease of Substitution. *Ortho-para* orienting groups promote substitution; *meta* orienting groups hinder it and make it more difficult. The rule may be stated otherwise: that substitution under the influence of *ortho-para* orienting groups occurs under less vigorous conditions of temperature, concentration of reagents, etc., than it does with the unsubstituted aromatic hydrocarbon itself; under the influence of *meta* orienting groups more vigorous conditions than with the unsubstituted hydrocarbon are necessary for its successful accomplishment. The rule may also be stated that *ortho-para* substitution is easier than *meta*. In this last form it fails to make comparison with substitution in the simple hydrocarbon, but does point clearly to the implication, or corollary, that the orienting effect of an *ortho-para* orienting group dominates over that of one which orients *meta*. To the rule in any of these forms, we must add that, when more than one group is already present on the nucleus, the effect of the groups is additive.

Toluene nitrates more easily than benzene; aniline and phenol more easily still. Higher temperature and stronger acid are needed for the introduction of a second nitro group into benzene than for the introduction of the first, for the second is introduced under the influence of the *meta*-orienting first nitro group which tends to make further substitution more difficult. The inhibitory effect of two nitro groups is so great that the nitration of dinitrobenzene to the trinitro compound is extremely difficult. It is more difficult to nitrate benzoic acid than to nitrate nitrobenzene. The common experience of organic chemists indicates that the order of the groups in promoting substitution is about as follows:

$$—OH > —NH_2 > —CH_3 > —Cl > —H > —NO_2 > —SO_2(OH) > —COOH$$

Any one of these groups makes substitution easier than the groups which are printed to the right of it.

Xylene nitrates more easily than toluene. Two methyl groups promote substitution more than one methyl group does, and this appears to be true whether or not the methyl groups agree among themselves in respect to the positions which they activate. Although a nitro group may be said to "activate" a particular position, inasmuch as it points to that position as the one in which substitution will next occur, it nevertheless makes substitution more difficult in that position, as well as in all other positions on

129

the nucleus. The nitroanilines are more difficult to nitrate than aniline because of their inhibiting nitro group, and more easy to nitrate than nitrobenzene because of their promoting amino group. In *o-* and *p*-nitroaniline the amino and nitro groups agree in activating the same positions, and both substances yield 2,4,6-trinitroaniline when they are nitrated. In *m*-nitroaniline, the nitro group "activates" the 5-position, while the amino group activates the 2-, 4-, and 6-positions. Nitration takes place under the influence of the *ortho-para*-orienting amino group, and 2,3,4,6-tetranitroaniline results.

Utilization of Coal Tar

The principal source of aromatic compounds is coal tar, produced as a by-product in the manufacture of coke. Gas tar, of which much smaller quantities are produced, also contains these same materials. Aromatic hydrocarbons occur in nature in Borneo and other petroleums, and they may be prepared artificially by stripping hydrogen atoms from the cycloparaffins which occur in Caucasus petroleum and elsewhere. They are also produced from paraffin hydrocarbons by certain processes of cracking, and it is to be expected that in the future aromatic compounds will be produced in increasing quantity from petroleum which does not contain them in its natural state.

Coal yields about 6 per cent of its weight of tar. One ton of tar on distillation gives:

Light Oil—yielding about 32 lb. of benzene, 5 lb. of toluene, and 0.6 lb. of xylene.
Middle Oil—yielding about 40 lb. of phenol and cresols, and 80-120 lb. of naphthalene.
Heavy Oil—yielding impure cresols and other phenols.
Green Oil—yielding 10-40 lb. of anthracene.
Pitch—1000-1200 lb.

Naphthalene is the most abundant pure hydrocarbon obtained from coal tar. It takes on three nitro groups readily, and four under vigorous conditions, but ordinarily yields no product which is suitable by itself for use as an explosive. Nitrated naphthalenes, however, have been used in smokeless powder and, when mixed with ammonium nitrate and other materials, in high explosives for shells and for blasting.

The phenol-cresol fraction of coal tar yields phenol on distillation, which is convertible to picric acid, and the cresols, of which

130

m-cresol is the only one which yields a trinitro derivative directly. Moreover, synthetic phenol from benzene, through chlorobenzene by the Dow process, is purer and probably cheaper in times of stress.

Of the hydrocarbons toluene is the only one which nitrates sufficiently easily and yields a product which has the proper physical and explosive properties. Trinitrotoluene is the most widely used of the pure aromatic nitro compounds. It melts at such temperature that it can be loaded by pouring. It is easily and surely detonated, and is insensitive to shock, though not insensitive enough to penetrate armor-plate without exploding until afterwards. It is powerful and brisant, but less so than trinitrobenzene which would offer certain advantages if it could be procured in sufficient quantity.

Of the xylenes, the *meta* compound yields a trinitro derivative more readily than toluene does, but trinitro-*m*-xylene (TNX) melts somewhat higher than is desirable and is not quite powerful enough when used alone. It has been used in shells in mixtures with TNT and with ammonium nitrate. The other xylenes yield only dinitro derivatives by direct nitration. A mixture of *o*- and *p*-xylene may be converted into an explosive—an oily mixture of a large number of isomers, which has been used in the composition of non-freezing dynamites—by chlorinating at an elevated

CH_3, CH_3 → CH_2—Cl, CH_3, Cl → CH_2—Cl, NO_2, CH_3, NO_2, Cl →
CH_2—OH, NO_2, CH_3, NO_2, OH → CH_2—ONO_2, NO_2, CH_3, NO_2, OH

temperature in the presence of a catalyst (whereby chlorine is substituted both in the side chain and on the nucleus), then nitrating, then hydrolyzing (whereby both chlorines are replaced by hydroxyl groups, the nuclear chlorine being activated by the nitro groups), and finally nitrating once more.

131

In each step several isomers are formed—only one of the possibilities in each case is indicated above—and the *ortho* and *para* compounds both go through similar series of reactions. The product is too sensitive and in the wrong physical state (liquid) for use as a military explosive. In short, for the manufacture of

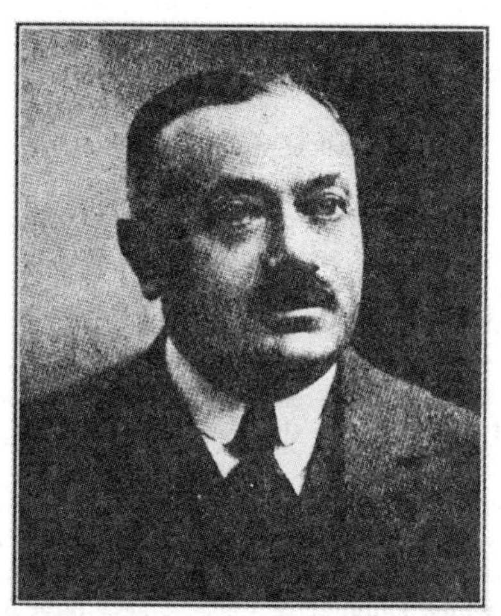

FIGURE 45. Marius Marqueyrol, Inspecteur-Général des Poudres, France. 1919. Author of many researches on aromatic nitro compounds, nitrocellulose, smokeless powder, stabilizers and stability, chlorate explosives, etc.—published for the most part in the *Mémorial des poudres* and in the *Bulletin de la société chimique de France*.

military explosives toluene is the most valuable of the materials which occur in coal tar.

In time of war the industries of a country strive to produce as much toluene as possible. The effort results in the production also of increased quantities of other aromatic hydrocarbons, particularly of benzene, and these become cheaper and more abundant. Every effort is made to utilize them profitably for military purposes. As far as benzene is concerned, the problem has been solved through chlorobenzene, which yields aniline and phenol by the Dow process, and hence picric acid, and which gives dinitrochlorobenzene on nitration which is readily convertible, as will be described later, into picric acid and tetryl and several other

132

explosives that are quite as necessary as TNT for military purposes.

Effects of Substituents on Explosive Strength

Bomb experiments show that trinitrobenzene is the most powerful explosive among the nitrated aromatic hydrocarbons. One methyl group, as in TNT, reduces its strength; two, as in TNX, reduce it further; and three, as in trinitromesitylene, still further yet. The amino and the hydroxyl groups have less effect than the methyl group; indeed, two hydroxyl groups have less effect than one methyl—and trinitroresorcinol is a stronger explosive than TNT, though weaker than TNB. TNT is stronger than trinitrocresol, which differs from it in having an hydroxyl group. The figures given below were determined by exploding the materials.

loaded at the density indicated, in a small bomb, and measuring the pressure by means of a piston and obturator. *Density of loading* is grams of explosive per cubic centimeter of bomb capacity.

	Pressure: Kilograms per square centimeter		
Density of loading:	0.20	0.25	0.30
Trinitrobenzene	2205	3050	4105
Trinitrotoluene	1840	2625	3675
Trinitro-*m*-xylene	1635	2340	2980
Trinitromesitylene	1470	2200	2780
Trinitrophenol (picric acid)	2150	3055	3865
Trinitroresorcinol (styphinic acid)	2080	2840	....
Trinitroaniline (picramide)	2080	2885	3940
Trinitro-*m*-cresol	1760	2480	3360
Trinitronaphthalene	....	2045	2670

Similar inferences may be made from the results of lead block tests. Fifteen grams of the explosives produced the expansions indicated below, each figure representing the average from twenty or more experiments:
133

Trinitrobenzene	480 cc.
Trinitrotoluene	452 cc.
Picric acid	470 cc.
Trinitrocresol	384 cc.
Trinitronaphthalene	166 cc.

Mono- and Di-Nitrobenzene

Nitrobenzene is a pale yellow liquid, b.p. 208.0°, which is poisonous and has an almondlike odor closely resembling that of benzaldehyde (which is not poisonous). It is used as a component of certain Sprengel explosives and as a raw material for the preparation of aniline and of intermediates for the manufacture of dyestuffs and medicinals. Its preparation, familiar to every student of organic chemistry, is described here in order that the conditions for the substitution of one nitro group in benzene may serve us more conveniently as a standard for judging the relative ease and difficulty of the nitration of other substances.

Preparation of Nitrobenzene. One hundred and fifty grams of concentrated sulfuric acid (*d.* 1.84) and 100 grams of nitric acid (*d.* 1.42) are mixed in a 500-cc. flask and cooled to room temperature, and 51 grams of benzene is added in small portions at a time with frequent shaking. Shaking at this point is especially necessary lest the reaction suddenly become violent. If the temperature of the mixture rises above 50-60°, the addition of the benzene is interrupted and the mixture is cooled at the tap. After all the benzene has been added, an air condenser is attached to the flask and the material is heated in the water bath for an hour at 60° (thermometer in the water). After cooling, the nitrobenzene (upper layer) is separated from the spent acid, washed once with water (the nitrobenzene is now the lower layer), then several times with dilute sodium carbonate solution until it is free from acid, then once more with water, dried with calcium chloride, and distilled (not quite to dryness). The portion boiling at 206-208° is taken as nitrobenzene.

m-Dinitrobenzene, in accordance with the rule of Crum Brown and Gibson, is the only product which results ordinarily from the nitration of nitrobenzene. Small amounts of the *ortho* and *para* compounds have been procured, along with the *meta*, from the nitration of benzene in the presence of mercuric nitrate. Dinitrobenzene has been used in high explosives for shells in mixtures with more powerful explosives or with ammonium nitrate. Its use
134
as a raw material for the manufacture of tetranitroaniline is now no longer important.

Preparation of Dinitrobenzene. A mixture of 25 grams of concentrated sulfuric acid (*d.* 1.84) and 15 grams of nitric acid (*d.* 1.52) is heated in an open flask in the boiling water bath in the hood, and 10 grams of nitrobenzene is added gradually during the course of half an hour. The mixture is cooled somewhat, and drowned in cold water. The dinitrobenzene separates as a solid. It is crushed with water, washed with water, and recrystallized from alcohol or from nitric acid. Dinitrobenzene crystallizes from nitric acid in beautiful needles which are practically colorless, m.p. 90°.

Trinitrobenzene

1,3,5-Trinitrobenzene (*sym*-trinitrobenzene, TNB) may be prepared only with the greatest difficulty by the nitration of *m*-dinitrobenzene. Hepp first prepared it by this method, and Hepp and Lobry de Bruyn improved the process, treating 60 grams of *m*-dinitrobenzene with a mixture of 1 kilo of fuming sulfuric acid and 500 grams of nitric acid (*d.* 1.52) for 1 day at 100° and for 4 days at 110°. Claus and Becker obtained trinitrobenzene by the action of concentrated nitric acid on trinitrotoluene. Trinitrobenzoic acid is formed first, and this substance in the hot liquid loses carbon dioxide from its carboxyl group.

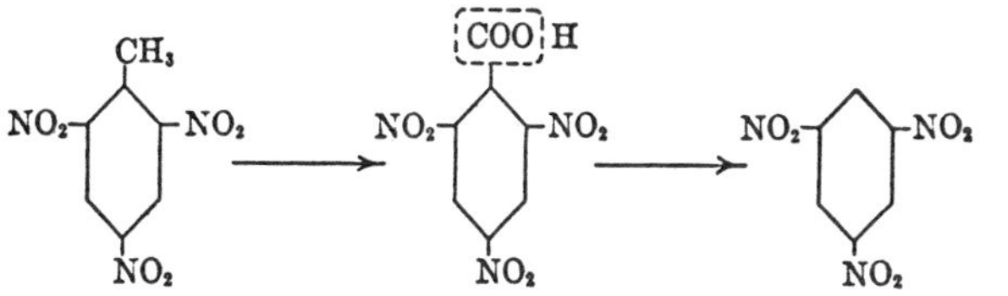

CH_3, NO_2, NO_2, NO_2 → COOH, NO_2, NO_2, NO_2 → NO_2, NO_2, NO_2

For commercial production the Griesheim Chem. Fabrik is reported to have used a process in which 1 part of TNT is heated at 150-200° with a mixture of 5 parts of fuming nitric acid and 10 parts of concentrated sulfuric acid. In a process devised by J. Meyer, picryl chloride (2,4,6-trinitrochlorobenzene) is reduced by means of copper powder in hot aqueous alcohol. The reported details are 25 kilos of picryl chloride, 8 kilos of copper
135
powder, 250 liters of 95 per cent alcohol, and 25 liters of water, refluxed together for 2 hours and filtered hot; the TNB crystallizes out in good yield when the liquid is cooled.

The nitration of *m*-dinitrobenzene is too expensive of acid and of heat for practical application, and the yields are poor. Toluene and chlorobenzene are nitrated more easily and more economically, and their trinitro compounds are feasible materials for the preparation of TNB. Oxidation with nitrosulfuric acid has obvious disadvantages. The quickest, most convenient, and cheapest method is probably that in which TNT is oxidized by means of chromic acid in sulfuric acid solution.

Preparation of Trinitrobenzene. A mixture of 30 grams of purified TNT and 300 cc. of concentrated sulfuric acid is introduced into a tall beaker, which stands in an empty agateware basin, and the mixture is stirred actively by means of an electric stirrer while powdered sodium dichromate ($Na_2Cr_2O_7 \cdot 2H_2O$) is added in small portions at a time, care being taken that no lumps are formed and that none floats on the surface of the liquid. The temperature of the liquid rises. When it has reached 40°, cold water is poured into the basin and the addition of dichromate is continued, with stirring, until 45 grams has been added, the temperature being kept always between 40° and 50°. The mixture is stirred for 2 hours longer at the same temperature, and is then allowed to cool and to stand over night, in order that the trinitrobenzoic acid may assume a coarser crystalline form and may be filtered off more readily. The strongly acid liquid is filtered through an asbestos filter; the solid material is rinsed with cold water and transferred to a beaker in which it is treated with warm water at 50° sufficient to dissolve all soluble material. The warm solution is filtered, and boiled until no more trinitrobenzene precipitates. The crystals of TNB growing in the hot aqueous liquid often attain a length of several millimeters. When filtered from the cooled liquid and rinsed with water, they are practically pure, almost colorless or greenish yellow leaflets, m.p. 121-122°.

Trinitrobenzene is only moderately soluble in hot alcohol, more readily in acetone, ether, and benzene. Like other polynitro aromatic compounds it forms colored molecular compounds with many aromatic hydrocarbons and organic bases. The compound with aniline is bright red;[136] that with naphthalene, yellow. The compounds with amines are beautifully crystalline substances, procurable by warming the components together in alcohol, and are formed generally in the molecular proportions 1 to 1, although diphenylamine and quinoline form compounds in which two molecules of TNB are combined with one of the base.

Trinitrobenzene gives red colors with ammonia and with aqueous alkalies. On standing in the cold with methyl alcoholic sodium methylate, it yields 3,5-dinitroanisol by a metathetical reaction.

$$C_6H_3(NO_2)_3 + CH_3ONa \longrightarrow C_6H_3(OCH_3)(NO_2)_2 + NaNO_2$$

On boiling with alcoholic soda solution it undergoes a partial reduction to form 3,3',5,5'-tetranitroazoxybenzene.

$$(NO_2)_2C_6H_3{-}N(=O){=}N{-}C_6H_3(NO_2)_2$$

The first product, however, of the reaction of methyl alcoholic caustic alkali on TNB is a red crystalline addition product having the empirical composition $TNB{\cdot}CH_3ONa{\cdot}\frac{1}{2}H_2O$, isolated by Lobry de Bruyn and van Leent in 1895. The structure of this substance has been discussed by Victor Meyer, by Angeli, by Meisenheimer, and by Schlenck, and is probably best represented by the formula which Meisenheimer suggested.[137] It is thus

$$C_6H_3(NO_2)_3 \xrightarrow{+CH_3ONa} C_6H_3(OCH_3)(NO_2)_2{=}N(O)ONa$$

probably the product of the 1,6-addition of sodium methylate to the conjugate system which runs through the ring and terminates in the oxygen of the nitro group. Busch and Kögel have prepared di- and tri-alcoholates of TNB, and Giua has isolated a compound of the empirical composition $TNB{\cdot}NaOH$, to which he ascribed a structure similar to that indicated above. All these compounds when dry are dangerous primary explosives. They are soluble in water, and the solutions after acidification contain red, water-soluble acids which yield sparingly soluble salts with copper and other heavy metals, and the salts are primary explosives. The acids, evidently having the compositions $TNB{\cdot}CH_3OH$, $TNB{\cdot}H_2O$, etc., have not been isolated in a state of purity, and are reported to decompose spontaneously in small part into TNB, alcohol, water, etc., and in large part into oxalic acid, nitrous fumes, and colored amorphous materials which have not been identified. All the polynitro aromatic hydrocarbons react similarly with alkali, and the use of alkali in any industrial process for their purification is bad practice and extremely hazardous.

Trinitrobenzene reacts with hydroxylamine in cold alcohol solution, picramide being formed by the direct introduction of an amino group.

$$C_6H_3(NO_2)_3 + NH_2{-}OH \longrightarrow C_6H_2(NH_2)(NO_2)_3 + H_2O$$

Two or three nitro groups on the aromatic nucleus, particularly those in the 2,4-, 2,6-, and 2,4,6-positions, have a strong effect in increasing the chemical activity of the group or atom in the 1-position.[138] Thus, the hydroxyl group of trinitrophenol is acidic, and the substance is called picric acid. A chlorine atom in the same position is like the chlorine of an acid chloride (picryl chloride), an amino group like the amino of an acid amide (trinitroaniline is picramide), and a methoxy like the methoxy of an ester (trinitroanisol has the reactions of methyl picrate). In general the picryl group affects the activity of the atom or group to which it is attached in the same way that the acyl or R—CO— group does. If the picryl group is attached to a carboxyl, the carboxyl will be expected to lose CO_2 readily, as pyruvic acid, $CH_3{-}CO{-}COOH$, does when it is heated with dilute sulfuric acid, and this indeed happens with the trinitrobenzoic acid from which TNB is commonly prepared. TNB itself will be expected to exhibit some of the properties of an aldehyde, of which the aldehydic hydrogen atom is readily oxidized to an acidic hydroxyl group, and it is in fact oxidized to picric acid by the action of potassium ferricyanide in mildly alkaline solution. We shall see many examples of the same principle throughout the chemistry of the explosive aromatic nitro compounds.

Trinitrobenzene is less sensitive to impact than TNT, more powerful, and more brisant. The detonation of a shell or bomb, loaded with TNB, in the neighborhood of buildings or other construction which it is desired to destroy, creates a more damaging explosive wave than an explosion of TNT, and is more likely to cause the collapse of walls, etc., which the shell or bomb has failed to hit. Drop tests carried out with a 5-kilogram weight falling upon several decigrams of each of the various explosives contained in a small cup of iron (0.2 mm. thick), covered with a small iron disc of the same thickness, gave the following figures for the distances through which the weight must fall to cause explosion in 50 per cent of the trials.

	Centimeters
Trinitrobenzene	150
Trinitrotoluene	110
Hexanitrodiphenylamine ammonium salt	75
Picric acid	65
Tetryl	50
Hexanitrodiphenylamine	45

According to Dautriche,[139] the density of compressed pellets of

TNB is as follows:

Pressure: Kilos per Square Centimeter	Density
275	1.343
685	1.523
1375	1.620
2060	1.641
2750	1.654
3435	1.662

The greatest velocity of detonation for TNB which Dautriche found, namely 7347 meters per second, occurred when a column of 10 pellets, 20 mm. in diameter and weighing 8 grams each, density 1.641 or 1.662, was exploded in a paper cartridge by means of an initiator of 0.5 gram of mercury fulminate and 80 grams of dynamite. The greatest which he found for TNT was 7140 meters per second, 10 similar pellets, density 1.60, in a paper cartridge exploded by means of a primer of 0.5 gram of fulminate and 25 grams of dynamite. The maximum value for picric acid was 7800 meters per second; a column of pellets of the same sort, density 1.71, exploded in a copper tube 20-22 mm. in diameter, by means of a primer of 0.5 gram of fulminate and 80 grams of dynamite. The highest velocity with picric acid in paper cartridges was 7645 meters per second with pellets of densities 1.73 and 1.74 and the same charge of initiator.

Velocity of detonation, other things being equal, depends upon the physical state of the explosive and upon the nature of the envelope which contains it. For each explosive there is an optimum density at which it shows its highest velocity of detonation. There is also for each explosive a minimum priming charge necessary to insure its complete detonation, and larger charges do not cause it to explode any faster. Figures for the velocity of detonation are of little interest unless the density is reported or unless the explosive is cast and is accordingly of a density which, though perhaps unknown, is easily reproducible. The cordeau of the following table was loaded with TNT which was subsequently pulverized *in situ* during the drawing down of the lead tube: [140]

	Meters per Second
Cast trinitrobenzene	7441
Cast tetryl	7229
Cast trinitrotoluene	7028
Cast picric acid	6777
Compressed trinitrotoluene (*d.* 0.909)	4961
Compressed picric acid (*d.* 0.862)	4835
Cordeau	6900

Nitration of Chlorobenzene

The nitration of chlorobenzene is easier than the nitration of benzene and more difficult than the nitration of toluene. Trinitrochlorobenzene (picryl chloride) can be prepared on the plant scale by the nitration of dinitrochlorobenzene, but the process is expensive of acid and leads to but few valuable explosives which cannot be procured more cheaply and more simply from dinitrochlorobenzene by other processes. Indeed, there are only two important explosives, namely TNB and hexanitrobiphenyl, for the preparation of which picryl chloride could be used advantageously if it were available in large amounts. In the laboratory, picryl chloride is best prepared by the action of phosphorus pentachloride on picric acid.

During the early days of the first World War in Europe, electrolytic processes for the production of caustic soda were yielding in this country more chlorine than was needed by the chemical industries, and it was necessary to dispose of the excess. The pressure to produce toluene had made benzene cheap and abundant. The chlorine, which would otherwise have become a nuisance and a menace, was used for the chlorination of benzene. Chlorobenzene and dichlorobenzene became available, and dichlorobenzene since that time has been used extensively as an insecticide and moth exterminator. Dinitrodichlorobenzene was tried as an explosive under the name of *parazol*. When mixed with TNT in high-explosive shells, it did not detonate completely, but presented interesting possibilities because the unexploded portion, atomized in the air, was a vigorous itch-producer and lachrymator, and because the exploded portion yielded phosgene. The chlorine atom of chlorobenzene is unreactive, and catalytic processes[22] for replacing it by hydroxyl and amino groups had

[22] Steam and silica gel to produce phenol from chlorobenzene, the Dow process with steam and a copper salt catalyst, etc. [141]

not yet been developed. In dinitrochlorobenzene, however, the chlorine is active. The substance yields dinitrophenol readily by hydrolysis, dinitroaniline by reaction with ammonia, dinitromethylaniline more readily yet by reaction with methylamine. These and similar materials may be nitrated to explosives, and the third nitro group may be introduced on the nucleus much more readily, after the chlorine has been replaced by a more strongly *ortho-para* orienting group, than it may be before the chlorine has been so replaced. Dinitrochlorobenzene thus has a definite advantage over picryl chloride. It has the advantage also over phenol, aniline, etc. (from chlorobenzene by catalytic processes), that explosives can be made from it which cannot be made as simply or as economically from these materials. Tetryl and hexanitrodiphenylamine are examples. The possibilities of dinitrochlorobenzene in the explosives industry have not yet been fully exploited.

Preparation of Dinitrochlorobenzene. One hundred grams of chlorobenzene is added drop by drop to a mixture of 160 grams of nitric acid (*d.* 1.50) and 340 grams of sulfuric acid (*d.* 1.84) while the mixture is stirred mechanically. The temperature rises because of the heat of the reaction, but is not allowed to go above 50-55°. After all the chlorobenzene has been added, the temperature is raised slowly to 95° and is kept there for 2 hours longer while the stirring is continued. The upper layer of light yellow liquid solidifies when cold. It is removed, broken up under water, and rinsed. The spent acid, on dilution with water, precipitates an additional quantity of dinitrochlorobenzene. All the product is brought together, washed with cold water, then several times with hot water while it is melted, and finally once more with cold water under which it is crushed. Then it is drained and allowed to dry at ordinary temperature. The product, melting at about 50°, consists largely of 2,4-dinitrochlorobenzene, m.p. 53.4°, along with a small quantity of the 2,6-dinitro compound, m.p. 87-88°. The two substances are equally suitable for the manufacture of explosives. They yield the same trinitro compound, and the same final products by reaction with methylamine, aniline, etc., and subsequent nitration of the materials which are first formed. Dinitrochlorobenzene causes a severe itching of the skin, both by contact with the solid material and by exposure to its vapors.

Trinitrotoluene (TNT, trotyl, tolite, triton, tritol, trilite, etc.)

When toluene is nitrated, about 96 per cent of the material behaves in accordance with the rule of Crum Brown and Gibson. [142] In industrial practice the nitration is commonly carried out in three stages, the spent acid from the trinitration being used for the next dinitration, the spent acid from this being used for the mononitration, and the spent acid from this either being fortified

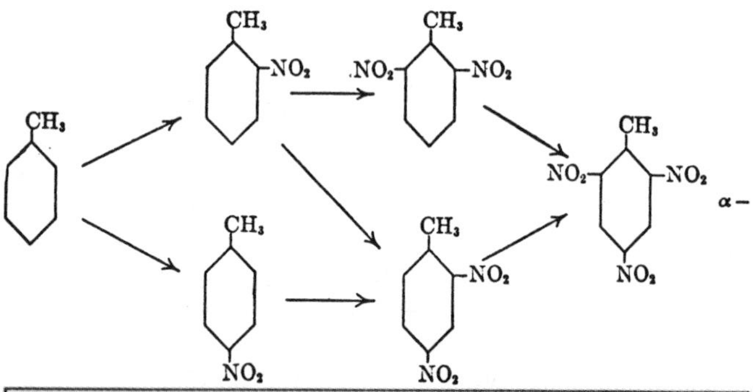

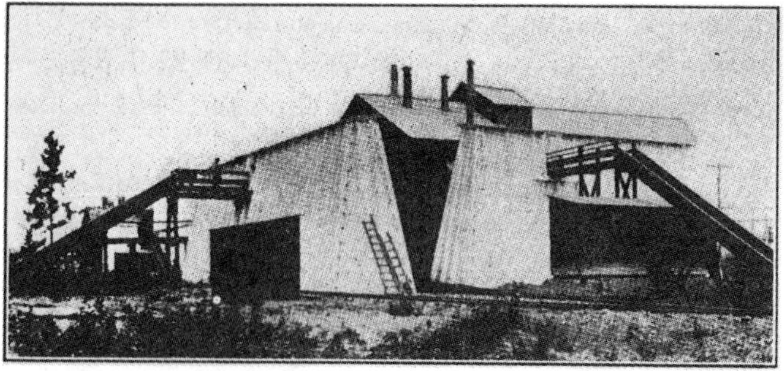

FIGURE 46. TNT Manufacturing Building, Showing Barricades and Safety Chutes. (Courtesy E. I. du Pont de Nemours and Company, Inc.)

for use again or going to the acid-recovery treatment. The principal products of the first stage are *o*- (b.p. 222.3°) and *p*-nitrotoluene (m.p. 51.9°) in relative amounts which vary somewhat according to the temperature at which the nitration is carried out. During the dinitration, the *para* compound yields only 2,4-dinitrotoluene (m.p. 70°), while the *ortho* yields the 2,4- and the 2,6- (m.p. 60.5°). Both these in the trinitration yield 2,4,6-trinitrotoluene or α-TNT. 2,4-Dinitrotoluene predominates in the product of the dinitration, and crude TNT generally contains a

143

small amount, perhaps 2 per cent, of this material which has escaped further nitration. The substance is stable and less reactive even than α-TNT, and a small amount of it in the purified TNT, if insufficient to lower the melting point materially, is not regarded as an especially undesirable impurity. The principal impurities arise from the *m*-nitrotoluene (b.p. 230-231°) which is formed to the extent of about 4 per cent in the product of the mononitration. We omit discussion of other impurities, such as the nitrated xylenes which might be present in consequence of impurities in the toluene which was used, except to point out that the same considerations apply to trinitro-*m*-xylene (TNX) as apply to 2,4-dinitrotoluene—a little does no real harm—while the nitro derivatives of *o*- and *p*-xylene are likely to form oils and are extremely undesirable. In *m*-nitrotoluene, the nitro group inhibits further substitution, the methyl group promotes it, the two groups disagree in respect to the positions which they activate, but substitution takes place under the orienting influence of the methyl group.

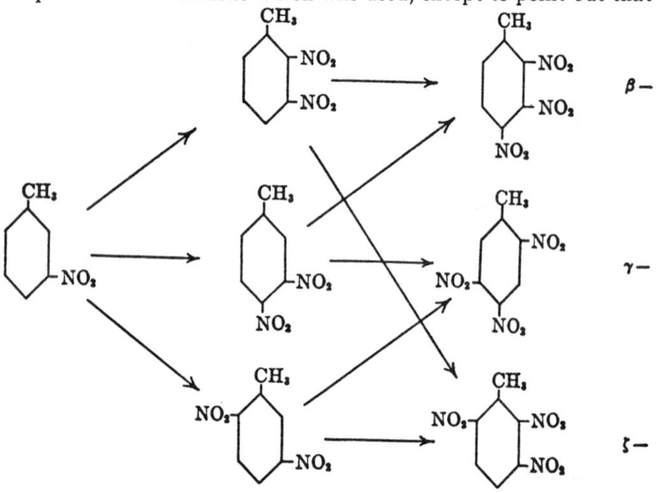

β-TNT or 2,3,4-trinitrotoluene (m.p. 112°) is the principal product of the nitration of *m*-nitrotoluene; γ-TNT or 2,4,5-trinitrotoluene (m.p. 104°) is present in smaller amount; and of ζ-TNT or 2,3,6-trinitrotoluene (m.p. 79.5°), the formation of

144

which is theoretically possible and is indicated above for that reason, there is not more than a trace.[23] During the trinitration a small amount of the α-TNT is oxidized to trinitrobenzoic acid, finally appearing in the finished product in the form of TNB, which, however, does no harm if it is present in small amount. At the same time some of the material is destructively oxidized and nitrated by the strong mixed acid to form tetranitromethane, which is driven off with the steam during the subsequent boiling and causes annoyance by its lachrymatory properties and unpleasant taste. The product of the trinitration is separated from the spent acid while still molten, washed with boiling water until free from acid, and grained—or, after less washing with hot water, subjected to purification by means of sodium sulfite.

[23] 3,5-Dinitrotoluene, in which both nitro groups are *meta* to the methyl, is probably not formed during the dinitration, and δ- and ε-TNT, namely 3,4,5- and 2,3,5-trinitrotoluene, are not found among the final products of the nitration of toluene.

In this country the crude TNT, separated from the wash water, is generally grained by running the liquid slowly onto the refrigerated surface of an iron vessel which surface is continually scraped by mechanical means. In France the material is allowed to cool slowly under water in broad and shallow wooden tubs, while it is stirred slowly with mechanically actuated wooden paddles. The cooling is slow, for the only loss of heat is by radiation. The French process yields larger and flatter crystals, flaky, often several millimeters in length. The crystallized crude TNT is of about the color of brown sugar and feels greasy to the touch. It consists of crystals of practically pure α-TNT coated with an oily (low-melting) mixture of β- and γ-TNT, 2,4-dinitrotoluene, and possibly TNB and TNX. It is suitable for many uses as an explosive, but not for high-explosive shells. The oily mixture of impurities segregates in the shell, and sooner or later exudes through the thread by which the fuze is attached. The exudate is disagreeable but not particularly dangerous. The difficulty is that exudation leaves cavities within the mass of the charge, perhaps a central cavity under the booster which may cause the shell to fail to explode. There is also the possibility that the shock of setback across a cavity in the rear of the charge may cause the shell to explode prematurely while it is still within the barrel of the gun.

The impurities may be largely removed from the crude TNT,

145

with a corresponding improvement in the melting point and appearance of the material, by washing the crystals with a solvent. On a plant scale, alcohol, benzene, solvent naphtha (mixed xylenes), carbon tetrachloride, and concentrated sulfuric acid have all been used. Among these, sulfuric acid removes dinitrotoluene most readily, and organic solvents the β- and γ-TNT, but all of them dissolve away a portion of the α-TNT with resulting loss. The material dissolved by the sulfuric acid is recovered by diluting with water. The organic solvents are recovered by distillation, and the residues, dark brown liquids known as "TNT oil," are used in the manufacture of non-freezing dynamite. The best process of purification is that in which the crude TNT is agitated with a warm solution of sodium sulfite. A 5 per cent solution is used, as much by weight of the solution as there is of the crude TNT. The sulfite leaves the α-TNT (and any TNB, TNX, and 2,4-dinitrotoluene) unaffected, but reacts rapidly and completely with the β- and γ-TNT to form red-colored materials

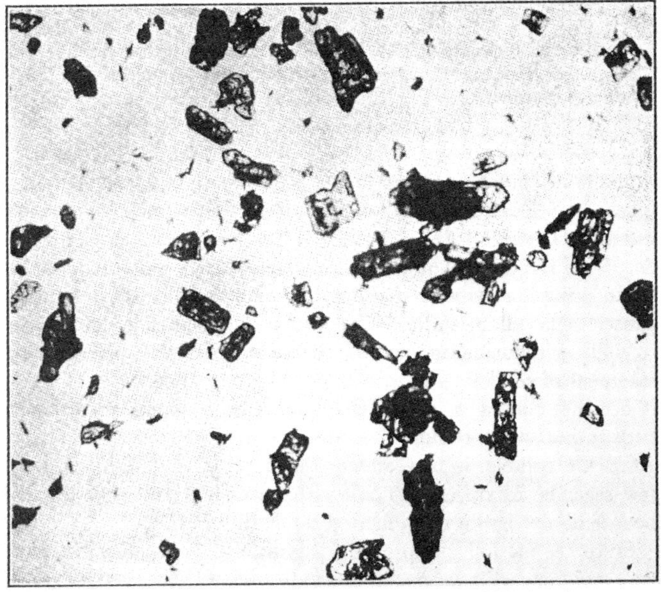

FIGURE 47. Commercial Sample of Purified TNT (25×).

[146] which are readily soluble in water. After the reaction, the purified material is washed with water until the washings are colorless.

Muraour believes the sulfite process for the purification of TNT to be an American invention. At any rate, the story of its discovery presents an interesting example of the consequences of working rightly with a wrong hypothesis. The nitro group in the *m*-position in β- and γ-TNT is *ortho*, or *ortho* and *para*, to two other nitro groups, and accordingly is active chemically. It is replaced by an amino group by the action of alcoholic ammonia both in the hot and in the cold, and undergoes similar reactions with hydrazine and with phenylhydrazine. It was hoped that it would be reduced more readily than the unactivated nitro groups of α- or symmetrical TNT, and that the reduction products could be washed away with warm water. Sodium polysulfide was tried and did indeed raise the melting point, but the treated material contained finely divided sulfur from which it could not easily be freed, and the polysulfide was judged to be unsuitable.

CH_3, $-NO_2$, $-NO_2$, NO_2 $\xrightarrow{+Na_2SO_3}$ CH_3, $-NO_2$, $-SO_2$—ONa, NO_2 + $NaNO_2$

and

CH_3, NO_2-, $-NO_2$, NO_2 ⟶ CH_3, NO_2-, $-SO_2$—ONa, NO_2

In seeking for another reducing agent, the chemist bethought himself of sodium sulfite, which, however, does not act in this case as a reducing agent, and succeeded perfectly in removing the β- and γ-TNT.

The reaction consists in the replacement of the nitro by a sodium sulfonate group: [147]

The soluble sulfonates in the deep red solution, if they are thrown into the sewer, represent a loss of about 4 per cent of all the toluene—a serious loss in time of war—as well as a loss of many pounds of nitro group nitrogen. The sulfonic acid group in these substances, like the nitro group which it replaced, is *ortho*, or *ortho* and *para*, to two nitro groups, and is active and still capable of undergoing the same reactions as the original nitro group. They may be converted into a useful explosive by reaction with methylamine and the subsequent nitration of the resulting dinitrotolylmethylamines, both of which yield 2,4,6-trinitrotolyl-3-methylnitramine or *m*-methyltetryl.

CH_3, $-NO_2$, $-SO_2$-ONa, NO_2 ⟶ CH_3, $-NO_2$, $-N(CH_3)(H)$, NO_2 ⟶ CH_3, NO_2-, $-NO_2$, $-N(CH_3)(NO_2)$, NO_2

CH_3, NO_2-, $-SO_2$-ONa, NO_2 ⟶ CH_3, NO_2-, $-N(CH_3)(H)$, NO_2 ⟶

m-Methyltetryl, pale yellow, almost white, crystals from alcohol, m.p. 102°, was prepared in 1884 by van Romburgh by the nitration of dimethyl-*m*-toluidine, and its structure was demonstrated fully in 1902 by Blanksma, who prepared it by the synthesis indicated on the next page.

β- and γ-TNT lose their active nitro group by the action of aqueous alkali and yield salts of dinitro-*m*-cresol. The mixed dinitro-*m*-cresols which result may be nitrated to trinitro-*m*-cresol, a valuable explosive. Their salts, like the picrates, are primary explosives and sources of danger. β- and γ-TNT react with lead oxide in alcohol to form lead dinitrocresolates, while α-TNT under the same conditions remains unaffected.

In plant-scale manufacture, TNT is generally prepared by a [148]

CH_3, $-OH$ ⟶ CH_3, $-OCH_3$ ⟶ CH_3, NO_2-, $-NO_2$, $-OCH_3$, NO_2 ⟶

CH_3, NO_2-, $-NO_2$, $-N(CH_3)(H)$, NO_2 ⟶ CH_3, NO_2-, $-NO_2$, $-N(CH_3)(NO_2)$, NO_2

three-stage process, but processes involving one and two nitrations have also been used.

Preparation of Trinitrotoluene (Three Stages). A mixture of 294 grams of concentrated sulfuric acid (*d.* 1.84) and 147 grams of nitric acid (*d.* 1.42) is added slowly from a dropping funnel to 100 grams of toluene in a tall 600-cc. beaker, while the liquid is stirred vigorously with an electric stirrer and its temperature is maintained at 30° to 40° by running cold water in the vessel in which the beaker is standing. The addition of acid will require from an hour to an hour and a half. The stirring is then continued for half an hour longer without cooling; the mixture is allowed to stand over night in a separatory funnel; the lower layer of spent acid is drawn off; and the crude mononitrotoluene is weighed. One-half of it, corresponding to 50 grams of toluene, is taken for the dinitration.

The mononitrotoluene (MNT) is dissolved in 109 grams of concentrated sulfuric acid (*d.* 1.84) while the mixture is cooled in running water. The solution in a tall beaker is warmed to 50°, and a mixed acid, composed of 54.5 grams each of nitric acid (*d.* 1.50) and sulfuric acid (*d.* 1.84), is added slowly drop by drop from a dropping funnel while the mixture is stirred mechanically. The heat generated by the reaction raises the temperature, and the rate of addition of the acid is regulated so that the temperature of the mixture lies always between 90° and 100°. The addition of the acid will require about 1 hour. After the acid has been added, the mixture is stirred for 2 hours longer at 90-100° to complete the nitration. Two layers separate on standing. The upper layer consists largely of dinitrotoluene (DNT), but probably contains a certain amount of TNT. The trinitration in the laboratory is conveniently carried out without separating the DNT from the spent acid.

While the dinitration mixture is stirred actively at a temperature of about 90°, 145 grams of fuming sulfuric acid (*oleum* containing 15 per [149] cent free SO_3) is added slowly by pouring from a beaker. A mixed acid, composed of 72.5 grams each of nitric acid (*d.* 1.50) and 15 per cent oleum, is now added drop by drop with good agitation while the heat of the reaction maintains the temperature at 100-115°. After about three-quarters of the acid has been added, it will be found necessary to apply external heat to maintain the temperature. After all the acid has been added (during 1½ to 2 hours), the heating and stirring are continued for 2 hours longer at 100-115°. After the material has stood over night, the upper TNT layer will be found to have solidified to a hard cake, and the lower layer of spent acid to be filled with crystals. The acid is filtered through a Büchner funnel (without filter paper), and the cake is broken up and washed with water on the same filter to remove excess of acid. The spent acid contains considerable TNT in solution; this is precipitated by pouring the acid into a large volume of water, filtered off, rinsed with water, and added to the main batch. All the product is washed three or four times by agitating it vigorously with hot water under which it is melted. After the last washing, the TNT is granulated by allowing it to cool slowly under hot water while the stirring is continued. The product, filtered off and dried at ordinary temperature, is equal to a good commercial sample of crude TNT. It may be purified by dissolving in warm alcohol at 60° and allowing to cool slowly, or it may be purified by digesting with 5 times its weight of 5 per cent sodium hydrogen sulfite solution at 90° for half an hour with vigorous stirring, washing with hot water until the washings are colorless, and finally granulating as before. The product of this last treatment is equal to a good commercial sample of purified TNT. Pure α-TNT, m.p. 80.8°, may be procured by recrystallizing this material once from nitric acid (*d.* 1.42) and once from alcohol.

Several of the molecular compounds of TNT with organic bases are listed below. TNT and diphenylamine give an orange-brown color when warmed together or when moistened with alcohol, and the formation of a labile molecular compound of the two substances has been demonstrated.

The compound of TNT with potassium methylate is a dark red powder which inflames or explodes when heated to 130-150°, and has been reported to explode spontaneously on standing at ordinary temperature. An aqueous solution of this compound, on the addition of copper tetrammine nitrate, gives a brick-red precipitate which, when dry, detonates violently at 120°. Pure TNT [150]

Molecular Proportions TNT:	Substance	M.P.	Description
1 : 1	Aniline	83–84°	Long brilliant red needles.
1 : 1	Dimethylaniline	...	Violet needles.
1 : 1	*o*-Toluidine	53–55°	Light red needles.
1 : 1	*m*-Toluidine	62–63°	Light red needles.
1 : 1	α-Naphthylamine	141.5°	Dark red needles.
1 : 1	β-Naphthylamine	113.5°	Bright red prismatic needles.
1 : 1	β-Acetnaphthalide	106°	Yellow needles.
1 : 1	Benzyl-β-naphthylamine	106.5°	Brilliant crimson needles.
1 : 1	Dibenzyl-β-naphthylamine	108°	Deep brick-red needles.
2 : 1	Benzaldehydephenylhydrazone	84°	Dark red needles.
1 : 1	2-Methylindole	110°	Yellow needles.
3 : 2	Carbazole	160°	Yellow needles.
1 : 1	Carbazole	140–200°	Dark yellow needles.

explodes or inflames when heated to about 230°, but Dupré found that the addition of solid caustic potash to TNT at 160° caused immediate inflammation or explosion. A mixture of powdered solid caustic potash and powdered TNT inflames when heated, either slowly or rapidly, to 80°. A similar mixture with caustic soda inflames at 80° if heated rapidly, but may be heated to 200° without taking fire if the heating is slow. If a small fragment of solid caustic potash is added to melted TNT at 100°, it becomes coated with a layer of reaction product and nothing further happens. If a drop of alcohol, in which both TNT and KOH are soluble, is now added, the material inflames within a few seconds. Mixtures of TNT with potassium and sodium carbonate do not ignite when heated suddenly to 100°.

Since the methyl group of TNT is attached to a picryl group, we should expect it in some respects to resemble the methyl group of a ketone. Although acetone and other methyl ketones brominate with great ease, TNT does not brominate and may even be recrystallized from bromine. The methyl group of TNT, however, behaves like the methyl group of acetone in certain condensation reactions. In the presence of sodium carbonate TNT condenses with *p*-nitrosodimethylaniline to form the dimethylaminoanilide of trinitrobenzaldehyde, from which trinitrobenzaldehyde and N,N-dimethyl-*p*-diaminobenzene are produced readily by acid hydrolysis. [151]

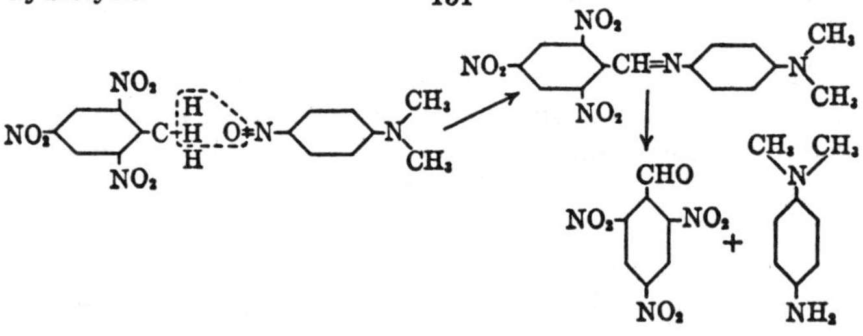

If a drop of piperidine is added to a pasty mixture of TNT and benzaldehyde, the heat of the reaction is sufficient to cause the material to take fire. The same substances in alcohol or benzene solution condense smoothly in the presence of piperidine to form trinitrostilbene.

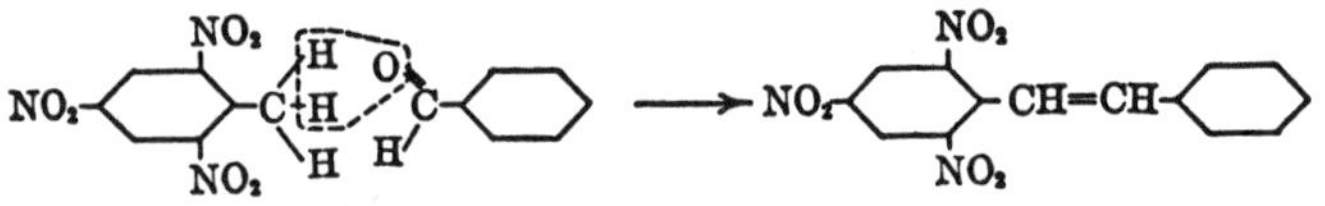

Preparation of Trinitrostilbene. To 10 grams of TNT dissolved in 25 cc. of benzene in a 100-cc. round-bottom flask equipped with a reflux condenser, 6 cc. of benzaldehyde and 0.5 cc. of piperidine are added, and the mixture is refluxed on the water bath for half an hour. The material, while still hot, is poured into a beaker and allowed to cool and crystallize. The crystals, collected on a filter, are rinsed twice with alcohol and recrystallized from a mixture of 2 volumes of alcohol and 1 of benzene. Brilliant yellow glistening needles, m.p. 158°.

Trinitrotoluene, in addition to the usual reactions of a nitrated hydrocarbon with alkali to form dangerous explosive materials, has the property that its methyl group in the presence of alkali condenses with aldehydic substances in reactions which produce heat and which may cause fire. Aldehydic substances from the action of nitrating acid on wood are always present where TNT is being manufactured, and alkali of all kinds ought to be excluded rigorously from the premises.

Giua reports that TNT may be distilled in vacuum without the slightest trace of decomposition. It boils at 210-212° at 10-20 mm. When heated for some time at 180-200°, or when exposed to sunlight[152] in open tubes, it undergoes a slow decomposition with a consequent lowering of the melting point. Exposure to sunlight in a vacuum in a sealed tube has much less effect. Verola has found that TNT shows no perceptible decomposition at 150°, but that it evolves gas slowly and regularly at 180°. At ordinary temperatures, and even at the temperatures of the tropics, it is stable in light-proof and air-tight containers—as are in general all the aromatic nitro explosives—and it does not require the same surveillance in storage that nitrocellulose and smokeless powder do.

The solubility of trinitrotoluene in various solvents is tabulated below.

Solubility of Trinitrotoluene

(Grams per 100 grams of solvent)

Temp.	Water	CCl_4	Benzene	Toluene	Acetone	95% Alcohol	$CHCl_3$	Ether
0°	0.0100	0.20	13	28	57	0.65	6	1.73
5°	0.0105	0.25	24	32	66	0.75	8.5	2.08
10°	0.0110	0.40	36	38	78	0.85	11	2.45
15°	0.0120	0.50	50	45	92	1.07	15	2.85
20°	0.0130	0.65	67	55	109	1.23	19	3.29
25°	0.0150	0.82	88	67	132	1.48	25	3.80
30°	0.0175	1.01	113	84	156	1.80	32.5	4.56
35°	0.0225	1.32	144	104	187	2.27	45	...
40°	0.0285	1.75	180	130	228	2.92	66	...
45°	0.0360	2.37	225	163	279	3.70	101	...
50°	0.0475	3.23	284	208	346	4.61	150	...
55°	0.0570	4.55	361	272	449	6.08	218	...
60°	0.0675	6.90	478	367	600	8.30	302	...
65°	0.0775	11.40	665	525	843	11.40	442	...
70°	0.0875	17.35	1024	826	1350	15.15	...	...
75°	0.0975	24.35	2028	1685	2678	19.50	...	...
80°	0.1075	...	...	...	...	...	...	...
85°	0.1175	...	...	...	...	...	...	...
90°	0.1275	...	...	...	...	...	...	...
95°	0.1375	...	...	...	...	...	...	...
100°	0.1475	...	...	...	...	...	...	...

Dautriche[153] found the density of powdered and compressed TNT to be as follows:

Pressure: Kilos per Square Centimeter	Density
275	1.320
685	1.456
1375	1.558
2060	1.584
2750	1.599
3435	1.602
4125	1.610

Trinitrotoluene was prepared by Wilbrand in 1863 by the nitration of toluene with mixed acid, and in 1870 by Beilstein and Kuhlberg by the nitration of *o*- and *p*-nitrotoluene, and by Tiemann by the nitration of 2,4-dinitrotoluene. In 1891 Haussermann with the Griesheim Chem. Fabrik undertook its manufacture on an industrial scale. After 1901 its use as a military explosive soon became general among the great nations. In the first World War all of them were using it.

Trinitroxylene (TNX)

In *m*-xylene the two methyl groups agree in activating the same positions, and this is the only one of the three isomeric xylenes which can be nitrated satisfactorily to yield a trinitro derivative. Since the three isomers occur in the same fraction of coal tar and cannot readily be separated by distillation, it is necessary to separate them by chemical means. When the mixed xylenes are treated with about their own weight of 93 per cent sulfuric acid for 5 hours at 50°, the *o*-xylene (b.p. 144°) and the *m*-xylene (b.p. 138.8°) are converted into water-soluble sulfonic acids, while the *p*-xylene (b.p. 138.5°) is unaffected. The aqueous phase is removed, diluted with water to about 52 per cent acidity calculated as sulfuric acid, and then heated in an autoclave at 130° for 4 hours. The *m*-xylene sulfonic acid is converted to *m*-xylene, which is removed. The *o*-xylene sulfonic acid, which remains in solution, may be converted into *o*-xylene by autoclaving at a higher temperature. The nitration of *m*-xylene is conveniently carried out in three steps.[154] The effect of the two methyl groups is so considerable that the introduction of the third nitro group may be accomplished without the use of fuming sulfuric acid. Pure TNX, large almost colorless needles from benzene, melts at 182.3°.

Trinitroxylene is not powerful enough for use alone as a high explosive, and it does not always communicate an initial detonation throughout its mass. It is used in commercial dynamites, for which purpose it does not require to be purified and may contain an oily mixture of isomers and other nitrated xylenes. Its large excess of carbon suggests that it may be used advantageously in conjunction with an oxidizing agent. A mixture of 23 parts of TNX and 77 parts of ammonium nitrate, ground intimately together in a black powder mill, has been used in high-explosive shells. It was loaded by compression. Mixtures, about half and half, of TNX with TNT and with picric acid are semi-solid when warm and can be loaded by pouring. The eutectic of TNX and TNT contains between 6 and 7 per cent of TNX and freezes at 73.5°. It is substantially as good an explosive as TNT. A mixture of 10 parts TNX, 40 parts TNT, and 50 parts picric acid can be melted readily under water. In explosives such as these the TNX helps by lowering the melting point, but it also attenuates the power of the more powerful high explosives with which it is mixed. On the other hand, these mixtures take advantage of the explosive power of TNX, such as that power is, and are themselves sufficiently powerful and satisfactory for many purposes—while making use of a raw material, namely *m*-xylene, which is not otherwise applicable for use in the manufacture of military explosives.

Nitro Derivatives of Naphthalene

Naphthalene nitrates more readily than benzene, the first nitro group taking the α-position which is *ortho* on one nucleus to the side chain which the other nucleus constitutes. The second nitro group takes one or another of the expected positions, either the position *meta* to the nitro group already present or one of the α-positions of the unsubstituted nucleus. The dinitration of naphthalene in actual practice thus produces a mixture which consists almost entirely of three isomers. Ten different isomeric dinitronaphthalenes are possible, seven of which are derived from α-nitronaphthalene, seven from β-nitronaphthalene, and four from both the α- and the β-compounds.[155] After two nitro groups have been introduced, conflicts of orienting tendencies arise and polynitro compounds are formed, among others, in which nitro groups occur *ortho* and *para* to one another. Only four nitro groups can be introduced into naphthalene by direct nitration.

The mononitration of naphthalene takes place easily with a mixed acid which contains only a slight excess of one equivalent of HNO_3.

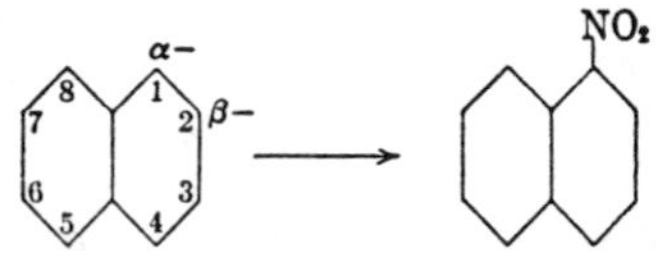

For the di-, tri-, and tetranitrations increasingly stronger acids and higher temperatures are necessary. In the tetranitration oleum is commonly used and the reaction is carried out at 130°.

The nitration of α-nitronaphthalene (m.p. 59-60°) yields a mixture of α- or 1,5-dinitronaphthalene (silky needles, m.p. 216°), β- or 1,8-dinitronaphthalene (rhombic leaflets, m.p. 170-172°), and γ- or 1,3-dinitronaphthalene (m.p. 144-145°).

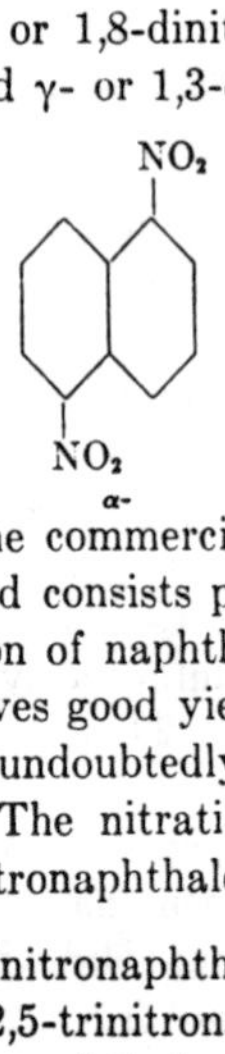

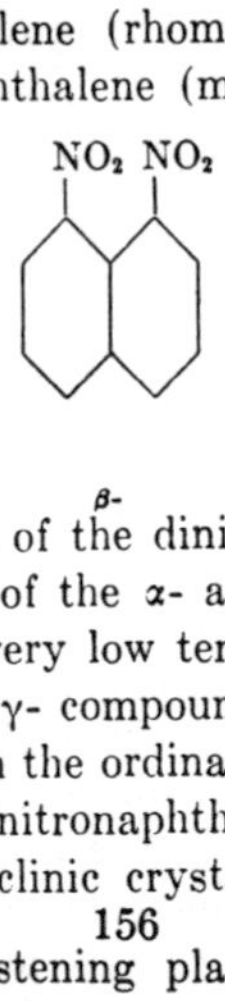

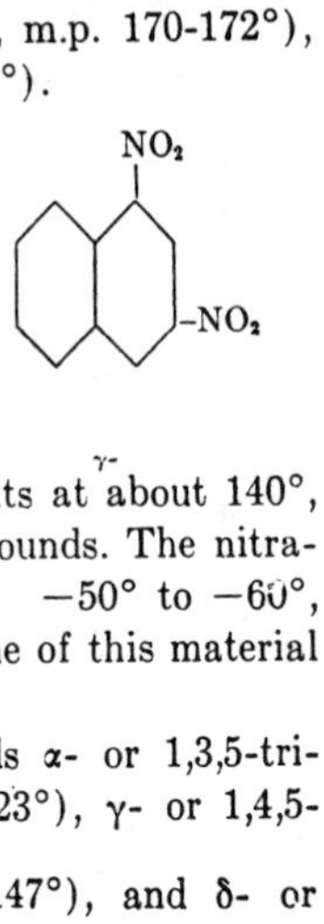

The commercial product of the dinitration melts at about 140°, and consists principally of the α- and β-compounds. The nitration of naphthalene at very low temperatures, −50° to −60°, gives good yields of the γ- compound, and some of this material is undoubtedly present in the ordinary product.

The nitration of α-dinitronaphthalene yields α- or 1,3,5-trinitronaphthalene (monoclinic crystals, m.p. 123°), γ- or 1,4,5-trinitronaphthalene (glistening plates, m.p. 147°),[156] and δ- or 1,2,5-trinitronaphthalene (m.p. 112-113°). The nitration of β-dinitronaphthalene yields β- or 1,3,8-trinitronaphthalene (monoclinic crystals, m.p. 218°), and the same substance, along with some α-trinitronaphthalene, is formed by the nitration of γ-dinitronaphthalene.

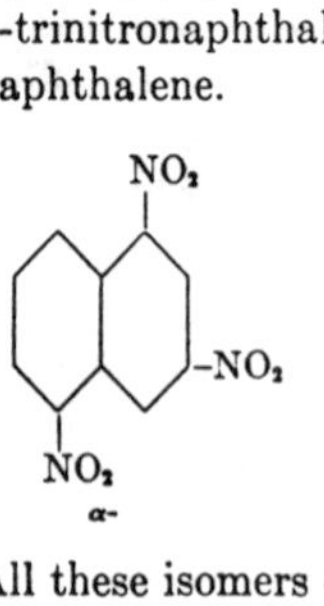

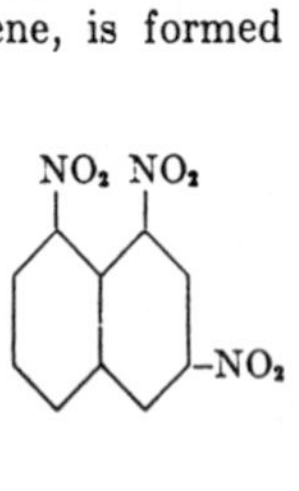

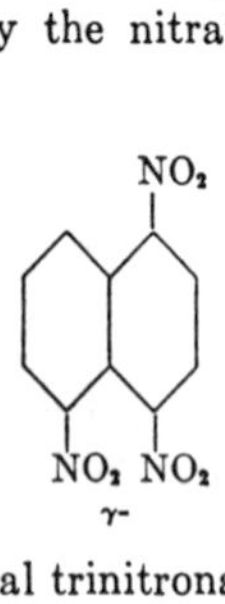

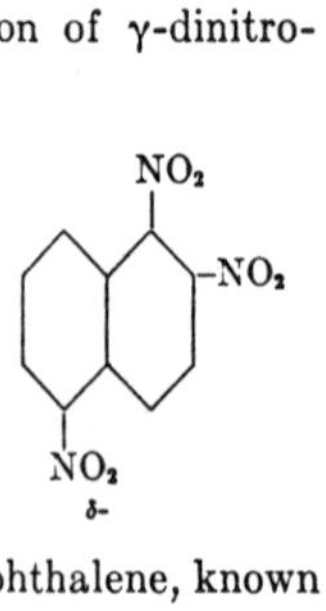

All these isomers occur in commercial trinitronaphthalene, known as *naphtite*, which melts at about 110°.

The nitration of α-, β-, and γ-trinitronaphthalene yields γ- or 1,3,5,8-tetranitronaphthalene (glistening tetrahedrons, m.p. 194-195°). The nitration of the β-compound also yields β- or 1,3,6,8-tetranitronaphthalene (m.p. 203°), and that of the δ-trinitro compound yields δ- or 1,2,5,8-tetranitronaphthalene (glistening prisms which decompose at 270° without melting), a substance which may be formed also by the introduction of a fourth nitro group into γ-trinitronaphthalene. The nitration of 1,5-dinitronaphthalene yields α-tetranitronaphthalene (rhombic crystals, m.p. 259°) (perhaps 1,3,5,7-tetranitronaphthalene), and this substance is also present in the crude product of the tetranitration, which, however, consists largely of the β-, γ-, and δ-isomers.

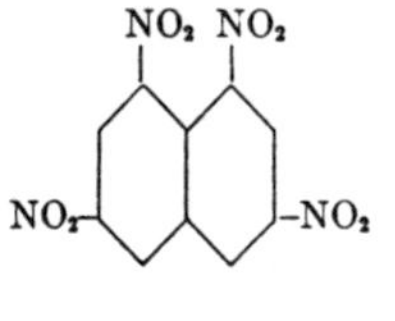

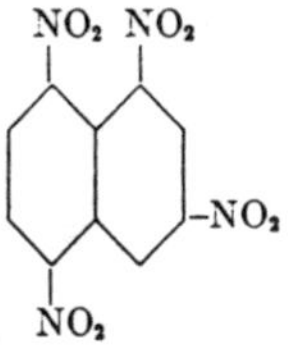

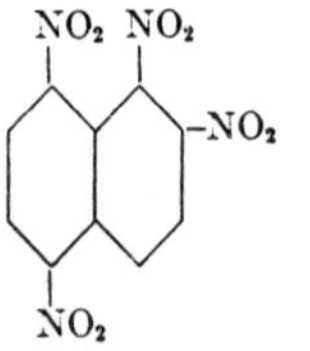

The crude product is impure and irregular in its appearance; it is commonly purified by recrystallization from glacial acetic acid[157] The purified material consists of fine needle crystals which melt at about 220° and have the clean appearance of a pure substance but actually consist of a mixture of isomers.

None of the nitrated naphthalenes is very sensitive to shock. α-Nitronaphthalene is not an explosive at all and cannot be detonated. Dinitronaphthalene begins to show a feeble capacity for explosion, and trinitronaphthalene stands between dinitrobenzene and dinitrotoluene in its explosive power. Tetranitronaphthalene is about as powerful as TNT, and distinctly less sensitive to impact than that explosive. Vennin and Chesneau report that the nitrated naphthalenes, charged in a manometric bomb at a density of loading of 0.3, gave on firing the pressures indicated below.

	KILOS PER SQUARE CENTIMETER
Mononitronaphthalene	1208
Dinitronaphthalene	2355
Trinitronaphthalene	3275
Tetranitronaphthalene	3745

The nitrated naphthalenes are used in dynamites and safety explosives, in the Favier powders, *grisounites*, and *naphtalites* of France, in the *cheddites* which contain chlorate, and for military purposes to some extent in mixtures with ammonium nitrate or with other aromatic nitro compounds. Street, who proposed their use in cheddites, also suggested a fused mixture of mononitronaphthalene and picric acid for use as a high explosive. *Schneiderite*, used by France and by Italy and Russia in shells during the first World War, consisted of 1 part dinitronaphthalene and 7 parts ammonium nitrate, intimately incorporated together by grinding in a black powder mill, and loaded by compression. A mixture (MMN) of 3 parts mononitronaphthalene and 7 parts picric acid, fused together under water, was used in drop bombs and was insensitive to the impact of a rifle bullet. A mixture (MDN) of 1 part dinitronaphthalene and 4 parts picric acid melts at about 105-110°; it is more powerful than the preceding and is also less sensitive to shock than picric acid alone.[158] The Germans used a mine explosive consisting of 56 per cent potassium perchlorate, 32 per cent dinitrobenzene, and 12 per cent dinitronaphthalene. Their *Tri-Trinal* for small-caliber shells was a compressed mixture of 2 parts of TNT (*Tri*) with 1 of trinitronaphthalene (*Trinal*), and was used with a booster of compressed picric acid.

Trinitronaphthalene appears to be a genuine stabilizer for nitrocellulose, a true inhibitor of its spontaneous decomposition. Marqueyrol found that a nitrocellulose powder containing 10 per cent of trinitronaphthalene is as stable as one which contains 2 per cent of diphenylamine. The trinitronaphthalene has the further effect of reducing both the hygroscopicity and the temperature of combustion of the powder.

Hexanitrobiphenyl

2,2′,4,4′,6,6′-Hexanitrobiphenyl was first prepared by Ullmann and Bielecki by boiling picryl chloride in nitrobenzene solution with copper powder for a short time. The solvent is necessary in order to moderate the reaction, for picryl chloride and copper powder explode when heated alone to about 127°. Ullmann and Bielecki also secured good yields of hexanitrobiphenyl by working in toluene solution, but found that a small quantity of trinitrobenzene was formed (evidently in consequence of the presence of moisture). Hexanitrobiphenyl crystallizes from toluene in light-yellow thick crystals which contain ½ molecule of toluene of crystallization. It is insoluble in water, and slightly soluble in alcohol, acetone, benzene, and toluene, m.p. 263°. It gives a yellow color with concentrated sulfuric acid, and a red with alcohol to which a drop of ammonia water or aqueous caustic soda has been added. It is neutral, of course, and chemically unreactive toward metals, and is reported to be non-poisonous.

Hexanitrobiphenyl cannot[50] be prepared by the direct nitration

[50] The effect may be steric, although there is evidence that the dinitrophenyl group has peculiar orienting and resonance effects. Rinkenbach and Aaronson, *J. Am. Chem. Soc.*, **52**, 5040 (1930), report that *sym*-diphenylethane yields only very small amounts of hexanitrodiphenylethane under the most favorable conditions of nitration.

159

of biphenyl. The most vigorous nitration of that hydrocarbon yields only 2,2′,4,4′-tetranitrobiphenyl, yellowish prisms from benzene, m.p. 163°.

Jahn in a patent granted in 1918 states that hexanitrobiphenyl is about 10 per cent superior to hexanitrodiphenylamine. Fifty grams in the lead block produced a cavity of 1810 cc., while the same weight of hexanitrodiphenylamine produced one of 1630 cc. Under a pressure of 2500 atmospheres, it compresses to a density of about 1.61.

Picric Acid (melinite, lyddite, pertite, shimose, etc.)

The *ortho-para* orienting hydroxyl group of phenol promotes nitration greatly and has the further effect that it "weakens" the ring and makes it more susceptible to oxidation. Nitric acid attacks phenol violently, oxidizing a portion of it to oxalic acid, and produces resinous by-products in addition to a certain amount of the expected nitro compounds. The carefully controlled action of mixed acid on phenol gives a mixture of *o*-nitrophenol (yellow crystals, m.p. 45°, volatile with steam) and *p*-nitrophenol (white crystals, m.p. 114°, not volatile with steam), but the yields are not very good. When these mononitrophenols are once formed, their nitro groups "activate" the same positions as the hydroxyls do, but the nitro groups also inhibit substitution, and their further nitration may now be carried out more smoothly. *p*-Nitrophenol yields 2,4-dinitrophenol (m.p. 114-115°), and later picric acid. *o*-Nitrophenol yields 2,4- and 2,6-dinitrophenol (m.p. 63-64°), both of which may be nitrated to picric acid, but the nitration of *o*-nitrophenol is invariably accompanied by losses resulting from its volatility. The straightforward nitration of phenol cannot be carried out successfully and with satisfying yields. In practice the phenol is sulfonated first, and the sulfonic acid is then nitrated. The use of sulfuric acid (for the sulfonation) in this process amounts to its use as an inhibitor or moderator of the nitration, for the *meta* orienting sulfonic acid group at first slows down the introduction of nitro groups until it is itself finally replaced by one of them.

160

OH → OH, SO_2-OH → OH, NO_2, SO_2-OH → OH, NO_2, NO_2 / OH, NO_2, NO_2, SO_2-OH → OH, NO_2, NO_2, NO_2

The sulfonation of phenol at low temperatures produces the *o*-sulfonic acid, and at high temperatures the *p*-sulfonic acid along with more or less of the di- and even of the trisulfonic acids according to the conditions of the reaction. All these substances yield picric acid as the final product of the nitration.

Unless carefully regulated the production of picric acid from phenol is accompanied by losses, either from oxidation of the material with the production of red fumes which represent a loss of fixed nitrogen or from over sulfonation and the loss of unconverted water-soluble nitrated sulfonic acids in the mother liquors. Olsen and Goldstein have described a process which yields 220 parts of picric acid from 100 parts of phenol. In France, where dinitrophenol was used during the first World War in mixtures with picric acid which were loaded by pouring, Marqueyrol and his associates have worked out the details of a four-stage process from the third stage of which dinitrophenol may be removed if it is desired. The steps are: (1) sulfonation; (2) nitration to the water-soluble mononitrosulfonic acid; (3) nitration to dinitrophenol, which is insoluble in the mixture and separates out, and to the dinitrosulfonic acid which remains in solution; and (4) further nitration to convert either the soluble material or both of the substances to picric acid. The process is economical of acid and gives practically no red fumes, but the reported yields are inferior to those reported by Olsen and Goldstein. The

161

dinitrophenol as removed contains some picric acid, but this is of no disadvantage because the material is to be mixed with picric acid anyway for use as an explosive.

Preparation of Picric Acid (Standard Method). Twenty-five grams of phenol and 25 grams of concentrated sulfuric acid (*d.* 1.84) in a round-bottom flask equipped with an air condenser are heated together for 6 hours in an oil bath at 120°. After the material has cooled, it is diluted with 75 grams of 72 per cent sulfuric acid (*d.* 1.64). To the resulting solution, in an Erlenmeyer flask in the hood, 175 cc. of 70 per cent nitric acid (*d.* 1.42) is added slowly, a drop at a time, from a dropping funnel. When all the nitric acid has been added and the vigorous reaction has subsided, the mixture is heated for 2 hours on the steam bath to complete the nitration. The next morning the picric acid will be found to have separated in crystals. These are transferred to a

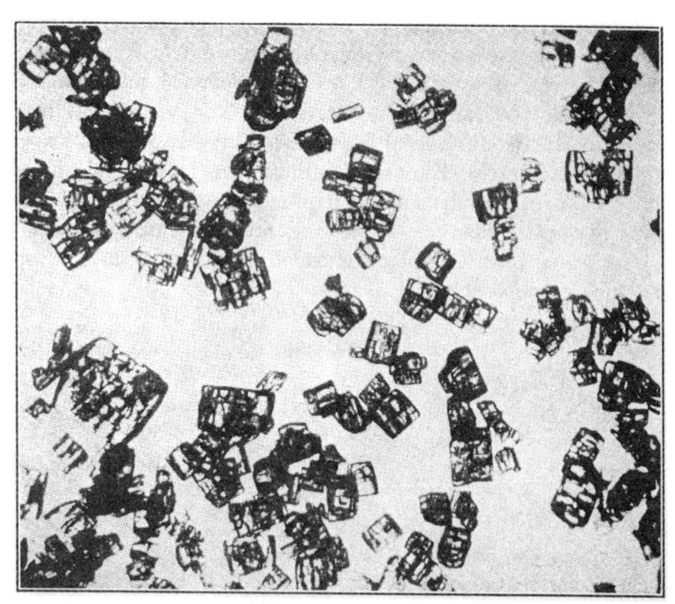

FIGURE 48. Commercial Sample of Picric Acid (25×).

porcelain filter, washed with small portions of water until the washings are free from sulfate, and dried in the air. The crude product, which is equal in quality to a good commercial sample, is purified by boiling it with water, in the proportion of 15 grams to the liter,[162] filtering hot, and allowing to cool slowly. The heavy droplets of brown oil which dissolve only slowly during this boiling ought to be discarded. Pure picric acid crystallizes from water in pale yellow flat needles, m.p. 122.5°. It may be obtained in crystals which are almost white by recrystallizing from aqueous hydrochloric acid.

The best process for the production of dinitrophenol is probably the autoclaving of dinitrochlorobenzene with aqueous caustic soda. The product is obtained on acidification and is used as such, or is nitrated to picric acid for the commercial production of that material by the so-called synthetic process.

The "catalytic process" for the production of picric acid directly from benzene in one step by the action of nitric acid in the presence of mercuric nitrate has much theoretical interest and has been applied, though not extensively, in plant-scale manufacture. It yields about as much picric acid as is procurable from the same weight of benzene by the roundabout method of sulfonating the benzene, converting the benzene sulfonic acid into phenol, and nitrating the phenol to picric acid—and the benzene which is not converted to picric acid is for the most part recovered as such or as nitrobenzene. The first mention of the process appears to be in the patent of Wolffenstein and Boeters.

Preparation of Picric Acid (Catalytic Process). Two hundred grams of benzene in a 2-liter round-bottom flask equipped with a sealed-on condenser is refluxed on the sand bath for 7 hours with 600 cc. of nitric acid (*d.* 1.42) in which 10 grams of mercuric nitrate has been dissolved. The material is then transferred to another flask and distilled with steam. Benzene comes over, then nitrobenzene, then finally and slowly a mixture of dinitrobenzene and dinitrophenol. The distillation is continued until all volatile matter has been removed. The liquid in the flask is filtered hot and allowed to crystallize. If the picric acid is not sufficiently pure, it is recrystallized from hot water.

Mercuric nitrate combines with benzene to form a deep-brown or black addition compound, the probable structure of which is indicated below. This material when warmed with nitric acid is oxidized with the production of red fumes and the formation of[163] a yellow nitrophenolate of mercuric nitrate. By the continued action of the acid this is nitrated to the trinitrophenolate and decomposed with the formation of picric acid and the regeneration of mercuric nitrate.

The addition of mercuric nitrate is here written as a 1,4-addition, but 1,2-addition would give the same final product, and there is no evidence in the facts concerning benzene which enables us to choose between the alternative hypotheses. Toluene yields trinitro-*m*-cresol by a similar series of reactions, and it is clear that the nitro group in the addition product of mercuric nitrate and toluene has taken either the 2-, the 4-, or the 6-position, that is, one or the other of the positions activated by the methyl group. In the addition of mercuric nitrate to naphthalene, the nitro group correspondingly may be supposed to go to the active α-position. If the addition is 1,2-, the product on oxidation will yield a derivative of β-naphthol. If it is 1,4-, it will yield a derivative of α-naphthol. The two possibilities are indicated below.

Gentle treatment of naphthalene with nitric acid containing mercuric nitrate yields, 2,4-dinitro-α-naphthol in conformity with the belief that the first addition product is 1,4- as represented by the second of the above formulations.

Picric acid was obtained in 1771 by Woulff, who found that[164] the action of nitric acid on indigo yielded a material which dyed silk yellow. Hausmann isolated the substance in 1778, and reported further studies upon it in 1788, noting particularly its bitter taste. Welter in 1799 obtained picric acid by the action of nitric acid on silk, and the material came to be known generally as "Welter's bitter." Its preparation from indigo, aloes, resin, and other organic substances was studied by many chemists, among them Fourcroy and Vauquelin, Chevreul, Liebig, Wöhler, Robiquet, Piria, Delalande, and Stenhouse. Its preparation from oil of eucalyptus was suggested during the first World War. It was given the name of *acide picrique* by Dumas; *cf.* Greek πικρός = bitter, old English *puckery*. Its relation to phenol was demonstrated in 1841 by Laurent, who prepared it by the nitration of that substance, and its structure was proved fully by Hepp, who procured it by the oxidation of *sym*-trinitrobenzene.

Picric acid is a strong acid; it decomposes carbonates and may be titrated with bases by the use of sodium alizarine sulfonate as an indicator. It is a fast yellow dye for silk and wool. It attacks the common metals, except aluminum and tin, and produces dangerously explosive salts. *Cordeau Lheure,* which was long used extensively in France, was made by filling a tin pipe with fused picric acid and later drawing down to the desired diameter. It had the disadvantage that the metal suffered from the "tin disease," became unduly brittle, and changed to its gray allotropic modification. Picric acid and nitrophenols, when used in ammunition, are not allowed to come in contact with the metal parts. Shells which are to be loaded with these explosives are first plated on the inside with tin or painted with asphaltum varnish or Bakelite.

Dupré in 1901 reported experiments which indicated that the picrates of calcium, lead, and zinc, formed *in situ* from melted picric acid are capable of initiating the explosion of that material. Kast found that the dehydrated picrates are more sensitive than those which contain water of crystallization. The data tabulated below have been published recently by J. D. Hopper.[165] Explosion temperature was determined as the temperature necessary to cause ignition or explosion in exactly 5 seconds when a thin-walled copper shell containing a few milligrams of the explosive was dipped into a molten metal bath to a constant depth. The minimum drop test was taken as the least distance through which a 2-kilogram weight must fall, in a standard apparatus, to produce detonation or ignition in one or more instances among ten trials.

Substance	Degree of Hydration	Temperature of Drying, °C.	Minimum Drop Test 2-kilo Weight, Inches	Explosion Temperature, °C.
Mercury fulminate	Anhydrous	...	2	210
Tetryl	Anhydrous	...	8	260
TNT	Anhydrous	...	14	470
Picric acid	Anhydrous	...	14	320
Ammonium picrate	Anhydrous	...	17	320
Sodium picrate	1 H_2O	50	17	360
Sodium picrate	Anhydrous	150	15	...
Sodium dinitrophenolate	1 H_2O	100	16	370
Sodium dinitrophenolate	Anhydrous	150	15	...
Copper picrate	3 H_2O	25	19	300
Copper picrate	Anhydrous	150	12	...
Zinc picrate	6 H_2O	25	34	310
Zinc picrate	Anhydrous	150	12	...
Cadmium picrate	8 H_2O	25	35	340
Cadmium picrate	Anhydrous	150	12	...
Nickel picrate	6 H_2O	25	26	390
Nickel picrate	....	100	9	...
Nickel picrate	Anhydrous	150	4	...
Aluminum picrate	10 H_2O	25	36	360
Aluminum picrate	2 H_2O	80	16	...
Aluminum picrate	....	100	16	...
Chromium picrate	13 H_2O	25	36	330
Chromium picrate	....	80	10	...
Chromium picrate	1 H_2O	100	8	...
Ferrous picrate	8 H_2O	25	36	310
Ferrous picrate	....	100	14	...
Ferric picrate	x H_2O	25	36	295
Ferric picrate	....	80	8	...
Ferric picrate	....	100	7	...
Ferric picrate	....	150	6	...

Cast picric acid has a density of about 1.64. The density of pellets of compressed picric acid, according to Dautriche,[166] is as follows.

Pressure: Kilos per Square Centimeter	Density
275	1.315
685	1.480
1375	1.614
2060	1.672
2750	1.714
3435	1.731
4125	1.740

The use of picric acid as an explosive appears to have been suggested first in 1867 by Borlinetto, who proposed a mixture of picric acid 35 per cent, sodium nitrate 35 per cent, and potassium chromate 30 per cent for use in mining. Sprengel in 1873 reported that picric acid in conjunction with suitable oxidizing agents is a powerful explosive. In 1885 Turpin patented its use, both compressed and cast, in blasting cartridges and in shells, and shortly thereafter the French government adopted it under the name of *mélinite*. In 1888 Great Britain commenced to use it under the name of *lyddite*. Cast charges require a booster, for which purpose compressed picric acid or tetryl is generally used. The loading of picric acid into shells by pouring is open to two objections, which, however, are not insuperable, namely, the rather high temperature of the melt and the fact that large crystals are formed which may perhaps cause trouble on setback. Both difficulties are met by adding to the picric acid another explosive substance which lowers its melting point. Mixtures are preferred which melt between 70° and 100°, above 70° in order that exudation may be less likely and below 100° in order that the explosive may be melted by hot water. The mixtures are not necessarily eutectics. Two of the favorite French explosives have been DD 60/40, which consists of 60 parts picric acid and 40 parts dinitrophenol; and *crésylite* 60/40, 60 parts trinitro-*m*-cresol and 40 parts picric acid. Others are MDPC, picric acid 55 parts, dinitrophenol 35, and trinitro-*m-cresol* 10; and MTTC, which has the same composition as MDPC except that TNT is used instead of dinitrophenol. All these mixtures melt between 80° and 90° and are prepared[167] by putting the materials together under water in wooden tanks and blowing in live steam. The water is sometimes acidulated with sulfuric acid to insure the removal of all metallic picrates. An explosive made by mixing 88 parts of picric acid with 12 parts of melted paraffin or stearic acid, and then rolling and graining, gives a compact charge when loaded by compression. It is nearly as powerful and brisant

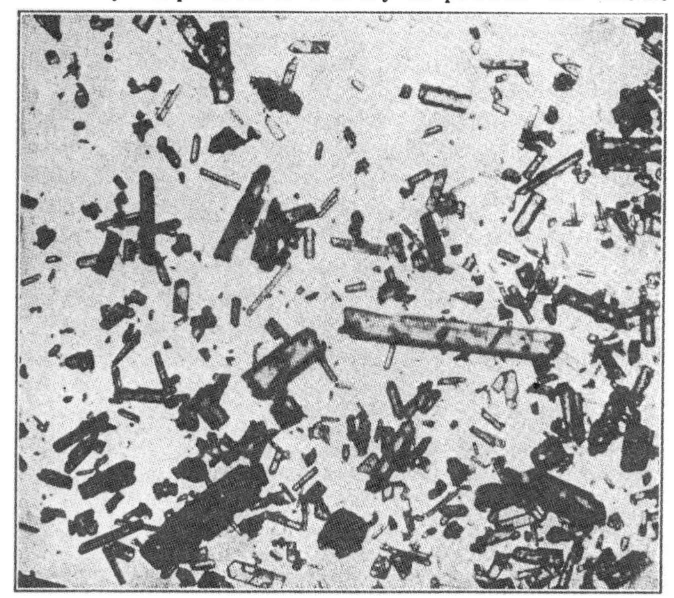

Figure 49. Commercial Sample of Ammonium Picrate (25×).

as picric acid, and responds satisfactorily to the impulse of the detonator, but is distinctly less sensitive to mechanical shock.

Ammonium Picrate

Ammonium picrate is less sensitive to shock than picric acid. It is not easily detonated by fulminate, but is commonly used with a booster of powdered and compressed picric acid or tetryl. The pure substance occurs in two forms, a stable form which is of a
168
bright lemon yellow color and a meta-stable form which is a brilliant red. These differ slightly in their crystal angles but show no detectable difference in their explosive properties. Thallium picrate similarly exists in two forms.

Ammonium picrate is prepared by suspending picric acid in a convenient quantity of hot water, adding strong ammonia water until everything goes into solution and a large excess of ammonia is present, and allowing to cool. The crystals which separate are the red form. A dry sample of this material in a stoppered bottle will remain without apparent change for many years. In contact with its saturated aqueous solution it changes to the yellow form during several months. The yellow form of ammonium picrate is best procured by recrystallizing the red form several times from water.

Pure ammonium picrate melts with decomposition at 265-271°. It is more soluble in warm alcohol than guanidine picrate is, and more soluble in acetone than in alcohol, but it goes into solution very slowly in alcohol and crystallizes out again very slowly when the liquid is allowed to stand.

SOLUBILITY OF AMMONIUM PICRATE

(Grams per 100 cc. of solution)

Temperature, °C.	Ethyl Acetate	Ethyl Alcohol
0	0.290	0.515
10	0.300	0.690
20	0.338	0.850
30	0.380	1.050
40	0.420	1.320
50	0.450	1.890
60	0.500	2.165
70	0.540	2.760
80	0.560	3.620

Guanidine Picrate

Guanidine picrate is procured as a yellow, finely crystalline precipitate by mixing warm solutions of guanidine nitrate and ammonium picrate. It is even less sensitive to blow and to shock than ammonium picrate; it is not detonated by fulminate and is used with a picric acid booster. The pure material, recrystallized from alcohol or from water, in both of which solvents it is sparingly soluble, melts with decomposition at 318.5-319.5°.
169

SOLUBILITY OF GUANIDINE PICRATE

(Grams per 100 cc. of solution)

Temperature, °C.	Water	Ethyl Alcohol	Acetone
0	0.005	0.077	0.455
10	0.038	0.093	0.525
20	0.070	0.122	0.605
30	0.100	0.153	0.695
40	0.150	0.200	0.798
50	0.230	0.255	0.920
60	0.350	0.321	1.075
70	0.480	0.413	...
80	0.700	0.548	...
90	1.010	...	...
100	1.380	...	...

Trinitrocresol (cresylite)

This explosive is prepared from *m*-cresol by a process entirely similar to that by which picric acid is prepared from phenol. The pure material is readily soluble in alcohol, ether, and acetone, soluble in 449 parts of water at 20° and in 123 parts at 100°, yellow needles from water, m.p. 107°. The ammonium salt, which is sparingly soluble in water, has been used in the composition of certain ammonium nitrate explosives, and it was adopted by the Austrian monarchy under the name of *ecrasite* as an explosive for shells of large caliber.

Trinitroresorcinol (styphnic acid)

Resorcinol nitrates readily to the trinitro compound, yellow prisms from water or alcohol, m.p. 175.5°. Styphnic acid is more expensive and less powerful than picric acid. Liouville found that styphnic acid exploded in a manometric bomb, at a density of loading of 0.2, gave a pressure of 2260 kilos per sq. cm., whereas picric acid under the same conditions gave a pressure of 2350 kilos per sq. cm. It did not agglomerate to satisfactory pellets under a pressure of 3600 kilos per sq. cm. It is a fairly strong dibasic acid, and its salts are notably more violent explosives than the picrates. Lead styphnate has been used to facilitate the ignition of lead azide in detonators.

Trinitroanisol and Trinitrophenetol

2,4,6-Trinitroanisol (2,4,6-trinitrophenyl methyl ether, methyl picrate) has explosive properties comparable with those of picric
170
acid and trinitrocresol, but it contains no hydroxyl group and does not attack metals readily with the formation of dangerously explosive salts. In actual use, however, it reacts slowly with moisture and yields some picric acid. It has been colloided with nitrocellulose in the form of a strip powder, flashless and of low hygroscopicity, but the powder in the course of time developed enough picric acid to stain the fingers and to give a yellow solution with water. Its relatively low melting point, 67-68°, gives it an advantage over picric acid for certain purposes. Methyl alcohol is needed for its synthesis, and the present availability of this substance cheaply from high-pressure synthesis further commends it. While anisol is an expensive raw material, and has the further disadvantage that its direct nitration is dangerous, trinitroanisol may be prepared, without it, economically and easily from benzene through the use of dinitrochlorobenzene.

Trinitroanisol was prepared by Cahours in 1849 by the direct nitration of anisol, and the same process has been studied more recently by Broadbent and Sparre. The strongly *ortho-para* orienting methoxy group promotes substitution greatly, the first products of the nitration are explosive, and the temperature of the reaction mixture during the first stages ought never to be allowed to rise above 0°. A small drop of anisol, or of phenetol or other aromatic-aliphatic ether, added to 10 cc. of nitric acid (*d.* 1.42) in a test tube and shaken, causes a remarkable series of color changes; the liquid turns yellow, then green, then blue, and finally reddish purple. A batch of anisol which was being nitrated at ordinary temperature in the author's laboratory detonated without warning and without provocation while showing a bluish-purple color. Small pieces of the 2-liter flask which had contained the mixture were propelled so violently that they punctured the plate-glass windows of the laboratory without, however, breaking or cracking them.

Trinitroanisol may also be prepared by the interaction of methyl iodide and silver picrate, and by the nitration of anisic acid, during which the carboxyl group is lost, but the most convenient method appears to be that of Jackson and his collaborators by which a methoxy group is substituted for chlorine in a nucleus already nitrated. A methyl alcohol solution of picryl chloride,[171] treated with an excess of sodium methylate or of strong caustic soda solution, turns dark red and deposits handsome brilliant red crystals of the empirical composition, trinitroanisol·$NaOCH_3$. The probable constitution of these crystals is indicated below. On treatment with acid the substance yields trinitroanisol.

Cl Na OCH₃ — NO_2, NO_2, NO_2 $\xrightarrow{NaOCH_3}$ CH_3O OCH_3, NO_2, NO_2, N(O)ONa $\xrightarrow{+HCl}$ OCH_3, NO_2, NO_2, NO_2 $+ NaCl + CH_3OH$

The red material is sparingly soluble in alcohol and in water, and is easily decomposed by aqueous acids. It is a primary explosive, stable to moderate heating but decomposing at 165° and exploding violently when introduced into a flame. It is not altered by dry air, but water decomposes it slowly to form first trinitroanisol and later picric acid. On boiling with ethyl alcohol, it yields the sodium ethylate addition product of trinitrophenetol—an interesting reaction analogous to the *ester interchange* in the aliphatic series.

Preparation of Trinitroanisol. Thirty-five grams of picryl chloride is dissolved in 400 cc. of methyl alcohol with warming under reflux, and the solution is allowed to cool to 30-35°. A solution of 23 grams of sodium hydroxide in 35 cc. of water is added slowly through the condenser, while the liquid is cooled, if need be, to prevent it from boiling. The mixture is allowed to stand for an hour or two. The red precipitate is filtered off, washed with alcohol, and stirred up with water while strong hydrochloric acid is added until all red color has disappeared. The slightly yellowish, almost white, precipitate, washed with water for the removal of sodium chloride, dried, and recrystallized from methyl alcohol, yields pale yellow leaflets of trinitroanisol, m.p. 67-68°. From anhydrous solvents the substance separates in crystals which are practically white.

Since the methoxy group exercises a greater effect in promoting substitution than the chlorine atom does, it is to be expected that dinitroanisol would take on a third nitro group more easily than dinitrochlorobenzene (to form picryl chloride), and with less expense for acid and for heat. The reactions indicated below are probably the best for the large-scale commercial production of trinitroanisol.[172]

Cl $\xrightarrow{\text{nitration}}$ Cl, NO_2, NO_2 $\xrightarrow[\text{then acid}]{CH_3ONa}$ OCH_3, NO_2, NO_2 $\xrightarrow{\text{nitration}}$ OCH_3, NO_2, NO_2, NO_2

During the first World War the Germans used a mixture of trinitroanisol and hexanitrodiphenyl sulfide in bombs.

Trinitrophenetol or ethyl picrate, m.p. 78°, is prepared by the same methods as trinitroanisol. The explosive properties of the two substances have been studied by Desparmets and Calinaud, and by Desvergnes, who has reported the results of the earlier workers together with data of his own and discussions of methods of manufacture and of the explosive properties of mixtures with picric acid, ammonium nitrate, etc. Drop test with a 5-kilogram weight were as follows:

	Height of Drop, Centimeters	Per Cent Explosion
Picric acid.........	30	50
Trinitroanisol......	100	20
Trinitroanisol......	110	30
Trinitrophenetol....	100	10
Trinitrophenetol....	110	10

Velocities of detonation (densities not reported) were trinitroanisol 7640 meters per second, trinitrophenetol 6880, and, for comparison, TNT 6880 meters per second. Pellets of the compressed explosives fired in the manometric bomb gave the results tabulated below.

	Density of Loading	Pressure: Kilos Per Square Centimeter
Picric acid...........	0.20	2310
Picric acid...........	0.20	2350
Picric acid...........	0.20	2210
Trinitroanisol........	0.20	2222
Trinitroanisol........	0.20	2250
Trinitroanisol........	0.20	2145
Trinitrophenetol......	0.20	1774
Picric acid...........	0.25	3230
Trinitroanisol........	0.25	2850
Trinitrophenetol......	0.25	2490
Trinitrophenetol......	0.30	3318

Both trinitroanisol and trinitrophenetol[173] were found to be as satisfactory as compressed TNT for use as a booster charge in 75-mm. shells loaded with *schneiderite.*

Trinitroaniline (picramide)

2,4,6-Trinitroaniline, orange-red crystals from alcohol, m.p. 186°, has but little interest as an explosive for the reason that other more powerful and more valuable explosives may be prepared from the same raw materials. It may be prepared by nitrating aniline in glacial acetic acid solution or by the use of mixed nitric-sulfuric acid in which no large excess of sulfuric acid is present. The presence of nitrous acid must be avoided, as this attacks the amino group, replaces it by hydroxyl, and results in the formation of picric acid. The nitration of aniline in the presence of a large amount of concentrated sulfuric acid yields *m*-nitroaniline and later the nitro compounds which are derived from it.

Tetranitroaniline (TNA)

2,3,4,6-Tetranitroaniline, discovered by Flurscheim, has interesting explosive properties but is such a reactive chemical substance that, when all things are considered, it is unsuitable for use. It was used to some extent during the first World War and was studied very thoroughly at that time.

Flurscheim prepared TNA by a one-stage nitration of *m*-nitroaniline sulfate, that substance being procured by the reduction of *m*-dinitrobenzene with sodium polysulfide. The nitration proceeds smoothly, and the entering groups take the positions indicated by the strongly ortho-para orienting amino group. The yield is about 120 per cent of the weight of the *m*-nitroaniline.[174]

Pure TNA, yellowish-brown or greenish-brown crystals from

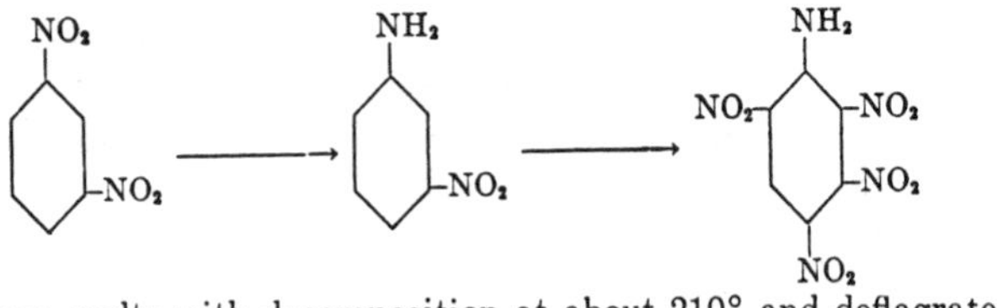

acetone, melts with decomposition at about 210° and deflagrates at about 226°. It is soluble in glacial acetic acid (1 part in 24 at boiling temperature), readily in acetone (1 in 6 at boiling temperature), and sparingly in benzene, ligroin, and chloroform. If a small amount of water is added to an acetone solution of TNA and the liquid is refluxed, the nitro group in the 3-position, having other nitro groups *ortho* and *para* to it, is replaced rapidly by hydroxyl. The resulting trinitroaminophenol, m.p. 176°, is capable of attacking metals to form dangerous explosive salts which are similar to the picrates. If TNA is boiled with aqueous sodium carbonate or bicarbonate both the amino group and the nitro group in the 3-position are hydrolyzed, and trinitroresorcinol is formed.

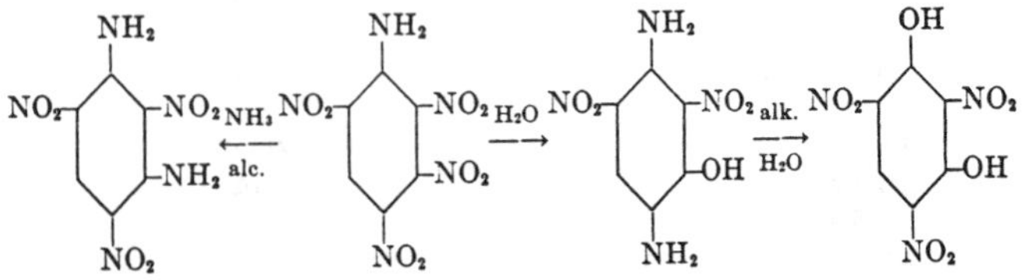

With alcoholic ammonia TNA yields trinitro-*m*-phenylenediamine, m.p. 288°. Its nitro group in the 3-position reacts with primary and secondary amines, with sodium acid sulfite, etc., in the same way that the *meta* nitro groups of β- and γ-trinitrotoluene do. Marqueyrol found that TNA is attacked rapidly by boiling water, about half of it being converted into trinitroaminophenol, the other half being destroyed with the evolution of gases, largely carbon dioxide and nitrogen along with smaller quantities of carbon monoxide, hydrocyanic acid, and nitric oxide. At 75° the reaction between water and TNA is complete after 4 days; at 60° it is about half complete after 7 days; at 40° it is appreciable after 10 days. Any decomposition of this sort, of course, is too much for an explosive intended for military use.

175

TNA shows about the same sensitivity as tetryl in the drop test. Lead block experiments have been reported which showed that 10 grams of TNA produced a net expansion of 430 cc., TNT 254 cc., picric acid 297 cc., tetryl 375 cc., guncotton 290 cc., and 75 per cent dynamite 300 cc.[76] Experiments with the manometric bomb gave the results indicated below.

[76] From the pamphlet "Tetra-Nitro-Aniline 'Flurscheim,'" Verona Chemical Company, sole licensed manufacturers for the United States, North Newark, New Jersey, 1917(?), p. 4. Giua, *op. cit.*, p. 317, states that the force of TNA measured in the lead block is 420 compared with picric acid 297.

	Density of Loading	Pressure: Kilos Per Square Centimeter
TNA	0.20	2356
TNA	0.25	3110
Tetryl	0.20	2423
Tetryl	0.25	3243

Since these data show that tetryl is slightly more powerful than TNA, the superiority of TNA in the lead block test must be interpreted as indicating that TNA has the higher velocity of detonation.

Tetryl (tetralite, pyronite)

Tetryl or 2,4,6-trinitrophenylmethylnitramine was first described by Michler and Meyer in 1879, and was studied soon thereafter by van Romburgh and by Mertens. Van Romburgh proved its structure by synthesizing it from picryl chloride and potassium methylnitramine.

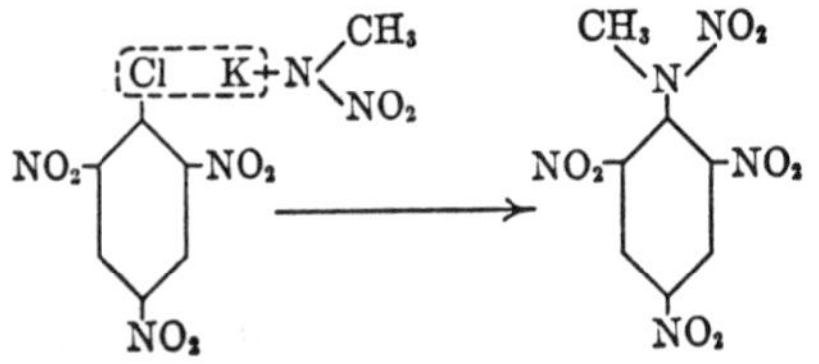

In the early literature of the subject, and to some extent at present, the substance is wrongly designated as tetranitromethylaniline. It results from the nitration of monomethyl- and of

176

dimethylaniline, and is prepared industrially by the nitration of the latter. The course of the reactions is first the introduction of two nitro groups in the nucleus, then the removal of one of the

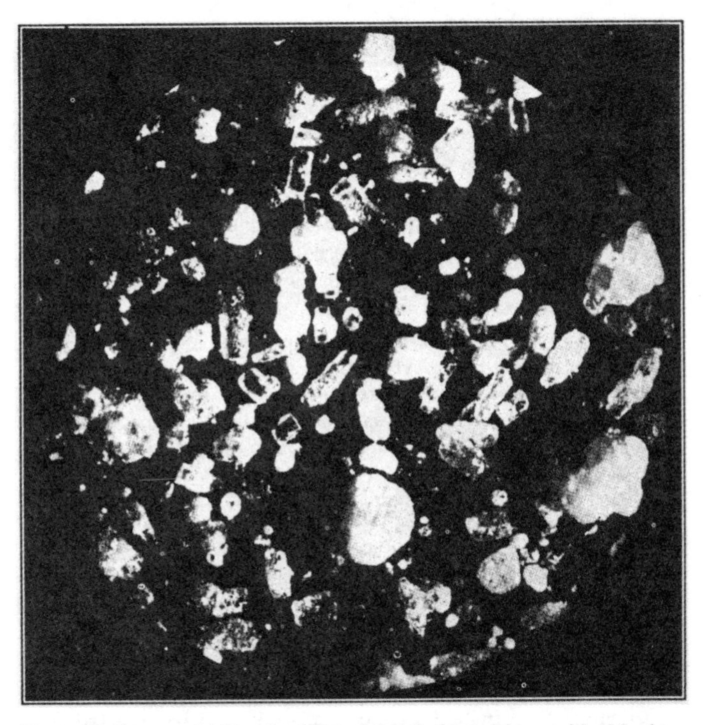

Figure 50. Commercial Sample of Tetryl (20×). Material crystallized in this form pours easily and may be made into pellets by machinery.

methyl groups by oxidation, then the introduction of a third nitro group in the nucleus, and finally the replacement of the amino hydrogen by a nitro group.

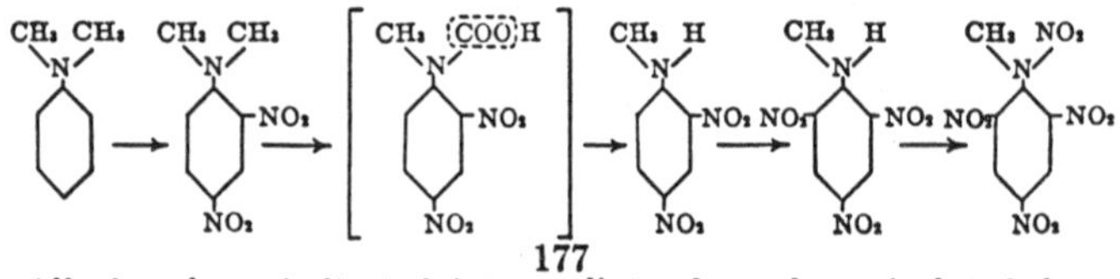

177

All the above-indicated intermediates have been isolated from the reaction. The last step is interesting because it is a reversible nitration. If tetryl is dissolved in concentrated (95 per cent) sulfuric acid and allowed to stand, the nitro group on the nitrogen is replaced by hydrogen, and nitric acid and trinitromethylaniline (methylpicramide), m.p. 111.8-112.4°, are formed. Tetryl accordingly gives up this nitro group, and only this one, in the nitrometer. In the industrial preparation of tetryl, the usual method is to dissolve the dimethylaniline in concentrated sulfuric acid and then to carry out all the reactions in one stage. The process has been the subject of many careful studies, among which those of Langenscheidt, van Duin, Knowles, Wride, Desvergnes, and Bain are especially to be noted. The crude tetryl contains impurities which must be removed by boiling the finely comminuted substance in water, and by dissolving the crude material in benzene and filtering for the removal of insoluble materials. For the industrial crystallization of tetryl, either acetone or benzene is commonly used.

Preparation of Tetryl. Twenty grams of dimethylaniline is dissolved in 240 grams of concentrated sulfuric acid (*d.* 1.84), the temperature being kept below 25°, and the solution is allowed to run from a separatory funnel drop by drop into 160 grams of 80 per cent nitric acid (*d.* 1.46), previously warmed to 55° or 60°, while this is stirred continuously and kept at a temperature between 65° and 70°. The addition requires about an hour. After all has been added, the stirring is continued while the temperature of the mixture is maintained at 65° to 70°. The material is allowed to cool; the solid matter is collected on an asbestos filter, washed with water, and boiled for an hour with 240 cc. of water while further water is added from time to time to replace that which boils away. The crude tetryl is filtered off, ground under water to pass a 150-mesh sieve, and boiled twice for 4 hours each time with 12 times its weight of water. The solid is dried and treated with benzene sufficient to dissolve all readily soluble material. The solution is filtered and allowed to evaporate spontaneously, and the residue is recrystallized from alcohol. Pure tetryl melts [178] at about 129.4°; a good commercial sample, at about 128.5°.

The nitration of aniline in the presence of a large amount of strong sulfuric acid results wholly in the formation of *m*-nitroaniline, but the similar nitration of dimethylaniline gives principally a mixture of the *ortho*- and *para*-derivatives. Monomethylaniline stands between aniline and dimethylaniline in respect to the orienting effect of its amino group; it yields a considerable amount of the *m*-nitro- compound—and dimethylaniline is preferred for the preparation of tetryl. Commercial dimethylaniline contains a certain amount of monomethylaniline, from which it is extremely difficult to free it, and this in the manufacture of tetryl is converted in part into 2,3,4,6-tetranitrophenylmethylnitramine, or *m*-nitrotetryl, pale yellow, almost white, crystals from benzene, m.p. 146-147.°[87]

[87] Van Romburgh, *Rec. trav. chim.*, **8**, 274 (1889). Van Romburgh and Schepers, *Versl. Kon. Akad. Wetenschapen*, **22**, 293 (1913), also prepared this substance by the nitration of dimethylaniline (in 20 times its weight of concentrated sulfuric acid).

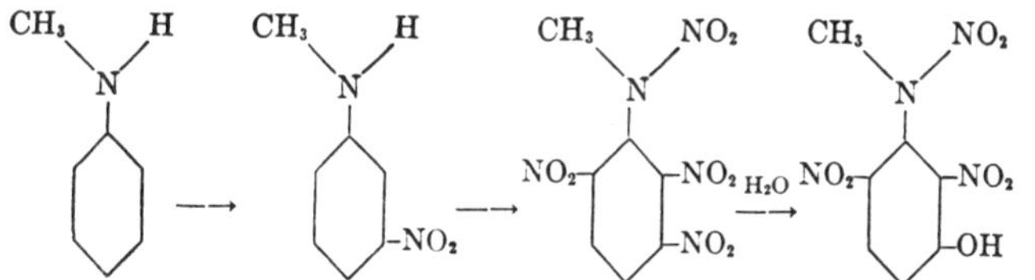

No *m*-nitrotetryl is produced if pure dimethylaniline is used in the usual process for the manufacture of tetryl. The amount of this impurity in the usual process depends upon the amount of monomethylaniline which may be present. A large excess of sulfuric acid tends toward the production of *m*-nitro compounds, but a reduction in the amount of sulfuric acid is not feasible for this increases the amount of benzene-insoluble material. *m*-Nitrotetryl reacts with water, as TNA does; the nitro group in the 3-position is replaced by hydroxyl, and *m*-hydroxytetryl or 2,4,6-trinitro-3-methylnitraminophenol, yellow crystals from water, m.p. 183°, is formed. This substance resembles picric acid and forms explosive salts. It is [179] readily soluble in water, and *m*-nitrotetryl is effectively removed from crude tetryl by boiling the finely powdered solid with water.

Crude tetryl commonly contains a small quantity of amorphous-appearing, buff-colored material of high melting point which is insoluble in benzene. The amount of this material is increased by the presence of larger amounts of water in the nitrating acid. Michler and Pattinson found that tetramethylbenzidine is produced when dimethylaniline is heated with concentrated sulfuric acid. The same material is evidently formed during the preparation of tetryl and gives rise to the three substances indicated below, which constitute the benzene-insoluble impurity.

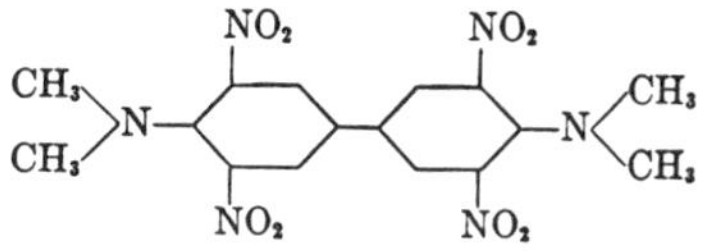

I

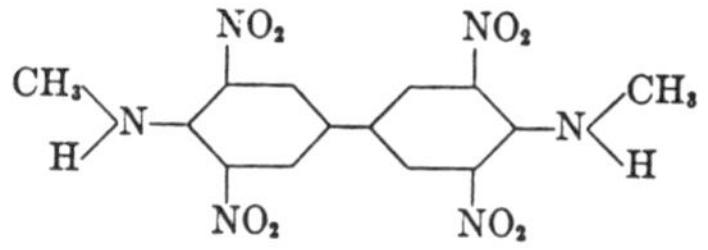

II

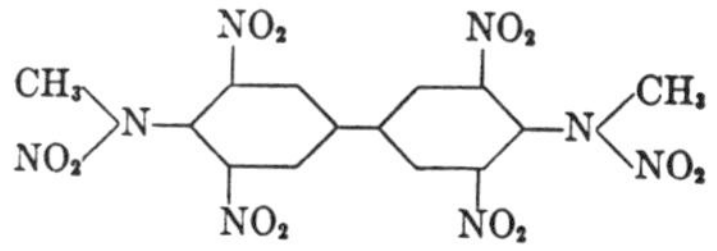

III

These substances were prepared by Mertens in 1886 by the action of nitric acid on dimethylaniline (I, II, and III) and on monomethylaniline (II and III). Van Romburgh in the same year proved them to be derivatives of benzidine, and at a much later time summarized the work which had been done upon them and synthesized the substances in such manner as to prove the position of the nitro groups. [180]

If the benzene-insoluble material from crude tetryl is dissolved in hot fuming nitric acid and allowed to cool, glistening yellow crystals are procured. These, recrystallized from nitric acid and then from acetone with the addition of two volumes of ligroin, yield cream-colored small crystals of the third of the above-indicated substances, 3,3′,5,5′-tetranitro-4,4′-di-(methylnitramino)-biphenyl, or 3,3′,5,5′-tetranitrodimethylbenzidinedinitramine. The material decomposes with foaming at 229-230° if its temperature is raised at the rate of 6° per minute. If it is heated more slowly, at 2° per minute, it melts partially and decomposes at 222° with preliminary softening and darkening. Like tetryl and other nitroamines, it gives a blue color with the diphenylamine reagent. Although Willstätter and Kalk have found that monomethylaniline is not convertible into a benzidine derivative by Michler's method, it is nevertheless true that the benzene-insoluble by-products are produced during the preparation of tetryl from monomethylaniline, as indeed Mertens first procured them by the action of nitric acid on that substance.

The usual process for the preparation of tetryl from dimethylaniline has the disadvantage that the by-products, namely, the *m*-nitrotetryl and the benzene-insoluble material, necessitate a rather elaborate purification, and it has the further disadvantage that one of the methyl groups of the dimethylaniline is destroyed by oxidation (expense) with the production of red fumes (nuisance) and the consequent loss of valuable combined nitrogen. All these disadvantages find their origin at points in the reaction earlier than the formation of dinitromonomethylaniline. 2,4-Dinitromonomethylaniline, orange-yellow crystals, m.p. 174°, nitrates smoothly to form tetryl without the production of by-products or red fumes. Synthetic methyl alcohol is now available cheaply and in a quantity which is limited only by the will of the manufacturers to produce it. It reacts with ammonia (from the fixation of nitrogen) at elevated temperatures in the presence of a thorium oxide catalyst to form methylamine, and methylamine reacts with dinitrochlorobenzene to form dinitromonomethylaniline. There seems every reason to believe that tetryl in the future will be manufactured chiefly, or wholly, from dinitrochlorobenzene.

[181]

The solubility of tetryl in various solvents is tabulated below.

SOLUBILITY OF TETRYL

(Grams per 100 grams of solvent)

Temperature, °C.	Water	95% Alcohol	Carbon Tetrachloride	Chloroform	Carbon Disulfide	Ether
0	0.0050	0.320	0.007	0.28	0.0090	0.188
5	0.0058	0.366	0.011	0.33	0.0120	0.273
10	0.0065	0.425	0.015	0.39	0.0146	0.330
15	0.0072	0.496	0.020	0.47	0.0177	0.377
20	0.0075	0.563	0.025	0.57	0.0208	0.418
25	0.0080	0.65	0.031	0.68	0.0244	0.457
30	0.0085	0.76	0.039	0.79	0.0296	0.493
35	0.0094	0.91	0.048	0.97	0.0392	...
40	0.0110	1.12	0.058	1.20	0.0557	...
45	0.0140	1.38	0.073	1.47	0.0940	...
50	0.0195	1.72	0.095	1.78	...	...
55	0.0270	2.13	0.124	2.23	...	...
60	0.0350	2.64	0.154	2.65	...	...
65	0.0440	3.33	0.193	...	...	...
70	0.0535	4.23	0.241	...	...	...
75	0.0663	5.33	0.297	...	...	...
80	0.0810	...	...	...	...	...
85	0.0980	...	...	...	...	...
90	0.1220	...	...	...	...	...
95	0.1518	...	...	...	...	...
100	0.1842	...	...	...	...	...

Tetryl is hydrolyzed rapidly by boiling aqueous sodium carbonate to form sodium picrate, sodium nitrite, and methylamine which escapes. It is not affected by prolonged boiling with dilute sulfuric acid. It reacts with aniline in benzene solution at ordinary temperature; red crystals of 2,4,6-trinitrodiphenylamine, m.p. 179.5-180°, separate after the liquid has stood for a few hours, and extraction of the liquid with water yields an aqueous solution of methylnitramine.

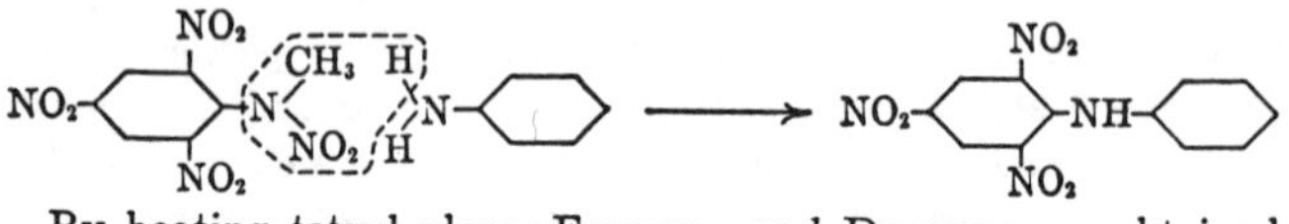

$$NO_2\text{-}C_6H_2(NO_2)_2\text{-}N(CH_3)NO_2 + H\text{-}NH\text{-}C_6H_5 \longrightarrow (NO_2)_3C_6H_2\text{-}NH\text{-}C_6H_5$$

By heating tetryl alone, Farmer and Desvergnes obtained picric acid, and by heating tetryl in high-boiling solvents Mertens,[96] van Romburgh,[96] and Davis and Allen[96] obtained methylpicramide. [182] When refluxed in xylene solution, tetryl gives off nitrous fumes and is converted into a tarlike mass from which picric acid and methylpicramide may be isolated, along with a third, unidentified, buff-colored finely crystalline substance which melts at 240.5°. If pure tetryl is kept at 100°, it gives off nitrous fumes and a small quantity of formaldehyde, and yields after 40 days a mass which remains semi-liquid at ordinary temperature. By heating at 125° it is converted into a viscous liquid after about the same number of hours.

At ordinary temperatures tetryl appears to be perfectly stable. Current methods of purification insure the absence of occluded acid. It is more powerful and more brisant than TNT and picric acid, though distinctly more sensitive to shock, and is probably the best of all the common explosives for use in boosters and reinforced detonators. Koehler reports pressures in the manometric bomb (density of loading = 0.3) and temperatures produced by the explosions, as follows:

	Pressure: Kilos per Square Centimeter	Temperature, °C.
Tetryl	4684	2911
Picric acid	3638	2419
TNT	3749	2060
TNB	3925	2356

Aranaz reports that the explosion of tetryl produces a temperature of 3339°. Tetryl is slightly more sensitive than picric acid, and considerably more sensitive than TNT, in the drop test. Experimenting with a 5-kilogram weight, Koehler found that a drop of 150 cm. caused the detonation of tetryl 10 times out of 10 trials, a drop of 100 cm. 9 times out of 10, of 50 cm. 5 times out of 10, and of 40 cm. 3 times out of 10. Martin has determined the minimum charges of various primary explosives necessary for the detonation of TNT and tetryl. The explosives were loaded into detonator capsules, and the initiators were compressed upon them at a pressure of 1100 kilos per square centimeter.

[183]

	Minimum Charge for Detonation of TNT	Tetryl
Mercuric fulminate	0.36	0.29
Silver fulminate	0.095	0.02
Cadmium fulminate	0.11	0.008
Mercurous azide	0.145	0.045
Silver azide	0.07	0.02
Lead azide	0.09	0.025
Cadmium azide	0.04	0.01

With each of the initiators which was tried, tetryl was more easily detonated than TNT. Taylor and Cope have determined the minimum charges of fulminate-chlorate (90:10) necessary to cause the complete detonation of various mixtures of TNT and tetryl, as follows:

Mixture of TNT-Tetryl		Weight of Initiator, Grams
100	0	0.25
90	10	0.22
80	20	0.21
50	50	0.20
0	100	0.19

"Ethyl Tetryl." 2,4,6-Trinitrophenylethylnitramine

The ethyl analogue of tetryl was first prepared by van Romburgh, who procured it both by nitrating monoethylaniline and by nitrating diethylaniline, and reported that it melts at 96°. The present writer has found that the pure material, recrystallized twice from nitric acid (*d*. 1.42) and once from alcohol, melts at 94°. It is comparable to tetryl in its chemical reactions and in its explosive properties.

"Butyl Tetryl." 2,4,6-Trinitrophenyl-*n*-butylnitramine

The *n*-butyl analogue of tetryl has been prepared by two methods: (*a*) by condensing 2,4-dinitrochlorobenzene with *n*-butylamine to form 2,4-dinitro-*n*-butylaniline,[103] and by the nitration of this product; and (*b*) by the nitration in one step of *n*-butylaniline. The pure substance crystallizes from alcohol in

[103] Pure 2,4-dinitro-*n*-butylaniline crystallizes from alcohol in deep yellow or orange needles, m.p. 92.5-93.0°.

184

lemon-yellow plates which melt at 97.5-98.0°. It is readily soluble in benzene, ethyl acetate, alcohol and acetone, and is insoluble in petroleum ether. It yields sodium picrate when boiled with sodium carbonate solution.

Butyl tetryl is suitable for use in boosters, reinforced detonators, detonating fuse, primer caps, etc. For the detonation of 0.4 gram, it requires 0.19 gram of mercury fulminate. It has a slightly greater shattering effect than TNT in the sand test and shows about the same sensitivity as tetryl in the drop test. It explodes spontaneously at 210°.

Hexanitrodiphenylamine

2,2',4,4',6,6'-Hexanitrodiphenylamine (hexil, hexite, hexamin, etc.) is another explosive which can be prepared most conveniently from dinitrochlorobenzene. Its ammonium salt has been used under the name of *aurantia* as a yellow dye for silk and wool. It has valuable explosive properties but is more poisonous than nitroglycerin and attacks the skin, causing severe blisters which resemble burns. Its dust is injurious to the mucous membranes of the mouth, nose, and lungs. Mertens[104] in 1878 prepared hexanitrodiphenylamine by the nitration of diphenylamine with fuming nitric acid in concentrated sulfuric acid solution. Its behavior as a pseudo-acid has been studied by Alexandrov and by Hantzsch and Opolski. Hausermann in 1891 reported upon its explosive power as compared with trinitrotoluene, and a patent granted in 1909 to Otto Freiherr von Schroetter described an explosive consisting of 80 parts of hexanitrodiphenylamine and 20 parts of trinitrotoluene. The large-scale preparation by the direct nitration of diphenylamine was reported in 1910, and the process from dinitrochlorobenzene, originally described in a patent to the Griesheim Chem. Fabrik, was reported by

[104] *Ber.*, **11**, 843 (1878). Austen, *ibid.*, **7**, 1249 (1874), reported the formation of the substance by the nitration of picryl-*p*-nitroaniline, and Gnehm, *ibid.*, **7**, 1399 (1874), by the nitration of methyldiphenylamine.

185

Carter in 1913 and studied further by Hoffman and Dame in 1919 and by Marshall in 1920.

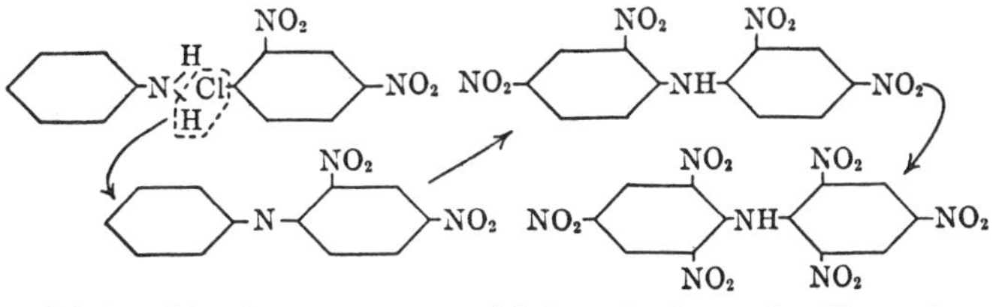

Dinitrochlorobenzene reacts with 2 equivalents of aniline, when the materials are warmed together in the absence of solvent or when they are stirred together vigorously with water 80-90°, to form dinitrodiphenylamine in practically quantitative yield, along with 1 equivalent of aniline hydrochloride. The use of the second molecule of aniline to combine with the hydrogen chloride involves unnecessary expense, and the same results may be accomplished by means of some mineral alkali or acid-neutralizing substance like sodium acetate or sodium or calcium carbonate. The product, which is insoluble in water, separates in bright red needles. Pure 2,4-dinitrodiphenylamine, recrystallized from alcohol or from benzene, melts at 156-157°. The crude product is nitrated in one or in two stages to the hexanitro compound.

Preparation of Hexanitrodiphenylamine (Two-Stage Nitration). Seventy grams of aniline and 32 grams of precipitated calcium carbonate are stirred up together with water in such manner as to form a homogeneous suspension, and the mixture is heated to about 60°. Dinitrochlorobenzene, 150 grams, previously melted, is poured in slowly in a fine stream while the stirring is continued and the mixture is heated gradually to about 90°, the rate of heating being regulated by the progress of the reaction. The product is washed with hydrochloric acid to free it from aniline and calcium carbonate, then with water until free from chlorides, and dried in the oven at 100°.

Fifty grams of finely powdered dinitrodiphenylamine is added in small portions at a time to 420 grams of nitric acid (*d.* 1.33), which is stirred vigorously while the temperature is maintained at 50-60°. The progress of the nitration is followed by observing the color change from

186

the red of the dinitro compound to the yellow of the tetranitrodiphenylamine. After all has been added, the temperature is raised to 80-90° and kept there for 2 hours longer while the stirring is continued. After the mixture has cooled, the product is filtered off directly, washed with water until free from acid, and dried in the air or in the oven at 100°.

Fifty grams of the tetranitrodiphenylamine is added slowly, with stirring, during an hour, to a mixture of 250 grams of nitric acid (*d.* 1.50) and 250 grams of sulfuric acid (*d.* 1.83). After all has been added, the mixture is allowed to stand for 3 hours at laboratory temperature, and is then drowned in ice water. The hexanitrodiphenylamine is filtered off, washed thoroughly with water, dried in the air, and recrystallized from acetone with the addition of petroleum ether.

Pure hexanitrodiphenylamine, small yellow needles, melts with decomposition at 243.0-244.5°. It is insoluble in chloroform, sparingly soluble in ether and in cold acetic acid, fairly soluble in alcohol, and readily soluble in cold acetone and in warm acetic and nitric acids.

Marshall reports minimum priming charges of fulminate-chlorate (90:10) necessary for the complete detonation of the indicated explosives to be as follows:

	Grams
Hexanitrodiphenylamine	0.18
Tetryl	0.20
Tetranitroaniline	0.20
Trinitrotoluene	0.25

He found hexanitrodiphenylamine to be slightly less sensitive in the drop test than tetryl and tetranitroaniline. When 1 pound of the explosive was loaded into a 3.5-inch cubical box of cardboard or tin and fired at with a U.S. Army rifle from a distance of 30 yards, hexanitrodiphenylamine gave no detonations in the cardboard boxes, and 7 detonations and 1 failure in tin; TNT gave no detonation in cardboard, fire and detonation in tin; and tetryl and tetranitroaniline gave detonations in every case with either kind of container. Marshall reported the velocity of detonation of hexanitrodiphenylamine to be 6898 meters per second at density 1.58, and 7150 meters per second at density 1.67. Pellets of the explosive, mixed with 1 per cent of stearic acid, compressed at 5000 pounds per square inch, had a density 1.43; at 10,000

[187]
pounds per square inch, density 1.56; at 15,000 pounds per square inch, density 1.59; and at 20,000 pounds per square inch, density 1.60. The pellets which showed the best homogeneity and the least tendency to crumble were those of density 1.56.

Hexanitrodiphenyl Sulfide

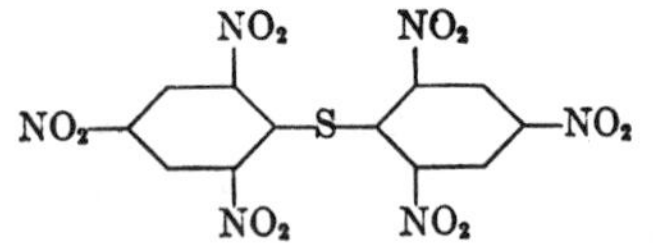

Hexanitrodiphenyl sulfide (picryl sulfide) is formed by the interaction of picryl chloride and sodium thiosulfate in alcohol solution in the presence of magnesium carbonate. It is sparingly soluble in alcohol and ether, more readily in glacial acetic acid and acetone, golden-yellow leaflets from alcohol-acetone, m.p. 234°. It does not stain the fingers yellow and is said to be non-poisonous. Its explosive properties are comparable to those of hexanitrodiphenylamine. Its use in reinforced detonators has been suggested, and the fact that its explosion produces sulfur dioxide has commended it for use in projectiles intended to make closed spaces, such as casemates, holds of ships, etc., untenable. During the first World War the Germans used drop bombs loaded with a mixture of equal parts of TNT and hexanitrodiphenyl sulfide.

Hexanitrodiphenyl Sulfone

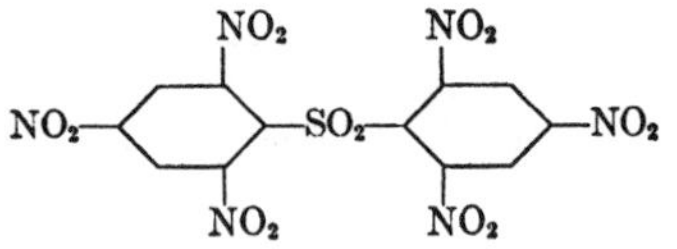

The action of nitric acid on hexanitrodiphenyl sulfide yields a substance, faintly yellowish crystals, m.p. 307°, which Stettbacher believes to be the sulfone, not the peroxide as the patent states, for the reason that it is stable at elevated temperatures [188] and is less sensitive to shock than the sulfide. It is a more powerful explosive than hexanitrodiphenyl sulfide.

Hexanitro-oxanilide

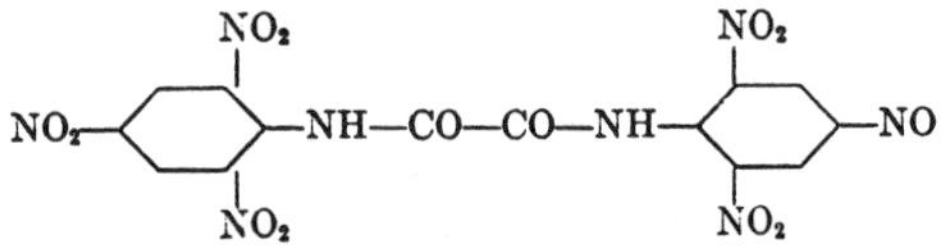

This substance, m.p. 295-300°, results from the direct nitration of oxanilide. It is stable and about as powerful as TNT, and is reported to explode with the production of a temperature which is distinctly lower than that produced by many high explosives.

Hexanitrocarbanilide

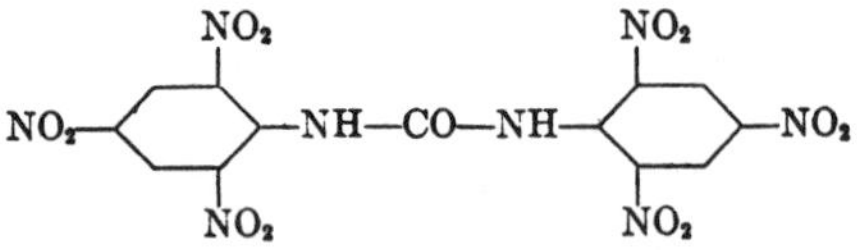

2,2',4,4',6,6'-Hexanitro-N,N'-diphenylurea (hexanitrocarbanilide or *sym*-dipicrylurea) may be prepared by the nitration of carbanilide (*sym*-diphenylurea) in one, in two, or in three stages. It is of interest because of its explosive properties and because it supplies one way in which benzene may be converted into an explosive which is valuable both for military and for civil uses. Carbanilide may be prepared by the interaction of aniline and phosgene but is most conveniently and economically procured by heating aniline and urea together at 160-165°.

Preparation of Hexanitrocarbanilide (Two Stages). Forty grams of carbanilide is dissolved in 60 cc. of concentrated sulfuric acid (*d.* 1.84), and the solution is added drop by drop during 4 hours to 96 cc. of nitric acid (*d.* 1.51) while the mixture is stirred vigorously with a mechanical stirrer and its temperature is maintained at 35° to 40°. After all has been added, the stirring is continued and the temperature is raised to 60° during half an hour and maintained at 60° for another hour. The mixture is cooled to room temperature, allowed to stand over night, then treated with cracked ice and water, and filtered. The crude tetra- [189] nitrocarbanilide is washed thoroughly with water and allowed to dry in the air.

Ten grams of crude tetranitrocarbanilide is added to a mixture of 16 grams of concentrated sulfuric acid (*d.* 1.84) and 24 grams of nitric acid (*d.* 1.51), and the material is heated on the steam bath for 1 hour with constant stirring. The mixture, after cooling, is treated with cracked ice and water, and filtered. The product, washed with 500 cc. of cold water, then with 500 cc. of hot water, and dried in the air, is hexanitrocarbanilide of satisfactory quality for use as an explosive.

Pure hexanitrocarbanilide crystallizes from acetone-ligroin in pale yellow rosettes which soften and darken at 204° and melt at 208-209° with decomposition. It yields picric acid when warmed with dilute sulfuric acid, and trinitroaniline when boiled with strong ammonia water. A deep ruby-red color is developed when hexanitrocarbanilide is allowed to stand at ordinary temperatures in contact with strong ammonia water. Tetranitrocarbanilide, dinitroaniline, trinitroaniline, picric acid, and dinitrophenol do not give this color.

Hexanitrocarbanilide is a brisant high explosive suitable for use in boosters, reinforced detonators, detonating fuse, primer caps, etc. For the detonation of 0.4 gram, it requires 0.19 gram of mercury fulminate. It is slightly stronger than TNT in the sand test and of about the same sensitivity as tetryl in the drop test. It explodes spontaneously at 345°.

Hexanitroazobenzene

Hexanitroazobenzene may be prepared from dinitrochlorobenzene and hydrazine by the reactions indicated below:

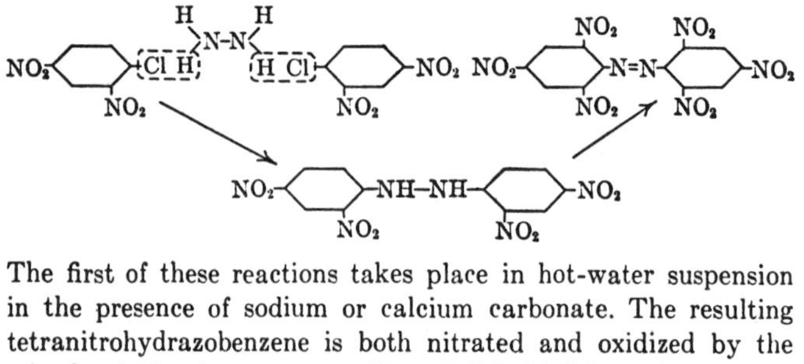

The first of these reactions takes place in hot-water suspension in the presence of sodium or calcium carbonate. The resulting tetranitrohydrazobenzene is both nitrated and oxidized by the mixed acid in the next step. Pure 2,2',4,4',6,6'-hexanitroazoben- [190] zene crystallizes from acetone in handsome orange-colored needles which melt at 215°. The explosive properties of the substance have not been reported in detail. The azo group makes it more powerful and more brisant than hexanitrodiphenylamine. The accessibility of the raw materials and the simplicity of its preparation commend it for use in boosters and compound detonators.

CHAPTER V [191]

NITRIC ESTERS

Nitric esters or *organic nitrates* contain the nitrate radical, $—O—NO_2$, attached to a carbon atom, or, to express the same idea in a different way, they contain the nitro group, $—NO_2$, attached to an oxygen atom which is attached to a carbon. In *nitro compounds,* strictly so called, the nitro group is attached directly to a carbon; in *nitroamines* or *nitramines* it is attached to an amino nitrogen atom, that is, to a nitrogen which is attached to a carbon. In the nitric esters and in the nitroamines alike, a single atom stands between the nitro group and the carbon atom of the organic molecule. Substances of the two classes are alike in their most characteristic reaction, namely, they are formed by the reversible nitration of alcohols and amines respectively.

During the nitration of glycerin by the action of strong nitric acid or of strong mixed acid upon it, nitro groups are introduced in place of three of the hydrogen atoms of the original molecule. There is therefore a certain propriety in thinking of the product as a nitro compound, and a reasonable warrant for the common practice of calling it by the name of trinitroglycerin or, more commonly, of *nitroglycerin.* The hydrogen atoms which are replaced were attached to oxygen atoms; the product is really a nitric ester, and its proper name is *glyceryl trinitrate.* Similarly, the substances which are commonly called nitroglycol, nitrostarch, nitrosugar, nitrolactose, nitrocotton, etc., are actually nitric esters.

The physical properties of the nitric esters resemble in a general way the physical properties of the alcohols from which they are derived. Thus, methyl and ethyl nitrate, like methyl and ethyl alcohol, are volatile liquids; nitroglycerin is a viscous oil, more viscous and less volatile than glycol dinitrate as glycerin is more viscous and less volatile than glycol. Nitrocellulose from [192] fibrous cellulose yields a tough and plastic colloid, but nitrostarch remains from the evaporation of its solutions as a mass which is brittle and friable.

Methyl Nitrate

Methyl nitrate is a powerful explosive although its physical properties are such that it is not of practical use, and it is of interest only because it is the simplest of the nitric esters. Like ethyl and *n*-propyl nitrates, it may be prepared by the careful distillation of the alcohol with concentrated nitric acid (*d.* 1.42) from which, however, the last traces of nitrous acid must first have been removed by the addition of urea. It may also be prepared by adding the alcohol to strong mixed acid at low temperature, stirring, and separating and washing the product without distillation, by a process similar to that which is used for the preparation of nitroglycerin and nitroglycol except that the volatility of the product requires the stirring to be done by mechanical means and not by compressed air. It is a colorless limpid liquid somewhat less viscous than water, boiling point 65–66°, specific gravity 1.2322 at 5°, 1.2167 at 15°, and 1.2032 at 25°. Its vapors have a strongly aromatic odor resembling that of chloroform, and cause headache if they are inhaled. It dissolves collodion nitrocotton to form a jelly from which the methyl nitrate evaporates readily.

Methyl nitrate has a slightly higher energy content than nitroglycerin and a slightly greater explosive effect. Naoúm reports that 10 grams of methyl nitrate in the Trauzl test with water tamping caused an expansion of 615 cc., while 10 grams of nitroglycerin under the same conditions gave 600 cc. Methyl nitrate is very much more sensitive to initiation than nitroglycerin, a fact which, like its higher velocity of detonation, is probably associated with its lower viscosity. It is less sensitive than nitroglycerin to the mechanical shock of the drop test. In the small lead block test, or lead block compression test, 100 grams of methyl nitrate under slight confinement in a shell of sheet lead 1 mm. thick and tamped with thin cork plates, gave a compres- [193] sion of 24.5 mm. while nitroglycol similarly gave 30 mm. and nitroglycerin 18.5 mm.

Methyl nitrate is easily inflammable and burns in an open dish with a large non-luminous flame. Its vapors explode when heated to about 150°.

Berthelot measured the velocity of detonation of methyl nitrate in tubes of such small diameter that the maximum velocity of detonation was not secured, but he was able to make certain interesting inferences both as to the effect of the envelope and as to the effect of the physical state of the explosive. Some of his results are summarized in the table below. The data indicate

Tube of	Internal Diameter, Millimeters	External Diameter, Millimeters	Velocity of Detonation, Meters per Second
Rubber, canvas covered	5	12	1616
Glass	3	12	2482
Glass	3	7	2191
Glass	5	7	1890
Britannia metal	3	12.6	1230
Steel	3	15	2084
Steel	3	15	2094

that with tubes of the same internal diameter the velocity of detonation is greater in those cases in which the rupture of the tube is more difficult; it is greater in the tubes which have thicker walls and in the tubes which are made of the stronger materials. The extent to which the velocity of detonation builds up depends in some measure upon the pressure which builds up before the container is ruptured. By comparing these results with those from other explosive substances, Berthelot was able to make further inductions.

> In fact, nitroglycerin in lead tubes 3 mm. internal diameter gave velocities in the neighborhood of 1300 meters per second, while dynamite in similar metallic tubes attained 2700 meters per second. This sets in evidence the influence of the structure of the explosive substance upon the velocity of propagation of the explosion, pure nitroglycerin, a viscous liquid, transmitting the shock which determines the detonation much more irregularly than the silica impregnated in [194] a uniform manner with the same liquid. Mica dynamite according to my observations produces effects which are still more considerable, a fact which could be foreseen from the crystalline structure of the mica, a substance which is less deformable than amorphous silica.
>
> This last induction is confirmed by observations on nitromannite, a crystalline solid which appears by reason of this circumstance better suited than liquid methyl nitrate for transmitting detonation. It has in fact given practically constant velocities of 7700 meters per second in lead tubes of 1.9 mm. internal diameter at a density of loading of 1.9.

Likewise picric acid, also crystalline, 6500 meters per second. . . .

The influence of the structure of the explosive substance on the course of the detonation being thus made evident, let us cite new facts which show the effect due to the containing envelope. . . . Compressed guncotton at such densities of loading as 1.0 and 1.27 in lead tubes 3.15 mm. internal diameter gave velocities of 5400 meters per second, while at a density of loading of practically one-half less (0.73) in a lead tube 3.77 mm. internal diameter, a velocity of 3800 meters per second was observed—a difference which is evidently due to the reduced continuity of the material. In supple cordeau, slightly resistant, formed by a single strand or braid, with a density of loading of 0.65, the velocity falls even to 2400 meters per second. But the feeble resistance of the envelope may be compensated by the mass of the explosive which opposes itself, especially in the central portion of the mass, to the instantaneous escape of the gas. Abel, in fact, with cartridges of compressed guncotton, of ten times the diameter of the above-mentioned cordeau, placed end to end, in the open air, has observed velocities of 5300 to 6000 meters per second.

Other Alkyl Nitrates

Ethyl nitrate is a colorless liquid of agreeable odor, boiling point 87°, specific gravity (15°/15°) 1.1159 at 15°, and 1.1044 (25°/25°) at 25°. It has a less favorable oxygen balance than methyl nitrate, and is much less sensitive to initiation than the latter substance. It has only about 48% of the energy content of nitroglycerin, but its lower viscosity tends to give it a higher initial velocity of detonation than nitroglycerin and it performs about 58% as well as nitroglycerin in the sand test. A No. 8 [195] blasting cap will not detonate ethyl nitrate unless the explosive is tamped or confined. Mixed with fuller's earth in the proportion 70/30 or 60/40, it yields a brisant explosive which may be detonated without confinement.

n-Propyl nitrate, like ethyl nitrate, can be prepared by mixing the alcohol with nitric acid of density 1.42 or thereabouts, and carefully distilling the mixture. Ethyl alcohol and *n*-propyl alcohol, which contain the methylene group, are easily oxidized; if they are added to nitric acid of greater strength than density 1.42, or if they are added to strong mixed acid, they are likely to react with explosive violence and the abundant production of nitrous fumes, no matter how efficient the cooling. *n*-Propyl nitrate has a pleasant ethereal odor, boiling point 110.5°, specific gravity (15°/15°) 1.0631 at 15°, and (25°/25°) 1.0531 at 25°. It is less sensitive to detonation than ethyl nitrate. Ten grams in a Trauzl block, with water tamping and with a No. 8 blasting cap, detonated only partially and gave an expansion of 45 cc., or 15 cc. more than the cap alone, but 10 grams of it, mixed with 4 grams of fuller's earth to form a moist powder and exploded with a No. 8 cap, gave a sharp explosion and a net expansion of 230 cc.

Isopropyl nitrate, b.p. 101–102°, specific gravity 1.054 at 0°, 1.036 at 19°, is prepared by the interaction of isopropyl iodide and silver nitrate. The hydrogen atom which is attached in isopropyl alcohol to the carbon atom carrying the hydroxyl group is so easily oxidized that it is not feasible to prepare the compound by the action of nitric acid on the alcohol.

Nitroglycerin (Glyceryl trinitrate, NG)

Nitroglycerin was first prepared late in the year 1846 or early in 1847 by the Italian chemist, Ascanio Sobrero (1812–1888), who was at the time professor of applied chemistry at the University of Torino. Sobrero had studied medicine in the same city, and in 1834 had been authorized to practice as a physician. After that he studied with Pelouze in Paris and served as his assistant in his private laboratory from 1840 to 1843. In 1843 he left Paris, studied for several months with Liebig at Giessen, and returned to Torino where he took up the duties of a teacher and in 1845 [196] built and equipped a modest laboratory of his own. The earliest printed account of nitroglycerin appears in a letter which Sobrero wrote to Pelouze and which Pelouze caused to be published in *L'Institut* of February 15, 1847. In the same month Sobrero presented to the Academy of Torino a paper, *Sopra alcuni nuovi composti fulminanti ottenuti col mezzo dell'azione dell'acido nitrico sulle sostanze organiche vegetali,* in which he described nitroglycerin, nitromannite, and nitrated lactose. Later in the year he presented another paper, *Sulla Glicerina Fulminante o Piroglycerina,* before the chemistry section of the Ninth Italian Scientific Congress at Venice.

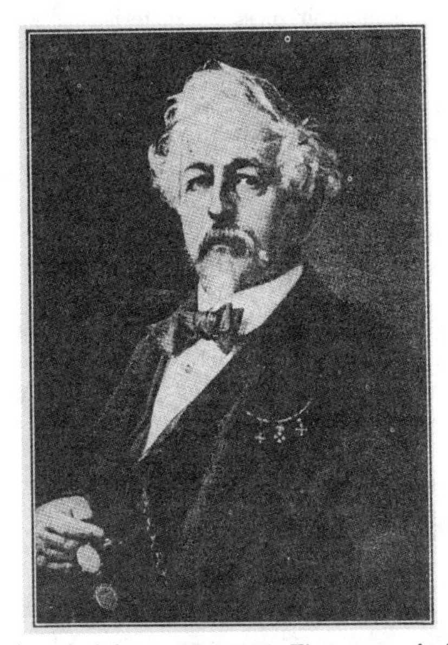

FIGURE 51. Ascanio Sobrero (1812-1888). First prepared nitroglycerin, nitromannite, and nitrolactose, 1846-1847.

Sobrero found that, if concentrated nitric acid or strong mixed acid is added to glycerin, a violent reaction ensues and red fumes [197] are evolved, but that, if syrupy glycerin is added to a mixture of two volumes of sulfuric acid (*d.* 1.84) and one volume of nitric acid (*d.* 1.50) with stirring while the mixture is kept below 0°, then the results are entirely different, the glycerin dissolves, and the solution when poured into water gives an oily precipitate of nitroglycerin. He collected the oil, washed it with water until free from acid, dried in a vacuum over sulfuric acid, and procured a transparent liquid of the color and appearance of olive oil. (Pure nitroglycerin is water-white.) Sobrero reported a value for the density which is very close to that which is now generally accepted, observed the ready solubility of nitroglycerin in alcohol and its reprecipitation by water, and reported a number of its chemical reactions—its comportments with acid and with alkali, that

It detonates when brought into contact with metallic

> potassium, and evolves oxides of nitrogen in contact with phosphorus at 20° to 30°C., but at higher temperatures it ignites with an explosion. . . . When heated, nitroglycerin decomposes. A drop heated on platinum foil ignites and burns very fiercely. It has, however, the property of detonating under certain circumstances with great violence. On one occasion a small quantity of an ethereal solution of nitroglycerin was allowed to evaporate in a glass dish. The residue of nitroglycerin was certainly not more than 2 or 3 centigrams. On heating the dish over a spirit lamp a most violent explosion resulted, and the dish was broken to atoms. . . . The safest plan for demonstrating the explosive power of nitroglycerin is to place a drop upon a watch glass and detonate it by touching it with a piece of platinum wire heated to low redness. Nitroglycerin has a sharp, sweet, aromatic taste. It is advisable to take great care in testing this property. A trace of nitroglycerin placed upon the tongue, but not swallowed, gives rise to a most violent pulsating headache accompanied by great weakness of the limbs.

For many years Sobrero kept in his laboratory and guarded jealously a sample of the original nitroglycerin which he had prepared in 1847. In 1886 he washed this material with a dilute solution of sodium bicarbonate and took it to the Nobel-Avigliana factory, of which he was a consultant, where he gave verbal testimony of its authenticity and where it has since been stored in one of the magazines. Molinari and Quartieri [198] in a book published in 1913 state that the sample, consisting of about 200 cc. under water in a bottle, was at that time unaltered and that analyses gave values for nitrogen in the neighborhood of 18.35%, close to the theoretical.

Sobrero seems originally to have thought more highly of the solid crystalline nitromannite, which he thought might be used in percussion caps, than of the liquid nitroglycerin, but a spontaneous explosion of 400 grams of the former substance in the laboratory of the arsenal of Torino in 1853 and the extensive damage which resulted caused him to lose interest in the material. After Nobel's invention of dynamite and of the blasting cap had made the use of nitroglycerin safe and practical, Sobrero attempted in 1873 to establish a factory to be operated by Italian capital for the manufacture of an explosive called *melanina*, which was a kind of dynamite formed by absorbing nitroglycerin in a mixture of powdered charcoal and the silicious earth of Santa Fiora in Tuscany. The project did not succeed. Shortly afterwards Sobrero accepted a position as consultant to the Nobel-Avigliana factory, a position which paid a generous salary during his life and a pension to his widow after his death. The high regard in which he was held by the Nobel company is indicated further by the bust of him which was unveiled in 1879 in the Avigliana factory.

Glycerin (glycerol) is a by-product of soap manufacture. All natural fats, whether of animal or vegetable origin, whether solid like beef suet or liquid like olive oil, are glyceryl esters of long-chain fatty acids containing an even number of carbon atoms. When they are warmed with an aqueous solution of strong alkali, they are saponified; soap, which is the alkali salt of the acids of the fats, is formed, and glycerin is produced which remains dissolved in the liquid. Glycerin is also formed from fats by the action of steam; the fatty acids, insoluble in water and generally of higher melting point than the fats, are formed at the same time.

Glycerin is a viscous liquid, colorless and odorless when pure, and possessing a sweet taste. It is hygroscopic, will absorb more [199] than half its own weight of moisture from the air, and does not evaporate. Glycerin will solidify in a freezing mixture, and when once frozen melts again at about 17°. It boils at atmospheric pressure at 290° with slight decomposition, and is best purified by distillation in vacuum. Its specific gravity is 1.265 at 15°. Perfectly pure and colorless glycerin yields a water-white nitroglycerin. Dynamite glycerin is a distilled product of high purity, density 1.262 or higher, and contains at least 99% of glycerin and less than 1% of water. It varies in color from pale yellow to dark brown, generally has a faint odor resembling that of burnt sugar, and yields a nitroglycerin of a pale yellow or pale brown color. The explosives makers consider a test nitration on a laboratory scale to be the surest way of estimating the quality of a sample of dynamite glycerin.

Small amounts of glycerin are produced during an ordinary alcoholic fermentation, but the quantity is greatly increased if a considerable amount of sodium sulfite is present. A commercial process based upon this principle was developed and used in Germany during the first World War, when the supply of glycerin from fats was insufficient to fill the needs of the explosives manufacturers, and similar processes have been used to some extent elsewhere and since that time. At the beginning of the second World War an effort was made to increase the production of whale oil for the manufacture of glycerin. Modern methods—harpoons shot from guns, fast Diesel-propelled steel ships—resulted immediately in a tremendous slaughter of whales, and whale oil again has become difficult to procure. Recent advances in synthetic chemistry make it probable that glycerin in the future will be prepared in large quantity from petroleum.

Cracking gas, which is produced when heavy petroleum is cracked to produce gasoline, consists in large part of olefins, particularly ethylene and propylene, and is being used more and more for the manufacture of such materials as glycol and glycerin, glycol dinitrate and nitroglycerin, mustard gas, ethanolamine and pentryl. The olefins under ordinary conditions combine with two atoms of chlorine, adding them readily to the unsaturated linkage, and thereafter react with chlorine no further. It has been found that chlorine does not add to hot propylene in the gas phase, but substitutes instead, one of the hydrogen atoms of the methyl group being replaced [200] and allyl chloride being formed. This at a lower temperature adds chlorine normally to

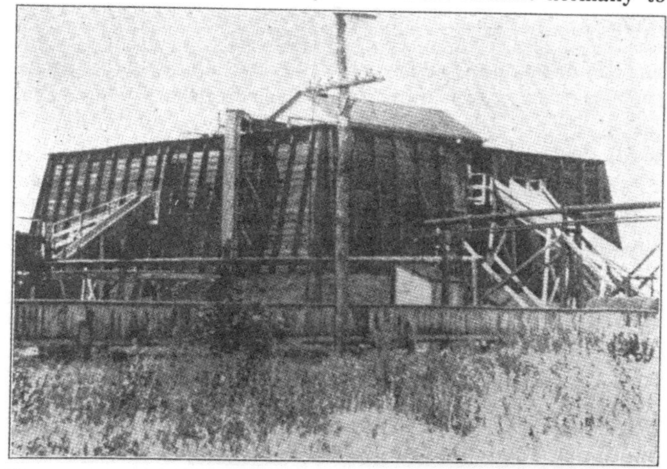

FIGURE 52. Nitroglycerin Nitrating House.

form 1,2,3-trichloropropane which gives glycerin on hydrolysis.

$$
\begin{array}{ccccccccc}
CH_3 & & CH_2{-}Cl & & CH_2{-}Cl & & CH_2{-}OH & & CH_2{-}ONO_2 \\
| & & | & & | & & | & & | \\
CH & \longrightarrow & CH & \longrightarrow & CH{-}Cl & \longrightarrow & CH{-}OH & \longrightarrow & CH{-}ONO_2 \\
\| & & \| & & | & & | & & | \\
CH_2 & & CH_2 & & CH_2{-}Cl & & CH_2{-}OH & & CH_2{-}ONO_2
\end{array}
$$

Nitroglycerin is formed and remains in solution if glycerin is added to a large excess of strong nitric acid. Heat is evolved, and cooling is necessary. The nitroglycerin is thrown out as a heavy oil when the solution is diluted with water. A further quantity of the substance is procured by extracting the dilute acid liquors with chloroform. Naoúm reports that 100 grams of glycerin treated in this manner with 1000 grams of 99% nitric acid yields 207.2 grams of nitroglycerin analyzing 18.16% nitrogen (calc. 18.50% N) and containing a small amount of dinitroglycerin (glyceryl dinitrate). The yield of the trinitrate may be improved by the addition to the nitric acid of dehydrating agents such as phosphorus pentoxide, calcium nitrate, or strong sulfuric acid.

201

Thus, if 100 grams of glycerin is added with cooling to a solution of 150 grams of phosphorus pentoxide in the strongest nitric acid, phosphoric acid precipitates as a heavy syrupy layer and the supernatant acid liquid on dilution yields about 200 grams of nitroglycerin. The yield is substantially the same if the glycerin is first dissolved in the nitric acid alone and if the phosphorus pentoxide is added afterwards. One hundred grams of glycerin in 500 grams of the strongest nitric acid, 400 grams of anhydrous

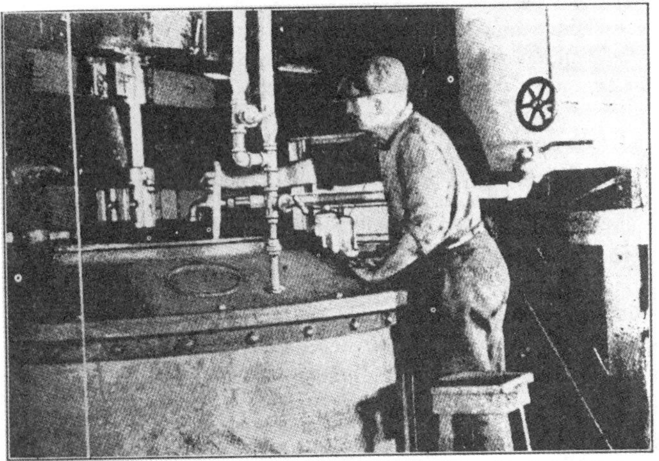

FIGURE 53. Nitroglycerin Nitrator. (Courtesy E. I. du Pont de Nemours and Company, Inc.)

calcium nitrate being added and the mixture allowed to stand for some hours, gives on drowning and purification 220 grams of nitroglycerin which contains about 10% of glyceryl dinitrate.

All these methods are too expensive, for the excess of nitric acid is lost or has to be recovered from dilute solution. A process in which the nitroglycerin comes out as a separate phase without the spent acid being diluted is preferable—and it is indeed true that the addition of strong sulfuric acid to a solution of glycerin in strong nitric acid completes the esterification and causes the nitroglycerin to separate out. Since the strongest nitric acid is expensive to manufacture, and since a mixture of less strong nitric acid with oleum (sulfuric acid containing free sulfur trioxide)

202

may be identical in all respects with a mixture of strong nitric and strong sulfuric acids, glycerin is universally nitrated in commercial practice by means of acid already mixed, and the nitroglycerin is procured by means of gravity separation of the phases. One hundred parts by weight of glycerin yield 225 to 235 parts of nitroglycerin.

One part of glycerin is nitrated with about 6 parts of mixed acid, made up by the use of oleum and containing about 40.0%

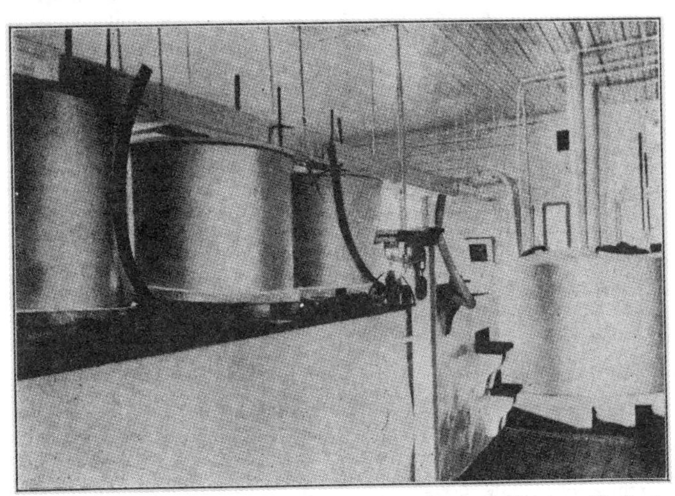

FIGURE 54. Interior of Nitroglycerin Storage House. (Courtesy E. I. du Pont de Nemours and Company, Inc.)

of nitric acid, 59.5% of sulfuric acid, and 0.5% of water. The nitration in this country is carried out in cast iron or steel nitrators, in Europe in nitrators of lead. The glycerin is commonly added from a cock, controlled by hand, in a stream about the size of a man's finger. The mixture is stirred by compressed air, and the temperature is controlled carefully by means of brine coils, there being usually two thermometers, one in the liquid, one in the gas phase above it. In Great Britain the temperature of the nitration mixture is not allowed to rise above 22°C., in this country generally not above 25°. If the temperature for any reason gets out of control, or if the workman sees red fumes through the window in the nitrator, then the charge is dumped

203

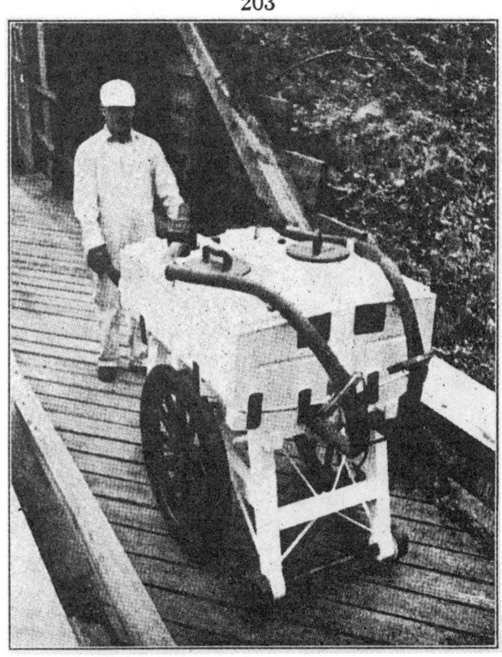

FIGURE 55. Nitroglycerin Buggy. (Courtesy Hercules Powder Company.) For transporting nitroglycerin from the storage house to the house where it is mixed with the other ingredients of dynamite. Note the absence of valves and the use of wooden hose clamps as a safety precaution.

quickly into a drowning tank and the danger is averted. The safety precautions which are everywhere exercised are such that the explosion of a nitroglycerin plant is a rare occurrence. After all the glycerin has been added to the nitrator, agitation and cooling are continued until the temperature drops to about 15°, and the mixture is then run off to the *separator* where the nitroglycerin rises to the top. The spent acid contains 9 to 10% of nitric acid, 72 to 74% of sulfuric acid, and 16 to 18% of water.

The nitroglycerin from the separator contains about 10% of its weight of dissolved acid (about 8% nitric and about 2% sulfuric). Most of this is removed by a *drowning wash* or *prewash* carried out, in Europe with water at about 15°, in this

204

country with water at 38° to 43°, while the mixture is agitated with compressed air. The higher temperature reduces the viscosity of the nitroglycerin and increases greatly the efficiency of the washing. The nitroglycerin is heavier than water and sinks rapidly to the bottom. It is washed again with water, then with sodium carbonate solution (2 or 3%), and then with water until the washings give no color with phenolphthalein and the nitroglycerin itself is neutral to litmus paper. In this country the nitroglycerin is sometimes given a final wash with a concentrated solution of common salt. This reduces the moisture which is suspended in it, to about the same extent as the filtration to which it is commonly subjected in European practice. The nitroglycerin then goes to storage tanks in a heated building where there is no danger of freezing. It has a milky appearance at first, but this quickly disappears. After one day of storage it generally contains not more than 0.3 or 0.4% of moisture, and this amount does not interfere with its use for the manufacture of dynamite.

Pure nitroglycerin is odorless at ordinary temperatures, but has a faint and characteristic odor at temperatures above 50°. Its specific gravity is 1.6009 at 15° and 1.5910 at 25°. It contracts on freezing. Its vapor pressure has been reported by Marshall and Peace to be 0.00025 mm. at 20°, 0.00083 mm. at 30°, 0.0024 at 40°, 0.0072 at 50°, 0.0188 at 60°, 0.043 at 70°, 0.098 at 80°, and 0.29 mm. at 93.3°. About 5 cc. of nitroglycerin passes over with one liter of water in a steam distillation. Snelling and Storm heated nitroglycerin at atmospheric pressure in a distillation apparatus behind an adequate barricade. They reported that

> Nitroglycerin begins to decompose at temperatures as low as 50° or 60°C. . . . At a temperature of about 135°C. the decomposition of nitroglycerin is so rapid as to cause the liquid to become of a strongly reddish color, owing to the absorption of the nitrous fumes resulting from that which is decomposed; and at a temperature of about 145°C. the evolution of decomposition products is so rapid that, at atmospheric pressures, ebullition begins, and the liquid
>
> 205
>
> "boils" strongly. This "boiling" is due in part to the evolution of decomposition products (mainly oxides of nitrogen and water vapor) and in part to the actual volatilization of nitroglycerin itself.

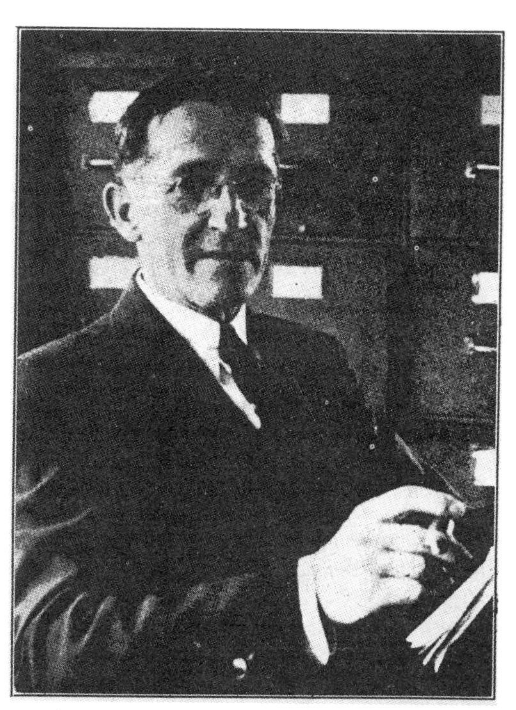

FIGURE 56. C. G. Storm. Author of numerous articles and government publications on the properties, testing, and analysis of smokeless powder and high explosives. Explosives Chemist at Navy Powder Works, 1901-1909, at U. S. Bureau of Mines, 1909-1915; Directing Chemist, Aetna Explosives Company, 1915-1917; Major and Lieutenant-Colonel, Ordnance Department, 1917-1919; Research Chemist, Trojan Powder Company, 1919; Chief Explosives Chemical Engineer, Office of the Chief of Ordnance, War Department, 1919-1942; since early in 1942, Technical Director, National Fireworks, Inc.

> . . . At temperatures between 145° and 215°C. the ebullition of nitroglycerin becomes more and more violent; at higher temperatures the amount of heat produced by the
>
> 206
>
> decomposing liquid becomes proportionately greater, and at about 218°C. nitroglycerin explodes.
>
> When nitroglycerin is maintained at a temperature between 145° and 210°C., its decomposition goes on rapidly, accompanied by much volatilization, and under these conditions nitroglycerin may be readily distilled. The distillate consists of nitroglycerin, nitric acid, water, and other decomposition products. The residue that remains after heating nitroglycerin under such conditions for some time probably consists mainly of glycerin, with small amounts of dinitroglycerin, mononitroglycerin, and other decomposition products. These substances are far less explosive than ordinary nitroglycerin, and accordingly by heating nitroglycerin slowly it can be caused to "boil" away until the residue consists of products that are practically non-explosive. In a number of experiments nitroglycerin was thus heated, and a copious residue was obtained. By carefully raising the

	B.P. (2 mm.) Experimental, °C.	B.P. (50 mm.) Experimental, °C.	B.P. (760 mm.) Most Probable Value, °C.	Ignition Temperature, °C.
Methyl nitrate	...	5	66	...
Glycol dinitrate	70	125	197 ± 3	195–200
TNT	190	245–250	300 ± 10	295–300
Picric acid	195	255	325 ± 10	300–310
TNB	175	250	315 ± 10	...
PETN	160	180	200 ± 10	215
Nitroglycerin	125	180	245 ± 5	200

temperature this residue could be made to char without explosion.

Belyaev and Yuzefovich heated nitroglycerin and other explosives in vacuum, and procured the results summarized in the following table. The fact that ignition temperatures are fairly close to probable boiling points indicates that high concentrations of vapor exist at the moment when the substances ignite. The authors point out that TNT, PETN, and picric acid neither detonate nor burn in vacuum and suggest that this is probably [207] because the boiling points in vacuum are considerably below the ignition temperatures.

Nitroglycerin crystallizes in two forms, a stable form, dipyramidal rhombic crystals, which melt or freeze at 13.2–13.5°, and a labile form, glassy-appearing triclinic crystals, m.p. 1.9–2.2°. It does not freeze readily or quickly. When cooled rapidly, it becomes more and more viscous and finally assumes the state of a hard glassy mass, but this is not true freezing, and the glassy mass becomes a liquid again at a temperature distinctly below the melting point of the crystalline substance. Nitroglycerin in dynamite freezes in crystals if the explosive is stored for a considerable length of time at low temperatures, the form in which it solidifies being determined apparently by the nature of the materials with which it is mixed. If liquid nitroglycerin is cooled strongly, say to $-20°$ or $-60°$, stirred with a glass rod, and seeded with particles of one or the other form, then it crystallizes in the form with which it has been seeded. If the solid is melted by warming, but not warmed more than a few degrees above its melting point, it will on being cooled solidify in the form, whether labile or stable, from which it had been melted. If, however, it is warmed for some time at 50°, it loses all preference for crystallizing in one form rather than in the other, and now shows the usual phenomena of supercooling when it is chilled. Crystals of the labile form may be preserved sensibly unchanged for a week or two, but gradually lose their transparency and change over to the stable form. Crystals of the stable form cannot be changed to the labile form except by melting, warming above the melting point, and seeding with the labile form.

Nitroglycerin is miscible in all proportions at ordinary temperatures with methyl alcohol, acetone, ethyl ether, ethyl acetate, glacial acetic acid, benzene, toluene, nitrobenzene, phenol, chloroform, and ethylene chloride, and with homologous nitric esters such as dinitroglycerin, dinitrochlorohydrin, nitroglycol, and trimethyleneglycol dinitrate. Absolute ethyl, propyl, isopropyl, and amyl alcohols mix with nitroglycerin in all proportions if they are hot, but their solvent power falls off rapidly at lower temperatures. One hundred grams of absolute ethyl alcohol dissolves [208] 37.5 grams of nitroglycerin at 0°, 54.0 grams at 20°. One hundred grams of nitroglycerin on the other hand dissolves 3.4 grams of ethyl alcohol at 0°, 5.5 grams at 20°.

Nitroglycerin dissolves aromatic nitro compounds, such as dinitrotoluene and trinitrotoluene, in all proportions when warm. When the liquids are cooled, 100 grams of nitroglycerin at 20° still holds in solution 35 grams of DNT or 30 grams of TNT. Both nitroglycerin and the polynitro aromatic compounds are solvents or gelatinizing agents for nitrocellulose.

Nitroglycerin dissolves in concentrated sulfuric acid with the liberation of its nitric acid, and may therefore be analyzed by means of the nitrometer (see below).

Nitroglycerin is destroyed by boiling with alcoholic sodium or potassium hydroxide, but glycerin is not formed; the reaction appears to be in accordance with the following equation.

$$C_3H_5(ONO_2)_3 + 5KOH \longrightarrow KNO_3 + 2KNO_2 + H\text{—}COOK + CH_3\text{—}COOK + 3H_2O$$

This however is not the whole story, for resinous products, oxalic acid, and ammonia are also formed. If the reaction with caustic alkali is carried out in the presence of thiophenol, some glycerin is formed and the thiophenol is oxidized to diphenyl sulfide. Alkali sulfides, K_2S, KHS, and CaS, also yield glycerin.

Nitroglycerin vapors cause severe and persistent headache. A workman who is exposed to them constantly soon acquires an immunity. If he is transferred to another part of the plant, he may retain his immunity by paying a short visit every few days to the area in which the nitroglycerin is being used. Workmen appear to suffer no ill effects from handling the explosive continually with the naked hands. Nitroglycerin relaxes the arteries, and is used in medicine under the name of *glonoin. Spirit of glonoin* is a 1% solution of nitroglycerin in alcohol. The usual dose for angina pectoris is one drop of this spirit taken in water, or one lactose or dextrose pellet, containing 1/100 grain (0.0006 gram) of nitroglycerin, dissolved under the tongue.

Nitroglycerin is not easily inflammable. If a small quantity is ignited, it burns with a slight crackling and a pale green flame—and may be extinguished readily before all is burned. If a larger amount is burned in such manner that the heat accumulates and [209] the temperature rises greatly, or if local overheating occurs as by burning in an iron pot, then an explosion ensues. The explosion of nitroglycerin by heat is conveniently demonstrated by heating a stout steel plate to dull redness, removing the source of heat, and allowing the nitroglycerin to fall drop by drop slowly onto the plate while it is cooling. At first the drops assume the spheroidal condition when they strike the plate and deflagrate or burn with a flash, but when the plate cools somewhat each drop yields a violent explosion.

Nitroglycerin is very sensitive to shock, and its sensitivity is greater if it is warm. A drop of the liquid on a steel anvil, or a drop absorbed by filter paper and the paper placed upon the anvil, is detonated by the blow of a steel hammer. The shock of iron striking against stone, or of porcelain against porcelain, also explodes nitroglycerin, that of bronze against bronze less readily, and of wood against wood much less so. Stettbacher reports drop tests with a 2-kilogram weight: mercury fulminate 4.5 cm., lead azide 9 cm., nitroglycerin 10–12 cm., blasting gelatin 12–15 cm., and tetryl 30–35 cm. He also reports the observations of Kast and Will and of Will that nitroglycerin at 90° requires only half as much drop to explode it as nitroglycerin at ordinary temperature, while the frozen material requires about three times as much.

Nitroglycerin and nitroglycerin explosives, like all other high explosives, show different velocities of detonation under different conditions of initiation and loading. They are sometimes described as having low and high velocities of detonation. Berthelot found for nitroglycerin a velocity of 1300 meters per second in lead or tin tubes of 3 mm. internal diameter. Abel found 1525 meters per second in lead pipe 30 mm. internal diameter, while Mettegang found 2050 meters per second in iron pipes of the same internal diameter. Comey and Holmes working with pipes of 25–37.5 mm. internal diameter found values varying from 1300–1500 to 8000–8500 meters per second, and, with especially strong detonators, they regularly found velocities between 6700 and 7500 meters per second. Naoúm[210] reports that blasting gelatin (92–93% NG, 7–8% collodion nitrocotton) has a low velocity of 1600–2000 meters per second and a high velocity of about 8000. Blasting gelatin filled with air bubbles always shows the higher velocity, while clear and transparent blasting gelatin almost always shows the lower velocity of detonation. Frozen dynamite is more difficult to initiate, but always detonates at the high velocity.

Certain properties of nitroglycerin and of other explosives, reported by Brunswig, are tabulated below and compared in a manner to show the relative power of the substances. The spe-

	Specific Volume, Liters	Explosion Temperature, °C.	Heat of Explosion, Calories	Characteristic Product
Nitroglycerin	712	3470	1580	1,125,000
Nitromannite	723	3430	1520	1,099,000
Blasting gelatin (93% NG, 7% NC)	710	3540	1640	1,164,000
75% Guhr dynamite	628	3160	1290	810,000
Nitrocotton (13% N)	859	2710	1100	945,000
Picric acid	877	2430	810	710,000
Black powder	285	2770	685	195,000
Ammonium nitrate	937	2120	630	590,000
Mercury fulminate	314	3530	410	129,000

cific volume is the volume, at 0° and 760 mm., of the gaseous products of the explosion. This number multiplied by the heat of explosion gives the *characteristic product* which Berthelot considered to be a measure of the mechanical work performed by the explosion. The mechanical work has also been estimated, differently, in kilogram-meters by multiplying the heat of explosion by 425, the mechanical equivalent of heat.

Naoúm reports the results of his own experiments with nitroglycerin and with other explosives in the Trauzl lead block test (sand tamping), 10-gram samples, as shown below. The Trauzl test is essentially a measure of brisance, but for explosives of similar velocities of detonation it supplies[211] a basis for the comparison of their total energies.

	Expansion, Cubic Centimeters
Nitroglycerin	550
Nitromannite	560
Compressed guncotton (13.2% N)	420
Blasting gelatin	580
65% Gelatin dynamite	410
75% Guhr dynamite	325
Tetryl	360
Picric acid	300
Trinitrotoluene	285
Mercury fulminate	150

For several years after the discovery of nitroglycerin, the possibility of using it as an explosive attracted very little interest. Indeed, it first came into use as a medicine, and the first serious study on its preparation, after the work of Sobrero, was made by J. E. de Vrij, professor of chemistry in the Medical School at Rotterdam, and published in the Dutch journal of pharmacy, *Tijdschrift voor wetensch. pharm.*, in 1855. The next significant work was done by Alfred Nobel who in 1864 patented improvements both in the process of manufacturing nitroglycerin and in the method of exploding it. No liquid explosive had been successful in practical use. Nobel believed that he had solved the difficulty by taking advantage of the property of nitroglycerin of exploding from heat or from the shock of an explosion. A small glass vessel containing black powder was to be immersed in the nitroglycerin and exploded. Another method was by the local heat of an electric spark or of a wire electrically heated under the surface of the nitroglycerin. And another was the percussion cap. Nobel used black powder first in glass bulbs, later in hollow wooden cylinders closed with cork stoppers, then a mixture of black powder and mercury fulminate, and later fulminate in small lead capsules and finally in the copper detonators which are still in general use. The invention of the blasting cap depended upon the discovery of the phenomenon of initiation, and signalized the beginning of a new era in the history of explosives.[212] Blasting caps were used first for the safe and certain explosion of the dangerous liquid nitroglycerin, but presently they were found to be exactly what was needed for the explosion of the safer and less sensitive dynamites which Nobel also invented.

The first establishment for the manufacture of nitroglycerin in industrial quantities was a laboratory set up by Alfred Nobel and his father, Immanuel Nobel, probably in the autumn of 1863, near the latter's home at Heleneborg near Stockholm. An explosion which occurred there in September, 1864, cost the life of Alfred's younger brother, Emil, and of four other persons. The manufacture of nitroglycerin was prohibited within the city area, but the explosive was already in practical use for the tunnelling operations of the State Railway, and it was desirable to continue its manufacture. The manufacture was removed to a pontoon moored in Malar Lake and was continued there during the late autumn of 1864 and during the following winter until March, 1865, when it was transferred to a new factory, the first real nitroglycerin factory in the world, at Winterwik near Stockholm. Later in the same year the Nobel company commenced manufacturing nitroglycerin in Germany, at a plant near Hamburg, and within a few years was operating explosives factories in the United States and in all the principal countries of Europe.

The first considerable engineering operation in the United States to be accomplished by means of nitroglycerin was the blasting out of the Hoosac tunnel in Massachusetts. The work had been progressing slowly until George M. Mowbray, an "operative chemist" of North Adams, was engaged to manufacture nitroglycerin at the site of the work and to supervise its use. Twenty-six feet of tunnel was driven during May, 1868, 21 during June, 47 during July when the use of nitroglycerin commenced, 44 during August, and 51 feet during September. Mowbray profited by the observation of W. P. Granger that frozen nitroglycerin could not be detonated, and accordingly transported his[213] material in safety in the frozen condition.[29] He described an explosion which occurred in December, 1870, in which the life of a foreman was lost, and another in March, 1871, in which a large amount of frozen nitroglycerin failed to explode.

[29] During the severe winter of 1867 and 1868, the Deerfield dam became obstructed with ice, and it was important that it should be cleared out without delay. W. P. Granger, Esq., engineer in charge, determined

to attempt its removal by a blast of nitroglycerine. In order to appreciate the following details, it must be borne in mind that the current literature of this explosive distinctly asserted that, when congealed, the slightest touch or jar was sufficient to explode nitroglycerine. Mr. Granger desired me to prepare for him ten cartridges, and, as he had to carry them in his sleigh from the west end of the tunnel to the east end or Deerfield dam, a distance of nine miles over the mountain, he requested them to be packed in such a way that they would not be affected by the inclement weather. I therefore caused the nitroglycerine to be warmed up to ninety degrees, warmed the cartridges, and, after charging them, packed them in a box with sawdust that had been heated to the same temperature; the box was tied to the back of the sleigh, with a buffalo robe thrown over it. In floundering across the divide where banks, road, hedge and water courses were indistinguishable beneath the drifted snow, horse, sleigh and rider were upset, the box of cartridges got loose, and were spread indiscriminately over the snow. After rectifying this mishap, picking up the various contents of the sleigh, and getting ready to start again, it occurred to Mr. Granger to examine his cartridges; his feelings may be imagined when he discovered the nitroglycerine frozen solid. To have left them behind and proceeded to the dam, where miners, engineers and laborers were waiting to see this then much dreaded explosive, would never do; so accepting the situation, he replaced them in the case, and, laying it between his feet, proceeded on his way, thinking a heap but saying nothing. Arrived, he forthwith attached fuse, exploder, powder and some guncotton, and inserted the cartridge in the ice. Lighting the fuse, he retired to a proper distance to watch the explosion. Presently a sharp crack indicated that the fuse had done its work, and, on proceeding to the hole drilled in the ice, it was found that fragments of the copper cap were imbedded in the solid cylinder of congealed nitroglycerine, which was driven through and out of the tin cartridge into the anchor ice beneath, but not exploded. A second attempt was attended with like results. Foiled in attempting to explode the frozen nitroglycerine, Mr. Granger thawed the contents of another cartridge, attached the fuse and exploder as before; this time the explosion was entirely successful. From that day I have never transported nitroglycerine except in a frozen condition, and to that lesson are we indebted for the safe transmission of more than two hundred and fifty thousand pounds of this explosive, over the roughest roads of New Hampshire, Vermont, Massachusetts, New York, and the coal and oil regions of Pennsylvania, in spring wagons with our own teams.

The new magazine had hardly been completed, and stored with nitroglycerine, when, on Sunday morning, at half past six o'clock, March twelfth, 1871, the neighborhood was startled by another explosion of sixteen hundred pounds of nitroglycerine. The cause of this last explosion was continuous overheating of the magazine. . . . The watchman con-

214

fessed he had neglected to examine the thermometer, made his fire under the boiler, and gone to bed. . . . Fortunately, this accident involved no damage to life or limb, whilst a very instructive lesson was taught in the following circumstance: Within twelve feet of the magazine was a shed, sixteen feet by eight, containing twelve fifty-pound cans of congealed nitroglycerine ready for shipment. This shed was utterly destroyed, the floor blasted to splinters, the joists rent to fragments, the cans of congealed nitroglycerine driven into the ground, the tin of which they were composed perforated, contorted, battered, and portions of tin and nitroglycerine sliced off but not exploded. Now, this fact proves one of two things: Either that the tri-nitroglycerine made by the Mowbray process, differs from the German nitroglycerine in its properties, or the statements printed in the foreign journals, as quoted again and again, that nitroglycerine, when congealed, is more dangerous than when in the fluid state, are erroneous.

Mowbray used his nitroglycerin in the liquid state, either loaded in cylindrical tin cannisters or cartridges, or poured directly into the bore hole, and exploded it by means of electric detonators. The electric detonators were operated by means of a static electric machine which caused a spark to pass between points of insulated wire; the spark set fire to a priming mixture made from copper sulfide, copper phosphide, and potassium chlorate; and this fired the detonating charge of 20 grains of mercury fulminate contained in a copper capsule, the whole being waterproofed with asphaltum varnish and insulated electrically with gutta-percha. The devices were so sensitive that they could be exploded by the static electricity which accumulated on the body of a miner operating a compressed air drill, and they required corresponding precautions in their use.

Liquid nitroglycerin is still used as an explosive to a limited extent, particularly in the blasting of oil wells, but its principal use is in the manufacture of dynamite and of the propellants, ballistite and cordite.

Dinitroglycerin (Glyceryl dinitrate)

Dinitroglycerin does not differ greatly from nitroglycerin in its explosive properties. It is appreciably soluble in water, and more expensive and more difficult to manufacture than nitrogly-

215

cerin. It mixes with the latter substance in all proportions and lowers its freezing point, and was formerly used in Germany in such mixtures in non-freezing dynamites. It has now been superseded entirely for that purpose by dinitrochlorohydrin which is insoluble in water, and cheaper and more convenient to manufacture.

Dinitroglycerin is never formed alone by the nitration of glycerin but is always accompanied by the trinitrate or the mononitrate or both. If the nitration is carried out in a manner to give the best yields of the dinitrate, then considerable trinitrate is formed: if the process is modified to reduce the yield of trinitrate, then the yield of dinitrate is also reduced and some mononitrate is formed. If 3 or 4 parts by weight of nitric acid is added slowly to 1 part of glycerin, so that the glycerin or its nitrated product is always in excess, then the dinitrate is the principal product. If the order of mixing is reversed, so that the glycerin dissolves first in the strong nitric acid, then the yield of trinitrate is more considerable. Dinitroglycerin is formed if glycerin is added to mixed acid which is low in nitric acid or high in water, or which contains insufficient sulfuric acid for the necessary dehydrating action. It is also one of the products of the hydrolysis of nitroglycerin by cold concentrated (95%) sulfuric acid, the trinitrate by this reagent being in part dissolved and in part converted to the dinitrate, the mononitrate, and to glyceryl sulfate according to the relative amount of sulfuric acid which is used. Dinitroglycerin is separated from its mixture with nitroglycerin and obtained pure by treating the oil with about 15 volumes of water, separating the insoluble trinitrate, extracting the aqueous solution with ether, washing the ether with dilute sodium carbonate solution, and evaporating. The resulting dinitroglycerin gives a poor heat test because of the peroxide which it contains from the ether. Material which gives an excellent heat test may be procured by evaporating the aqueous solution in vacuum.

The dinitroglycerin obtained by the nitration of glycerin is a colorless, odorless oil, more viscous and more volatile than nitroglycerin. It causes the same kind of a headache. It has a specific gravity of 1.51 at 15°, boils at 146–148° at 15 mm. with only slight decomposition, and solidifies at $-40°$ to a glassy solid which melts if the temperature is raised to $-30°$. It is readily

216

soluble in alcohol, ether, acetone, and chloroform, somewhat less soluble than nitroglycerin in benzene, and insoluble in carbon tetrachloride and ligroin. It consists of a mixture of the two possible structural isomers, the 1,2- or α,β-dinitrate, known also as "dinitroglycerin F," and the 1,3- or α,α'-dinitrate or "dinitroglycerin K." Both are uncrystallizable oils, and both are hygroscopic and take up about 3% of their weight of moisture from the air. They are separated by virtue of the fact that the α,α'-dinitrate, forms a hydrate with one-third of a molecule of water, $C_3H_6O_7N_2 + \frac{1}{3} H_2O$, water-clear prisms, m.p. 26°. No hydrate of the α,β-dinitrate has ever been isolated in the state of a crystalline solid. If a test portion of the moist mixture of the isomers is mixed with fuller's earth and chilled strongly, it deposits crystals; and if these are used for seeding the principal quantity of the moist dinitroglycerin, then the hydrate of the α,α′-dinitrate crystallizes out. It may be recrystallized from water, or from alcohol, ether, or benzene without losing its water of crystallization, but it yields the anhydrous α,α′-dinitrate if it is dried over sulfuric acid or warmed in the air at 40°.

The chemical relationships between the mononitroglycerins and dinitroglycerins supply all the evidence which is needed for inferring the identities of the isomers. Of the two mononitrates, the β-compound obviously cannot yield any α,α′-dinitrate by nitration; it can yield only the α,β-. That one of the two isomers which yields only one dinitrate is therefore the β-mononitrate, and the dinitrate which it yields is the α,β-dinitrate. The α-mononitrate on the other hand yields both the α,β- and the α,α′-dinitrates.

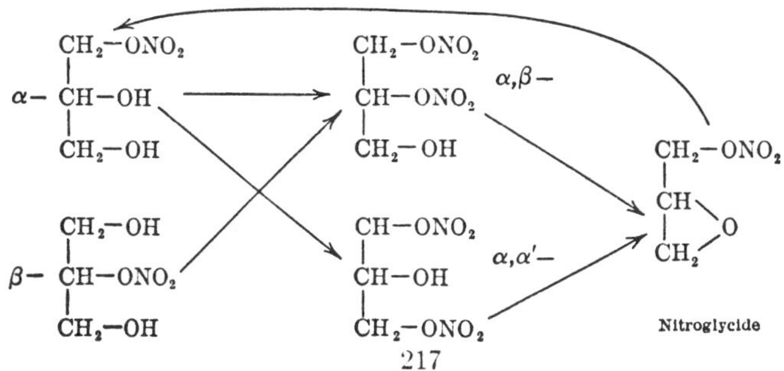

[217]

Both of the dinitroglycerins on treatment with 30% sodium hydroxide solution at room temperature yield nitroglycide, and this substance on boiling with water gives α-mononitroglycerin, a series of reactions which demonstrates the identity of the last-named compound.

Dinitroglycerin is a feeble acid and gives a wine-red color with blue litmus, but none of its salts appear to have been isolated and characterized. It does not decompose carbonates, but dissolves in caustic alkali solutions more readily than in water. One hundred parts of water alone dissolves about 8 parts at 15° and about 10 parts at 50°.

Dinitroglycerin gelatinizes collodion nitrocotton rapidly at ordinary temperature. The gel is sticky, less elastic, and more easily deformed than a nitroglycerin gel. Unlike the latter it is hygroscopic, and becomes softer and greasier from the absorption of moisture from the air. Water dissolves out the dinitroglycerin and leaves the nitrocellulose as a tough, stiff mass.

Dinitroglycerin has about the same sensitivity to initiation as nitroglycerin, only slightly less sensitivity to shock, and offers no marked advantages from the point of view of safety. It shows a greater stability in the heat test, and a small amount can be evaporated by heat without explosion or deflagration. It gives off red fumes above 150°, and at 170° decomposes rapidly with volatilization and some deflagration, or in larger quantities shows a tendency to explode.

Naoúm reports that a 10-gram sample of dinitroglycerin in the Trauzl test with water tamping gave a net expansion of about 500 cc., or 83.3% as much as the expansion (600 cc.) produced by 10 grams of nitroglycerin under the same conditions. He points out that the ratio here is almost the same as the ratio between the heats of explosion, and that in this case the Trauzl test has supplied a fairly accurate measure of the relative energy contents of the two explosives. In the small lead block test the effect of the greater brisance and higher velocity of detonation of nitroglycerin becomes apparent; 100 grams of dinitroglycerin gave a compression of 21 mm. while the same amount of nitroglycerin gave one of 30 mm.[218]

Mononitroglycerin (Glyceryl mononitrate)

Mononitroglycerin is a by-product in the preparation of dinitroglycerin and is separated from the latter substance by its greater solubility in water. It is usually obtained as a colorless oil, density 1.417 at 15°, more viscous than dinitroglycerin and less viscous than nitroglycerin. This oil is a mixture of the two isomers which are crystalline when separate but show little tendency to crystallize when they are mixed. α-Mononitroglycerin when pure consists of colorless prisms, m.p. 58–59°, specific gravity 1.53 at 15°; it yields both of the dinitrates on nitration. The β-compound crystallizes in dendrites and leaflets, m.p. 54°, and is more readily soluble in ether than the α-compound; it yields only the α,β-dinitrate on nitration. Both isomers boil at 155–160° at 15 mm.

Mononitroglycerin resembles glycerin in being very hygroscopic and miscible in all proportions with water and alcohol, and in being only slightly soluble in ether, but it differs from glycerin in being freely soluble in nitroglycerin. It does not form a satisfactory gel with collodion cotton. Its aqueous solution reacts neutral. It appears to be perfectly stable on moderate heating, but decomposes to some extent at 170°, gives off gas, and turns yellow.

Mononitroglycerin is insensitive to shock. In the form of oil it is not detonated by a No. 8 blasting cap in the Trauzl test. If the oil is absorbed in fuller's earth, 10 grams gives a net expansion of 75 cc. The crystalline material, however, detonates easily; 10 grams gives an expansion of 245 cc. It is interesting to compare these results, reported by Naoúm, with the results which the same author reports for nitroglycide which is the anhydride of mononitroglycerin. Ten grams of liquid nitroglycide with water tamping and a No. 8 detonator gave a net expansion of 430 cc.; 10 grams absorbed in fuller's earth, with sand tamping, gave 310 cc.; and 10 grams gelatinized with 5% collodion nitrocotton, with sand tamping, gave 395 cc.

Nitroglycide

This substance cannot be prepared by the nitration of glycide, for the action of acids upon that substance opens the ethylene[219] oxide ring, and mononitroglycerin is formed. Nitroglycide was first prepared by Naoúm in 1907 by shaking dinitroglycerin at room temperature with a 30% aqueous solution of sodium hydroxide. The clear solution presently deposited a colorless oil, and this, washed with water and dried in a desiccator, constituted a practically quantitative yield of nitroglycide.

Nitroglycide is a very mobile liquid with a faint but pleasant aromatic odor, specific gravity 1.332 at 20°. It does not freeze at −20°. It boils at 94° at 20 mm., and with some decomposition at 174–175° at atmospheric pressure. It is not hygroscopic but is distinctly soluble in water, 5 grams in 100 cc. at 20°. Ether will extract nitroglycide from the cool aqueous solution; if the solution is boiled, however, the nitroglycide is hydrated to mononitroglycerin. Nitroglycide is miscible in all proportions with alcohol, ether, acetone, ethyl acetate, and nitroglycerin. It gelatinizes collodion nitrocotton and even guncotton rapidly at ordinary temperature. It explodes in contact with concentrated sulfuric acid. If dissolved in dilute sulfuric acid and then treated with strong sulfuric acid, it gives off nitric acid. It is converted into dinitroglycerin and nitroglycerin by the action of nitric acid. It dissolves in concentrated hydrochloric acid with the evolution of considerable heat, and the solution on dilution with water gives a precipitate of monochlorohydrin mononitrate. Nitroglycide reduces ammoniacal silver nitrate slowly on gentle warming; glycide reduces the same reagent in the cold.

When heated rapidly in a test tube nitroglycide explodes with a sharp report at 195–200°. It is more easily detonated than liquid nitroglycerin. Naoúm believes that its great sensitivity results mainly from the easy propagation of the wave of detonation by a liquid of low viscosity. He points out further that mononitroglycerin has 69.5% of the energy content (i.e., heat of explosion) of nitroglycide, but as a crystal powder in the Trauzl test it gives only about 62% as much net expansion, whence it is to be inferred that nitroglycide has the higher velocity of detonation. Nitroglycide has only 52% of the energy content of nitroglycerin, but produces 72% as much effect in the Trauzl test. It is therefore "relatively more brisant than nitroglycerin."

[220]

Dinitrochlorohydrin (Glycerin chlorohydrin dinitrate)

Among the various substances which may be used in admixture with nitroglycerin for the purpose of lowering its freezing point, dinitrochlorohydrin is preferred in Germany but has not found favor in the United States. Since dinitrochlorohydrin is distinctly safer to prepare than nitroglycerin, it is most commonly prepared by itself, that is, by the nitration of chlorohydrin which is substantially pure and contains not more than a small amount of glycerin. The product is used directly for the preparation of certain explosives, or it is mixed with nitroglycerin for the manufacture of non-freezing dynamites.

Chlorohydrin is prepared by autoclaving glycerin with concentrated hydrochloric acid or by treating it at moderate temperature with sulfur chloride. In the former process, in order to avoid the formation of dichlorohydrin, only enough hydrochloric acid is used to convert about 75% of the glycerin. The product is procured by a vacuum distillation. The monochlorohydrin, which consists almost entirely of the α-compound, comes over between 130° and 150° at 12–15 mm. and the unchanged glycerin between 165° and 180°. It is nitrated with the same mixed acid as is used for the preparation of nitroglycerin; less acid is needed of course, less heat is produced, and the process is safer and more rapid.

$$\begin{array}{l} CH_2-OH \\ | \\ CH-OH \\ | \\ CH_2-OH \end{array} \longrightarrow \begin{array}{l} CH_2-Cl \\ | \\ CH-OH \\ | \\ CH_2-OH \end{array} \longrightarrow \begin{array}{l} CH_2-Cl \\ | \\ CH-ONO_2 \\ | \\ CH_2-ONO_2 \end{array}$$

If a mixture of chlorohydrin and glycerin is nitrated, the resulting mixture of nitrates contains relatively more nitroglycerin than the original mixture contained of glycerin, for the relative increase of molecular weight during the nitration of glycerin is greater.

Commercial dinitrochlorohydrin is usually yellowish or brownish in color, specific gravity about 1.541 at 15°. It boils at atmospheric pressure with decomposition at about 190°. It may be distilled at 13 mm. at 121.5°, or at 10 mm. at 117.5°, but some decomposition occurs for the distillate is acid to litmus.

Dinitrochlorohydrin is non-hygroscopic, distinctly more volatile than nitroglycerin, and it has similar physiological effects. It can be frozen only with great difficulty,[221] shows a strong tendency to supercool, and can be kept for a long time at −20° without depositing crystals. The solubility of dinitrochlorohydrin and nitroglycerin in each other is so great that only small quantities of nitroglycerin can be frozen out from the mixtures, even after seeding, at winter temperatures. A mixture of 75 parts of nitroglycerin and 25 parts of dinitrochlorohydrin is practically non-freezing, and yields a dynamite which is not significantly less strong than one made from straight nitroglycerin.

Dinitrochlorohydrin does not take fire readily, and, if ignited, burns rather slowly without detonating and with but little of the sputtering which is characteristic of nitroglycerin mixtures. "Even larger quantities of pure dinitrochlorohydrin in tin cans burn without explosion when in a fire, so that liquid dinitrochlorohydrin is permitted on German railroads in tin cans holding 25 kg., as a safe explosive for limited freight service in the 200 kg. class, while liquid nitroglycerin is absolutely excluded." Dinitrochlorohydrin is more stable toward shock than nitroglycerin. Naoúm, working with a pure sample, was not able to secure a first-rate explosion in the drop test. A 2-kilogram weight dropped from a height of 40 cm. or more gave a very slight partial decomposition and a slight report, from a height of 75 cm. or more, a somewhat more violent partial deflagration but in no case a sharp report, and even a 10-kilogram weight dropped from a height of 10 or 15 cm. gave a very weak partial decomposition. The substance, however, is detonated readily by fulminate. It gives in the Trauzl test a net expansion of 475 cc., or 79% of the 600-cc. expansion given by nitroglycerin, although its heat of explosion is only about 71% of the heat of explosion of nitroglycerin.

Dinitrochlorohydrin produces hydrogen chloride when it explodes. This would tend to make it unsuitable for use in mining explosives were it not for the fact that the incorporation into the explosives of potassium or sodium nitrate sufficient to form chloride with the chlorine of the dinitrochlorohydrin prevents it altogether—and this amount of the nitrate is usually present anyway for other reasons. [222]

Acetyldinitroglycerin (monoacetin dinitrate) and formyldinitroglycerin (monoformin dinitrate) have been proposed by Vender for admixture with nitroglycerin in non-freezing dynamite. The former substance may be prepared by nitrating monoacetin or by acetylating dinitroglycerin. The latter substance may be procured already mixed with nitroglycerin by warming glycerin with oxalic acid, whereby monoformin (glyceryl monoformate) is formed, and nitrating the resulting mixture of monoformin and glycerin. Formyldinitroglycerin has apparently not yet been isolated in the pure state. These substances are satisfactory explosives but are more expensive to manufacture than dinitrochlorohydrin over which they possess no distinct advantage, and they have not come into general use.

Tetranitrodiglycerin (Diglycerin tetranitrate)

If glycerin is heated with a small amount of concentrated

sulfuric acid, ether formation occurs, water splits out, and diglycerin and polyglycerin are formed. If the heating is carried out in the absence of acids, and in such a way that the water which is formed is allowed to escape while the higher-boiling materials are condensed and returned, especially if a small amount of alkali, say 0.5%, or of sodium sulfite is present as a catalyst, then the principal product is diglycerin and not more than a few per cent of polyglycerin is formed. It is feasible for example to convert glycerin into a mixture which consists of 50–60% diglycerin, 4–6% polyglycerin, and the remainder, 34–46%, unchanged glycerin. The diglycerin is ordinarily not isolated in the pure state. The mixture, either with or without the addition of glycerin, is nitrated directly to form a mixture of tetranitrodiglycerin and nitroglycerin which is used for the manufacture of non-freezing dynamite.

Diglycerin when obtained pure by a vacuum distillation is a water-white liquid, more viscous and more dense than glycerin, sweet-tasting, very hygroscopic, b.p. 245–250° at 8 mm. It is nitrated with the same mixed acid as glycerin, although a smaller

223

amount is necessary. Salt solutions are always used for washing the nitrated product, otherwise the separation of the phases is extremely slow.

```
CH2-OH          CH2-OH          CH2-ONO2
|               |               |
CH-OH           CH-OH           CH-ONO2
|               |               |
CH2-O[H]        CH2\            CH2\
      :    --->     O    --->       O
CH2-[OH]        CH2/            CH2/
|               |               |
CH-OH           CH-OH           CH-ONO2
|               |               |
CH2-OH          CH2-OH          CH2-ONO2
```

Tetranitrodiglycerin is a very viscous oil, non-hygroscopic, insoluble in water, and readily soluble in alcohol and in ether. It has not been obtained in the crystalline state. It is not a good gelatinizing agent for collodion cotton when used alone. Its mixture with nitroglycerin gelatinizes collodion cotton more slowly than nitroglycerin alone but gives a satisfactory gel. It is less sensitive to mechanical shock than nitroglycerin, about the same as dinitroglycerin, but is readily exploded by fulminate. According to Naoúm 75% tetranitrodiglycerin guhr dynamite gave in the Trauzl test a net expansion of 274 cc. or 85.6% of the expansion (320 cc.) produced by 75% nitroglycerin guhr dynamite.

Nitroglycol (Ethylene glycol dinitrate, ethylene dinitrate)

Nitroglycol first found favor in France as an ingredient of non-freezing dynamites. It has many of the advantages of nitroglycerin and is safer to manufacture and handle. Its principal disadvantage is its greater volatility. Formerly the greater cost of procuring glycol, which is not as directly accessible as glycerin but has to be produced by synthesis from ethylene, was an impediment to its use, but new sources of ethylene and new methods of synthesis have reduced its cost and increased its accessibility.

Ethylene was formerly procured from alcohol (itself produced from raw material which was actually or potentially a foodstuff) by warming with sulfuric acid, by passing the vapors over heated coke impregnated with phosphoric acid, or by comparable methods. Ethylene combines with bromine to give ethylene dibromide,

224

which yields glycol by hydrolysis, but bromine is expensive. Ethylene also combines readily with chlorine, but, even if care is exercised always to have the ethylene present in excess, substitution occurs, and tri- and tetrachloroethane are formed along with the ethylene dichloride, and these do not yield glycol by hydrolysis. Ethylene is now produced in large quantities during the cracking of petroleum. Its comportment with chlorine water has been found to be much more satisfactory for purposes of synthesis than its comportment with chlorine gas. Chlorine water contains an equilibrium mixture of hydrogen chloride and hypochlorous acid.

$$Cl_2 + H_2O \leftrightarrows HCl + HOCl$$

Ethylene adds hypochlorous acid more readily than it adds either moist chlorine or hydrogen chloride. Bubbled into chlorine water, it is converted completely into ethylene chlorohydrin, and by the hydrolysis of this substance glycol is obtained. Ethylene chlorohydrin is important also because of its reaction with ammonia whereby mono-, di-, and triethanolamine are formed, substances which are used in the arts and are not without interest for the explosives chemist. Ethylene may be oxidized catalytically in the gas phase to ethylene oxide which reacts with water to form glycol and with glycol to form diglycol which also is of interest to the dynamite maker.

```
              CH2-Cl          CH2-OH          CH2-OH
            / |       --->    |       --->    |
           /  CH2-OH          CH2-OH          CH2\
CH2       /                   Glycol   /          O
||                              /     /       CH2/
CH2       \                    /     /        |
           \  CH2\            /     /         CH2-OH
            \ |   O  --------      /
              CH2/  -------------              Diglycol
```

Glycol is a colorless liquid (bluer than water in thick layers), syrupy, sweet tasting, less viscous than glycerin, specific gravity 1.1270 at 0°, 1.12015 at 10°, and 1.11320 at 20°. It shows a tendency to supercool but freezes at temperatures between −13° and −25°, and melts again at −11.5°. It boils at 197.2° at atmospheric pressure. It is very hygroscopic, miscible in all pro-

225

portions with water, alcohol, glycerin, acetone, and acetic acid, and not miscible with benzene, chloroform, carbon disulfide, and ether.

Nitroglycol is manufactured with the same mixed acid and with the same apparatus as nitroglycerin. Somewhat more heat is produced by the nitration reaction, and, as glycol is less viscous than glycerin, it is feasible to conduct the operation at a lower temperature. The washing is done with cold water and with less agitation by compressed air, and smaller amounts of wash water are used than are used with nitroglycerin, for nitroglycol is appreciably more volatile and more soluble in water. The tendency of the partially washed product to undergo an acid-catalyzed decomposition is less in the case of nitroglycol than in the case of nitroglycerin.

Nitroglycol is a colorless liquid, only slightly more viscous than water, specific gravity ($x°/15°$) 1.5176 at 0°, 1.5033 at 10°, and 1.4890 at 20°. It freezes at about −22.3°. Rinkenbach reports the index of refraction of nitroglycol for white light to be 1.4452 at 22.3°, and that of a commercial sample of nitroglycerin under the same conditions to be 1.4713. The same author reports the vapor pressure of nitroglycol to be 0.007 mm. of mercury at 0° and 0.0565 mm. at 22°, and points out that its vapor pressure at 22° is approximately 150 times as great as the vapor pressure, 0.00037 mm., reported by Peace and Marshall for nitroglycerin at 22°. Nitroglycol produces a headache similar to that produced by nitroglycerin, but, corresponding to its greater volatility, the headache is more violent and does not last so long. Nitroglycol is non-hygroscopic. Its comportment with organic solvents is similar to that of nitroglycerin, but it is distinctly more soluble in water than that substance. Naoúm reports that 1 liter of water at 15° dissolves 6.2 grams of nitroglycol, at 20° 6.8 grams of nitroglycol or 1.8 grams of nitroglycerin, and at 50° 9.2 grams of nitroglycol.

Nitroglycol has a slightly larger energy content than nitroglycerin. In the Trauzl test with 10-gram samples and water tamping, Naoúm found that nitroglycol gave a net expansion [226] of 650 cc. and nitroglycerin one of 590 cc. Nitroglycol, like nitroglycerin, burns with sputtering and explodes if local overheating occurs, but nitroglycol and nitroglycol explosives in general burn more quietly and show less tendency to explode from heat than the corresponding nitroglycerin preparations. Nitroglycol explodes with a sharp report if heated rapidly to 215°. It is less sensitive to mechanical shock than nitroglycerin. Naoúm reports the height of drop necessary to cause explosion, with a 2-kilogram weight, as follows.

	Height of Drop, Centimeters	
	Nitroglycol	Nitroglycerin
Drop absorbed on filter paper	20–25	8–10
Blasting gelatin	25–30	12
Guhr dynamite	15	5

Rinkenbach reports tests with a small drop machine having a weight of 500 grams, nitroglycol 110 cm., nitroglycerin 70 cm., and a commercial mixture of nitroglycerin and nitropolyglycerin 90 cm.

Nitroglycol gelatinizes collodion cotton much faster than nitroglycerin and acts at ordinary temperatures, while nitroglycerin requires to be warmed. The greater volatility of nitroglycol does not affect its usefulness in gelatin dynamite, especially in temperate climates, but renders it unsuitable for use during the warm season of the year in ammonium nitrate explosives which contain only a few per cent of the oily nitric ester. It is too volatile for use in double-base smokeless powder, for its escape by evaporation affects the ballistic properties.

Dinitrodiglycol (Diethylene glycol dinitrate)

A study of the preparation and properties of dinitrodiglycol was reported by Rinkenbach in 1927 and a further study of the nitration of diethylene glycol by Rinkenbach and Aaronson in 1931. Dinitrodiglycol is a viscous, colorless, and odorless liquid, specific gravity ($x°/15°$) 1.4092 at 0°, 1.3969 at 10°, and 1.3846 at 20°, freezing point −11.5°. It is completely miscible at ordinary temperatures with nitroglycerin, nitroglycol, ether, acetone, [227] methyl alcohol, chloroform, benzene, and glacial acetic acid. It is immiscible, or only slightly soluble, in ethyl alcohol, carbon tetrachloride, and carbon disulfide. It is slightly hygroscopic and is soluble in water to the extent of about 4.1 grams per liter of water at 24°. It can be ignited only with difficulty, and in small quantity is not readily exploded by heat. It is less sensitive than nitroglycol in the drop test. It is so insensitive to initiation that it will not propagate its own detonation under conditions where nitroglycol and nitroglycerin will do it. In 50/50 mixture however with either of these substances it detonates satisfactorily "and shows an explosive effect but little less than that of either of these compounds." It has a vapor pressure of about 0.007 mm. of mercury at 22.4°, and produces headaches similar to those produced by nitroglycerin.

Trinitrophenoxyethyl Nitrate

Another explosive which is preparable from glycol and which may perhaps be of interest for special purposes in the future is the β-2,4,6-trinitrophenoxyethyl nitrate described by Wasmer in 1938. Glycol is converted into its monosodium derivative, and this is made to react with dinitrochlorobenzene at 130° for the production of β-dinitrophenoxyethyl alcohol which gives the explosive by nitration with mixed acid.

$$CH_2OH\text{—}CH_2OH \longrightarrow CH_2ONa\text{—}CH_2OH \longrightarrow CH_2\text{—}O\text{—}C_6H_3(NO_2)_2\text{—}CH_2OH \longrightarrow CH_2\text{—}O\text{—}C_6H_2(NO_2)_3\text{—}CH_2\text{—}ONO_2$$

Trinitrophenoxyethyl nitrate is procured as a white powder, m.p. 104.5°, insoluble in water and readily soluble in acetone. It gelatinizes collodion nitrocotton, and is intermediate between picric acid and tetryl in its sensitivity to mechanical shock.

[228]

Nitration of Ethylene

By passing ethylene into a mixture of concentrated nitric and sulfuric acids Kekulé obtained an oil, specific gravity 1.47, which broke down when distilled with steam to give glycollic acid, oxalic acid, nitric oxide, and nitric acid. On reduction with sodium amalgam it yielded glycol and ammonia among other products. Wieland and Sakellarios distilled the Kekulé oil in steam and then in vacuum, and obtained nitroglycol, b.p. 105° at 19 mm., and β-nitroethyl nitrate, b.p. 120–122° at 17 mm. These two substances are evidently formed from ethylene by the reactions indicated below.

$$CH_2{=}CH_2 + HO\text{—}NO_2 \longrightarrow CH_2OH\text{—}CH_2NO_2 \xrightarrow{+\,HNO_3} H_2O + \underset{\beta\text{-Nitroethyl nitrate}}{CH_2ONO_2\text{—}CH_2NO_2}$$

$$CH_2{=}CH_2 + 3HNO_3 \longrightarrow HONO + H_2O + \underset{\text{Nitroglycol}}{CH_2ONO_2\text{—}CH_2ONO_2}$$

A considerable amount of nitrous acid is present in the spent acid. β-Nitroethyl nitrate is feebly acidic and dissolves in dilute alkali solutions with a yellow color. It is not sufficiently stable for use in commercial explosives. On digestion with warm water or on slow distillation with steam it undergoes a decomposition or sort of hydrolysis whereby nitrous acid and other materials are produced. Numerous patents have been issued for processes of procuring pure nitroglycol from the Kekulé oil. One hundred parts of the last-named material yield about 40 parts of nitroglycol, and the economic success of the process depends upon the recovery of valuable by-products from the β-nitroethyl nitrate which is destroyed.

Öhman in Sweden has developed an ingenious electrolytic

process for the production of nitric esters direct from ethylene. The discharge of the nitrate ion (NO_3^-) at the anode liberates the free nitrate radical (NO_3) which in part combines directly with ethylene to form nitroglycol.

$$\begin{matrix} CH_2 \\ \| \\ CH_2 \end{matrix} + 2NO_3 \longrightarrow \begin{matrix} CH_2\text{—}ONO_2 \\ | \\ CH_2\text{—}ONO_2 \end{matrix}$$

Another portion of the free nitrate radical apparently reacts with itself and with water as indicated below, and the oxygen which becomes available enters into the reaction with the consequent formation of dinitrodiglycol.[229]

$$\begin{cases} 2NO_3 \longrightarrow N_2O_5 + [O] \\ N_2O_5 + H_2O \longrightarrow 2HNO_3 \end{cases}$$

$$\begin{matrix} CH_2 \\ \| \\ CH_2 \end{matrix} + [O] + 2NO_3 \longrightarrow \begin{matrix} CH_2\text{—}ONO_2 \\ | \\ CH_2 \\ \diagdown \\ O \\ \diagup \\ CH_2 \\ | \\ CH_2\text{—}ONO_2 \end{matrix}$$

A platinum gauze anode is used. It is immersed in an acetone solution of calcium nitrate which is kept continuously saturated with ethylene which is bubbled through in such manner that it sweeps over the surface of the platinum gauze. An aluminum cathode is used, in a catholyte consisting of a nitric acid solution of calcium nitrate, and the cathode compartment is filled to a higher level since the liquid moves into the anode compartment as the electrolysis progresses. After the electrolysis, the cathode liquid is fortified with nitric acid for use again. The anode liquid is neutralized with slaked lime, and distilled in vacuum for the recovery of the acetone, and the residue, after the removal of calcium nitrate, washing, and drying, consists of a mixture of nitroglycol and dinitrodiglycol and is known as *Oxinite*. Dynamites made from Oxinite differ but little from those made from nitroglycerin.

Pentryl

Pentryl, or 2,4,6-trinitrophenylnitraminoethyl nitrate, is another explosive which is derived from ethylene. It is a nitric ester, an aromatic nitro compound, and a nitroamine. The substance was described in 1925 by Moran who prepared it by the action of mixed acid on 2,4-dinitrophenylethanolamine (large orange-yellow crystals from alcohol, m.p. 92°) procured by the interaction of dinitrochlorobenzene with ethanolamine. von Herz later prepared pentryl by the nitration of β-hydroxyethylaniline, a material which is more commonly called phenylethanolamine and is now available commercially in this country, and was granted British and German patents[230] for its use for certain military purposes. The genesis of pentryl from ethylene, through the intermediacy both of ethanolamine and of phenylethanolamine, is indicated below. The preparation and properties of pentryl have been studied extensively by LeRoy V. Clark at the U. S. Bureau of Mines. By the reaction of dinitrochlorobenzene in the presence of sodium hydroxide with ethanolamine in alcohol solution at 70–80° he procured dinitrophenylethanolamine in 70% yield. The alcohol solution was filtered for the removal of sodium chloride, which was found to be mixed with a certain quantity of the by-product tetranitrodiphenylethanolamine (lemon-yellow fine powder, m.p. 222°); it was then concentrated to about one-third its volume, and deposited crystals of the product on cooling. This material, dissolved in concentrated sulfuric acid and nitrated by

$CH_2{=}CH_2 \rightarrow CH_2\text{–}Cl/CH_2\text{–}OH$ (ethylene chlorohydrin) $\xrightarrow{\text{aniline}}$ $H\text{–}N\text{–}CH_2\text{–}CH_2\text{–}OH$ (phenylethanolamine) $\longrightarrow$ $NO_2\text{–}N\text{–}CH_2\text{–}CH_2\text{–}ONO_2$ with ring NO_2 at 2,4,6 (Pentryl)

$CH_2\text{–}Cl/CH_2\text{–}OH \rightarrow CH_2\text{–}NH_2/CH_2\text{–}OH$ (ethanolamine) $\xrightarrow{\text{dinitrochlorobenzene}}$ $H\text{–}N\text{–}CH_2\text{–}CH_2\text{–}OH$ with ring NO_2 at 2,4 $\longrightarrow$ Pentryl

adding the solution to nitric acid and heating, gave pentryl in yields of about 90%, minute cream-colored crystals from benzene, m.p. 128°.

Clark reports that pentryl has an absolute density of 1.82 and an apparent density of only 0.45. When compressed in a detonator shell at a pressure of 3400 pounds per square inch, it has an apparent density of 0.74. It is soluble to some extent in most of the common organic solvents, and is very readily soluble in nitroglycerin. In the drop test with a 2-kilogram weight, 0.02 gram of pentryl was exploded by a drop of 30 cm., a similar sample of[231] tetryl by one of 27.5 cm., and one of picric acid by a drop of 42.5 cm., while TNT was not exploded by a drop of 100 cm. It is somewhat more sensitive to friction than tetryl, and much more sensitive than picric acid and TNT. Pentryl explodes in 3 seconds at 235°.

The results of Clark's experiments to determine the minimum amounts of primary explosive necessary to initiate the explosion of pentryl and of other high explosives are tabulated below. For

	Minimum Initiating Charge (Grams) of		
	Diazodinitrophenol	Mercury Fulminate	Lead Azide
Pentryl	0.095	0.150	0.025
Picric acid	0.115	0.225	0.12
TNT	0.163	0.240	0.16
Tetryl	0.075	0.165	0.03
Trinitroresorcinol	0.110	0.225	0.075
Trinitrobenzaldehyde	0.075	0.165	0.05
Tetranitroaniline	0.085	0.175	0.05
Hexanitrodiphenylamine	0.075	0.165	0.05

the purpose of these experiments a half-gram portion of the high explosive was weighed into a No. 8 detonator shell, a weighed amount of primary explosive was introduced on top of it, and both were compressed under a reenforcing capsule at a pressure of 3400 pounds per square inch. Without the reenforcing capsule diazodinitrophenol did not cause detonation, and pentryl required 0.035 gram of lead azide and more than 0.4 gram of fulminate. The results show that pentryl has about the same sensitivity to initiation as tetryl and hexanitrodiphenylamine.

In the small Trauzl test pentryl caused an expansion of 15.8 cc., while the same weight of tetryl caused one of 13.8 cc., TNT 12.2 cc., and picric acid 12.4 cc. In the small lead block compression test, in which 50 grams of the explosive was exploded by means of a detonator on top of a lead cylinder 64 mm. long, it was found that pentryl produced a shortening of the block of 18.5 mm., tetryl 16.6 mm., picric acid 16.4 mm., TNT 14.8 mm., and diazodinitrophenol 10.5 mm. Determinations of velocity of detonation made with half-meter lengths, the explosives being contained in extra light lead tubing ½ inch internal diameter and weighing 12 ounces to the foot, gave the following figures. [232]

	Density	Velocity of Detonation (Meters per second)
Pentryl	0.80	5000
Tetryl	0.90	5400
Picric acid	0.98	4970
TNT	0.90	4450

These are not however the maximum velocities of detonation of the substances.

Hexanitrodiphenylaminoethyl Nitrate

This substance also has been studied by LeRoy V. Clark who prepared it by the nitration with mixed acid of tetranitrodiphenylethanolamine, a by-product from the preparation of pentryl.

$$2\ C_6H_3Cl(NO_2)_2 \xrightarrow{NH_2-CH_2-CH_2-OH} [C_6H_3(NO_2)_2]_2N-CH_2-CH_2-OH \rightarrow [C_6H_2(NO_2)_3]_2N-CH_2-CH_2-ONO_2$$

He procured the pure substance in the form of pale yellow glistening plates, m.p. 184° (corr.), precipitated from acetone solution by the addition of alcohol. Its explosive properties are not widely different from those of pentryl. Its response to initiation [233] is about the same; it is slightly less sensitive to impact, about 7% less effective in the sand test, and about 3% more effective in the small Trauzl test. In compound detonators it is somewhat better than TNT and somewhat poorer than pentryl, tetryl, and picric acid, as indicated by the lead plate test. When heated rapidly, it ignites at 390–400°.

Trimethylene Glycol Dinitrate

Trimethylene glycol occurs in the glycerin which is produced by fermentation. There is no harm in leaving it in glycerin which is to be used for the manufacture of explosives. It may however be separated by fractional distillation. When pure it is a colorless, odorless, syrupy liquid, specific gravity ($x°/4°$) 1.0526 at 18°. It mixes with water in all proportions and boils at atmospheric pressure at 211° without decomposition. At temperatures above 15° or so, it is oxidized rapidly by nitric acid or by mixed acid. It is accordingly nitrated at 0–10° under conditions similar to those which are used in the preparation of ethyl nitrate and other simple aliphatic nitric esters (except methyl nitrate).

$$CH_2OH-CH_2-CH_2OH \longrightarrow CH_2ONO_2-CH_2-CH_2ONO_2$$

Trimethylene glycol dinitrate is a water-white liquid, very mobile, and scarcely more viscous than nitroglycol, specific gravity (20°/4°) 1.393 at 20°. It boils at 108° at 10 mm. without decomposition. It is less volatile than nitroglycol and more volatile than nitroglycerin. It has about the same solubility relationships as nitroglycerin, and forms a good gelatin with collodion nitrocotton. It causes headache by contact with the skin. When heated slowly it takes fire with a puff and burns tranquilly or decomposes at about 185° and deflagrates at about 225°. It is much less sensitive to shock than nitroglycerin and is much more stable in storage. Naoúm reports that a 10-gram sample in the Trauzl test with water tamping gave an expansion of 540 cc. or about 90% of the expansion produced by nitroglycerin. The calculated energy content of trimethylene glycol dinitrate is only [234] about 77% of that of nitroglycerin, but the relatively greater brisance results from the low viscosity of the substance which gives it a higher velocity of detonation. Naoúm also reports that a 93% trimethylene glycol dinitrate gelatin with 7% collodion cotton gave an expansion of 470 cc. or about 80% as much as a similar nitroglycerin gelatin.

Propylene Glycol Dinitrate (Methylglycol dinitrate, methylnitroglycol)

Propylene occurs along with ethylene in cracking gas. Its use as a raw material for the synthesis of glycerin has already been mentioned in the section on nitroglycerin. It yields propylene glycol when subjected to the same chemical processes as those which are used for the preparation of glycol from ethylene.[59] Propylene glycol shows the same tendency toward oxidation during nitration that trimethylene glycol does, but to a less extent; noticeable decomposition occurs only above 30°.

[59] Symmes, in a footnote, p. 375, in his English translation of Naoúm's book, *op. cit.*, cites U. S. patents 1,307,032, 1,307,033, 1,307,034, and 1,371,215 which describe a method for the manufacture of mixed ethylene and propylene glycols from cracking gas, satisfactory methods for the nitration of the mixture and for the stabilization of the mixed nitric esters, and explosives made from the products "which practical tests in actual use showed could not be frozen even at temperatures prevailing in winter along the Canadian border, or −10° to −30° F."

$$CH_3-CH=CH_2 \xrightarrow{HOCl} CH_3-CH(OH)-CH_2Cl \xrightarrow{HOH} CH_3-CH(OH)-CH_2OH \xrightarrow{nitration} CH_3-CH(ONO_2)-CH_2ONO_2$$

Propylene glycol dinitrate is a colorless liquid of characteristic aromatic odor, more volatile and less viscous than trimethylene glycol dinitrate with which it is isomeric. Its specific gravity (20°/4°) is 1.368 at 20°. It boils at 92° at 10 mm., and does not freeze at −20°. Its solubilities, gelatinizing power, and explosive properties are substantially the same as those of its isomer. Indeed, Naoúm reports that it gave exactly the same expansion as trimethylene glycol dinitrate in the Trauzl lead block test, namely, 540 cc. [235]

Butylene Glycol Dinitrate

Of the four isomeric butylene glycols, the 1,3-compound appears to be the only one which has attracted any interest as a raw material for the preparation of explosives. Its dinitrate, either alone or in admixture with nitroglycerin, has been proposed for use in non-freezing dynamites. The preparation of the glycol from acetaldehyde has been suggested, the acetaldehyde being condensed to aldol and the aldol reduced to glycol. Since acetaldehyde is produced commercially by the catalyzed hydration of acetylene, then butylene glycol-1,3 can be procured by synthesis from coke.

Coke → CaC_2 → CH≡CH → CH_3–CHO → CH_3–CH(OH)–CH_2–CHO → CH_3–CH(OH)–CH_2–CH_2–OH → CH_3–CH(ONO_2)–CH_2–CH_2–ONO_2

Butylene glycol shows a strong tendency to oxidize during nitration, and ought to be nitrated at a temperature of −5° or lower. Butylene glycol dinitrate is a colorless liquid, intermediate in volatility between nitroglycol and nitroglycerin, possessing a specific gravity of 1.32 at 15°. It does not freeze at temperatures as low as −20°. It yields a good gelatin with collodion nitrocotton. It deflagrates feebly if heated suddenly. It is very insensitive to mechanical shock but detonates easily by initiation. Naoúm reports that a mixture of 75% butylene glycol dinitrate and 25% kieselguhr gave about 240 cc. expansion in the Trauzl test, and that a gelatin containing 90% butylene glycol dinitrate and 10% collodion nitrocotton gave about 370 cc.

Nitroerythrite (Erythritol tetranitrate)

NO_2—O—CH_2—(CH—ONO_2)$_2$—CH_2—ONO_2

i-Erythrite occurs in algae and in lichens. It is a white, crystalline, sweet-tasting substance, very readily soluble in water, m.p. 120°, b.p. 330°, specific gravity 1.59. The tetranitrate is prepared [236] by dissolving erythrite in strong nitric acid with cooling, and then precipitating by the addition of concentrated sulfuric acid. It crystallizes from alcohol in colorless plates, m.p. 61°. Its use as an addition to smokeless powder has been suggested, but it is as powerful as nitroglycerin, and has the advantage over it that it is a solid, and it would be suitable, if it were cheaper, for the same uses as nitromannite.

Nitromannite (Mannitol hexanitrate)

NO_2—O—CH_2—(CH—ONO_2)$_4$—CH_2—ONO_2

d-Mannitol occurs fairly widely distributed in nature, particularly in the *Fraxinus ornus*, the sap of which is *manna*. It may also be procured by the reduction of *d*-mannose either electrolytically or by means of sodium amalgam, or along with *d*-sorbite by the reduction of *d*-fructose. It may be nitrated satisfactorily with the same mixed acid as is used for the nitration of glycerin, or more conveniently, because the mass of crystals is so voluminous, by dissolving in strong nitric acid and precipitating by the addition of concentrated sulfuric acid.

Preparation of Nitromannite. Fifty grams of nitric acid (specific gravity 1.51) is cooled thoroughly in a 300-cc. Erlenmeyer pyrex flask immersed in a freezing mixture of ice and salt. Ten grams of mannite is then introduced in small portions at a time while the flask is tilted from side to side and the contents is stirred gently with a thermometer, care being taken that the temperature does not rise above 0°. After all is dissolved, 100 grams of sulfuric acid (specific gravity 1.84) is added slowly from a dropping funnel while the liquid is stirred and the temperature is maintained below 0°. The porridge-like mass is filtered on a sinter-glass filter, or on a Büchner funnel with a hardened filter paper, washed with water, then with dilute sodium bicarbonate solution, then finally again with water. The crude product is dissolved in boiling alcohol; the solution is filtered if need be, and on cooling deposits white needle crystals of nitromannite, m.p. 112-113°. A second crop of crystals may be obtained by warming the alcoholic mother liquors to boiling, adding water while still boiling until a turbidity appears, and allowing to cool. Total yield about 23 grams.

Nitromannite is readily soluble in ether and in hot alcohol, only slightly soluble in cold alcohol, and insoluble in water. [237] While its stability at ordinary temperatures is such that it can be used commercially, at slightly elevated temperatures it is distinctly less stable than nitroglycerin. Nitroglycerin will tolerate heating in a covered glass vessel for several days at 75° before it begins to give off acid fumes; nitroglycol, methylglycol dinitrate, and trimethylene glycol dinitrate are more stable yet, but nitromannite decomposes after a few hours and evolves red fumes. If a small quantity is heated, it decomposes at once at about 150° with copious evolution of nitrous fumes but ordinarily does not deflagrate. With larger samples deflagration occurs at 160–170°.

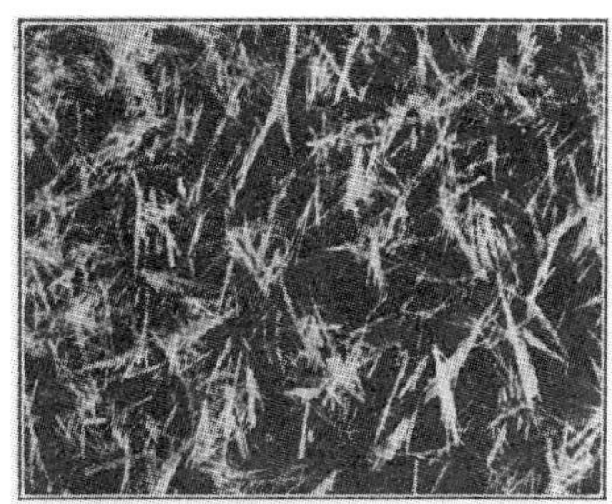

FIGURE 57. Nitromannite, Crystals from Alcohol (5×). (Courtesy Atlas Powder Company.)

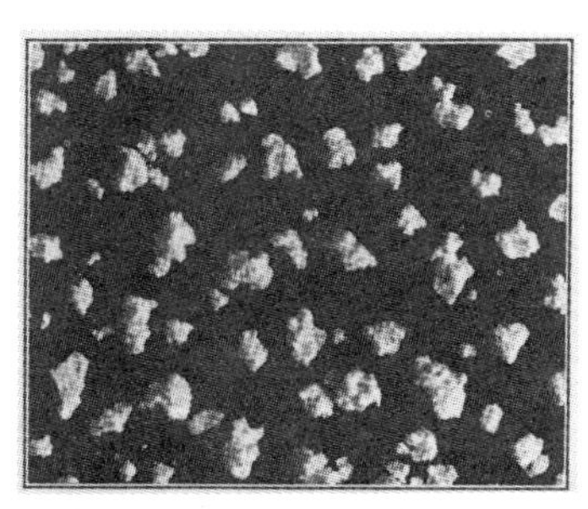

FIGURE 58. Nitromannite, in Grained Form for Charging Detonators (5×). (Courtesy Atlas Powder Company.)

Kast [238] has reported a velocity of detonation of 8260 meters per second for nitromannite compressed to a density of 1.73 in a column 12.8 mm. in diameter.

Nitromannite is about as sensitive as nitroglycerin to shock and to friction. It detonates under a 4-cm. drop of a 2-kilogram weight, and may be exploded readily on a concrete surface by a blow of a carpenter's hammer. It is not fired by the spit of a fuse, but is made to detonate by the flame of a match which causes local overheating. It is almost, but not quite, a primary explosive. It is used as the high-explosive charge in compound detonators which contain the relatively safe diazodinitrophenol as the primary explosive. A mixture of nitromannite and tetracene is a powerful and brisant primary explosive which detonates from moderate heat.

Nitrodulcite (Dulcitol hexanitrate)

Dulcite is obtained from Madagascar manna by extraction with water and recrystallizing, large monoclinic prisms, m.p. 188°, less soluble than mannite. It may also be procured by the action of sodium amalgam on aqueous solutions of lactose and of *d*-galactose. Nitrodulcite, isomeric with nitromannite, crystallizes from alcohol in needles which melt at 94–95°.

Nitrosorbite (Sorbitol hexanitrate)

d-Sorbite occurs in the berries of the mountain ash, but is more readily procured by the electrolytic reduction of *d*-glucose. It crystallizes with one molecule of water in small crystals which lose their water when heated and melt at about 110°. Nitrosorbite, isomeric with nitromannite, exists as a viscous liquid and has never been obtained in the crystalline state. It is used in non-freezing dynamites.

Nitrated Sugar Mixtures

The sugars are polyhydric alcohols which contain an aldehyde or a ketone group or a cyclic acetal or ketal arrangement within the molecule. They yield nitric esters which are perhaps less stable than the nitric esters of the simple polyhydric alcohols but which probably owe part of their reputation for instability to the

239

fact that they are difficult to purify. The nitrosugars resemble the sugars from which they are derived in the respect that often they do not crystallize rapidly and easily. When warmed gently, they frequently soften and become sticky and resinous. In this condition they retain within their masses traces of decomposition products by which further decomposition is provoked; they cannot be washed free from acid, and in the solid or semi-solid state are impossible to stabilize. The stabilization however may be accomplished easily if the nitrosugar is in solution.

A mixture of nitrosucrose and nitroglycerin, prepared by nitrating a solution of 20 parts of cane sugar in 80 parts of glycerin, or of 25 parts in 75, has been used in this country under the name of *nitrohydrene*. It is suitable for use in non-freezing dynamites, and is cheaper than nitroglycerin to the extent that sugar is cheaper than glycerin. The nitrated product is much more viscous than nitroglycerin and forms emulsions readily. It requires repeated washings with soda solution to insure a satisfactory heat test, and then washings with concentrated salt solutions to facilitate the separation of the phases. Nitrohydrene 80/20 (from 80 parts of glycerin and 20 parts of cane sugar) consists of about 86% nitroglycerin and 14% nitrosucrose, and nitrohydrene 75/25 of about 82% nitroglycerin and 18% nitrosucrose. Naoúm reports the following data. The stability of nitro-

	Specific Gravity at 20°	Lead Block Expansion, 10-Gram Sample in Glass Tube: Sand Tamping, cc.	Water Tamping, cc.
Nitroglycerin	1.596	550	595
Nitrohydrene 80/20	1.605	533	560
Nitrohydrene 75/25	1.612	514	535

hydrene is distinctly poorer than that of nitroglycerin and appears to depend upon the proportion of nitrosucrose which it contains, for nitrohydrene 75/25 gives a poorer heat test than nitrohydrene 80/20 which contains less nitrosucrose. Naoúm points out that the wood meal, etc., which is contained in dynamite made from nitrohydrene apparently acts as a stabilizer and

240

absorbs or reacts chemically with the first decomposition products and destroys them. He says:

> Better still, are very small additions of diphenylamine, which is admirably suited for the stabilization of smokeless powder, since it readily takes up the nitrous acid. Nitrohydrene 80/20 or 75/25, containing only 0.1 to 0.2 per cent of diphenylamine, was stored for seventy-five days at 55°C. without undergoing decomposition. The samples merely showed a coloration and became dark green, a phenomenon which also occurred but to a less extent with a check sample of nitroglycerin containing the same quantity of diphenylamine. After seventy-five days the nitroglycerin still had a slight odor of diphenylamine, but the nitrohydrene smelled slightly acid, somewhat like sour milk, but not like nitrous or nitric acid.
>
> Similar samples of 100 grams each of the above nitrohydrene containing 0.1 per cent diphenylamine have been stored by the author for more than eight years in diffuse daylight at room temperatures, about 20°C. So far they have remained unchanged, have no acid odor, and show no signs of decomposition. . . . From this it is evident that nitrosugar dissolved in nitroglycerin, although its stability does not reach that of the latter, is sufficiently stable for practical purposes, particularly in the presence of stabilizers.

The individual nitrosugars are stabilized similarly by diphenylamine, and certain ones of them, specifically nitromaltose, nitrolactose, and nitrosucrose, have been able by means of that substance to find a limited industrial application.

Solutions of cane sugar in glycol, and of glucose and lactose in glycerin, have been nitrated to produce mixtures of nitric esters comparable to nitrohydrene.

Nitroarabinose (*l*-Arabinose tetranitrate), $C_5H_6O(ONO_2)_4$

Nitroarabinose is prepared, as indeed the highly nitrated sugars in general may be prepared, by adding concentrated sulfuric acid drop by drop to a solution of the corresponding sugar in concentrated nitric acid at 0°. It consists of colorless monoclinic crystals which melt at 85° and decompose at 120°. It is readily soluble in alcohol, acetone, and acetic acid, and insoluble in water and ligroin. It reduces Fehling's solution on warming. It is but little stable above 50°, and is easily exploded by shock.

241

Nitroglucose (*d*-Glucose pentanitrate), $C_6H_7O(ONO_2)_5$

d-Glucose pentanitrate[69] is a colorless viscous syrup, insoluble in water and in ligroin, readily soluble in alcohol. It becomes hard at 0°. It is unstable above 50°, and if heated slowly to a higher temperature decomposes rapidly at about 135°. It reduces Fehling's solution on warming. *Glucosan trinitrate,* $C_6H_7O_2(ONO_2)_3$, is produced by the nitration of α-glucosan and by the action for several days of mixed acid on *d*-glucose. It is readily soluble in alcohol and insoluble in water. It has been obtained in the form of aggregates or crusts of crystals which melted not sharply at about 80° and which were probably not entirely free from glucose pentanitrate.

Nitromannose (*d*-Mannose pentanitrate), $C_6H_7O(ONO_2)_5$

d-Mannose pentanitrate,[69] transparent rhombic needles from alcohol, melts at 81–82° and decomposes at about 124°. It is soluble in alcohol and insoluble in water and reduces Fehling's solution slowly on warming. It undergoes a rapid decomposition if stored at 50°.

Nitromaltose (Maltose octonitrate), $C_{12}H_{14}O_3(ONO_2)_8$

Maltose octonitrate,[69] glistening needles from methyl alcohol, melts with decomposition at 164–165°. If heated quickly, it puffs off at 170–180°. It decomposes slowly at 50°. If fused and allowed to solidify, it has a specific gravity of 1.62. It is readily soluble in methyl alcohol, acetone, and acetic acid, difficultly soluble in ethyl alcohol, and insoluble in water. It reduces warm Fehling's solution more rapidly than nitrosucrose.

Nitrolactose (Lactose octonitrate), $C_{12}H_{14}O_3(ONO_2)_8$

Lactose octonitrate,[69] monoclinic needles from methyl or ethyl alcohol, melts at 145–146° with decomposition. Its specific gravity is 1.684. It is readily soluble in methyl alcohol, hot ethyl alcohol, acetone, and acetic acid, difficultly soluble in cold ethyl alcohol, and insoluble in water. It reduces Fehling's solution on warming.

242

Lactose hexanitrate, $C_{12}H_{16}O_5(ONO_2)_6$, has been found in the alcoholic mother liquors from the crystallization of the octonitrate, white, amorphous material melting not sharply at about 70°.

Crater in 1934 described explosives containing nitrolactose, one consisting, say, of nitrolactose 25%, ammonium nitrate 65%, sodium nitrate 6%, and vegetable absorbent material 4%, another made by treating wood pulp with an acetone solution of nitrolactose and dinitrotoluene and containing about 78% nitrolactose, about 9% DNT, and about 13% wood pulp. For this use the nitrolactose ought to be stabilized with diphenylamine.

Nitrosucrose (Sucrose octonitrate), $C_{12}H_{14}O_3(ONO_2)_8$

The nitration of cane sugar[69] yields sucrose octonitrate, white glistening needles, which melt at 85.5°. If heated slowly, nitrosucrose decomposes at about 135° and if heated rapidly deflagrates at about 170°. The fused and solidified material has a specific gravity of 1.67. It is readily soluble in methyl alcohol, ether, and nitrobenzene, difficultly soluble in ethyl alcohol and benzene, and insoluble in water and in petroleum ether. It reduces Fehling's solution on warming. It is relatively stable when pure. Monasterski reports that it gives a feeble puff under a 20-cm. drop of a 2-kilogram weight, a puff with one of 25 cm., and a detonation with one of 30 cm. He states that samples of 10 grams in the Trauzl test gave average net expansions of 296 cc.

Other Nitrosugars

The nitration of *d*-xylose[69] yields *d-xylose tetranitrate*, $C_5H_6O(ONO_2)_4$, an oily substance insoluble in water, and a crystalline by-product, m.p. 141°, insoluble in water, which is evidently the *trinitrate*, $C_5H_7O_2(ONO_2)_3$. *Xylosan dinitrate*, $C_5H_6O_2(ONO_2)_2$, has been prepared by the action of mixed acid on *d*-xylose. It consists of little spherical crystal aggregates, soluble in alcohol and melting at 75–80°.

l-Rhamnose tetranitrate,[69] $C_6H_8O(ONO_2)_4$, crystallizes in compact short rhombs which melt with decomposition at 135°. It is

243

readily soluble in acetone, acetic acid, and in methyl and ethyl alcohol, and is relatively stable. It reduces Fehling's solution on warming. *l-Rhamnose trinitrate*, $C_6H_9O_2(ONO_2)_3$, results from the action of mixed acid on *l*-rhamnose. It is a white amorphous material, melting below 100°, readily soluble in alcohol and insoluble in water. It explodes feebly under a hammer blow.

α-Methylglucoside tetranitrate,[69] $C_7H_{10}O_2(ONO_2)_4$, crystallizes from alcohol in quadrilateral plates which melt at 49–50° and decompose at 135°. It is more stable than the nitrate of the free sugar. It reduces Fehling's solution slowly on warming.

α-Methylmannoside tetranitrate,[69] $C_7H_{10}O_2(ONO_2)_4$, from the nitration of *d*-α-methylmannoside, crystallizes in fine asbestos-like needles which melt at 36°. It is relatively stable at 50°.

d-Galactose pentanitrate α, $C_6H_7O(ONO_2)_5$, from the nitration of *d*-galactose[69] crystallizes in bundles of transparent needles which melt at 115–116° and decompose at 126°. It is sparingly soluble in alcohol. It decomposes slowly at 50°, and reduces Fehling's solution slowly on warming. The alcoholic mother liquors from the α-form yield *d-galactose pentanitrate β*, transparent monoclinic needles which melt at 72–73° and decompose at 125°. This substance is readily soluble in alcohol, decomposes rapidly at 50°, and reduces hot Fehling's solution. *Galactosan trinitrate*, $C_6H_7O_2(ONO_2)_3$, results from the action during several days of mixed acid on *d*-galactose. It is deposited from alcohol in crusts of small crystals.

Fructosan trinitrate α, $C_6H_7O_2(ONO_2)_3$, is produced by the action of mixed acid at 0–15° on *d*-fructose or on laevulosan, colorless, quickly effluorescing needles from alcohol, which melt at 139–140° and decompose at about 145°. It is readily soluble in methyl and ethyl alcohol, acetic acid, and acetone, and insoluble in water. It is relatively stable at 50°. It reduces hot Fehling's solution. The alcoholic mother liquors from the α-form yield *fructosan trinitrate β*, crusts of white crystals which melt at 48–52° and decompose at 135°. The material decomposes slowly at 50°. It reduces Fehling's solution rapidly on warming.

The action of mixed acid on *d*-sorbose at 15° yields *sorbosan trinitrate*, $C_6H_7O_2(ONO_2)_3$, a crystalline substance which melts not sharply at 40–45°.

244

d-α-Glucoheptose hexanitrate, $C_7H_8O(ONO_2)_6$, from the nitration of *d*-α-glucoheptose,[69] crystallizes from alcohol in transparent needles which melt at 100°. It reduces Fehling's solution on warming.

Trehalose octonitrate, $C_{12}H_{14}O_3(ONO_2)_8$, from the nitration of trehalose,[69] crystallizes from alcohol in birefringent pearly leaflets which melt at 124° and decompose at 136°. It reduces Fehling's solution on warming.

Raffinose hendecanitrate, $C_{18}H_{21}O_5(ONO_2)_{11}$, from the nitration of raffinose,[69] exists in the form of amorphous aggregates which melt at 55–65° and decompose at 136°. It reduces Fehling's solution on warming. It decomposes rapidly when kept at 50°.

α-Tetraamylose octonitrate, $[C_6H_8O_3(ONO_2)_2]_4$, from α-tetraamylose,[76] crystallizes from acetic acid in fine glistening needles which decompose at 204°. It is readily soluble in ethyl acetate, amyl acetate, pyridine, and nitrobenzene, and sparingly soluble or insoluble in alcohol, ether, benzene, and water. *α-Diamylose hexanitrate*,[76] $[C_6H_7O_2(ONO_2)_3]_2$, prepared from α-diamylose or as the final product of the nitration of tetraamylose, crystallizes from acetone in plates which puff off at 206–207°. It is difficultly soluble in acetic acid, and is reported to be but little stable. The alcohol extract of the crude hexanitrate yields a certain amount of the amorphous *tetranitrate*. *β-Triamylose hexanitrate*,

$[C_6H_8O_3(ONO_2)_2]_3$, is procured by dissolving either β-triamylose or β-hexaamylose in strong nitric acid at 0° and adding concentrated sulfuric acid drop by drop, and extracting the crude product with alcohol. It crystallizes from the alcoholic extract in aggregates of microscopic cubes, m.p. 203°. The residue which is insoluble in hot alcohol is recrystallized from acetic acid and yields crystalline crusts of *β-triamylose enneanitrate,*[76] $[C_6H_7O_2(ONO_2)_3]_3$, m.p. 198°.

Early History of Nitrated Carbohydrates

The history of modern explosives commenced with the discoveries of nitroglycerin and of nitrocellulose. At about the time that Sobrero first prepared nitroglycerin, Schönbein at Basel and Böttger at Frankfort-on-the-Main independently of each other nitrated cotton, perceived the possibilities in the product, and

245

soon cooperated with each other to exploit its use in artillery. Pelouze had nitrated paper at an earlier time, and the question may indeed be raised whether he was not the first discoverer of nitrocellulose. Before that, Braconnot, professor of chemistry at Nancy, had prepared a nitric ester from starch. The principal events in the early history of these substances are summarized below.

1833. Braconnot found that starch dissolved in concentrated nitric acid and that the liquid on dilution with water gave a curdy precipitate of material which, after washing, dried out to a white, pulverulent, tasteless, and neutral mass. The product gave a brown color with a solution of iodine. It was not affected by bromine. It did not dissolve in boiling water but softened to a sticky mass. Dilute sulfuric acid did not affect it. Concentrated sulfuric acid dissolved it, and the solution gave no precipitate if it was diluted with water. The material, to which Braconnot gave the name of *xyloïdine,* dissolved in acetic acid very readily on heating, and the solution, if evaporated slowly, gave a transparent film which retained its transparency when placed in water. Applied to paper or cloth it yielded a brilliant, varnish-like coating which was impervious to water. Xyloïdine took fire very readily. It carbonized and liquefied if heated upon a piece of cardboard or heavy paper while the cardboard or paper, though exposed directly to the heat, was not appreciably damaged. Sawdust, cotton, and linen yielded products which Braconnot considered to be identical with the xyloïdine from starch.

1838. Pelouze studied xyloïdine further. He found that if starch was dissolved in concentrated nitric acid and if the solution was diluted immediately with water, xyloïdine precipitated and the acid filtrate on evaporation yielded practically no residue. If the solution of starch in nitric acid was allowed to stand before being precipitated with water, then the amount of xyloïdine was less. If it was allowed to stand for 2 days, or perhaps only for some hours, the xyloïdine was entirely destroyed, a new acid was formed, no precipitate appeared when the solution was diluted,

246

and the liquid on evaporation gave the new acid in the form of a solid, white, non-crystalline, deliquescent mass of considerably greater weight than the starch which was taken for the experiment. Neither carbon dioxide nor oxalic acid was produced during the reaction, but the new acid on long standing, or on boiling, with nitric acid was converted to oxalic acid without the formation of carbon dioxide. Pelouze considered xyloïdine to be a nitrate of starch. He observed that it was readily combustible, that it ignited at a temperature of 180° and burned with very

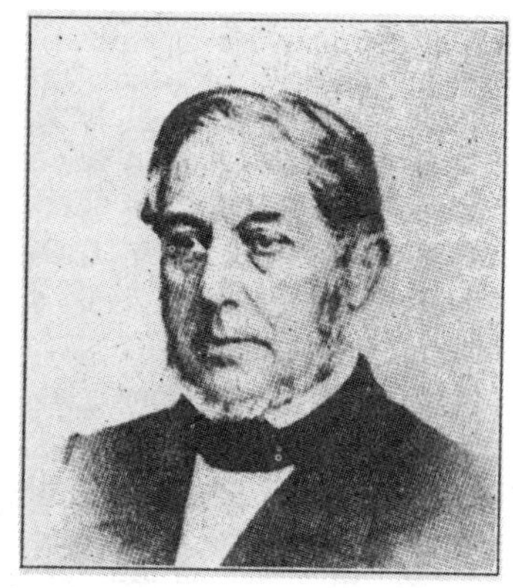

FIGURE 59. Théophile-Jules Pelouze (1807-1867). (Courtesy E. Berl.) Made many important contributions to organic and inorganic chemistry—ethereal salts, the first nitrile, borneol, glyceryl tributyrate, pyroxylin, improvements in the manufacture of plate glass. He nitrated paper in 1838 and was thus probably the first to prepare nitrocellulose. Reproduced from original in Kekulé's portrait album.

considerable violence leaving practically no residue. The observation, he says, led him to make certain experiments which, he believed, might have practical application in artillery. Paper, dipped into nitric acid of specific gravity 1.5 and left there long enough for the acid to penetrate into it (generally 2 or 3 minutes), removed, and washed thoroughly, gave a parchment-like material which was impervious to moisture and was extremely combustible. Pelouze had nitrocellulose in his hands, but evidently did not recognize that the material, which had not changed greatly in its physical form, was nevertheless nitrated through-

247

out its mass, for he believed that the products which he obtained from paper and from cotton and linen fabrics owed their new properties to the xyloïdine which covered them.

1846. Schönbein announced his discovery of guncotton at a meeting of the Society of Scientific Research at Basel on May 27, 1846. In an article, probably written in 1847 but published in the *Archives des sciences physiques et naturelles* of 1846, he described some of his experiences with the material and his efforts

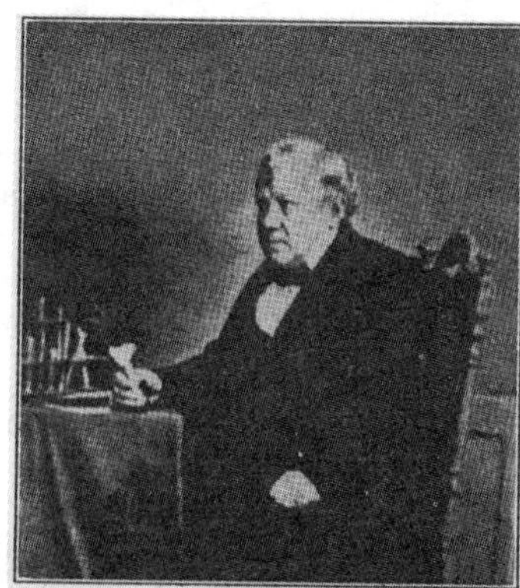

FIGURE 60. Christian Friedrich Schönbein (1799-1868). (Courtesy E. Berl.) Discovered guncotton, 1846. Discovered ozone, worked on hydrogen peroxide, auto-oxidation, the passivity of iron, hydrosulfites, catalysts, and prussic acid. Professor of Chemistry at Basel from 1829 until the time of his death. He published more than 300 papers on chemical subjects. Reproduced from original in Kekulé's portrait album.

to put it to practical use and discussed the controversial question of priority of discovery; he described the nitration of cane sugar but deliberately refrained from telling how he had prepared his nitrocellulose. He was led to perform the experiments by certain theoretical speculations relative to ozone which he had discovered a few years before. One volume of nitric acid (1.5) and 2 volumes of sulfuric acid (1.85) were mixed and cooled to 0°, finely powdered sugar was stirred in so as to form a paste, the stirring was continued, and after a few minutes a viscous mass separated from the acid liquid without the disengagement of gas. The pasty mass was washed with boiling water until free from acid, and was [248] dried at a low temperature. The product was brittle at low temperatures, could be molded like jalap resin at slightly elevated ones, was semi-fluid at 100°, and at high temperatures gave off red fumes. When heated more strongly, it deflagrated suddenly and with violence. Schönbein also experimented with other organic substances, and states that in experiments carried out during December, 1845, and the first few months of 1846 he discovered, one after another, all those substances about which so much had lately been said in the French Academy. In March he sent specimens of the new compounds, among them guncotton, to several of his friends, notably, Faraday, Herschel, and Grove.

About the middle of April, 1846, Schönbein went to Württemberg where he carried out experiments with guncotton at the arsenal at Ludwigsburg in the presence of artillery officers and at Stuttgart in the presence of the king. During May, June, and July he experimented at Basel with small arms, mortars, and cannon. On July 28 he fired for the first time a cannon which was loaded with guncotton and with a projectile. Shortly afterward he used guncotton to blast rocks at Istein in the Grand Duchy of Baden and to blow up some old walls in Basel.

In the middle of August Schönbein received news from Professor Böttger of Frankfort-on-the-Main that he too had succeeded in preparing guncotton, and the names of the two men soon became associated in connection with the discovery and utilization of the material. There were, moreover, several other chemists who at about the same time, or within a few months, also worked out methods of preparing it. In a letter to Schönbein dated November 18, 1846, Berzelius congratulated him on the discovery as interesting as it was important, and wrote, "Since Professor Otto of Brunswick made known a method of preparing the guncotton, this discovery has perhaps occupied a greater number of inquisitive persons than any other chemical discovery ever did. I have likewise engaged in experiments upon it."

In August Schönbein went to England where, with the help of the engineer Richard Taylor of Falmouth, he carried out experiments with guncotton in the mines of Cornwall. He also demonstrated his material successfully with small arms and with artillery at Woolwich, at Portsmouth, and before the British [249] Association. He did not apply for an English patent in his own name but communicated his process to John Taylor of Adelphi, Middlesex, who was granted English patent 11,407, dated October 8, 1846, for "Improvements in the Manufacture of Explosive Compounds, communicated to me from a certain foreigner residing abroad." He entered into an agreement for three years with Messrs. John Hall & Sons of Faversham that they should have the sole right in England to manufacture guncotton by his process and in return should pay him one-third of the net profit with a minimum of £1000 down and the same each year. The first factory for the manufacture of guncotton was erected at Faversham. On July 14, 1847, within less than a year, the factory was

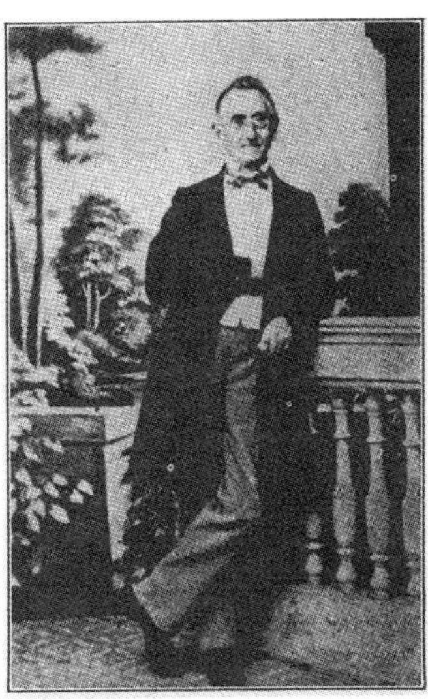

FIGURE 61. Rudolf Böttger (1806-1887). (Courtesy E. Berl.) Professor at Frankfort-on-the-Main. Discovered guncotton independently of Schönbein but somewhat later, in the same year, 1846. He also invented matches, and made important studies on the poisoning of platinum catalysts. Reproduced from original in Kekulé's portrait album.

destroyed by an explosion with the loss of twenty-one lives. After this, Messrs. John Hall & Sons refused to continue the manu- [250] facture. About the same time disastrous guncotton explosions occurred at Vincennes and at Le Bouchet, and these produced such an unfavorable effect that no more guncotton was manufactured in England or in France for about sixteen years.

Schönbein offered his process to the Deutscher Bund for 100,000 thalers, and a committee was formed to consider the matter, Liebig representing the state of Hesse and Baron von Lenk, who was secretary, representing Austria. The committee continued to sit until 1852 when it finally decided to take no action. At the suggestion of von Lenk, Austria then acquired the process for 30,000 gulden.

1846. The *Comptes rendus* of 1846 contains several papers on the nitration of cellulose, which papers were presented to the French Academy before the details of Schönbein's process were yet known. Among these, the papers by Dumas and Pelouze are especially interesting. Dumas stated that certain details of the manufacture of guncotton had already been published in Germany. Professor Otto of Brunswick dipped the cotton for half a minute in concentrated fuming nitric acid, pressed between two pieces of glass, washed until free from acid, and afterwards dried.

> The explosive property can be considerably increased by several dippings, and I have found that a product of extreme force is obtained after an immersion of 12 hours. A point of extreme importance is the care which ought to be exercised in washing the cotton. The last traces of acid are very difficult to remove, and should any remain it will be found that, on drying, the substance smells strongly of oxides of nitrogen, and when ignited also produces a strong acid smell. The best test of a sample of guncotton is to ignite it upon a porcelain plate. Should it burn slowly, leaving a residue upon the plate, it must be considered as unsatisfactory. A good guncotton burns very violently without leaving any residue. It is also of very great importance that when the guncotton is withdrawn from the acid, it should be washed immediately in a large quantity of water. Should small quantities of water be used it will be found that the guncotton becomes very hot, and that spots of a blue or green color are produced, which

are very difficult to remove, and the guncotton is very impure.

Dr. Knopp of the University of Leipzig used a mixture of equal parts of concentrated sulfuric and nitric acids, and immersed the cotton in it for several minutes[251] at ordinary temperature. Dumas stated that satisfactory guncotton could be obtained without observing any great exactitude in the proportion of the two acids or in the duration of the immersion. Dr. Bley of Bernberg had discovered that sawdust, treated in the same way as cotton, yielded an explosive which, he believed, might replace gunpowder in firearms and in blasting.

1846. Pelouze made clear distinction between xyloïdine and guncotton. "I shall call *pyroxyline* or *pyroxyle* the product of the action of monohydrated nitric acid on cotton, paper, and ligneous substances, when this action has taken place without having caused the solution of the cellulose." Braconnot in 1833 had prepared xyloïdine from starch; Pelouze had prepared pyroxylin in 1838. He pointed out that xyloïdine dissolves readily in strong nitric acid and, in the course of a day, is destroyed by it and converted to a deliquescent acid. Pyroxylin does not dissolve in concentrated nitric acid. Xyloïdine is very inflammable and explodes when struck, but it leaves a considerable residue of carbon when heated in a retort and may be analyzed like an ordinary organic substance by heating with copper oxide. Pyroxylin explodes when heated to 175° or 180° and cannot be distilled destructively. Pelouze found that 100 parts of starch, dissolved in nitric acid and precipitated immediately, yielded at most 128 to 130 parts of xyloïdine. One hundred parts of cotton or paper, after a few minutes' or after several days' immersion in concentrated nitric acid, yielded 168 to 170 parts of washed and dried pyroxylin. The acid mother liquors, both from the nitration of the starch and from the nitration of the cotton, contained not more than mere traces of organic matter.

1846. Schönbein's process soon became known through the publication of the English patent to John Taylor (cited above). He carried out the nitration by means of a mixture of 1 volume of strong nitric acid (1.45 to 1.5) and 3 volumes of strong sulfuric acid (1.85). The cotton was immersed in this acid at 50–60°F. for 1 hour, and was then washed in a stream of running water until free from acid. It was pressed to remove as much water as possible, dipped in a very dilute solution of potassium carbonate (1 ounce to the gallon), and again pressed as dry as possible.[252] It was then rinsed with a very dilute solution of potassium nitrate (1 ounce to the gallon). The patent states that "the use of this solution appears to add strength to the compound, but the use of this solution and also potassium carbonate are not essential and may be dispensed with." The product is pressed, opened out, and dried at 150°F., and when dried it is fit for use. The patent also covers the possibility of using instead of cotton "other matters of vegetable origin and the possibility of carrying out the nitration with nitric acid alone or with mixed acids of inferior strength."

1846. Teschemacher studied the preparation of guncotton and demonstrated that no sulfuric acid is consumed by the reaction.

1847. Gladstone by exercising special precautions was able to carry out combustion analyses of xyloïdine and of pyroxylin prepared according to the directions of Schönbein. Nitrogen was determined by the differential method. The pyroxylin was found to contain 12.75% nitrogen and was thought to correspond to a pentanitrate while the xyloïdine corresponded more nearly to a trinitrate.

1847. Crum nitrated cotton until he could introduce no further nitrogen into the molecule, and analyzed the product for nitric acid by the method which is used in the nitrometer. His result calculated as nitrogen gives a figure of 13.69%. It is interesting to note that Crum's cotton was "bleached by boiling in caustic soda and put in a solution of bleaching powder; then caustic soda again, and afterwards weak nitric acid. It was well washed and beaten in a bag with water after each operation. . . . The cotton, dried and carded after bleaching, was exposed in parcels of 10 grains each for several hours to the heat of a steam bath, and each parcel was immersed, while hot, into a 1 oz. measure of the following mixture: Sulphuric acid (1.84) 1 measure, and 3 measures of pale lemon-colored nitric acid (1.517). After one hour it was washed in successive portions of water until no trace of acid remained, and was then dried in the open air"—or, for analysis, was dried completely in a vacuum desiccator over sulfuric acid.[253]

1852. The Austrian government acquired the use of Schönbein's process (as mentioned above) and the Emperor of Austria appointed a committee to investigate the use of guncotton for military purposes. This committee, of which von Lenk was the leading spirit, continued to function with some interruptions until 1865. In 1853 a factory was erected at Hirtenberg for the manufacture of guncotton by the method of von Lenk which involved a more elaborate purification than Schönbein's original process. The product was washed for 3 weeks, then boiled with dilute potassium carbonate solution for 15 minutes, washed again for several days, impregnated with water glass, and finally dried. Von Lenk constructed 12-pounder guns which were shot with guncotton cartridges, but they were much damaged by the firing. About 1860 he tried bronze guns, which were less likely to burst than iron ones, and with propelling charges of guncotton fired from them shells which were filled with bursting charges of guncotton. The shells often burst within the barrel, for the acceleration produced by the propelling charge of guncotton was much too sudden and shocking. They could be shot out without exploding when a propelling charge of black gunpowder was used. On July 20, 1863, the magazine at Hirtenberg exploded, and the Austrian government thereupon decided to abandon the use of guncotton as a propellent explosive. Von Lenk was permitted to communicate his process to other nations. In 1862 and 1863, under the name of Révy, he took out English patents to protect his method of purification. In 1863 he visited England and described his process to a committee of the British Association. In the same year Messrs. Prentice and Co. commenced the manufacture of guncotton at Stowmarket by von Lenk's process, but an explosion soon occurred at their establishment. In 1865 a guncotton magazine at Steinfelder Heath, near Vienna, exploded, and on October 11 of that year the manufacture of guncotton in Austria was officially forbidden.

1862. Tonkin's English patent deserves our notice because it mentions the pulping of guncotton—and it was the pulping of guncotton, introduced later by Abel, which remedied in large measure the difficulties of stability which had given guncotton a bad repute and brought it back again to the favorable consideration[254] of the users of explosives. The patent describes the nitration of the cotton with mixed acid, the washing with running water, the pressing, and the dipping in a very dilute solution of potassium carbonate. "The fibre is then taken in the wet state and converted into pulp in the same manner as is practiced by paper-makers, by putting the fibre into a cylinder, having knives revolving rapidly, working close to fixed knives." The patent makes no claim to the pulping of guncotton, but only claims the use of pulped guncotton in an explosive consisting of sodium nitrate 65%, charcoal 16%, sulfur 16%, and guncotton pulp 3%.

1865. Abel's patent for "Improvements in the Preparation and Treatment of Guncotton" claims the pulping and the pressing of it into sheets, discs, cylinders, and other forms and was probably designed to cover the process of getting it into a state where it would burn less violently in the gun. The compressed blocks were an improvement over the yarn of von Lenk, but they were still much too fast; they damaged the guns and were not ballistically uniform in performance. The blocks of compressed guncotton, however, have continued to find use in blasting. And the outstanding advantage of Abel's pulping was that it converted the guncotton into a state where the impurities were more easily washed out of it, and resulted thereby in a great improvement in stability.

1866–1867. Abel's "Researches on Guncotton" demonstrated that guncotton, after proper purification, is far more stable than it had been thought to be. Moisture does not harm it, or exposure to sunlight, and it decomposes only slowly at elevated temperatures; the principal cause of its decomposition is acid, and this is removed by the pulping. Abel wrote:

> In reducing the material to a very fine state of division by means of the ordinary beating and pulping machines, the capillary power of the fibre is nearly destroyed, and the guncotton is, for a considerable period, very violently agitated in a large volume of water. It would be very difficult to devise a more perfect cleansing process than that to which the guncotton is submitted; and the natural result of its application is that the material thus additionally purified acquires considerably increased powers of resisting the destructive effects of heat.[255] Samples of the pulped guncotton, even in the most porous conditions, have been found to resist change perfectly upon long-continued exposure to temperatures which developed marked symptoms of decomposition in the guncotton purified only as usual. The pulping process applied to guncotton affords, therefore, important additional means of purifying the material, the value of which may be further enhanced by employing a slightly alkaline water in the pulping machine. The slightest change sustained by guncotton is attended by the development of free acid, which, if it accumulates in the material, even to a very trifling extent, greatly promotes decomposition.
>
> Numerous experimental data have been collected with respect to the establishment and acceleration of decomposition in guncotton by free acid whilst exposed to light or elevated temperature. This acid is present either in the imperfectly purified material or has been developed by decomposition of guncotton or its organic impurities. Samples of guncotton which, by exposure to elevated temperatures or for considerable periods to strong daylight, had sustained changes resulting in a considerable development of acid, have afterwards been thoroughly purified by washing. When exposed to light for months, and in some instances for two or three years (up to the present time), they have undergone no further change, while corresponding samples confined in close vessels without being purified, have continued, in some instances, to undergo decomposition, and the original substance has been completely transformed into the products repeatedly spoken of.

Abel found that the guncotton regularly produced at Waltham Abbey contained a small amount of material soluble in ether-alcohol, an average amount of 1.62% in the guncotton which was made by treating cotton with 18 times its weight of mixed acid, and an average of 2.13% in the guncotton which was made by the use of 10 parts of acid. "The employment of the higher proportion of acid furnished results more nearly approaching perfection than those obtained when the guncotton was left in contact with a smaller proportion of the acid mixture. As far as can be judged at present, however, from the general properties of the products, the difference observed when the larger or the smaller proportion of acid is used, is not of sufficient importance to render necessary the consumption of the larger quantity of acid in the manufacture." Abel was able to carry out satisfactory combustion analyses, with the following average results:[256]

Material soluble in ether-alcohol, C 30.50%; H 2.91%; N 11.85%;
Material insoluble in ether-alcohol, C 24.15%; H 2.46%; N 13.83%.

He concluded that the different analytical results which had been procured with different samples of guncotton resulted from the samples containing different amounts of the ether-alcohol soluble material, and judged that completely nitrated guncotton is the trinitrate of cellulose, $[C_6H_7O_2(ONO_2)_3]_n$, as had been first suggested by Crum. This substance contains theoretically 14.14% nitrogen.

1868. E. A. Brown, assistant to Abel, discovered that dry compressed guncotton could be made to detonate very violently by the explosion of a fulminate detonator such as Nobel had already used for exploding nitroglycerin. Shortly afterwards he made the further important discovery that wet guncotton could be exploded by the explosion of a small quantity of dry guncotton (the principle of the booster). This made it possible to use large blocks of wet guncotton in naval mines with comparative safety.

Nitrocellulose (NC)

Cellulose occurs everywhere in the vegetable kingdom; it is wood fiber and cell wall, the structural material of all plants. Cotton fiber is practically pure cellulose, but cellulose of equal purity, satisfactory in all respects for the manufacture of explosives and smokeless powder, may be produced from wood. Cellulose and starch both yield glucose on hydrolysis, and the molecules of both these substances are made up of anhydroglucose units linked together.

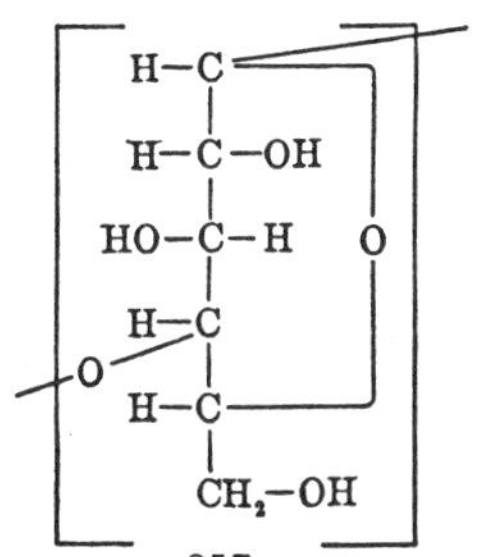

```
 [    H—C———————┐   ]
        |       |
      H—C—OH    |
        |       |
     HO—C—H     O
        |       |
      H—C       |
  —O/   |       |
      H—C———————┘
        |
        CH2—OH
 [                  ]
```

[257] The two substances differ in the configuration of the number 1 carbon atom. In cellulose this atom has the β-configuration; 2000 or 3000 anhydroglucose units are linked together in long, straight, threadlike masses which are essentially one dimensional. In starch the number 1 carbon atom has the α-configuration which leads to spiral arrangements essentially three dimensional,

and the molecule contains not more than 25 or 30 anhydroglucose units.

Cellulose contains 3 hydroxyl groups per anhydroglucose unit, and yields a trinitrate on complete nitration (14.14% N). An absolutely complete nitration is difficult to secure, but a product containing 13.75% nitrogen may be produced commercially. If the conditions of nitration, concentration of acid, temperature, and duration of the reaction, are less severe, less nitrogen is introduced, and products ranging all the way from a few per cent of nitrogen upward, and differing widely in solubilities and viscosities, may be secured. In the cellulose nitrates which contain less than enough nitrogen to correspond to the trinitrate, the nitrate groups are believed to be distributed at random among the three possible positions, and no definite structural formulas can be assigned to the materials. Nor is it to be supposed that a sample which may correspond in empirical composition to cellulose mononitrate or dinitrate really represents a single chemical individual.

Collodion is a nitrocellulose which is soluble in ether-alcohol and contains, according to the use for which it is destined, from 8%, more or less, of nitrogen to 12% or thereabouts. The name of *pyroxylin* is now generally applied to collodion of low nitrogen content intended for use in pharmacy, in the making of lacquers or of photographic film, or intended in general for industrial uses outside of the explosives industry. In 1847 Maynard discovered that nitrocellulose existed which was soluble in a mixture of ether and alcohol although it would not dissolve in either of these solvents taken singly.[92] The discovery soon led to the invention of collodion photography by Archer in 1851. Chardonnet's first patent for artificial silk was granted in 1884. *Celluloid,* made by dissolving collodion nitrocellulose in camphor with the use of

[92] After the material is dissolved, the solution may be diluted either with alcohol or with ether without precipitating.

258

heat and pressure, was patented by J. W. and I. S. Hyatt in 1870. Worden states that collodion for the manufacture of celluloid is made by nitrating tissue paper with a mixed acid which contains nitric acid 35.4%, sulfuric acid 44.7%, and water 19.9%. Twenty-two pounds of acid are used per pound of paper. The nitration is carried out at 55° for 30 minutes, and the product contains 11.0–11.2% nitrogen. Ether-alcohol solutions of collodion, to which camphor and castor oil have been added in order that they may yield tough and flexible films on evaporation, are used in pharmacy for the application of medicaments to the skin in cases where prolonged action is desired. Two per cent of salicylic acid, for example, in such a mixture makes a "corn remover." Collodion for use with nitroglycerin to make blasting gelatin is generally of higher nitrogen content. Here the desideratum is that the jelly should be stiff, and the higher nitrogen content tends in that direction, but the collodion dissolves in the nitroglycerin more slowly, and the product becomes stiffer on prolonged storage, and less sensitive, and may cause misfires. The nitrogen content of collodion for use in the manufacture of blasting explosives is generally between 11.5 and 12.0%. The official definition in England of collodion for this purpose gives an upper limit of 12.3% nitrogen.

Two kinds of nitrocellulose were used in France at the time of the first World War, *coton-poudre No. 1* (CP_1), insoluble in ether-alcohol and containing about 13% nitrogen, and *coton-poudre No. 2* (CP_2), soluble in ether-alcohol and containing about 12% nitrogen.[96] CP_1 thus contained a little less nitrogen than the material which we are accustomed to call guncotton, and CP_2 contained a little more than the material which we are accustomed to call collodion. CP_1 and CP_2 were not respectively wholly insoluble and wholly soluble in ether-alcohol; their compositions were approximate, and CP_2 always contained a certain amount of material soluble in alcohol alone. A mixture of CP_1 and CP_2 colloided with ether-alcohol was used for making *pou-*

[96] The French are accustomed to report their analyses of nitrocellulose, not as per cent nitrogen, but as cubic centimeters of NO (produced in the nitrometer and measured under standard conditions) per gram of sample. Per cent nitrogen times 15.96 equals number of cubic centimeters of NO per gram of nitrocellulose.

259

dre B. Either CP_1 with nitroglycerin and an acetone solvent or both with nitroglycerin and an ether-alcohol solvent were used for making ballistite, and both of them with nitroglycerin and with non-volatile solvents were used in attenuated ballistite. CP_2 was also used in France for the manufacture of blasting gelatin.

Mendeleev studied the nitration of cellulose during the years 1891 to 1895 in an effort to prepare a nitrocellulose which should have the largest content of nitrogen (and hence the greatest explosive power) compatible with complete solubility in ether-alcohol. He produced *pyrocellulose* containing 12.60% nitrogen. Russia adopted a military smokeless powder made from pyrocellulose by colloiding with ether-alcohol, and the United States in 1898 was using a similar powder in the Spanish-American War.

The word *guncotton* has about the same meaning in English and in American usage, namely, nitrocellulose containing 13% or more of nitrogen, usually 13.2–13.4%, insoluble in ether-alcohol and soluble in acetone and in ethyl acetate. One American manufacturer prefers to call guncotton *high-grade nitrocellulose.*

Preparation of Pyrocellulose. Equal volumes of sulfuric acid (1.84) and nitric acid (1.42) are mixed by pouring the sulfuric acid with stirring into the nitric acid, and the mixture is allowed to cool to room temperature. Five grams of absorbent cotton, previously dried at 100° for 2 hours, is thrust quickly into 150 cc. of this mixed acid and allowed to remain there for 30 minutes while it is stirred occasionally with a glass rod. The cotton is removed, freed as much as possible from acid by pressing against the side of the vessel, and introduced quickly into a large beaker of cold water where it is stirred about in such manner as to accomplish the prompt dilution of the acid with which it is saturated. The product is washed thoroughly in running water, and boiled for an hour with distilled water in a large beaker, then boiled three times with fresh portions of distilled water for a half hour each time. If the water from the last boiling shows the slightest trace of acidity to litmus paper, the pyrocellulose ought to be rinsed and boiled once more with distilled water. Finally, the excess of water is wrung out, and the pyrocellulose is dried in a paper tray for 48 hours at room temperature.

Pyrocellulose is made commercially from purified cotton *linters* or *hull shavings* or wood cellulose, most commonly by the mechanical dipper process. The thoroughly dry cellulose is introduced into the mixed acid contained in an iron or stainless steel

260

nitrator which is equipped with two paddles revolving vertically in opposite directions and designed to thrust the cotton quickly under the surface of the acid. For 32 pounds of cellulose a charge of about 1500 pounds of mixed acid is used. This contains approximately 21% nitric acid, 63% sulfuric acid, and 16% water. It may contain also a small amount, say 0.5%, of nitrous acid, NO_2 or N_2O_4, which, however, is calculated as being equivalent to a like amount of water and is not reckoned as any part of the *nitrating total* of actual nitric and sulfuric acids. The sulfuric acid content of the nitrating acid is kept as constant as possible in practice; the nitric acid content may vary somewhat, less than 1%, however, for slightly more nitric acid is necessary in warm weather to offset the tendency toward denitration which exists at that time. At the start the acid has a temperature of about 30°, the introduction of the cellulose requires about 4 minutes, and the nitration is continued for 20 minutes longer while the mixture is stirred mechanically with the paddles and the temperature is kept between 30° and 34°. When the nitration is complete, a valve in the bottom of the nitrator is opened and the slurry is allowed to run into a centrifuge on the floor below. Here the crude nitrocellulose is separated quickly from the spent acid which is fortified for use again or, in part, goes to the acid recovery plant. Wringer fires are by no means uncommon, especially on damp days, for the air which is sucked through the acid-soaked material in the centrifuge gives up its moisture to the strong acid and dilutes it with the development of considerable heat. The nitrated product is forked through an orifice in the bottom of the wringer and falls into an immersion basin below, where it is *drowned* by being mixed rapidly with a swiftly moving stream of water. Thence it proceeds on its way down the *guncotton line* where it is *stabilized* or purified and then prepared for shipment or for use.

The crude nitrocellulose contains certain amounts of cellulose sulfate, of nitrate of oxycellulose, and possibly of some cellulose nitrate which is less stable than the ordinary, all of which are capable of being hydrolyzed by long-continued boiling with slightly acidified water. Guncotton requires a longer stabilizing boil than pyrocellulose. After the boiling the acid is washed off and removed from the nitrocellulose, yielding a product which is now stabilized because it contains neither free acid nor compo-
261
nent materials which are prone to decompose with the formation of acid.

The *preliminary boiling* or *sour boiling* is carried out in large wooden tubs heated by means of steam. At the beginning the nitrocellulose is boiled with water which contains 0.25% to 0.50% of acidity calculated as sulfuric acid. The first boil lasts usually for 16 hours during which time the acidity of the solution increases. The increase is due largely to actual sulfuric acid. After 16 hours the steam is shut off, the solution is decanted from the nitrocellulose, the tub is filled with fresh water, and the material is boiled again for 8 hours. The boiling is repeated until each tubful has been boiled for 40 hours with at least 4 changes of water.
262
The hollow fibers still contain an acid solution within them. In order that this acid may be washed out, they are *pulped* or broken up into short lengths by means of apparatus like that which is used in the manufacture of paper. A Jordan mill cuts the fibers off rather sharply, leaving square ends, but a beater tears

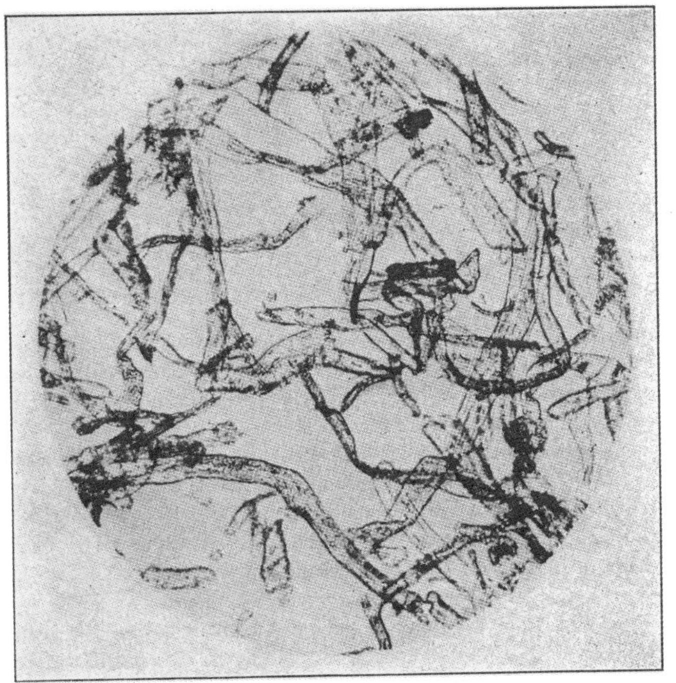

FIGURE 62. Nitrocellulose Fibers before Beating (132×).

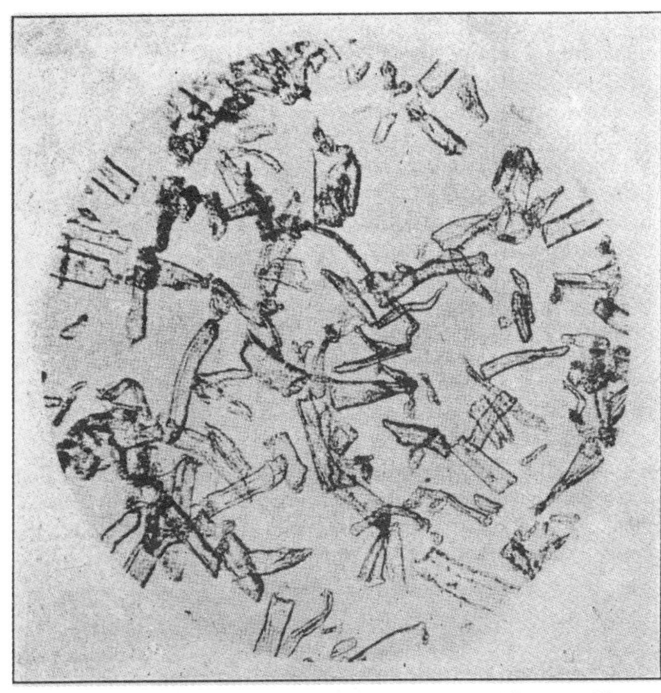

FIGURE 63. Nitrocellulose Fibers after Beating (132×). (Courtesy Western Cartridge Company.)

them, leaving ends which appear rough and shredded under the microscope and which result on the whole in the better opening up of the tubular fibers. The two machines are usually used in series. A weak solution of sodium carbonate is added during the pulping to neutralize the acid which is liberated. The pulping is continued until the desired fineness has been attained as shown by laboratory test.
263
The pulped fibers still retain acid adsorbed or occluded on their surface. This is removed by *poaching* the nitrocellulose, by boiling it again, first for 4 hours with fresh water with or without the addition of dilute sodium carbonate solution,[97] then for 2 hours with water without addition of soda, then twice with water for 1 hour each time. The material is then washed at least 8 times by thorough agitation with cold water, and by decantation each time of at least 40% of the liquid. After the washing, the material undergoes *screening,* where it passes through apertures 0.022 inch in width, *wringing,* whereby its moisture content is reduced

to 26–28%, and finally *packing* for shipment or for storage in containers which are hermetically sealed.

[97] Not more than 10 gallons of sodium carbonate solution (1 pound per gallon) for every 2000 pounds of nitrocellulose (dry weight).

Guncotton is made in substantially the same way as pyrocellulose except that a stronger mixed acid containing approximately 24% nitric acid, 67% sulfuric acid, and 9% water is used. Long-fiber high-grade guncotton is usually manufactured by the pot process and with the use of mixed acid which is nearly anhydrous. Iron pots are generally used. For the nitration of 4 pounds of dry cotton, 140 pounds of acid is introduced into the pot and the cotton is immersed in it, pressed down, and allowed to digest for 20 or 30 minutes. The contents of several pots are centrifuged at once, and the product is stabilized in the same way as pyrocellulose except that it is not pulped.

There can be no doubt that, in the standard method of stabilizing nitrocellulose, there are, among the results which the poaching accomplishes, at least some which would have been accomplished much earlier during the boiling if the material at that time had been pulped. This seems especially evident with respect to the hydrolysis of easily hydrolyzed material adjacent to the inner wall of the tubular fibers. Olsen, discussing the standard method, has written, "The preliminary boiling tub treatment reduced the acidity of the fibers and of the interstitial material, but the pulping process, by macerating these fibers, has set free an additional amount of acid. It is, therefore, necessary to repurify the pyrocotton by boiling." He discovered that a marked reduction in time and in cost could be secured by carrying out the pulping operation prior to the hydrolyzing boils. If the pulping is done at the outset,[264] "less than half of the 16 hours sour boiling usually employed will suffice for obtaining the desired degree of purity when followed by alternating boils in fresh water and washes with cold fresh water, again less than half of the amount of boiling being sufficient." With less than 20 hours total time of purification, he obtained results as good as are ordinarily procured by the 52 hours of the standard method.

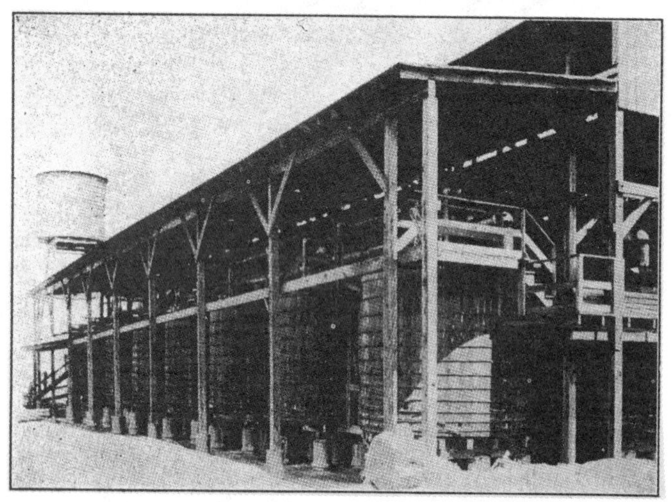

Figure 64. Boiling Tubs for Purification of Nitrocellulose.

Olsen's quick stabilization process is the result of further thinking along this same line and represents an ingenious application of a simple principle of colloid chemistry. After the nitrocellulose has been thoroughly pulped, and after the easily decomposed cellulose sulfate, etc., have been hydrolyzed, there remains only the necessity for removing the acid which clings to the fiber. The acid, however, is adsorbed on the nitrocellulose, or bound to it, in such manner that it is not easily washed away by water or even by dilute soda solution; many boilings and washings are necessary to remove it. Olsen has found that the acid is removed rapidly and completely if the nitrocellulose is digested or washed with a solution of some substance[265] which is adsorbed by nitrocellulose with greater avidity than the acid is adsorbed, that is, with a solution of some substance which has, as he says, a greater *adhesion tension* for nitrocellulose than the acid has. Such substances are aniline red, Bismarck brown, methyl orange,

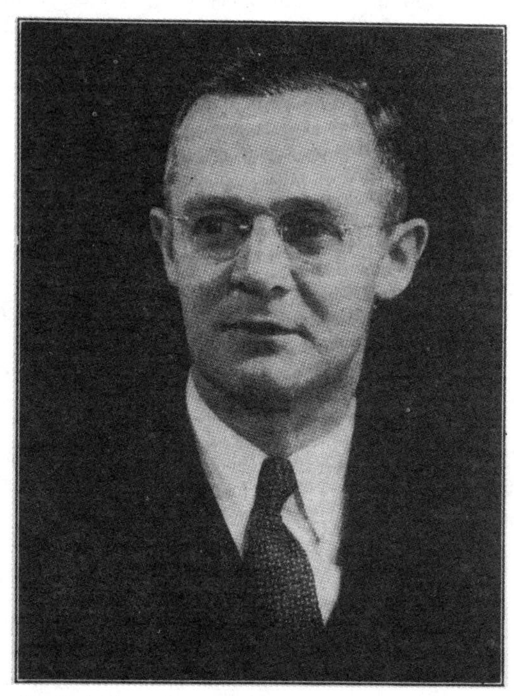

Figure 65. Fred Olsen. Has done important work on cellulose and has made many improvements in detonating explosives, high explosives, and smokeless powder; in particular, has invented processes for the quick stabilization of nitrocellulose and for the production of ball-grain powder. Chief of Chemical Research, Aetna Explosives Company, 1917-1919; Chemical Adviser, Picatinny Arsenal, 1919-1928; Technical Director, Western Cartridge Company, 1929—.

m-phenylenediamine, urea, substituted ureas such as diethyldiphenylurea, and diphenylamine. A 0.5% solution of urea in water may be used. A half-hour washing with a 0.5% solution of diphenylamine in alcohol was more effective in producing stability[266] than 20 hours of boiling with water. A solution of 0.1 gram of Bismarck brown in 300 cc. of water gave better stabilization of 30 grams of nitrocellulose in 1 hour than 10 boilings of 1 hour each with separate 300-cc. portions of water.

Nitrocellulose, like all other nitric esters with the possible exception of PETN, is intrinsically unstable, even at ordinary temperatures. Yet the decomposition of a thoroughly purified sample is remarkably slow. Koehler and Marqueyrol have made a careful study of the decomposition of nitrocellulose at various temperatures in the vacuum of a mercury pump. They found that it evolved gas at the rate of about 0.7 cc. per gram per day at 100°, 0.01 cc. per gram per day at 75°, and 0.0001 cc. per gram per day at 40°.

A sample of CP_1 was freed from carbonate by digestion with carbonated water and subsequent washing; it was dried thoroughly, and 35.152 grams of the material (analyzing 211.2 cc. NO per gram) was heated in vacuum at 75°. The results are summarized in the following table, where all gas volumes have been reduced to 0° and 760 mm. The residual gas, insoluble both

Duration of Heating at 75°	Total Volume, Cubic Centimeters	Cubic Centimeters per Gram per Day	Composition of Gas, % NO	CO_2	Residue
1st period (5 days)	2.25	0.0128	62.5	16.7	20.8
2nd period (56 days)	17.29	0.0088	63.2	19.5	17.3
3rd period (56 days)	18.25	0.00927	60.8	21.5	17.6
4th period (56 days)	18.34	0.0080	65.5	18.0	16.5
5th period (56 days)	18.19	0.0079	60.0	20.7	19.6
6th period (56 days)	18.3	0.0084	61.2	20.4	18.3

in ferrous sulfate and in caustic soda solution, was analyzed and was found to consist approximately of 46% carbon monoxide, 18% nitrous oxide, 35% nitrogen, and a trace of hydrocarbons. After 309 days of heating at 75°, the temperature of the oven was reduced, and the same sample of nitrocellulose was heated in vacuum at 40° for 221 days. During this time it evolved a total of 0.697 cc. of gas or 0.0001154 cc. per gram per day. The same sample was then heated in vacuum at 100°, as follows.

267

Duration of Heating at 100°	Total Volume, Cubic Centimeters	Cubic Centimeters per Gram per Day	Composition of Gas, % NO	CO_2	Residue
1st period (30 hrs.)	29.09	0.662	51.9	24.1	24.0
2nd period (8.5 hrs.)	8.57	0.689	68.1	17.6	14.3
3rd period (9 hrs.)	8.09	0.614			

The residual gas, neither NO nor CO_2, was found to contain about 64% of carbon monoxide, the remainder being nitrous oxide and nitrogen with a trace of hydrocarbons. The nitrocellulose left at the end of the experiment weighed 34.716 grams corresponding to a loss of 1.24% of the weight of the original material. It gave on analysis 209.9 cc. NO per gram corresponding to a denitration per gram of 2.2 cc.

The gases from the decomposition of nitrocellulose in vacuum contain nothing which attacks nitrocellulose. If the decomposition occurs in air, the nitric oxide which is first produced combines with oxygen to form nitrogen dioxide, and the red fumes, which are acidic in the presence of moisture, attack the nitrocellulose and promote its further decomposition. The decomposition then, if it occurs in the presence of air or oxygen, is self-catalyzed. The amount of nitric oxide which is produced if the decomposition occurs in the absence of air, or the amount of nitrogen dioxide which is produced in the first instance if the decomposition occurs in the presence of air, is a function solely of the mass of the sample. The extent to which the red fumes attack the nitrocellulose depends, on the other hand, upon the concentration of the gases and upon the area of the surface of the sample which is accessible to their attack. The greater the density of loading of the sample, the greater will be the concentration of the red fumes. For the same density of loading, the finer the state of subdivision of the sample, the greater will be the surface. Pellets of compressed nitrocellulose, heated in the air, decompose more rapidly than the same nitrocellulose in a fluffier condition. The pellets give a poorer heat test (see below) but obviously consist of material which has the same stability. Likewise, nitrocellulose which has been dissolved in ether-alcohol and precipitated by the addition of water, decomposes in the air more

268

rapidly than the original, bulkier material. Straight nitrocellulose powder always gives a better heat test than the nitrocellulose from which it was made. If small grains and large grains of smokeless powder are made from the same nitrocellulose, the large grains will give the better heat test.

In this country the most common heat tests which are made regularly upon nitrocellulose and smokeless powder are the 65.5° KI starch test and the 134.5° methyl violet test. In the former of these, five several portions of the material under test, differing in their moisture content from nearly dry to thoroughly dry, are heated in test tubes in a bath warmed by the vapors of boiling methyl alcohol. Within each tube, a strip of potassium iodide starch paper, spotted with a 50% aqueous solution of glycerin, hangs from a hook of platinum wire a short distance above the sample, the hook itself being supported from a glass rod through a cork stopper. The tubes are examined constantly, and the time needed for the first appearance of any color on the test paper in any one of the tubes is reported.

In the 134.5° methyl violet test, heavy glass test tubes about a foot long are used. They are closed loosely at their upper ends with perforated or notched cork stoppers, and are heated for almost their whole length in a bath which is warmed by the vapors of boiling xylene. Two tubes are used. The samples occupy the lower 2 inches of the tubes, strips of methyl violet paper are inserted and pushed down until their lower ends are about 1 inch above the samples, the tubes are heated and examined every 5 minutes, and the times are noted which are necessary for the test papers to be turned completely to a salmon-pink color, for the first appearance of red fumes, and for explosion. The explosion usually manifests itself by the audible popping of the cork from the tube, but causes no other damage. A test similar to this one, but operated at 120°, using blue litmus paper and reporting the time necessary for the paper to be reddened completely, is sometimes used.

In the Bergmann-Junk test the number of cubic centimeters of nitrogen dioxide produced by heating a 5-gram sample for 5 hours at 132° is reported. The determination was originally made by absorbing the gas in ferrous sulfate solution, liberating the nitric oxide by warming, and measuring its volume. A method based

269

upon the absorption of the gas in caustic soda solution and the titration of its acidity is now often used instead.

There are many other variations of the heat test. They are sometimes called *stability tests*, but most of them, it will be noted, involve the self-catalyzed decomposition of the sample in an atmosphere of air or of red fumes. They indicate the comparative stability only of materials which are physically alike. True indications of the stability of nitric esters are to be secured only by studying the decomposition of the substances in vacuum. For this purpose the 120° vacuum stability test is most generally preferred.

Ash in nitrocellulose is determined by gelatinizing the sample with acetone which contains 5% of castor oil, setting fire to the colloid, allowing it to burn tranquilly, and igniting the charred residue to constancy of weight. It is sometimes determined as sulfate by dissolving the sample in pure concentrated sulfuric acid and igniting to constant weight.

Nitrogen in nitrocellulose is determined by means of the *nitrometer*, an instrument of great usefulness to the chemist who is working with nitric esters or with nitroamines.

Determination of Nitrogen

Nitric acid and organic and inorganic nitrates, and in general all substances which contain free nitric acid or yield nitric acid when they are treated with concentrated sulfuric acid, are analyzed by means of the nitrometer. The method depends upon the measurement of the volume of the nitric oxide which is produced when concentrated sulfuric acid acts upon the sample in the presence of mercury. It is satisfactory also for the determination of nitro group nitrogen in certain nitroamines, in nitroguanidine and in tetryl but not in methylnitramine. It is not satisfactory in the presence of mononitro aromatic compounds or of other substances which are nitrated readily by a solution of nitric acid in concentrated sulfuric acid.[270]

Cold concentrated sulfuric acid does not attack mercury. Cold nitric acid acts upon mercury to form mercurous nitrate with the evolution of nitric oxide. If concentrated sulfuric acid is present, mercurous nitrate cannot form, and the nitric acid is converted by the mercury quantitatively into nitric oxide. The method appears to have been used for the first time by Walter Crum who applied it at an early date to the analysis of guncotton.

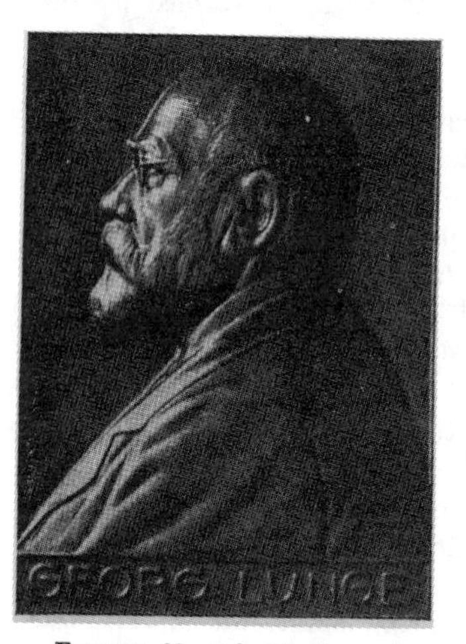

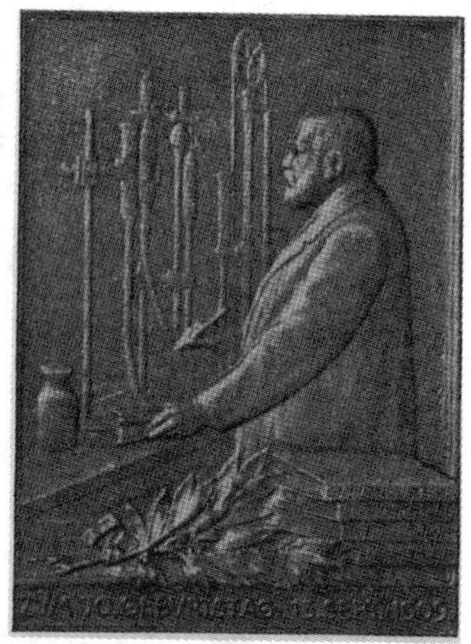

FIGURES 66 and 67. Georg Lunge and His Nitrometer. Obverse and reverse of commemorative bronze plaquette by Hans Frei in celebration of Lunge's seventieth birthday.

He introduced the sample of guncotton into a eudiometer filled with mercury and inverted in that liquid, and carried out the reaction and measured the gas volume in the same eudiometer. Since he was unable to separate the guncotton from the air entangled with it, the measured gas volume was too large. The true volume of nitric oxide was determined by admitting a solution of ferrous sulfate to the eudiometer and noting the volume of gas which was absorbed.

The Lunge nitrometer is so designed that the nitrate or nitric ester is dissolved first in concentrated sulfuric acid and the solution, without entrained gas, is afterwards admitted to the reaction vessel.[271] In the usual form of the instrument as used in Europe, the gas from the reaction is measured in cubic centimeters at atmospheric pressure, the barometer and the thermometer are read, and the weight of the nitrogen in the nitric oxide and the percentage of nitrogen in the sample are calculated.

In the extremely ingenious DuPont nitrometer, a 1-gram sample is used for the analysis, and the gas is collected in a measuring tube which has been graduated to read, at a certain temperature and pressure, the correct percentage of nitrogen in the 1-gram sample. By means of a compensating bulb and leveling device, the gas in the measuring tube is brought to the volume which it would occupy if it were confined at the temperature and pressure at which the graduations are correct, and the percentage of nitrogen is then read off directly. The DuPont nitrometer was invented by Francis I. DuPont about 1896. It quickly came into general use in the United States, and represents the form of the nitrometer which is preferred and generally used in this country. Lunge in 1901 claimed that it differs in no significant respect from the "gasvolumeter" or "five-part nitrometer" which he had described in 1890.

Calibration and Use of the DuPont Nitrometer. The five essential parts of the DuPont nitrometer are illustrated in Figure 68. The graduations on the measuring bulb correspond to dry nitric oxide measured at 20° and 760 mm., which nitric oxide contains the indicated number of centigrams of nitrogen. Thus, the point marked 10 indicates the volume which would be occupied under the standard conditions of temperature and pressure by the quantity of dry nitric oxide which contains 0.10 gram of nitrogen, that is, by the nitric oxide produced in the nitrometer reaction from a 1-gram sample of nitrate containing 10% nitrogen. The point marked 12 corresponds to 12/10 of this volume, that marked 14 to 14/10, and so on. And the tube reads correctly the per cent of nitrogen in a 1-gram sample provided the gas is measured at 20° and 760 mm.

In setting up the instrument, dry air is introduced into the compensating bulb and the outlet at the upper end of the bulb is sealed. Dry air is introduced into the measuring bulb, the outlet is connected to a sulfuric acid manometer, and the mercury reservoir and the compensating bulb are raised or lowered until the portions of air confined in both bulbs are at atmospheric pressure.[272] The stopcock is closed, the volume in the measuring bulb is read, thermometer and barometer are noted, the volume which the air in the measuring bulb would occupy at 20° and 760 mm. is calculated, and the mercury reservoir and the bulbs are adjusted until the air in the measuring bulb occupies this

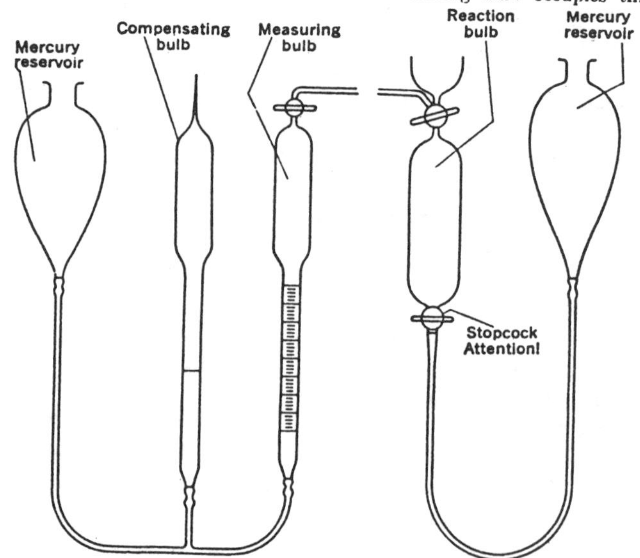

FIGURE 68. Du Pont Nitrometer.

calculated volume and until the air in the compensating bulb is at exactly the same pressure as that in the measuring bulb. A glass tube bent twice at right angles and containing some water is used for leveling the mercury in the two bulbs. The position of the mercury in the compensating bulb is now marked by means of a strip of paper glued to the glass. Whenever in the future the gas in the compensating bulb is again confined in this same volume, and whenever the nitric oxide in the measuring bulb is confined at the same pressure as the gas in the compensating bulb, then the nitric oxide will occupy the volume which it would occupy if confined at 20° and 760 mm., and, if a 1-gram sample was taken for the analysis, the reading will indicate correctly the nitrogen content. If a sample larger or smaller than 1 gram was taken, then the reading is to be corrected accordingly.

273

At the beginning of an analysis, the reaction bulb and the measuring bulb and the capillary tubes at the tops of the bulbs are completely filled with mercury. A sample of about 1 gram of nitrocellulose is weighed in a small weighing bottle, dried for an hour and a half at 100°, cooled in a desiccator, and weighed accurately. A little 95% sulfuric acid is poured onto the nitrocellulose and the whole is washed into the reaction bulb. The weighing bottle is rinsed out with several small portions of sulfuric acid, the same acid is used for rinsing the cup and is finally introduced into the reaction bulb, until altogether about 20 cc. of acid has been used, care being taken that no air is introduced. The mercury reservoir is lowered to give a reduced pressure in the reaction bulb and the bulb is shaken gently, *the stopcock at its bottom being open,* until the generation of gas has practically ceased. The bulb is then raised until the level of the mercury drops nearly to its lower shoulder, the stopcock is closed, and the bulb is shaken vigorously for 3 minutes. The cock is opened and the apparatus is allowed to stand for several minutes. The mercury level is then adjusted as before, the cock is closed, and the shaking is repeated for another 3 minutes. Finally the gas is transferred to the measuring bulb and allowed to stand for about 20 minutes. The measuring bulb and the compensating bulb are then adjusted in such fashion that the mercury in both stands at the same level and that the mercury in the compensating bulb stands at the point indicated by the paper strip. The volume in the measuring bulb is then read. After each determination the reaction bulb is rinsed out twice with concentrated sulfuric acid.

In practice it is convenient to standardize the nitrometer from time to time by means of a sample of pure potassium nitrate (13.85% N) or of nitrocellulose of known nitrogen content.

The nitrometer is dangerous to one who does not understand it fully. The closing at the wrong time of the stopcock at the bottom of the reaction bulb may result in the explosion of that vessel and the throwing about of glass and of acid.

Nitrostarch

Nitrostarch is manufactured and used in the United States, but has not found favor in other countries. In all the early attempts to manufacture nitrostarch, the starch was dissolved in strong nitric acid and the nitric ester was precipitated by mixing the solution with sulfuric acid or with the spent acid from some

274

other nitration, as from the nitration of glycerin. The product resembled the xyloïdine of Braconnot, showed a very poor stability, and could not be stored or handled safely in the dry condition. The pulverulent, dusty form of the dry material probably also contributed to the disrepute into which it fell in Europe. In this country starch is nitrated with mixed acid in which it does not dissolve, and the product retains the appearance of ordinary starch, as guncotton retains the appearance of cotton.

Cassava or tapioca starch was preferred at first, for it was claimed that it contained less fat than corn starch and that the

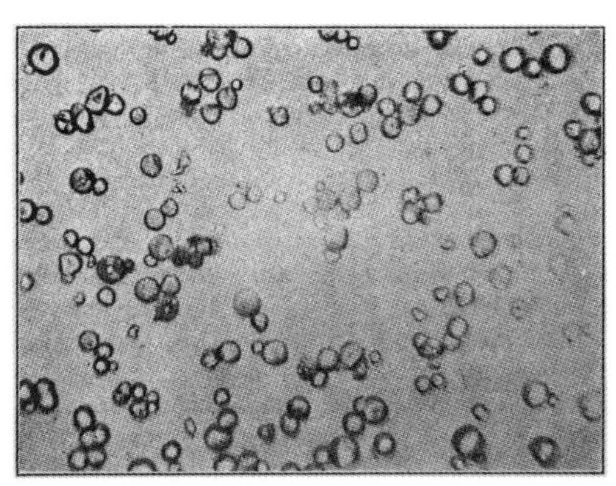

FIGURE 69. Nitrostarch Granules (about 30×).

granules, being smaller than those of corn and potato starch, permitted a more uniform nitration and a more efficient purification. Since 1917 corn starch has been used in this country. The starch is first freed from fats and from pectic acid by washing with dilute caustic soda or ammonia solution and then with water, and it is dried until it contains less than 0.5% of moisture. In one process which produced a nitrostarch containing 12.75% nitrogen, a mixed acid containing 38% of nitric acid and 62% of sulfuric acid was used, 800 pounds of the acid in a single nitrator for 200 pounds of starch. The initial temperature of the acid was 32°, the mixture was agitated by a mechanical stirrer having a downward pitch, and the temperature during the nitration was kept between 38° and 40°. At the end of the nitration

275

the contents of the nitrator was drowned in a small tub of water. The product was purified entirely by cold-water washings, without boiling. Ammonia was used to neutralize the acidity during the preliminary washing, and it is probable that this use of ammonia determined the stability of the product, perhaps because ammonia was preferentially adsorbed, instead of acid, by the material of the nitrostarch granules. The product was dried at 35–40°.

Nitrostarch gives no color with iodine. It is insoluble in water and does not gelatinize to form a paste as starch does when it is boiled with water. It is not notably hygroscopic, but may take up 1 or 2% of moisture from a damp atmosphere. It is soluble in acetone. The varieties of nitrostarch which are soluble in ether-alcohol contain about the same amounts of nitrogen as the varieties of nitrocellulose which dissolve in that mixed solvent. Nitrostarch does not form a good film or tough colloid as nitrocellulose does.

During the first World War a *Trojan explosive* which contained nitrostarch was used in trench mortar shells and in hand and rifle grenades. Its composition was as follows.

	Not Less Than	Not More Than
Nitrostarch	23.0%	27.0%
Ammonium nitrate	31.0	35.0
Sodium nitrate	36.0	40.0
Charcoal	1.5	2.5
Heavy hydrocarbons	0.5	1.5
Anti-acid	0.5	1.5
Diphenylamine	0.2	0.4
Moisture	....	1.2

All the *dope materials* were first ground to the desired fineness and dried, and then turned over in a large mixing barrel while the dry nitrostarch was added. Trench mortar shells were loaded by *stemming*, but the explosive was *jarred* into the grenades through small funnel-shaped openings. Another nitrostarch explosive, which was used only in grenades, was called *Grenite* and consisted almost entirely of nitrostarch (about 97%) with small amounts (about 1.5% each) of petroleum oil and of gum arabic. It was made by spraying the dry materials with a solution of the binder[276] while the mixture was stirred in a rotary mixer. The resulting granules were dried and screened, and yielded a free-running explosive which could be loaded easily by machine.

Three United States patents granted in 1916 to Bronstein and Waller describe several nitrostarch blasting explosives, of which the following table reports typical examples. In actual use,

	I	II	III	IV	V	VI
Nitrostarch	30.0%	39.0%	30.0%	40.0%	40.0%	40.0%
Ammonium nitrate TNT mixture	15.0	20.0	...	...	...	20.0
Sodium nitrate	46.8	37.25	58.0	37.7	34.7	17.7
Barium nitrate	...	...	...	20.0	20.0	20.0
Carbonaceous material	3.0	...	5.0	...	...	...
Paraffin oil	0.7	0.75	0.5	0.8	0.8	0.8
Sulfur	3.0	2.0	5.0	...	3.0	...
Calcium carbonate	1.5	1.0	1.5	1.5	1.5	1.5

these explosives would also contain a small amount of some stabilizer, say 0.2% of diphenylamine or of urea.

Utilization of Formaldehyde

At the time of the first World War the methyl alcohol which was needed for the preparation of tetryl was procured from the distillation of wood. It was expensive and limited in amount. Formaldehyde was produced then, as it is now, by the oxidation of methyl alcohol, and a demand for it was a demand upon the wood-distillation industry. Formaldehyde was the raw material from which methylamine was produced commercially, and the resulting methylamine could be used for the preparation of tetryl by the alternative method from dinitrochlorobenzene. It was also the raw material from which certain useful explosives could be prepared, but its high price and its origin in the wood-distillation industry deprived the explosives in question of all but an academic interest. With the commercial production of synthetic methyl alcohol, the same explosives are now procurable from a raw material which is available in an amount limited only by the will of the manufacturers to produce it.

Carbon monoxide and hydrogen, heated under pressure in the presence of a suitable catalyst, combine to form methyl alcohol. A mixture of zinc oxide and chromium oxide has been used as a catalyst[277] for the purpose. Carbon monoxide and hydrogen (equimolecular amounts of each) are produced as *water gas* when steam is passed over hot coke.

$$C + H_2O \longrightarrow CO + H_2$$

Additional hydrogen, from the action of iron on steam or from the electrolysis of water, is added to the water gas to provide the mixture which is needed for the synthesis of methyl alcohol.

$$CO + 2H_2 \longrightarrow CH_3\text{—}OH$$

It is evident that carbon dioxide may be used instead of the monoxide if a correspondingly larger amount of hydrogen is also used.

$$CO_2 + 3H_2 \longrightarrow CH_3\text{—}OH + H_2O$$

Methyl alcohol in fact is made in this manner from the carbon dioxide which results from certain industrial fermentations. When methyl alcohol vapor is mixed with air and passed over an initially heated catalyst of metallic copper or silver gauze, oxidation occurs, sufficient heat is evolved to maintain the catalyst at a bright red, and formaldehyde is formed.

$$2CH_3\text{—}OH + O_2 \longrightarrow 2H_2O + 2\,H_2C{=}O$$

Of the several explosives which are preparable from formaldehyde, two are the most powerful and brisant of the solid high explosives which are suitable for military use. One of these, *cyclotrimethylenetrinitramine* or *cyclonite*, is a nitroamine and is discussed in the chapter which is devoted to those substances. The other, *pentaerythrite tetranitrate* or PETN, is a nitric ester. Both may be prepared from coke and air.

Formaldehyde enters readily into combination with substances which add to its unsaturated carbonyl group. If a substance containing an active hydrogen adds to formaldehyde or condenses with it, the active hydrogen attaching itself to the oxygen of the formaldehyde and the rest of the molecule attaching itself to the carbon, the result is that the position originally occupied by the active hydrogen is now occupied by a $\text{—}CH_2\text{—}OH$ or methylol group. Hydrogens which are active in condensation reactions are those which are α- to a carbonyl, a nitro, or a cyano group, etc., that is, they are attached to a carbon atom[278] to which a carbonyl, a nitro, or a cyano group is also attached and are in general the hydrogen atoms which are involved in the phenomena of tautomerism. The condensation of formaldehyde with acetaldehyde, with nitromethane, with cyclopentanone, and with cyclohexanone thus leads to polyhydric primary alcohols the nitric esters of which are useful explosives.

Pentaerythrite Tetranitrate (PETN, penta, niperyth, penthrit)

Four equivalents of formaldehyde in warm aqueous solution in the presence of calcium hydroxide react with one equivalent of acetaldehyde to form pentaerythrite. Three of the four react with the three α-hydrogens of the acetaldehyde, the fourth acts as a reducing agent, converts the —CHO group to $\text{—}CH_2\text{—}OH$, and is itself oxidized to formic acid.

$$3\,H_2C{=}O + CH_3\text{—}CHO \longrightarrow [(HOCH_2)_3C\text{—}CHO]$$

$$[(HOCH_2)_3C\text{—}CHO] + H_2C{=}O \longrightarrow H\text{—}COOH + C(CH_2OH)_4 \text{ (PE)}$$

$$C(CH_2OH)_4 \longrightarrow C(CH_2\text{—}ONO_2)_4 \text{ (PETN)}$$

The name, pentaerythrite, indicates that the substance contains five carbon atoms and (like erythrite) four hydroxyl groups. In commercial practice the reaction is carried out at 65–70°. After 2 hours at this temperature, the calcium is precipitated by means of sulfuric acid, the mixture is filtered, and the filtrate is concentrated and crystallized by evaporation in vacuum. Penta-

[279] erythrite crystallizes from water in white tetragonal crystals, m.p. 253°. One part requires 18 parts of water at 15° for its solution.

PETN may be prepared, according to Naoúm, by adding 100 grams of finely powdered pentaerythrite to 400 cc. of nitric acid (1.52) while the temperature is maintained between 25° and 30° by efficient cooling. Toward the end of the nitration a certain amount of the tetranitrate crystallizes out. The separation of the product is completed by the gradual addition of 400 cc. of concentrated sulfuric acid (1.84) while the stirring and cooling are continued. The mixture is not drowned, but the crude PETN (85–90% of the theory) is filtered off directly, and washed first with 50% sulfuric acid and then with water. It still contains some occluded acid and is purified, according to Naoúm, by dissolving in hot acetone to which a little ammonium carbonate is added, and filtering the hot solution into twice its volume of 90% alcohol by which the PETN is precipitated in fine needles.

Pentaerythrite may also be nitrated satisfactorily, and probably in better yield, without the use of sulfuric acid and with the use of nitric acid from which the nitrous acid has been removed.

Preparation of Pentaerythrite Tetranitrate. Four hundred cc. of strong *white* nitric acid—prepared by adding a little urea to fuming nitric acid, warming, and blowing dry air through it until it is completely decolorized—is cooled in a 600-cc. beaker in a freezing mixture of ice and salt. One hundred grams of pentaerythrite, ground to pass a 50-mesh sieve, is added to the acid a little at a time with efficient stirring while the temperature is kept below 5°. After all has been added, the stirring and the cooling are continued for 15 minutes longer. The mixture is then drowned in about 3 liters of cracked ice and water. The crude product, amounting to about 221 grams or 95% of the theory, is filtered off, washed free from acid, digested for an hour with a liter of hot 0.5% sodium carbonate solution, again filtered off and washed, dried, and finally recrystallized from acetone. A good commercial sample of PETN melts at 138.0–138.5°. The pure material melts at 140.5–141.0°, short prismatic needles, insoluble in water, difficultly soluble in alcohol and ether.

Pentaerythrite tetranitrate is the most stable and the least reactive of the explosive nitric esters. It shows no trace of decomposition if stored for a very long time at 100°. While nitrocellulose [280] is destroyed within a few minutes by boiling with a 2.5% solution of caustic soda, PETN requires several hours for its complete decomposition. Ammonium sulfide solution attacks PETN slowly at 50°, and a boiling solution of ferrous chloride decomposes it fairly rapidly. It does not reduce Fehling's solution even on boiling, and differs in this respect from erythrite tetranitrate.

PETN does not take fire from the spit of a fuse. If a small quantity is submitted to the action of a flame, it melts and takes fire and burns quietly with a slightly luminous flame without smoke. Above 100° it begins to show appreciable volatility, and at 140–145°, or at temperatures slightly above its melting point, it shows red fumes within half an hour. It inflames spontaneously at about 210°. It is relatively insensitive to friction but makes a loud crackling when rubbed in a rough porcelain mortar. It may be exploded readily by pounding with a carpenter's hammer on a concrete floor. In the drop test it is detonated by a 20-cm. drop of a 2-kilogram weight, sometimes by a drop of 10 or 15 cm.

Naoúm reports that 10 grams of PETN in the Trauzl test with sand tamping gave a net expansion of about 500 cc., with water tamping one of 560 cc. The same investigator found a velocity of detonation of 5330 meters per second for the material, only slightly compressed, at a density of loading of 0.85 in an iron pipe 25 mm. in internal diameter. For PETN compressed to a density of 1.62 Kast found a velocity of detonation of 8000 meters per second.

PETN is extraordinarily sensitive to initiation. It is detonated by 0.01 gram of lead azide, whereas tetryl requires 0.025 gram of lead azide for its certain detonation. This sensitivity and its great brisance combine to make PETN exceptionally serviceable in compound detonators.

Under high pressure powdered PETN agglomerates to a mass which has the appearance of porcelain, but which, when broken up into grains, is a very powerful smokeless powder functioning satisfactorily with the primers which are commonly used in small arms ammunition. The powder is hot and unduly erosive, but cooler powders have been prepared by incorporating and compressing PETN in binary or in ternary mixtures with TNT, [281] nitroguanidine, and guanidine picrate. A mixture of PETN with guanidine picrate is less sensitive to heat and to shock than ordinary colloided smokeless powder, and is stable at all temperatures which are likely to be encountered. PETN does not colloid with nitrocellulose. It dissolves readily in warm trinitrotoluene, and mixtures may be prepared which contain 65% or more of PETN. The richer mixtures may be used as propellent powders. The less-rich mixtures are brisant and powerful high explosives comparable in their behavior and effects to TNB.

Stettbacher in 1931 described several dynamite-like explosives which contained both PETN and nitroglycerin. He called them by the general name of *Penthrinit*, and described simple penthrinit, *gelatin penthrinit*, and *ammonpenthrinit*. Naoúm later in the same year reported comparative tests of ammonpenthrinit and gelatin dynamite, as follows.

	Ammonpenthrinit	Gelatin Dynamite
Composition		
PETN	37%	....
Nitroglycerin	10%	63%
Collodion nitrocotton	....	2%
Dinitrotoluene	5%	....
Wood meal	....	5%
Ammonium nitrate	48%	30%
Trauzl test (average)	430 cc.	465 cc.
Velocity of detonation (average)	6600 meters per sec.	7025 meters per sec.
At density of loading	1.36	1.47

A Swiss patent of 1932 to Stettbacher covers the conversion of PETN into a plastic mass by means of 10–30% of a fluid nitric ester such as nitroglycerin or nitroglycol. It states that a mixture of 80% PETN and 20% nitroglycerin is a plastic mass, density 1.65, which does not separate into its components and which is suitable for loading shells and detonators. For the latter purpose it is initiated with 0.04 gram of lead azide.

Dipentaerythrite Hexanitrate (Dipenta)

The formation of a certain amount of dipentaerythrite is unavoidable during the preparation of pentaerythrite. It is nitrated [282] along with the latter substance, and, unless a special purification is made, remains in the PETN where its presence is undesirable because of its lower stability.

Dipentaerythrite hexanitrate is procured in the pure state by the fractional crystallization from moist acetone of the crude PETN which precipitates when the nitration mixture is drowned in water, white crystals, m.p. 72°. The crystals have a specific

$$HO-CH_2-C(CH_2OH)_2-CH_2-OH \quad + \quad HO-CH_2-C(CH_2OH)_2-CH_2-OH \longrightarrow HO-CH_2-C(CH_2OH)_2-CH_2-O-CH_2-C(CH_2OH)_2-CH_2-OH$$

Dipentaerythrite

$$\longrightarrow NO_2-O-CH_2-C(CH_2ONO_2)_2-CH_2-O-CH_2-C(CH_2ONO_2)_2-CH_2-ONO_2$$

Dipentaerythrite hexanitrate

gravity of 1.630 at 15°, after being fused and solidified 1.613 at 15°. The substance is less sensitive to friction, less sensitive to the mechanical shock of the drop test, and less sensitive to temperature than PETN, but it is less stable and decomposes much more rapidly at 100°.

Brün[283] reports measurements by the Dautriche method of the velocities of detonation of several explosives loaded in copper tubes 10 mm. in diameter and compressed under a pressure of 2500 kilograms per square centimeter.

Explosive	Density	Velocity of Detonation, Meters per Second
Dipentaerythrite hexanitrate	1.589	7370
	1.589	7450
Pentaerythrite tetranitrate	1.712	8340
	1.712	8340
Tetryl	1.682	7530
	1.682	7440
Trinitrotoluene	1.615	7000
	1.615	7000

He also reports that a 10-gram sample of dipentaerythrite hexanitrate in the Trauzl test gave a net expansion of 283 cc. (average of 2), and PETN under the same conditions gave a net expansion of 378 cc. (average of 3).

Trimethylolnitromethane Trinitrate (Nitroisobutanetriol trinitrate, nitroisobutylglycerin trinitrate, nib-glycerin trinitrate)[118]

[118] The first two of these names are scientifically correct. The third is not correct but is used widely. The trihydric alcohol from which the nitric ester is derived is not an isobutylglycerin. In the abbreviated form of this name, the syllable, nib, stands for nitro-iso-butyl and is to be pronounced, not spelled out like TNT and PETN.

This explosive was first described in 1912 by Hofwimmer[284] who prepared it by the condensation of three molecules of formaldehyde with one of nitromethane in the presence of potassium bicarbonate, and by the subsequent nitration of the product.

$$3\ H_2C{=}O \ + \ H_3C-NO_2 \longrightarrow NO_2-C(CH_2OH)_2-CH_2-OH \longrightarrow NO_2-C(CH_2ONO_2)_2-CH_2-ONO_2$$

At a time when the only practicable methods for the preparation of nitromethane were the interaction of methyl iodide with silver nitrite and the Kolbe reaction from chloracetic acid, the explosive was far too expensive to merit consideration. The present cheap and large scale production of nitromethane by the vapor-phase nitration of methane and of ethane has altered the situation profoundly. Trimethylolnitromethane trinitrate is an explosive which can now be produced from coke, air, and natural gas. Nitromethane too has other interest for the manufacturer of explosives. It may be used as a component of liquid explosives, and it yields on reduction methylamine which is needed for the preparation of tetryl.

The crude trimethylolnitromethane from the condensation commonly contains a small amount of mono- and dimethylolnitromethane from reactions involving one and two molecules of formaldehyde respectively. It is recrystallized from water to a melting point of 150°, and is then nitrated. Stettbacher reports that the pure substance after many recrystallizations melts at 164–165°. The nitration is carried out either with the same mixed acid as is used for the nitration of glycerin (40% nitric acid, 60% sulfuric acid) or with very strong nitric acid, specific gravity 1.52. If the trihydric alcohol has been purified before nitration, there is but little tendency for the nitrate to form emulsions during the washing, and the operation is carried out in the same way as with nitroglycerin. In the laboratory preparation, the nitric ester is taken up in ether, neutralized with ammonium carbonate, dried with anhydrous sodium sulfate, and freed from solvent in a vacuum desiccator.

The explosive is procured as a yellow oil, more viscous than nitroglycerin, density 1.68 at ordinary temperature. It has but little tendency to crystallize at low temperatures. A freezing point of −35° has been reported. It is very readily soluble in ether and in acetone, readily soluble in alcohol, in benzene, and in chloroform, and insoluble in ligroin. It is less soluble in water and less volatile than nitroglycerin. Because it is less volatile, it is slower to cause headaches, and for the same reason the headaches are slower to go away. It is distinctly inferior to nitroglycerin as a gelatinizing agent for collodion nitrocotton. The nitro group attached directly to an aliphatic carbon atom appears to have an unfavorable effect on stability, for trimethylolnitromethane trinitrate gives a poorer potassium iodide 65.5° heat test than nitroglycerin. Naoúm[285] reports the data which are tabulated below.

	Trimethylolnitromethane Trinitrate	Nitroglycerin
Trauzl test: 75% kieselguhr dynamite	325 cc.	305 cc.
93% blasting gelatin	580 cc.	600 cc.
Drop test, 2-kilogram weight	6 cm.	2 cm.

Nitropentanone and Related Substances

Cyclopentanone and cyclohexanone contain four active hydrogen atoms and condense with formaldehyde to form substances which contain four $-CH_2-OH$ groups. The latter may be converted directly into explosive tetranitrates or they may be reduced, the carbonyl groups yielding secondary alcohol groups, and the products then may be nitrated to pentanitrates.

Cyclopentanone (CH₂ ring with C=O) → tetramethylolcyclopentanone [$C(CH_2-OH)_2$, $C=O$, $C(CH_2-OH)_2$] → Tetramethylolcyclopentanone tetranitrate [$C(CH_2-ONO_2)_2$, $C=O$, $C(CH_2-ONO_2)_2$]

Tetramethylolcyclopentanone ↓ tetramethylolcyclopentanol [$C(CH_2-OH)_2$, $CH-OH$, $C(CH_2-OH)_2$] → Tetramethylolcyclopentanol pentanitrate [$C(CH_2-ONO_2)_2$, $CH-ONO_2$, $C(CH_2-ONO_2)_2$]

The explosives derived in this way from cyclopentanone and cyclohexanone were patented in 1929 by Friederich and Flick. They [286] are less sensitive to mechanical shock than PETN, and three out of four of them have conveniently low melting points which permit them to be loaded by pouring. *Tetramethylolcyclopentanone tetranitrate,* called *nitropentanone* for short, melts at 74°. *Tetramethylolcyclopentanol pentanitrate* is called *nitropentanol* and melts at 92°. *Tetramethylolcyclohexanone tetranitrate,* m.p. 66°, is called *nitrohexanone,* and *tetramethylolcyclohexanol pentanitrate,* m.p. 122.5°, *nitrohexanol.* They are less brisant than PETN. Wöhler and Roth have measured their velocities of detonation at various densities of loading, as follows.

Explosive	Density of Loading	Velocity of Detonation, Meters per Second
Nitropentanone	1.59	7940
	1.44	7170
	1.30	6020
	1.13	4630
Nitropentanol	1.57	7360
	1.51	7050
	1.29	6100
	1.11	5940
	1.01	5800
	0.91	5100
	0.75	5060
Nitrohexanone	1.51	7740
	1.42	7000
	1.25	5710
Nitrohexanol	1.44	7670
	1.28	6800
	1.00	5820
	0.81	5470

[287]

CHAPTER VI

SMOKELESS POWDER

An account of smokeless powder is, in its main outlines, an account of the various means which have been used to regulate the temperature and the rate of the burning of nitrocellulose. After the degree of nitration of the nitrocellulose, other factors which influence the character of the powder are the state of aggregation of the nitrocellulose, whether colloided or in shreds, the size and shape of the powder grains, and the nature of the materials other than nitrocellulose which enter into its composition.

Bulk Powder

The first successful smokeless powder appears to have been made by Captain Schultze of the Prussian Artillery in 1864. At first he seems only to have impregnated little grains of wood with potassium nitrate, but afterwards he purified the wood by washing, boiling, and bleaching, then nitrated it, purified the nitrated product by a method similar to that which had been used by von Lenk, and finally impregnated the grains with potassium nitrate alone or with a mixture of that salt and barium nitrate. The physical structure of the wood and the fact that it contained material which was not cellulose both tended to make the nitrated product burn more slowly than guncotton. The added nitrates further reduced the rate of burning, but Schultze's powder was still too rapid for use in rifles. It found immediate favor for use in shot guns. It was manufactured in Austria by a firm which in 1870 and 1871 took out patents covering the partial gelatinization of the powder by treatment with a mixture of ether and alcohol. The improved powder was manufactured between 1872 and 1875 under the name of *Collodin,* but the Austrian gov- [288] ernment stopped its manufacture on the grounds that it infringed the government's gunpowder monopoly. A company was formed in England in 1868 to exploit Schultze's invention, a factory was established at Eyeworth in the New Forest in 1869, and the

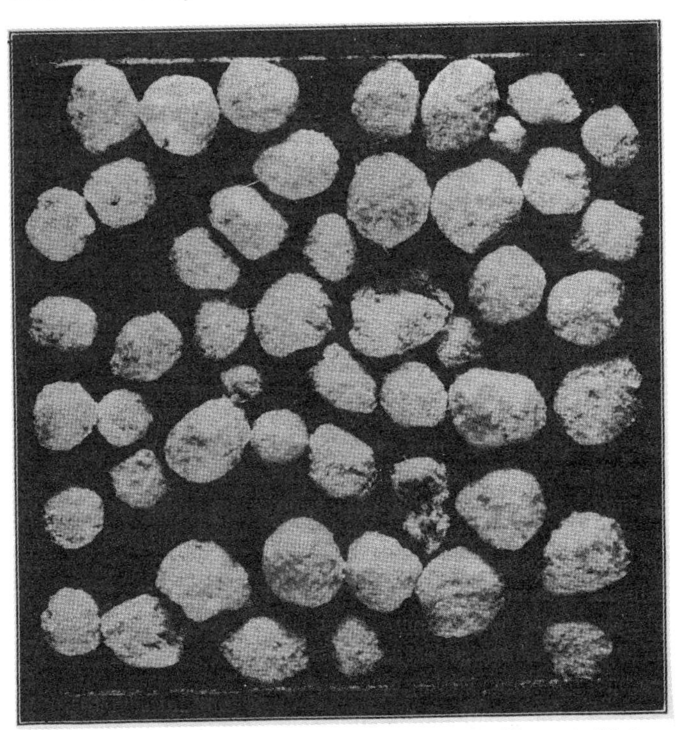

FIGURE 70. Shreddy Grains of Bulk Powder (25×). (Courtesy Western Cartridge Company.)

methods of manufacture were later improved by Griffiths and achieved great success. In 1883 Schultze entered into a partnership in Germany and started a factory at Hetzbach in Hesse-

Darmstadt.

The next successful smokeless powder was invented at the works of the Explosives Company at Stowmarket in England. It

289

was called E. C. powder (Explosives Company), and consisted of nitrocotton mixed with potassium and barium nitrates with the addition of coloring matter and small amounts of other organic material. It was made into grains which were hardened by being partially gelatinized with ether-alcohol. A separate company was organized to develop the invention, and the manufacture was started at Green Street Green, near Dartford, in Kent.

Schultze powder and E. C. powder are known as *bulk sporting* powders, either because they are loaded by bulk or because, for the same bulk, they have about the same power as black powder. Bulk powders burn quickly. They are used in shot guns, in hand grenades, in blank cartridges, and occasionally in the igniter charges which set fire to the dense colloided propellent powder which is used in artillery.

Bulk powders are made in considerable variety, but they consist always of nitrocellulose fibers which are stuck together but are not completely colloided. Some contain little else but nitrocellulose; others contain, in addition to potassium and barium nitrates, camphor, vaseline, paraffin, lampblack, starch, dextrine, potassium dichromate or other oxidizing or deterrent salts, and diphenylamine for stabilization, and are colored in a variety of brilliant hues by means of coal-tar dyes. In the United States bulk powders are manufactured by one or the other of two processes, either one of which, however, may be modified considerably; the materials are incorporated under wooden wheels, grained, and partially gelatinized, or the grains are formed in a still where a water suspension of pulped nitrocellulose is stirred and heated with a second liquid, a solvent for nitrocellulose which is volatile and immiscible with water.

Three typical bulk powders are made up according to the approximate formulas tabulated below. The nitrogen content of

Nitrocellulose	84.0	87.0	89.0
% N in nitrocellulose	13.15	12.90	12.90
Potassium nitrate	7.5	6.0	6.0
Barium nitrate	7.5	2.0	3.0
Starch	....	....	1.0
Paraffin oil	....	4.0	....
Diphenylamine	1.0	1.0	1.0

the nitrocellulose is an average secured by mixing pyrocellulose and guncotton. A batch usually amounts to 200 pounds, 100

290

pounds of water is added and about 90 grams of rosaniline or some other, generally bright-colored, water-soluble dyestuff, and the charge is incorporated by milling for about 45 minutes in a wheel mill which is built like a black-powder mill but is smaller and has light wooden wheels. The charge is then run through a mechanical rubber, which consists of wooden blocks rubbing with a reciprocating motion on a perforated zinc plate; the larger lumps are broken up and the material is put into proper condition for granulating. For this purpose about 50 pounds is placed in a copper pan or "sweetie barrel" which is revolving in a vat of hot water and is heated by that means. The pan rotates fairly rapidly, say at about 15 r.p.m., and carries the powder up along its sloping side to a point where it is scraped off by suitably arranged wooden scrapers and falls back again. It thus receives a rolling motion which has the effect of granulating the powder into spherical grains. The operation requires about 40 minutes, and its completion is indicated by the failure of the powder to carry up on the pan because of the loss of moisture.

After it has been granulated, the powder is given a preliminary screening with a 12-mesh sieve. The material which is retained on the sieve is returned to the wheel mill. That which passes through is hardened. It is put into a horizontal revolving cylinder and a mixed solvent, consisting of about 1 part of acetone and 6 parts of alcohol, is added in the proportion of 1 gallon of solvent to 15 pounds of powder. Acetone dissolves nitrocellulose, alcohol does not; the mixed solvent swells and softens the fibers and makes them stick together. The cylinder is rotated, while hot air is blown through, until the solvent has been volatilized. During this process the temperature is allowed to rise as high as 50° or 55°. The product, which consists of grains now more or less completely agglutinated, is given a final screening. In a typical case, the portion passed by a 12-mesh sieve and retained by a 50-mesh sieve is taken; it is given a final drying and is ready for use.

In a typical example of the still process for the manufacture of bulk sporting powder, 500 pounds of pulped nitrocellulose (12.60% N) is placed in a vertical cast-iron still along with 700 gallons of water containing 2% of potassium nitrate and 6% of barium nitrate dissolved in it. The material is mixed thoroughly

291

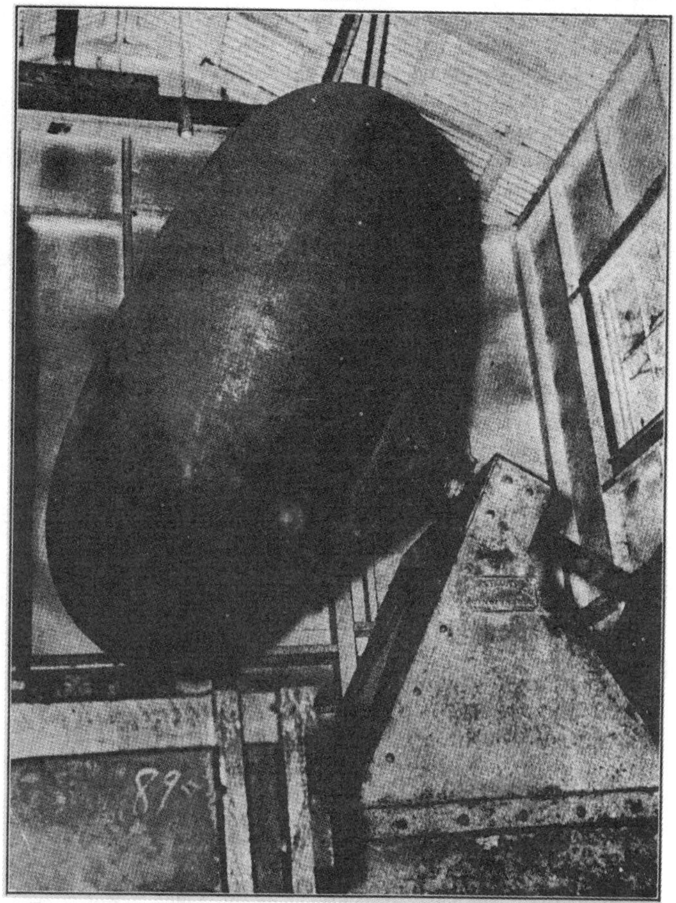

FIGURE 71. Sweetie Barrel. (Courtesy Western Cartridge Company.) The moist and mixed ingredients of bulk powder, tumbled in this apparatus, take on the form of grains. Similar equipment is used for sugar-coating pills and for applying a deterrent coating or a graphite glaze to grains of colloided smokeless powder.

292

and agitated actively by mechanical stirrers while 145 gallons of mixed solvent (2 parts butyl acetate, 3 parts benzene) containing about 3 pounds of diphenylamine dissolved in it is pumped in. The stirring is violent enough to break the solvent phase up into many small droplets, and around each droplet a globular cluster of nitrocellulose shreds builds up. The mixture is stirred continuously and distilled in vacuum at a temperature of about 30°. The distillate is collected in a separating device in such manner that the solvent is drawn off while the water is returned to the still. At the end of the process the contents of the still consists of water with potassium and barium nitrates in solution along with granules of the wet but otherwise finished powder. The individual grains of the powder are broken apart by a very violent stirring, filtered off in a centrifuge, and dried. The finished powder contains about 1 or 1.5% of potassium nitrate and about 3.5% of barium nitrate.

Early History of Colloided Powders

1884. The first smokeless powder which was satisfactory for use in rifled guns was the dense, colloided *poudre B*,[3] invented by the French physicist, Paul Vieille, and adopted immediately for the use of the French army and navy. It was made by treating a mixture of soluble and insoluble nitrocotton with ether-alcohol, kneading to form a stiff jelly, rolling into thin sheets, cutting into squares and drying, or, in later practice, extruding through a die in the form of a strip, cutting to length, and drying. The results of the first proof firing of this powder, made with a 65-mm. cannon, were communicated to the Minister of Armaments on December 23, 1884.

> It was then established that the new processes would permit the ballistic effect of black powder to be secured with the same pressure and with the charge reduced to about a third, and that the power of the arms could be increased notably, with a slight reduction of the charge, while still keeping to the ordinary pressures. The standard powder for the model 1886 rifle was determined in the early months of the year 1885. . . . The standard powder made possible an increase of velocity of 100 meters per second for the same pressures.

[3] *Poudre blanche*, white powder in contradistinction to *poudre N*, *poudre noire*, black powder.

293

> . . . This substitution has had the foreseen consequence of suppressing the smoke from the shooting.

The author of the note in the *Mémorial des poudres* in which the above-quoted public announcement was made concerning the new powder was so impressed by the importance of the invention that he concludes the note by saying:

> It results from this that the adaptation to firearms of any other explosive known at the present time would be able to bring to the armament only a perfectioning of detail, and that a new progress, comparable to that which has been realized recently, cannot be made except by the discovery of explosives of a type entirely different from those which chemistry today puts at our disposition.

French powder for the military rifle consists of small square flakes lightly glazed with graphite. The glazing serves to retard slightly the rate of burning of the surface layer, and, more important, it serves to make the powder electrically conducting and to prevent the accumulation of a static charge during the blending of small lots of the powder into a single, ballistically uniform large lot. For guns the powder consists of unglazed strips. The squares and strips, ignited over their entire surfaces, burn for lengths of time which depend upon their thicknesses, and they retain, during the burning, surfaces which change but little in area until at the end the grains are completely consumed.

1888. The second successful dense smokeless powder was the *ballistite* which was invented by Alfred Nobel. This was a stiff gelatinous mixture of nitroglycerin and soluble nitrocellulose in proportions varying between 1 to 2 and 2 to 1, prepared with the use of a solvent which was later removed and recovered. Nobel appears to have been led to the invention by thinking about celluloid, for the patent specification states that the substitution of almost all the camphor in celluloid by nitroglycerin yields a material which is suitable for use as a propellant. In the method of manufacture first proposed, camphor was dissolved in nitroglycerin, benzene was added, and then dry, pulped, soluble nitrocellulose; the mixture was kneaded, the benzene was allowed to evaporate, and the material was rolled between warm rollers

294

to make it completely homogeneous. It was rolled into thin sheets which were cut with a knife or scissors into the desired shape and size. The use of nitrostarch instead of part of the nitrocellulose, and the addition of pulverized chlorate or picrate in various proportions, were also mentioned in the patent.

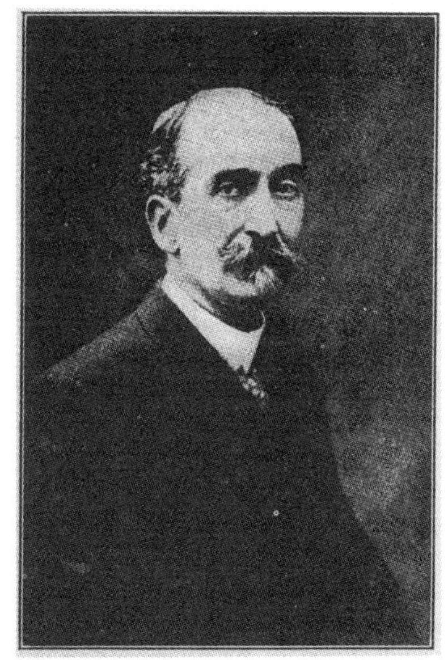

FIGURE 72. Paul Vieille (1854-1934). Inventor of *poudre B*, the first progressive-burning smokeless powder, 1884. Author of classic researches on erosion. Secretary and later, as successor to Berthelot, President of the French Powder and Explosives Commission.

1889. Nobel soon discovered that the use of soluble nitrocellulose made it possible to manufacture ballistite without using camphor or any other solvent. The nitroglycerin and soluble nitrocellulose were brought together under water. As soon as the nitroglycerin had been absorbed by the nitrocellulose, the mass was heated to 80° to complete the gelatinization, and was then rolled and cut up in the usual way. In an alternative process the gelatinization was hastened by using more nitroglycerin than was

desired in the powder, and the excess was removed by means of 75% methyl alcohol by which it was extracted while the nitrocellulose was unaffected by that solvent.

1889. Lundholm and Sayers devised a better process of incorporating the materials. The nitroglycerin and the soluble nitrocellulose were brought together under hot water and stirred by means of compressed air. The nitroglycerin presently gelatinized, or dissolved in, the nitrocellulose. The doughlike mass was removed, and passed between rollers heated to 50° or 60° whereby the water was pressed out. The sheet was folded over and passed through the rolls again, and the process was repeated until a uniform colloid resulted. It was rolled to the desired thickness and cut into squares which were generally glazed with graphite and finally blended.

1889. At about the time that Vieille was developing *poudre B*, the British government appointed a committee to investigate and report upon a smokeless powder for the use of the British service. Samples of ballistite and other smokeless powders were procured, the patent specifications relative to them were studied, and the decision was reached to use a powder which differed from Nobel's ballistite in being made from insoluble nitrocellulose containing more nitrogen than the soluble material which he used. The guncotton and nitroglycerin were incorporated together by means of acetone, mineral jelly (vaseline) was added, the colloid was pressed through dies into the form of cords of circular or oval cross section, and the acetone was evaporated off. The product was called *cordite*. The experimental work in connection with its development was done mostly in Abel's laboratory, and mostly by Kellner who later succeeded Abel as War Department chemist. Patents in the names of Abel and Dewar, members of the committee, were taken out on behalf of the government in 1889, and later in the same year the manufacture of cordite was commenced at the royal gunpowder factory at Waltham Abbey.

The mineral jelly was added to cordite originally with the idea that it would lubricate the barrel of the gun, but it seems to have no such effect. Actually it is consumed during the combustion. Because of it the powder gases contain a larger number of mols

at a lower temperature, and produce, with less erosion, substantially the same ballistic effect as the same weight of powder made up without mineral jelly. The original cordite Mk. I. contained guncotton 37%, nitroglycerin 58%, and mineral jelly 5%. This produced such serious erosion of the guns in the British South African war that the composition was modified; the relative amount of nitroglycerin was reduced for the purpose of making it cooler. Cordite M. D. (modified) consists of guncotton 65%, nitroglycerin 30%, and mineral jelly 5%.

Mineral jelly in cordite has a distinct stabilizing action. The material is known to take up nitric oxide in the nitrometer and to cause a falsely low nitrogen analysis if it is present in the material which is being analyzed.

Any distinction between cordite and ballistite which is based upon the methods by which the materials are manufactured is now no longer valid. Certain cordites are made without the use of a volatile solvent. Ballistites are made from soluble and from insoluble nitrocellulose, with and without the use of acetone, ethyl acetate, or other volatile solvent. Cordite is the name of the propellant which is used by the British armed forces. Ballistite, generally in flakes, sometimes in cords and in single-perforated tubes, is the preferred military powder of Italy, Germany, and the Scandinavian countries.

1891. Charles E. Munroe commenced investigations of smokeless powder at the Naval Torpedo Station, Newport, Rhode Island, about 1886, and about 1891 invented *indurite*. This was made from guncotton, freed from lower nitrates by washing with methyl alcohol, and colloided with nitrobenzene. The colloid was rolled to the desired thickness and cut into squares or strips which were hardened or indurated by the action of hot water or steam. Most of the nitrobenzene was distilled out by this treatment, and the colloid was left as a very hard and tough mass. Indurite was manufactured which gave satisfactory tests in guns ranging in caliber from the one-pounder to the six inch.

1895–1897. After Munroe's resignation from the Torpedo Station, Lieutenant John B. Bernadou, U. S. Navy, took up the

work on smokeless powder and in 1895 patented a powder consisting of a mixture of guncotton, collodion cotton, and potassium nitrate, colloided with acetone, and in 1897 an improved powder made from nitrocellulose alone colloided with ether-alcohol. The nitrocellulose first used contained approximately 12.45% nitrogen, but this was later replaced by pyrocellulose, 12.60% nitrogen. The powder was made in multiperforated cylindrical grains, and was substantially the same as was used by the United States in the first World War. Patents covering various improvements in the manufacture of pyrocellulose powder were taken out in the names of Lieutenant Bernadou and Captain Converse, U. S. Navy, and were licensed or sold to private interests, the United States government retaining the right to manufacture under these patents powder for its own use.

1900–1907. About 1900 the Navy Department built the Naval Powder Factory at Indian Head, Maryland. The plant was capable of producing several thousand pounds of smokeless powder per day, and was enlarged during the course of a few years to a capacity of about 10,000 pounds daily. About 1907 the Ordnance Department, U. S. Army, built at Picatinny Arsenal, Dover, New Jersey, a powder plant with a capacity of several thousand pounds per day.

Classification of Colloided Nitrocellulose Powders

American pyrocellulose powder and French *poudre B* are *straight nitrocellulose* or *single-base* powders. They are made by the use of a volatile solvent, generally ether-alcohol, which solvent is removed wholly or in large part during the process of manufacture. They are the simplest of colloided powders, the pyrocellulose powder being really the simpler of the two, for it is made from one single kind of nitrocellulose. Modified forms of these powders are made by incorporating into the colloid non-volatile solvents (i.e. solvents which remain in the finished powder) which may be either explosive or non-explosive or by distributing throughout the colloid as a separate phase materials, either explosive or non-explosive, which affect the rate or the temperature of the burning or the strength of the powder. Aromatic nitro compounds, such as DNT, TNX oil, etc., dissolve nitrocellulose or are dissolved by it, and thus constitute themselves non-volatile solvents, but they are also explosives in their

own right, and a nitrocellulose powder which contains one of them might, it would seem, be designated with propriety as a *double-base powder*. This, however, is not in accordance with prevailing usage. The name of double-base powder is reserved for such powders as ballistite and cordite which contain nitrocellulose and nitroglycerin (or perhaps some substitute for nitroglycerin such as nitroglycol). Double-base powders are made both with and without volatile solvent, and are also capable of being modified in all of the ways in which a single base powder may be modified. We have, therefore, colloided powder of various kinds, as follows.

I. Nitrocellulose powder without nitroglycerin
  a. with volatile solvent,
  b. with non-explosive non-volatile solvent,
  c. with explosive non-volatile solvent,
  d. with non-explosive non-volatile non-solvent,
  e. with explosive non-volatile non-solvent.
II. Nitrocellulose powder with nitroglycerin
  a. with volatile solvent,
  b. with non-explosive non-volatile solvent,
  c. with explosive non-volatile solvent,
  d. with non-explosive non-volatile non-solvent,
  e. with explosive non-volatile non-solvent.
III. Coated and laminated powders the grains of which are non-homogeneous combinations of the powders above classified.

This classification is offered, not in any belief that it clarifies a matter which is otherwise difficult to understand, but because it directs attention to the various possibilities and displays their relationships to one another. Some of the possibilities correspond to powders which are or have been used in this country or in Europe, and which are sufficiently described for our present purpose if they are mentioned specifically. Others will be discussed at greater length in the sections, below, which are concerned with the absorption of moisture, with gelatinizing agents, and with flashless charges and flashless powder. All the possibilities are actually exploited, though not always separately.

Cordite MD, it may be noted, is a double base powder made with volatile solvent and containing a non-volatile, non-explosive non-solvent, namely mineral jelly, and is classified in class II *a d*,

299

while a flashless ballistite of class II *b c* is made by incorporating centralite and DNX oil with nitroglycerin and nitrocellulose, and one of class II *b e* by mixing centralite and nitroguanidine with nitroglycerin and nitrocellulose. The nitroguanidine does not dissolve in the colloid but is distributed through it in a state of fine subdivision. Ten or 15 parts of nitroguanidine incorporated with 90 or 85 parts of pyrocellulose colloided with ether-alcohol gives a mixture which may be extruded through dies and yields a powder (I *a e*) which is flashless. PETN is another substance, insoluble in nitrocellulose colloids, which in the state of a fine powder may be incorporated in single-base or in double-base mixtures to yield powders (I *a e* and II *a e*) which are hotter and more powerful than otherwise.

Manufacture of Single-Base Powder

The operations in the manufacture of smokeless powder from pyrocellulose, briefly, are as follows.

1. *Dehydrating.* The pulped pyrocellulose contains about 25% moisture when it arrives at the smokeless powder plant. Most of this is squeezed out by pressing with a moderate pressure, say 250 pounds per square inch, for a few moments. The pressure is then released, alcohol in an amount at least equal to the dry weight of the pyrocellulose is forced into the mass by means of a pump, and the pressure is increased to about 3500 pounds per square inch. The process is managed in such fashion that the resulting cylindrical block consists of pyrocellulose moistened with exactly the amount of alcohol which is needed for the formation of the colloid. The requisite amount of ether is added later. The solvent consists altogether of 1 part by weight of alcohol and 2 parts of ether, 105 pounds of the mixed solvent for every 100 pounds of pyrocellulose if the colloid is to be made into 0.30-caliber powder, 100 parts if into powder of which the web thickness is approximately 0.025 inch, and 85 parts for powder having a web thickness of 0.185 inch. The block is received in a cannister of vulcanized fiber and is covered over in order that loss of solvent by evaporation may be reduced to a minimum. From this point on, in fact, the material is kept and is moved from one operation to another in covered cannisters at all times except when it is being worked.

300

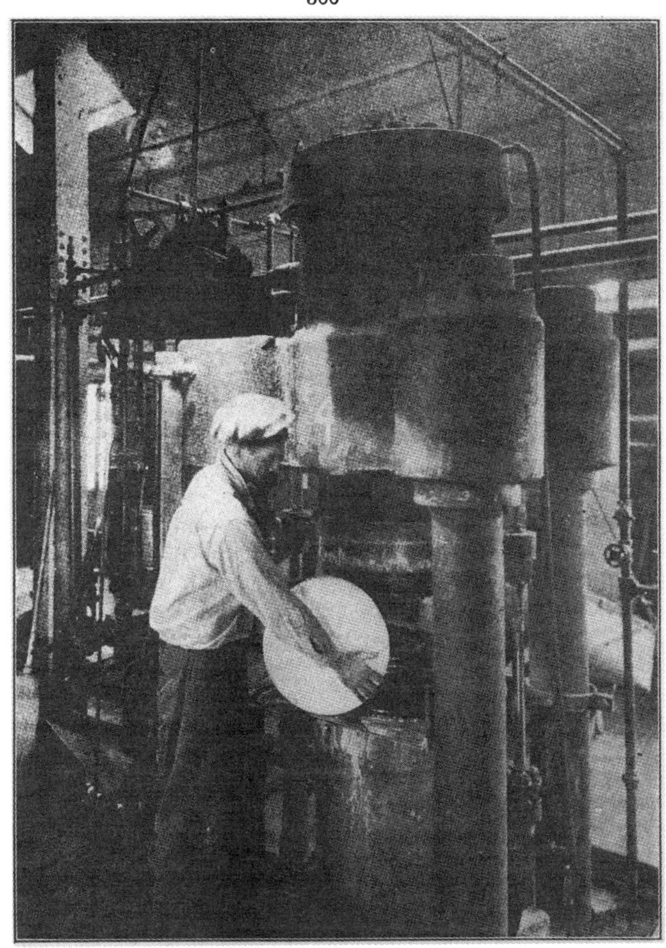

FIGURE 73. Smokeless Powder Manufacture. (Courtesy E. I. du Pont de Nemours and Company, Inc.) Dehydrating Press. The nitrocellulose comes from the dehydrating press in the form of a cylindrical block, impregnated with alcohol, ready for the mixer where ether is added and where it is colloided.

301

FIGURE 74. Smokeless Powder Manufacture. (Courtesy E. I. du Pont de Nemours and Company, Inc.) Smokeless Powder Mixer—open to show the crumbly, partially colloided material. In use, the apparatus is closed tightly to prevent the loss of volatile solvent.

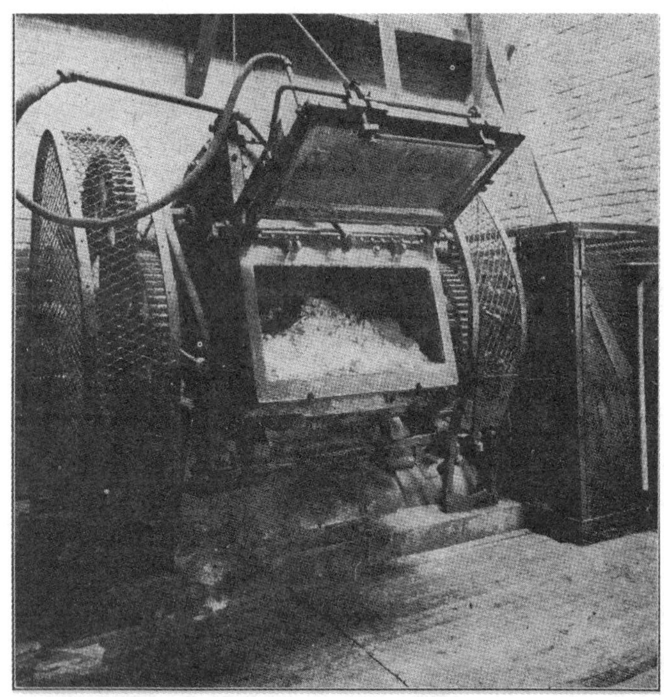

302

2. *Mixing or incorporating.* The compressed block from the dehydrating press is broken up by hand against the blades of the mixing machine. This is similar to the bread-mixing machines which are used in large commercial bakeries, and consists of a water-cooled steel box in which two shafts carrying curved blades rotate in opposite directions and effectively knead the material. The ether is added rapidly and mixed in as fast as possible. Diphenylamine sufficient to constitute 0.9–1.1% of the weight of the finished powder is previously dissolved in the ether, and is thus distributed uniformly throughout the colloid. The incorporated material has an appearance similar to that of a mass of brown sugar which has been churned; it is soft enough to be deformed between the fingers, and, when squeezed, welds together in the form of a film or colloid.

3. *Pressing.* The loose and not yet completely colloided material is pressed into a compact cylindrical mass by means of a pressure of about 3500 pounds per square inch in the *preliminary blocking press.* The *preliminary block* is then placed in the *macaroni press* where it is pressed or strained through 1 12-mesh steel plate, 2 sheets of 24-mesh and 1 sheet of 36-mesh steel wire screen, and through the perforations in a heavy plate of brass from which it emerges in wormlike pieces resembling macaroni. A pressure of 3000 to 3500 pounds per square inch is commonly used. The material drops directly into the cylinder of the *final blocking press,* where it is squeezed into a compact cylindrical block of the right size to fit the graining press. A pressure of about 3500 pounds per square inch is maintained for 1 or 2 minutes, and completes the colloiding of the pyrocellulose. The *final block* is dense, tough, elastic, light brown or amber colored, and translucent.

4. *Graining and cutting.* The colloid is forced by an hydraulic press through dies by which it is formed into single-perforated or into multiperforated tubes. For the formation of a single-perforated tube, the plastic mass is forced in the die into the space which surrounds a centrally fixed steel wire; it is then squeezed past the wire through a circular hole and emerges in the form of a tube. For the formation of a multiperforated tube, 7 such wires are accurately spaced within the die. A pressure of 2500 to 3800 pounds per square inch is used. For small arms powder the head of the press may contain as many as 36 dies, for large-

303

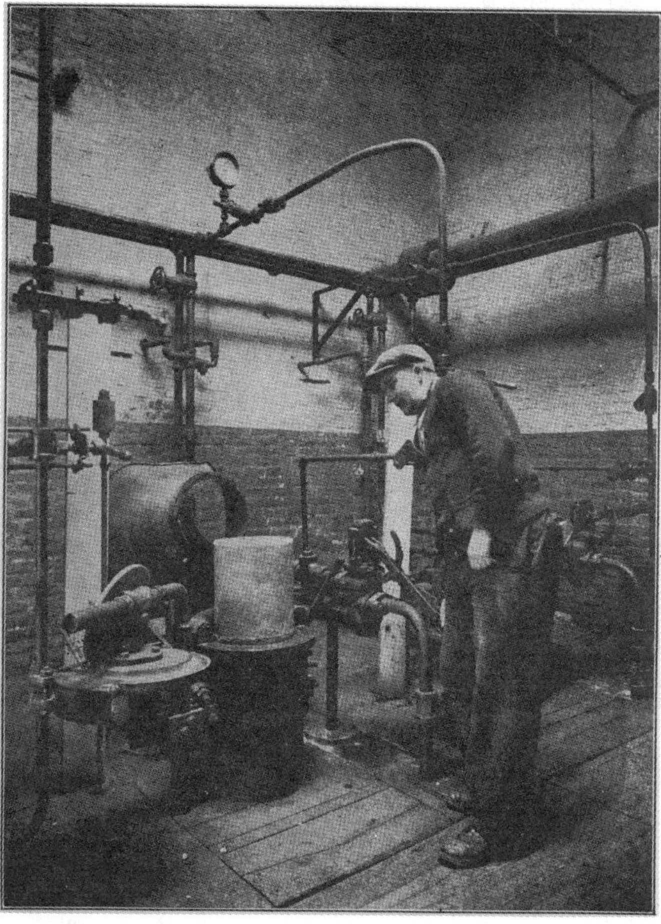

FIGURE 75. Smokeless Powder Manufacture. (Courtesy E. I. du Pont de Nemours and Company, Inc.) Blocking Press.

304

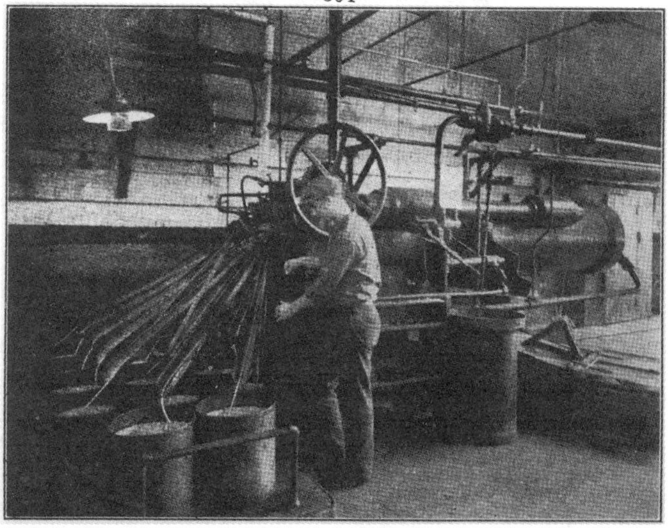

FIGURE 76. Smokeless Powder Manufacture. (Courtesy E. I. du Pont de Nemours and Company, Inc.) Finishing Press. The colloid is extruded

in the form of a perforated cylinder which is later cut into pieces or grains.

caliber powder, such as that for the 16-inch gun, it usually contains only one. The cord or rope of powder as it comes from the press is passed over pulleys or through troughs to a rotary cutter where it is cut into short cylinders about 2.1 to 2.5 times as long as their diameters or it is coiled up in a fiber cannister in which it is taken to another room for cutting. In France the colloid is pressed through slots from which it emerges in the form of ribbons which are cut into strips of a length convenient for loading into the gun for which the powder is intended.

5. *Solvent recovery.* The *green powder* contains a large amount of ether and alcohol which presents a twofold problem: (1) the recovery of as much of the valuable volatile solvent as is economically feasible, and (2) the removal of the solvent to such an extent that the finished powder will not be disposed either to give off or to take up much volatile matter or moisture under changing atmospheric conditions. For the recovery of the solvent, the pow-

305

der is put into a closed system and warm air at 55–65° is circulated through it; the air takes up the alcohol and ether from the powder and deposits much of it again when it is passed through a condenser. It is then heated and again passed through the powder. In some European plants the air, after refrigeration, is passed upward through an absorption tower down which cresol or other suitable liquid is trickling. This removes the ether which was not condensed out by the cooling, and the ether is recovered from it by distillation. The whole process of solvent recovery requires careful control, for the colloid on drying tends to form a skin on its surface (the way a pot of glue does when drying) and the skin tends to prevent the escape of volatile matter from the interior of the powder grain.

6. *Water-drying.* Powder is now most commonly dried by the rapid water-drying process whereby the formation of a skin upon its surface is prevented and certain other advantages are gained. Water at 65° is circulated throughout the powder. The water causes the production of microscopic cracks and pores through which the alcohol and ether escape more freely. These substances leave the powder to dissolve in the water, and then the ether in particular evaporates out from the water. When the volatile solvent content of the powder is sufficiently reduced, the powder grains are taken out and the water with which they are superficially covered is removed in a dry-house or in a continuous dryer at 55–65°. The finished powder contains 3.0 to 7.5% of volatile solvent in the interior of the grain, the amount depending upon the thickness of the web, and 0.9 to 1.4% of *external moisture,* mostly water actually resident in the cracks or pores of the surface. The amount of moisture which the powder thus holds upon its surface is an important factor in maintaining its ballistic stability under varying atmospheric conditions. The amount ought to be such that there is no great tendency for the moisture to evaporate off in dry weather, and such also that there is no great tendency for the powder to take up moisture in damp weather. The importance of surface moisture is so considerable that the French powder makers, long before there was any thought of using warm water to dry the powder, were accustomed to submit it to a *trempage* or tempering by immersion in water for several days. Later, periods of air-drying were alternated

306

with periods of *trempage* in warm water at temperatures sometimes as high as 80°.

Powder for small arms is generally *glazed* with graphite, by which treatment its attitude toward the loss and absorption of moisture is improved, and by which also it is made electrically conducting so that it can be *blended* without danger from static

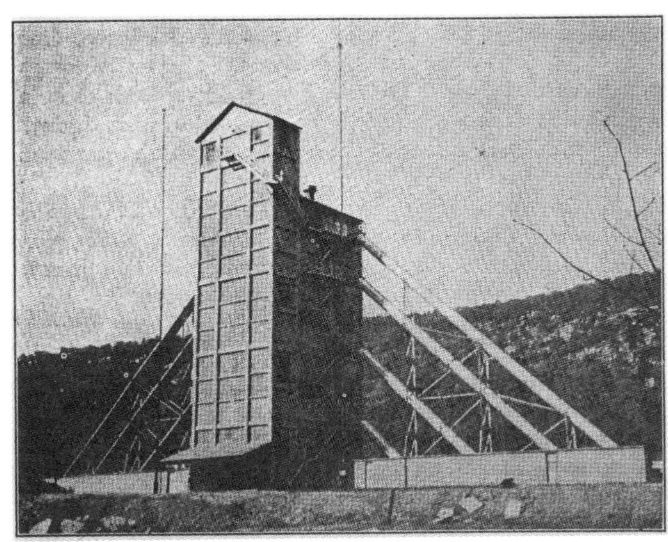

FIGURE 77. Smokeless Powder Blending Tower. The powder is blended by being made to flow through troughs and bins. Lots as large as 50,000 pounds of rifle powder and 125,000 pounds of cannon powder have been blended in this tower.

electricity and loaded satisfactorily by a volumetric method. The powder is blended in order that large lots can be made up which will be ballistically uniform, and hence that the proof firing, the operations of loading, and the calculations of the artilleryman may all be either simplified in kind or reduced in amount. Powder in short cylindrical grains, such as is used in the United States, is particularly easy to blend, but the blending of strips, or of long tubes or cords, is obviously difficult or impracticable. The finished powder is stored and shipped in airtight boxes which contain 110–150 pounds.

307

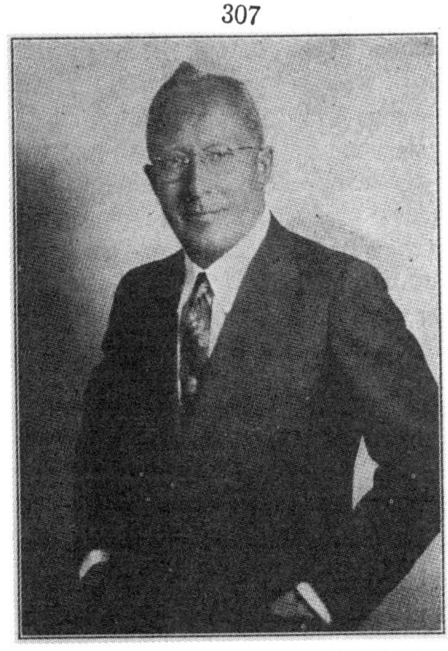

FIGURE 78. Bernhart Troxler. (Greystone Studios, Inc.) Introduced many innovations into the manufacture of smokeless powder and improved the design of equipment in such manner as to increase production while re-

ducing the hazard—the steam-air-dry process for double-base powder, methods of coating, apparatus for solvent recovery, water drying, and air drying of single-base powder without transferring the powder during the three operations. His whole professional life has been devoted to smokeless powder, with the Laflin and Rand Powder Company until 1913, and afterwards with the Hercules Powder Company from the time when that company was organized and built its first smokeless powder line.

Stabilizers

The spontaneous decomposition of nitrocellulose in the air produces nitrous and nitric acids which promote a further decomposition. If these products however are removed continuously, the uncatalyzed decomposition is extremely slow, and smokeless powder may be stabilized by the addition to it of a substance which reacts with these acids and removes them, provided neither the substance itself nor the products of its reaction with the acids attacks the nitrocellulose.

Vieille suggested the use of amyl alcohol as a stabilizer, and powder containing this material was used in France until 1911

308

when, in consequence of the disastrous explosion of the battleship *Jena* in 1907 and of the battleship *Liberté* in 1911, both ascribed to the spontaneous inflammation of the powder, and in consequence of the researches of Marqueyrol, its use was discontinued entirely. Indeed no powder containing amyl alcohol was manufactured in France after October, 1910. Freshly manufactured *poudre BAm* smelled of amyl alcohol; the alcohol was converted by the products of the decomposition into the nitrous and nitric esters, and these soon broke down to produce red fumes anew and evil-smelling valerianic acid. The presence of the latter in the powder was easily detected, and was taken as evidence that the powder had become unstable. The Italians early used aniline as a stabilizer for their military ballistite. This forms nitro derivatives of aniline and of phenol, but it attacks nitrocellulose and is now no longer used. As early as 1909, diphenylamine was being used in the United States, in France, and in Germany, and, at the present time, it is the most widely used stabilizer in smokeless powder. The *centralites* (see below) also have a stabilizing action in smokeless powder but are used primarily as non-volatile solvents and deterrent coatings.

Calcium carbonate, either powdered limestone or precipitated chalk, is used as an anti-acid in dynamite where it serves as a satisfactory stabilizer. Urea is used in dynamite and in celluloid. It reacts with nitrous acid to produce nitrogen and carbon dioxide, and is unsuitable for use in smokeless powder because the gas bubbles destroy the homogeneity of the colloid and affect the rate of burning. The small gas bubbles however commend it for use in celluloid, for they produce an appearance of whiteness and counteract the yellowing of age.

In addition to the ability of certain substances to combine with the products of the decomposition of nitrocellulose, it is possible that the same or other substances may have a positive or a negative catalytic effect and may hasten or retard the decomposition by their presence. But it has not yet been made clear what types of chemical substance hasten the decomposition or why they do so. Nitrogen dioxide hastens it. Pyridine hastens it, and a powder containing 2 or 3% of pyridine will inflame spontaneously if heated for half an hour at 110°. Powders containing tetryl are very unstable, while those containing 10% of trinitronaphthalene (which does not react with the products of decomposition) are as

309

stable as those containing 2% of diphenylamine (which does react).

In a series of researches extending over a period of 15 years Marqueyrol has determined the effect of various substances, particularly naphthalene, mononitronaphthalene, diphenylbenzamide, carbazol, diphenylamine, and diphenylnitrosamine, upon the stability of smokeless powder at 110°, 75°, 60°, and 40°. Samples of *poudre BF* [12] were made up containing different amounts of each stabilizer, and were subjected to dry heat in open vessels and in vessels closed with cork stoppers. Samples were removed from time to time and the nitrogen content of their nitrocellulose was determined. A sample of the powder was taken up in a solvent, and precipitated in a granular state; the precipitate was washed with cold chloroform until a fresh portion of chloroform was no longer colored by 18 hours contact with it, and was dried, and analyzed by the nitrometer. It was necessary to isolate the pure nitrocellulose and to separate it from the stabilizer, for the reason that otherwise the stabilizer would be nitrated in the nitrometer and a low result for nitrogen would be secured. A selected portion of Marqueyrol's results, from experiments carried out by heating in open vessels, are shown in the tables on

[12] F = *fusil*, rifle.

Days of heating at 40°	0	387	843	1174	2991	3945	4016
Analysis:							
no stabilizer	201.8	....	199.5	*147.8*	....	....	....
2% amyl alcohol	202.2	....	198.7	200.6	199.2	....	172.9
8% " "	201.4	....	199.2	200.8	198.9	....	198.2
1% diphenylamine	201.3	....	199.5	201.0	200.9	....	201.0
2% "	199.5	....	198.2	199.2	199.4	....	200.2
5% "	200.1	201.2	....	....	....	197.6	....
10% "	200.1	199.0	198.2	....	....	....	....

Days of heating at 60°	0	146	295	347	1059	2267	3935
Analysis:							
no stabilizer	201.8	*146.5*	....	....	....	....	....
2% amyl alcohol	202.2	197.4	....	*147.2*	....	....	....
8% " "	201.4	197.3	....	198.3	159.5	....	....
1% diphenylamine	201.3	197.6	....	200.0	....	....	....
2% "	199.5	196.1	....	198.3	....	....	....
5% "	200.1	....	196.0	....	....	....	185.7
10% "	200.1	....	192.3	....	....	....	173.0

310

Days of heating at 75°	0	86	231	312	516	652	667
Analysis:							
2% amyl alcohol	203.1	*191.4*	....	....	....	....	....
1% diphenylamine	201.3	196.0	....	198.0	190.9	....	....
2% "	199.5	194.7	....	198.1	....	192.1	....
5% "	200.1	....	192.8	....	....	....	186.2
10% "	200.1	....	184.2	....	....	....	175.9

Days of heating at 75°	0	55	146	312	419	493	749
Analysis:							
1% diphenylnitrosamine	200.4	197.9	198.4	199.2	197.5	198.2	194.0
2% "	200.0	201.5	198.3	198.5	197.6	171.5	....
10% "	201.5	195.3	194.1	193.0	190.6	187.3	184.3

Days of heating at 75°	0	60	85	108	197	377	633
Analysis:							
2% amyl alcohol	200.9	198.9	*196.9*	....	....	....	....
1.25% carbazol	200.6	199.4	....	199.1	*182.8*	....	....
10% "	200.3	198.7	....	197.7	198.2	193.0	190.2

Days of heating at 75°	0	31	50	62	87	227	556
Analysis:							
1.5% diphenylbenzamide	200.2	199.3	*186.1*	....	....	....	....
10% "	200.2	198.1	....	....	200.3	....	....
1.5% mononitronaphthalene	202.4	199.8	....	....	....	....	....

10% mononitronaphthalene	202.0	198.1	....	*193.0*	....	....	....
1.5% naphthalene	202.3	200.2	194.8	....	....	....	....
10% "	201.8	199.2	....	....	....	199.1	200.2

pages 309–310, where the numbers representing *analyses* indicate the nitrogen contents as usually reported in France, namely, cubic centimeters of nitric oxide per gram of nitrocellulose. When the numbers are printed in italics, the samples which were taken for analysis were actively giving off red nitrous fumes.

Diphenylnitrosamine, which is always present in powders made from diphenylamine, is decomposed at 110°, and that temperature therefore is not a suitable one for a study of the stability of smokeless powder. At 75° diphenylnitrosamine attacks nitrocellulose less rapidly than diphenylamine itself, but this is not true at lower temperatures (40° and 60°) at which there is no appreciable difference between the two substances. Carbazol at 110° is an excellent stabilizer but at 60° and 75° is so poor as to
311
deserve no further consideration. Ten per cent of diphenylamine gives unstable smokeless powder. Powder containing 40% of diphenylamine inflames spontaneously when heated in an open vessel at 110° for an hour and a half. Diphenylamine attacks nitrocellulose, but it does not attack it as rapidly as do the products themselves of the decomposition of nitrocellulose in air; and 1 or 2% of the substance, or even less, in smokeless powder is as good a stabilizer as has yet been found.

Transformations of Diphenylamine During Aging of Powder

Desmaroux, Marqueyrol and Muraour, and Marqueyrol and Loriette have studied the diphenylamine derivatives which give a dark color to old powder, and have concluded that they are produced by impurities in the ether which is used in the manufacture or by the oxidizing action of the air during drying and storage. Their presence is not evidence that the powder has decomposed, but indicates that a certain amount of the diphenylamine has been consumed and that correspondingly less of it remains available for use as a stabilizer.

The transformations of diphenylamine in consequence of its reaction with the products of the decomposition of nitrocellulose are indicated by the following formulas. None of these substances imparts any very deep color to the powder.

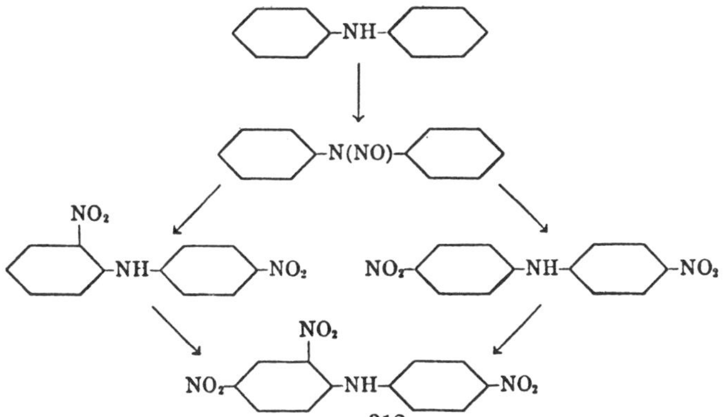

-NH-

-N(NO)-

NO_2 -NH- -NO_2 NO_2- -NH- -NO_2

NO_2 NO_2- -NH- -NO_2

312

The diphenylamine is converted first into diphenylnitrosamine which is as good a stabilizer as diphenylamine itself. Since both of these substances may be detected by simple tests upon an alcoholic extract of a sample of the powder, the fitness of the powder for continued storage and use may be easily demonstrated. A strip of filter paper on which the alcoholic extract has been allowed to evaporate is colored blue by a drop of ammonium persulfate solution if unchanged diphenylamine is present. Likewise the extract, if it contains diphenylamine, is colored blue by the addition of a few drops of a saturated aqueous solution of ammonium persulfate. Since the alcoholic extract is often colored, the test is best carried out by comparing the colors of two equal portions of the extract, one with and one without the addition of ammonium persulfate. Diphenylnitrosamine gives no color with ammonium persulfate. One-tenth of a milligram of diphenylnitrosamine imparts an intense blue color to a few cubic centimeters of cold concentrated sulfuric acid. It gives no color with a cold 1% alcoholic solution of α-naphthylamine, but an orange color if the solution is heated.[17] None of the other diphenylamine derivatives which occur in smokeless powder give these tests.

Diphenylnitrosamine rearranges under the influence of mineral acids to form *p*-nitrosodiphenylamine. The latter substance is evidently formed in smokeless powder and is oxidized and nitrated by the products of the decomposition to form 2,4′- and 4,4′-dinitrodiphenylamine. Davis and Ashdown have isolated both of these substances from old powder, and have also prepared them by the nitration of diphenylnitrosamine in glacial acetic acid solution. Both substances on further nitration yield 2,4,4′-trinitrodiphenylamine, which represents the last stage in the nitration of diphenylamine by the products of the decomposition of smokeless powder. This material has been isolated from a sample of U. S. pyrocellulose powder which was kept at 65° in a glass-stoppered bottle for 240 days after the first appearance of red fumes. The several nitro derivatives of diphenylamine may be distinguished by color reactions with alcoholic solutions of ammonia, sodium hydroxide, and sodium cyanide, and some insight into the past history of the powder may be gained from tests on the alcohol extract with these reagents, but their pres-
313
ence is evidence of instability, and no powder in which the diphenylnitrosamine is exhausted is suitable for further storage and use.

Absorption of Moisture

Nitrocellulose itself is hygroscopic, but its tendency to take up moisture is modified greatly by other substances with which it is incorporated. Colloided with nitroglycerin in the absence of solvent, it yields a product which shows no tendency to take up moisture from a damp atmosphere. Colloided with ether-alcohol, as in the case of the *poudre B* and the straight pyrocellulose powders which were used in the first World War, it yields a powder which is hygroscopic both because of the hygroscopicity of the nitrocellulose itself and because of the hygroscopicity of the alcohol and ether which it contains. In water-dried powder the alcohol and ether of the surface layer have been largely removed or replaced with water, the hygroscopicity of the surface layer is reduced, and the interior of the grain is prevented to a considerable extent from attracting to itself the moisture which it would otherwise attract. In certain coated and *progressive burning* powders, the surface layers are made up of material of greatly reduced hygroscopicity and the interiors are rendered inaccessible to atmospheric influences.

The tendency of straight nitrocellulose powder to take up moisture and the effect of the absorbed moisture in reducing the ballistic power of the powder are shown by the table below.

Period of exposure, hrs.	0	24	48	72	96
Total volatiles, %	3.26	3.55	3.71	3.84	3.93
External moisture, %	1.02	1.15	1.40	1.47	1.57
Residual solvent, %	2.24	2.40	2.31	2.37	2.35
Velocity, ft. per sec.	1706.6	1699.0	1685.4	1680.4	1669.0
Pressure, lb. per sq. in.	31,100	31,236	30,671	29,636	28,935

A sample of water-dried powder was exposed to an atmosphere practically saturated with water vapor. Portions were removed each day; one part was fired in the gun, and another part was analyzed for *total volatile* matter (TV) and for volatile matter driven off by an hour's heating at 100° (*external moisture*, EM).

314

The amount of total volatile matter increased regularly during the period of exposure, as did also the amount of volatile matter resident at or near the surface of the powder grains. The amount of volatile matter in the interior of the powder grains (*residual solvent*, RS) did not alter materially during the experiment.

Total volatiles in powder is determined by dissolving the sample in a solvent, precipitating in a porous and granular condition, evaporating off the volatile matter, and drying the residue to constant weight. External moisture is the amount of volatile matter which is driven off by some convenient method of desiccation. The difference between the two is residual solvent, $TV - EM = RS$, and is supposed to correspond to volatile matter resident within the interior of the grain and not accessible to desiccating influences. Various methods of determining external moisture have been in use among the nations which use straight nitrocellulose powder and in the same nation among the manufacturers who produce it. At the time of the first World War, for example, external moisture was determined in Russia by heating the sample at 100° for 6 hours, in France by heating at 60° for 4 hours, and in the United States by heating at 60° in a vacuum for 6 hours. These several methods, naturally, all give different results for external moisture and consequently different results for residual solvent.

There appears really to be no method by which true external moisture may be determined, that is, no method by which only the surface moisture is removed in such fashion that the residual solvent in the powder is found to be the same both before and after the powder has been allowed to take up moisture. Samples of powder were taken and residual solvent was determined by the several methods indicated in the next table. The samples were exposed 2 weeks to an atmosphere practically saturated with water vapor, and residual solvent was again determined as before. The surprising result was secured in every case, as indicated, that the amount of residual solvent was less after the powder had been exposed to the moist atmosphere than it was before it had been exposed. Yet the powder had taken up large quantities of moisture during the exposure. It is clear that the exposure to the moist atmosphere had made the volatile matter of the interior of the grains more accessible to desiccating influ-

315

ences. Evidently the moisture had opened up the interior of the grains, presumably by precipitating the nitrocellulose and producing minute cracks and pores in the colloid. Verification of this explanation is found in the effect of alcohol on colloided pyrocellulose powder. The powder took up alcohol from an atmosphere saturated with alcohol vapor, but alcohol does not precipitate the colloid, it produces no cracks or pores, and in every case residual solvent was found to be greater after the powder had been exposed to alcohol vapor than it had been before such exposure. The following table shows data for typical samples of powder before and after exposures of 2 weeks to atmospheres saturated respectively with water and with alcohol.

Method of Determining External Moisture and Residual Solvent	Exposure to Water Residual solvent			Exposure to Alcohol Residual solvent		
	Before	After	Difference	Before	After	Difference
1 hr. at 100° in open oven	3.12	2.82	−0.30	2.41	4.57	+2.16
6 hrs. at 100° in open oven	2.81	2.36	−0.45	2.22	3.92	+1.70
6 hrs. at 55° in vacuum	2.91	2.54	−0.37	2.27	4.10	+1.83
55° to constant weight in open oven	3.00	2.72	−0.28	2.58	4.25	+1.67
Over sulfuric acid to constant weight	2.95	2.39	−0.56	2.32	4.10	+1.78

Samples of pyrocellulose powder, varying in size from 0.30 caliber single-perforated to large multiperforated grains for the 10-inch gun, were exposed to a moist atmosphere until they no longer gained any weight. They were then desiccated by the rather vigorous method of heating for 6 hours at 100°. All the samples lost more weight than they had gained. As the exposures to moisture and subsequent desiccations were repeated, the differences between the weights gained by taking up moisture and the weights lost by drying became less and less until finally the powders on desiccation lost, within the precision of the experiments, exactly the amounts of volatile matter which they had taken up. At this point it was judged that all residual solvent had

316

been driven out of the powder and that further treatment would produce no additional cracks and pores in the grains. The gain or loss (either one, for the two were equal) calculated as per cent of the weight of the desiccated sample gave the apparent hygroscopicities listed below. Since all the powders were made from the

Caliber	Apparent Hygroscopicity, %
0.30	3.00
75 mm.	2.75
4.7 inches	2.42
6 inches	2.41
10 inches	2.11

same material, namely, straight pyrocellulose, the differences in the apparent hygroscopicity are presumed to be caused by the drying treatment not being vigorous enough to drive out all the moisture from the interior of the grains of greater web thickness. The drying, however, was so vigorous that the powders became unstable after a few more repetitions of it. The losses on desiccation became greater because of decomposition, and the gains on exposure to moisture became greater because of the hygroscopicity of the decomposition products.

Although hygroscopicity determined in this way is apparent and not absolute, it supplies nevertheless an important means of estimating the effects both of process of manufacture and of composition upon the attitude of the powder toward moisture. Thus, samples of pyrocellulose powder for the 4.7-inch gun, all of them being from the same batch and pressed through the same die, one air-dried, one water-dried, one dried under benzene at 60°, and one under ligroin at 60°, showed apparent hygroscopicities of 2.69%, 2.64%, 2.54%, and 2.61%, which are the same within the experimental error. Milky grains [19] of 75-mm. powder showed an apparent hygroscopicity of 2.79%, compared with 2.75% for the normal amber-colored grains. The experiment with this powder was continued until considerable decomposition was evident; the successive gains and losses were as follows, calculated as per cent of the original weight of the sample.

[19] Grains which had a milky appearance because of the precipitation of the colloid during the water-dry treatment. This result follows if the grains contain more than 7 or 7.5% of ether-alcohol when they are submitted to water-drying.

317

Gain, %	Loss, %
2.315	3.030
2.439	2.623
2.259	2.337
2.279	2.319
2.179	2.577
2.448	2.554
2.325	2.630
2.385	3.022

Experiments with 75-mm. powders, made from pyrocellulose with the use of ether-alcohol and with various other substances incorporated in the colloids, gave the following results for hygroscopicity. Hydrocellulose does not dissolve in the nitrocellulose

Pyrocellulose with	
5% hydrocellulose	2.79%
10% crystalline DNX	2.09%
10% DNX oil	1.99%
10% crystalline DNT	1.93%
15% " "	1.41%
20% " "	1.23%
25% " "	1.06%

colloid, and does not affect its hygroscopicity. The aromatic nitro compounds dissolve, and they have a marked effect in reducing the absorption of moisture. They are explosive non-volatile solvents and contribute to the energy of the powder.

Other non-volatile solvents which are not explosive are discussed below in the section on gelatinizing agents. These tend to reduce the potential of the powder, but their action in this respect is counteracted in practice by using guncotton in place of part or all the nitrocellulose. The guncotton is colloided by the gelatinizing agent, either in the presence or in the absence of a volatile solvent, and the resulting powder is non-hygroscopic and as strong or stronger than straight pyrocellulose powder.

Control of Rate of Burning

Cordite is *degressive* burning, for its burning surface decreases as the burning advances. Powder in strips, in flakes, and in single-perforated tubes has a burning surface which is very nearly constant if the size of the strips or flakes, or the length of the tubes, is large relative to their thickness. Multiperforated grains are *progressive* burning, for their burning surface actually increases

318

nitroglycerin and 50% soluble nitrocellulose, made without volatile solvent, and sandwiched between two thin strips of powder made, without volatile solvent, from 50% soluble nitrocellulose and 50% crystalline dinitrotoluene. The two compositions were rolled to the desired thicknesses separately between warm rolls, as the burning advances, and, other things in the gun being equal, they produce gas at a rate which accelerates more rapidly and, in consequence, gives a greater velocity to the projectile.

A progressive burning strip ballistite was used to some extent by the French in major caliber guns during the first World War. It consisted of a central thick strip or slab of ballistite, 50%

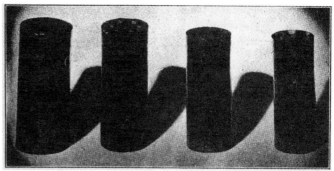

Figure 79. Progressive Burning Colloided Smokeless Powder. 12-Inch powder at different stages of its burning. A grain of 12-inch powder, such as appears at the left, was loaded into a 75-mm. gun along with the usual charge of 75-mm. powder (of the same form as the 12-inch grain but of less web thickness). When the gun was fired, a layer of colloid having a thickness equal to one-half the web of the 75-mm. powder was burned off from every grain in the gun. This consumed the 75-mm. powder completely. The 12-inch grain was extinguished when thrown from the muzzle of the gun; it was picked up from the ground—and is the second grain in the above picture. The next grain was shot twice from a 75-mm. gun, the last grain three times. After three shootings, the perforations are so large that a fourth shooting would cause them to meet one another, and the grain to fall apart, leaving slivers.

and were then combined into the laminated product by pressing between warm rolls. The outer layers burned relatively slowly with a temperature of about 1500°; the inner slab burned rapidly with a temperature of about 3000°.

319

Progressive burning *coated powders*, usually flakes or single-perforated short cylinders, are made by treating the grains with a gelatinizing agent, or non-volatile, non-explosive solvent for nitrocellulose, dissolved in a volatile liquid, generally benzene or acetone, tumbling them together in a sweetie barrel or similar device, and evaporating off the volatile liquid by warming while the tumbling is continued. The material which is applied as a coating is known in this country as a *deterrent*, in England as a

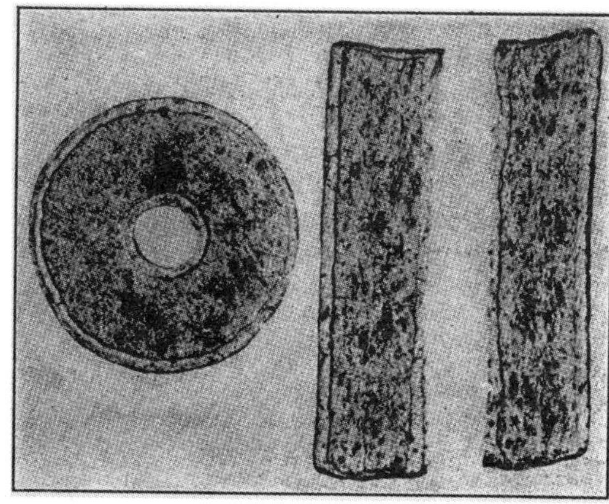

Figure 80. Cross Section and Longitudinal Section of a Grain of .50 Caliber Extruded Smokeless Powder, Deterrent Coated (25×). (Courtesy Western Cartridge Company.)

moderant. At the time of the first World War *sym*-dimethyldiphenylurea was already used widely as a deterrent in rifle powder intended for use in shooting matches and in military propellants designed to produce especially high velocities. The substance was called *centralite* because its use had been developed in Germany at the Central War Laboratory at Spandau. The ethyl analog, diethyldiphenylurea, at first known as *ethyl centralite*, is usually called Centralite No. 1 and has generally superseded the methyl compound (or Centralite No. 2) for use in smokeless powder. Although many other substances have been tried and have been patented, this remains the most widely used of any. *Butyl centralite* is a better gelatinizing agent for nitrocellulose than either the methyl or the ethyl compound,[320] and is likely to find more extensive use in the future.

Gelatinizing Agents

Gelatinizing agents, of which the centralites are examples, are often incorporated in colloided straight nitrocellulose and double-base powders where they cause the materials to burn more slowly, where they serve as flash reducing agents, and where they reduce the tendency of the powders to take up moisture. They reduce the amount of volatile solvent which is needed in the manufacture of nitrocellulose powders, and facilitate the manufacture of double-base powders without any volatile solvent at all. The centralites happen also to be effective stabilizers, but this is not a general property of gelatinizing agents.

Marqueyrol and Florentin have published a list of patents for gelatinizing agents, esters, amides, urea derivatives, halogen compounds, ketones, and alcohols, and have reported their study of many of them with respect to their effectiveness on the CP_1 and CP_2, insoluble and soluble nitrocellulose respectively, which were standard in the French service. To a weighed quantity of the dry nitrocellulose a dilute solution of the gelatinizing agent in 95% alcohol was added in portions of 1 cc. at a time, the alcohol was then evaporated at a temperature of 35–40°, more of the alcohol solution was added, and the evaporation was repeated until gelatinization was complete. The results with the best gelatinizing agents are shown in the table below, where the numbers

	CP_1 (Insoluble)	CP_2 (Soluble)
Ethyl sebacate	320	65
Dimethylphenyl-o-tolylurea	260	65
Dimethyldiphenylurea	...	80
Ethyl succinate	400	90
Ethyl phthalate	360	95

represent the amounts by weight of the several substances which were needed for the complete gelatinization of 100 parts of the nitrocellulose. Ninety parts of ethyl citrate or of benzyl benzoate almost completely gelatinized 100 parts of CP_2, 90 of ethyl malonate incompletely, 90 of ethyl oxalate or of ethyl stearate more incompletely, and 90 of ethyl acetoacetate or of ethyl ricinoleate[321] but very little. Four hundred parts of triphenyl phosphate almost completely gelatinized 100 parts of CP_1, and 400 of ethyl malonate or of ethyl oxalate produced only incomplete gelatinization.

Marqueyrol and Florentin point out that the lower members of the series of esters, the acetates, butyrates, valerates, etc., are good solvents for nitrocellulose—ethyl and amyl acetate have long been used for the purpose—but the higher members, the stearates and oleates, gelatinize nitrocellulose but very little. To the esters of the dibasic acids the opposite rule appears to apply; the higher members are better than the lower. Acetone is a well-known solvent both for soluble and for "insoluble" nitrocellulose, but acetophenone gelatinizes even soluble nitrocellulose only feebly.

Experiments by the present writer with a variety of other gelatinizing agents have shown that the amounts necessary to produce complete gelatinization of pyrocellulose are different if different solvents are used for applying them. In general they are more effective in benzene than in alcohol, and more in alcohol than in ligroin. Half-gram samples of dry pyrocellulose were treated in 30-cc. beakers with known quantities of the gelatinizing agents dissolved in convenient volumes (15–30 cc.) of alcohol, benzene, or ligroin. The volatile liquids were evaporated off slowly at 60°, the residues were warmed at 60° for 10 minutes longer (during which time a considerable improvement in the gelatinization was generally observed), and were then examined to determine their condition. If complete gelatinization had not occurred, other experiments were carried out with fresh samples. The results, summarized in the table on page 322, are accurate to the nearest 10%. They support several conclusions. *Sym*-dialkyl ureas are excellent gelatinizing agents for nitrocellulose, and the property remains if additional aliphatic or aromatic groups are introduced into the molecule. The heavier the alkyl groups, the greater appears to be the gelatinizing power. Of the aromatic substituted ureas, those in which there are less than three aromatic groups appear to be without action. Among the alkyl esters of sebacic and phthalic acids, those which contain the heavier alkyl groups are generally the better gelatinizing agents. The alkyl esters of aliphatic and of aromatic substituted carbamic acids are excellent gelatinizing agents, but the aromatic esters appear to be without action unless the total number of aromatic groups is equal to three.

[322]

Parts by Weight Necessary for the Complete Gelatinization of 100 Parts of Pyrocellulose

	In Alcohol	In Benzene	In Ligroin
Methylurea	No action with 100 parts		
Ethyleneurea	No action with 100 parts		
Sym-dimethylurea	60	70	...
Sym-diethylurea	50	50	...
Unsym-dimethylurea	No action with 100 parts		
Tetramethylurea	80	...	...
Benzylurea	No action with 100 parts		
Sym-diphenylurea	No action with 100 parts		
Sym-di-*p*-tolylurea	No action with 100 parts		
Unsym-diphenylurea	No action with 100 parts		
Triphenylurea	...	35	...
α,α-diphenyl-*p*-tolylurea	...	40	...
Tetraphenylurea	No action with 160 parts	30	...
Ethyltriphenylurea	80	...	...
Sym-dimethyldiphenylurea	70	25	...
Sym-diethyldiphenylurea	70	30	...
Sym-di-*n*-butyldiphenylurea	60	20	...
Unsym-dimethyldiphenylurea	60	...	...
Carbamic acid ethyl ester	140	80	...
Methylcarbamic acid ethyl ester	90	60	...
Ethylcarbamic acid ethyl ester	90	60	...
Phenylcarbamic acid ethyl ester	20	90	...
Phenylcarbamic acid phenyl ester	No action with 200 parts		
Phenylcarbamic acid benzyl ester	No action with 100 parts		
Diphenylcarbamic acid phenyl ester	80	70	...
Methyl sebacate	80	70	105
Ethyl sebacate	80	50	90
Iso-amyl sebacate	70	95	90
Methyl phthalate	95	70	115
Ethyl phthalate	95	50	100
Iso-amyl phthalate	95	50	80
DNX oil	120	130	330
Trinitrotoluene	...	300	...

Flashless Charges and Flashless Powder

The discharge of a machine gun shooting ordinary charges of smokeless powder produces bright flashes from the muzzle which [323] at night disclose the position of the gun to the enemy. When a large gun is fired, there is a large and dazzlingly bright muzzle flash, from a 12-inch gun for example a white-hot flame 150 feet or more in length. The light from such a flame reflects from the heavens at night and is visible for a distance of as much as 30 miles, much farther than the sound from the gun may be heard. The enemy by the use of appropriate light-ranging apparatus may determine the position of the flash, and may undertake to bombard and destroy the battery from a great distance.

Smokeless powder, burning in the chamber of the gun at the expense of its own combined oxygen, produces gas which contains hydrogen, carbon monoxide, carbon dioxide, etc., and this gas, being both hot and combustible, takes fire when it emerges from the muzzle and comes into contact with the fresh oxygen supply of the outer air. One part of the brilliancy of the flash is the result of the emergent gas being already preheated, often to a temperature at which it would be visible anyway, generally to a point far above the temperature of its inflammation in air. In thinking about this latter temperature, it is necessary to take account of the fact that, other things being equal, a small cloud of gas from a small gun loses its temperature more quickly and becomes completely mixed with the air more rapidly than a large cloud of gas from a large gun. The gas emerging from a small gun would need to be hotter in the first place if it is to inflame than gas of the same composition emerging from a large gun. It is for this reason perhaps that it is easier to secure flashless discharges with guns of small caliber (not over 6 inch) than with those of major caliber.

There are four ways, distinguishably different in principle, by which flashlessness has been secured, namely,

(1) by the addition to the charge of certain salts, particularly potassium chloride or potassium hydrogen tartarate, or by the use of powdered tin or of some other substance which, dispersed throughout the gas from the powder, acts as an anti-oxidant and prevents its inflammation;

(2) by incorporating carbonaceous material in the smokeless powder, by which means the composition of the gas is altered and [324] the number of mols of gas is actually increased while the temperature is lowered;

(3) by incorporating in the powder a *cool explosive*, such as ammonium nitrate, guanidine nitrate, or nitroguanidine, which explodes or burns with the production of gas notably cooler than the gas from the combustion of ordinary smokeless powder; and

(4) by contriving the ignition of the powder, the acceleration of its burning rate, and the design of the gun itself, any or all these factors, in such fashion that the projectile takes up energy from the powder gas more quickly and more effectively than is ordinarily the case, and thereby lowers the temperature of the gas to a point where the flash is extinguished.

The first of these methods is applicable to all calibers; the second and the third are successful only with calibers of less than 6 inches; the fourth has not yet been sufficiently studied and exploited. It is true, however, that an improved igniter, with the same gun and with the same powder, may determine the difference between a flash and a flashless discharge.

The use of salts to produce flashlessness appears to derive from an early observation of Dautriche that a small amount of black powder, added to the smokeless powder charge of small-arms ammunition, makes the discharge flashless. During the first World War the French regularly loaded a part of their machine gun ammunition with a propellant consisting of 9 parts of smokeless powder and 1 of black powder.

The Germans in their cannon used *anti-flash bags* or *Vorlage*, loaded at the base of the projectiles, between the projectiles and the propelling charges. These consisted of two perforated discs of artificial silk or cotton cloth sewed together in the form of doughnut-shaped bags. The bags were filled with coarsely pulverized potassium chloride. The artillerymen were not informed of the nature of the contents of the bags but were advised against using any whose contents had hardened to a solid cake, and were instructed in their tactical use as follows.

> In firing with *Vorlage*, there is produced a red fire [a red glow] at the muzzle and in front of the piece. The smoke is colored red [by the glow]. This light however gives no reflection in the heavens. In fact it is visible and appreciable at a distance only if the piece is placed in such a way that [325] the enemy can see its muzzle. In the daytime, *Vorlage* must be used only when the weather is so dark that the flashes of the shots without them are more visible than the clouds of smoke which they produce. The opaqueness of the background against which the battery stands out or the obscurity of the setting which surrounds it are also at times of a kind to justify the use of *Vorlage* in the daytime.

The anti-flash bags reduced the range by 4.5 to 8%.

Fauveau and Le Paire studied the anti-flash effect of potassium chloride and of other salts and concluded that the lowering of the temperature of the gas which undoubtedly results from their volatiliz tion and dissociation is insufficient to account for the extinction of the flash. Prettre found that the chlorides of sodium and of lithium, and other alkali metal salts which are volatile, had the same effect as potassium chloride. He found that small amounts of potassium chloride, volatilized in mixtures of carbon monoxide and air, had a powerful anti-oxidant action and a correspondingly large effect in raising the temperature of inflammation of the gas. Some of his results are shown in the table below. He found that potassium chloride was without effect

Milligrams of KCl per Liter of Gaseous Mixture	Temperature (°C.) of Inflammation of Air Containing		
	24.8% CO	44.1% CO	67.3% CO
0.0	656	657	680
0.4	...	750	800
0.5	730	...	820
0.7	...	810	900
1.0	790	850	1020
1.3	810	...	...
2.0	890	950	...
2.5	...	1000	...
3.0	970	...	...
3.5	1010	...	...

upon the temperature of inflammation of mixtures of hydrogen and air.

The French have used anti-flash bags (*sachets antilueurs*) filled with the crude potassium hydrogen tartarate (about 70% [326] pure) or *argols* which is a by-product of the wine industry. The flat, circular, cotton bags containing the argols were assembled along with the smokeless powder and black powder igniter in silk cartridge bags to make up the complete charge. Since the anti-flash material tended to reduce the ballistic effect of the charge, it was necessary when firing flashless rounds to add an *appoint* or additional quantity of smokeless powder. Thus, for ordinary firing of the 155-mm. gun, the charge consisted of 10 kilograms of *poudre BM7* along with an igniter system containing a total of 115 grams of black powder. For a flashless round, 3 *sachets* containing 500 grams of argols each were used and an additional 305 grams of smokeless powder to restore the ballistics to normal.

Another method of securing flashlessness was by the use of pellets (*pastilles*) of a compressed intimate mixture of 4 parts of potassium nitrate and 1 part of crystalline DNT. Pellets for use in the 155-mm. gun weighed 1 gram each, and were about 2 mm. thick and 15 mm. in diameter. Two or three hundred of these were sewed up in a silk bag which was loaded into the gun along with the bag containing the powder. The pellets burned with the same velocity as *poudre B*, and had but very little effect upon the ballistics. They of course produced a certain amount of smoke and the discharge gave a red glow from the muzzle of the gun.

Oxanilide functions well as an anti-flash agent if it is distributed throughout the powder charge, but not if it is loaded into the gun in separate bags like the materials which have just been mentioned. It is made into a thick paste with glue solution, the paste is extruded in the form of little worms or pellets, and these are dried. Pellets to the amount of 15% of the powder charge produce flashlessness in the 6-inch gun, but the charge is more difficult to light than ordinarily and requires a special igniter.

Oxanilide and many other carbonaceous materials, incorporated in the grains of colloided powder, yield powders which are flashless in guns of the smaller calibers and, in many cases, are as powerful, weight for weight, as powders which contain none of the inert, or at least non-explosive, ingredients. If nitrocellulose burning in the gun produces 1 mol of carbon dioxide and a certain amount of other gaseous products, then nitrocellulose plus 1 mol of carbon under the same conditions will produce 2 mols of

327

carbon monoxide along with substantially the same amount of the other gaseous products. There will be more gas and cooler gas. A colloided powder made from pyrocellulose 85 parts and hydrocellulose 15 parts is flashless in the 75-mm. gun, and gives practically the same ballistic results as a hotter and more expensive powder made from straight nitrocellulose. The strength of the powder may be increased without affecting its flashlessness by substituting part of the pyrocellulose by guncotton of a higher nitrogen content.

Among the materials which have been incorporated into colloided powder for the purpose of reducing or extinguishing the flash are (1) substances, such as starch, hydrocellulose, and anthracene, which are insoluble in the colloid and are non-explosive. They, of course, must exist in a state of fine subdivision to be suitable for this use. Other anti-flash agents are (2) solid or liquid non-explosive substances, such as diethyldiphenylurea and dibutyl phthalate, which are solvents for nitrocellulose and dissolve in the colloid. They reduce the hygroscopicity of the powder and they reduce the amount of volatile solvent which is needed for the manufacture. Still others are (3) the explosive solid and liquid aromatic nitro compounds which are solvents for nitrocellulose and are effective in reducing both the flash and the hygroscopicity. All or any of the substances in these three classes may be used either in a straight nitrocellulose or in a nitrocellulose-nitroglycerin powder. Several flashless powders have been described in the section on the "Classification of Smokeless Powders." Many varieties have been covered by numerous patents. We cite only a single example, for a smokeless, flashless, non-hygroscopic propellent powder made from about 76–79% nitrocellulose (of at least 13% nitrogen content), about 21–24% dinitrotoluene, and about 0.8–1.2% diphenylamine. During the first World War the French and the Italians used a *superattenuated* ballistite, made without volatile solvent, and containing enough aromatic dinitro compound (in place of part of the nitroglycerin) to make it flashless. In a typical case the powder was made from 30 parts CP_1, 30 CP_2, 15 DNT, and 25 nitroglycerin.

328

Ball-Grain Powder

The process for the manufacture of ball-grain powder which Olsen and his co-workers have devised combines nicely with Olsen's process for the quick stabilization of nitrocellulose to form a sequence of operations by which a finished powder may be produced more rapidly and more safely than by the usual process. It supplies a convenient means of making up a powder which contains non-volatile solvents throughout the mass of the grains or deterrent or accelerant coatings upon their surface.

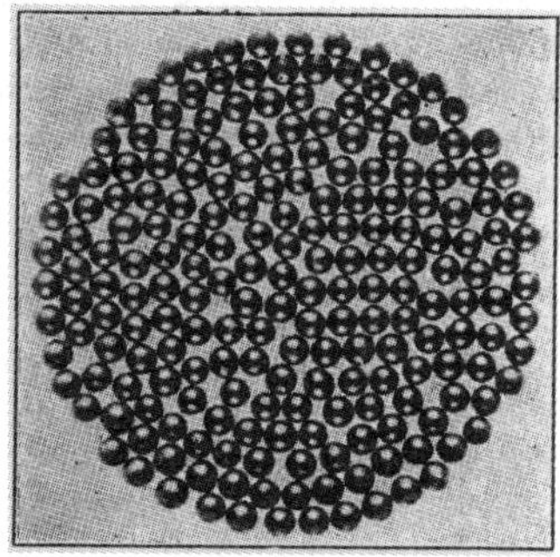

FIGURE 81. Ball Grains (Smokeless Powder) (3×). (Courtesy Western Cartridge Company.)

Nitrocellulose, pulped and given a preliminary or sour boiling, may be used directly without poaching. Deteriorated smokeless powder, containing nitro derivatives of diphenylamine and acidic decomposition products, may be reduced to a coarse powder under water in a hammer mill, and may then be used. Whichever is used, the first necessity is to stabilize it by complete removal of the acid. For this purpose, the material in the presence of water (which may contain a little chalk in suspension or urea in solution) is introduced into a still where it is dissolved with agitation in ethyl acetate to form a heavy syrup or lacquer, and is treated with some substance which is adsorbed by nitrocellulose more readily than acid is adsorbed. It is a curious fact that nitrocellulose is dissolved or dispersed by ethyl acetate much more readily

329

in the presence of water than when water is absent. Diphenylamine is dissolved in the ethyl acetate before the latter is added to the water and nitrocellulose in the still. At the same time, centralite or DNT or any other substance which it may be desired to incorporate in the powder is also dissolved and added. The water phase and the lacquer are then stirred for 30 minutes by which operation the nitrocellulose is stabilized.[27] Starch or gum arabic solution to secure the requisite colloidal behavior is then introduced into the still, the still is closed, the temperature is raised so that the lacquer becomes less viscous, and the mixture

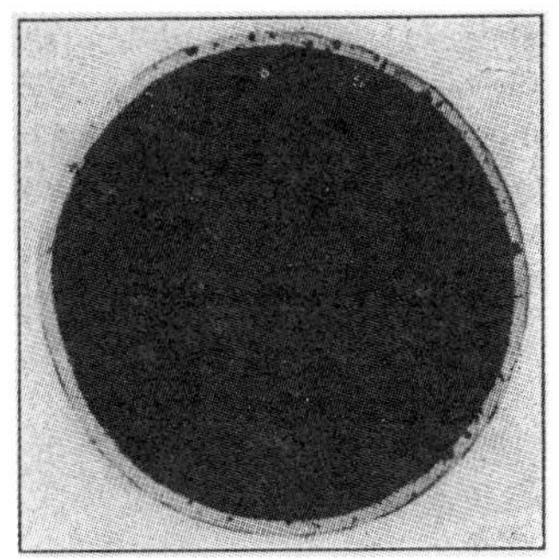

FIGURE 82. Cross Section of Ball Grain, Double Base, Deterrent Coated (112×). (Courtesy Western Cartridge Company.)

under pressure is agitated vigorously until the lacquer is broken up into small globules of the correct size. The pressure is then reduced, and the ethyl acetate is distilled off and recovered. If the distillation is carried out too rapidly, the grains are shaped like kernels of popcorn. If it is carried out at such a rate that the volatile solvent is evaporated from the surface of the globules no faster than it moves from the interior to the surface, if the distillation is slow at first and more rapid afterwards, then smooth ball grains are formed, dense and of homogeneous structure.

[27] Diphenylamine in the presence of water thus has an action beyond that which it has when it is added to the nitrocellulose gel (in the absence of a separate water phase) during the manufacture of smokeless powder by the usual process. Being preferentially adsorbed by the nitrocellulose, it drives any acid which may be present out of the nitrocellulose and into the water. After that it fulfils its usual function in the powder.

330

After the material has cooled, the powder grains are transferred in a slurry to another still and are treated with an emulsion of nitroglycerin dissolved in toluene, or of some other coating agent dissolved in a solvent in which nitrocellulose itself is insoluble, and the volatile solvent is distilled off, leaving the nitroglycerin or other material deposited on the surface of the grains. As much nitroglycerin as 15% of the weight of the powder may be applied in this way. A coating of centralite may, if desired, be put on top of it. The grains are sieved under water and are then dried for use in shotguns. If the powder is to be used in rifles, it is passed in a slurry between warm steel rollers by which all the grains are reduced to the same least dimension or web thickness. Previous to the drying, all the operations in the manufacture of ball-grain powder are carried out under water, and are safe. After the drying, the operations involve the same hazards, by no means insurmountable, as are involved in the ordinary process. The grains are glazed with graphite and blended.

331

CHAPTER VII

DYNAMITE AND OTHER HIGH EXPLOSIVES

Invention of Dynamite

Dynamite and the fulminate blasting cap both resulted from Alfred Nobel's effort to make nitroglycerin more safe and more convenient to use. Having discovered that nitroglycerin is exploded by the explosion of a small firecracker-like device filled with black powder, he tried the effect of mixing the two materials, and in 1863 was granted a patent which covered the use of a liquid explosive, such as nitroglycerin or methyl or ethyl nitrate, in mixture with gunpowder in order to increase the effectiveness of the latter. The amount of the liquid was limited by the requirement that the mixtures should be dry and granular in character. The explosives were supposed to be actuated by fire, like black powder, but the liquid tended to slow down the rate of burning, and they were not notably successful. The same patent also covered the possibility of substituting a part of the saltpeter by nitroglycerin. Because this substance is insoluble in water and non-hygroscopic, it acts as a protective covering for the salt and makes the use of sodium nitrate possible in these mixtures.

Nobel's next patent, granted in 1864, related to improvements in the manufacture of nitroglycerin and to the exploding of it by heating or by means of a detonating charge. He continued his experiments and in 1867 was granted a patent for an explosive prepared by mixing nitroglycerin with a suitable non-explosive, porous absorbent such as charcoal or siliceous earth. The resulting material was much less sensitive to shock than nitroglycerin. It was known as *dynamite,* and was manufactured and sold also

332

under the name of Nobel's Safety Powder. The absorbent which was finally chosen as being most satisfactory was diatomaceous earth or kieselguhr (guhr or fuller's earth). Nobel believed that dynamite could be exploded by a spark or by fire if it was confined closely, but preferred to explode it under all conditions by means of a special exploder or cap containing a strong charge of

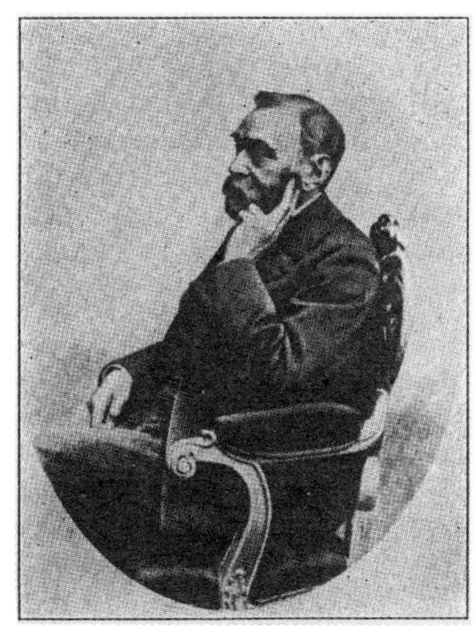

FIGURE 83. Alfred Nobel (1833-1896). First manufactured and used nitroglycerin commercially, 1863; invented dynamite and the fulminate blasting cap, 1867; straight dynamite, 1869; blasting gelatin and gelatin dynamite, 1875; and ballistite, 1888. He left the major part of his large fortune for the endowment of prizes, now known as the Nobel Prizes, for notable achievements in physics, in chemistry, in physiology and medicine, in literature, and in the promotion of peace.

mercury fulminate, crimped tightly to the end of the fuse in order that it might detonate more strongly. He stated that the form of the cap might be varied greatly but that its action depended upon the sudden development of an intense pressure or shock.

Dynamite with an inactive base (guhr dynamite) is not manufactured commercially in this country. Small quantities are used for experimental purposes where a standard of comparison is needed in studies on the strength of various explosives.[333]

The next important event in the development of these explosives was Nobel's invention of *dynamite with an active base*, an explosive in which the nitroglycerin was absorbed by a mixture of materials which were themselves not explosive separately, such as potassium, sodium, or ammonium nitrate mixed with wood meal, charcoal, rosin, sugar, or starch. The nitroglycerin formed a thin coating upon the particles of the solid materials, and caused them to explode if a fulminate cap was used. The patent suggested a mixture of barium nitrate 70 parts, rosin or charcoal 10, and nitroglycerin 20, with or without the addition of sulfur, as an example of the invention. Nitroglycerin alone was evidently not enough to prevent the deliquescence of sodium and ammonium nitrate in these mixtures, for a later patent of Nobel claimed the addition of small amounts of paraffin, ozokerite, stearine, naphthalene, or of any similar substance which is solid at ordinary temperatures and is of a fatty nature, as a coating for the particles to prevent the absorption of moisture by the explosive and the resulting danger from the exudation of nitroglycerin.

Dynamite with an active base is manufactured and used extensively in this country and in Canada and Mexico. It is known as *straight dynamite*, or simply as dynamite, presumably because its entire substance contributes to the energy of its explosion. The standard 40% straight dynamite which is used in comparative tests at the U. S. Bureau of Mines contains nitroglycerin 40%, sodium nitrate 44%, calcium carbonate (anti-acid) 1%, and wood pulp 15%. Since the time when this standard was adopted, the usage of the term "straight" has altered somewhat in consequence of changes in American manufacturing practice, with the result that this standard material is now better designated as 40% straight nitroglycerin (straight) dynamite. This name distinguishes it from 40% l. f. or 40% low-freezing (straight) dynamite which contains, instead of straight nitroglycerin, a mixture of nitric esters produced by nitrating a mix-[334]ture of glycerin and glycol or of glycerin and sugar. Practically all active-base dynamites now manufactured in the United States, whether straight or ammonia or gelatin, are of this l. f. variety. American straight dynamites contain from 20 to 60% of mixed nitric esters absorbed on wood pulp and mixed with enough sodium or potassium nitrate to maintain the oxygen balance and to take care of the oxidation of part or occasionally of all the wood pulp.

Judson powder is a special, low-grade dynamite in which 5 to 15% of nitroglycerin is used as a coating on a granular *dope* made by mixing ground coal with sodium nitrate and sulfur, warming the materials together until the sulfur is melted, forming into grains which harden on cooling and are screened for size. It is intermediate in power between black powder and ordinary dynamite and is used principally for moving earth and soft rock in railroad work.

Nobel's inventions of *blasting gelatin* and *gelatin dynamite* are both covered by the same patent. Seven or 8% of collodion cotton dissolved in nitroglycerin converted it to a stiff jelly which was suitable for use as a powerful high explosive. Solvents, such as acetone, ether-alcohol, and nitrobenzene, facilitated the incorporation of the two substances in the cold, but Nobel reported that collodion cotton dissolved readily in nitroglycerin without additional solvent if the nitroglycerin was warmed gently on the water bath. A cheaper explosive of less power could be made by mixing the gelatinized nitroglycerin with black powder or with mixtures composed of an oxidizing agent, such as a nitrate or chlorate, and a combustible material, such as coal dust, sulfur, sawdust, sugar, starch, or rosin. A typical gelatin dynamite consists of nitroglycerin 62.5%, collodion cotton 2.5%, saltpeter 27.0%, and wood meal 8%. A softer jelly is used for making gelatin dynamite than is suitable for use by itself as a blasting gelatin, and somewhat less collodion is used in proportion to the amount of nitroglycerin.

All straight nitroglycerin explosives can be frozen. Straight dynamite when frozen becomes less sensitive to shock and to initiation, but blasting gelatin becomes slightly more sensitive.[335] When the explosives are afterwards thawed, the nitroglycerin shows a tendency to exude.

Invention of Ammonium Nitrate Explosives

In 1867 two Swedish chemists, C. J. Ohlsson and J. H. Norrbin, patented an explosive, called *ammoniakkrut*, which consisted of ammonium nitrate either alone or in mixture with charcoal, sawdust, naphthalene, picric acid, nitroglycerin, or nitrobenzene. Theoretical calculations had shown that large quantities of heat and gas were given off by the explosions of these mixtures. The proportions of the materials were selected in such manner that all the carbon should be converted to carbon dioxide and all the hydrogen to water. Some of these explosives were difficult to ignite and to initiate, but the trouble was remedied by including some nitroglycerin in their compositions and by firing them with fulminate detonators. They were used to some extent in Sweden. Nobel purchased the invention from his fellow-countrymen early in the 1870's, and soon afterwards took out another patent in connection with it, but still found that the hygroscopicity of the ammonium nitrate created real difficulty. He was not able to deal satisfactorily with the trouble until after the invention of gelatin dynamite. In present manufacturing practice in this country the tendency of the ammonium nitrate to take up water is counteracted by coating the particles with water-repelling substances, oils, or metallic soaps.

In 1879 Nobel took out a Swedish patent for *extra-dynamite* (ammon-gelatin-dynamit), one example of which was a fortified gelatin dynamite consisting of nitroglycerin 71%, collodion 4%, charcoal 2%, and ammonium nitrate 23%. Another contained much less nitroglycerin, namely, 25%, along with collodion 1%, charcoal 12%, and ammonium nitrate 62%, and was crumbly and plastic between the fingers rather than clearly gelatinous.

In these explosives, and in the ammonium nitrate *permissible* explosives which contain still less nitroglycerin, it is supposed that the nitroglycerin or the nitroglycerin jelly, which coats the particles of ammonium nitrate, carries the explosive impulse originating in the detonator, that this causes the ammonium nitrate to decompose explosively to produce nitrogen and water[336] and oxygen, the last named of which enters into a further explosive reaction with the charcoal or other combustible material. Other explosive liquids or solids, such as liquid or solid DNT,

TNT, or TNX, nitroglycol, nitrostarch, or nitrocellulose, may be used to sensitize the ammonium nitrate and to make the mixture more easily detonated by a blasting cap. Non-explosive combustible materials, such as rosin, coal, sulfur, cereal meal, and paraffin, also work as sensitizers for ammonium nitrate, and a different hypothesis is required to explain their action.

Guhr Dynamite

Guhr dynamite is used rather widely in Europe. It is not hygroscopic. Liquid water however, brought into contact with it, is absorbed by the kieselguhr and displaces the nitroglycerin which separates in the form of an oily liquid. The nitroglycerin thus set free in a wet bore hole might easily seep away into a fissure in the rock where it would later be exploded accidentally by a drill or by the blow of a pick. Water does not cause the separation of nitroglycerin from blasting gelatin or gelatin dynamite. It tends to dissolve the soluble salts which are present in straight dynamite and to liberate in the liquid state any nitroglycerin with which they may be coated.

Guhr dynamite, made from 1 part of kieselguhr and 3 parts of nitroglycerin, is not exploded by a blow of wood upon wood, but is exploded by a blow of iron or other metal upon iron. In the drop test it is exploded by the fall of a 1-kilogram weight through 12 to 15 cm., or by the fall of a 2-kilogram weight through 7 cm. The frozen material is less sensitive: a drop of more than 1 meter of the kilogram weight or of at least 20 cm. of the 2-kilogram weight is necessary to explode it. Frozen or unfrozen it is exploded in a paper cartridge by the impact of a bullet from a military rifle. A small sample will burn quietly in the open, but will explode if it is lighted within a confined space. A cartridge explodes if heated on a metal plate.

The velocity of detonation of guhr dynamite varies with the density of loading and with the diameter of the charge, but does not reach values equal to the maxima under best conditions for nitroglycerin and blasting gelatin. Velocities of 6650 to 6800 meters per second, at a density of loading of 1.50 (the highest [337] which is practical) have been reported. Naoúm, working with charges in an iron pipe 34 mm. in internal diameter and at a density of loading of 1.30, found for nitroglycerin guhr dynamite a velocity of detonation of 5650 meters per second, and, under the same conditions, for nitroglycol guhr dynamite one of 6000 meters per second.

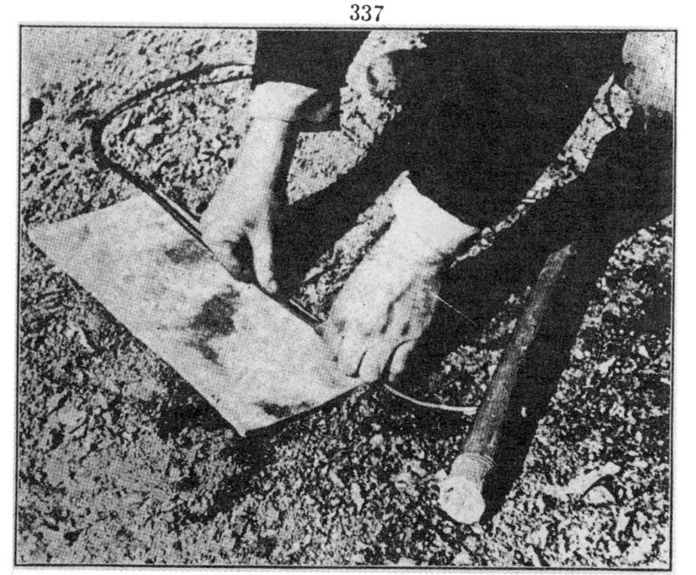

FIGURE 84. Determination of the Velocity of Detonation of Dynamite by the Dautriche Method. (Courtesy Hercules Powder Company.) Compare Figure 9, page 17.

Dynamites, like guhr dynamite and straight dynamite, which contain nitroglycerin in the subdivided but liquid state communicate explosion from cartridge to cartridge more readily, and in general are more easy to initiate, than blasting gelatin and gelatin dynamite in which no liquid nitroglycerin is present. A cartridge of guhr dynamite 30 mm. in diameter will propagate its explosion through a distance of 30 cm. to a similar cartridge.[338]

Straight Dynamite

Straight dynamite containing 60% or less of mixed nitric esters—but not more because of the danger of exudation—is used extensively in the United States, but has found little favor in Europe. It is made simply by mixing the explosive oil with the absorbent materials; the resulting loose, moist-appearing or greasy mass, from which oil ought not to exude under gentle pressure, is put up in cartridges or cylinders wrapped in paraffined paper and dipped into melted paraffin wax to seal them against moisture.

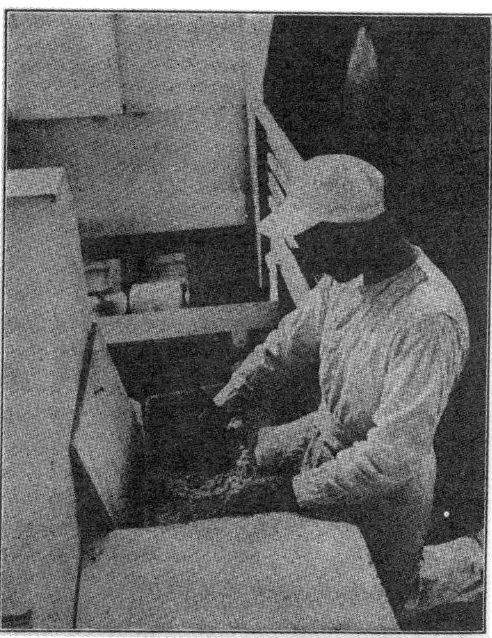

FIGURE 85. Dynamite Manufacture. (Courtesy Hercules Powder Company.) Rubbing the dry ingredients of dynamite through a screen into the bowl of a mixing machine.

The strength of straight nitroglycerin dynamite is expressed by the per cent of nitroglycerin which it contains. Thus, "40% straight nitroglycerin dynamite" contains 40% of nitroglycerin,[339] but "40% ammonia dynamite," "40% gelatin dynamite," etc., whatever their compositions may be, are supposed to have the same strength or explosive force as 40% straight nitroglycerin dynamite. Munroe and Hall in 1915 reported for typical straight nitroglycerin dynamites the compositions which are shown in the following table. Although these dynamites are not now manufactured commercially in the United States, their explosive properties, studied intensively at the U. S. Bureau of

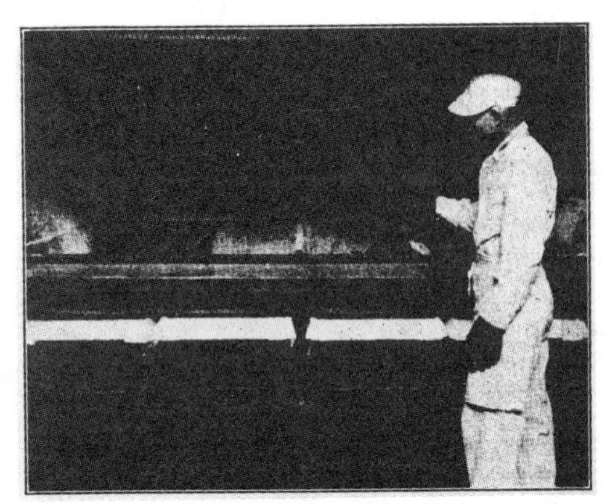

FIGURE 86. Dynamite Manufacture. (Courtesy Hercules Powder Company.) Hoppers underneath the mixing machine, showing the buggies which carry the mixed dynamite to the packing machines.

	STRENGTH									
	15%	20%	25%	30%	35%	40%	45%	50%	55%	60%
Nitroglycerin	15	20	25	30	35	40	45	50	55	60
Combustible material	20	19	18	17	16	15	14	14	15	16
Sodium nitrate......	64	60	56	52	48	44	40	35	29	23
Calcium or magnesium carbonate...	1	1	1	1	1	1	1	1	1	1

Mines and reported as a matter of interest, do not differ greatly from those of the l. f. dynamites by which they have been superseded in common use. The combustible material stated to be used in these compositions consists[340] of a mixture of wood pulp, flour, and brimstone for the grades below 40% strength, wood pulp alone for the 40% and stronger. In commercial practice the dope sometimes contains coarse combustible material, like rice hulls, sawdust, or bran, which makes the explosive more bulky and has the effect of reducing the velocity of detonation. Tests at the U. S. Bureau of Mines on standard straight dynamites in cartridges 1¼ inches in diameter showed for the 30% grade a velocity of detonation of 4548 meters per second, for the 40%

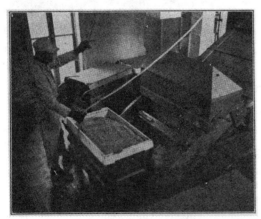

FIGURE 87. Dynamite Manufacture. (Courtesy Hercules Powder Company.) Dumping the mixed dynamite onto the conveyor belt which raises it to the hopper of the semi-automatic packing machine.

grade 4688 meters per second, and for the 60% grade 6246 meters per second. The 40% dynamite was exploded in one case out of three by an 11-cm. drop of a 2-kilogram weight, in no case out of five by a 10-cm. drop. Cartridges 1¼ inches in diameter and 8 inches long transmitted explosion from one to another through a distance of 16 inches once in two trials, but not through a distance of 17 inches in three trials. The 40% dynamite gave a small lead block compression of 16.0 mm., and an expansion (average of three) in the Trauzl test of 278 cc.

Munroe and Hall[341] also reported the following compositions for typical ordinary and low-freezing ammonia dynamites, the combustible material in each case being a mixture of wood pulp, flour, and brimstone. Low-freezing dynamites at present in use in this country contain nitroglycol or nitrosugar instead of the above-mentioned nitrosubstitution compounds. In Europe dinitrochlorohydrin, tetranitrodiglycerin, and other nitric esters are used.

Strength	Ordinary					Low-Freezing				
	30%	35%	40%	50%	60%	30%	35%	40%	50%	60%
Nitroglycerin............	15	20	22	27	35	13	17	17	21	27
Nitrosubstitution compounds...............	..	..	..	..	..	3	4	4	5	6
Ammonium nitrate.......	15	15	20	25	30	15	15	20	25	30
Sodium nitrate..........	51	48	42	36	24	53	49	45	36	27
Combustible material....	18	16	15	11	10	15	14	13	12	9
Calcium carbonate or zinc oxide................	1	1	1	1	1	1	1	1	1	1

Three of the standard French ammonia dynamites, according to Naoúm, have the compositions and explosive properties listed below.

Nitroglycerin	40	20	22
Ammonium nitrate	45	75	75
Sodium nitrate	5	...	...
Wood or cereal meal	10	5	...
Charcoal	...	...	3
Lead block expansion	400.0 cc.	335.0 cc.	330.0 cc.
Lead block crushing	22.0 mm.	15.5 mm.	16.0 mm.
Density	1.38	1.20	1.33

Taylor and Rinkenbach report typical analyses of American ammonium nitrate dynamite (I below) and ammonium nitrate sodium nitrate dynamite (II below). These formulas really represent ammonium nitrate permissible explosives, very close in their compositions to Monobel (III below) which is permissible in this country for use in coal mines. Naoúm[342] reports that this

	I	II	III
Nitroglycerin	9.50	9.50	10.0
Ammonium nitrate	79.45	69.25	80.0
Sodium nitrate	...	10.20	...
Carbonaceous combustible material[17]	9.75	9.65	...
Wood meal	...	...	10.0
Anti-acid	0.40	0.50	...
Moisture	0.90	0.90	...

[17] The carbonaceous combustible material contains 0.40% grease or oil which was added to the ammonium nitrate to counteract its hygroscopicity. Note that the figures in the first two columns of the table represent results of analyses; those in the third column represent the formula according to which the explosive is mixed.

Monobel (density about 1.15) gives a lead block expansion of about 350 cc. and a lead block crushing of 12 mm. He states that Monobel belongs to the class of typical ammonium nitrate explosives rather than to the dynamites, and points out that no specific effect can be ascribed to the 10% nitroglycerin which it contains, for an explosive containing only a small quantity, say 4%,

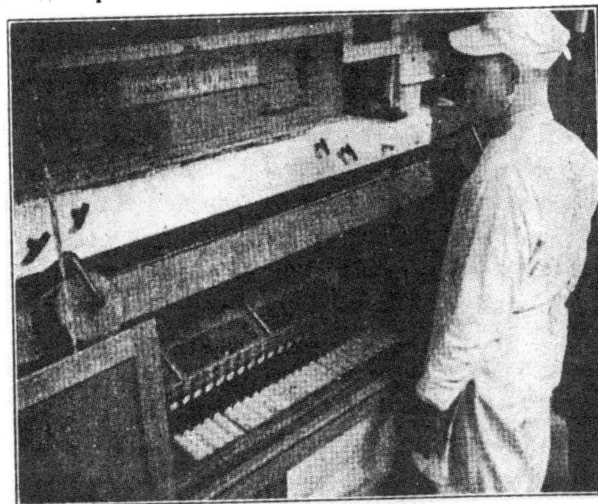

FIGURE 88. Dynamite Manufacture. (Courtesy Hercules Powder Company.) Cartridges of dynamite as they come from the semi-automatic packing machine.

343

of nitroglycerin, or none at all, will give essentially the same performance. But the ammonium nitrate explosive with no nitroglycerin in it is safer to handle and more difficult to detonate.

Blasting Gelatin

Blasting gelatin exists as a yellowish, translucent, elastic mass of density about 1.63. Strong pressure does not cause nitroglycerin to exude from it. Its surface is rendered milky by long contact with water, but its explosive strength is unaffected. It is less sensitive to shock, blows, and friction than nitroglycerin, guhr dynamite, and straight dynamite, for its elasticity enables it more readily to absorb the force of a blow, and a thin layer explodes under a hammer more easily than a thick one. Blasting gelatin freezes with difficulty. When frozen, it loses its elasticity and flexibility, and becomes a hard, white mass. Unlike guhr dynamite and straight dynamite, it is more sensitive to shock when frozen than when in the soft and unfrozen state.

Unlike nitroglycerin, blasting gelatin takes fire easily from a flame or from the spark of a fuse. Its combustion is rapid and violent, and is accompanied by a hissing sound. If a large quantity is burning, the combustion is likely to become an explosion, and the same result is likely to follow if even a small quantity of the frozen material is set on fire.

Pulverulent explosives or explosive mixtures are easier to initiate and propagate detonation for a greater distance than liquid explosives, especially viscous ones, and these are easier to detonate and propagate more readily than colloids. The stiffer the colloid the more difficult it becomes to initiate, until, with increasingly large proportions of nitrocellulose in the nitroglycerin gel, tough, horny colloids are formed, like ballistite and cordite, which in sizable aggregates can be detonated only with difficulty. Blasting gelatin is more difficult to detonate than any of the forms of dynamite in which the nitroglycerin exists in the liquid state. Naoúm reports that a freshly prepared blasting gelatin made from 93 parts of nitroglycerin and 7 parts of collodion cotton is exploded by a No. 1 (the weakest) blasting cap and propagates detonation even in 25-mm. cartridges across a gap of about 10 mm. A blasting gelatin containing 9% of collodion cotton requires a No. 4 blasting cap to make it explode and propagates

344

its explosion to an adjacent cartridge only when initiated by a No. 6 blasting cap.

Blasting gelatin and gelatin dynamite on keeping become less sensitive to detonation, and, after long storage in a warm climate, may even become incapable of being detonated. The effect has been thought to be due to the small air bubbles which make newly prepared blasting gelatin appear practically white but which disappear when the material is kept in storage and becomes translucent and yellowish. But this cannot be the whole cause of the effect, for the colloid becomes stiffer after keeping. The loss of sensitivity is accompanied by a rapid dropping off in the velocity of detonation and in the brisance. According to Naoúm, blasting gelatin containing 7% collodion cotton when newly prepared gave a lead block expansion of 600 cc., after 2 days 580 cc., and one containing 9% collodion gave when freshly made an expansion of 580 cc., after 2 days 545 cc.

Blasting gelatin under the most favorable conditions has a velocity of detonation of about 8000 meters per second. In iron pipes it attains this velocity only if its cross section exceeds 30 mm. in diameter, and it attains it only at a certain distance away from the point of initiation, so that in the Dautriche method where short lengths are used lower values are generally obtained. In tubes of 20–25 mm. diameter, and with samples of a sensitivity reduced either by storage or by an increased toughness of the colloid, values as low as 2000–2500 meters per second have been observed.

Gelatin Dynamite

Blasting gelatin is not used very widely in the United States; the somewhat less powerful gelatin dynamite, or simply gelatin as it is called, is much more popular. Gelatin dynamite is essentially a straight dynamite in which a gel is used instead of the liquid nitroglycerin or l. f. mixture of nitric esters. It is a plastic mass which can be kneaded and shaped. The gel contains between 2 and 5.4% collodion cotton, and is not tough and really elastic like blasting gelatin. Correspondingly it is initiated more easily and has a higher velocity of detonation and better propagation. The gel is prepared by mixing the nitroglycerin and collodion cotton, allowing to stand at 40–45°C. for some hours or over

345

night, and then incorporating mechanically with the dope materials which have been previously mixed together. Munroe and Hall in 1915 gave the compositions listed below as typical of gelatin dynamites offered for sale at that time in this country. Instead of straight nitroglycerin, l. f. mixtures of nitric esters are now used.

	Strength						
	30%	35%	40%	50%	55%	60%	70%
Nitroglycerin	23.0	28.0	33.0	42.0	46.0	50.0	60.0
Nitrocellulose	0.7	0.9	1.0	1.5	1.7	1.9	2.4
Sodium nitrate	62.3	58.1	52.0	45.5	42.3	38.1	29.6
Combustible material [21]	13.0	12.0	13.0	10.0	9.0	9.0	7.0
Calcium carbonate	1.0	1.0	1.0	1.0	1.0	1.0	1.0

21 Wood pulp was used in the 60% and 70% grades. Flour, wood pulp, and, in some examples, rosin and brimstone were used in the other grades.

The three standard explosives which are used in Great Britain are called respectively blasting gelatin, gelatin dynamite, and *Gelignite*. Gelignite, let us note, is a variety of gelatin dynamite as the latter term is used in this country. It is the most widely used of the three and may indeed be regarded as the standard explosive.

	Blasting Gelatin	Gelatin Dynamite	Gelignite
Nitroglycerin	92	75	60
Collodion cotton	8	5	4

Wood meal	5	8
Potassium nitrate	15	28

The gelatin dynamites most widely used in Germany contain about 65 parts of gelatinized nitroglycerin and about 35 parts of dope or absorbent material. The dope for an explosive for domestic use consists of 76.9% sodium nitrate, 22.6% wood meal, and 0.5% chalk, and for one for export of 80% potassium nitrate, 19.5% wood meal, and 0.5% chalk. A weaker *Gelignite II* and certain high-strength gelatin dynamites, as tabulated below, are also manufactured for export.

	Gelignite	High-Strength	Gelatin	Dynamite
	II	80%	81%	75%
Nitroglycerin	47.5	75	75.8	70.4
Collodion cotton	2.5	5	5.2	4.6
Potassium nitrate	37.5	15	15.2	19.3
Wood meal with chalk......	3.5	5	3.8	5.7
Rye meal	9.0	..	...	...

346

The gelatin dynamites manufactured in Belgium are called *Forcites*. The reported compositions of several of them are tabulated below. *Forcite extra* is an ammonia gelatin dynamite.

	Forcite extra	Forcite Superieure	Forcite Super Forcite	Forcite No. 1	Forcite No. 1P	Forcite No. 2	Forcite No. 2P
Nitroglycerin	64	64	64	49	49	36	36
Collodion cotton	3.5	3	3	2	2	3	2
Sodium nitrate	..	24	..	36	..	35	..
Potassium nitrate	..	..	23	..	37	..	46
Ammonium nitrate	25	..	..	..	..	..	..
Wood meal	6.5	8	9	13	11	11	..
Bran	..	..	..	..	..	14	15
Magnesium carbonate	1	1	1	1	1	1	1

In France gelatin dynamites are known by the names indicated in the following table where the reported compositions of several of them are tabulated.

	Dynamite-gomme-extra-forte	Dynamite-gomme-potasse	Dynamite-gomme-soude	Gélatine A	Gélatine B-potasse	Gélatine B-soude	Gomme E	Gélignite
Nitroglycerin..........	92–93	82–83	82–83	64	57.5	57	49	58
Collodion cotton.......	8–7	6–5	6–5	3	2.5	3	2	2
Potassium nitrate......	...	9–10	...	..	32.0	..	36	28
Sodium nitrate........	...	...	9–10	24	..	34	..	..
Wood meal...........	...	2–3	2–3	8	8.0	6	10	9
Flour.................	...	...	...	..	..	..	3	3
Magnesium carbonate..	...	...	...	1	..	..	..	..

Permissible Explosives

The atmosphere of coal mines frequently contains enough methane (fire damp) to make it explode from the flame of a black powder or dynamite blast. Dust also produces an explosive atmosphere, and it may happen, if dust is not already present,
347
that one blast will stir up clouds of dust which the next blast will cause to explode. Accidents from this cause became more and more frequent as the industrial importance of coal increased during the nineteenth century and as the mines were dug deeper and contained more fire damp, until finally the various nations which were producers of coal appointed commissions to study and develop means of preventing them. The first of these was appointed in France in 1877, the British commission in 1879, the Prussian commission in 1881, and the Belgian and Austrian commissions at later dates. The Pittsburgh testing station of the U. S. Geological Survey was officially opened and regular work was commenced there on December 3, 1908, with the result that the first American list of explosives permissible for use in gaseous and dusty coal mines was issued May 15, 1909. On July 1, 1909, the station was taken over by the U. S. Bureau of Mines, which, since January 1, 1918, has conducted its tests at the Explosives Experiment Station at Bruceton, not far from Pittsburgh, in Pennsylvania.

Explosives which are approved for use in gaseous and dusty coal mines are known in this country as *permissible* explosives, in England as *permitted* explosives, and are to be distinguished from *authorized* explosives which conform to certain conditions with respect to safety in handling, in transport, etc. Explosives which are safe for use in coal mines are known in France as *explosifs antigrisouteux*, in Belgium as *explosifs S. G. P.* (*sécurité, grisou, poussière*), in Germany as *schlagwettersichere Sprengstoffe* while the adjective *handhabungssichere* is applied to those which are safe in handling. Both kinds, permissible and authorized, are *safety explosives, explosifs de sûreté, Sicherheitssprengstoffe*.

A mixture of air and methane is explosive if the methane content lies between 5 and 14%. A mixture which contains 9.5% of methane, in which the oxygen exactly suffices for complete combustion, is the one which explodes most violently, propagates the explosion most easily, and produces the highest temperature. This mixture ignites at about 650° to 700°. Since explosives in general produce temperatures which are considerably above 1000°, explo-
348
sive mixtures of methane and air would always be exploded by them if it were not for the circumstance, discovered by Mallard and Le Chatelier, that there is a certain delay or period of induction before the gaseous mixture actually explodes. At 650° this amounts to about 10 seconds, at 1000° to about 1 second, and at 2200° there is no appreciable delay and the explosion is presumed to follow instantaneously after the application of this temperature however momentary. Mallard and Le Chatelier concluded that an explosive having a temperature of explosion of 2200° or higher would invariably ignite fire damp. The French commission which was studying these questions at first decided that the essential characteristic of a permissible explosive should be that its calculated temperature of explosion should be not greater than 2200°, and later designated a temperature of 1500° as the maximum for explosives permissible in coal seams and 1900° for those intended to be used in the accompanying rock.

The flame which is produced by the explosion of a brisant explosive is of extremely short duration, and its high temperature continues only for a small fraction of a second, for the hot gases by expanding and by doing work immediately commence to cool themselves. If they are produced in the first place at a temperature below that of the instantaneous inflammation of fire damp, they may be cooled to such an extent that they are not sufficiently warm for a sufficiently long time to ignite fire damp at all. Black powder, burning slowly, always ignites explosive gas mixtures. But any high explosive may be made safe for use in gaseous mines by the addition to it of materials which reduce the initial temperature of the products of its explosion. Or, in cases where this initial temperature is not too high, the same safety may be secured by limiting the size of the charge and by firing the shot in a well-tamped bore hole under such conditions that the gases are obliged to do more mechanical work and are cooled the more in consequence.

Permissible explosives may be divided into two principal classes: (1) those which are and (2) those which are not based upon a high explosive which is cool in itself, such as ammonium nitrate, or guanidine nitrate, or nitroguanidine. The second class may be subdivided further, according to composition, into as

349

many classes as there are varieties in the compositions of high explosives, or it may be subdivided, irrespective of composition, according to the means which are used to reduce the explosion temperature. Thus, an explosive containing nitroglycerin, nitrostarch, chlorate or perchlorate, or tetranitronaphthalene, or an explosive which is essentially black powder, may have its temperature of explosion reduced by reason of the fact that (*a*) it contains an excess of carbonaceous material, (*b*) it contains water physically or chemically held in the mixture, or (*c*) it contains volatile salts or substances which are decomposed by heat. Ammonium nitrate may also be used as a means of lowering the temperature of explosion, and thus defines another subdivision (*d*) which corresponds to an overlapping of the two principal classes, (*a*) and (*b*).

Ammonium nitrate, although it is often not regarded as an explosive, may nevertheless be exploded by a suitable initiator. On complete detonation it decomposes in accordance with the equation

$$2NH_4NO_3 \longrightarrow 4H_2O + 2N_2 + O_2$$

but the effect of feeble initiation is to cause decomposition in another manner with the production of oxides of nitrogen. By using a booster of 20–30 grams of Bellite (an explosive consisting of a mixture of ammonium nitrate and dinitrobenzene) and a detonator containing 1 gram of mercury fulminate, Lobry de Bruyn succeeded in detonating 180 grams of ammonium nitrate compressed in a 8-cm. shell. The shell was broken into many fragments. A detonator containing 3 grams of mercury fulminate, used without the booster of Bellite, produced only incomplete detonation. Lheure secured complete detonation of cartridges of ammonium nitrate loaded in bore holes in rock by means of a trinitrotoluene detonating fuse which passed completely through them.

The sensitiveness of ammonium nitrate to initiation is increased by the addition to it of explosive substances, such as nitroglycerin, nitrocellulose, or aromatic nitro compounds, or of

350

non-explosive combustible materials, such as rosin, sulfur, charcoal, flour, sugar, oil, or paraffin. Substances of the latter class react with the oxygen which the ammonium nitrate would otherwise liberate; they produce additional gas and heat, and increase both the power of the explosive and the temperature of its explosion. Pure ammonium nitrate has a temperature of explosion of about 1120° to 1130°. Ammonium nitrate explosives permissible in the United States generally produce instantaneous temperatures between 1500° and 2000°.

Among the first permissible explosives developed in France were certain ones of the Belgian Favier type which contained no nitroglycerin and consisted essentially of ammonium nitrate, sometimes with other nitrates, along with a combustible material such as naphthalene or nitrated naphthalene or other aromatic nitro compounds. These explosives have remained the favorites in France for use in coal mines. The method of manufacture is simple. The materials are ground together in a wheel mill, and the mass is broken up, sifted, and packed in paraffined paper cartridges. The compositions of the mixtures are those which calculations show to give the desired temperatures of explosion. *Grisounites roches*, permissible for use in rock, have temperatures of explosion between 1500° and 1900°; *Grisounites couches*, for use in coal, below 1500°. Several typical compositions are listed below.

	Grisou-naphtalite-roche	Grisou-naphtalite-roche salpêtrée	Grisou-naphtalite-couche	Grisou-naphtalite-couche salpêtrée	Grisou-tétrylite-couche
Ammonium nitrate......	91.5	86.5	95	90	88
Potassium nitrate......	..	5.0	..	5	5
Dinitronaphthalene.	8.5	8.5	..	..	..
Trinitronaphthalene.	..	..	5	5	..
Tetryl........	..	..	..	..	7

351

The French also have permissible explosives containing both ammonium nitrate and nitroglycerin (gelatinized), with and without saltpeter. These are called *Grisou-dynamites* or *Grisoutines.*

	Grisou-dynamite-roche	Grisou-dynamite-roche salpêtrée	Grisou-dynamite-couche	Grisou-dynamite-couche salpêtrée
Nitroglycerin......	29.0	29.0	12.0	12.0
Collodion cotton....	1.0	1.0	0.5	0.5
Ammonium nitrate.	70.0	65.0	87.5	82.5
Potassium nitrate...	..	5.0	..	5.0

The effect of ammonium nitrate in lowering the temperature of explosion of nitroglycerin mixtures is nicely illustrated by the data of Naoúm who reports that guhr dynamite (75% actual nitroglycerin) gives a temperature of 2940°, a mixture of equal amounts of guhr dynamite and ammonium nitrate 2090°, and a mixture of 1 part of guhr dynamite and 4 of ammonium nitrate 1468°.

In ammonium nitrate explosives in which the ingredients are not intimately incorporated as they are in the Favier explosives, but in which the granular particles retain their individual form, the velocity of detonation may be regulated by the size of the nitrate grains. A relatively slow explosive for producing lump coal is made with coarse-grained ammonium nitrate, and a faster explosive for the procurement of coking coal is made with fine-grained material.

The first explosives to be listed as permissible by the U. S. Bureau of Mines were certain *Monobels* and *Carbonites,* and

Monobels are still among the most important of American permissibles. Monobels contain about 10% nitroglycerin, about 10% carbonaceous material, wood pulp, flour, sawdust, etc., by the physical properties of which the characteristics of the explosive are somewhat modified, and about 80% ammonium nitrate of which, however, a portion, say 10%, may be substituted by a volatile salt such as sodium chloride.

[352]

In Europe the tendency is to use a smaller amount of nitroglycerin, say 4 to 6%, or, as in the Favier explosives, to omit it altogether. Ammonium nitrate permissible explosives which contain nitroglycerin may be divided broadly into two principal classes, those of low ammonium nitrate content in which the oxygen is balanced rather accurately against the carbonaceous material and which are cooled by the inclusion of salts, and those which have a high ammonium nitrate content but whose temperature of explosion is low because of an incomplete utilization of the oxygen by a relatively small amount of carbonaceous material. Explosives of the latter class are more popular in England and in Germany. Several examples of commercial explosives of each sort are listed in the following table.

	I	II	III	IV	V	VI	VII	VIII
Ammonium nitrate	52.0	53.0	60.0	61.0	66.0	73.0	78.0	83.0
Potassium nitrate	21.0	...	...	...	...	2.8	5.0	7.0
Sodium nitrate	...	12.0	5.0	3.0	...	...	...	...
Barium nitrate	...	...	...	...	...	...	...	2.0
Na or K chloride	...	...	21.0	20.5	22.0	15.0	8.0	...
Hydrated ammonium oxalate	16.0	19.0	...	...	...	...	...	...
Ammonium chloride	6.0	...	...	...	...	...	...	...
Cereal or wood meal	...	4.0	4.0	7.5	2.0	1.0	5.0	2.0
Glycerin	...	...	...	3.0	...	...	...	...
Powdered coal	...	...	...	...	4.0	...	...	...
Nitrotoluene	...	...	6.0	1.0	...	...	...	...
Dinitrotoluene	...	...	...	...	...	5.0	...	...
Trinitrotoluene	...	6.0	...	...	...	...	...	2.0
Nitroglycerin	5.0	5.0	4.0	4.0	4.0	3.2	4.0	4.0

The *Carbonites* which are permissible are straight dynamites whose temperatures of explosion are lowered by the excess of carbon which they contain. As a class they merge, through the *Ammon-Carbonites,* with the class of ammonium nitrate explosives. The Carbonites, have the disadvantage that they produce gases which contain carbon monoxide, and for that reason have largely given way for use in coal mines to ammonium nitrate permissibles which contain an excess of oxygen. Naoúm reports the compositions and explosive characteristics of four German Carbonites as follows.

[353]

	I	II	III	IV
Nitroglycerin	25.0	25.0	25.0	30.0
Potassium nitrate	30.5	34.0	...	...
Sodium nitrate	...	...	30.5	24.5
Barium nitrate	4.0	1.0	...	...
Spent tan bark meal	40.0	1.0	...	...
Meal	...	38.5	39.5	40.5
Potassium dichromate	...	...	5.0	5.0
Sodium carbonate	0.5	0.5	...	...
Heat of explosion, Cal./kg.	576	506	536	602
Temperature of explosion	1874°	1561°	1666°	1639°
Velocity of detonation, meters/sec.	2443	2700	3042	2472
Lead block expansion	235 cc.	213 cc.	240 cc.	258 cc.

The salts which are most frequently used in permissible explosives are sodium chloride and potassium chloride, both of which are volatile (the potassium chloride more readily so), ammonium chloride and ammonium sulfate, which decompose to form gases, and the hydrated salts, alum $Al_2(SO_4)_3 \cdot K_2SO_4 \cdot 24H_2O$; ammonium alum $Al_2(SO_4)_3 \cdot (NH_4)_2SO_4 \cdot 24H_2O$; chrome alum $Cr_2(SO_4)_3 \cdot K_2SO_4 \cdot 24H_2O$; aluminum sulfate $Al_2(SO_4)_3 \cdot 18H_2O$; ammonium oxalate $(NH_4)_2C_2O_4 \cdot H_2O$; blue vitriol $CuSO_4 \cdot 5H_2O$; borax $Na_2B_4O_7 \cdot 10H_2O$; Epsom salt $MgSO_4 \cdot 7H_2O$; Glauber's salt $Na_2SO_4 \cdot 10H_2O$; and gypsum $CaSO_4 \cdot 2H_2O$, all of which give off water, while the ammonium salts among them yield other volatile products in addition. Hydrated sodium carbonate is not suitable for use because it attacks both ammonium nitrate and nitroglycerin.

Sprengel Explosives

Explosives of a new type were introduced in 1871 by Hermann Sprengel, the inventor of the mercury high-vacuum pump, who patented a whole series of mining explosives which were prepared by mixing an oxidizing substance with a combustible one "in such proportions that their mutual oxidation and de-oxidation should be theoretically complete." The essential novelty of his invention lay in the fact that the materials were mixed just before the explosive was used, and the resultant explosive mixture was [354] fired by means of a blasting cap. Among the oxidizing agents which he mentioned were potassium chlorate, strong nitric acid, and liquid nitrogen dioxide; among the combustible materials nitrobenzene, nitronaphthalene, carbon disulfide, petroleum, and picric acid.[31] Strong nitric acid is an inconvenient and unpleasant material to handle. It can eat through the copper capsule of a blasting cap and cause the fulminate to explode. Yet several explosives containing it have been patented, *Oxonite,* for example, consisting of 58 parts of picric acid and 42 of fuming nitric acid, and *Hellhoffite,* 28 parts of nitrobenzene and 72 of nitric acid. These explosives are about as powerful as 70% dynamite, but are distinctly more sensitive to shock and to blows. Hellhoffite was sometimes absorbed on kieselguhr to form a plastic mass, but it still had the disadvantage that it was intensely corrosive and attacked paper, wood, and the common metals.

[31] Sprengel was aware in 1871 that picric acid alone could be detonated by means of fulminate but realized also that more explosive force could be had from it if it were mixed with an oxidizing agent. Picric acid alone was evidently not used practically as an explosive until after Turpin in 1886 had proposed it as a bursting charge for shells.

The peculiarities of the explosives recommended by Sprengel so set them apart from all others that they define a class; explosives which contain a large proportion of a liquid ingredient and which are mixed *in situ* immediately before use are now known as Sprengel explosives. They have had no success in England, for the reason that the mixing of the ingredients has been held to constitute manufacture within the meaning of the Explosives Act of 1875 and as such could be carried out lawfully only on licensed premises. Sprengel explosives have been used in the United States, in France, and in Italy, and were introduced into Siberia and China by American engineers when the first railroads were built in those countries. *Rack-a-rock,* patented by S. R. Divine, is particularly well known because it was used for blasting out Hell Gate Channel in New York Harbor. On October 10, 1885, 240,399 pounds of it, along with 42,331 pounds of dynamite, was exploded for that purpose in a single blast. It was prepared for use by adding 21 parts of nitrobenzene to 79 parts of potassium chlorate contained in water-tight copper cartridges.

The *Prométhées*, authorized in France[355] under the name of *explosifs O No. 3*, are prepared by dipping cartridges of a compressed oxidizing mixture of potassium chlorate 80 to 95% and manganese dioxide 5 to 20% into a liquid prepared by mixing nitrobenzene, turpentine, and naphtha in the proportions 50/20/30 or 60/15/25. The most serious disadvantage of these explosives was an irregularity of behavior resulting from the circumstance that different cartridges absorbed different quantities of the combustible oil, generally between 8 and 13%, and that the absorption was uneven and sometimes caused incomplete detonation. Similar explosives are those of Kirsanov, a mixture of 90 parts of turpentine and 10 of phenol absorbed by a mixture of 80 parts of potassium chlorate and 20 of manganese dioxide, and of Fielder, a liquid containing 80 parts of nitrobenzene and 20 of turpentine absorbed by a mixture of 70 parts of potassium chlorate and 30 of potassium permanganate.

The *Panclastites*, proposed by Turpin in 1881, are made by mixing liquid nitrogen dioxide with such combustible liquids as carbon disulfide, nitrobenzene, nitrotoluene, or gasoline. They are very sensitive to shock and must be handled with the greatest caution after they have once been mixed. In the first World War the French used certain ones of them, under the name of *Anilites*, in small bombs which were dropped from airplanes for the purpose of destroying personnel. The two liquids were enclosed in separate compartments of the bomb, which therefore contained no explosive and was safe while the airplane was carrying it. When the bomb was released, a little propeller on its nose, actuated by the passage through the air, opened a valve which permitted the two liquids to mix in such fashion that the bomb was then filled with a powerful high explosive which was so sensitive that it needed no fuze but exploded immediately upon impact with the target.

Liquid Oxygen Explosives

Liquid oxygen explosives were invented in 1895 by Linde who had developed a successful machine for the liquefaction of gases. The *Oxyliquits*, as he called them, prepared by impregnating cartridges of porous combustible material with liquid oxygen or liquid air are members of the general class of Sprengel explosives, and have the unusual advantage[356] from the point of view of safety that they rapidly lose their explosiveness as they lose their liquid oxygen by evaporation. If they have failed to fire in a bore hole, the workmen need have no fear of going into the place with a pick or a drill after an hour or so has elapsed.

Liquid oxygen explosives often explode from flame or from the spurt of sparks from a miner's fuse, and frequently need no detonator, or, putting the matter otherwise, some of them are themselves satisfactory detonators. Like other detonating explosives, they may explode from shock. Liquid oxygen explosives made from carbonized cork and from kieselguhr mixed with petroleum were used in the blasting of the Simplon tunnel in 1899. The explosive which results when a cartridge of spongy metallic aluminum absorbs liquid oxygen is of theoretical interest because its explosion yields no gas; it yields only solid aluminum oxide and heat, much heat, which causes the extremely rapid gasification of the excess of liquid oxygen and it is this which produces the explosive effect. Lampblack is the absorbent most commonly used in this country.

Liquid oxygen explosives were at first made up from liquid air more or less self-enriched by standing, the nitrogen (b.p. −195°) evaporating faster than the oxygen (b.p. −183°), but it was later shown that much better results followed from the use of pure liquid oxygen. Rice reports that explosives made from liquid oxygen and an absorbent of crude oil on kieselguhr mixed with lampblack or wood pulp and enclosed in a cheesecloth bag within a corrugated pasteboard insulator were 4 to 12% stronger than 40% straight nitroglycerin dynamite in the standard Bureau of Mines test with the ballistic pendulum. They had a velocity of detonation of about 3000 meters per second. They caused the ignition of fire damp and produced a flame which lasted for 7.125 milliseconds as compared with 0.342 for an average permissible explosive (no permissible producing a flame of more than 1 millisecond duration). The length of the flame was 2½ times that of the flame of the average permissible. In the Trauzl lead block an explosive made up from a liquid air (i.e., a mixture of liquid oxygen and liquid nitrogen)[357] containing 33% of oxygen gave no explosion; with 40% oxygen an enlargement of 9 cc.; with 50% 80 cc., with 55% 147 cc.; and with 98% oxygen an enlargement of 384 cc., about 20% greater than the enlargement produced by 60% straight dynamite. The higher temperatures of explosion of the liquid oxygen explosives cause them to give higher results in the Trauzl test than correspond to their actual explosive power.

Liquid oxygen explosives are used in this country for open-cut mining or strip mining, not underground, and are generally prepared near the place where they are to be used. The cartridges are commonly left in the "soaking box" for 30 minutes, and on occasions have been transported in this box for several miles.

One of the most serious faults of liquid oxygen explosives is the ease with which they inflame and the rapidity with which they burn, amounting practically and in the majority of cases to their exploding from fire. Denues[34] has found that treatment of the granular carbonaceous absorbent with an aqueous solution of phosphoric acid results in an explosive which is non-inflammable by cigarettes, matches, and other igniting agents. Mono- and diammonium phosphate, ammonium chloride, and phosphoric acid were found to be suitable for fireproofing the canvas wrappers. Liquid oxygen explosives made up from the fireproofed absorbent are still capable of being detonated by a blasting cap. Their strength, velocity of detonation, and length of life after impregnation are slightly but not significantly shorter than those of explosives made up from ordinary non-fireproofed absorbents containing the same amount of moisture.

Chlorate and Perchlorate Explosives

The history of chlorate explosives goes back as far as 1788 when Berthollet attempted to make a new and more powerful gunpowder by incorporating in a stamp mill a mixture of potassium chlorate with sulfur and charcoal. He used the materials in the proportion 6/1/1. A party had been organized to witness the manufacture, M. and Mme. Lavoisier, Berthollet, the Commissaire M. de Chevraud and his daughter, the engineer M. Lefort, and others. The mill was started, and the party went away for breakfast.[358] Lefort and Mlle. de Chevraud were the first to return. The material exploded, throwing them to a considerable distance and causing such injuries that they both died within a few minutes. In 1849 the problem of chlorate gunpowder was again attacked by Augendre who invented a *white powder* made from potassium chlorate 4 parts, cane sugar 1 part, and potassium ferrocyanide 1 part. However, no satisfactory propellent powder for use in guns has yet been made from chlorate. Chlorate powders are used in toy salutes, maroons, etc., where a sharp explosion accompanied by noise is desired, and chlorate is used in primer compositions and in practical high explosives of the Sprengel type (described above) and in the Cheddites and Silesia explosives.

Many chlorate mixtures, particularly those which contain sulfur, sulfides, and picric acid, are extremely sensitive to blows and to friction. In the *Street explosives*, later called Cheddites because they were manufactured at Chedde in France, the chlorate is phlegmatized by means of castor oil, a substance which appears to have remarkable powers in this respect. The French *Commission des Substances Explosives* in 1897 commenced its first investigation of these explosives by a study of those which are listed below, and concluded that their sensitivity to shock is

	I	II	III
Potassium chlorate	75.0	74.6	80.0
Picronitronaphthalene	20.0	...	...
Nitronaphthalene	...	5.5	12.0
Starch	...	14.9	...
Castor oil	5.0	5.0	8.0

less than that of No. 1 dynamite (75% guhr dynamite) and that when exploded by a fulminate cap they show a considerable brisance which however is less than that of dynamite. Later studies showed that the Cheddites had slightly more force than No. 1 dynamite, although they were markedly less brisant because of their lower velocity of detonation. After further experimentation four Cheddites were approved for manufacture in France, but the output of the Poudrerie de Vonges where they were made consisted principally of Cheddites No. 1 and No. 4.

	O No. 1 Formula 41	O No. 1 Formula 60 *bis*	O No. 2 Formula 60 *bis* M Cheddite No. 4	O No. 5 Cheddite No. 1
Potassium chlorate	80	80	79	..
Sodium chlorate	..	..	..	79
Nitronaphthalene	12	13	1	..
Dinitrotoluene	..	2	15	16
Castor oil	8	5	5	5

The Cheddites are manufactured by melting the nitro compounds in the castor oil at 80°, adding little by little the pulverized chlorate dried and still warm, and mixing thoroughly. The mixture is emptied out onto a table, and rolled to a thin layer which hardens on cooling and breaks up under the roller and is then sifted and screened.

Sodium chlorate contains more oxygen than potassium chlorate, but has the disadvantage of being hygroscopic. Neither salt ought to be used in mixtures which contain ammonium nitrate or ammonium perchlorate, for double decomposition might occur with the formation of dangerous ammonium chlorate. Potassium chlorate is one of the chlorates least soluble in water, potassium perchlorate one of the least soluble of the perchlorates. The latter salt is practically insoluble in alcohol. The perchlorates are intrinsically more stable and less reactive than the chlorates, and are much safer in contact with combustible substances. Unlike the chlorates they are not decomposed by hydrochloric acid, and they do not yield an explosive gas when warmed with concentrated sulfuric acid. The perchlorates require a higher temperature for their decomposition than do the corresponding chlorates.

SOLUBILITY: PARTS PER 100 PARTS OF WATER

	$KClO_3$	$NaClO_3$	$KClO_4$	NH_4ClO_4
At 0°	3.3	82.	0.7	12.4
At 100°	56.	204.	18.7	88.2

Mixtures of aromatic nitro compounds with chlorate are dangerously sensitive unless they are phlegmatized with castor oil or a similar material, but there are other substances, such as

rosin, animal and vegetable oils, and petroleum products, which give mixtures which are not unduly sensitive to shock and friction and may be handled with reasonable safety. Some of these, such as *Pyrodialyte* and the *Steelites*, were studied by the *Commission des Substances Explosives*. The former consisted of 85 parts of potassium chlorate and 15 of rosin, 2 parts of alcohol being used during the incorporation. The latter, invented by Everard Steele of Chester, England, contained an oxidized rosin (*résidée* in French) which was made by treating a mixture of 90 parts of colophony and 10 of starch with 42 Bé nitric acid. After washing, drying, and powdering, the *résidée* was mixed with powdered potassium chlorate, moistened with methyl alcohol, warmed, and stirred gently while the alcohol was evaporated. *Colliery Steelite*

	STEELITE No. 3	STEELITE No. 5	STEELITE No. 7	COLLIERY STEELITE
Potassium chlorate	75	83.33	87.50	72.5–75.5
Résidée	25	16.67	12.50	23.5–26.5
Aluminum	..	5.00	...	...
Castor oil	..	....	....	0.5–1.0
Moisture	..	....	....	0–1

passed the Woolwich test for safety explosives and was formerly on the British permitted list but failed in the Rotherham test. In Germany the *Silesia* explosives have been used to some extent. *Silesia No. 4* consists of 80 parts of potassium chlorate and 20 of rosin, and *Silesia IV 22*, 70 parts of potassium chlorate, 8 of rosin, and 22 of sodium chloride, is cooled by the addition of the volatile salt and is on the permissible list.

The *Sebomites*, invented by Eugène Louis, contained animal fat which was solid at ordinary temperature, and were inferior to the Cheddites in their ability to transmit detonation. *Explosifs P* (*potasse*) and *S* (*soude*) and the *Minélites*, containing petroleum hydrocarbons, were studied in considerable detail by Dautriche, some of whose results for velocities of detonation are reported in the table on pages 362–363 where they are compared with

his results for Cheddite 60, fourth formula.[41] His experimental results[42] illustrate very clearly the principle that there is an optimum density of loading at which the velocity of detonation is greatest and that at higher densities the velocity drops and the detonation is incomplete and poorly propagated. The Cheddite 60,

	EXPLOSIFS P	EXPLOSIFS S	MINÉLITES A	MINÉLITES B	MINÉLITES C
Potassium chlorate	90	..	90	90	89
Sodium chlorate	..	89	..	..	..
Heavy petroleum oil	..	..	3	..	..

Vaseline	..	..	..	3	4
Paraffin	10	11	7	7	5
Pitch	..	..	..	..	2

fourth formula, when ignited burns slowly with a smoky flame. *Explosifs P* and *S* and the *Minélites* burn while the flame of a Bunsen burner is played upon them but, in general, go out when the flame is removed. *Minélite B,* under the designation *O No. 6 B,* was used by the French during the first World War in grenades and mines. A similar explosive containing 90 parts of sodium chlorate instead of 90 of potassium chlorate was used in grenades and in trench mortar bombs.

[41] The composition of this explosive was the same as that which is given in the table on page 359 as that of *O* No. 2, formula 60 *bis* M, or Cheddite No. 4.

[42] In several cases Dautriche reported temperatures, but the velocity of detonation appears to be unaffected by such temperature variations as those between summer and winter.

Chlorate explosives which contain aromatic nitro compounds have higher velocities of detonation and are more brisant than those whose carbonaceous material is merely combustible. The addition of a small amount of nitroglycerin increases the velocity of detonation still farther. Brisant chlorate explosives of this sort were developed in Germany during the first World War and were known as *Koronit* and *Albit* (*Gesteinskoronit, Kohlenkoronit, Wetteralbit,* etc.). They found considerable use for a time but have now been largely superseded by low-percentage dynamites and by perchlorate explosives. Two of them, manufactured by the Dynamit A.-G., had according to Naoúm the compositions and explosive characteristics which are indicated

362

Explosive	In Tubes of	Diameter	Density of Loading	Velocity of Detonation, M./Sec.
Explosif P	copper	20–22 mm.	0.62	2137
			1.00	3044
			1.05	3185
			1.36	3621
			1.48	3475
			1.54	Incomplete
			0.99	2940
			1.24	3457
			1.45	3565
			1.59	Incomplete
Explosif P	paper	29 mm.	0.95	2752
			1.30	3406
			1.35	3340
			0.90	2688
			1.21	3308
			1.36	3259
			1.41	Incomplete
Explosif S	copper	20–22 mm.	0.88	2480
			1.25	2915
			0.81	2191
			0.92	2457
			1.33	2966
			1.45	2940
			1.54	2688
			1.56	Incomplete
			1.58	Incomplete
Explosif S	paper	29 mm.	1.05	2335
			1.16	2443
			1.29	2443
			1.39	Incomplete
			1.47	Incomplete
Cheddite 60 4th formula	copper	20–22 mm.	1.51	3099
			1.62	2820
			0.84	2457
			1.39	3045
			1.48	3156
Cheddite 60 4th formula	paper	29 mm.	1.25	2774
			1.31	2915
			1.40	2843
			1.50	Incomplete

363

Explosive	In Tubes of	Diameter	Density of Loading	Velocity of Detonation, M./Sec.
Minélite A in powder	copper	20–22 mm.	0.87	2800
			0.99	2930
			1.17	3125
			1.24	3235
			1.38	Incomplete
			1.52	Incomplete
			0.89	2435
			0.95	2835
			1.20	3235
			1.39	3125
			1.45	Incomplete
			0.87	2395
			1.27	3355
			1.39	Incomplete
Minélite A in powder	paper	29 mm.	1.08	2670
			1.19	2835
			1.25	Incomplete
			1.28	Incomplete
			1.19	2895
			1.24	Incomplete
Minélite A in grains	copper	20–22 mm.	0.87	2150
			1.12	2415
			1.20	2550
			1.29	3025
			1.33	2480
			1.35	Incomplete
			1.30	2895
			0.85	2100
			1.17	2415
			1.27	2750
Minélite B in powder	copper	20–22 mm.	0.97	2350
			1.07	2895
			1.24	3235
			1.33	3090
			1.45	Incomplete
			1.57	Incomplete
			1.00	2925
			1.12	2925
			1.26	3165
			1.02	2585
			1.14	2910
			1.30	3180
			1.41	Complete
			1.38	3160
Minélite C in powder	copper	20–22 mm.	1.28	3125
			1.37	Incomplete
			1.48	Incomplete

364

below. It is interesting that the explosive which contained a small amount of nitroglycerin was more brisant, as well as softer and more plastic, and less sensitive to shock, to friction, and to initiation than the drier explosive which contained no nitroglycerin. It required a No. 3 blasting cap to explode it, but the material which contained no nitroglycerin was exploded by a weak No. 1.

	Gesteins-Koronit T1	Gesteins-Koronit T2
Sodium chlorate	72.0	75.0
Vegetable meal	1.0–2.0	1.0–2.0
Di- and trinitrotoluene	20.0	20.0
Paraffin	3.0–4.0	3.0–4.0
Nitroglycerin	3.0–4.0	...

Heat of explosion, Cal./kg.	1219.0	1241.0
Temperature of explosion	3265.0°	3300.0°
Velocity of detonation, m./sec.	5000.0	4300.0
Density of cartridge	1.57	1.46
Lead block expansion	290.0 cc.	280.0 cc.
Lead block crushing	20.0 mm.	19.5 mm.

During the first World War when Germany needed to conserve as much as possible its material for military explosives, blasting explosives made from perchlorate came into extensive use. The Germans had used in their trench mortar bombs an explosive, called *Perdit,* which consisted of a mixture of potassium perchlorate 56%, with dinitrobenzene 32% and dinitronaphthalene 12%. After the War, the perchlorate recovered from these bombs and that from the reserve stock came onto the market, and perchlorate explosives, *Perchlorit, Perchloratit, Persalit, Perkoronit,* etc., were used more widely than ever. The sale of these explosives later ceased because the old supply of perchlorate became exhausted and the new perchlorate was too high in price. Each of these explosives required a No. 3 cap for its initiation. Perchlorate explosives in general are somewhat less sensitive to initiation than chlorate explosives. A small amount of nitroglycerin in perchlorate explosives plays a significant part in propagating the explosive wave and is more important in these compositions than it is in ammonium nitrate explosives. Naoúm[365] reports the following particulars concerning two of the Perkoronites.

	Perkoronit A	Perkoronit B
Potassium perchlorate	58	59
Ammonium nitrate	8	10
Di- and trinitrotoluene, vegetable meal	30	31
Nitroglycerin	4	..
Heat of explosion, Cal./kg.	1170.0	1160.0
Temperature of explosion	3145.0°	3115.0°
Velocity of detonation, m./sec.	5000.0	4400.0
Density of cartridge	1.58	1.52
Lead block expansion	340.0 cc.	330.0 cc.
Lead block crushing	20.0 mm.	18.0 mm.

Potassium perchlorate and ammonium perchlorate permissible explosives, cooled by means of common salt, ammonium oxalate, etc., and containing either ammonium nitrate or alkali metal nitrate with or without nitroglycerin, are used in England, Belgium, and elsewhere. They possess no novel features beyond the explosives already described. Explosives containing ammonium perchlorate yield fumes which contain hydrogen chloride. Potassium perchlorate produces potassium chloride.

Early in the history of these explosives the French *Commission des Substances Explosives* published a report on two ammonium perchlorate Cheddites.[366] The manufacture of these explosives,

	I	II
Ammonium perchlorate	82	50
Sodium nitrate	..	30
Dinitrotoluene	13	15
Castor oil	5	5

however, was not approved for the reason that the use of castor oil for phlegmatizing was found to be unnecessary. Number I took fire easily and burned in an 18-mm. copper gutter at a rate of 4.5 mm. per second, and produced a choking white smoke. Cheddite 60, for comparison, burned irregularly in the copper gutter, with a smoke which was generally black, at a rate of 0.4–0.5 mm. per second. Number II took fire only with the greatest difficulty, and did not maintain its own combustion. The maximum velocities of detonation in zinc tubes 20 mm. in diameter were about 4020 meters per second for No. I and about 3360 for No. II.

The *Commission* published in the same report a number of interesting observations on ammonium perchlorate. Pieces of cotton cloth dipped into a solution of ammonium perchlorate and dried were found to burn more rapidly than when similarly treated with potassium chlorate and less rapidly than when similarly treated with sodium chlorate. Ammonium perchlorate inflamed in contact with a hot wire and burned vigorously with the production of choking white fumes, but the combustion ceased as soon as the hot wire was removed. Its sensitivity to shock, as determined by the drop test, was about the same as that of picric acid, but its sensitivity to initiation was distinctly less. A 50-cm. drop of a 5-kilogram weight caused explosions in about 50% of the trials. A cartridge, 16 cm. long and 26 mm. in diameter, was filled with ammonium perchlorate gently tamped into place (density of loading about 1.10) and was primed with a cartridge of the same diameter containing 25 grams of powdered picric acid (density of loading about 0.95) and placed in contact with one end of it. When the picric acid booster was exploded, the cartridge of perchlorate detonated only for about 20 mm. of its length and produced merely a slight and decreasing furrow in the lead plate on which it was resting. When a booster of 75 grams of picric acid was used, the detonation was propagated in the perchlorate for 35 mm. The temperature of explosion of ammonium perchlorate was calculated to be 1084°.

The French used two ammonium perchlorate explosives during the first World War.

	I	II
Ammonium perchlorate	86	61.5
Sodium nitrate	..	30.0
Paraffin	14	8.5

The first of these was used in 75-mm. shells, the second in 58-mm. trench mortar bombs.

Hydrazine perchlorate melts at 131–132°, burns tranquilly, and explodes violently from shock.

Guanidine perchlorate is relatively stable to heat and to mechanical shock but possesses extraordinary explosive power and sensitivity to initiation. Naoúm[367] states that it gives a lead block expansion of about 400 cc. and has a velocity of detonation of about 6000 meters per second at a density of loading of 1.15.

Ammonium Nitrate Military Explosives

The *Schneiderite* (*Explosif S* or *Sc*) which the French used during the first World War in small and medium-size high-explosive shells, especially in the 75 mm., was made by incorporating 7 parts of ammonium nitrate and 1 of dinitronaphthalene in a wheel mill, and was loaded by compression. Other mixtures, made in the same way, were used in place of Schneiderite or as a substitute for it.

	NX	*NT*	*NTN*	*NDNT*	*N2TN*
Ammonium nitrate	77	70	80	85	50
Sodium nitrate	..	..	..	..	30
Trinitrotoluene	..	30	..	5	..
Trinitroxylene	23	..	..	..	..
Dinitronaphthalene	..	..	..	10	..
Trinitronaphthalene	..	..	20	..	20

Amatol, developed by the British during the first World War, is made by mixing granulated ammonium nitrate with melted trinitrotoluene, and pouring or extruding the mixture into the shells where it solidifies. The booster cavity is afterwards drilled out from the casting. The explosive can be cut with a hand saw. It is insensitive to friction and is less sensitive to initiation and more sensitive to impact than trinitrotoluene. It is hygroscopic, and in the presence of moisture attacks copper, brass, and bronze.

Amatol is made up in various proportions of ammonium nitrate to trinitrotoluene, such as 50/50, 60/40, and 80/20. The granulated, dried, and sifted ammonium nitrate, warmed to about 90°, is added to melted trinitrotoluene at about 90°, and the warm mixture, if 50/50 or 60/40, is ladled into the shells which have been previously warmed somewhat in order that solidification may not be too rapid, or, if 80/20, is *stemmed* or extruded into the shells by means of a screw operating within a steel tube. Synthetic ammonium nitrate is preferred for the preparation of amatol. The pyridine which is generally present in gas liquor and tar liquor ammonia remains in the ammonium nitrate which is made from these liquors and causes frothing and the formation of bubbles in the warm amatol—with the consequent probability of cavitation in the charge. Thiocyanates which are often present in ammonia from the same sources likewise cause frothing, and phenols if present tend to promote exudation.

The velocity of detonation of TNT-ammonium nitrate mixtures decreases regularly with increasing amounts of ammonium
368
nitrate, varying from about 6700 meters per second for TNT to about 4500 meters per second for 80/20 amatol. The greater the proportion of ammonium nitrate the less the brisance and the greater the heaving power of the amatol. 50/50 Amatol does not contain oxygen enough for the complete combustion of its trinitrotoluene, and gives a smoke which is dark colored but less black than the smoke from straight TNT. 80/20 Amatol is less brisant than TNT. It gives an insignificant white smoke. Smoke boxes are usually loaded with 80/20 amatol in order that the artilleryman may observe the bursting of his shells. The best smoke compositions for this purpose contain a large proportion of aluminum and provide smoke by day and a brilliant flash of light by night.

The name of *ammonal* is applied both to certain blasting explosives which contain aluminum and to military explosives, based upon ammonium nitrate, which contain this metal. Military ammonals are brisant and powerful explosives which explode with a bright flash. They are hygroscopic, but the flake aluminum which they contain behaves somewhat in the manner of the shingles on a roof and helps materially to exclude moisture. At the beginning of the first World War the Germans were using in major caliber shells an ammonal having the first of the compositions listed below. After the War had advanced and TNT

	German Ammonal I	German Ammonal II	French Ammonal
Ammonium nitrate	54	72	86
Trinitrotoluene	30	12	..
Aluminum flakes	16	16	8
Stearic acid	..	..	6

had become more scarce, ammonal of the second formula was adopted. The French also used ammonal in major caliber shells during the first World War. All three of the above-listed explosives were loaded by compression. Experiments have been tried with an ammonal containing ammonium thiocyanate; the mixture was melted, and loaded by pouring but was found to be unsatisfactory because of its rapid decomposition. Ammonal yields a flame which is particularly hot, and consequently gives an unduly high result in the Trauzl lead block test.

369

CHAPTER VIII

NITROAMINES AND RELATED SUBSTANCES

The nitroamines are substituted ammonias, substances in which a nitro group is attached directly to a trivalent nitrogen atom. They are prepared in general either by the nitration of a nitrogen base or of one of its salts, or they are prepared by the splitting off of water from the nitrate of the base by the action of concentrated sulfuric acid upon it. At present two nitroamines are of particular interest to the explosives worker, namely, nitroguanidine and cyclotrimethylenetrinitramine (cyclonite). Both are produced from synthetic materials which have become available in large commercial quantities only since the first World War, the first from cyanamide, the second from formaldehyde from the oxidation of synthetic methyl alcohol.

Nitroamide (Nitroamine)

Nitroamide, the simplest of the nitroamines, is formed by the action of dilute acid on potassium nitrocarbamate, which itself results from the nitration of urethane and the subsequent hydrolysis of the nitro ester by means of alcoholic potassium hydroxide.

$$NH_2-COOC_2H_5 \rightarrow NO_2-NH-COOC_2H_5 \rightarrow NO_2-NH-COOK \rightarrow [NO_2-NH-COOH] \rightarrow NH_2-NO_2 + CO_2$$

Nitroamide is strongly acidic, a white crystalline substance, melting at 72–73° with decomposition, readily soluble in water, alcohol, and ether, and insoluble in petroleum ether. It explodes on contact with concentrated sulfuric acid. The pure material decomposes slowly on standing, forming nitrous oxide and water; it cannot be preserved for more than a few days. When an aqueous solution of nitroamide is warmed, gas bubbles begin to
370
come off at about 60–65°, and decomposition is complete after boiling for a short time.

The solution which results when ammonium nitrate is dissolved in a large excess of concentrated sulfuric acid evidently contains nitroamide. If the solution is warmed directly, no nitric acid distils from it but at about 150° it gives off nitrous oxide which corresponds to the dehydration of the nitroamide by the action of the strong acid. The nitroamide moreover, by the action of the same acid, may be hydrated to yield nitric acid, slowly if the solution is digested at 90° to 120°, under which conditions the nitric acid distils out, and rapidly at ordinary temperature in the nitrometer where mercury is present which reacts with the nitric acid as fast as it is formed.

$$NH_3 \cdot HONO_2 \text{ minus } H_2O \longrightarrow NH_2-NO_2 \begin{cases} \text{minus } H_2O \longrightarrow N_2O \\ \text{plus } H_2O \longrightarrow NH_3 + HONO_2 \end{cases}$$

The two reactions, hydration and dehydration, or, more exactly, the formation of nitrous oxide and of nitric acid, are more or less general reactions of the substituted nitroamines. The extent to which one or the other occurs depends largely upon the groups which are present in the molecule. Thus, tetryl on treatment with concentrated sulfuric acid forms nitric acid, and it gives up one and only one of its nitro groups in the nitrometer, but the reaction is not known by which nitrous oxide is eliminated from it. Methylnitramine, on the other hand, gives nitrous oxide readily enough but shows very little tendency to produce nitric acid.

Solutions of nitrourea and nitroguanidine in concentrated sulfuric acid contain actual nitroamide, and these substances give up their nitro group nitrogen in the nitrometer. Nitroamide has been isolated both from an aqueous solution of nitrourea and from a solution of the same substance in concentrated sulfuric acid.

$$NH_2—CO—NH—NO_2 \rightleftharpoons HNCO + NH_2—NO_2$$

The reaction is reversible, for nitroamide in aqueous solution combines with cyanic acid to form nitrourea.

371

Methylnitramine

Methylnitramine is produced when aniline reacts with tetryl in benzene solution, and when ammonia water or barium hydroxide solution acts upon dinitrodimethyloxamide. The structure of tetryl was first proved by its synthesis from picryl chloride and the potassium salt of methylnitramine.

Methylnitramine is a strong monobasic acid, very readily soluble in water, alcohol, chloroform, and benzene, less soluble in ether, and sparingly soluble in petroleum ether. It crystallizes from ether in flat needles which melt at 38°. It is not decomposed by boiling in aqueous solution even in the presence of an excess of alkali. On distillation it yields dimethylnitramine, m.p. 57°, methyl alcohol, nitrous oxide and other products. Methylnitramine owes its acidity to the fact that it is tautomeric.

$$CH_3—N\begin{matrix}\diagup H \\ \diagdown NO_2\end{matrix} \rightleftharpoons CH_3—N{=}N\begin{matrix}\diagup O \\ \diagdown OH\end{matrix}$$

Dimethylnitramine, in which there is no hydrogen atom attached to the atom which carries the nitro group, cannot tautomerize, and is not acidic.

Methylnitramine decomposes explosively in contact with concentrated sulfuric acid. If the substance is dissolved in water, and if concentrated sulfuric acid is added little by little until a considerable concentration is built up, then the decomposition proceeds more moderately, nitrous oxide is given off, and dimethyl ether (from the methyl alcohol first formed) remains dissolved in the sulfuric acid. The same production of nitrous oxide occurs even in the nitrometer in the presence of mercury. If methylnitramine and a small amount of phenol are dissolved together in water, and if concentrated sulfuric acid is then added little by little, a distinct yellow color shows that a trace of nitric acid has been formed. The fact that methylnitramine gives a blue color with the diphenylamine reagent shows the same thing.

Methylnitramine is conveniently prepared by nitrating methylurethane with absolute nitric acid, drowning in water, neutralizing with sodium carbonate, extracting with ether, and

372

then passing ammonia gas into the ether solution of methylnitrourethane.

$$CH_3-NH-COOC_2H_5 \rightarrow CH_3-\underset{NO_2}{\underset{|}{N}}-COOC_2H_5 \rightarrow CH_3-\underset{NO_2}{\underset{|}{N}}\overset{H-NH_2}{\vdots}COOC_2H_5 + NH_3 \rightarrow CH_3-NH-NO_2{\cdot}NH_3 \rightarrow CH_3-N\begin{matrix}\diagup H \\ \diagdown NO_2\end{matrix}$$

A white crystalline precipitate of the ammonium salt of methylnitramine is deposited. This is dissolved in alcohol, and the solution is boiled—whereby ammonia is driven off—and concentrated to a small volume. The product is procured by completing the evaporation in a vacuum desiccator over sulfuric acid.

The heavy metal salts of methylnitramine are primary explosives, but have not been investigated extensively.

Urea Nitrate

Although urea has the properties of an amide (carbamide) rather than those of an amine, it nevertheless acts as a monoacid base in forming salts among which the nitrate and the oxalate are noteworthy because they are sparingly soluble in cold water, particularly in the presence of an excess of the corresponding acid. The nitrate, white monoclinic prisms which melt at 152° with decomposition, is procured by adding an excess of nitric acid (1.42) to a strong aqueous solution of urea. The yield is increased if the mixture is chilled and allowed to stand for a time. Urea nitrate is stable and not deliquescent. It has interest as a powerful and cool explosive, but suffers from the disadvantage that it is corrosively acidic in the presence of moisture.

Pure urea is manufactured commercially by pumping ammonia and carbon dioxide into an autoclave where they are heated together under pressure while more of each gas is pumped in. Ammonium carbamate is formed at first, this loses water from its molecule to form urea, and the autoclave finally becomes

373

filled with a strong solution of urea which is drawn off and crystallized.

$$2NH_3 + CO_2 \longrightarrow NH_3{\cdot}HO—CO—NH_2 \longrightarrow H_2O + NH_2—CO—NH_2$$

Urea is sometimes incorporated in blasting explosives for the purpose of lowering the temperature of explosion. Its use as a stabilizer has already been mentioned.

Nitrourea

Nitrourea is a cool but powerful explosive, and would be useful if it were not for the fact that it tends to decompose spontaneously in the presence of moisture. The mechanism of its reactions is the same as that of the reactions of nitroguanidine, which differs from it in containing an >NH group where nitrourea contains a >CO, but the reactions of nitrourea are very much more rapid. The nitro group promotes the *urea dearrangement,* so that nitrourea when dissolved in water or when warmed breaks down into cyanic acid and nitroamide much more readily than urea breaks down under like conditions into cyanic acid and ammonia. The imido group in place of the carbonyl hinders it; guanidine dearranges less readily than urea, and nitroguanidine is substantially as stable as urea itself.

Nitrourea is prepared by adding dry urea nitrate (200 grams) in small portions at a time with gentle stirring to concentrated sulfuric acid (1.84) (300 cc.) while the temperature of the mixture is kept below 0°. The milky liquid is poured without delay into a mixture of ice and water (1 liter), the finely divided white precipitate is collected on a filter, sucked as dry as may be, and, without washing, is immediately dissolved while still wet in boiling alcohol.[4] The liquid on cooling deposits pearly leaflets of nitrourea. It is chilled and filtered, and the crystals are rinsed with cold alcohol and dried in the air. The product, which melts at 146° to 153° with decomposition, is sufficiently pure for use in synthesis, and may be preserved for several years unchanged in hard glass bottles. If slightly moist nitrourea is allowed to stand in contact with soft glass, that is, in contact with a trace

[4] The product at this point contains acid enough to prevent it from decomposing in boiling alcohol. For a second recrystallization it is unsafe to heat the alcohol above 60°.

374

of alkali, it decomposes completely within a short time forming water, ammonia, nitrous oxide, urea, biuret, cyanuric acid, etc. Pure nitrourea, recrystallized from benzene, ether, or chloroform, in which solvents it is sparingly soluble, melts with decomposition at 158.4–158.8°.

In water and in hydrophilic solvents nitrourea dearranges rapidly into cyanic acid and nitroamide. Alkalis promote the reaction. If an aqueous solution of nitrourea is warmed, bubbles of nitrous oxide begin to come off at about 60°. If it is allowed to stand over night at room temperature, the nitrourea disappears completely and the liquid is found to be a solution of cyanic acid. Indeed, nitrourea is equivalent to cyanic acid for purposes of synthesis. It reacts with alcohols to form carbamic esters (urethanes) and with primary and second amines to form mono- and *unsym*-di-substituted ureas.

Guanidine Nitrate

Guanidine nitrate is of interest to us both as an explosive itself and a component of explosive mixtures, and as an intermediate in the preparation of nitroguanidine. All other salts of guanidine require strong mixed acid to convert them to nitroguanidine, but the nitrate is converted by dissolving it in concentrated sulfuric acid and pouring the solution into water.

Guanidine is a strong monoacid base, indistinguishable from potassium hydroxide in an electrometric titration. There is considerable evidence which indicates that the charge of the guanidonium ion resides upon its carbon atom.

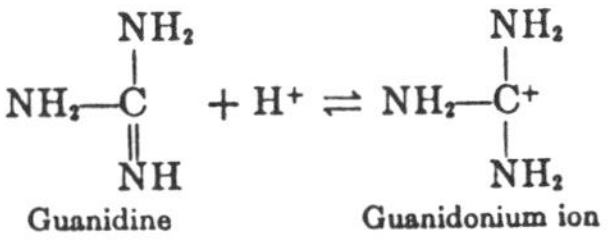

$$\underset{\text{Guanidine}}{NH_2-C(NH_2)=NH} + H^+ \rightleftharpoons \underset{\text{Guanidonium ion}}{NH_2-C^+(NH_2)-NH_2}$$

Guanidine itself is crystalline, deliquescent, and strongly caustic, and takes up carbon dioxide from the air.

Guanidine was first obtained by Strecker in 1861 by the oxidation with hydrochloric acid and potassium chlorate of guanine (a substance found in guano and closely related to uric acid).

375

Guanidine or its salts may be prepared, among other ways, by the interaction (1) of orthocarbonic ester or (2) of chloropicrin

$$1.\ CCl_3\cdot NO_2 + 3NH_3 \longrightarrow NH_2-C(NH)-NH_2 + HNO_2 + 3HCl$$

$$2.\ C(OC_2H_5)_4 + 3NH_3 \longrightarrow NH_2-C(NH)-NH_2 + 4C_2H_5-OH$$

with aqueous ammonia at 150°, by the interaction (3) of carbon tetrabromide with alcoholic ammonia in a sealed tube at 100°,

$$3.\ CBr_4 + 3NH_3 \longrightarrow NH_2-C(NH)-NH_2 + 4HBr$$

by the interaction (4) of cyanogen iodide with alcoholic ammonia in a sealed tube at 100°, whereby cyanamide and ammonium iodide are formed first and then combine with one another to

$$4.\ I-C\equiv N + 2NH_3 \longrightarrow NH_2-C\equiv N + NH_3\cdot HI \longrightarrow NH_2-C(NH)-NH_2\cdot HI$$

form guanidine iodide, by the combination (5) of cyanamide, already prepared, with an ammonium salt by heating the materials with alcohol in a sealed tube at 100°, and (6) by heating

$$6.\ NH_4NCS \rightleftharpoons NH_3 + HNCS \rightleftharpoons NH_2-CS-NH_2 \rightleftharpoons NH_2-C\equiv N + H_2S$$

$$NH_4NCS + NH_2-C\equiv N \longrightarrow NH_2-C(NH)-NH_2\cdot HNCS$$

ammonium thiocyanate at 170–190° for 20 hours, or until hydrogen sulfide no longer comes off, whereby the material is converted into guanidine thiocyanate. The reaction depends upon the fact that the ammonium thiocyanate is in part converted into thiourea, and that this breaks down into hydrogen sulfide, which escapes, and cyanamide which combines with the unchanged ammonium thiocyanate to form the guanidine salt. The yield from this process is excellent.

For many years guanidine thiocyanate was the most easily prepared and the most commonly used of the salts of guanidine. Other salts were made from it by metathetical reactions. Nitroguanidine, prepared from the thiocyanate by direct nitration with mixed acids, was found to contain traces of sulfur compounds which attacked nitrocellulose and affected the stability of smokeless powder, and this is one of the reasons why nitroguanidine powders did not come into early use. Guanidine thiocyanate is deliquescent. Strong solutions of it dissolve filter paper.

376

Cyanamide itself is not a suitable raw material for the preparation of guanidine salts, for it is difficult to prepare and to purify, and it polymerizes on keeping. The evaporation of an aqueous solution of cyanamide yields the dimer, dicyandiamide, and the heating, or even the long keeping, of the dry substance produces the trimer, melamine.

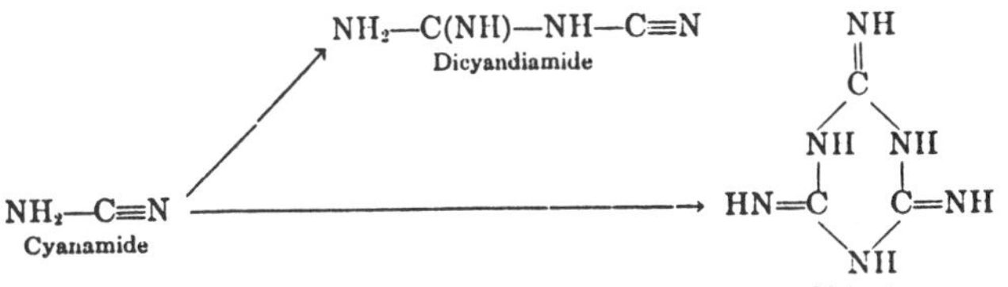

$$\underset{\text{Cyanamide}}{NH_2-C\equiv N} \longrightarrow \underset{\text{Dicyandiamide}}{NH_2-C(NH)-NH-C\equiv N}$$

$$\underset{\text{Cyanamide}}{NH_2-C\equiv N} \longrightarrow \underset{\text{Melamine}}{HN=C\langle NH-C(=NH)-NH \rangle C=NH \ (\text{ring closed by } NH)}$$

Cyanamide, colorless crystals, m.p. 40°, is readily soluble in water, alcohol, and ether. An aqueous solution of cyanamide gives a black precipitate of copper cyanamide with ammoniacal copper sulfate solution, and a yellow precipitate of silver cyanamide with ammoniacal silver nitrate. The precipitates are almost unique among the compounds of copper and silver in the respect that they are insoluble in ammonia water.

Before the development of the cyanamide process for the fixation of nitrogen, cyanamide was prepared by the interaction of cyanogen chloride or bromide (from the action of the halogen on potassium cyanide) with ammonia in water or ether solution.

$$KCN + Cl_2 \longrightarrow KCl + Cl-CN$$

$$2NH_3 + Cl-CN \longrightarrow NH_4Cl + NH_2-CN$$

If the reaction, say, with cyanogen chloride, is carried out in ether solution, ammonium chloride precipitates and is filtered off, and the cyanamide is procured as a syrup by allowing the ether solution to evaporate spontaneously and later as crystals by allowing the syrup to stand over sulfuric acid in a desiccator. Cyanamide may also be prepared by removing the component atoms of hydrogen sulfide from thiourea by means of mercuric oxide. Thionyl chloride effects the corresponding removal of water from urea.

$$NH_2—CS—NH_2 \text{ minus } H_2S\ (HgO) \longrightarrow NH_2—CN + HgS + H_2O$$

$$NH_2—CO—NH_2 \text{ minus } H_2O\ (Cl_2SO) \longrightarrow NH_2—CN + SO_2 + 2HCl$$

377

The cyanamide process has made cyanamide and its derivatives more easily available for commercial synthesis. Coke and limestone are heated together in the electric furnace for the production of calcium carbide. This substance, along with a small amount of calcium chloride which acts as a catalyst, is then heated at 800–1000° in a stream of nitrogen gas.

$$2CaCO_3 + 5C \longrightarrow 2Ca\langle{}^{C}_{C}\ (\equiv) + 3CO_2$$

$$Ca\langle{}^{C}_{C}\ (\equiv) + N_2 \longrightarrow CaNCN + C$$

The resulting dark-colored mixture of calcium cyanamide and carbon is known as *lime nitrogen* (*Kalkstickstoff*) and is used in fertilizers. If steam is passed through it, it yields ammonia.

$$CaNCN + 3H_2O\ (\text{steam}) \longrightarrow CaCO_3 + 2NH_3$$

Water, whether cool or warm, produces some cyanamide, which is readily soluble, and some calcium hydrogen cyanamide, white, microcrystalline, and sparingly soluble, but water plus acid for the removal of the calcium (sulfuric acid, oxalic acid, or carbon dioxide) yields a solution of cyanamide which is directly applicable for use in certain reactions.

$$2CaNCN + 2H_2O \longrightarrow Ca(OH)_2 + Ca\langle{}^{NH—CN}_{NH—CN}$$

$$Ca\langle{}^{NH—CN}_{NH—CN} + CO_2 + H_2O \longrightarrow CaCO_3 + 2NH_2—CN$$

On hydrolysis with dilute sulfuric acid it yields urea. On treatment with ammonium sulfide it prefers to react with the hydrogen sulfide part of the molecule to form thiourea, not with the ammonia part to form guanidine, and the reaction is the commercial source of many tons of thiourea for the rubber industry. On evaporation for crystals, the solution yields dicyandiamide which constitutes a convenient source for the preparation of guanidine nitrate.

Dicyandiamide crystallizes from water in handsome flat needles or plates which melt at 208.0–208.1° and decompose if heated slightly above the melting point. A saturated aqueous solution contains—

378

Temperature, °C.	Grams per 100 cc. of Solution
0	1.3
10	2.0
20	3.4
30	5.0
40	7.6
50	11.4
60	16.1
70	22.5
80	30.0
90	37.9
100	46.7

The preparation of guanidine nitrate from dicyandiamide by the action of aqua regia has been patented, but the reaction evidently depends solely upon the hydrolysis of the cyan group and does not require the use of a vigorous oxidizing agent. Marqueyrol and Loriette in a French patent of September 26, 1917, described a process for the preparation of nitroguanidine direct from dicyandiamide without the isolation of any intermediate products. The process depends upon the hydrolysis of the dicyandiamide by means of 61% sulfuric acid to form guanylurea or dicyandiamidine (sulfate) which is then further hydrolyzed to form carbon dioxide, which escapes, and guanidine and ammonia, which remain in the reaction mixture in the form of sulfates.

$$\underset{\text{Dicyandiamide}}{NH_2—C(NH)—NH—CN} + H_2O \longrightarrow$$

$$\underset{\text{Guanylurea}}{NH_2—C(NH)—NH—CO—NH_2} + H_2O \longrightarrow$$

$$\underset{\text{Guanidine}}{NH_2—C(NH)—NH_2} + CO_2 + NH_3$$

The guanidine sulfate, without removal from the mixture, is then nitrated to nitroguanidine.[7] The process yields a nitroguanidine which is suitable for use in nitrocellulose powder, but it suffers from the disadvantages that the dicyandiamide, which corresponds after all to two molecules of cyanamide, yields in theory only one molecular equivalent of guanidine, that the actual yield is considerably less than the theory because of the loss of guanidine by hydrolysis to carbon dioxide and ammonia, and that the final nitration of the guanidine sulfate, which is carried out in the presence of water and of ammonium sulfate, requires strong and expensive mixed acid.

[7] The procedure, under conditions somewhat different from those described in the patent, is illustrated by our process for the preparation of β-nitroguanidine; see page 383.

379

Werner and Bell reported in 1920 that dicyandiamide heated for 2 hours at 160° with 2 mols of ammonium thiocyanate gives 2 mols of guanidine thiocyanate in practically theoretical yield. Ammonium thiocyanate commends itself for the reaction because it is readily fusible. The facts suggest that another fusible ammonium salt might work as well, ammonium nitrate melts at about 170°, and, of all the salts of guanidine, the nitrate is the one which is most desired for the preparation of nitroguanidine. When dicyandiamide and 2 mols of ammonium nitrate are mixed and warmed together at 160°, the mixture first melts to a colorless liquid which contains biguanide (or guanylguanidine) nitrate, which presently begins to deposit crystals of guanidine nitrate, and which after 2 hours at 160° solidifies completely to a mass of that substance. The yield is practically theoretical. The reaction consists, first, in the addition of ammonia to the cyan group of the dicyandiamide, then in the ammoniolytic splitting of the biguanide to form two molecules of guanidine.

$$\underset{\text{Dicyandiamide}}{NH_2—C(NH)—NH—CN} + NH_3 \cdot HNO_3 \longrightarrow$$

$$\underset{\text{Biguanide nitrate}}{NH_2—C(NH)—NH—C(NH)—NH_2 \cdot HNO_3} + NH_3 \cdot HNO_3 \longrightarrow$$

$$2\underset{\text{Guanidine nitrate}}{NH_2—C(NH)—NH_2 \cdot HNO_3}$$

The nitric acid of the original 2 mols of ammonium nitrate is exactly sufficient for the formation of 2 mols of guanidine nitrate. But the intermediate biguanide is a strong diacid base; the ammonium nitrate involved in its formation supplies only one equivalent of nitric acid; and there is a point during the early part of the process when the biguanide mononitrate tends to attack the unchanged ammonium nitrate and to liberate ammonia from it. For this reason the process works best if a small excess of

380

ammonium nitrate is used. The preparation may be carried out by heating the materials together either in the dry state or in an autoclave in the presence of water or of alcohol.

Guanidine nitrate is not deliquescent. It is readily soluble in alcohol, very readily in water, and may be recrystallized from either solvent. The pure material melts at 215–216°.

Preparation of Guanidine Nitrate. An intimate mixture of 210 grams of dicyandiamide and 440 grams of ammonium nitrate is placed in a 1 liter round-bottom flask, and the flask is arranged for heating in an oil bath which has a thermometer in the oil. The oil bath is warmed until the thermometer indicates 160°, and the temperature is held at this point for 2 hours. At the end of that time the flask is removed and allowed to cool, and its contents is extracted on the steam bath by warming with successive portions of water. The combined solution is filtered while hot for the removal of white insoluble material (ammeline and ammelide), concentrated to a volume of about a liter, and allowed to crystallize. The mother liquors are concentrated to a volume of about 250 cc. for a second crop, after the removal of which the residual liquors are discarded. The crude guanidine nitrate may be recrystallized by dissolving it in the least possible amount of boiling water and allowing to cool, etc., or it may be dried thoroughly and used directly for the preparation of nitroguanidine. A small amount of ammonium nitrate in it does not interfere with its conversion to nitroguanidine by the action of concentrated sulfuric acid.

Nitroguanidine

Nitroguanidine exists in two forms. The α-form invariably results when guanidine nitrate is dissolved in concentrated sulfuric and the solution is poured into water. It is the form which is commonly used in the explosives industry. It crystallizes from water in long, thin, flat, flexible, lustrous needles which are tough and extremely difficult to pulverize; $N_\alpha = 1.518$, N_β = a little greater than 1.668, N_γ = greater than 1.768, double refraction 0.250. When α-nitroguanidine is decomposed by heat, a certain amount of β-nitroguanidine is found among the products.

β-Nitroguanidine is produced in variable amount, usually along with some of the α-compound, by the nitration of the mixture of guanidine sulfate and ammonium sulfate which results from the hydrolysis of dicyandiamide by sulfuric acid. Conditions have

381

been found, as described later, which have yielded exclusively the β-compound in more than thirty trials. It crystallizes from water in fernlike clusters of small, thin, elongated plates; N_α = 1.525, N_β not determined, $N_\gamma = 1.710$, double refraction 0.185. It is converted into the α-compound by dissolving in concentrated sulfuric acid and pouring the solution into water.

Both α- and β-nitroguanidine, if dissolved in hot concentrated nitric acid and allowed to crystallize, yield the same nitrate, thick, rhomb-shaped prisms which melt at 147° with decomposition. The nitrate loses nitric acid slowly in the air, and gives α-nitroguanidine when recrystallized from water. Similarly, both forms recrystallized from strong hydrochloric acid yield a hydrochloride which crystallizes in needles. These lose hydrogen chloride rapidly in the air, and give α-nitroguanidine when recrystallized from water. The two forms are alike in all their chemical reactions, in their derivatives and color reactions.

Both forms of nitroguanidine melt at 232° if the temperature is raised with moderate slowness, but by varying the rate of heating melting points varying between 220° and 250° may be obtained.

Neither form can be converted into the other by solution in water, and the two forms can be separated by fractional crystallization from this solvent. They appear to differ slightly in their solubility in water, the two solubility curves lying close together but apparently crossing each other at about 25°, where the solubility is about 4.4 grams per liter, and again at about 100°, where the solubility is about 82.5 grams per liter. Between these temperatures the β-form appears to be the more soluble.

Preparation of α-Nitroguanidine. Five hundred cc. of concentrated sulfuric acid in a 1-liter beaker is cooled by immersing the beaker in cracked ice, and 400 grams of well-dried guanidine nitrate is added in small portions at a time, while the mixture is stirred with a thermometer and the temperature is not allowed to rise above 10°. The guanidine nitrate dissolves rapidly, with very little production of heat, to form a milky solution. As soon as all crystals have disappeared, the milky liquid is poured into 3 liters of cracked ice and water, and the mixture is allowed to stand with chilling until precipitation and crystallization are complete. The product is collected on a filter, rinsed with water for the removal of sulfuric acid, dissolved in boiling water

382

(about 4 liters), and allowed to crystallize by standing over night. Yield 300–310 grams, about 90% of the theory.

The rapid cooling of a solution of α-nitroguanidine produces small needles, which dry out to a fluffy mass but which are still too coarse to be incorporated properly in colloided powder. An

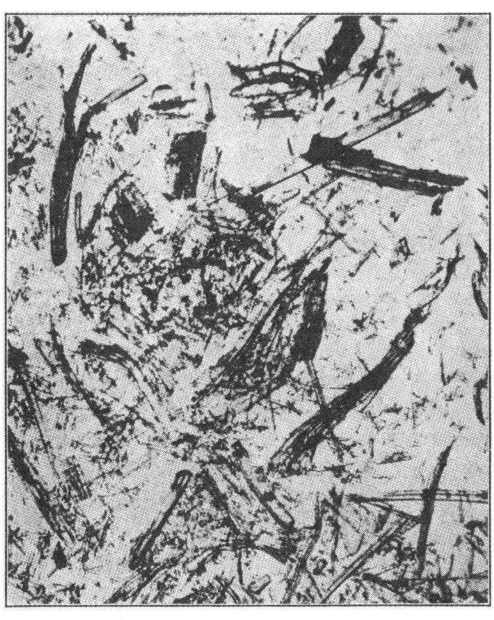

FIGURE 89. α-Nitroguanidine (25×). Small crystals from the rapid cooling of a hot aqueous solution.

extremely fine powder may be procured by the rapid cooling of a mist or spray of hot nitroguanidine solution, either by spraying it against a cooled surface from which the material is removed continuously, or by allowing the spray to drop through a tower up which a counter current of cold air is passing.

Preparation of β-Nitroguanidine. Twenty-five cc. of 61% aqueous sulfuric acid is poured upon 20 grams of dicyandiamide contained in a 300-cc. round-bottom flask equipped with a reflux condenser. The mixture warms up and froths considerably. After the first vigorous reaction has subsided, the material is heated for 2 hours in an oil bath at 140° (thermometer in the oil). The reaction mass, chilled in a freezing

383

mixture, is treated with ice-cold nitrating acid prepared by mixing 20 cc. of fuming nitric acid (1.50) with 10 cc. of concentrated sulfuric acid (1.84). After the evolution of red fumes has stopped, the mixture is heated for 1 hour in the boiling-water bath, cooled, and drowned in 300 cc. of cracked ice and water. The precipitate, collected on a filter, rinsed with water for the removal of acid, and recrystallized from water, yields about 6 grams of β-nitroguanidine, about 25% of the theory.

Saturated solutions of nitroguanidine in sulfuric acid of various concentrations contain the amounts indicated below.

Concentration of Solvent Sulfuric Acid, %	Nitroguanidine (Grams) per 100 cc. at 0°	at 25°
45	5.8	10.9
40	3.4	8.0
35	2.0	5.2
30	1.3	2.9
25	0.75	1.8
20	0.45	1.05
15	0.30	0.55
0	0.12	0.42

Nitroguanidine on reduction is converted first into nitrosoguanidine and then into aminoguanidine (or guanylhydrazine). The latter substance is used in the explosives industry for the preparation of tetracene. In organic chemical research it finds use because of the fact that it reacts readily with aldehydes and ketones to form products which yield crystalline and easily characterized nitrates.

$NO_2-NH-C(NH)-NH_2$ (Nitroguanidine) → $C_6H_5-CHO + H_2N-NH-C(NH)-NH_2$ (Aminoguanidine) → $C_6H_5-CH=N-NH-C(NH)-NH_2$ (Benzalaminoguanidine)

Preparation of Benzalaminoguanidine Nitrate (Benzaldehyde Guanylhydrazone Nitrate). Twenty-six grams of zinc dust and 10.4 grams of nitroguanidine are introduced into a 300-cc. Erlenmeyer flask, 150 cc. of water is added, then 42 cc. of glacial acetic acid at such a rate that the temperature of the mixture does not rise above 40°. The liquid at first turns yellow because of the formation of nitrosoguanidine but

384

becomes colorless again when the reduction is complete. After all the zinc has disappeared, 1 mol of concentrated nitric acid is added, then 1 mol of benzaldehyde, and the mixture is shaken and scratched to facilitate the separation of the heavy granular precipitate of benzalaminoguanidine nitrate. The product, recrystallized from water or from alcohol, melts when pure at 160.5°.

Nitroguanidine and nitrosoguanidine both give a blue color with the diphenylamine reagent, and both give the tests described below, but the difference in the physical properties of the substances is such that there is no likelihood of confusing them.

Tests for Nitroguanidine. To 0.01 gram of nitroguanidine in 4 cc. of cold water 2 drops of saturated ferrous ammonium sulfate solution is added, then 1 cc. of 6 *N* sodium hydroxide solution. The mixture is allowed to stand for 2 minutes, and is filtered. The filtrate shows a fuchsine color but fades to colorless on standing for half an hour. Larger quantities of nitroguanidine give a stronger and more lasting color.

One-tenth gram of nitroguanidine is treated in a test tube with 5 cc. of water and 1 cc. of 50% acetic acid, and the mixture is warmed at 40–50° until everything is dissolved. One gram of zinc dust is added, and the mixture is set aside in a beaker of cold water for 15 minutes. After filtering, 1 cc. of 6% copper sulfate solution is added. The solution becomes intensely blue, and, on boiling, gives off gas, becomes turbid, and presently deposits a precipitate of metallic copper. If, instead of the copper sulfate solution, 1 cc. of a saturated solution of silver acetate[12] is added, and the solution is boiled, then a precipitate of metallic silver is formed.

[12] Two grams of silver acetate, 2 cc. of glacial acetic acid, diluted to 100 cc., warmed, filtered, and allowed to cool.

Many of the reactions of nitroguanidine, particularly its decomposition by heat and the reactions which occur in aqueous and in sulfuric acid solutions, follow directly from its dearrangement. Nitroguanidine dearranges in two modes, as follows.

$$H_2N-C(NH)-NH-NO_2 \rightleftharpoons NH_2-NO_2 + HNCNH \rightleftharpoons NH_2CN \text{ (Cyanamide)}$$

$$H_2N-C(NH)-NH-NO_2 \rightleftharpoons NH_3 + HNCN-NO_2 \rightleftharpoons NC-NH-NO_2 \text{ (Nitrocyanamide)}$$

385

A solution of nitroguanidine in concentrated sulfuric acid comports itself as if the nitroguanidine had dearranged into nitroamide and cyanamide. When it is warmed, nitrous oxide containing a small amount of nitrogen comes off first (from the dehydration of the nitroamide) and carbon dioxide (from the hydrolysis of the cyanamide) comes off later and more slowly. Long-continued heating at an elevated temperature produces ammonia and carbon dioxide quantitatively according to the equation,

$$NH_2-C(NH)-NH-NO_2 + H_2O \longrightarrow N_2O + 2NH_3 + CO_2$$

The production of nitrous oxide is not exactly quantitative because of secondary reactions. A solution of nitroguanidine in concentrated sulfuric acid, after standing for some time, no longer gives a precipitate of nitroguanidine when it is diluted with water.

A freshly prepared solution of nitroguanidine in concentrated sulfuric acid contains no nitric acid, for none can be distilled out of it, but it is ready to produce nitric acid (by the hydration of the nitroamide) if some material is present which will react with it. Thus, it gives up its nitro group quantitatively in the nitrometer, and it is a reagent for the nitration of such substances as aniline, phenol, acet-*p*-toluide, and cinnamic acid which are conveniently nitrated in sulfuric acid solution.

In aqueous solution nitroguanidine dearranges in both of the above-indicated modes, but the tendency toward dearrangement is small unless an acceptor for the product of the dearrangement is present. It results that nitroguanidine is relatively stable in aqueous solution; after many boilings and recrystallizations the same solution finally becomes ammoniacal. Ammonia, being alkaline, tends to promote the decomposition of nitroamide in aqueous solution. Also, because of its mass action effect, it tends to inhibit dearrangement in the second mode which produces ammonia. If nitroguanidine is warmed with aqueous ammonia, the reaction is slow. But, if it is warmed with water and a large excess of ammonium carbonate, nitrous oxide comes off rapidly, the ammonia combines with the cyanamide from the dearrangement, and guanidine carbonate is formed in practically quantitative amount.

Preparation of Guanidine Carbonate from Nitroguanidine. Two hundred and eight grams of nitroguanidine, 300 grams of ammonium carbonate, and 1 liter of water are heated together in a 2-liter flask in the

386

water bath. The flask is equipped with a reflux condenser and with a thermometer dipping into the mixture. When the thermometer indicates 65–70°, nitrous oxide escapes rapidly, and it is necessary to shake the flask occasionally to prevent the undissolved nitroguanidine from being carried up into the neck. The temperature is raised as rapidly as may be done without the reaction becoming too violent. After all the material has gone into solution, the flask is removed from the water bath and the contents boiled under reflux for 2 hours by the application of a free flame. The liquid is then transferred to an evaporating dish and evaporated to dryness on the steam or water bath. During this process all the remaining ammonium carbonate ought to be driven off. The residue is taken up in the smallest possible amount of cold water, filtered for the removal of a small amount of melamine, and the filtrate is stirred up with twice its volume of 95% alcohol which causes the precipitation of guanidine carbonate (while the traces of urea which will have been formed remain in solution along with any ammonium carbonate which may have survived the earlier treatment). The guanidine carbonate is filtered off, rinsed with alcohol, and dried. The filtrate is evaporated to dryness, taken up in water, and precipitated with alcohol for a second crop—total yield about 162 grams or 90% of the theory. The product gives no color with the diphenylamine reagent; it is free from nitrate and of a quality which would be extremely difficult to procure by any process involving the double decomposition of guanidine nitrate.

In the absence of ammonia and in the presence of a primary aliphatic amine, nitroguanidine in aqueous solution dearranges in the second of the above-indicated modes, ammonia is liberated, and the nitrocyanamide combines with the amine to form an alkylnitroguanidine.

$$\underset{\text{Nitrocyanamide}}{HNCN{-}NO_2} + CH_3{-}NH_2 \longrightarrow \underset{\text{Methylnitroguanidine}}{CH_3{-}NH{-}C(NH){-}NH{-}NO_2}$$

The structure of the N-alkyl,N′-nitroguanidine is demonstrated by the fact that it yields the amine and nitrous oxide on hydrolysis, indicating that the alkyl group and the nitro group are attached to different nitrogen atoms.

$$CH_3{-}NH{-}C(NH){-}NH{-}NO_2 + H_2O \longrightarrow CH_3{-}NH_2 + NH_3 + N_2O + CO_2$$

The same N-alkyl,N′-nitroguanidines are produced by the nitration of the alkyl guanidines.

387

Nitroguanidine, warmed with an aqueous solution of hydrazine, yields N-amino,N′-nitroguanidine, white crystals from water, m. p. 182°. This substance explodes on an iron anvil if struck with a heavy sledge hammer allowed to drop through a distance of about 8 inches. It may perhaps have some interest as an explosive.

Flashless colloided powder containing nitroguanidine produces a considerable amount of gray smoke made up of solid materials from the decomposition of the substance. The gases smell of ammonia. The powder produces more smoke than the other flashless powders which are used in this country.

Nitroguanidine decomposes immediately upon melting and cannot be obtained in the form of a liquid, as can urea, dicyandiamide, and other substances which commence to decompose when heated a few degrees above their melting points. A small quantity heated in a test tube yields ammonia, water vapor, a white sublimate in the upper part of the tube, and a yellow residue of mellon which is but little affected if warmed to a bright red heat. The products which are formed are precisely those which would be predicted from the dearrangements, namely, water and nitrous oxide (from nitroamide), cyanamide, melamine (from the polymerization of cyanamide), ammonia, nitrous oxide again and cyanic acid (from nitrocyanamide), cyanuric acid (from the polymerization of cyanic acid), ammeline and ammelide (from the co-polymerization of cyanic acid and cyanamide) and, from the interaction and decomposition of these substances, carbon dioxide, urea, melam, melem, mellon, nitrogen, prussic acid, cyanogen, and paracyanogen. All these substances have been detected in, or isolated from, the products of the decomposition of nitroguanidine by heat.

There is no doubt whatever that nitroguanidine is a cool explosive, but there appears to be a disagreement as to the temperature which it produces. A package of nitroguanidine, exploded at night by means of a blasting cap, produces no visible flash. If 10 or 15% of the substance is incorporated in nitrocellulose powder, it makes the powder flashless. Vieille found that the gases from the explosion of nitroguanidine were much less erosive

388

than those from other explosives of comparable force, and considered the fact to be in harmony with his general conclusion that the hotter explosives are the more erosive. In his experiments the explosions were made to take place in a steel bomb equipped with a crusher gauge and with a removable, perforated, steel plug through the perforation in which the hot gases from the explosion were allowed to escape. They swept away, or eroded off, a certain amount of the metal. The plug was weighed before and after the experiment, its density had been determined, and the number of cubic millimeters of metal lost was reported as a measure of the erosion. Some of Vieille's results are indicated in the following table.

Explosive	Charge (Grams)	Pressure (Kg./sq. cm.)	Erosion	Erosion per Gram		Force
Poudre BF	3.45	2403	20.3	5.88		
	3.50	2361	22.7	6.58		
	3.55	2224	24.7	6.96	6.4	9,600
	3.55	2253	25.5	7.19		
	3.55	2143	20.1	5.66		
Cordite	3.55	2500	64.2		18.1	10,000
Ballistite VF	3.47	2509	84.5	24.3		
	3.51	2370	83.2	23.7		
	3.55	2542	90.2	25.4	24.3	10,000
	3.55	2360	85.9	24.2		
	3.55	2416	84.5	23.8		
Black military	10.00	2167	22.3		2.2	3,000
Black sporting	8.88	1958	40.0		4.5	3,000
Blasting gelatin	3.35	2458	105.0		31.4	10,000
Nitromannite	3.54	2361	83.5		23.6	10,000
Nitroguanidine	3.90	2019	8.8		2.3	9,000

These experiments [18] were carried out in a bomb of 17.8 cc. capacity, which corresponds, for the example cited, to a density of loading of 0.219 for the nitroguanidine which was pulverulent

[18] The cordite used in these experiments was made from 57% nitroglycerin, 5% vaseline, and 38% high nitration guncotton colloided with acetone; the ballistite VF of equal amounts by weight of nitroglycerin and high nitration guncotton colloided with ethyl acetate. The black military powder was made from saltpeter 75, sulfur 10, and charcoal 15; the black sporting powder from saltpeter 78, sulfur 10, and charcoal 12. The blasting gelatin contained 94% nitroglycerin and 6% soluble nitrocotton.

389

material "firmly agglomerated in a manner to facilitate the naturally slow combustion of that substance."

An experiment with 18.11 grams nitroguanidine in a bomb of 75.0 cc. capacity (density of loading 0.241) showed an erosion of 2.29 per gram of explosive.

The temperature (907°) which Vieille accepted as the temperature produced by the explosion of nitroguanidine had been determined earlier by Patart who published in 1904 an account of manometric bomb experiments with guanidine nitrate and with nitroguanidine. The explosives were agglomerated under a pressure of 3600 kilograms per square centimeter, broken up into grains 2 or 3 mm. in diameter, and fired in a bomb of 22 cc. capacity. Some of Patart's experimental results are tabulated below. Calculated from these data, Patart reported for guanidine

Density of Loading	Pressure, Kilograms per Square Centimeter: Guanidine Nitrate		Nitroguanidine	
0.15	1128	1083	1304	1435
	1038		1584	
	...		1416	
0.20	1556	1486	2060	2091
	1416		2122	
0.25	2168	2098	3092	3080
	2028		3068	
0.30	3068	2941	4118	4078
	2814		4038	
0.35	3668	3699	...	
	3730		...	

nitrate, covolume 1.28, force 5834, and temperature of explosion 929°; for nitroguanidine, covolume 1.60, force 7140, and temperature of explosion 907°. He appears to have felt that these calculated temperatures of explosion were low, for he terminated his article by calling attention to the extraordinary values of the covolume deduced from the pressures in the closed vessel, and subpended a footnote:

> It may be questioned whether the rapid increase of the pressure with the density of loading, rather than being the consequence of a constant reaction giving place to a considerable covolume, is not due simply to the mode of de-
>
> 390
>
> composition being variable with the density of loading and involving a more and more complete decomposition of the explosive. Only an analysis of the gases produced by the reaction can determine this point, as it also can determine the actual temperature of the deflagration.

The later studies of Muraour and Aunis have shown that the temperature of explosion of nitroguanidine may be much higher than Patart calculated, and have given probability to his hypothesis that the density of loading has an effect upon the mode of the explosive decomposition. These investigators found that a platinum wire 0.20 mm. in diameter, introduced into the bomb along with the nitroguanidine, was melted by the heat of the explosion—a result which indicates a temperature of at least 1773°C. They pointed out that nitroguanidine, if compressed too strongly, may take fire with difficulty and may undergo an incomplete decomposition, and hence at low densities of loading may produce unduly low pressures corresponding to a covolume which is too large and to a temperature of explosion which is too low. The pressure of 3600 kilograms per square centimeter, under which Patart compressed his nitroguanidine, is much too high. Nitroguanidine compressed under 650 kilograms per square centimeter, and fired in a manometric bomb of 22 cc. capacity, at a density of loading of 0.2, and with a primer of 1 gram of black powder, gave a pressure of 1737 kilograms per square centimeter; compressed under 100 kilograms per square centimeter and fired in the same way nitroguanidine gave a pressure of 1975 kilograms per square centimeter, or a difference of 238 kilograms. In an experiment with a bomb of 139 cc. capacity, density of loading 0.2, Muraour and Aunis observed a pressure which, correction being made for various heat losses, corresponded to a temperature of 1990°.

Assuming that nitroguanidine explodes to produce carbon dioxide, water, carbon monoxide, hydrogen, and nitrogen,[21] assuming that the equilibrium constant for the reaction, $CO + H_2O \rightleftharpoons CO_2 + H_2$, is 6, and that the molecular heat of formation at con-

[21] This assumption however is not true, for powder which contains nitroguanidine produces a gray smoke consisting of solid decomposition products and yields gases which smell of ammonia.

391

stant volume of nitroguanidine is 17.9 Calories, and taking the values of Nernst and Wohl for the specific heats of the various gases, Muraour and Aunis calculated the following values for the explosion of nitroguanidine, temperature 2098°, covolume 1.077, force 9660, and pressure (at density of loading 0.20) 2463 kilograms per square centimeter. They have also calculated the temperature of explosion of ammonium nitrate 1125°, of "explosive NO" (ammonium nitrate 78.7, trinitrotoluene 21.3) 2970°, and of explosive N4 (ammonium nitrate 90, potassium nitrate 5, trinitronaphthalene 5) 1725°, and have found by experiment that the last named of these explosives, fired at a density of loading of 0.30, did not fuse a platinum wire (0.06-mm. diameter) which had been introduced along with it into the bomb.

Nitroguanidine detonates completely under the influence of a detonator containing 1.5 gram of fulminate. According to Patart 40 grams exploded on a lead block 67 mm. in diameter produced a shortening of 7 mm. Picric acid under the same conditions produced a shortening of 10.5 mm., and Favier explosive (12% dinitronaphthalene, 88% ammonium nitrate) one of 8 mm. Muraour and Aunis experimented with nitroguanidine compressed under 100 kilograms per square centimeter and with trinitrotoluene compressed under 1000 kilograms per square centimeter, in a manometric bomb of 22-cc. capacity and at densities of loading of 0.13, 0.20, 0.25, and 0.30, and reported that the two explosives gave the same pressures.

During the first World War the Germans used in trench mortar bombs an explosive consisting of nitroguanidine 50%, ammonium nitrate, 30%, and paraffin 20%.

Nitrosoguanidine

Nitrosoguanidine is a cool and flashless primary explosive, very much more gentle in its behavior than mercury fulminate and lead azide. It is a pale yellow crystalline powder which explodes on contact with concentrated sulfuric acid or on being heated in a melting point tube at 165°. It explodes from the blow of a car-

392

penter's hammer on a concrete block. Its sensitivity to shock, to friction, and to temperature, and the fact that it decomposes slowly in contact with water at ordinary temperatures, militate against its use as a practical explosive. It may be kept indefinitely in a stoppered bottle if it is dry.

The reactions of nitrosoguanidine in aqueous solution are similar to those of nitroguanidine except that nitrogen and nitrous acid respectively are formed under conditions which correspond to the formation of nitrous oxide and nitric acid from nitroguanidine. It dearranges principally as follows.

$$NH_2—C(NH)—NH—NO \rightleftharpoons NH_2—NO + HNCNH \rightleftharpoons NH_2—CN$$

If it is warmed in aqueous solution, the nitrosoamide breaks down into water and nitrogen, and the cyanamide polymerizes to dicyandiamide. The evaporation of the solution yields crystals of the latter substance. A cold aqueous solution of nitrosoguanidine acidified with hydrochloric acid yields nitrous acid, and may be used for the introduction of a nitroso group into dimethylaniline or some similar substance which is soluble in the acidified aqueous liquid.

Preparation of Nitrosoguanidine. Twenty-one grams of nitroguanidine, 11 grams of ammonium chloride, 18 grams of zinc dust, and 250 cc. of water in an 800-cc. beaker are stirred together mechanically while external cooling is applied to prevent the temperature from rising above 20–25°. After 2 hours or so the gray color of the zinc disappears, the mixture is yellow, and on settling shows no crystals of nitroguanidine. The mixture is then cooled to 0° or below by surrounding the beaker with a mixture of cracked ice and salt; it is filtered, and the filtrate is discarded. The yellow residue, consisting of nitrosoguanidine mixed with zinc oxide or hydroxide and basic zinc chloride, is extracted with 4 successive portions of 250 cc. each of water at 65°. The combined extracts, allowed to stand over night at 0°, deposit nitrosoguanidine which is collected, rinsed with water, and dried at 40°. Yield 8.0–9.2 grams, 45–52% of the theory.

The flashlessness of nitrosoguanidine may be demonstrated safely by igniting about 0.5 gram of it on the back of the hand. The experiment is most striking if carried out in a darkened room. The sample being poured out in a conical heap on the back of the left hand, a match held in the right hand is scratched and allowed to burn until the mate-

393

rial which composes the burnt head of the match has become thoroughly heated, it is extinguished by shaking, and the burnt head is then touched to the heap of nitrosoguanidine. The nitrosoguanidine explodes with a zishing sound and with a cloud of gray smoke, but with no visible flash whatsoever. The place on the hand where the nitrosoguanidine was fired will perhaps itch slightly, and the next day will perhaps show a slight rash and peeling of the skin. There is no sensation of being burned, and the explosion is so rapid that the hand remains steady and makes no reflex movement.

Ethylenedinitramine

Ethylenedinitramine, m.p. 174–176° with decomposition, is produced when dinitroethyleneurea is refluxed with water, or it

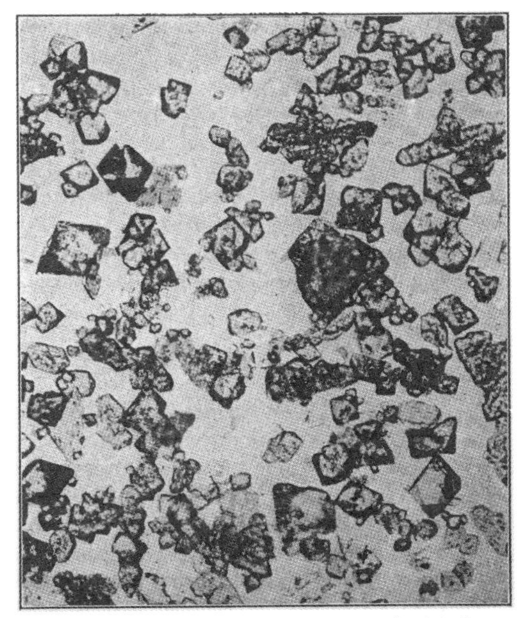

FIGURE 90. Ethylenedinitramine Crystals (60×).

may be prepared directly, without isolating this intermediate, by the nitration of ethyleneurea with mixed acid.

394

$$\begin{array}{c}CH_2-NH \\ | \\ CH_2-NH\end{array}\!\!>CO \;\text{(Ethyleneurea)} \longrightarrow \begin{array}{c}CH_2-N(NO_2) \\ | \\ CH_2-N(NO_2)\end{array}\!\!>CO \;\text{(Dinitroethyleneurea)} \longrightarrow \begin{array}{c}CH_2-NH-NO_2 \\ | \\ CH_2-NH-NO_2\end{array} \;\text{(Ethylenedinitramine)}$$

It is a dibasic acid and forms neutral salts, the silver salt a pulverulent precipitate, the potassium salt needles from alcohol. It is sparingly soluble in water, about 1 part in 200 at 25°, and is not affected by refluxing with this solvent. On refluxing with dilute sulfuric acid it gives nitrous oxide, acetaldehyde, and glycol. Hale has reported that it explodes spontaneously when heated to 180°, in which respect it resembles mercury fulminate and nitroglycerin, but that it corresponds in resistance to shock more nearly to the relatively insensitive high explosives, like TNT and picric acid, which are used as the bursting charges of shells. He found that it is exploded by a 10-inch drop of a 2-kilogram weight, the same as picric acid, and reported that it withstands the standard 120° stability test as well as tetryl.

Dinitrodimethyloxamide

This substance was prepared by Franchimont by dissolving dimethyloxamide in very strong nitric acid (specific gravity 1.523) without cooling, allowing to stand, and pouring into water, and by Thiele and Meyer by dissolving dimethyloxamide in crude nitric acid, adding fuming sulfuric acid to the chilled solution, and pouring onto ice. Dimethyloxamide is prepared readily by the interaction of methylamine with an ester of oxalic acid.

$$\begin{array}{c}COOR \\ | \\ COOR\end{array} + 2NH_2-CH_3 \longrightarrow \begin{array}{c}CO-NH-CH_3 \\ | \\ CO-NH-CH_3\end{array} \;\text{(Dimethyloxamide)} \longrightarrow \begin{array}{c}CO-N(NO_2)-CH_3 \\ | \\ CO-N(NO_2)-CH_3\end{array} \;\text{(Dinitrodimethyloxamide)}$$

Dinitrodimethyloxamide is very slightly soluble in water, sparingly in ether and chloroform, and soluble in alcohol from which it crystallizes in needles which melt at 124° and decompose at a higher temperature. By reduction with zinc and acetic acid in alcohol solution it yields dimethyloxamide. It is not destroyed by refluxing with concentrated hydrochloric acid. Concentrated sulfuric acid splits off nitric acid, and the substance accordingly

395

gives up its nitro group in the nitrometer. On treatment with an excess of aqueous ammonia or on refluxing with a slight excess of barium hydroxide solution, it yields the corresponding salt of methylnitramine. Haid, Becker, and Dittmar have reported that dinitrodimethyloxamide, like PETN, tetryl, TNT, and picric acid, gives no red fumes after 30 days at 100° while nitrocellulose in their experiments gave red fumes after 36 hours and dipentaerythrite hexanitrate after 8 days.

Dinitrodimethyloxamide has interesting explosive properties, but it is limited in its use because it develops an acidity when wet with water. It has been reported that 30 parts of dinitrodimethyloxamide and 70 parts of PETN yield a eutectic which melts at 100° and can be poured as a homogeneous liquid. The cast explosive has a velocity of detonation of 8500 meters per second which is equal to that of PETN under the best conditions. The further addition of dimethyl oxalate or of camphor lowers the melting point still more and affects the brisance only slightly but has a significant phlegmatizing action. A mixture of PETN 60%, dinitrodimethyloxamide 30%, and dimethyl oxalate 10% melts at 82°, and has, when cast, a velocity of detonation of 7900 meters per second which is higher than the velocity of detonation of cast picric acid.

Dinitrodimethylsulfamide

This substance was first prepared by Franchimont by dissolving 1 part of dimethylsulfamide in 10 parts of the strongest nitric acid, and drowning in water. Dimethylsulfamide is prepared by the interaction of methylamine and sulfuryl chloride in chilled absolute ether solution.

$$O_2S(Cl)_2 + 2NH_2{-}CH_3 \longrightarrow O_2S(NH{-}CH_3)_2 \longrightarrow O_2S(N(NO_2){-}CH_3)_2$$

Dimethylsulfamide   Dinitrodimethylsulfamide

Dinitrodimethylsulfamide is very slightly soluble in water, very readily in hot alcohol, and moderately in chloroform and benzene. Crystals from benzene, m.p. 90°. The vapor of the substance [396] explodes if heated to about 160°. Dinitrodimethylsulfamide has been suggested as an addition to PETN for the preparation of a fusible explosive which can be loaded by pouring.

Cyclotrimethylenetrinitramine (Cyclonite, Hexogen, T4).

The name of *cyclonite,* given to this explosive by Clarence J. Bain because of its cyclic structure and cyclonic nature, is the one by which it is generally known in the United States. The Germans call it *Hexogen,* the Italians *T4.*

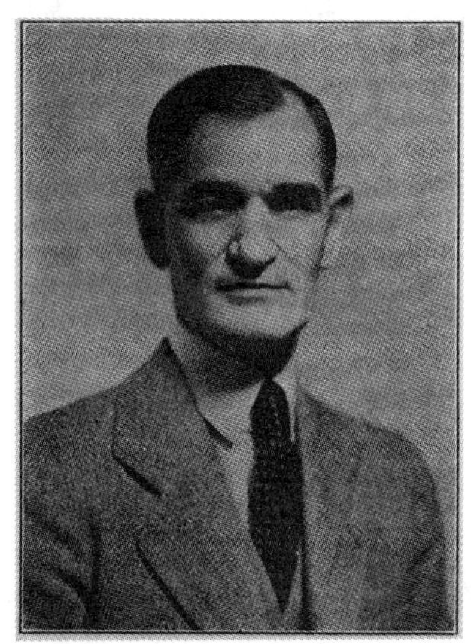

FIGURE 91. George C. Hale. Has studied cyclonite, ethylenedinitramine, and many other explosives. Author of numerous inventions and publications in the field of military powder and explosives. Chief Chemist, Picatinny Arsenal, 1921-1929; Chief of the Chemical Department, Picatinny Arsenal, 1929—.

Cyclonite, prepared by the nitration of hexamethylenetetramine, is derived ultimately from no other raw materials than coke, air, and water. It has about the same power and brisance as PETN, and a velocity of detonation under the most favorable conditions of about 8500 meters per second.

Hexamethylenetetramine, $C_6H_{12}N_4$, is obtained in the form of colorless, odorless, and practically tasteless crystals by the evapo- [397] ration of an aqueous solution of formaldehyde and ammonia. It is used in medicine under the names of *Methenamine, Hexamine, Cystamine, Cystogen,* and *Urotropine,* administered orally as an antiseptic for the urinary tract, and in industry in the manufacture of plastics and as an accelerator for the vulcanization of rubber. It has feebly basic properties and forms a nitrate, $C_6H_{12}N_4 \cdot 2HNO_3$, m.p. 165°, soluble in water, insoluble in alcohol, ether, chloroform, and acetone. The product, $C_3H_6O_6N_6$, prepared by nitrating this nitrate and patented by Henning for possible use in medicine, was actually cyclonite. Herz later patented the same substance as an explosive compound, cyclotrimethylenetrinitramine, which he found could be prepared by treating hexamethylenetetramine directly with strong nitric acid. In his process the tetramine was added slowly in small portions at a time to nitric acid (1.52) at a temperature of 20–30°. When all was in solution, the liquid was warmed to 55°, allowed to stand for a few minutes, cooled to 20°, and the product precipitated by the addition of water. The nitration has been studied further by Hale who secured his best yield, 68%, in an experiment in which 50 grams of hexamethylenetetramine was added during 15 minutes to 550 grams of 100% nitric acid while the temperature was not allowed to rise above 30°. The mixture was then cooled to 0°, held there for 20 minutes, and drowned.

$$C_6H_{12}N_4 + 3HNO_3 \longrightarrow (CH_2)_3(N{-}NO_2)_3 + 3CH_2O + NH_3$$

Hexamethylenetetramine   Cyclotrimethylenetrinitramine

The formaldehyde which is liberated by the reaction tends to be oxidized by the nitric acid if the mixture is allowed to stand or is warmed. It remains in the spent acid after drowning and interferes with the recovery of nitric acid from it.

[398] Cyclonite is a white crystalline solid, m.p. 202°. It is insoluble in water, alcohol, ether, ethyl acetate, petroleum ether, and carbon tetrachloride, very slightly soluble in hot benzene, and soluble 1 part in about 135 parts of boiling xylene. It is readily soluble in hot aniline, phenol, ethyl benzoate, and nitrobenzene, from all of which it crystallizes in needles. It is moderately soluble in hot acetone, about 1 part in 8, and is conveniently recrystallized from this solvent from which it is deposited in beautiful, transparent, sparkling prisms. It dissolves very slowly in cold concentrated sulfuric acid, and the solution decomposes on standing. It dissolves readily in warm nitric acid (1.42 or stronger) and separates only partially again when the liquid is cooled. The chemical reactions of cyclonite indicate that the cyclotrimethylenetrinitramine formula which Herz suggested for it is probably correct.

Cyclonite is hydrolyzed slowly when the finely powdered material is boiled with dilute sulfuric acid or with dilute caustic soda solution.

$$C_3H_6O_6N_6 + 6H_2O \longrightarrow 3NH_3 + 3CH_2O + 3HNO_3$$

Quantitative experiments have shown that half of its nitrogen appears as ammonia. If the hydrolysis is carried out in dilute sulfuric acid solution, the formaldehyde is oxidized by the nitric acid and nitrous acid is formed.

If cyclonite is dissolved in phenol at 100° and reduced by means of sodium, it yields methylamine, nitrous acid, and prussic acid. Finely powdered cyclonite, suspended in 80% alcohol and treated with sodium amalgam, yields methylamine, ammonia, nitrous acid, and formaldehyde, a result which probably indicates that both hydrolysis and reduction occur under these conditions.

When a large crystal of cyclonite is added to the diphenylamine reagent, a blue color appears slowly on the surface of the crystal. Powdered cyclonite gives within a few seconds a blue color which rapidly becomes more intense. If cinnamic acid is dissolved in concentrated sulfuric acid, and if finely powdered cyclonite is added while the mixture is stirred, gas comes off at a moderate rate, and the mixture, after standing over night and drowning, gives a precipitate which contains a certain amount of *p*-nitrocinnamic acid.

In the drop test cyclonite is exploded by a 9-inch drop of a 2-kilogram weight. For the detonation of 0.4 gram, the explosive
399
requires 0.17 gram of mercury fulminate. It fails to detonate when struck with a fiber shoe, and detonates when struck with a steel shoe, in the standard frictional impact test of the U. S. Bureau of Mines. In 5 seconds it fumes off at 290°, but at higher temperatures, even as high as 360°, it does not detonate.
400

CHAPTER IX

PRIMARY EXPLOSIVES, DETONATORS, AND PRIMERS

Primary explosives explode from shock, from friction, and from heat. They are used in primers where it is desired by means of shock or friction to produce fire for the ignition of powder, and they are used in detonators where it is desired to produce shock for the initiation of the explosion of high explosives. They are also used in toy caps, toy torpedoes, and similar devices for the making of noise. Indeed, certain primary explosives were used for this latter purpose long before the history of modern high explosives had yet commenced.

Discovery of Fulminating Compounds

Fulminating gold, silver, and platinum (Latin, *fulmen*, lightning flash, thunderbolt) are formed by precipitating solutions of these metals with ammonia. They are perhaps nitrides or hydrated nitrides, or perhaps they contain hydrogen as well as nitrogen and water of composition, but they contain no carbon and must not be confused with the fulminates which are salts of fulminic acid, HONC. They are dangerously sensitive, and are not suited to practical use.

Fulminating gold is described in the writings of the pseudonymous Basil Valentine,[1] probably written by Johann Thölde (or Thölden) of Hesse and actually published by him during the years 1602–1604. The author called it *Goldkalck*, and prepared it by dissolving gold in an *aqua regia* made by dissolving sal ammoniac in nitric acid, and then precipitating by the addition of potassium carbonate solution. The powder was washed by decantation 8 to 12 times, drained from water, and dried in the air where no sunlight fell on it, "and not by any means over the
401
fire, for, as soon as this powder takes up a very little heat or warmth, it kindles forthwith, and does remarkably great damage, when it explodes with such vehemence and might that no man would be able to restrain it." The author also reported that warm distilled vinegar converted the powder into a material which was no longer explosive. The name of *aurum fulminans* was given to the explosive by Beguinus who described its preparation in his *Tyrocinium Chymicum*, printed in 1608.

Fulminating gold precipitates when a solution of pure gold chloride is treated with ammonia water. The method of preparation described by Basil Valentine succeeds because the sal ammoniac used for the preparation of the *aqua regia* supplies the necessary ammonia. If gold is dissolved in an *aqua regia* prepared from nitric acid and common salt, and if the solution is then treated with potassium carbonate, the resulting precipitate has no explosive properties. Fulminating gold loses its explosive properties rapidly if it is allowed to stand in contact with sulfur.

Fulminating gold was early used both for war and for entertainment. The Dutch inventor and chemist, Cornelis Drebbel, being in the service of the British Navy, devoted considerable time to the preparation of fulminating gold and used his material as a detonator in petards and torpedoes in the English expedition against La Rochelle in 1628. Pepys, in his diary for November 11, 1663, reports a conversation with a Dr. Allen concerning *aurum fulminans* "of which a grain . . . put in a silver spoon and fired, will give a blow like a musquett and strike a hole through the silver spoon downward, without the least force upward."

Fulminating silver was prepared in 1788 by Berthollet who precipitated a solution of nitrate of silver by means of lime water, dried the precipitated silver oxide, treated it with strong ammonia water which converted it into a black powder, decanted the liquid, and left the powder to dry in the open air. Fulminating silver is more sensitive to shock and friction than fulminating gold. It explodes when touched; it must not be enclosed in a bottle or transferred from place to place, but must be left in the vessel, or better upon the paper, where it was allowed to dry.

The black material which deposits in a reagent bottle of ammoniacal silver nitrate, and sometimes collects on the rim and
402
around the stopper, contains fulminating silver. Explosions are reported to have been caused by the careless turning of the glass stopper of a bottle containing this reagent. After a test (for aldehyde, for example) has been made with ammoniacal silver nitrate solution, the liquid ought promptly to be washed down the sink, and all insoluble matter left in the vessel ought to be dissolved out with dilute nitric acid.

Fulminating platinum was first prepared by E. Davy, about 1825, by adding ammonia water to a solution of platinum sulfate, boiling the precipitate with a solution of potash, washing, and allowing to dry. It was exploded by heat, but not easily by percussion or friction.

Fourcroy prepared a *fulminating mercury* by digesting red oxide of mercury in ammonia water for 8 or 10 days. The material became white and finally assumed the form of crystalline scales. The dried product exploded loudly from fire, but underwent a spontaneous decomposition when left to itself. At slightly elevated temperatures it gave off ammonia and left a residue of mercury oxide.

In the *Journal de physique* for 1779 the apothecary, Bayen, described a fulminating mercurial preparation of another kind. Thirty parts of precipitated, yellow oxide of mercury, washed and dried, was mixed with 4 or 5 parts of sulfur; the mixture exploded with violence when struck with a heavy hammer or when heated on an iron plate. Other mixtures which react explosively when initiated by percussion have been studied more recently, metallic sodium or potassium in contact with the oxide or the chloride of silver or of mercury or in contact with chloroform or carbon tetrachloride.

The explosion of chloroform in contact with an alkali metal may be demonstrated by means of the apparatus illustrated in Figure 92. About 0.3 gram of sodium or of potassium or of the liquid alloy of the two is introduced into a thin-wall glass tube, or, better yet, is sealed up in a small glass bulb, 6 to 8 mm. in diameter, which has a capillary 15 to 20 mm. in length. The tube or bulb containing the alkali metal is placed in the bottom of a narrow test tube into which 1 or 2 cc. of chloroform has already been introduced, and the apparatus is then

403

ready for the experiment. Or, if it is desired to prepare in advance an explosive capsule which can safely be kept as long as desired, then the bulb is held in place at the bottom of the test tube by a collar of glass (a section of glass tubing) sintered to the inner wall of the test tube, and the top of the test tube is drawn down and sealed. When the prepared test tube or capsule is dropped onto a concrete pavement from

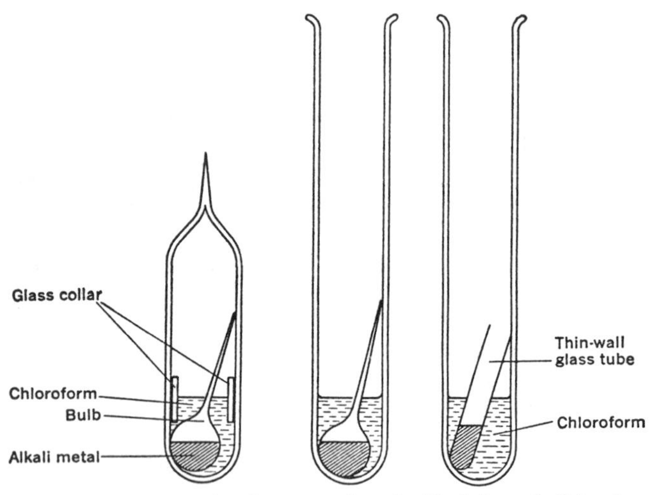

FIGURE 92. Apparatus for Demonstrating the Explosion of Chloroform with an Alkali Metal.

a height of 6 feet, a loud explosion is produced accompanied by a bright flash which is visible even in the direct sunlight. The chemical reaction is as follows, each one of the three chlorine atoms of the chloroform reacting in a different manner.

$$6CHCl_3 + 6Na \longrightarrow 6NaCl + 6HCl + C_6Cl_6$$

Mercury fulminate appears to have been prepared for the first time by Johann Kunckel von Löwenstern (1630–1703), the same chemist who discovered phosphorus and applied the purple of

404

Cassius practically to the manufacture of ruby glass. In his posthumous *Laboratorium Chymicum* he says:

> Further evidence that mercury is cold is to be seen when you dissolve it in *aqua fortis* (nitric acid), evaporate the solution to dryness, pour highly rectified *spiritum vini* (alcohol) over the residue, and then warm it slightly so that it begins to dissolve. It commences to boil with amazing vigor. If the glass is somewhat stopped up, it bursts into a thousand pieces, and, in consequence, it must by no means be stopped up. I once dissolved silver and mercury together in *aqua fortis* and poured over it an excess of *spiritum vini*, and set the mixture to putrify *in fimum equinum* (horse manure) after having stopped up the glass with mere sealing wax only. When it happened a few days later that the manure became a little warm, it made such a thunder-crack, with the shattering of the glass, that the stable-servant imagined, since I had put it in a box, either that someone had shot at him through the window or that the Devil himself was active in the stable. As soon as I heard this news, I was able easily to see that the blame was mine, that it must have been my glass. Now this was with silver and mercury, 2 *loth* of each. Mercury does the same thing[4] alone, but silver not at all.

[4] Kunckel's meaning in the last sentence is evidently that mercury nitrate reacts with alcohol on warming, and that silver nitrate does not react with alcohol under the same conditions.

The preparation and properties of mercury fulminate were described in much detail by Edward Howard in 1800 in a paper presented to the Royal Society of London. The method of preparation which he found to be most satisfactory was as follows: 100 grains of mercury was dissolved by heating in 1½ drams of nitric acid (specific gravity 1.3), the solution was cooled and added to 2 ounces of alcohol (specific gravity 0.849) in a glass vessel, the mixture was warmed until effervescence commenced, the reaction was allowed to proceed to completion, and the precipitate which formed was collected on a filter, washed with distilled water, and dried at a temperature not exceeding that of the water bath. Howard found that the fulminate was exploded by means of an electric spark or by concentrated sulfuric acid brought into contact with it. When a few grains were placed on a

405

cold anvil and struck with a cold hammer, a very stunning disagreeable noise was produced and the faces of the hammer and anvil were indented. A few grains floated in a tinfoil capsule on hot oil exploded at 368°F. (186.7°C.). When a mixture of fine- and coarse-grain black powder was placed on top of a quantity of fulminate and the fulminate was fired, the black powder was blown about but it was not ignited and was recovered unchanged. Howard also attempted by means of alcohol to produce fulminating compounds from gold, platinum, antimony, tin, copper, iron, lead, nickel, bismuth, cobalt, arsenic, and manganese, but silver was the only one of these metals with which he had any success.

Brugnatelli in 1802 worked out a satisfactory method for the preparation of silver fulminate by pouring onto 100 grains of powdered silver nitrate first an ounce of alcohol and then an ounce of nitric acid. After the fulminate had precipitated, the mixture was diluted with water to prevent it from dissolving again and immediately filtered. Silver fulminate explodes more easily from heat and from friction than mercury fulminate and is more spectacular in its behavior. It quickly became an object of amateur interest and public wonderment, one of the standard exhibits of street fakirs and of mountebanks at fairs. Liebig, who was born in 1803, saw a demonstration of silver fulminate in the market place at Darmstadt when he was a boy. He watched the process closely, recognized by its odor the alcohol which was used, went home, and succeeded in preparing the substance for himself. He retained his interest in it, and in 1823 carried out studies on the fulminates in the laboratory of Gay-Lussac at Paris.

Mercury Fulminate

The commercial preparation of mercury fulminate is carried out by a process which is essentially the same as that which Howard originally recommended. Five hundred or 600 grams of mercury is used for each batch, the operation is practically on the laboratory scale, and several batches are run at the same time. Since the reaction produces considerable frothing, capacious glass balloons are used. The fumes, which are poisonous and inflammable, are passed through condensers, and the condensate, which contains alcohol, acetaldehyde, ethyl nitrate, and ethyl nitrite, is utilized by mixing it with the alcohol for the next batch.

406

Pure fulminate is white, but the commercial material is often grayish in color. The color is improved if a small amount of cupric chloride is added to the nitric acid solution of mercury before it is poured into the alcohol in the balloon, but the resulting white fulminate is actually less pure than the unbleached material.

Preparation of Mercury Fulminate. Five grams of mercury is added to 35 cc. of nitric acid (specific gravity 1.42) in a 100-cc. Erlenmeyer

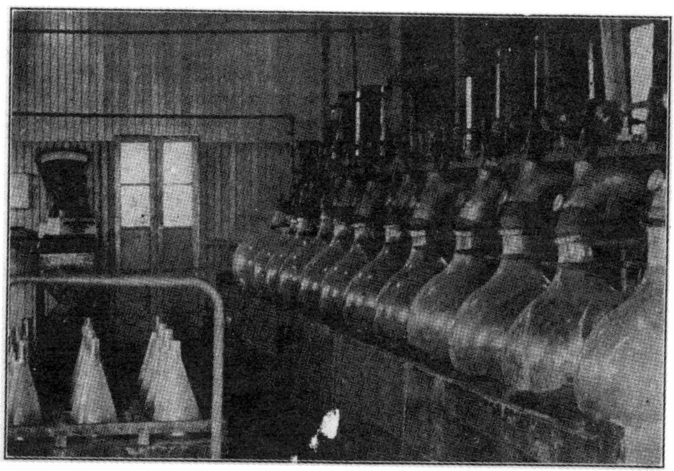

FIGURE 93. Fulminate Manufacture. (Courtesy Atlas Powder Company.) At left, flasks in which mercury is dissolved in nitric acid. At right, balloons in which the reaction with alcohol occurs.

flask, and the mixture is allowed to stand without shaking until the mercury has gone into solution. The acid liquid is then poured into 50 cc. of 90% alcohol in a 500-cc. beaker in the hood. The temperature of the mixture rises, a vigorous reaction commences, white fumes come off, and crystals of fulminate soon begin to precipitate. Red fumes appear and the precipitation of the fulminate becomes more rapid, then white fumes again as the reaction moderates. After about 20 minutes the reaction is over; water is added, and the crystals are washed with water repeatedly by decantation until the washings are no longer acid to litmus. The product consists of grayish-yellow crystals, and corresponds to a good grade of commercial fulminate. It may be obtained white and entirely pure by dissolving in strong ammonia

407

water, filtering, and reprecipitating by the addition of 30% acetic acid. The pure fulminate is filtered off, washed several times with cold water, and stored under water, or, if a very small amount is desired for experimental purposes, it is dried in a desiccator.

The chemical reactions in the preparation appear to be as follows. (1) The alcohol is oxidized to acetaldehyde, and (2) the nitrous acid which is formed attacks the acetaldehyde to form a nitroso derivative which goes over to the more stable, tautomeric, isonitroso form.

$$CH_3{-}CH_2{-}OH \rightarrow CH_3{-}CHO \longrightarrow \underset{\text{Nitrosoacetaldehyde}}{\begin{matrix} CH_2{-}CHO \\ | \\ NO \end{matrix}} \rightleftharpoons \underset{\text{Isonitrosoacetaldehyde}}{\begin{matrix} CH{-}CHO \\ \| \\ N{-}OH \end{matrix}}$$

(3) The isonitrosoacetaldehyde is oxidized to isonitrosoacetic acid, and (4) this is nitrated by the nitrogen dioxide which is present to form nitroisonitrosoacetic acid.

$$\begin{matrix} CH{-}CHO \\ \| \\ N{-}OH \end{matrix} \longrightarrow \underset{\text{Isonitrosoacetic acid}}{\begin{matrix} CH{-}COOH \\ \| \\ N{-}OH \end{matrix}} \longrightarrow \underset{\text{Nitroisonitrosoacetic acid}}{\begin{matrix} NO_2 \\ | \\ C{-}COOH \\ \| \\ N{-}OH \end{matrix}}$$

(5) The nitroisonitrosoacetic acid loses carbon dioxide to form formonitrolic acid which (6) decomposes further into nitrous acid and fulminic acid, and (7) the fulminic acid reacts with the mercury nitrate to form the sparingly soluble mercury fulminate which precipitates.

$$\begin{matrix} NO_2 \\ | \\ C{-}\boxed{COO}H \\ \| \\ N{-}OH \end{matrix} \longrightarrow \underset{\text{Formonitrolic acid}}{\begin{matrix} \boxed{NO_2} \\ | \\ C\boxed{H} \\ \| \\ N{-}OH \end{matrix}} \longrightarrow HONC \longrightarrow \underset{\text{Mercury fulminate}}{Hg(ONC)_2}$$

Fulminate can be prepared from acetaldehyde instead of from alcohol, and from substances which are convertible into acetaldehyde, such as paraldehyde, metaldehyde, dimethyl- and diethylacetal. Methyl alcohol, formaldehyde, propyl alcohol, butyraldehyde, glycol, and glyoxal do not yield fulminate.

Fulminate can, however, be prepared from a compound which contains only one carbon atom. The sodium salt of nitromethane gives with an aqueous solution of mercuric chloride at 0° a white

408

precipitate of the mercuric salt of nitromethane which gradually becomes yellow and which, digested with warm dilute hydrochloric acid, yields mercury fulminate.

$$CH_2{=}N{\overset{\nearrow O}{\searrow ONa}} \longrightarrow C\boxed{H_2{=}N}{\overset{\nearrow O}{\searrow OHgO}}{\overset{\swarrow}{}}N{=}C\boxed{H_2} \longrightarrow Hg{\overset{\nearrow ONC}{\searrow ONC}}$$

Sodium fulminate, soluble in water, has a molecular weight which corresponds to the simple monomolecular formula, NaONC. These facts, taken together with the fact that mercury fulminate warmed with concentrated aqueous hydrochloric acid yields hydroxylamine and formic acid, prove that fulminic acid is the oxime of carbon monoxide.

$$HO{-}N{=}C\langle \; + 2H_2O \longrightarrow HO{-}NH_2 + H{-}COOH$$

Mercury fulminate dissolves readily in an aqueous solution of potassium cyanide to form a complex compound from which it is reprecipitated by the addition of strong acid. It dissolves in pyridine and precipitates again if the solution is poured into water. A sodium thiosulfate solution dissolves mercury fulminate with the formation of mercury tetrathionate and other inert compounds, and this reagent is used both for the destruction of fulminate and for its analysis. The first reaction appears to be as follows.

$$Hg(ONC)_2 + 2Na_2S_2O_3 + H_2O \longrightarrow HgS_4O_6 + 2NaOH + NaCN + NaNCO$$

The cyanide and cyanate are salts of weak acids and are largely hydrolyzed, and the solution, if it is titrated immediately, appears to have developed four molecules of sodium hydroxide for every molecule of mercury in the sample which was taken. If the solution is allowed to stand, the alkalinity gradually decreases because of a secondary reaction whereby sulfate and thiocyanate are formed.

409

$$HgS_4O_6 + NaCN + NaNCO + 2NaOH \longrightarrow HgSO_4 + Na_2SO_4 + 2NaNCS + H_2O$$

This reaction is restrained by a large excess of thiosulfate, and even more effectively by potassium iodide. A moderate excess of thiosulfate is commonly used, and an amount of potassium iodide

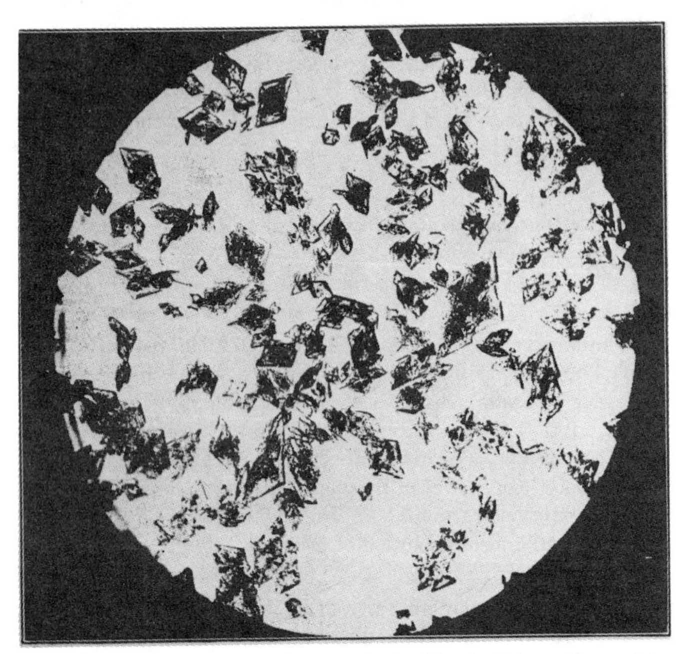

FIGURE 94. Mercury Fulminate Crystals for Use in Primer Composition (30×).

equal to 10 times the weight of the fulminate, and the titration for acidity (methyl orange indicator) is made as rapidly as possible. After that, the same solution is titrated with iodine (starch indicator) to determine the amount of unused thiosulfate and hence, by another method, the amount of actual fulminate in the sample. Speed is not essential in the second titration, for the iodine value does not change greatly with time as does the alkalinity. Blank determinations ought to be made because of the possibility that the iodide may contain iodate, and the apparent analytical results ought to be corrected accordingly.[410]

Mercury fulminate has a specific gravity of 4.45, but a mass of the crystals when merely shaken down has an apparent density (gravimetric density) of about 1.75. In detonators the material is usually compressed to a density of about 2.5, but densities as high as 4.0 have been obtained by vigorous compression. Mercury fulminate crystallizes from water in crystals which contain $\frac{1}{2}H_2O$, from alcohol in crystals which are anhydrous. One liter of water at 12° dissolves 0.71 gram, at 49° 1.74 grams, and at 100° 7.7 grams.

Mercury fulminate is usually stored under water, or, where there is danger of freezing, under a mixture of water and alcohol. When wet it is not exploded by a spark or by ordinary shock, but care must be taken that no part of the individual sample is allowed to dry out, for wet fulminate is exploded by the explosion of dry fulminate. It is not appreciably affected by long storage, either wet or dry, at moderate temperatures. At the temperature of the tropics it slowly deteriorates and loses its ability to explode. At 35°C. (95°F.) it becomes completely inert after about 3 years, at 50°C. (122°F.) after about 10 months. The heavy, dark-colored product of the deterioration of fulminate is insoluble in sodium thiosulfate solution.

When loaded in commercial detonators mercury fulminate is usually compressed under a pressure of about 3000 pounds per square inch, and in that condition has a velocity of detonation of about 4000 meters per second, explodes from a spark, and, in general, has about the same sensitivity to fire and to shock as the loosely compressed material. When compressed under greater and greater pressures, it gradually loses its property of detonating from fire. After being pressed at 25,000–30,000 pounds per square inch, mercury fulminate becomes "dead pressed" and no longer explodes from fire but merely burns. Dead-pressed fulminate however is exploded by loosely pressed fulminate or other initial detonating agent, and then shows a higher velocity of detonation than when compressed at a lower density.

The temperature at which mercury fulminate explodes depends upon the rate at which it is heated and, to some extent, upon the state of subdivision of the sample. Wöhler and Matter[411] experimented with small particles of various primary explosives, heated in copper capsules in a bath of Wood's metal. If a sample did not explode within 20 seconds, the temperature of the bath was raised 10° and a new sample was tried. The temperatures at which explosions occurred were as follows.

Mercury fulminate	190°
Sodium fulminate	150°
Nitrogen sulfide	190°
Benzenediazonium nitrate	90°
Chloratotrimercuraldehyde	130°
Silver azide	290°
Basic mercury nitromethane	160°

In a later series of experiments Wöhler and Martin studied a large number of fulminates and azides. The materials were in the form of microcrystalline powders, and all were compressed under the same pressure into pellets weighing 0.02 gram. The temperatures at which explosions occurred within 5 seconds were as follows.

Mercury fulminate	215°
Silver fulminate	170°
Copper fulminate	205°
Cadmium fulminate	215°
Sodium fulminate	215°
Potassium fulminate	225°
Thallium fulminate	120°
Cobalt azide	148°
Barium azide	152°
Calcium azide	158°
Strontium azide	169°
Cuprous azide	174°
Nickel azide	200°
Manganese azide	203°
Lithium azide	245°
Mercurous azide	281°
Zinc azide	289°
Cadmium azide	291°
Silver azide	297°
Lead azide	327°

Wöhler and Martin in the same year also reported determinations of the smallest amounts of certain fulminates and azides necessary to cause the detonation of various high explosives.[412]

Smallest Amount (Grams) Which Will Cause Detonation of:	Tetryl	Picric Acid	Trinitro-toluene	Trinitro-anisol	Trinitro-xylene
Cadmium azide	0.01	0.02	0.04	0.1	..
Silver azide	0.02	0.035	0.07	0.26	0.25
Lead azide	0.025	0.025	0.09	0.28	..
Cuprous azide	0.025	0.045	0.095	0.375	0.40
Mercurous azide	0.045	0.075	0.145	0.55	0.50
Thallium azide	0.07	0.115	0.335	...	..
Silver fulminate	0.02	0.05	0.095	0.23	0.30
Cadmium fulminate	0.008	0.05	0.11	0.26	0.35
Copper fulminate	0.025	0.08	0.15	0.32	0.43
Mercury fulminate	0.29	0.30	0.36	0.37	0.40
Thallium fulminate	0.30	0.43	...	...	..

From these data it is apparent that mercury fulminate is by no means the most efficient initiating agent among the fulminates and azides. Silver fulminate is about 15 times as efficient as mercury fulminate for exploding tetryl, but only about 4/3 as efficient for exploding trinitroxylene. Mercury fulminate however will tolerate a higher temperature, and is much less sensitive to shock and friction, than silver fulminate. Lead azide, which has about the same initiating power as silver fulminate, has an explosion temperature more than 100° higher than that of mercury fulminate. Many other interesting inferences are possible from the data. Among them we ought especially to note that the order of the several fulminates and azides with respect to their efficiency in detonating one explosive is not always the same as their order with respect to their efficiency in detonating another.

Silver Fulminate

Silver fulminate is so sensitive and so dangerous to handle that it has not been used for practical purposes in blasting or in the military art. It early found use in toys, in tricks, and in such devices for entertainment as those which Christopher Grotz described in 1818 in his book on "The Art of Making Fireworks, Detonating Balls, &c."

413

> Amusements with Fulminating Silver. . . .
> Segars.
> Are prepared by opening the smoking end, and inserting a little of the silver; close it carefully up, and it is done.
> Spiders.
> A piece of cork cut into the shape of the body of a spider, and a bit of thin wire for legs, will represent with tolerable exactness this insect. Put a small quantity of the silver underneath it; and on any female espying it, she will naturally tread on it, to crush it, when it will make a loud report.

Silver fulminate is still used for similar purposes in practical jokes, in toy torpedoes (see Vol. I, p. 106), and in the snaps or pull-crackers which supply the noise for bon-boms, joy-boms, and similar favors.

Silver fulminate is insoluble in nitric acid, and is decomposed by hydrochloric acid. It darkens on exposure to light. One liter of water at 13° dissolves 0.075 gram of the salt, and at 30° 0.18 gram. The double fulminate of silver and potassium, AgONC·KONC, is soluble in 8 parts of boiling water.

Detonators

The discovery of the phenomenon of initiation by Alfred Nobel and the invention of the blasting cap stand at the beginning of the development of modern explosives, perhaps the most important discovery and invention in the history of the art. The phenomenon has supplied a basis for the definition of high explosives, that is to say, of those explosives, whether sensitive or insensitive, which are incapable, without the invention, of being used safely and controllably or perhaps even of being used at all.

Nobel's experiments quickly led him to the form of the blasting cap which is now in use, a cylindrical capsule, generally of copper but sometimes of aluminum or zinc, filled for about half of its length with a compressed charge of primary explosive. The charge is fired either by an electric igniter or by a fuse, crimped into place, its end held firmly against the charge in order that the chances of a misfire may be reduced. Its action depends upon the development of an intense pressure or shock. Fulminate of mercury was the only substance known at the time of Nobel's invention which could be prepared and loaded for the purpose with reasonable safety, and caps loaded with straight fulminate were the first to

414

be manufactured. The original fulminate detonators were numbered according to the amount of fulminate which they contained,

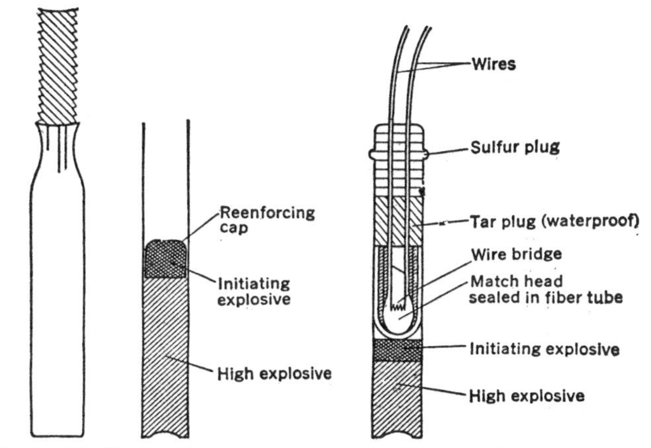

Figure 95. Blasting Caps. Detonator crimped to miner's fuse. Compound detonator. Compound electric detonator.

the same numbers being used throughout the world. The charges of fulminate for the various sizes are shown in the following table,

Detonator	Weight of Mercury Fulminate		External Dimensions of Capsule	
	Grams	Grains	Diameter, mm.	Length, mm.
No. 1	0.30	4.6	5.5	16
No. 2	0.40	6.2	5.5	22
No. 3	0.54	8.3	5.5	26
No. 4	0.65	10.0	6	28
No. 5	0.80	12.3	6	30–32
No. 6	1.00	15.4	6	35
No. 7	1.50	23.1	6	40–45
No. 8	2.00	30.9	6–7	50–55

along with the usual (but not universal) dimensions of the cylindrical copper capsules. The same numbers are now applied to commercial blasting caps of the same sizes, whatever the weights and

415

characters of the charges. A No. 6 cap, for example, is a cap of the same size as one which contains 1 gram of straight fulminate. No. 6 caps of different manufacturers may differ in their power

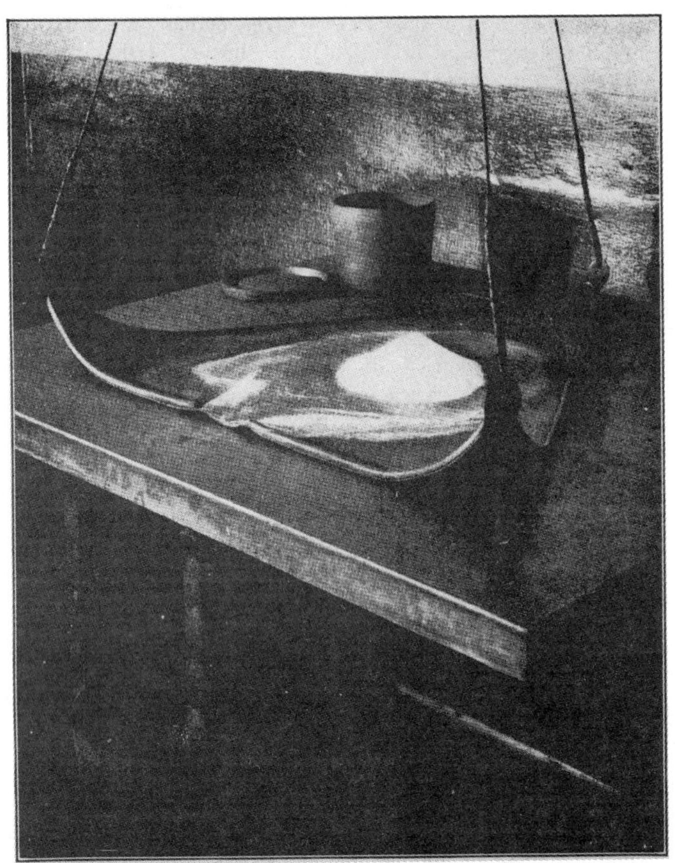

FIGURE 96. Manufacture of Detonators. (Courtesy Hercules Powder Company.) The safe mixing of the primary explosive charge for blasting caps is accomplished mechanically behind a concrete barricade by lifting slowly and then lowering first one corner of the triangular rubber tray, then the next corner, then the next, and so on. In the background, the rubber bowl or box in which the mixed explosive is carried to the building where it is loaded into caps. [416]

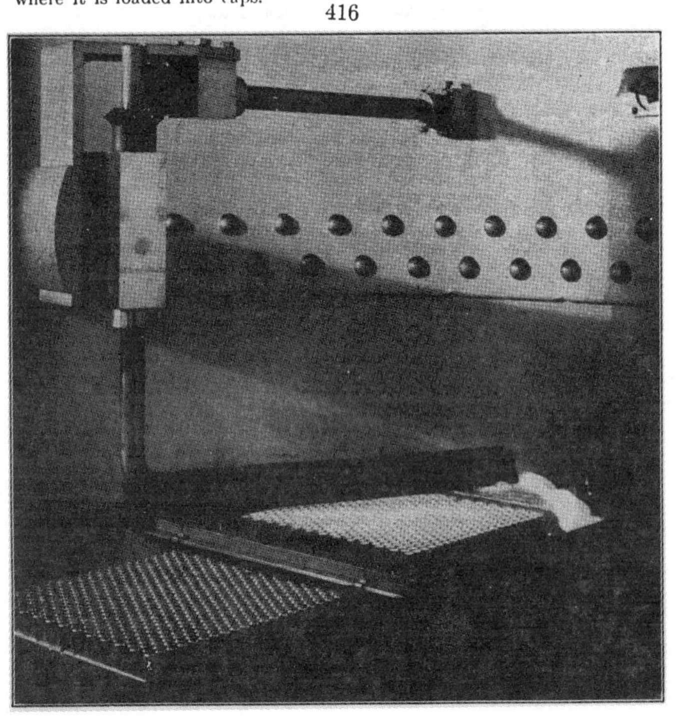

FIGURE 97. Manufacture of Detonators. (Courtesy Hercules Powder Company.) Charging the capsules. Each of the holes in the upper steel plate (*charging plate*) is of the right size to contain exactly enough explosive for the charging of one detonator. The mixed explosive is emptied onto the plate, the rubber-faced arm sweeps the material over the charging plate filling all the holes and throwing the excess into the box at the right. Under the charging plate is the thin *indexing plate* which supplies a bottom to all the holes in the charging plate. The detonator capsules, seen at the left, are placed under the indexing plate and in line with the holes in the charging plate; the indexing plate is then removed, the explosive falls down into the capsules, exactly the right amount into each, and is later pressed into place.

as they differ in their composition. No. 6, 7, and 8 caps are the only ones which are manufactured regularly in the United States, and the No. 6 cap is the one which is most commonly used.

The fulminate in detonators was first modified by mixing it with black powder, then with potassium nitrate, and later with [417] potassium chlorate.[15] The chlorate mixtures soon attained commercial importance in the United States, and by 1910 had largely displaced straight fulminate. Detonators containing them dominated the market until recently, and are now largely, but not yet wholly, displaced by compound detonators in which use is made of the principle of the booster. Mixtures of fulminate and potassium chlorate are distinctly more hygroscopic than straight fulminate, but are cheaper and slightly safer to handle and to load. Weight for weight they make better detonators. Storm and Cope in a series of experiments in the sand test bomb found that 80/20 fulminate-chlorate pulverizes more sand than the same weight of the 90/10 mixture and that this pulverizes more than straight fulminate. The results show that the sand test is an instrument of considerable precision. A difference of $\frac{1}{40}$ gram in the size of the charge of fulminate generally caused a difference of more than 1 gram in the weight of sand which was pulverized.

[15] Detonators were manufactured abroad and sold for a time under Nobel's patent, A. V. Newton (from A. Nobel, Paris), Brit. Pat. 16,919 (1887), covering the use, instead of fulminate, of a granulated mixture of lead picrate, potassium picrate, and potassium chlorate, but the invention apparently contributed little to the advance of the explosives art.

WEIGHT OF SAND (GRAMS) PULVERIZED FINER THAN 30-MESH BY

WEIGHT OF CHARGE, GRAMS	Mercury Fulminate	90/10 Fulminate-Chlorate	80/20 Fulminate-Chlorate
2.0000	56.94	58.57	59.68
1.5000	47.71	51.11	52.54
1.0000	38.33	40.13	41.42
0.7500	29.65	32.30	34.28
0.5000	22.45	23.07	23.22
0.4000	17.91	17.90	18.13
0.3500	14.16	15.13	15.94
0.3250	12.20	12.90	13.13
0.3000	10.01	12.71	12.61
0.2500	8.84	9.57	11.94
0.2250	6.93	8.71	10.29
0.2000	5.48	8.33	9.44

Storm and Cope [418] also used the sand test to determine the minimum amounts of fulminate and of the fulminate-chlorate mixtures which were necessary to detonate several high explosives in reenforced detonators. It is necessary to specify that the tests were made with reenforced detonators, for the results would have been quite different if reenforcing caps had not been used. In an ordinary detonator TNA required 0.3125 gram of 80/20 fulminate-chlorate instead of the 0.1700 gram which was sufficient when a reenforced detonator was used.

Primary Explosive	Minimum Initiating Charge (Grams) Necessary for Explosion of 0.4 Gram of		
	TNT	TNA	Picric Acid
Mercury fulminate	0.26	0.20	0.25
90/10 Fulminate-chlorate	0.25	0.17	0.23
80/20 Fulminate-chlorate	0.24	0.17	0.22

The reenforced detonators which were used in this work were made by introducing the weighed charge of high explosive into the detonator shell and the weighed charge of primary explosive into the small reenforcing cap while the latter was held in a cavity in a brass block which served to prevent the explosive from falling through the hole in the end of the cap. The primary explosive was then pressed down gently by means of a wooden rod, the cap was filled by adding a sufficient quantity of the high explosive from the detonator shell, this was similarly pressed down, and the reenforcing cap was then removed from the brass block and inserted carefully in the detonator shell with its perforated end upward. The detonator was then placed in a press block, a plunger inserted, and the contents subjected to a pressure of 200 atmospheres per square inch maintained for 1 minute. The pressure expanded the reenforcing cap against the detonator shell and fixed it firmly in place.

The minimum initiating charge was determined as follows. The amount of sand pulverized by a detonator loaded, say, with TNT and with fulminate insufficient to explode the TNT was determined. Another experiment with a slightly larger amount of fulminate was tried. If this showed substantially the same amount of sand pulverized, then the charge of fulminate was increased still further, and so on, until a sudden large increase

419

in the amount of sand pulverized showed that the TNT had detonated. After this point had been reached, further increases in the amount of fulminate caused only slight increases in the amount of sand pulverized. The magnitude of the effects, and the definiteness of the results, are shown by the following data of Storm and Cope.

Primary Explosive	Weight of Sand (Grams) Pulverized Finer than 30-Mesh by Reenforced Detonator Containing 0.40 Gram TNT and a Priming Charge (Grams) of					
	0.3000	0.2800	0.2600	0.2500	0.2400	0.2300
Mercury fulminate	34.20	34.70	33.00	13.55	12.60	...
	...	...	31.50	...	...	...
	...	...	30.00	...	...	...
	...	...	32.70	...	...	...
	...	...	32.00	...	...	...
90/10 Fulminate-chlorate	...	...	33.55	34.45	32.95	13.90
	...	...	34.05	34.67	13.20	...
	...	...	34.35	34.07	...	...
	...	...	34.42	35.07	...	...
	...	...	34.70	33.80	...	...
80/20 Fulminate-chlorate	...	...	...	...	34.40	16.80
	...	...	...	...	34.60	...
	...	...	...	...	34.60	...
	...	...	...	...	33.80	...
	...	...	...	...	34.85	...

Fulminate owes its success as an initiating agent primarily to the fact that it explodes easily from fire—and it catches the fire more readily than do lead azide and many another primary explosive—to the fact that it quickly attains its full velocity of detonation within a very short length of material, and probably also to the fact that the heavy mercury atom which it contains enables it to deliver an especially powerful blow. Its maximum velocity of detonation is much lower than that of TNT and similar substances, and its power to initiate the detonation of high explosives is correspondingly less. Wöhler in 1900 patented detonators in which a main charge of TNT or other nitro compound is initiated by a relatively small charge of fulminate.

420

Detonators which thus make use of the principle of the booster are known as compound detonators and are made both with and without reenforcing caps. Some manufacturers insert the reenforcing cap with the perforated end down, others with the perforated end up.[20]

[20] In addition to its other functions, the reenforcing cap tends toward greater safety by preventing actual contact between the primary explosive and the squarely cut end of the miner's fuse to which the detonator is crimped.

Not long after Curtius had discovered and described hydrazoic (hydronitric) acid and its salts, Will and Lenze experimented with the azides (hydronitrides, hydrazotates) at the military testing station at Spandau, but a fatal accident put an end to their experiments and their results were kept secret by the German war office. Wöhler and Matter later studied several primary explosives in an effort to find a substitute for fulminate, and in 1907, in ignorance of the earlier work of Will and Lenze, published experiments which demonstrated the great effectiveness of the azides. At about the same time, the first attempt to use lead azide practically in the explosives industry was made by F. Hyronimus in France who secured a patent in February, 1907, for the use of lead azide in detonators, to replace either wholly or in part the mercury fulminate which had theretofore been used, and this whether or not the fulminate would ordinarily be used alone or in conjunction with some other explosive substance such as picric acid or trinitrotoluene. In March of the same year Wöhler in Germany patented,[25] as a substitute for fulminate, the heavy metal salts of hydrazoic acid, "such as silver and mercury azides." He pointed out, as the advantages of these substances, that a smaller weight of them is necessary to produce detonation than is necessary of mercury fulminate, as, for example, that a No. 8 blasting cap containing 2 grams of mercury fulminate can be replaced, for use in detonating explosives, by a No. 8 copper capsule containing 1 gram of picric acid on top of which 0.023 gram of silver azide has been com-

421

pressed. In February of the next year Wöhler was granted a French patent in which lead azide was specifically mentioned, but the use of this substance had already been anticipated by the patent of Hyronimus. Lead azide was soon afterwards manufactured commercially in Germany and in France, and compound detonators containing this material were used fairly generally in Europe at the time of the first World War. A few years later the manufacture of lead azide detonators was commenced in the United States. In this country compound detonators having a base charge of tetryl and primed with 80/20 fulminate-chlorate or with lead azide have been superseded in part by detonators loaded with a more powerful high-explosive charge of nitromannite, PETN, or diazodinitrophenol and primed with lead azide, alone or sensitized to flame by the addition of lead styphnate or tetracene, or with diazodinitrophenol as the primary explosive.

Testing of Detonators

Among the tests which are used for determining the relative efficiency of detonators, the lead block or small Trauzl test, in which the detonators are fired in holes drilled in lead blocks and the resulting expansions of the holes are measured, and the lead or aluminum plate test in which the detonators are stood upright upon the plates and fired, and the character and extent of the effects upon the plates are observed, have already been mentioned. The first of these gives results which are expressible by numbers, and in that sense quantitative, and it is evident that both methods may be applied, for example, to the determination of the minimum amount of primary explosive necessary for the initiation of a high explosive, for both show notably different effects according as the high explosive explodes or not. Another useful test is the determination of the maximum distance through which the detonator is capable of initiating the explosion of some standard material, say, a piece of cordeau loaded with TNT. In the *nail test,* a wire nail is fastened to the side of the detonator, the detonator is fired, and the angle of the bend which the explosion imparts to the nail is measured.[422] The sand test, in which the detonator is fired in the center of a mass of carefully screened sand contained in a suitable bomb and the sand which has been pulverized is screened off and weighed, is the most precise and significant of the tests on detonators. It is a real test of brisance, and its usefulness is not limited to the study of detonators but may be extended to the study of high explosives as well. Thus, two explosives may be compared by loading equal amounts in detonator shells, priming with equal amounts of the same initiator, firing in the sand test bomb, and comparing the amounts of sand pulverized.

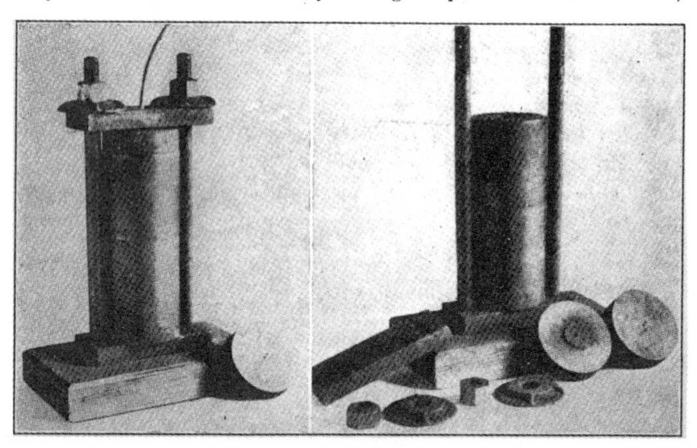

FIGURE 98. U. S. Bureau of Mines Sand Test Bomb No. 1. (Courtesy U. S. Bureau of Mines.) At left, assembled for making the test. At right, disassembled showing the parts. Two covers, one with a single hole for miner's fuse, the other with two holes for the two wires of an electric detonator.

The sand test was devised in 1910 by Walter O. Snelling, explosives chemist of the U. S. Bureau of Mines, who worked out the technique of its operation and designed the standard Bureau of Mines sand test bomb No. 1 which was used in his own investigations and in those of Storm and Cope.[423] Munroe and Taylor later recommended a bomb of larger diameter, Bureau of Mines sand test bomb No. 2, as being able to differentiate more exactly between the different grades of detonators in commercial use. The test grew out of an earlier test which Snelling had developed in 1908 for measuring the strength of detonating agents. Starting with the thought that true explosives, when subjected to a sufficiently strong initiating influence, detonate in such manner as to set free more energy than that which had been applied to them by the initiating charge, he tested several materials which failed to be true explosives and, although decomposed by the detonating agent, did not give off energy enough to continue their own decomposition and to propagate a detonation wave. Copper oxalate was the best of the "near explosives" which he tried.[424] He found it possible to measure the initiating effect of mercury fulminate and of other initial detonators by firing them in compositions consisting partly or wholly of copper oxalate, and then by chemical means determining the amount of the oxalate which had been decomposed. The experiments were carried out in a small steel bomb, the detonator was placed in the middle of a mass of oxalate or of oxalate composition, and sand was put in on top to fill the bomb completely. The fact that part of the sand was pulverized by the force of the explosion suggested that the mechanical effect of the initiator might perhaps serve as an approximate measure of the detonating efficiency; the oxalate was omitted, the bomb was filled entirely with sand, and the sand test was devised. Before Snelling left the Bureau of Mines in 1912 he had made about 40 tests on ordinary and electric detonators. Storm and Cope extended the usefulness of the test and applied it not only to the study of detonators but also to the study of the materials out of which detonators are constructed, both initial detonating agents and high explosives.

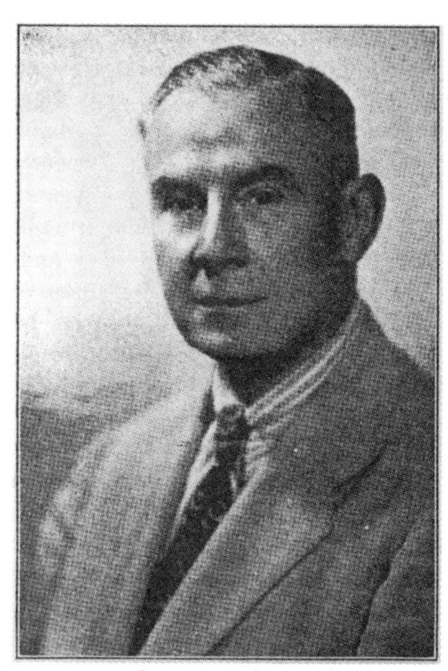

FIGURE 99. Walter O. Snelling. (Metzger & Son.) Devised the sand test. Has worked extensively with nitrostarch explosives and has patented many improvements in military and in mining explosives. Chemist at the U. S. Bureau of Mines, 1908-1916; Director of Research, Trojan Powder Company, 1917—.

Lead Azide

Lead azide is a more efficient detonating agent than mercury fulminate. It requires a higher temperature for its spontaneous explosion, and it does not decompose on long continued storage at moderately elevated temperatures. It cannot be dead-pressed by any pressure which occurs in ordinary manufacturing operations. Lead azide pressed into place in a detonator capsule takes the fire less readily, or explodes from spark less readily, than mercury fulminate. For this reason the main initiating charge of lead azide in a blasting cap is generally covered with a layer of lead styphnate, or of styphnate-azide mixture or other *sensitizer*, which explodes more easily, though less violently, from fire, and serves to initiate the explosion of the azide.

Lead azide is not used in primers where it is desired to produce fire or flame from impact. Fulminate mixtures and certain mixtures which contain no fulminate are preferred for this purpose. Lead azide is used where it is desired to produce, either from flame or from impact, an initiatory shock for the detonation of a high explosive—in compound detonators as already described, and in the detonators of artillery fuzes. For the latter purpose, caps containing azide and tetryl (or other booster explosive) are

425

used; the azide is exploded by impact, and the tetryl communicates the explosion to the booster or perhaps to the main charge of the shell.

Lead azide is produced as a white precipitate by mixing a solution of sodium azide with a solution of lead acetate or lead nitrate. It is absolutely essential that the process should be carried out in such manner that the precipitate consists of very small particles. The sensitivity of lead azide to shock and to friction increases rapidly as the size of the particles increases. Crystals 1 mm. in length are liable to explode spontaneously because of the internal stresses within them. The U. S. Ordnance Department specifications require that the lead azide shall contain no needle-shaped crystals more than 0.1 mm. in length. Lead azide is about as sensitive to impact when it is wet as when it is dry. Dextrinated lead azide can apparently be stored safely under water for long periods of time. The belief exists, however, that crystalline "service azide" becomes more sensitive when stored under water because of an increase in the size of the crystals.

The commercial preparation of lead azide is carried out on what is practically a laboratory scale, 300 grams of product constituting an ordinary single batch. There appear to be diverse opinions as to the best method of precipitating lead azide in a finely divided condition. According to one, fairly strong solutions are mixed while a gentle agitation is maintained, and the precipitate is removed promptly, and washed, and dried. According to another, dilute solutions ought to be used, with extremely violent agitation, and a longer time ought to be devoted to the process. The preparation is sometimes carried out by adding one solution to the other in a nickel vessel, which has corrugated sides, and is rotated around an axis which makes a considerable angle with the vertical, thereby causing turbulence in the liquid. The precipitation is sometimes carried out in the presence of dissolved colloidal material, such as gelatin or dextrin, which tends to prevent the formation of large crystals. Sometimes the lead azide is precipitated on starch or wood pulp, either of which will take up about 5 times its own weight of the material, and the impregnated starch is worked up, say, by tumbling in a sweetie barrel with a little dextrine, to form a free-flowing granular mass which can conveniently be loaded into detonators, or the impregnated wood pulp is converted into pasteboard which is cut into discs

426

for loading. A small amount of basic salt in the lead azide makes it somewhat less sensitive to impact and slightly safer to handle, but has no appreciable effect upon its efficacy as an initiator.

The commercial preparation of the azides is carried out either by the interaction of hydrazine with a nitrite or by the interaction of sodamide with nitrous oxide. The first of these methods

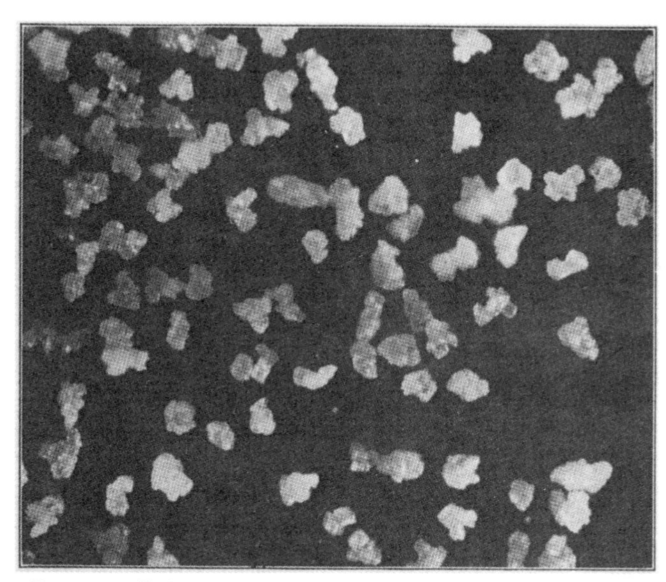

FIGURE 100. Technical Lead Azide, 90-95% pure (75×). For use in detonators. Precipitated in the presence of dextrin, it shows no crystal faces under the microscope.

follows from the original work of Curtius, the second from a reaction discovered by Wislicenus in 1892 and later developed for plant scale operation by Dennis and Browne. Curtius first prepared hydrazoic acid by the action of aqueous or alcoholic alkali or ammonia on acyl azides prepared by the action of nitrous acid on acyl hydrazides. The hydrazides are formed by

427

the interaction of hydrazine with esters just as the amides are formed by the corresponding interaction of ammonia.

$$R{-}COOC_2H_5 + NH_2{-}NH_2 \longrightarrow C_2H_5OH + \underset{\text{Acyl hydrazide}}{R{-}CO{-}NH{-}NH_2}$$

$$R{-}CO{-}NH{-}NH_2 + HONO \longrightarrow 2H_2O + \underset{\text{Acyl azide}}{R{-}CO{-}N_3}$$

$$R{-}CO{-}N_3 + H_2O \longrightarrow R{-}COOH + HN_3$$

$$R{-}CO{-}N_3 + NH_3 \longrightarrow R{-}CO{-}NH_2 + \underset{\text{Hydrazoic acid}}{HN_3}$$

By acidifying the hydrolysis mixture with sulfuric acid and by fractionating the product, Curtius procured anhydrous hydrazoic as a colorless liquid which boils at 37°. Hydrazoic acid is intensely poisonous and bad smelling. It is easily exploded by flame, by a brisant explosive, or by contact with metallic mercury. The anhydrous substance is extremely dangerous to handle, but dilute solutions have been distilled without accident.

Angeli obtained a white precipitate of insoluble silver azide by mixing saturated solutions of silver nitrite and hydrazine sulfate and allowing to stand in the cold for a short time. Dennstedt and Göhlich later procured free hydrazoic acid by the interaction of hydrazine sulfate and potassium nitrite in aqueous solution.

$$\underset{\text{Hydrazine sulfate}}{NH_2{-}NH_2 \cdot H_2SO_4} + KONO \longrightarrow KHSO_4 + 2H_2O + HN_3$$

The yield from this reaction is greatest if the medium is alkaline, for nitrous acid attacks hydrazoic acid oxidizing it with the liberation of nitrogen. If hydrazine sulfate [37] is used in the mixture, the resulting hydrazoic acid is not available for the preparation of lead azide until it has been distilled out of the solution. (Lead ions added to the solution would cause the precipitation of lead sulfate.) The reaction mixture may be acidified with sulfuric acid, a little ammonium sulfate may be added in order that the

[37] Hydrazine is produced commercially by treating ammonia in aqueous solution with sodium hypochlorite to form chloramine, NH_2—Cl, and by coupling this with another molecule of ammonia to form hydrazine and hydrochloric acid. Sulfuric acid is added to the liquid, sparingly soluble hydrazine sulfate crystallizes out, and it is in the form of this salt that hydrazine generally occurs in commerce.

428

ammonia may react with any unchanged nitrous acid which may be present, and the hydrazoic acid may be distilled directly into a solution of a soluble lead salt; but methods involving the distillation of hydrazoic acid present many dangers and have not found favor for commercial production. The alternative is to work with materials which contain no sulfate, and to isolate the azide by precipitation from the solution, and it is by this method that sodium azide (for the preparation of lead azide) is generally manufactured in this country and in England.

Hydrazine [38] reacts in alcohol solution with ethyl nitrite [39] and caustic soda to form sodium azide which is sparingly soluble in alcohol (0.315 gram in 100 grams of alcohol at 16°) and precipitates out.

[38] Hydrazine hydrate is actually used. It is an expensive reagent procured by distilling hydrazine sulfate with caustic soda in a silver retort. It is poisonous, corrosive, strongly basic, and attacks glass, cork, and rubber. Pure hydrazine hydrate is a white crystalline solid which melts at 40° and boils at 118°, but the usual commercial material is an 85% solution of the hydrate in water.

[39] It is necessary to use ethyl nitrite or other alcohol-soluble nitrous ester, instead of sodium nitrite, in order that advantage may be taken of a solvent from which the sodium azide will precipitate out.

$$NH_2\text{—}NH_2 + C_2H_5ONO + NaOH \longrightarrow NaN_3 + C_2H_5OH + 2H_2O$$

The sodium azide is filtered off, washed with alcohol, and dried. It is soluble in water to the extent of 42 grams in 100 grams of water at 18°. It is not explosive, and requires no particular precaution in its handling.

Azide has been manufactured in France and in Germany by the sodamide process. Metallic sodium is heated at about 300° while dry ammonia gas is bubbled through the molten material.

$$2Na + 2NH_3 \longrightarrow 2NaNH_2 + H_2$$

The sodamide which is formed remains liquid (m.p. 210°) and does not prevent contact between the remaining sodium and the ammonia gas. The progress of the reaction is followed by passing the effluent gas through water which absorbs the ammonia and allows the hydrogen to pass; if there is unabsorbed gas which forms an explosive mixture with air, the reaction is not yet complete. For the second step, the sodamide is introduced into a nickel or nickel-lined, trough-shaped autoclave along the bottom

429

of which there extends a horizontal shaft equipped with teeth. The air in the apparatus is displaced with ammonia gas, the autoclave is heated to about 230°, and nitrous oxide is passed in while the horizontal stirrer is rotated. The nitrous oxide reacts with one equivalent of sodamide to form sodium azide and water. The water reacts with a second equivalent of sodamide to form sodium hydroxide and ammonia.

$$NaNH_2 + N_2O \longrightarrow NaN_3 + H_2O$$
$$NaNH_2 + H_2O \longrightarrow NaOH + NH_3$$

The reaction is complete when no more ammonia is evolved. The product, which consists of an equimolecular mixture of sodium hydroxide and sodium azide, may be taken up in water and neutralized carefully with nitric acid, and the resulting solution may be used directly for the preparation of lead azide, or the product may be fractionally crystallized from water for the production of sodium azide. The same material may be procured by washing the product with warm alcohol which dissolves away the sodium hydroxide.

The different methods by which hydrazoic acid and the azides may be prepared indicate that the acid may properly be represented by any one or by all of the following structural formulas.

$$H\text{—}N\langle{}^{N}_{N} \qquad H\text{—}N\langle{}^{N}_{N}\| \qquad H\text{—}N{=}N{\equiv}N$$

Hydrazoic acid is a weak acid; its ionization constant at 25°, 1.9×10^{-5}, is about the same as that of acetic acid at 25°, 1.86×10^{-5}. It dissolves zinc, iron, magesium, and aluminum, forming azides with the evolution of hydrogen and the production of a certain amount of ammonia. It attacks copper, silver, and mercury, forming azides without evolving hydrogen, and is reduced in part to ammonia and sometimes to hydrazine and free nitrogen. Its reaction with copper, for example, is closely analogous to the reaction of nitric acid with that metal.

$$Cu + 3HN_3 \longrightarrow Cu(N_3)_2 + N_2 + NH_3$$
$$3Cu + 8HNO_3 \longrightarrow 3Cu(NO_3)_2 + 2NO + 4H_2O$$

So also, like nitric acid, it oxidizes hydrogen sulfide with the liberation of sulfur.

430

$$H_2S + HN_3 \longrightarrow S + N_2 + NH_3$$
$$3H_2S + 2HNO_3 \longrightarrow 3S + 2NO + 4H_2O$$

Mixed with hydrochloric acid it forms a liquid, comparable to *aqua regia,* which is capable of dissolving platinum.

$$Pt + 2HN_3 + 4HCl \longrightarrow PtCl_4 + 2N_2 + 2NH_3$$
$$3Pt + 4HNO_3 + 12HCl \longrightarrow 3PtCl_4 + 4NO + 8H_2O$$

Hydrazoic acid and permanganate mutually reduce each other with the evolution of a mixture of nitrogen and oxygen. The acid and its salts give with ferric chloride solution a deep red coloration, similar to that produced by thiocyanates, but the color is discharged by hydrochloric acid.

The solubilities of the azides in general are similar to those of the chlorides. Thus, silver azide is soluble in ammonia water and insoluble in nitric acid. Lead azide, like lead chloride, is sparingly soluble in cold water, but hot water dissolves enough of it so that it crystallizes out when the solution is cooled. One hundred grams of water at 18° dissolve 0.03 gram, at 80° 0.09 gram.

The true density of lead azide is 4.8, but the loose powder has an apparent density of about 1.2.

Lead azide is dissolved by an aqueous solution of ammonium acetate, but it is not destroyed by it. The solution contains azide ions and lead ions, the latter quantitatively precipitable as lead chromate, $PbCrO_4$, by the addition of potassium dichromate solution. Lead azide in aqueous suspension is oxidized by ceric sulfate with the quantitative production of nitrogen gas which may be collected in an azotometer and used for the determination of the azide radical.

$$Pb(N_3)_2 + 2Ce(SO_4)_2 \longrightarrow PbSO_4 + 3N_2 + Ce_2(SO_4)_3$$

Nitrous acid oxidizes hydrazoic acid with the evolution of nitrogen. A dilute solution of nitric or acetic acid, in which a little sodium nitrite has been dissolved, dissolves and destroys lead azide. Such a solution may conveniently be used for washing floors, benches, etc., on which lead azide may have been spilled.

Silver Azide

Silver azide is a more efficient initiator than mercury fulminate, and about as efficient as lead azide. It melts at 251° and decomposes rapidly above its melting point into silver and nitrogen. Its [431] temperature of spontaneous explosion varies somewhat according to the method of heating, but is considerably higher than that of mercury fulminate and slightly lower than that of lead azide. Taylor and Rinkenbach reported 273°. Its sensitivity to shock, like that of lead azide, depends upon its state of subdivision.

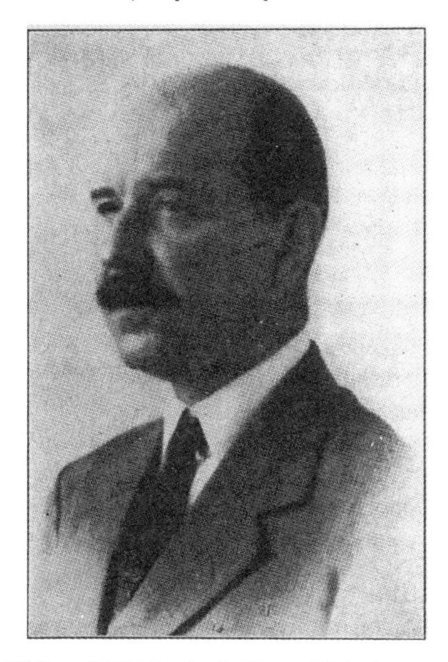

FIGURE 101. William H. Rinkenbach. Has published many studies on the physical, chemical, and explosive properties of pure high-explosive substances and primary explosives. Research Chemist, U. S. Bureau of Mines, 1919-1927; Assistant Chief Chemist, Picatinny Arsenal, 1927-1929; Chief Chemist, 1929—.

Taylor and Rinkenbach prepared a "colloidal" silver azide which required a 777-mm. drop of a 500-gram weight to cause detonation. Mercury fulminate required a drop of 127 mm. According to the same investigators 0.05 gram of silver azide was necessary to cause the detonation of 0.4 gram of trinitrotoluene in a No. 6 detonator capsule, whether the charge was confined by a reenforcing cap or not, as compared with 0.24 gram of mercury fulminate when the charge was [432] confined by a reenforcing cap and 0.37 gram when it was not confined. They also measured the sand-crushing power of silver azide when loaded into No. 6 detonator capsules and compressed under a pressure of 1000 pounds per square inch, and compared it with that of mercury fulminate, with the results which are tabulated below. It thus appears that

	Weight of Sand Crushed (Grams) by	
Weight of Charge, Grams	Silver Azide	Mercury Fulminate
0.05	1.4	0.00
0.10	3.3	0.00
0.20	6.8	4.2
0.30	10.4	8.9
0.50	18.9	16.0
0.75	30.0	26.1
1.00	41.1	37.2

the sand-crushing power of silver azide is not as much greater than the sand-crushing power of mercury fulminate as the difference in their initiatory powers would suggest. Storm and Cope in their studies on the sand test found that the powers of fulminate and of fulminate-chlorate mixtures to crush sand were about proportional to the initiatory powers of these materials, but the present evidence indicates that the law is not a general one.

Cyanuric Triazide

Cyanuric triazide, patented as a detonating explosive by Erwin Ott in 1921, is prepared by adding powdered cyanuric chloride, slowly with cooling and agitation, to a water solution of slightly more than the equivalent quantity of sodium azide.

```
        Cl                                   N3
        |                                    |
        C                                    C
       / \\                                 / \\
      N    N                              N    N
      ||   |     + 3NaN3 ——→              ||   |      + 3NaCl
  Cl—C    C—Cl                       N3—C    C—N3
      \\  //                              \\  //
        N                                    N
```

[433] Cyanuric triazide

The best results are secured if pure and finely powdered cyanuric chloride is used, yielding small crystals of pure cyanuric triazide in the first instance, in such manner that no recrystallization, which might convert them into large and more sensitive crystals, is necessary. Cyanuric chloride, m.p. 146°, b.p. 190°, is prepared by passing a stream of chlorine into a solution of hydrocyanic acid in ether or chloroform or into liquid anhydrous hydrocyanic acid exposed to sunlight. It is also formed by distilling cyanuric acid with phosphorus pentachloride and by the polymerization of cyanogen chloride, Cl—CN, after keeping in a sealed tube.

Cyanuric triazide is insoluble in water, slightly soluble in cold alcohol, and readily soluble in acetone, benzene, chloroform, ether, and hot alcohol. It melts at 94°, and decomposes when heated above 100°. It may decompose completely without detonation if it is heated slowly, but it detonates immediately from flame or from sudden heating. The melted material dissolves TNT and other aromatic nitro compounds. Small crystals of cyanuric triazide are more sensitive than small crystals of mercury fulminate, and have exploded while being pressed into a detonator capsule. Large crystals from fusion or from recrystallization have detonated when broken by the pressure of a rubber policeman.

Cyanuric triazide is not irritating to the skin, and has no poisonous effects on rats and guinea pigs in fairly large doses.[43]

Taylor and Rinkenbach have reported sand test data which show that cyanuric triazide is much more brisant than mercury fulminate.[43]

	Weight of Sand Crushed (Grams) by	
Weight of Explosive, Grams	Cyanuric Triazide	Mercury Fulminate
0.050	2.6	...
0.100	4.8	...
0.200	12.2	3.8
0.400	33.2	12.2
0.600	54.4	20.1
0.800	68.9	28.2
1.000	78.6	36.8

In conformity with these results are the findings of Kast and

Haid who reported that cyanuric triazide has a higher velocity of detonation than mercury fulminate. They made their measure-
434
ments on several primary explosives loaded into detonator capsules 7.7 mm. in internal diameter and compressed to the densities which they usually have in commercial detonators.

Explosive	Density	Velocity of Detonation, Meters per Second
Cyanuric triazide	1.15	5545
Lead azide	3.8	4500
Mercury fulminate	3.3	4490
Mixture: $Hg(ONC)_2$ 85%, $KClO_3$ 15%	3.1	4550
Lead styphnate	2.6	4900

Taylor and Rinkenbach found that cyanuric triazide is a more efficient initiator of detonation than mercury fulminate. This result cannot properly be inferred from its higher velocity of detonation, for there is no direct correlation between that quality and initiating efficiency. Lead azide is also a much more efficient initiator than mercury fulminate but has about the same velocity of detonation as that substance. The following results were secured by loading 0.4 gram of the high explosive into detonator capsules, pressing down, adding an accurately weighed amount of the initiator, covering with a short reenforcing cap, and pressing with a pressure of 200 atmospheres per square inch. The size of the initiating charge was reduced until it was found that a further reduction resulted in a failure of the high explosive to detonate.

High Explosive	Minimum Initiating Charge (Grams) of Cyanuric Triazide	Mercury Fulminate
Trinitrotoluene	0.10	0.26
Picric acid	0.05	0.21
Tetryl	0.04	0.24
Tetranitroaniline	0.09	0.20
Ammonium picrate	0.15	0.85

Cyanuric triazide is slightly more hygroscopic and distinctly more sensitive in the drop test than fulminate of mercury.[44] It is slightly volatile, and must be dried at as low a temperature as possible, preferably in vacuum. Detonators in which it is used
435

Temperature of Explosion

Explosive	When temperature is raised 20° per minute in Glass Tube	Iron Tube	In Iron Tube Temp., °C.	Elapsed time, seconds
Cyanuric triazide	206°	205°	200	40, 2
	208°	207°	205	0,
Lead azide	338°	337°	335	12, 9
			340	5, 7
			345	7, 6
			350	4, 5
			355	0
			360	0
Mercury fulminate	175°	166°	145	480, 331
			150	275, 255
			155	135, 165
			160	64, 85
			170	40, 35
			180	15, 13
			190	10, 8
			195	8, 7
			200	7, 8
			205	5, 5
			210	1, 3
			215	0
Mixture:	168°	169°	145	370, 365
$Hg(ONC)_2$ 85%	171°	170°	150	210, 215
$KClO_3$ 15%			155	155, 145
			160	125, 74
			170	45, 50
			180	23, 22
			190	8, 8
			195	7, 7
			200	7, 8
			205	7, 6
			210	4, 3
			215	0
Lead styphnate	276°	275°	250	90, 85
	277°	276°	265	65, 45
		275°	270	0

436
must be manufactured in such a way that they are effectively sealed.

Kast and Haid have determined the temperatures at which cyanuric triazide and certain other initiators explode spontaneously, both by raising the temperature of the samples at a constant rate and by keeping the samples at constant temperatures and noting the times which elapsed before they exploded. When no measurable time elapsed, the temperature was "the temperature of instantaneous explosion." Their data are especially interesting because they show the rate of deterioration of the materials at various temperatures.[44]

Trinitrotriazidobenzene

1,3,5-Trinitro-2,4,6-triazidobenzene is prepared from aniline by the reactions indicated below.

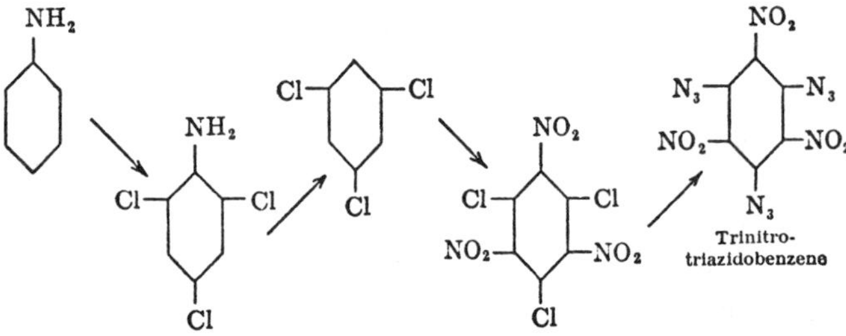

Trinitro-triazidobenzene

Aniline is chlorinated to form trichloroaniline. The amino group is eliminated from this substance by means of the diazo reaction, and the resulting *sym*-trichlorobenzene is nitrated. The nitration, as described by Turek, is carried out by dissolving the material in warm 32% oleum, adding strong nitric acid, and heating at 140–150° until no more trinitrotrichlorobenzene, m.p. 187°, precipitates out. The chlorine atoms of this substance are then replaced by azido groups. This is accomplished by adding an acetone solution of the trinitrotrichlorobenzene, or better, the powdered substance alone, to an actively stirred solution of sodium azide in moist alcohol. The precipitated trinitrotriazidobenzene is filtered off, washed with alcohol and with water, and, after drying, is sufficiently pure for technical purposes. It may be

[437] purified further by dissolving in chloroform and allowing to cool, greenish-yellow crystals, m.p. 131° with decomposition. It is decomposed slowly by boiling in chloroform solution.

Trinitrotriazidobenzene is readily soluble in acetone, moderately soluble in chloroform, sparingly in alcohol, and insoluble in water. It is not hygroscopic, is stable toward moisture, and does not attack iron, steel, copper, or brass in the presence of moisture. It is not appreciably volatile at 35–50°. It darkens in color superficially on exposure to the light. It decomposes on melting with the evolution of nitrogen and the formation of hexanitrosobenzene.

$$C_6(NO_2)_3(N_3)_3 \longrightarrow 3N_2 + C_6(NO)_6$$

The same reaction occurs at lower temperatures: 0.665% of a given portion of the material decomposes in 3 years at 20°, 2.43% in 1 year at 35°, 0.65% in 10 days at 50°, and 100% during 14 hours heating at 100°. The decomposition is not self-catalyzed. The product, hexanitrosobenzene, m.p. 159°, is stable, not hygroscopic, not a primary explosive, and is comparable to tetryl in its explosive properties.

Trinitrotriazidobenzene, if ignited in the open, burns freely with a greenish flame; enclosed in a tube and ignited, it detonates with great brisance. It is less sensitive to shock and to friction than mercury fulminate. It gives a drop test of 30 cm., but it may be made as sensitive as fulminate by mixing with ground glass. The specific gravity of the crystalline material is 1.8054. Under a pressure of 3000 kilograms per square centimeter it yields blocks having a density of 1.7509, under 5000 kilograms per square centimeter 1.7526. One gram of TNT compressed in a No. 8 detonator shell under a pressure of 500 kilograms per square centimeter, with trinitrotriazidobenzene compressed on top of it under 300 kilograms per square centimeter, required 0.02 gram of the latter substance for complete detonation. Tetryl under similar conditions required only 0.01 gram. Trinitrotriazidobenzene[438] may be dead-pressed and in that condition burns or puffs when it is ignited. It is a practical primary explosive and is prepared for loading in the granular form by mixing the moist material with nitrocellulose, adding a small amount of amyl acetate, kneading, rubbing through a sieve, and allowing to dry.

In the Trauzl test, trinitrotriazidobenzene gives 90% as much net expansion as PETN; tetryl gives 70%, TNT 60%, mercury fulminate 23%, and lead azide 16%. Used as a high explosive in compound detonators and initiated with lead azide, trinitrotriazidobenzene is about as strong as PETN and is stronger than tetryl.

Nitrogen Sulfide

Nitrogen sulfide was first prepared by Soubeiran in 1837 by the action of ammonia on sulfur dichloride dissolved in benzene.

$$6SCl_2 + 16NH_3 \longrightarrow N_4S_4 + 2S + 12NH_4Cl$$

It is conveniently prepared by dissolving 1 volume of sulfur chloride in 8 or 10 volumes of carbon disulfide, cooling, and passing in dry ammonia gas until the dark brown powdery precipitate which forms at first has dissolved and an orange-yellow solution results which contains light-colored flocks of ammonium chloride. These are filtered off and rinsed with carbon disulfide, the solution is evaporated to dryness, and the residue is extracted with boiling carbon disulfide for the removal of sulfur. The undissolved material is crude nitrogen sulfide. The hot extract on cooling deposits a further quantity in the form of minute golden-yellow crystals. The combined crude product is recrystallized from carbon disulfide.

The same product is also produced by the action of ammonia on disulfur dichloride in carbon disulfide, benzene, or ether solution.

$$6S_2Cl_2 + 16NH_3 \longrightarrow N_4S_4 + 8S + 12NH_4Cl$$

Nitrogen sulfide has a density of 2.22 at 15°. It is insoluble in water, slightly soluble in alcohol and ether, somewhat more soluble in carbon disulfide and benzene. It reacts slowly with water at ordinary temperature with the formation of pentathionic acid, sulfur[439] dioxide, free sulfur, and ammonia. It melts with sublimation at 178°, and explodes at a higher temperature which, however, is variable according to the rate at which the substance is heated. Berthelot found that it deflagrates at 207° or higher, and remarked that this temperature is about the same as the temperature of combustion of sulfur in the open air. Berthelot and Vieille studied the thermochemical properties of nitrogen sulfide. Their data, recalculated to conform to our present notions of atomic and molecular weight, show that the substance is strongly endothermic and has a heat of formation of −138.8 Calories per mol. It detonates with vigor under a hammer blow, but is less sensitive to shock and less violent in its effects than mercury fulminate. Although its rate of acceleration is considerably less than that of mercury fulminate, it has been recommended as a filling for fuses, primers, and detonator caps, both alone and in mixtures with oxidizing agents such as lead peroxide, lead nitrate, and potassium chlorate.

Nitrogen selenide was first prepared by Espenschied by the action of ammonia gas on selenium chloride. His product was an orange-red, amorphous powder which exploded violently when heated and was dangerous to handle. Verneuil studied the substance further and supplied a sample of it to Berthelot and Vieille for thermochemical experiments. It detonates when brought into contact with a drop of concentrated sulfuric acid or when warmed to about 230°. It also detonates from friction, from a very gentle blow of iron on iron, and from a slightly stronger blow of wood on iron. It has a heat of formation of −169.2 Calories per mol, and, with nitrogen sulfide, illustrates the principle, as Berthelot pointed out, that in analogous series (such as that of the halides and that of the oxides, sulfides, and selenides) "the explosive character of the endothermic compounds becomes more and more pronounced as the molecular weight becomes larger."

Lead Styphnate (Lead trinitroresorcinate)[440]

Lead styphnate is commonly prepared by adding a solution of magnesium styphnate[52] at 70° to a well-stirred solution of lead acetate at 70°. A voluminous precipitate of the basic salt separates. The mixture is stirred for 10 or 15 minutes; then dilute

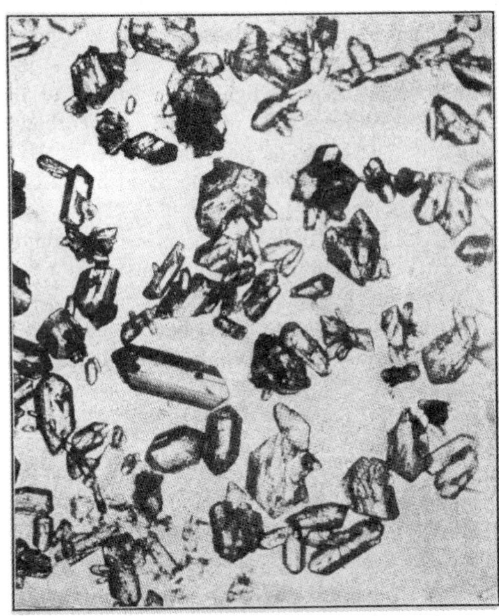

FIGURE 102. Lead Styphnate Crystals (90×).

nitric acid is added with stirring to convert the basic to the normal salt, and the stirring is continued while the temperature drops to about 30°. The product, which consists of reddish-brown, short, rhombic crystals, is filtered off, washed with water, sieved through silk, and dried.

52 Prepared by adding magnesium oxide to a suspension of styphnic acid in water until a clear solution results and only a very small portion of the styphnic acid remains undissolved.

Lead styphnate is a poor initiator, but it is easily ignited by fire or by a static discharge. It is used as an ingredient of the priming layer which causes lead azide to explode from a flash.[441] A 0.05-gram sample of lead styphnate in a test tube in a bath of Wood's metal heated at a rate of 20° per minute explodes at 267–268°.

Wallbaum determined the minimum charges of several primary explosives necessary for initiating the explosion of PETN. In the first series of tests, the PETN (0.4 gram) was tamped down or pressed loosely into copper capsules 6.2 mm. in inside diameter, and weighed amounts of the priming charges were pressed down loosely on top. The weights of the priming charges were decreased until one failure occurred in 10 tests with the same weight of charge. In later series, the PETN was compressed at 2000 kilograms per square centimeter. When the priming charges were pressed loosely on the compressed PETN, considerably larger amounts were generally necessary. One gram of lead styphnate, however, was not able to initiate the explosion of the compressed PETN. When the priming charges were pressed, on top of the already compressed PETN, with pressures of 500, 1000, and 1500 kilograms per square centimeter, then it was found that the tetracene and the fulminate were dead-pressed but that the amounts of lead azide and silver azide which were needed were practically the same as in the first series when both the PETN and the priming charge were merely pressed loosely. Wallbaum reports the results which are tabulated below.

Pressure on PETN, kg. per sq. cm.	0	2000	2000	2000	2000
Pressure on initiator, kg. per sq. cm.	0	0	500	1000	1500
PRIMARY EXPLOSIVE	MINIMUM INITIATING CHARGE, GRAMS				
Tetracene	0.16	0.250	dead-pressed		
Mercury fulminate (gray)	0.30	0.330	"	"	
Mercury fulminate (white)	0.30	0.340	"	"	
Lead styphnate	0.55	No detonation with 1 g.			
Lead azide (technical)	0.04	0.170	0.05	0.05	0.04
Lead azide (pure)	0.015	0.100	0.01	0.01	0.01
Silver azide	0.005	0.110	0.005	0.005	0.005

Diazonium Salts

Every student of organic chemistry has worked with diazonium salts in solution. The substances are commonly not isolated in the solid state, for the dry materials are easily exploded by shock and by friction, and numerous laboratory accidents have resulted from their unintended crystallization and drying.

The first volume of the *Mémorial des Poudres et Salpêtres* contains a report by Berthelot and Vieille[442] on the properties of benzenediazonium nitrate (diazobenzene nitrate). They prepared the material by passing nitrous gas into a cooled aqueous solution of aniline nitrate, diluting with an equal volume of alcohol, and precipitating in the form of white, voluminous flocks by the addition of an excess of ether.

$$2C_6H_5\text{—}NH_2 \cdot HNO_3 + N_2O_3 \longrightarrow 3H_2O + 2C_6H_5\text{—}\underset{\underset{N}{|||}}{N}\text{—}NO_3$$

The product was washed with ether, pressed between pieces of filter paper, and dried in a vacuum desiccator. In dry air and in the dark it could be kept in good condition for many months. In the daylight it rapidly turned pink, and on longer keeping, especially in a moist atmosphere, it turned brown, took on an odor of phenol, and finally became black and swelled up with bubbles of gas.

Benzenediazonium nitrate detonates easily from the blow of a hammer or from any rubbing which is at all energetic. It explodes violently when heated to 90°. Its density at 15° is 1.37, but under strong compression gently applied it assumes an apparent density of 1.0. Its heat of formation is −47.4 Calories per mol, heat of explosion 114.8 Calories per mol.

m-Nitrobenzenediazonium perchlorate was patented by Herz in 1911, and is reported to have been used in compound detonators with a high-explosive charge of nitromannite or other brisant nitric ester. It explodes spontaneously when heated to about 154°. It is sensitive to shock and to blow. Although it is very sparingly soluble in water and is stabilized to some extent by the nitro group on the nucleus, it is distinctly hygroscopic and is not exempt from the instability which appears to be characteristic of diazonium salts.

$$C_6H_4(NH_2)(NO_2) + HNO_2 + HClO_4 \longrightarrow 2H_2O + C_6H_4(N{\equiv}N\text{—}ClO_4)(NO_2)$$

Preparation of m-Nitrobenzenediazonium Perchlorate.[443] Half a gram of *m*-nitroaniline is suspended in 5 cc. of water in a wide test tube, and 0.5 cc. of concentrated hydrochloric acid and 2.2 cc. of 20% perchloric acid solution are added. After the nitraniline has dissolved, 15 cc. of water is added and the solution is cooled by immersing the test tube in a beaker filled with a slurry of cracked ice. One-quarter of a gram of sodium nitrite dissolved in 1 or 2 cc. of water is added in 3 or 4 portions, the mixture being shaken after each addition or stirred with a stirring rod the end of which is covered with a short piece of rubber tubing. After standing in the cold for 5 minutes, the material is transferred to a filter, and the feltlike mass of pale yellow needles is washed with cold water, with alcohol, and with ether. The product is dried in several small portions on pieces of filter paper.

Diazodinitrophenol (DDNP, Dinol)

4,6-Dinitrobenzene-2-diazo-1-oxide, or diazodinitrophenol as it is more commonly called, occupies a place of some importance in the history of chemistry, for its discovery by Griess led him to undertake his classic researches on the diazonium compounds and the diazo reaction. He prepared it by passing nitrous gas into an alcoholic solution of picramic acid, but it is more conveniently prepared by carrying out the diazotization in aqueous solution with sodium nitrite and hydrochloric acid.

Picric acid (OH; NO_2, NO_2, NO_2) —reduce→ Picramic acid (OH; NO_2, NH_2, NO_2) —diazotize→ Diazodinitrophenol ($O—N$, N; NO_2, NO_2)

Picramic acid, red needles, m. p. 169°, may be prepared by evaporating ammonium picrate in alcohol solution with ammonium sulfide.

Preparation of Diazodinitrophenol. Ten grams of picramic acid is suspended in 120 cc. of 5% hydrochloric acid in a beaker which stands in a basin of ice water, and the mixture is stirred rapidly with a mechanical stirrer. Sodium nitrite (3.6 grams) dissolved in 10 cc. of water is added all at once, and the stirring is continued for 20 minutes. The product is collected on a filter[444] and washed thoroughly with ice water. The dark brown granular material may be used as such, or it may be dissolved in hot acetone and precipitated by the addition of a large volume of ice water to the rapidly agitated liquid, a treatment which converts it into a brilliant yellow amorphous powder.

L. V. Clark, who has made an extensive study of the physical and explosive properties of diazodinitrophenol, reports that it has

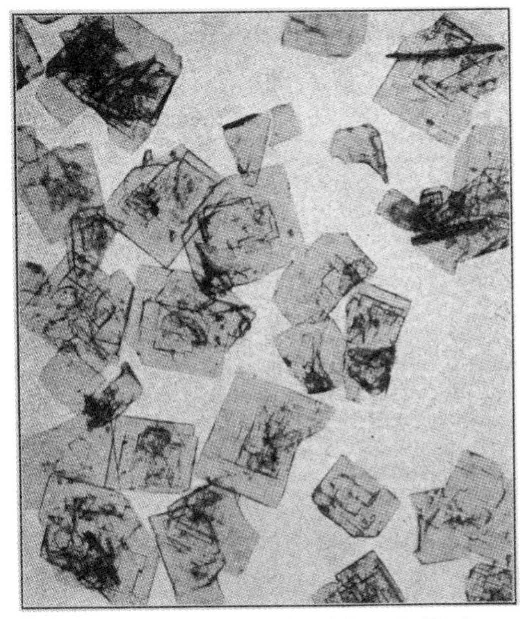

FIGURE 103. Diazodinitrophenol Crystals (90×).

a true density at 25°/4° of 1.63. Its apparent density after being placed in a tube and tapped is only 0.27, but, when compressed in a detonator capsule at a pressure of 3400 pounds per square inch (239 kilograms per square centimeter), it has an apparent density of 0.86. It is not dead-pressed by a pressure of 130,000 pounds per square inch (9139 kilograms per square centimeter). It is soluble in nitrobenzene, acetone, aniline, pyridine, acetic acid, strong hydrochloric acid, and nitroglycerin at ordinary temperatures. Its solubility at 50° in 100 grams of solvent is: in ethyl acetate 2.45 grams, in methyl alcohol 1.25 grams, in ethyl[445] alcohol 2.43 grams, in benzene 0.23 gram, and in chloroform 0.11 gram.

Diazodinitrophenol is less sensitive to impact than mercury fulminate and lead azide. Its sensitivity to friction is about the same as that of lead azide, much less than that of mercury fulminate. It detonates when struck a sharp blow, but, if it is ignited when it is unconfined, it burns with a quick flash, like nitrocellulose, even in quantities of several grams. This burning produces little or no local shock, and will not initiate the explosion of a high explosive. Commercial detonators containing a high-explosive charge of nitromannite and a primary explosive charge of diazodinitrophenol explode if they are crimped to a piece of miner's fuse and the fuse is lighted, but a spark falling into the open end has been reported to cause only the flashing of the diazodinitrophenol. Likewise, if an open cap of this sort falls into a fire, the diazodinitrophenol may flash, the nitromannite may later melt and run out and burn with a flash, and the detonator may be destroyed without exploding. While it is not safe to expect that this will always happen, it is an advantage of diazodinitrophenol that it sometimes occurs.

Diazodinitrophenol is darkened rapidly by exposure to sunlight. It does not react with water at ordinary temperatures, but is desensitized by it. It is not exploded under water by a No. 8 blasting cap.

Clark reports experiments with diazodinitrophenol, mercury fulminate, and lead azide in which various weights of the explosives were introduced into No. 8 detonator capsules, pressed under reenforcing caps at 3400 pounds per square inch, and fired in the No. 2 sand test bomb. His results, tabulated below, show that diazodinitrophenol is much more powerful than mercury fulminate and lead azide. Other experiments by Clark showed

	WEIGHT (GRAMS) OF SAND PULVERIZED FINER THAN 30-MESH BY		
WEIGHT (GRAMS) OF CHARGE	Diazo-dinitro-phenol	Mercury Fulminate	Lead Azide
0.10	9.1	3.1	3.5
0.20	19.3	6.5	7.2
0.40	36.2	17.0	14.2
0.60	54.3	27.5	21.5
0.80	72.1	38.0	28.7
1.00	90.6	48.4	36.0

that diazodinitrophenol in the[446] sand test has about the same strength as tetryl and hexanitrodiphenylamine.

Clark found that the initiatory power of diazodinitrophenol is about twice that of mercury fulminate and slightly less than that of lead azide. His experiments were made with 0.5-gram charges of the high explosives in No. 8 detonator capsules, with reenforcing caps, and with charges compressed under a pressure of 3400 pounds per square inch. He reported the results which are tabulated below.

High Explosive	Minimum Initiating Charge (Grams) of Mercury Fulminate	Diazo-dinitrophenol	Lead Azide
Picric acid	0.225	0.115	0.12
Trinitrotoluene	0.240	0.163	0.16
Tetryl	0.165	0.075	0.03
Trinitroresorcinol	0.225	0.110	0.075
Trinitrobenzaldehyde	0.165	0.075	0.05
Tetranitroaniline	0.175	0.085	0.05
Hexanitrodiphenylamine	0.165	0.075	0.05

One gram of diazodinitrophenol in a No. 8 detonator capsule, compressed under a reenforcing cap at a pressure of 3400 pounds per square inch, and fired in a small Trauzl block, caused an expansion of 25 cc. Mercury fulminate under the same conditions caused an expansion of 8.1 cc., and lead azide one of 7.2 cc.

Clark determined the ignition temperature of diazodinitrophenol by dropping 0.02-gram portions of the material onto a heated bath of molten metal and noting the times which elapsed between the contacts with the hot metal and the explosions: 1 second at 200°, 2.5 seconds at 190°, 5 seconds at 185°, and 10.0 seconds at 180°. At 177° the material decomposed without an explosion.

Tetracene

1-Guanyl-4-nitrosoaminoguanyltetrazene, called tetracene for short, was first prepared by Hoffmann and Roth. Hoffmann and his co-workers studied its chemical reactions and determined 447 its structure. It is formed by the action of nitrous acid on aminoguanidine, or, more exactly, by the interaction of an aminoguanidine salt with sodium nitrite in the absence of free mineral acid.

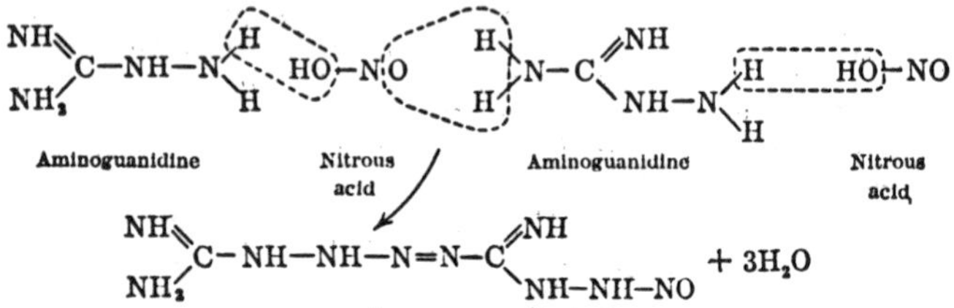

$$(NH)(NH_2)C-NH-NH_2 \ (\text{Aminoguanidine}) + HO-NO \ (\text{Nitrous acid}) + H_2N-NH-C(NH)-NH_2 \ (\text{Aminoguanidine}) + HO-NO \ (\text{Nitrous acid}) \longrightarrow (NH)(NH_2)C-NH-NH-N{=}N-C(NH)-NH-NH-NO + 3H_2O$$

1-Guanyl-4-nitrosoaminoguanyltetrazene

Tetracene is a colorless or pale yellow, fluffy material which is practically insoluble in water, alcohol, ether, benzene, and carbon tetrachloride. It has an apparent density of only 0.45, but yields a pellet of density 1.05 when it is compressed under a pressure of 3000 pounds per square inch. Tetracene forms explosive salts, among which the perchlorate is especially interesting. It is soluble in strong hydrochloric acid; ether precipitates the hydrochloride from the solution, and this on treatment with sodium acetate or with ammonia gives tetracene again. With an excess of silver nitrate it yields the double salt, $C_2H_7N_{10}OAg \cdot AgNO_3 \cdot 3H_2O$. Tetracene is only slightly hygroscopic. It is stable at ordinary temperatures both wet and dry, but is decomposed by boiling water with the evolution of $2N_2$ per molecule. On hydrolysis with caustic soda it yields ammonia, cyanamide, and triazonitrosoaminoguanidine which can be isolated in the form of a bright blue precipitate of the explosive copper salt by the addition of copper acetate to the alkaline solution. The copper salt on treatment with acid yields tetrazolyl azide (5-azidotetrazole).

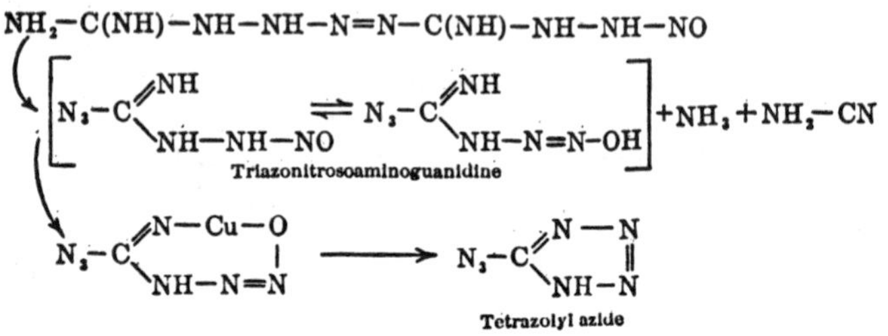

$$NH_2-C(NH)-NH-NH-N{=}N-C(NH)-NH-NH-NO \longrightarrow \left[N_3-C(NH)-NH-NH-NO \rightleftharpoons N_3-C(NH)-NH-N{=}N-OH \right] + NH_3 + NH_2-CN$$

Triazonitrosoaminoguanidine

$$N_3-C{\scriptstyle (=N-Cu-O)(-NH-N{=}N)} \longrightarrow N_3-C{\scriptstyle (=N-N{=}N-NH)}$$

Tetrazolyl azide

448

In the presence of mineral acids, sodium nitrite reacts in a different manner with aminoguanidine, and guanyl azide is formed.

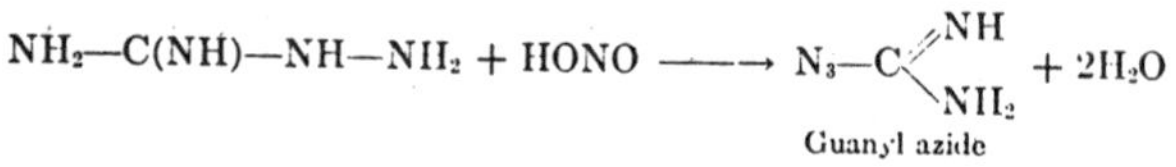

$$NH_2-C(NH)-NH-NH_2 + HONO \longrightarrow N_3-C(NH)-NH_2 + 2H_2O$$

Guanyl azide

This substance forms salts with acids, and was first isolated in the form of its nitrate. The nitrate is not detonated by shock but undergoes a rapid decomposition with the production of light when it is heated. The picrate and the perchlorate explode violently from heat and from shock. Guanyl azide is not decomposed by boiling water. On hydrolysis with strong alkali, it yields the alkali metal salt of hydrazoic acid. It is hydrolyzed by ammoniacal silver nitrate in the cold with the formation of silver azide which remains in solution and of silver cyanamide which appears as a yellow precipitate. By treatment with acids or weak bases it is converted into 5-aminotetrazole.

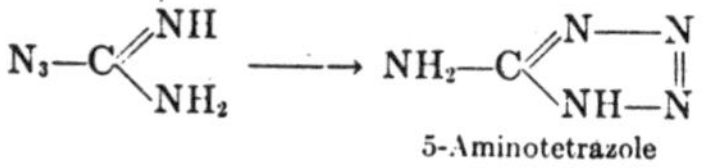

$$N_3-C(NH)-NH_2 \longrightarrow NH_2-C{\scriptstyle (=N-N{=}N-NH)}$$

5-Aminotetrazole

When the reaction between aminoguanidine and sodium nitrite occurs in the presence of an excess of acetic acid, still another product is formed, namely, 1,3-ditetrazolyltriazine, the genesis of which is easily understood from a consideration of the reactions already mentioned. 5-Aminotetrazole is evidently formed first; the amino group of one molecule of this substance is diazotized by the action of the nitrous acid, and the resulting diazonium salt in the acetic acid solution couples with a second molecule of the aminotetrazole.

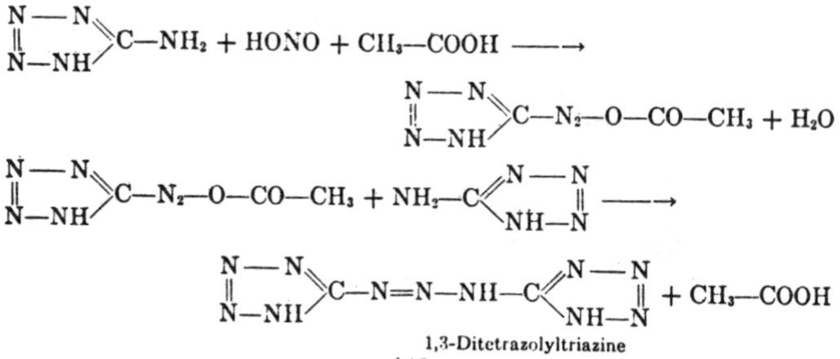

$$(N{-}N{=}\,,\,N{-}NH)\!>\!C-NH_2 + HONO + CH_3-COOH \longrightarrow (N{-}N{=}\,,\,N{-}NH)\!>\!C-N_2-O-CO-CH_3 + H_2O$$

$$(N{-}N{=}\,,\,N{-}NH)\!>\!C-N_2-O-CO-CH_3 + NH_2-C(=N-N{=}N-NH) \longrightarrow (N{-}N{=}\,,\,N{-}NH)\!>\!C-N{=}N-NH-C(=N-N{=}N-NH) + CH_3-COOH$$

1,3-Ditetrazolyltriazine

449

Preparation of Tetracene. Thirty-four grams of aminoguanidine bicarbonate, 2500 cc. of water, and 15.7 grams of glacial acetic acid are brought together in a 3-liter flask, and the mixture is warmed on the steam bath with occasional shaking until everything has gone into solution. The solution is filtered if need be, and cooled to 30° at the tap. Twenty-seven and sixth-tenths grams of solid sodium nitrite is added. The flask is swirled to make it dissolve, and is set aside at room temperature. After 3 or 4 hours, the flask is shaken to start precipitation of the product. It is allowed to stand for about 20 hours longer (22 to 24 hours altogether). The precipitate of tetracene is washed several times by decantation, transferred to a filter, and washed thoroughly with water. The product is dried at room temperature and is stored in a bottle which is closed by means of a cork or rubber stopper.

Tetracene explodes readily from flame without appreciable noise but with the production of much black smoke. Rinkenbach and Burton, who have made an extended study of the explosive properties of tetracene, report that it explodes in 5 seconds at 160° (mercury fulminate 190°). They found that it is slightly more sensitive to impact than mercury fulminate; an 8-inch drop of an 8-ounce weight was needed to explode it, a drop of 9–10 inches to explode fulminate.

The brisance of tetracene, if it is used alone and is fired by a fuse, is greatest when the explosive is not compressed at all. Thus, 0.4 gram of tetracene, if uncompressed, crushed 13.1 grams of sand in the sand test; if compressed under a pressure of 250 pounds per square inch, 9.2 grams; if under 500 pounds per square inch, 7.5 grams; and, if under 3000 pounds per square inch, 2.0 grams. The data show the behavior of tetracene as it approaches the condition of being dead-pressed.

In another series of experiments, Rinkenbach and Burton used charges of 0.4 gram of tetracene, compressed under a pressure of 3000 pounds per square inch and initiated with varying amounts of fulminate (loaded under the same pressure), and found that the tetracene developed its maximum brisance (21.1 grams of sand crushed) when initiated with 0.4 gram of fulminate. A compound primer of 0.15 gram of tetryl initiated with 0.25 gram of mercury fulminate caused 0.4 gram of tetracene to crush 22.6 grams, or substantially the same amount, of sand. It appears[450] then that tetracene is more brisant—and presumably explodes with a greater velocity of detonation—when initiated by fulminate or tetryl than when self-initiated by fire.

Tetracene is easily dead-pressed, its self-acceleration is low, and it is not suitable for use alone as an initiating explosive.

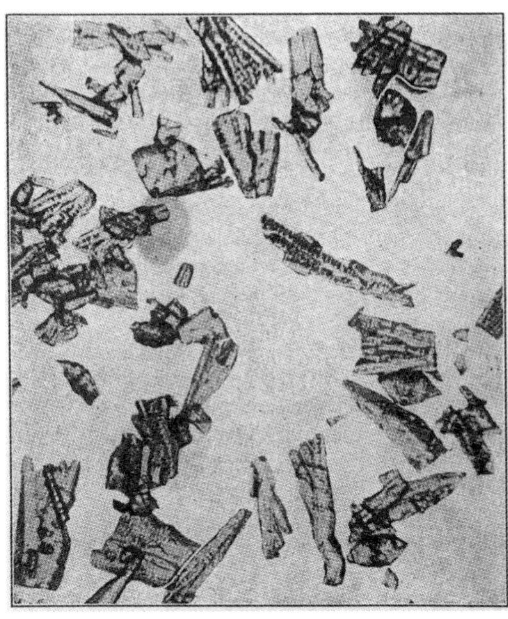

FIGURE 104. Tetracene Crystals (150×).

It is as efficient as fulminate only if it is externally initiated. It is used in detonators either initiated by another primary explosive and functioning as an intermediate booster or mixed with another primary explosive to increase the sensitivity of the latter to flame or heat. A recent patent recommends the use of a mixture of tetracene and lead azide in explosive rivets. Tetracene is used in primer caps where as little as 2% in the composition results in an improved uniformity of percussion sensitivity.

Hexamethylenetriperoxidediamine (HMTD)[451]

Hexamethylenetriperoxidediamine is the only organic peroxide which has been considered seriously as an explosive. Its explosive properties commend it, but it is too reactive chemically and too unstable to be of practical use. It is most conveniently prepared by treating hexamethylenetetramine with hydrogen peroxide in the presence of citric acid which promotes the reaction by combining with the ammonia which is liberated.

$$C_6H_{12}N_4 + 3H_2O_2 \longrightarrow N\begin{matrix} -CH_2-O-O-CH_2- \\ -CH_2-O-O-CH_2- \\ -CH_2-O-O-CH_2- \end{matrix}N + 2NH_3$$

Hexamethylenetriperoxidediamine

Preparation of Hexamethylenetriperoxidediamine. Fourteen grams of hexamethylenetetramine is dissolved in 45 grams of 30% hydrogen peroxide solution which is stirred mechanically in a beaker standing in a freezing mixture of cracked ice with water and a little salt. To the solution 21 grams of powdered citric acid is added slowly in small portions at a time while the stirring is continued and the temperature of the mixture is kept at 0° or below. After all the citric acid has dissolved, the mixture is stirred for 3 hours longer while its temperature is kept at 0°. The cooling is then discontinued, the mixture is allowed to stand for 2 hours at room temperature, and the white crystalline product is filtered off, washed thoroughly with water, and rinsed with alcohol in order that it may dry out more quickly at ordinary temperatures.

Hexamethylenetriperoxidediamine is almost insoluble in water and in the common organic solvents at room temperature. It detonates when struck a sharp blow, but, when ignited, burns with a flash like nitrocellulose. Taylor and Rinkenbach found its true density (20°/20°) to be 1.57, its apparent density after being placed in a tube and tapped 0.66, and its density after being compressed in a detonator capsule under a pressure of 2500 pounds per square inch only 0.91. They found that it required a 3-cm. drop of a 2-kilogram weight to make it explode, but that fulminate required a drop of only 0.25 cm. In the sand test it pulverized 2½ to 3 times as much sand as mercury fulminate, and slightly more sand than lead azide. It is not dead-pressed by a pressure of 11,000 pounds per square inch. It is considerably more effective than mercury fulminate[452] as an initiator of detonation. Taylor and Rinkenbach, working with 0.4-gram portions of the high explosives and with varying weights of the primary explosives, compressed in detonator capsules under a pressure of 1000 pounds per square inch, found the minimum charges necessary to produce detonation to be as indicated in the following table.

	MINIMUM INITIATING CHARGE (GRAMS) OF		
		Hexamethylenetriperoxidediamine	
HIGH EXPLOSIVE	Fulminate with Reenforcing Cap	With Reenforcing Cap	Without Reenforcing Cap
Trinitrotoluene	0.26	0.08	0.10
Picric acid	0.21	0.05	0.06
Tetryl	0.24	0.05	0.06
Ammonium picrate	0.8–0.9	0.30	0.30
Tetranitroaniline	0.20	0.05	0.05
Guanidine picrate	0.30	0.13	0.15

Trinitroresorcinol	0.20	0.08	0.10
Hexanitrodiphenylamine	...	0.05	0.05
Trinitrobenzaldehyde	...	0.08	0.10

Taylor and Rinkenbach found that 0.05-gram portions of hexamethylenetriperoxidediamine, pressed in No. 8 detonator capsules under a pressure of 1000 pounds per square inch and fired by means of a black-powder fuse crimped in the usual way, caused the detonation of ordinary 40% nitroglycerin dynamite and of a gelatin dynamite which had become insensitive after storage of more than a year. The velocity of detonation of HMTD, loaded at a density of 0.88 in a column 0.22 inch in diameter, was found by the U. S. Bureau of Mines Explosives Testing Laboratory to be 4511 meters per second.

A small quantity of HMTD decomposed without exploding when dropped onto molten metal at 190°, but a small quantity detonated instantly when dropped onto molten metal at 200°. A 0.05-gram sample ignited in 3 seconds at 149°. At temperatures which are only moderately elevated the explosive shows signs of volatilizing and decomposing. Taylor and Rinkenbach report the results of experiments in which samples on watch glasses were heated in electric ovens at various temperatures, and weighed and examined from time to time, as shown below. The sample

453

which had been heated at 60° showed no evidence of decomposition. The sample which had been heated at 75° was unchanged in color but had a faint odor of methylamine and appeared slightly moist. At 100° the substance gave off an amine odor. The residue which remained after 24 hours of heating at 100° consisted of a colorless liquid and needle crystals which were soluble in water.

% Weight Lost at	60°	75°	100°
In 2 hrs.	0.10	0.25	3.25
In 8 hrs.	0.35	0.60	29.60
In 24 hrs.	0.50	1.30	67.95
In 48 hrs.	0.50	2.25	....

When hexamethylenetriperoxidediamine is boiled with water, it disappears fairly rapidly, oxygen is given off, and the colorless solution is found to contain ammonia, formaldehyde, ethylene glycol, formic acid, and hexamethylenetetramine.

Friction Primers

Friction primers (friction tubes, friction igniters) are devices for the production of fire by the friction of the thrust, either push or pull, of a roughened rod or wire through a pellet of primer composition. They are used for firing artillery in circumstances where the propelling charge is loaded separately and is not enclosed in a brass case supplied with a percussion primer. They are sometimes crimped to an end of Bickford fuse for the purpose of lighting it. They are sometimes used for lighting flares, etc., which are thrown overboard from airplanes. For this use, the pull element of the primer is attached to the airplane by a length of twine or wire which the weight of the falling flare first pulls and then breaks off entirely.

The following table shows three compositions which have been widely used in friction primers for artillery. All the materials

Potassium chlorate	2	56.2	44.6
Antimony sulfide	1	24.6	44.6
Sulfur	..	9.0	3.6
Meal powder	..	...	3.6
Ground glass	..	10.2	3.6

are in the powdered condition except in the first mixture where half of the potassium chlorate is powdered and half of it is granu-

454

lar. The first mixture is probably the best. The sulfur which is contained in the second and third mixtures makes them more sensitive, but also makes them prone to turn sour after they have been wet-mixed, and these mixtures ought to be made up with a small amount of anti-acid (calcium carbonate, trimethylamine, etc., not mentioned in the table). All the mixtures are wet-mixed with 5% gum arabic solution, loaded wet, and dried out *in situ* to form pellets which do not crumble easily.

In a typical friction primer for an airplane flare, ignition is secured by pulling a loop of braided wire coated with red phosphorus and shellac through a pellet, made from potassium chlorate (14 parts) and charcoal (1.6 parts), hardened with dextrin (0.3 part).

Percussion Primers

Percussion primers produce fire or flame from the impact of the trigger or firing pin of a pistol, rifle, or cannon, or of the inertia-operated device in a fuze which functions when the projectile starts on its flight (the so-called concussion element, the primer of which is called a concussion primer) or of that which functions when the projectile strikes its target (the percussion element). A typical primer composition consists of a mixture of mercury fulminate (a primary explosive which produces the first explosion with heat and flame), antimony sulfide (a combustible material which maintains the flame for a longer time), and potassium chlorate (an oxidizing agent which supplies oxygen for the combustion). Sometimes no single primary explosive substance is present; the mixture itself is the primary explosive. Sometimes the compositions contain explosives such as TNT, tetryl, or PETN, which make them hotter, or ground glass which makes them more sensitive to percussion. Hot particles of solid (glass or heavy metal oxide) thrown out by a primer will set fire to black powder over a considerable distance, but they will fall onto smokeless powder without igniting it. The primers which produce the hottest gas are best suited for use with smokeless powder.

Primer compositions are usually mixed by hand on a glass-top table by a workman wearing rubber gloves and working alone in a small building remote from others. They are sometimes mixed dry, but in this country more commonly wet, with water

455

or with water containing gum arabic or gum tragacanth, with alcohol alone or with an alcohol solution of shellac. The caps are loaded in much the same manner that blasting caps are loaded, the mixture is pressed down by machine and perhaps covered with a disc of tinfoil, the anvil is inserted and pressed into place (unless the primer is to be used in a cartridge or fuze of which the anvil is already an integral part), and the caps are finally dried in a dry-house and stored in small magazines until needed for loading.

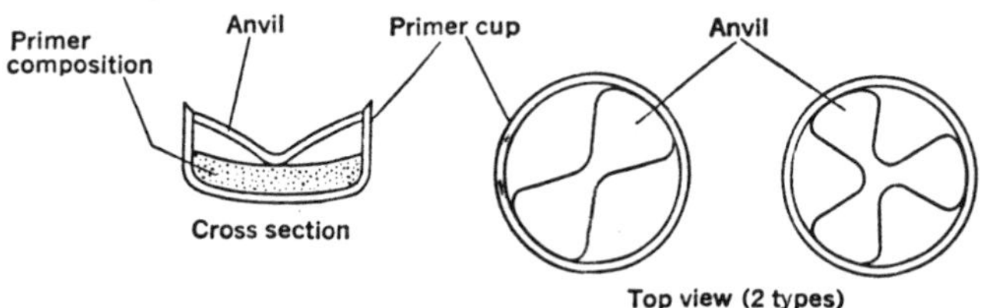

Figure 105. Primer Cap for Small Arms Cartridge.

For many years the standard mixture in France for all caps which were to be fired by the blow of a hammer was made from 2 parts of mercury fulminate, 1 of antimony sulfide, and 1 of saltpeter. This was mixed and loaded dry, and was considered to be safer to handle than similar mixtures containing potassium chlorate. Where a more sensitive primer was needed, the standard French composition for all concussion and percussion primers of fuzes was made from 5 parts of mercury fulminate and 9 parts each of antimony sulfide and potassium chlorate.

All the compositions listed in the following table (gum or shellac binder not included) have been used, in small arms primers or in fuze primers, by one or another of the great powers, and they illustrate the wide variations in the proportions of the ingredients which are possible or desirable according to the design of the device in which the primer is used.

Mercury fulminate	10.0	28.0	48.8	4	5	2	11.0	32	16.5	7	19.0
Potassium chlorate	37.0	35.5	24.4	2	9	3	52.5	45	50.0	21	33.0
Antimony sulfide	40.0	28.0	26.2	3	3	3	36.5	23	33.5	17	43.0
Sulfur	...	...	...	..	..	..	...	..	...	..	2.5
Meal powder	...	...	...	..	..	..	...	..	...	..	2.5
Ground glass	13.0	8.5	...	5	..	..	...	..	...	5	...
Ground coke	...	...	...	..	1	..	...	..	...	..	...
Tetryl	...	...	...	..	2	..	...	..	...	..	...

456

A non-fulminate primer composition is probably somewhat safer to mix than one which contains fulminate. It contains no single substance which is a primary explosive, only the primary explosive mixture of the chlorate with the appropriate combustible material, or, more exactly, the explosive which exists at the point of contact between particles of the two substances. For a non-fulminate primer to perform properly, it is necessary that the composition should be mixed thoroughly and very uniformly in order that dissimilar particles may be found in contact with each other beneath the point of the anvil and may be crushed together by the blow of the trigger. It is not absolutely essential that fulminate compositions should be mixed with the same uniformity. Even if no fulminate happens to lie beneath the point of the anvil, the trigger blow sufficiently crushes the sensitive material in the neighborhood to make it explode. For mechanical reasons, the ingredients of primer composition ought not to be pulverized too finely.

Several non-fulminate primer compositions are listed below.

Potassium chlorate	50	50.54	67	60	53
Antimony sulfide	20	26.31	..	30	17
Lead thiocyanate	..	...	..	..	25
Lead peroxide	25	...	..	..	..
Cuprous thiocyanate	..	...	15	3	..
TNT	5	...	..	..	5
Sulfur	..	8.76	16	7	..
Charcoal	..	...	2	..	..
Ground glass	..	12.39	..	..	..
Shellac	..	2.00	..	..	..

Sulfur ought not to be used in any primer composition, whether fulminate or non-fulminate, which contains chlorate unless an anti-acid is present. In a moist atmosphere, the sulfuric acid, which is inevitably present on the sulfur, attacks the chlorate, liberating chlorine dioxide which further attacks the sulfur, producing more sulfuric acid, and causing a self-catalyzed *souring* which results first in the primer becoming slow in its response to the trigger (hang fire) and later in its becoming inert (misfire). It is evident that the presence of fulminate in the composition will tend to nullify the effect of the souring, and that it

457

is safest to avoid the use of sulfur with chlorate especially in non-fulminate mixtures. The second of the above-listed compositions is an undesirable one in this respect. In the third and fourth compositions, the cuprous thiocyanate serves both as a combustible and as an anti-acid, and it helps, particularly in the third mixture, by supplying copper oxide which is a solid vehicle for the transfer of heat. The first and the last of the above-listed mixtures are the best. They contain no sulfur, and they contain lead enough to supply plenty of solid particles of hot material.

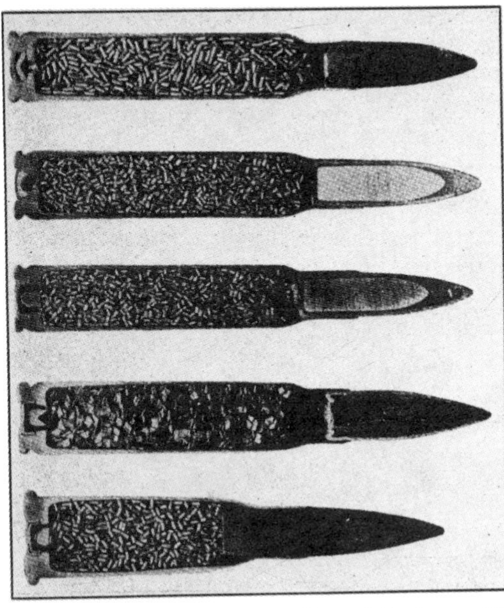

FIGURE 106. Longitudinal Sections of Military Rifle Ammunition of the First World War. (Courtesy Émile Monnin Chamot.) The cartridge at the bottom, French 9.0-mm. Lebel rifle, the one above it, German 7.9-mm. Mauser, and the one above that, Canadian .30 caliber, all have anvils of the Berdan type integrally one with the metal of the cartridge case.

Gunnery experts ascribe a large part of the erosion of shotgun and rifle barrels to the action of the soluble salts which are produced from the materials of the primer compositions, particularly

458

to the chlorides which come from the chlorate, and to the sulfates which result from the combustion of the antimony sulfide. The following table lists several non-chlorate, non-erosive primer compositions. They contain no compounds of chlorine. They contain either lead or barium or both, and both of these metals form sulfates which are insoluble in water. Moreover, the soluble portions of the residues from the primers which contain barium nitrate are alkaline and are even capable of neutralizing any acidity which might arise from the smokeless powder.

Mercury fulminate	36	40	25	20	39
Antimony sulfide	20	25	15	20	9
Barium nitrate	..	25	25	40	41
Lead peroxide	..	..	35	10	..
Lead chromate	40	..	..	..	..
Barium carbonate	..	6	..	..	..
Picric acid	..	..	..	..	5
Powdered glass	4	4	..	..	6
Calcium silicide	..	..	..	10	..

The Chemistry of Powder and Explosives

BY

TENNEY L. DAVIS, PH.D.

Emeritus Professor of Organic Chemistry
Massachusetts Institute of Technology
Director of Research and Development
National Fireworks, Inc.

COMPLETE IN ONE VOLUME

NEW YORK
JOHN WILEY & SONS, INC.
LONDON: CHAPMAN & HALL, LIMITED

INDEX OF SUBJECTS

D

E

F

G

U

V

W

X

Y

Z